Essentials of
PHYSICAL MEDICINE
and REHABILITATION

Musculoskeletal Disorders, Pain, and Rehabilitation

Essentials of
PHYSICAL MEDICINE
and REHABILITATION

Musculoskeletal Disorders, Pain, and Rehabilitation

SECOND EDITION

Walter R. Frontera, MD, PhD
Dean, School of Medicine
Professor, Departments of Physical
Medicine and Rehabilitation and
Physiology
University of Puerto Rico School of
Medicine
San Juan, Puerto Rico

Lecturer
Department of Physical Medicine
and Rehabilitation
Harvard Medical School
Boston, Massachusetts

Julie K. Silver, MD
Assistant Professor, Department of
Physical Medicine and Rehabilitation
Harvard Medical School

Associate in Physiatry
Massachusetts General Hospital,
Brigham and Women's Hospital, and
Spaulding Rehabilitation Hospital
Boston, Massachusetts

Thomas D. Rizzo, Jr., MD
Assistant Professor, Physical Medicine
and Rehabilitation
College of Medicine, Mayo Clinic

Consultant and Chair
Department of Physical Medicine
and Rehabilitation
Mayo Clinic
Jacksonville, Florida

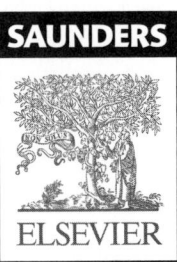

SAUNDERS
ELSEVIER

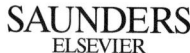

1600 John F. Kennedy Blvd.
Ste 1800
Philadelphia, PA 19103-2899

ESSENTIALS OF PHYSICAL MEDICINE AND REHABILITATION: ISBN: 978-1-4160-4007-1
MUSCULOSKELETAL DISORDERS, PAIN, AND REHABILITATION

Library of Congress Cataloging-in-Publication Data
Essentials of physical medicine and rehabilitation: musculoskeletal disorders, pain, and rehabilitation/
[edited by] Walter R. Frontera, Julie K. Silver, Thomas D. Rizzo Jr.—2nd ed.
   p. ; cm.
Includes bibliographical references and index.
ISBN 978-1-4160-4007-1
1. Medicine, Physical. 2. Medical rehabilitation. I. Frontera, Walter R., 1955- II. Silver, J. K. (Julie K.), 1965- III. Rizzo, Thomas D., 1959-
[DNLM: 1. Musculoskeletal Diseases—rehabilitation. WE 140 E782 2008]

RM700.E84 2008
617'.03—dc22

                                                                    2007045181

Acquisitions Editor: Dolores Meloni
Developmental Editor: Joan Ryan
Publishing Services Manager: Frank Polizzano
Project Manager: Rachel Miller
Design Direction: Steven Stave

Printed in Canada.

Last digit is the print number: 9 8 7 6 5 4 3 2 1

We dedicate this book to our mentors, teachers, colleagues,
and students who have encouraged us to pursue academic careers with their enthusiasm
for knowledge and learning; to our patients, who often are our greatest teachers;
and to our families, who support us and provide
the foundation for our pursuits.

Walter R. Frontera, MD, PhD
Julie K. Silver, MD
Thomas D. Rizzo, Jr., MD

Contents

Contents   vii
Contributors   xi
Preface   xix

PART 1: MUSCULOSKELETAL DISORDERS

Section 1: Head and Neck

1   Cervical Spondylotic Myelopathy   1
    Avital Fast, MD, and Miriam Segal, MD

2   Cervical Facet Arthropathy   7
    Ted A. Lennard, MD

3   Cervical Degenerative Disease   11
    Avital Fast, MD, and Miriam Segal, MD

4   Cervical Radiculopathy   17
    Isaac Cohen, MD, and Cristin Jouve, MD

5   Cervical Sprain or Strain   23
    *Thomas H. Hudgins, MD, Lena Shahban, MD,
    and Joseph T. Alleva, MD*

6   Cervical Stenosis   27
    Alec L. Meleger, MD

7   Cervicogenic Vertigo   33
    Joanne Borg-Stein, MD

8   Trapezius Strain   37
    Isaac Cohen, MD, and Cristin Jouve, MD

Section 2: Shoulder

9   Acromioclavicular Injuries   41
    Thomas D. Rizzo, Jr., MD

10 Adhesive Capsulitis   49
    *Brian J. Krabak, MD, MBA, and
    Norman L. Banks, MD, MS*

11 Biceps Tendinitis   55
    *Brian J. Krabak, MD, MBA, and
    William Moore, MD*

12 Biceps Tendon Rupture   59
    Michael F. Stretanski, DO

13 Glenohumeral Instability   63
    *William Micheo, MD, and
    Edwardo Ramos, MD*

14 Rotator Cuff Tendinitis   71
    Jay E. Bowen, DO, and Gerard A. Malanga, MD

15 Rotator Cuff Tear   77
    Gerard A. Malanga, MD, and Jay E. Bowen, DO

16 Scapular Winging   83
    Peter M. McIntosh, MD

17 Shoulder Arthritis   91
    Michael F. Stretanski, DO

Section 3: Elbow and Forearm

18 Elbow Arthritis   97
    Charles Cassidy, MD, and Chien Chow, MD

19 Epicondylitis   105
    Lyn D. Weiss, MD, and Jay M. Weiss, MD

20 Median Neuropathy   109
    *Francisco H. Santiago, MD, and
    Ramon Vallarino, Jr., MD*

21 Olecranon Bursitis   115
    Charles Cassidy, MD, and Sarah S. Banerjee, MD

22 Radial Neuropathy   121
    Lyn D. Weiss, MD, and Thomas E. Pobre, MD

23 Ulnar Neuropathy (Elbow)   125
    Lyn D. Weiss, MD, and Jay M. Weiss, MD

Section 4: Hand and Wrist

24 de Quervain Tenosynovitis   129
    Carina J. O'Neill, DO

25 Dupuytren Contracture   133
    Michael F. Stretanski, DO

26 Extensor Tendon Injuries   139
    Jeffrey S. Brault, DO, PT, and Gregory L. Umphrey, MD

27 Flexor Tendon Injuries   145
    *Jeffrey S. Brault, DO, PT, and
    Gregory L. Umphrey, MD*

28 Hand and Wrist Ganglia   149
    Charles Cassidy, MD, and Victor Chung, BS

29 Hand Osteoarthritis   155
    David Ring, MD, PhD

30 Hand Rheumatoid Arthritis   161
    David Ring, MD, PhD, and Jonathan Kay, MD

31 Kienböck Disease   167
    Charles Cassidy, MD, and Vivek M. Shah, MD

32 Median Neuropathy (Carpal Tunnel Syndrome)   173
    Meijuan Zhao, MD, and David Burke, MD, MA

33   Trigger Finger   179
      Julie K. Silver, MD

34   Ulnar Collateral Ligament Sprain   183
      Sheila Dugan, MD

35   Ulnar Neuropathy (Wrist)   187
      *Ramon Vallarino, Jr., MD, and
      Francisco H. Santiago, MD*

36   Wrist Osteoarthritis   193
      *José M. Nolla, MD, and Chaitanya S.
      Mudgal, MD, MS (Orth), MCh (Orth)*

37   Wrist Rheumatoid Arthritis   203
      *Brian T. Fitzgerald, MD, and Chaitanya S. Mudgal,
      MD, MS (Orth), MCh (Orth)*

Section 5: Mid Back

38   Thoracic Compression Fracture   213
      Toni J. Hanson, MD

39   Thoracic Radiculopathy   219
      Darren Rosenberg, DO

40   Thoracic Sprain or Strain   223
      *Alexios Carayannopoulos, DO, MPH,
      and Darren Rosenberg, DO*

41   Lumbar Degenerative Disease   229
      *Michael K. Schaufele, MD, and
      Aimee H. Walsh, MD*

42   Lumbar Facet Arthropathy   237
      Ted A. Lennard, MD

43   Lumbar Radiculopathy   241
      Maury Ellenberg, MD, and Joseph C. Honet, MD

44   Low Back Strain or Sprain   247
      Omar El Abd, MD

45   Lumbar Spondylolysis and Spondylolisthesis   253
      James Spinelli, DO, and James Rainville, MD

46   Lumbar Spinal Stenosis   259
      Zacharia Isaac, MD, and David Wang, DO

47   Sacroiliac Joint Dysfunction   267
      Zacharia Isaac, MD, and Jennifer Devine, MD

Section 6: Hip and Thigh

48   Hip Osteoarthritis   271
      Patrick M. Foye, MD, and Todd P. Stitik, MD

49   Femoral Neuropathy   277
      Earl J. Craig, MD, and Daniel M. Clinchot, MD

50   Lateral Femoral Cutaneous Neuropathy   283
      Earl J. Craig, MD, and Daniel M. Clinchot, MD

51   Piriformis Syndrome   287
      *Thomas H. Hudgins, MD, and
      Joseph T. Alleva, MD*

52   Quadriceps Contusion   291
      *Seneca A. Storm, MD, and
      J. Michael Wieting, DO*

53   Total Hip Replacement   295
      Robert S. Skerker, MD, and Gregory J. Mulford, MD

54   Trochanteric Bursitis   303
      Michael Fredericson, MD, and Kelvin Chew, MD

Section 7: Knee and Lower Leg

55   Anterior Cruciate Ligament Tear   307
      Eduardo Amy, MD, and William Micheo, MD

56   Baker's Cyst   315
      *Ed Hanada, MD, Meryl Stein, MD, and
      Darren Rosenberg, DO*

57   Collateral Ligament Sprain   319
      Paul Lento, MD, and Venu Akuthota, MD

58   Compartment Syndrome   325
      Karen P. Barr, MD

59   Hamstring Strain   331
      *Carole S. Vetter, MD, and
      Anne Z. Hoch, DO, PT*

60   Iliotibial Band Syndrome   337
      *Venu Akuthota, MD, Sonja K. Stilp, MD,
      Paul Lento, MD, and Peter Gonzalez, MD*

61   Knee Osteoarthritis   345
      *Allen N. Wilkins, MD, and
      Edward M. Phillips, MD*

62   Knee Bursitis   355
      *Ed Hanada, MD, Florian S. Keplinger, MD,
      and Navneet Gupta, MD*

63   Meniscal Injuries   359
      Paul Lento, MD, and Venu Akuthota, MD

64   Jumper's Knee   367
      Thomas H. Hudgins, MD

65   Patellofemoral Syndrome   371
      Thomas H. Hudgins, MD

66   Peroneal Neuropathy   375
      John C. King, MD

67   Posterior Cruciate Ligament Sprain   381
      *Christine Curtis, BS, Peter Bienkowski, MD,
      and Lyle J. Micheli, MD*

68   Quadriceps Tendinitis   387
      *Christine Curtis, BS, Peter Bienkowski, MD,
      and Lyle J. Micheli, MD*

69   Shin Splints   389
      Michael F. Stretanski, DO

70   Stress Fractures   393
      Sheila Dugan, MD

71   Total Knee Replacement   399
      Robert J. Kaplan, MD

Section 8: Foot and Ankle

72   Achilles Tendinitis   407
      Michael F. Stretanski, DO

73 Ankle Arthritis 411
*David Wexler, MD, FRCS (Tr, Orth), Dawn M.
Grosser, MD, and Todd A. Kile, MD*

74 Foot and Ankle Bursitis 415
*Allen N. Wilkins, MD, Daniel Sipple, DO,
and Thomas H. Hudgins, MD*

75 Ankle Sprain 421
Brian J. Krabak, MD, MBA, and Jennifer Baima, MD

76 Bunion and Bunionette 427
*David Wexler, MD, FRCS (Tr, Orth), Dawn M.
Grosser, MD, and Todd A. Kile, MD*

77 Chronic Ankle Instability 433
Michael D. Osborne, MD

78 Claw Toe 437
David Wang, DO

79 Corns 441
*Robert J. Scardina, DPM, and
Sammy M. Lee, DPM*

80 Foot and Ankle Ganglia 445
*Robert J. Krug, MD, Elliot Pollack, DPM, and
Jeffrey T. Brodie, MD*

81 Hallux Rigidus 449
*David Wexler, MD, FRCS (Tr, Orth), Dawn M.
Grosser, MD, and Todd A. Kile, MD*

82 Hammer Toe 453
*Robert J. Krug, MD, Elise H. Lee, MD,
Sheila Dugan, MD, and
Katherine Mashey, DPM*

83 Mallet Toe 457
Sandra Maguire, MD

84 Metatarsalgia 461
Sandra Maguire, MD

85 Morton Neuroma 465
*Robert J. Scardina, DPM, and
Sammy M. Lee, DPM*

86 Plantar Fasciitis 469
Paul F. Pasquina, MD, and Leslie S. Foster, DO

87 Posterior Tibial Tendon Dysfunction 475
*David Wexler, MD, FRCS (Tr, Orth),
Todd A. Kile, MD, and Dawn M. Grosser, MD*

88 Tibial Neuropathy (Tarsal Tunnel Syndrome) 479
David R. Del Toro, MD

PART 2: PAIN

89 Occipital Neuralgia 483
Aneesh Singla, MD, MPH

90 Trigeminal Neuralgia 491
Aneesh Singla, MD, MPH

91 Thoracic Outlet Syndrome 497
Karl-August Lindgren, MD, PhD

92 Chronic Pain Syndrome 505
S. Ali Mostoufi, MD

93 Complex Regional Pain Syndrome 511
*Allison Bailey, MD, and
Joseph F. Audette, MA, MD*

94 Headaches 519
Elizabeth Loder, MD, MPH

95 Fibromyalgia 525
Joanne Borg-Stein, MD

96 Myofascial Pain Syndrome 529
*Martin K. Childers, DO, PhD, Jeffery B.
Feldman, PhD, and H. Michael Guo, MD, PhD*

97 Repetitive Strain Injuries 539
Kelly McInnis, DO

98 Costosternal Syndromes 545
Marta Imamura, MD, and David A. Cassius, MD

99 Intercostal Neuralgia 549
Susan J. Dreyer, MD

100 Tietze Syndrome 555
*Marta Imamura, MD, and Satiko Tomikawa
Imamura, MD, PhD*

101 Postherpetic Neuralgia 561
Ariana Vora, MD, and Anita Thompson, PT

102 Arachnoiditis 565
Michael D. Osborne, MD

103 Coccydynia 571
Ariana Vora, MD

104 Phantom Limb Pain 575
Moon Suk Bang, MD, PhD, and Se Hee Jung, MD, MS

105 Cervical Dystonia 579
Moon Suk Bang, MD, PhD, and Shi-Uk Lee, MD, PhD

106 Post-Thoracotomy Pain Syndrome 585
Justin Riutta, MD

107 Post-Mastectomy Pain Syndrome 589
Justin Riutta, MD

PART 3: REHABILITATION

108 Upper Limb Amputations 593
*Timothy R. Dillingham, MD, and
Diane W. Braza, MD*

109 Lower Limb Amputations 599
Michelle Gittler, MD

110 Ankylosing Spondylitis 605
Steven E. Braverman, MD, MS

111 Burns 609
Jeffrey C. Schneider, MD

112 Cardiac Rehabilitation 615
Alan M. Davis, MD, PhD

113 Cancer 621
Andrea Cheville, MD, and Lora Beth Packel, PT, MS

114 Cerebral Palsy 627
Yong-Tae Lee, MD, and Patrick Brennan, MD

115 Chronic Fatigue Syndrome 635
Gerold R. Ebenbichler, MD

116 Chronic Kidney Disease 643
Ajay K. Singh, MD

117 Joint Contractures 651
Nancy Dudek, MD, MEd, and Guy Trudel, MD

118 Deep Venous Thrombosis 657
Jonas Sokolof, DO, and Ricardo Knight, MD, PT

119 Dementia 665
Jatin Dave, MD, MPH, and Melvyn Hecht, MD

120 Management of the Patient with a Foot at Risk:
Peripheral Arterial Disease and Diabetes 763
*Timothy R. Dillingham, MD, and
Diane W. Braza, MD*

121 Dysphagia 679
*Jeffrey B. Palmer, MD, and
Koichiro Matsuo, DDS, PhD*

122 Enteropathic Arthritides 685
Karen Atkinson, MD, MPH

123 Heterotopic Ossification 691
*Amanda L. Harrington, MD, Philip J. Blount, MD,
and William L. Bockenek, MD*

124 Lymphedema 697
*Mabel E. Caban, MD, Sandra S. Hatch, MD,
and Atul Patel, MD*

125 Motor Neuron Disease 705
Lisa S. Krivickas, MD

126 Movement Disorders 713
Kenneth H. Silver, MD

127 Multiple Sclerosis 719
Ann-Marie Thomas, MD, PT

128 Myopathies 729
Kristian Borg, MD, PhD, and Erik Ensrud, MD

129 Neurogenic Bladder 733
Ayal M. Kaynan, MD, and Inder Perkash, MD

130 Osteoarthritis 745
Allen N. Wilkins, MD, and Edward M. Phillips, MD

131 Osteoporosis 753
David M. Slovik, MD, and Jonas Sokolof, DO

132 Parkinson Disease 761
Nutan Sharma, MD, PhD

133 Peripheral Neuropathies 767
Seward B. Rutkove, MD

134 Plexopathy—Brachial 773
Erik Ensrud, MD, and John C. King, MD

135 Plexopathy—Lumbosacral 779
Hope S. Hacker, MD, and John C. King, MD

136 Polytrauma Rehabilitation 787
*Steven G. Scott, DO, Joel D. Scholten, MD,
Gail A. Latlief, DO, Faiza Humayun, MD,
Heather G. Belanger, PhD, and
Rodney D. Vanderploeg, PhD*

137 Post-Poliomyelitis Syndrome 793
Julie K. Silver, MD

138 Post-Concussion Disorders 801
Mel B. Glenn, MD

139 Psoriatic Arthritis 809
Mahboob U. Rahman, MD, PhD

140 Pressure Ulcers 813
Chester H. Ho, MD, and Kath Bogie, DPhil

141 Pulmonary Rehabilitation 823
John R. Bach, MD

142 Rheumatoid Arthritis 833
Karen Atkinson, MD, MPH, and Jonas Sokolof, DO

143 Scoliosis and Kyphosis 841
Mark A. Thomas, MD, and Yumei Wang, MD

144 Spasticity 849
Joel Stein, MD

145 Speech and Language Disorders 853
*Jason H. Kortte, MS, CCC-SLP, and
Jeffrey B. Palmer, MD*

146 Spinal Cord Injury (Cervical) 859
Sunil Sabharwal, MD

147 Spinal Cord Injury (Thoracic) 871
*Jane Wierbicky, RN, BSN, and
Shanker Nesathurai, MD*

148 Spinal Cord Injury (Lumbosacral) 879
Sunil Sabharwal, MD

149 Stroke 887
Joel Stein, MD

150 Stroke in Young Adults 893
Randie M. Black-Schaffer, MD, MA

151 Systemic Lupus Erythematosus 901
Mahboob U. Rahman, MD, PhD

152 Transverse Myelitis 907
Peter A.C. Lim, MD

153 Traumatic Brain Injury 913
David Burke, MD, MA

Contributors

Venu Akuthota, MD
Associate Professor of Physical Medicine and Rehabilitation, University of Colorado School of Medicine, Denver, Colorado

Joseph T. Alleva, MD
Assistant Professor, Northwestern University Medical School, Chicago, Illinois; Medical Director, Outpatient Services, Division of Physical Medicine and Rehabilitation, Evanston Northwestern Healthcare, Evanston, Illinois

Eduardo Amy, MD
Assistant Professor, Department of Physical Medicine, Rehabilitation, and Sports Medicine, University of Puerto Rico School of Medicine, San Juan, Puerto Rico; Orthopedic Surgeon, University Hospital, Ponce, Puerto Rico

Karen Atkinson, MD, MPH
Assistant Professor, Department of Medicine/Rheumatology, Emory University School of Medicine, Atlanta, Georgia; Chief of Rheumatology, Atlanta Veterans Affairs Medical Center, Decatur, Georgia

Joseph F. Audette, MA, MD
Assistant Professor, Harvard Medical School; Staff Physiatrist, Spaulding Rehabilitation Hospital, Boston, Massachusetts

John R. Bach, MD
Professor, Physical Medicine and Rehabilitation, Professor of Neurosciences, Department of Physical Medicine and Rehabilitation, University of Medicine and Dentistry of New Jersey–New Jersey Medical School; Associate Medical Director, Department of Physical Medicine and Rehabilitation, University Hospital, Newark, New Jersey

Allison Bailey, MD
Instructor, Harvard Medical School; Staff Physiatrist, Spaulding Rehabilitation Hospital, Boston, Massachusetts

Jennifer Baima, MD
Clinical Instructor, Harvard Medical School; Staff Physiatrist, Brigham and Women's Hospital; Staff Physiatrist, Spaulding Rehabilitation Hospital, Boston, Massachusetts

Sarah S. Banerjee, MD
Clinical Instructor, Department of Orthopaedic Surgery, Texas Tech University Health Sciences Center; Private Practice, El Paso, Texas

Moon Suk Bang, MD, PhD
Professor, Department of Rehabilitation Medicine, Seoul National University, College of Medicine; Professor, Department of Rehabilitation Medicine, Seoul National University Hospital, Seoul, South Korea

Norman L. Banks, MD, MS
Adjunct Clinical Professor, University of Southern California School of Biokinesiology and Physical Therapy, Los Angeles, California; Physician, Director of Chronic Pain Clinic, Palo Alto Medical Foundation, Department of Physical Medicine and Rehabilitation, Palo Alto, California

Karen P. Barr, MD
Associate Professor, Rehabilitation Medicine, University of Washington, Seattle, Washington

Heather G. Belanger, PhD
Assistant Professor, Psychology Department, University of South Florida; Staff Psychologist, James A. Haley Veterans' Hospital, Tampa, Florida

Peter Bienkowski, MD
Resident, Department of Orthopedics, Children's Hospital, Boston, Massachusetts

Randie M. Black-Schaffer, MD, MA
Assistant Professor, Department of Physical Medicine and Rehabilitation, Harvard Medical School; Lecturer, Department of Rehabilitation Medicine, Tufts University School of Medicine; Interim Director, Stroke Program, Medical Director, Young Adult Stroke Service, Spaulding Rehabilitation Hospital, Boston, Massachusetts

Philip J. Blount, MD
Assistant Professor of Medicine, Department of Orthopedics and Rehabilitation, University of Mississippi; Physiatrist, University of Mississippi Medical Center, Jackson, Mississippi

William L. Bockenek, MD
Adjunct Clinical Professor, University of North Carolina at Chapel Hill, Chapel Hill, North Carolina; Medical Director, Carolinas Rehabilitation, Chairman, Department of Physical Medicine and Rehabilitation, Carolinas Medical Center, Charlotte, North Carolina

Kath Bogie, DPhil
Senior Research Associate, Department of Orthopaedics, Case Western Reserve University, School of Medicine; Senior Research Scientist, Louis Stokes Cleveland Department of Veterans Affairs Medical Center, Cleveland, Ohio

Kristian Borg, MD, PhD
Professor, Karolinska Institute; Director, Rehabilitation Medicine, Department of Clinical Sciences, Danderyd Hospital; Senior Consultant, Department of Rehabilitation Medicine, Danderyd Hospital, Stockholm, Sweden

Joanne Borg-Stein, MD
Assistant Professor, Harvard Department of Physical Medicine and Rehabilitation, Harvard Medical School; Chief, Physical Medicine and Rehabilitation, Newton-Wellesley Hospital, Medical Director, Spaulding-Wellesley Rehabilitation Center, Medical Director, Newton-Wellesley Hospital Spine Center, Spaulding Rehabilitation Hospital, Harvard Medical School, Boston, Massachusetts

Jay E. Bowen, DO
Clinical Assistant Professor, Department of Physical Medicine and Rehabilitation, University of Medicine and Dentistry, New Jersey: New Jersey School of Medicine, Newark, New Jersey

Jeffrey S. Brault, DO, PT
Assistant Professor, Mayo Medical School; Consultant, Mayo Clinic, Rochester, Minnesota

Steven E. Braverman, MD, MS
Assistant Professor, Uniformed University of the Health Sciences, Bethesda, Maryland; Deputy Director, Health Policy and Services, Chief Consultant to the Army Surgeon General, United States Army Medical Command, Houston, Texas

Diane W. Braza, MD
Associate Professor, Department of Physical Medicine and Rehabilitation, Medical College of Wisconsin; Physiatrist and Interist, Froedtert Memorial Lutheran Hospital, Milwaukee, Wisconsin

Patrick Brennan, MD
Instructor, Department of Physical Medicine and Rehabilitation, Harvard Medical School; Physician, Spaulding Rehabilitation Hospital, Boston, Massachusetts

Jeffrey T. Brodie, MD
Attending Physician, Division of Orthopaedic Surgery, St. Joseph Medical Center, Baltimore, Maryland

David Burke, MD, MA
Professor, Emory University School of Medicine; Chairman, Department of Rehabilitation Medicine, Atlanta, Georgia

Mabel E. Caban, MD
Assistant Professor, University of Texas Medical Branch, Galveston, Texas

Alexios Carayannopoulos, DO, MPH
Medical Director, Spine Center, Department of Neurosurgery, Lahey Clinic, Burlington, Massachusetts

Charles Cassidy, MD
Henry H. Banks Associate Professor and Chairman, Department of Orthopaedic Surgery, Tufts University School of Medicine; Chairman, Department of Orthopaedic Surgery, Tufts-New England Medical Center, Boston, Massachusetts

David A. Cassius, MD
Private Practice, Broadway Sports and Internal Medicine, Seattle, Washington

Andrea Cheville, MD
Associate Professor, Physical Medicine and Rehabilitation, Mayo Clinic, Rochester, Minnesota

Kelvin Chew, MD
Director, Sports Medicine Center, Department of Orthopedics, Alexandria Hospital, Singapore

Martin K. Childers, DO, PhD
Associate Professor, Wake Forest University Health Sciences, Department of Neurology; Associate Professor, Wake Forest Institute for Regenerative Medicine, Winston-Salem, North Carolina

Chien Chow, MD
Associate Instructor of Surgery, Harvard School of Medicine; Surgical Intern, Beth Israel Deaconess Medical Center, Boston, Massachusetts

Victor Chung, BS
Medical Student, Tufts University School of Medicine, Boston, Massachusetts

Daniel M. Clinchot, MD
Residency Program Director, Department of Physical Medicine and Rehabilitation; Director, Medical Humanities, Ohio State University College of Medicine, Columbus, Ohio

Isaac Cohen, MD
Physiatrist, The Orthopaedic and Sports Medicine Center, Trumbull, Connecticut

Earl J. Craig, MD
Associate Professor, Department of Physical Medicine and Rehabilitation, Indiana University School of Medicine, Indianapolis, Indiana

Christine Curtis, BS
Research Coordinator, Children's Hospital of Boston, Division of Sports Medicine, Department of Orthopedics, Boston, Massachusetts

Jatin Dave, MD, MPH
Instructor, Department of Medicine, Harvard Medical School, Boston, Massachusetts; Director of Education, Division of Aging, Brigham and Women's Hospital, Boston, Massachusetts; Medical Director, Evercare Hospice and Palliative Care, Waltham, Massachusetts

Alan M. Davis, MD, PhD
Assistant Professor, Division of Physical Medicine and Rehabilitation, University of Utah School of Medicine; Medical Director, Salt Lake Regional Medical Center Rehabilitation; Chief of Staff, Promise Specialty Hospital, Salt Lake City, Utah

David R. Del Toro, MD
Associate Professor, Department of Physical Medicine and Rehabilitation, Medical College of Wisconsin; Medical Director, Comprehensive Inpatient Rehabilitation Unit, Froedtert Memorial Lutheran Hospital, Milwaukee, Wisconsin

Jennifer Devine, MD
Resident Physician, Spaulding Rehabilitation Hospital and Harvard Medical School, Boston, Massachusetts

Timothy R. Dillingham, MD
Professor and Chairman, Department of Physical Medicine and Rehabilitation, Froedtert Memorial Lutheran Hospital and the Medical College of Wisconsin, Milwaukee, Wisconsin

Susan J. Dreyer, MD
Associate Professor, Physical Medicine and Rehabilitation, Associate Professor, Orthopaedic Surgery, Emory University, School of Medicine; Physiatrist, Emory Orthopaedic and Spine Center, Atlanta, Georgia

Nancy Dudek, MD, MEd
Assistant Professor, University of Ottawa; Associate Staff, Ottawa Hospital, Ottawa, Ontario, Canada

Sheila Dugan, MD
Assistant Professor, Department of Physical Medicine and Rehabilitation, Rush Medical College; Medical Director, Department of Physical Medicine and Rehabilitation, Rush University Medical Center, Chicago, Illinois

Gerold R. Ebenbichler, MD
Research Associate Professor, Vienna Medical University; Senior Medical Specialist, University Clinics of Physical Medicine and Rehabilitation, Vienna General Hospital, Vienna, Austria

Omar El Abd, MD
Instructor, Harvard Medical School, Boston, Massachusetts; Interventional Spine Director, Newton-Wellesley Hospital, Newton, Massachusetts; Attending Physician, Spaulding Rehabilitation Hospital, Boston, Massachusetts

Maury Ellenberg, MD
Clinical Professor, Department of Physical Medicine and Rehabilitation; Wayne State University-School of Medicine; Chief, Department of Physical Medicine and Rehabilitation, Sinai Grace Hospital, Detroit, Michigan

Erik Ensrud, MD
Assistant Professor, Medicine/Neurology, University of Texas Health Science Center at San Antonio; Staff Physician, Neurology, University Health System, San Antonio, Texas

Avital Fast, MD
Professor and Chairman, Department of Physical Medicine and Rehabilitation, Albert Einstein College of Medicine, Bronx, New York; Professor and Chairman, Department of Physical Medicine and Rehabilitation, Montefiore Medical Center, Bronx, New York

Jeffery B. Feldman, PhD
Assistant Professor, Director of Occupational Rehabilitation Programs, Wake Forest University School of Medicine, Winston-Salem, North Carolina

Brian T. Fitzgerald, MD
Staff Orthopaedic Hand Surgeon, Naval Medical Center, San Diego, California

Leslie S. Foster, DO
Assistant Chief, Physical Medicine and Rehabilitation, Walter Reed Army Medical Center, Washington, DC

Patrick M. Foye, MD
Associate Professor of Physical Medicine and Rehabilitation, Co-Director, Musculoskeletal/Sports/Spine Fellowship, University of Medicine and Dentistry of New Jersey, New Jersey Medical School; Director, Coccyx Pain Service, Co-Director, Osteoarthritis and Back Pain Clinic, University Hospital, Newark, New Jersey

Michael Fredericson, MD
Associate Professor, Stanford University; Chief, Physical Medicine and Rehabilitation Clinics, Stanford Hospital, Stanford, California

Michelle Gittler, MD
Clinical Associate Professor, Department of Orthopedic Surgery and Rehabilitation Medicine, University of Chicago; Program Director, Associate Medical Director for Academic Affairs, Schwab Rehabilitation Hospital, Chicago, Illinois

Mel B. Glenn, MD
Associate Professor, Department of Physical Medicine and Rehabilitation, Harvard Medical School, Boston, Massachusetts; Director of Outpatient and Community Brain Injury Rehabilitation, Spaulding Rehabilitation Hospital, Boston, Massachusetts; Medical Director, MENTOR ABI, Braintree, Massachusetts; Clinical Medical Director, Community Rehabilitation Care, Newton, Massachusetts

Peter Gonzalez, MD
Assistant Professor of Physical Medicine and Rehabilitation, University of Colorado School of Medicine, Denver, Colorado

Dawn M. Grosser, MD
Orthopaedic Surgery, Christus Spohn Hospital, Corpus Christi Medical Center; Orthopaedic Associates of Corpus Christi, Corpus Christi, Texas

H. Michael Guo, MD, PhD
Assistant Professor, Wake Forest University Health Sciences; Assistant Professor, Wake Forest University Baptist Medical Center, Winston-Salem, North Carolina

Navneet Gupta, MD
Physician, Pain Medicine Associates, Johnson City, Tennessee

Hope S. Hacker, MD
Assistant Professor, University of Texas Health Science Center, San Antonio; Director, Electrodiagnostic Medicine, Rehabilitation Medicine Service, South Texas Veterans Health Care System, San Antonio, Texas

Ed Hanada, MD
Assistant Professor, Faculty of Medicine, Dalhousie University; Staff Physiatrist, Capital District Health Authority, Halifax, Nova Scotia, Canada

Toni J. Hanson, MD
Assistant Professor, Physical Medicine and Rehabilitation, Staff Physician, Department of Physical Medicine and Rehabilitation, Mayo Clinic, Rochester, Minnesota

Amanda L. Harrington, MD
Resident Physician, Department of Physical Medicine and Rehabilitation, Carolinas Rehabilitation, Carolinas Medical Center, Charlotte, North Carolina

Sandra S. Hatch, MD
Professor, Vice-Chairman, Department of Radiation Oncology, Residency Director, Radiation Oncology, University of Texas Medical Branch, Galveston, Texas

Melvyn L. Hecht, MD
Clinical Instructor, Department of Medicine, Harvard Medical School, Boston, Massachusetts; Beth Israel Deaconess Medical Center, Boston, Massachusetts; Chief Medical Officer, Youville Hospital and Rehabilitation Center, Cambridge, Massachusetts; Department of Medicine, Cambridge Hospital, Cambridge, Massachusetts; Spaulding Rehabilitation Hospital, Boston, Massachusetts

Chester H. Ho, MD
Assistant Professor, Department of Physical Medicine and Rehabilitation, Case Western Reserve University School of Medicine; Chief, Spinal Cord Injury, Louis Stokes Cleveland Department of Veterans Affairs Medical Center, Cleveland, Ohio

Anne Z. Hoch, DO, PT
Associate Professor, Physical Medicine and Rehabilitation; Associate Professor, Orthopedic Surgery; Director, Women's Sports Medicine Program, Medical College of Wisconsin, Milwaukee, Wisconsin

Joseph C. Honet, MD
Professor, Wayne State University, School of Medicine; Professor Emeritus, Department of Physical Medicine and Rehabilitation, Sinai Grace Hospital, Detroit Medical Center, Detroit, Michigan

Thomas H. Hudgins, MD
Assistant Professor, Northwestern University Medical School, Chicago, Illinois; Medical Director; Center for Sports and Spine Care, Division of Physical Medicine and Rehabilitation, Evanston Northwestern Healthcare, Evanston, Illinois

Faiza Humayun, MD
Staff Physician, James A. Haley Veterans' Hospital, Tampa, Florida

Marta Imamura, MD
Collaborative Professor, University of São Paulo School of Medicine; Attending Physician, Division of Physical Medicine and Rehabilitation, Department of Orthopaedics and Traumatology, University of São Paulo School of Medicine, São Paulo, Brazil

Satiko Tomikawa Imamura, MD, PhD
Professor, University of São Paulo School of Medicine; Coordinator, Pain Clinic, Division of Rehabilitation Medicine, University of São Paulo School of Medicine, São Paulo, Brazil

Zacharia Isaac, MD
Instructor, Physical Medicine and Rehabilitation, Harvard Medical School; Director, Interventional Physiatry, Medical Director, Brigham and Women's Hospital, Comprehensive Spine Care Center, Spaulding Rehabilitation Hospital, Brigham and Women's Hospital, Boston, Massachusetts

Cristin Jouve, MD
Clinical Instructor, Physical Medicine and Rehabilitation, Harvard Medical School; Physiatrist, New England Baptist Spine Center, Boston, Massachusetts

Se Hee Jung, MD, MS
Instructor, Department of Rehabilitation Medicine, Seoul National University College of Medicine; Clinical Assistant Professor, Department of Physical Medicine and Rehabilitation, Seoul Metropolitan Boramae Medical Center, Seoul, South Korea

Robert J. Kaplan, MD
Associate Professor, Rehabilitation Medicine, University of Kansas School of Medicine; Staff Physician, Kansas University Medical Center, Department of Rehabilitation Medicine, Kansas City, Kansas

Jonathan Kay, MD
Associate Clinical Professor of Medicine, Harvard Medical School; Director of Clinical Trials, Rheumatology Unit, Massachusetts General Hospital, Boston, Massachusetts

Ayal M. Kaynan, MD
Director, Minimally Invasive and Robotic Surgery, Morristown Memorial Hospital, Morristown, New Jersey

Florian S. Keplinger, MD
Assistant Professor, Department of Physical Medicine and Rehabilitation, University of Arkansas for Medical Sciences, Little Rock, Arkansas

Todd A. Kile, MD
Associate Professor of Orthopedic Surgery, Mayo Graduate School of Medicine; Chair, Division of Foot and Ankle Surgery, Consultant, Department of Orthopedic Surgery, Mayo Clinic, Scottsdale, Arizona

John C. King, MD
Professor, The University of Texas Health Science Center at San Antonio; Director of Reeves Rehabilitation Center at University Hospital, San Antonio, Texas

Ricardo Knight, MD, PT
Instructor, Department of Physical Medicine and Rehabilitation, Harvard Medical School; Spaulding Rehabilitation Hospital and Massachusetts General Hospital, Boston, Massachusetts

Jason H. Kortte, MS, CCC-SLP
Senior Speech-Language Pathologist, Good Samaritan Hospital, Baltimore, Maryland

Brian J. Krabak, MD, MBA
Clinical Associate Professor, University of Washington Medicine Sports and Spine Physicians, Rehabilitation, Orthopaedics, and Sports Medicine, University of Washington, Seattle, Washington; Team Physician, University of Washington, Medical Director, 4 Deserts Races

Lisa S. Krivickas, MD
Associate Professor, Physical Medicine and Rehabilitation, Harvard Medical School; Director, Electromyography, Spaulding Rehabilitation Hospital, Associate Chief, Physical Medicine and Rehabilitation, Massachusetts General Hospital, Boston, Massachusetts

Robert J. Krug, MD
Chairman and Director, Department of Rehabilitation Medicine, Saint Francis Hospital and Medical Center, Avon, Connecticut; Medical Director and Director of the Neuromuscular-Skeletal Program, Mount Sinai Rehabilitation Hospital, Hartford, Connecticut

Gail A. Latlief, DO
Assistant Professor, Internal Medicine, University of South Florida; Medical Director, Comprehensive Integrated Inpatient Rehabilitation Program, James A. Haley Veterans' Hospital, Tampa, Florida

Elise H. Lee, MD
Physical Medicine and Rehabilitation, Harvard Medical School; Spaulding Rehabilitation Hospital, Boston, Massachusetts

Sammy M. Lee, DPM
Attending Staff, Podiatry Service, Massachusetts General Hospital, Boston, Massachusetts

Shi-Uk Lee, MD, PhD
Assistant Professor, Department of Rehabilitation Medicine, Seoul National University College of Medicine; Chairman, Department of Physical Medicine and Rehabilitation, Seoul Metropolitan Boramae Medical Center, Seoul, South Korea

Yong-Tae Lee, MD
Instructor, Harvard Medical School; Attending Physician, Spaulding Rehabilitation Hospital, Boston, Massachusetts

Ted A. Lennard, MD
Clinical Assistant Professor, Department of Physical Medicine and Rehabilitation, University of Arkansas for Medical Sciences, Little Rock, Arkansas; Department of Physical Medicine and Rehabilitation, Springfield Neurological and Spine Institute, Springfield, Missouri

Paul Lento, MD
Assistant Professor, Northwestern University School of Medicine; Attending Physician, Rehabilitation Institute of Chicago, Spine and Sports Rehabilitation Center, Chicago, Illinois

Peter A.C. Lim, MD
Clinical Associate Professor, Department of Physical Medicine and Rehabilitation, Baylor College of Medicine, Houston, Texas; Head and Senior Consultant, Department of Rehabilitation Medicine, Singapore General Hospital, Singapore

Karl-August Lindgren, MD, PhD
Physician in Chief, Rehabilitation ORTON, Invalid Foundation, Helsinki, Finland

Elizabeth Loder, MD, MPH
Associate Professor of Neurology, Harvard Medical School, Boston, Massachusetts; Chief, Division of Headache and Pain, Department of Neurology, Brigham and Women's Hospital, Boston, Massachusetts; Clinical Editor, British Medical Journal, London, United Kingdom

Sandra Maguire, MD
Attending Physician, Physical Medicine and Rehabilitation, Compass Medical PC, East Bridgewater, Massachusetts

Gerard A. Malanga, MD
Clinical Professor, Physical Medicine and Rehabilitation, University of Medicine and Dentistry of New Jersey: New Jersey School of Medicine, Newark, New Jersey; Director, Pain Management, Department of Neuroscience, Overlook Hospital, Summit, New Jersey; Director, Sports Medicine Fellowship, Physical Medicine and Rehabilitation, Mountainside Hospital, Montclair, New Jersey; Physician, Atlantic Sports Health and Morristown Memorial Hospital, Morristown, New Jersey

Katherine Mashey, DPM
Assistant Director of the Podiatric Surgical Residency, Saint Francis Hospital and Medical Center, Hartford, Connecticut

Koichiro Matsuo, DDS, PhD
Assistant Professor, Department of Physical Medicine and Rehabilitation, Johns Hopkins University School of Medicine, Baltimore, Maryland

Kelly McInnis, DO
Sports Medicine Fellow, Spaulding Rehabilitation Hospital, Massachusetts General Hospital, Boston, Massachusetts

Peter M. McIntosh, MD
Clinical Instructor, Mayo Graduate School of Medicine; Consultant, Mayo Clinic, Jacksonville, Florida

Alec L. Meleger, MD
Clinical Instructor, Department of Physical Medicine and Rehabilitation, Harvard Medical School, Boston, Massachusetts; Director, Pain Medicine Fellowship, Spaulding Rehabilitation Hospital, Medford, Massachusetts; Interventional Physiatrist, Spine Center, Newton-Wellesley Hospital, Newton, Massachusetts

Lyle J. Micheli, MD
Clinical Professor of Orthopedic Surgery at Harvard Medical School; Director, Division of Sports Medicine Department of Orthopedics, Children's Hospital of Boston, Boston, Massachusetts

William Micheo, MD
Professor and Chairman, Department of Physical Medicine, Rehabilitation and Sports Medicine, University of Puerto Rico, School of Medicine, San Juan, Puerto Rico; Program Director, Physical Medicine and Rehabilitation, University Hospital, San Juan, Puerto Rico; Chief, Section of Physical Medicine and Rehabilitation, Department of Medicine, Hospital San Pablo, Bayamón, Puerto Rico; Chief, Section of Physical Medicine and Rehabilitation, Auxilio Mutuo Hospital, Hato Rey, Puerto Rico

William Moore, MD
Physician, Sports Medicine Department, Kaiser Permanente, Union City, California

S. Ali Mostoufi, MD
Interventional Physiatrist, Assistant Professor of Rehabilitation Medicine, Tufts University School of Medicine, Boston, Massachusetts; Medical Director, Cambridge Spine Center, Cambridge, Massachusetts

Chaitanya S. Mudgal, MD, MS (Orth), MCh (Orth)
Instructor, Department of Orthopaedic Surgery, Attending Staff, Orthopaedic Hand Service, Co-Director, Hand Surgery Fellowship, Harvard Medical School; Attending Staff, Orthopaedic Hand Service, Massachusetts General Hospital, Boston, Massachusetts

Gregory J. Mulford, MD
Clinical Associate Professor, Department of Physical Medicine and Rehabilitation, University of Medicine and Dentistry of New Jersey: New Jersey School of Medicine, Newark, New Jersey; Chairman, Department of Rehabilitation Medicine, Morristown Memorial Hospital; Medical Director, Atlantic Rehabilitation Services, Atlantic Health, Morristown, New Jersey

Shanker Nesathurai, MD
Assistant Professor, Physical Medicine and Rehabilitation, Harvard Medical School; Researcher, Spaulding Rehabilitation Hospital and Massachusetts General Hospital, Boston, Massachusetts

José M. Nolla, MD
Attending Orthopaedic/Hand Surgeon, St. Luke's Episcopal Hospital, Houston, Texas

Carina J. O'Neill, DO
Clinical Associate, Harvard Medical School, Boston, Massachusetts, Medical Director, Spaulding Rehabilitation Hospital, Braintree Massachusetts Outpatient Clinic, Braintree, Massachusetts

Michael D. Osborne, MD
Assistant Professor in Physical Medicine and Rehabilitation, Assistant Professor in Anesthesiology, Mayo Clinic; Consultant, Department of Physical Medicine and Rehabilitation, Consultant, Department of Pain Medicine, Mayo Clinic, Jacksonville, Florida

Lora Beth Packel, PT, MS
Assistant Professor in Physical Therapy, University of the Sciences in Philadelphia, Philadelphia, Pennsylvania

Jeffrey B. Palmer, MD
Lawrence Cardinal Sheham Professor and Director, Department of Physical Medicine and Rehabilitation, Professor, Otolaryngology–Head and Neck Surgery, Professor, Functional Anatomy and Evolution, Johns Hopkins University, School of Medicine; Physiatrist-in-Chief, Department of Physical Medicine and Rehabilitation, Johns Hopkins Hospital, Baltimore, Maryland

Paul F. Pasquina, MD
Chairman, Physical Medicine and Rehabilitation, Walter Reed Army Medical Center and National Naval Medical Center; Department of Orthopaedics and Rehabilitation, Walter Reed Army Medical Center, Washington, DC

Atul Patel, MD
Physician, Physical Medicine and Rehabilitation, Kansas City Bone and Joint Clinic, Overland Park, Kansas; Medical Director, Outpatient Rehabilitation, Research Brookside Campus, Kansas City, Missouri

Inder Perkash, MD
Professor of Urology, Stanford University School of Medicine, Stanford, California; Director, Regional Center for Spinal Cord Injuries, Veterans Affairs Palo Alto Health Care System, Palo Alto, California

Edward M. Phillips, MD
Instructor, Department of Physical Medicine and Rehabilitation, Harvard Medical School; Director, Outpatient Medical Services, Spaulding Rehabilitation Hospital Network, Boston, Massachusetts

Thomas E. Pobre, MD
Clinical Assistant Professor, Physical Medicine and Rehabilitation, State University of New York, Stony Brook, New York; Adjunct Clinical Assistant Professor, New York College of Osteopathic Medicine, Old Westbury, New York; Attending Physician, Physical Medicine and Rehabilitation, Nassau University Medical Center, East Meadow, New York

Elliot Pollack, DPM
Chief, Section of Podiatric Surgery, Saint Francis Hospital and Medical Center, Hartford, Connecticut; Private Practice, Hartford and East Granby, Connecticut

Mahboob U. Rahman, MD, PhD
Associate Professor (Adjunct), University of Pennsylvania School of Medicine, Philadelphia, Pennsylvania; Senior Director, Clinical Research and Development, Johnson & Johnson Centocor, Inc., Horsham, Pennsylvania

James Rainville, MD
Assistant Clinical Professor, Department of Physical Medicine, Harvard Medical School; Chief, Physical Medicine and Rehabilitation, New England Baptist Hospital, Boston, Massachusetts

Edwardo Ramos, MD
Department of Physical Medicine, Rehabilitation and Sports Medicine, University of Puerto Rico School of Medicine, San Juan, Puerto Rico; Physical Medicine and Rehabilitation Residency Program Director, University Hospital and Pediatric Hospital, Chief, Section of Physical Medicine and Rehabilitation, Department of Medicine, Hospital San Pablo, Bayamón, Puerto Rico

David Ring, MD, PhD
Assistant Professor of Orthopaedic Surgery, Harvard Medical School; Medical Director and Director of Research, Orthopaedic Hand and Upper Extremity Service, Massachusetts General Hospital, Boston, Massachusetts

Darren Rosenberg, DO
Instructor, Harvard Medical School, Boston, Massachusetts; Clinical Assistant Professor, University of New England College of Osteopathic Medicine, Biddeford, Maine; Medical Director, Department of Physical Medicine and Rehabilitation, Spaulding-Framingham Outpatient Center, Framingham, Massachusetts; Director, Osteopathic Manipulative Medicine, Spaulding Rehabilitation Hospital; Clinical Associate, Massachusetts General Hospital; Clinical Associate, Brigham and Women's Hospital, Boston, Massachusetts

Justin Riutta, MD
Director, Breast Cancer Rehabilitation; Director, Lymphedema Program, William Beaumont Hospital, Royal Oak, Michigan

Thomas D. Rizzo, Jr., MD
Assistant Professor, Physical Medicine and Rehabilitation, College of Medicine, Mayo Clinic; Consultant and Chair, Department of Physical Medicine and Rehabilitation, Mayo Clinic, Jacksonville, Florida

Seward B. Rutkove, MD
Associate Professor of Neurology, Harvard Medical School; Chief, Division of Neuromuscular Disease, Department of Neurology, Beth Israel Deaconess Medical Center, Boston, Massachusetts

Sunil Sabharwal, MD
Assistant Professor, Department of Physical Medicine and Rehabilitation, Harvard Medical School; Chief of Spinal Cord Injury, Veterans Affairs Boston Healthcare System, Boston, Massachusetts

Francisco H. Santiago, MD
Attending Physician, Rehabilitation Medicine, Bronx Lebanon Hospital, Bronx, New York

Robert J. Scardina, DPM
Clinical Instructor in Orthopaedic Surgery, Harvard Medical School; Chief, Podiatry Service, Residency Program Director, Podiatry Service, Massachusetts General Hospital, Boston, Massachusetts

Michael K. Schaufele, MD
Assistant Professor, Emory University, School of Medicine, Department of Orthopaedics, Department of Rehabilitation Medicine; Attending Physiatrist, Emory Spine Center, Atlanta, Georgia

Jeffrey C. Schneider, MD
Instructor, Department of Physical Medicine and Rehabilitation, Harvard Medical School; Medical Director, Burn Rehabilitation, Spaulding Rehabilitation Hospital, Massachusetts General Hospital, Boston, Massachusetts

Joel D. Scholten, MD
Assistant Professor, Internal Medicine, University of South Florida; Medical Director, Polytrauma Rehabilitation Center, James A. Haley Veterans' Hospital, Tampa, Florida

Steven G. Scott, DO
Assistant Professor, Internal Medicine, University of South Florida; Chief, Physical Medicine and Rehabilitation, Director, Polytrauma Rehabilitation Center, James A. Haley Veterans' Hospital, Tampa, Florida

Miriam Segal, MD
Attending Physician, Department of Physical Medicine and Rehabilitation, Albert Einstein College of Medicine, Bronx, New York; Attending Physician, Department of Physical Medicine and Rehabilitation, Montefiore Medical Center, Bronx, New York

Vivek M. Shah MD
Clinical Associate, Tufts University School of Medicine; Orthopaedic Resident, Tufts-New England Medical Center, Boston, Massachusetts

Lena Shahban, MD
Physiatrist, Interventional Pain Consultants, Oak Brook, Illinois

Nutan Sharma, MD, PhD
Assistant Professor of Neurology, Harvard Medical School, Cambridge, Massachusetts; Assistant Neurologist, Massachusetts General Hospital, Boston, Massachusetts; Associate Neurologist, Brigham and Women's Hospital, Boston, Massachusetts

Julie K. Silver, MD
Assistant Professor, Department of Physical Medicine and Rehabilitation, Harvard Medical School; Associate in Physiatry, Brigham and Women's Hospital and Spaulding Rehabilitation Hospital, Boston, Massachusetts

Kenneth H. Silver, MD
Associate Professor, Department of Physical Medicine and Rehabilitation, John Hopkins University School of Medicine; Chief, Rehabilitation Medicine Service, Good Samaritan Hospital, Baltimore, Maryland

Ajay K. Singh, MD
Associate Professor of Medicine, Harvard Medical School; Clinical Director, Renal Division, Brigham and Women's Hospital, Boston, Massachusetts

Aneesh Singla, MD, MPH
Instructor, Harvard Medical School; Assistant Anesthetist, Massachusetts General Hospital, Boston, Massachusetts

Daniel Sipple, DO
Attending Physiatrist, Rehabilitation Institute of Chicago Chronic Pain Care Center, Chicago, Illinois

Robert S. Skerker, MD
Associate Clinical Professor of Rehabilitation Medicine, University of Medicine and Dentistry of New Jersey: New Jersey School of Medicine, Newark, New Jersey; Attending Physiatrist, Atlantic Rehabilitation Institute, Morristown, New Jersey

David M. Slovik, MD
Associate Professor of Medicine, Harvard Medical School; Physician, Endocrine Unit, Massachusetts General Hospital, Boston, Massachusetts

Jonas Sokolof, DO
Clinical Fellow, Physical Medicine and Rehabilitation, Harvard Medical School; Resident Physician, Spaulding Rehabilitation Hospital, Boston, Massachusetts

James Spinelli, DO
Pain Management Fellow, Spaulding Rehabilitation Hospital, Harvard Medical School, Boston, Massachusetts

Joel Stein, MD
Associate Professor, Department of Physical Medicine and Rehabilitation, Harvard Medical School; Chief Medical Officer, Spaulding Rehabilitation Hospital, Boston, Massachusetts

Meryl Stein, MD
Resident Physician, Department of Physical Medicine and Rehabilitation, Harvard Medical School, Spaulding Rehabilitation Hospital, Boston, Massachusetts

Sonja K. Stilp, MD
Attending Physiatrist, Boulder Orthopedics, Boulder, Colorado

Todd P. Stitik, MD
Professor and Acting Director, Department of Physical Medicine and Rehabilitation-Sports Medicine, University of Medicine and Dentistry of New Jersey: New Jersey School of Medicine, Newark, New Jersey

Seneca A. Storm, MD
Clinical Assistant Professor, Department of Physical Medicine and Rehabilitation, Michigan State University, College of Osteopathic Medicine, East Lansing, Michigan; Private Practice, Lansing Spine and Extremity Rehabilitation, Lansing, Michigan

Michael F. Stretanski, DO
Clinical Assistant Professor, Ohio University College of Osteopathic Medicine, Columbus, Ohio; Fellowship Director, Interventional Spine and Pain Rehabilitation; President, Neurosciences Committee, MedCentral, Mansfield, Ohio; Fisher-Titus Medical Center, Norwalk, Ohio

Ann-Marie Thomas, MD, PT
Instructor, Harvard Medical School; Staff Physiatrist, Spaulding Rehabilitation Hospital; Clinical Associate, Massachusetts General Hospital; Associate Physiatrist in Medicine, Brigham and Women's Hospital, Boston, Massachusetts

Mark A. Thomas, MD
Associate Professor, Physical Medicine and Rehabilitation, Albert Einstein College of Medicine; Program Director, Physical Medicine and Rehabilitation, Associate Chairman, Department of Physical Medicine and Rehabilitation, Montefiore Medical Center, Bronx, New York

Anita Thompson, PT
Massachusetts General Hospital Institute for Health Professions, Charlestown, Massachusetts; Physical Therapy Supervisor, Spaulding Rehabilitation Hospital, Wellesley, Massachusetts

Guy Trudel, MD
Professor of Medicine and Surgery, University of Ottawa, Ottawa, Ontario, Canada

Gregory L. Umphrey, MD
Physician, Department of Physical Medicine and Rehabilitation, Mayo Clinic, Rochester, Minnesota

Roman Vallarino, Jr., MD
Assistant Clinical Professor, Physical Medicine and Rehabilitation, Albert Einstein School of Medicine, Bronx, New York; Attending Physician, Department of Neurosciences, New York Methodist Hospital, Brooklyn, New York

Rodney D. Vanderploeg, PhD
Associate Professor, Department of Psychology, University of South Florida; Staff Psychologist, Clinical Director of the Brain Injury Rehabilitation Program, James A. Haley Veterans' Hospital, Tampa, Florida

Carole S. Vetter, MD
Assistant Professor, Orthopaedic Surgery Associate Program; Director, Orthopaedic Surgery Residency, Medical College of Wisconsin, Milwaukee, Wisconsin

Ariana Vora, MD
Instructor, Harvard Medical School; Staff Physiatrist, Massachusetts General Hospital; Staff Physiatrist, Spaulding Rehabilitation Hospital, Boston, Massachusetts

Aimee H. Walsh, MD
Assistant Professor, University of Alabama at Birmingham, Department of Anesthesia; Medical Director, Pain Treatment Center, University of Alabama, Highlands Pain Treatment Clinic, Birmingham, Alabama

David Wang, DO
Instructor, Harvard Medical School; Staff Physiatrist, Spaulding Rehabilitation Hospital, Boston, Massachusetts

Yumei Wang, MD
Assistant Professor, Physical Medicine and Rehabilitation, Albert Einstein College of Medicine; Attending Physician, Montefiore Medical Center, Bronx, New York

Jay M. Weiss, MD
Assistant Professor of Clinical Physical Medicine and Rehabilitation, SUNY Stony Brook, Stony Brook, New York; Medical Director, Long Island Physical Medicine and Rehabilitation, Levittown, New York

Lyn D. Weiss, MD
Professor of Clinical Physical Medicine and Rehabilitation, SUNY Stony Brook, Stony Brook, New York; Chairman and Program Director, Department of Physical Medicine and Rehabilitation, Director, Electrodiagnostic Medicine, Nassau University Medical Center, East Meadow, New York

David Wexler, MD, FRCS (Tr, Orth)
Orthopaedic Surgeon, Millinocket Regional Hospital, Millinocket, Maine

Jane Wierbicky, RN, BSN
Health Services Coordinator, Department of Rehabilitation Medicine, Boston Medical Center, Boston, Massachusetts

J. Michael Wieting, DO
Professor of Physical Medicine and Rehabilitation and Osteopathic Principles and Practices, Medical Director of Sports Medicine, Lincoln Memorial University–De Busk College of Osteopathic Medicine, Harrogate, Tennessee

Allen N. Wilkins, MD
Chief Resident, Harvard Medical School; Chief Resident, Spaulding Rehabilitation Hospital, Boston, Massachusetts

Meijuan Zhao, MD
Instructor, Department of Physical Medicine and Rehabilitation, Harvard Medical School; Staff Physiatrist, Physical Medicine and Rehabilitation, Spaulding Rehabilitation Hospital, Boston, Massachusetts

Preface

From the beginning, it was our idea to create a book that covers a variety of medical conditions that the average internist/family practitioner, physiatrist, orthopedist, rheumatologist, and neurologist encounters in his or her medical practice. We particularly wanted to emphasize the outpatient aspects of both musculoskeletal injuries and chronic medical conditions requiring rehabilitation from the perspective of a practitioner in an ambulatory setting. In this new edition, we have added an entirely new section on the ambulatory management of pain conditions.

Essentials of Physical Medicine and Rehabilitation covers many diagnoses in a deliberately succinct and specific format. This book is now divided into three sections. The first section contains chapters on specific musculoskeletal diagnoses, organized anatomically. The second section describes the management of pain conditions. The third section covers common medical conditions that are typically chronic and benefit from rehabilitative as well as other interventions. Although some of these conditions require hospitalization, we have tried to focus on the rehabilitation that takes place in an ambulatory setting. Each chapter includes the same sections in the same order (Synonyms, ICD-9 Codes, Definition, Symptoms, Physical Examination, Functional Limitations, Diagnostic Studies, Differential Diagnosis, Treatment [Initial, Rehabilitation, Procedures, and Surgery], Potential Disease Complications, Potential Treatment Complications, and References). It is our hope that physicians in all specialties and allied health care providers will find that this book complements the excellent existing rehabilitation textbooks and that it will be an efficient and useful tool in the office setting.

We are extremely grateful for the hard work of our colleagues who authored these chapters and who represent many different specialties and come from excellent institutions. Their generous support of our work has made this book possible.

Finally, we would like to thank our editorial team at Elsevier. Their assistance was invaluable in bringing this book to publication.

Walter R. Frontera, MD, PhD
Julie K. Silver, MD
Thomas D. Rizzo, Jr., MD

MUSCULOSKELETAL DISORDERS

SECTION 1: Head and Neck

SECTION 2: Shoulder

SECTION 3: Elbow and Forearm

SECTION 4: Hand and Wrist

SECTION 5: Mid Back

SECTION 6: Hip and Thigh

SECTION 7: Knee and Lower Leg

SECTION 8: Foot and Ankle

Cervical Spondylotic Myelopathy

1

Avital Fast, MD, and Miriam Segal, MD

Synonyms

Cervical radiculitis
Degeneration of cervical intervertebral disc
Cervical spondylosis without myelopathy
Cervical pain

ICD-9 Codes

721.0   Cervical spondylosis without myelopathy
722.4   Degeneration of cervical intervertebral disc
723.3   Cervical pain
723.4   Cervical radiculitis

DEFINITION

Cervical spondylotic myelopathy (CSM) is a frequently encountered entity in middle-aged and elderly patients. The condition affects both men and women. Progressive degeneration of the cervical spine involves the discs, facet joints, joints of Luschka, ligamenta flava, and laminae, leading to gradual encroachment on the spinal canal and spinal cord compromise. CSM has a fairly typical clinical presentation and, frequently, a progressive and disabling course.

As a consequence of aging, the spinal column goes through a cascade of degenerative changes that tend to affect selective regions of the spine. The cervical spine is affected in most adults, most frequently at the C4-7 region.[1,2] Degeneration of the intervertebral discs triggers a cascade of biochemical and biomechanical changes, leading to decreased disc height among other changes. As a result, abnormal load distribution in the motion segments causes cervical spondylosis (i.e., facet arthropathy) and neural foraminal narrowing. Disc degeneration also leads to the development of herniations (soft discs), disc calcification, posteriorly directed bone ridges (hard discs), hypertrophy of the facet and the uncinate joints, and ligamenta flava thickening. On occasion, more frequently in Asians but not infrequently in white individuals, the posterior longitudinal ligament and the ligamenta flava ossify.[3] These degenerative changes narrow the dimensions and change the shape of the cervical spinal canal. In normal adults, the anteroposterior diameter of the subaxial cervical spinal canal measures 17 to 18 mm, whereas the spinal cord diameter in the same dimension is about 10 mm. Severe CSM gradually decreases the space available for the cord and brings about cord compression in the anterior-posterior axis. Cord compression usually occurs at the discal levels.[4-6]

The encroaching structures may also compress the anterior spinal artery, resulting in spinal cord ischemia that usually involves several cord segments beyond the actual compression site. Spinal cord changes in the form of demyelination, gliosis, myelomalacia, and eventually severe atrophy may develop.[4,7-9] Dynamic instability, which can be diagnosed in flexion or extension lateral x-ray views, further complicates matters. Disc degeneration leads to laxity of the supporting ligaments, bringing about anterolisthesis or retrolisthesis in flexion and extension, respectively. This may further compromise the spinal cord and intensify the presenting symptoms.[2,4]

SYMPTOMS

CSM develops gradually during a lengthy period of months to years. Not infrequently, the patient is unaware of any functional compromise, and the first person to notice that something is amiss may be a close family member. Whereas pain appears rather early in cervical radiculopathy and alerts the patient to the presence of a problem, this is usually not the case in CSM. A long history of neck discomfort and intermittent pain may frequently be obtained, but these are not prominent at the time of CSM presentation.

Most patients have a combination of upper motor neuron symptoms in the lower extremities and lower motor neuron symptoms in the upper extremities.[4] Patients frequently present with gait dysfunction resulting from a combination of factors, including ataxia due to impaired joint proprioception, hypertonicity, weakness, and muscle control deficiencies.

Studies have demonstrated that severely myelopathic patients display abnormalities of deep sensation, including vibration and joint position sense, which is

3

attributed to compression of the posterior columns.[10,11] Paresthesias and numbness may be frequently mentioned. Compression of the pyramidal and extrapyramidal tracts can lead to spasticity, weakness, and abnormal muscle contractions. These sensory and motor deficits result in an unstable gait. Patients may complain of stiffness in the lower extremities or plain weakness manifesting as foot dragging and tripping.[5] Symptoms related to the upper extremities are mostly the result of fine motor coordination deficits. Patients may have difficulties inserting keys, picking up coins, buttoning a shirt, or manipulating small objects. Handwriting may deteriorate. Patients may drop things from the hands and occasionally can complain of numbness affecting the fingers or the palms, mimicking peripheral neuropathy.[2,5,12-14] At times, the symptoms in the upper extremities are much more severe than those related to the lower extremities, attesting to central cord compromise.[4] Most patients do not have urinary symptoms. However, urinary symptoms (i.e., incontinence) may occasionally develop in patients with long-standing myelopathy.[15] As CSM develops in middle-aged and elderly patients, the urinary symptoms may be attributed to aging, comorbidities, and cord compression. Bowel incontinence is rare.

PHYSICAL EXAMINATION

Because of sensory ataxia, the patient may be observed walking with a wide-based gait. Some resort to a cane to increase the base of support and to enhance safety during ambulation. Patients with severe gait dysfunction frequently require a walker and cannot ambulate without one. Many patients lose the ability to tandem walk. The Romberg test result may become positive. Examination of the lower extremities may reveal muscle atrophy, increased muscle tone, abnormal reflexes—clonus or upgoing toes (Babinski sign), and abnormalities of position and vibration sense. Muscle fasciculations may be observed.

In the upper extremities, weakness and atrophy of the small muscles of the hands may be noted. The patient may have difficulties in fine motor coordination (e.g., unbuttoning the shirt or picking a coin off the table). The patient frequently displays difficulty in performing repetitive opening and closing of the fist. In normal individuals, 20 to 30 repetitions can be performed in 10 seconds.

Weakness can occasionally be documented in more proximal muscles and may appear symmetrically. Fasciculations may appear in the wasted muscles. Hypesthesia, paresthesia, or anesthesia may be documented. On occasion, the sensory findings in the hands are in a glove distribution. As in the lower extremities, the vibration and joint position senses may be disturbed. Hyporeflexia or hyperreflexia may be found. The Hoffmann response may become positive and can be facilitated in early myelopathy by cervical extension.[16] In some patients, severe atrophy of all the hand intrinsic muscles is observed.[1,5,14,17]

The neck range of motion may be limited in all directions. Many patients cannot extend the neck beyond neutral and may feel electric-like sensation radiating down the torso on neck flexion, known as the Lhermitte sign. Often, when a patient stands against the wall, the ack of the head stays an inch to several inches away, and the patient is unable to push the head backward to bring it to touch the wall.

FUNCTIONAL LIMITATIONS

Patients with CSM have difficulties with activities of daily living. They may have problems dressing and undressing and handling small objects. When weakness is a predominant feature, they will be unable to carry heavy objects. Unassisted ambulation may become difficult. The gait is slowed and becomes inefficient. In late stages of CSM, patients may become almost totally disabled and require assistance with most activities of daily living.

DIAGNOSTIC STUDIES

Plain radiographs usually reveal multilevel degenerative disc disease with cervical spondylosis. Dynamic studies (flexion and extension views) may reveal segmental instability with anterolisthesis on flexion and retrolisthesis on extension. In patients with ossification of the posterior longitudinal ligament, the ossified ligament may be detected on lateral plain films. The Torg-Pavlov ratio may help diagnose congenital spinal stenosis. This ratio can be obtained on plain films by dividing the anteroposterior diameter of the vertebral body by the anteroposterior diameter of the spinal canal at that level. The canal diameter can be measured from the posterior wall of the vertebra to the spinolaminar line.[18] A ratio of 0.8 and below confirms the presence of congenital spinal stenosis (Fig. 1-1).

Magnetic resonance imaging, the study of choice, provides critical information about the extent of stenosis and the condition of the compressed spinal cord. Sagittal and axial cuts clearly show the offending structures (discs, thickened ligamenta flava), and the cord shape and signal provide critical information about the extent of cord compression and the prognosis (Fig. 1-2). Increased cord signal on T2-weighted images is abnormal and points to the presence of edema, demyelination, myelomalacia, or gliosis. Severe cord atrophy denotes a poor prognosis even when decompressive surgery is performed.

Computed tomographic myelography provides fine and detailed information on the amount and location of neural compression and is frequently obtained before surgery. Electrodiagnostic studies play an important role, especially in diabetic patients with peripheral neuropathy, which may confound the clinical diagnosis.

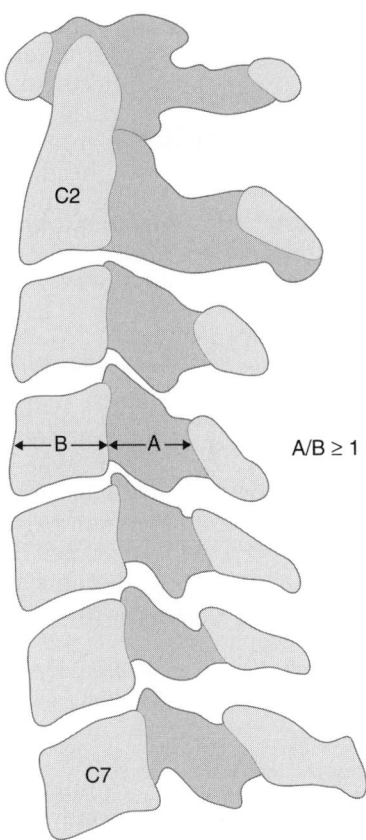

FIGURE 1-1. Schematic lateral view of the cervical spine. The canal diameter (A) can be measured by drawing a line between the posterior border of the vertebral body and the spinolaminar line. The vertebral diameter is reflected by line B. (Reprinted with permission from Fast A, Goldsher D. Navigating the Adult Spine. New York, Demos Medical Publishing, 2007.)

A/B ≥ 1

Differential Diagnosis

Amyotrophic lateral sclerosis

Multifocal motor neuropathy[19]

Multiple sclerosis

Syringomyelia

Peripheral neuropathy

TREATMENT

Initial

The treatment of CSM depends on the stage in which it is discovered. No conservative treatment can be expected to decompress the spinal cord. In the initial stages, education of the patient is of paramount importance. The patient is instructed to avoid cervical spinal hyperextension. As the cervical spinal canal diameter decreases and the spinal cord diameter increases during cervical hyperextension, this position may lead to further cord compression.[20] The patient is advised to drink with a straw, to avoid prolonged overhead activities, and to face the sink while getting the hair washed.

Rehabilitation

Because the course of CSM may be unpredictable and a significant percentage of patients deteriorate in a slow stepwise course, close monitoring of the patient's neurologic condition and spine is indicated. Patients with mild CSM may be managed conservatively. Biannual detailed neurologic examination and an annual magnetic resonance imaging evaluation are indicated. Special attention should be devoted to the cord cross-sectional area and the cord signal; these are important prognostic factors and may help determine whether surgery is indicated. In the interim, patients should be instructed in isometric neck exercises. Weak muscles in the upper or lower extremities should be strengthened. Judicial use of anti-inflammatory medications is called for, especially in elderly individuals. Soft cervical collars are frequently used (recommended by physicians or obtained by patients without the physician's recommendations) without a sound scientific basis. Assistive devices, such as a cane or walker, should be provided when ambulation safety is compromised.

Procedures

No existing procedures affect the course or symptoms of cervical myelopathy.

Surgery

Patients with moderate to severe progressive CSM (unsteady gait, limited function in the upper extremities) who have significant cord compression or cord signal

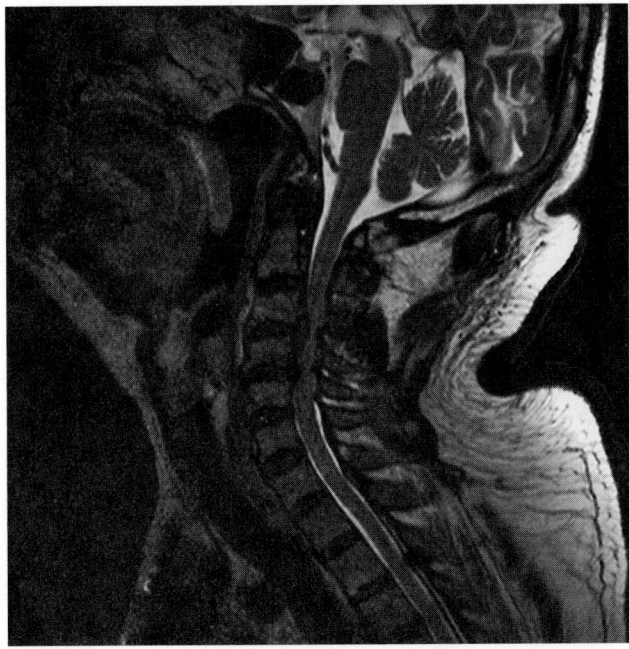

FIGURE 1-2. Sagittal T2-weighted image of the cervical spine showing degenerative disc disease involving the C4-5 and C5-6 intervertebral discs.

changes should be referred for decompressive surgery. Two main approaches exist—anterior and posterior.

Anterior Approach

The anterior approach is usually reserved for patients with myelopathy affecting up to three spinal levels. This approach allows adequate decompression of "anterior" disease. Anterior disease refers to pathologic changes that are anterior to the spinal cord (i.e., soft disc, hard disc, vertebral body spurs, and ossified posterior longitudinal ligament). Through this approach, the offending structures can be removed without disturbing the spinal cord. The anterior approach allows adequate decompression in patients with cervical kyphotic deformity. After anterior decompression (anterior cervical decompression and fusion, corpectomies), bone grafting and instrumentation ensure stabilization and fusion. This approach is not indicated in patients whose predominant pathologic process is posterior to the cord (i.e., hypertrophied ligamentum flavum) or in patients with disease affecting more than three or four segments because this may lead to an increased rate of complications, including pseudarthrosis.[6,17]

Posterior Approach

The posterior approach consists of two basic procedures, laminectomy and laminoplasty.

Cervical laminectomy can be easily performed by most spinal surgeons and is less technically demanding than anterior corpectomies are. This approach allows easy access to posterior disease, such as hypertrophied laminae and ligamenta flava. The main disadvantage of the laminectomy procedure is that it requires stripping of the paraspinal muscles and thus tends to destabilize the cervical spine. This may result in loss of the cervical lordosis or frank kyphotic deformity and instability (stepladder deformity), especially when it is performed over several spinal levels or when the facet joints have to be sacrificed.

Laminoplasty, another procedure performed through the posterior approach, has been developed in Japan and addresses some of the shortcomings of laminectomy. Unlike laminectomy, cervical laminoplasty preserves the cervical facets and the laminae. In this procedure, the laminae are hinged away (lifted by an osteotomy) from the site of main pathologic change, resulting in an increase of sagittal canal diameter.[21] Unilateral or bilateral hinges can be performed; the bilateral hinge approach allows symmetric expansion of the spinal canal. It is hoped that after posterior decompression, the spinal cord will "migrate" away from the anterior pathologic process, and thus cord decompression will be achieved.[17,22] This has been confirmed in magnetic resonance imaging studies after laminoplasty.

Regardless of the surgical approach, poor outcome can be expected in elderly patients with long-standing myelopathy and spinal cord atrophy.

POTENTIAL DISEASE COMPLICATIONS

Left untreated, a patient with progressive myelopathy may develop severe disability. Patients may become totally dependent and nonambulatory. In some cases, neurogenic bladder may develop and further compromise the quality of life.

POTENTIAL TREATMENT COMPLICATIONS

Pseudarthrosis, restenosis, spinal instability, postoperative radiculopathy, kyphotic deformity, and axial pain are among the surgical complications.[17]

References

1. Heller J. The syndromes of degenerative cervical disease. Orthop Clin North Am 1992;23:381-394.
2. Bernhardt M, Hynes RA, Blume HW, White AA III. Cervical spondylotic myelopathy. Current Concepts Review. J Bone Joint Surg Am 1993;75:119-128.
3. Yu YL, Leong JCY, Fang D, et al. Cervical myelopathy due to ossification of the posterior longitudinal ligament. A clinical, radiological and evoked potentials study in six Chinese patients. Brain 1988;111:769-783.
4. Rao R. Neck pain, cervical radiculopathy, and cervical myelopathy. Pathophysiology, natural history, and clinical evaluation. J Bone Joint Surg Am 2002;84:1872-1881.
5. Law MD, Bernhardt M, White AA III. Evaluation and management of cervical spondylotic myelopathy. Instr Course Lect 1995;44:99-110.
6. Truumees E, Herkowitz HN. Cervical spondylotic myelopathy and radiculopathy. Instr Course Lect 2000;49:339-360.
7. Taylor AR. Vascular factors in the myelopathy associated with cervical spondylosis. Neurology 1964;14:62-68.
8. Breig A, Turnbull I, Hassler O. Effects of mechanical stresses on the spinal cord in cervical spondylosis. J Neurosurg 1966;25:45-56.
9. Doppman JL. The mechanism of ischemia in anteroposterior compression of the spinal cord. Invest Radiol 1975;10:543-551.
10. Takayama H, Muratsu H, Doita M, et al. Impaired joint perception in patient with cervical myelopathy. Spine 2004;30:83-86.
11. Okuda T, Ochi M, Tanaka N, et al. Knee joint position sense in compressive myelopathy. Spine 2006;31:459-462.
12. Ono K, Ebara S, Fiji T, et al. Myelopathy hand. New clinical signs of cervical cord damage. J Bone Joint Surg Br 1987;69:215-219.
13. Ebara S, Yonenobu K, Fujiwara K, et al. Myelopathy hand characterized by muscle wasting. A different type of myelopathy hand in patients with cervical spondylosis. Spine 1988;13:785-791.
14. Dillin WH, Watkins RG. Cervical myelopathy and cervical radiculopathy. Semin Spine Surg 1989;1:200-208.
15. Misawa T, Kamimura M, Kinoshita T, et al. Neurogenic bladder in patients with cervical compressive myelopathy. J Spinal Disord Tech 2005;18:315-320.
16. Denno JJ, Meadows GR. Early diagnosis of cervical spondylotic myelopathy. A useful clinical sign. Spine 1991;16:1353-1355.
17. Edwards CC, Riew D, Anderson PA, et al. Cervical myelopathy: current diagnostic and treatment strategies. Spine J 2003;3:68-81.
18. Pavlov H, Torg JS, Robie B, Jahre C. Cervical spinal stenosis: determination with vertebral body ratio method. Radiology 1987;164:171-175.
19. Olney RK, Lewis RA, Putnam TD, Campellone JV Jr. Consensus criteria for the diagnosis of multifocal motor neuropathy. Muscle Nerve 2003;27:117-121.
20. Lauryssen C, Riew KD, Wang JC. Severe cervical stenosis: operative treatment or continued conservative care. SpineLine 2006;January/February:1-25.
21. Hirabayashi K, Watanabe K, Wakano K, et al. Expansive open-door laminoplasty for cervical spinal stenotic myelopathy. Spine 1983;8:693-699.
22. Aita I, Hayashi K, Wadano T, Yabuki T. Posterior movement and enlargement of the spinal cord after cervical laminoplasty. J Bone Joint Surg Br 1998;80:33-37.

Cervical Facet Arthropathy 2

Ted A. Lennard, MD

Synonyms

Apophyseal joint pain
Facet joint arthritis
Z-joint pain
Zygapophyseal joint pain
Posterior element disorder
Spondylosis

ICD-9 Codes

715.1 Osteoarthrosis, localized, primary
715.2 Osteoarthrosis, localized, secondary
719.4 Pain in joint
721.0 Cervical spondylosis without myelopathy
723.1 Cervicalgia
723.9 Unspecified musculoskeletal disorders and symptoms referable to neck
847.0 Neck: atlanto-occipital (joints), atlantoaxial (joints), whiplash injury

DEFINITION

Cervical facet joints are paired diarthrodial structures located in the posterior portion of the spinal axis. These synovium-lined joints contain highly innervated joint capsules[1-3] and allow mobility and stability to the head. Cervical facet arthropathy refers to any acquired, degenerative, or traumatic process that affects the normal function of the facet joints in the cervical region, often resulting in a source of neck pain and cervicogenic headaches. It may be a primary source of pain (e.g., after a whiplash injury) but often is secondary to a degenerative or injured cervical disc, fracture, or ligamentous injury. Common causes of cervical facet pain include acceleration-deceleration cervical injuries (whiplash), a sudden torque motion to the head and neck with extension and rotation, and a cervical compression force. In some cases, simply looking upward may cause facet pain. The cervical facet joints may also become painful in conjunction with a cervical disc herniation, after a cervical discectomy or fusion, or after a cervical compression fracture.

SYMPTOMS

Patients typically complain of suboccipital and generalized posterior neck pain but may present with localized tenderness over the posterolateral aspect of the neck. Pain provoked with cervical extension and axial rotation is common. These joints may refer pain anywhere from the midthoracic spine to the cranium and often in the suboccipital region.[4-6] Neurologic findings such as numbness, weakness, atrophy, and reflex changes in the upper extremities are not expected in patients with primary cervical facet pain. Concomitant nerve root or cord injury is suspected if these clinical findings are present.

PHYSICAL EXAMINATION

The essential element of the examination is manual palpation of the spinal segments and elicitation of reproducible pain over the involved joints.[7] The area of maximum tenderness is often over the paraspinal muscles, which overlie the facet joints, and is precipitated by excessive cervical lordosis, causing abnormal joint forces. The fluidity of motion of the involved spinal area–cervical region may suggest extension pain with relief on flexion. Patients may present with loss of cervical motion and paraspinal spasms. Unless cervical disc or nerve root disease is also present, the findings of the cervical examination are otherwise typically normal.

FUNCTIONAL LIMITATIONS

Cervical extension and rotation, overhead reaching, and overhead lifting may be difficult when the cervical spine is involved. This may interfere with activities such as driving, going to the theater, and brushing one's hair.

DIAGNOSTIC STUDIES

Fluoroscopically guided intra-articular arthrography-confirmed anesthetic injections are considered the "gold standard" for diagnosis (Fig. 2-1).[8-11] Abnormalities detected on radiography, computed tomography, or magnetic resonance imaging have not been shown to

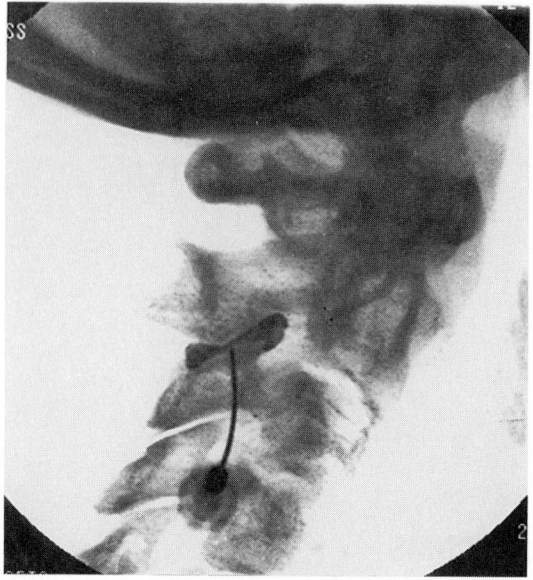

FIGURE 2-1. Lateral radiograph of a C2-3 Z-joint arthrogram by a lateral approach. (Reprinted with permission from Dreyfuss P, Kaplan M, Dreyer SJ. Zygapophyseal joint injection techniques in the spinal axis. In Lennard TA, ed. Pain Procedures in Clinical Practice, 2nd ed. Philadelphia, Hanley & Belfus, 2000:291.)

Differential Diagnosis

Disc herniation

Internal disc disruption

Degenerative disc disease

Myofascial pain syndrome

Nerve root compression

Cervical stenosis

Spondylolysis, spondylolisthesis

Infection

Tumor

Osteoid osteoma

correlate with facet joint pain. A single-photon emission computed tomographic scan can be used in refractory cases of suspected cervical facet disorders to rule out underlying bone processes that may mimic facet pain (e.g., spondylolysis, infection, tumor).[12] When an abnormality is detected, the scan may confirm the proposed diagnosis and determine which specific joint is affected.

TREATMENT

Initial

Initial treatment emphasizes local pain control with ice, nonsteroidal anti-inflammatory drugs and oral analgesics, topical creams, transcutaneous electrical nerve stimulation, local periarticular corticosteroid injections, and

avoidance of exacerbating activities.[13] Specialized pillows may be helpful, but rarely are cervical collars indicated.

Rehabilitation

Manual forms of therapy (i.e., myofascial release, soft tissue mobilization, muscle energy, and strain-counterstrain techniques) and low-velocity manipulations (e.g., osteopathic manipulation) may be useful to patients with isolated facet disorders. In healthy patients with no associated spinal disease (e.g., disc abnormalities, radiculopathy, stenosis, fracture), low-velocity manipulations may be used on a limited basis in cases unresponsive to routine conservative care.[14-16] Use in the cervical region should be approached with extreme caution and performed only by experienced practitioners.

Physical therapy may consist of passive modalities such as ultrasound, electrical stimulation including transcutaneous electrical nerve stimulation, traction, and diathermy to reduce local pain. However, these modalities have not been shown to change long-term outcomes.[14-17] Regional manual therapy with facet gapping techniques can be helpful. Advancement into a flexion-biased exercise program with regional stretching is the mainstay of rehabilitation. Cervical exercises include both isometric and isotonic resisted forward and lateral flexion movements. For recurrent episodes of pain, a change in daily and work activity or in sporting technique and other biomechanical adjustments may eliminate the underlying forces at the joint level.

Procedures

Intra-articular, fluoroscopically guided, contrast-enhanced facet injections are considered critical for proper diagnosis and can be instrumental in the treatment of facet joint arthropathies. Some centers use ultrasound guidance.[18] A patient can be examined both before and after injection to determine what portion of his or her pain can be attributed to the joints injected. Typically, small amounts of anesthetic or corticosteroid are injected directly into the joint. Another step may be to perform medial branch blocks of the affected joints with small volumes (0.1 to 0.3 mL) of anesthetic. If the facet joint is found to be the putative source of pain, a denervation procedure by use of radiofrequency, cryotherapy, or chemicals (e.g., phenol) may be considered.[19,20] Acupuncture may also be considered.[21]

Surgery

Surgery is rarely necessary in isolated facet joint arthropathies. Surgical spinal fusion may be performed for discogenic pain, which may affect secondary cases of facet joint arthropathies.

POTENTIAL DISEASE COMPLICATIONS

Because facet joint arthropathy is usually degenerative in nature, this disorder is often progressive, resulting in chronic, intractable spinal pain. It usually coexists with spinal disc abnormalities, further leading to chronic pain. This subsequently results in diminished spinal motion, weakness, and loss of flexibility.

POTENTIAL TREATMENT COMPLICATIONS

Treatment-related complications may be caused by medications; nonsteroidal anti-inflammatory drugs may cause gastrointestinal and renal problems, and analgesics may result in liver dysfunction and constipation. Local periarticular injections and acupuncture may cause local transient needle pain. Facet injections may cause transient local spinal pain, swelling, and possibly bruising. More serious injection complications may include infection, injury to a blood vessel or nerve, injury to the spinal cord, and allergic reaction to the medications.[11] Exacerbation of symptoms often transiently occurs after injection. Cervical injections may also precipitate headaches.

References

1. Lee KE, Davis MB, Mejilla RM, et al. In vivo cervical facet capsule distraction: mechanical implications for whiplash and neck pain. Stapp Car Crash J 2004;48:373-395.
2. Ebraheim NA, Patil V, Liu J, et al. Morphometric analyses of the cervical superior facets and implications for facet dislocation. Int Orthop 2006;Nov 17.
3. Zhou HY, Chen AM, Guo FJ, et al. Sensory and sympathetic innervation of cervical facet joint in rats. Chin J Traumatol 2006;9:377-380.
4. Bogduk N, Marsland A. The cervical zygapophyseal joints as a source of neck pain. Spine 1988;13:610-617.
5. Dwyer A, Aprill C, Bogduk N. Cervical zygapophyseal joint pain patterns 1: a study in normal volunteers. Spine 1990;15:453-457.
6. Fukui S, Ohseto K, Shiotani M. Referred pain distribution of the cervical zygapophyseal joints and cervical dorsal rami. Pain 1996;68:79-83.
7. King W, Lau P, Lees R, et al. The validity of manual examination in assessing patients with neck pain. Spine J 2007;7:22-26.
8. Bogduk N. International Spinal Injection Society Guidelines for the performance of spinal injection procedures. Part I. Zygapophysial joint blocks. Clin J Pain 1997;13:285-302.
9. Hechelhammer L, Pfirrmann CW, Zanetti M, et al. Imaging findings predicting the outcome of cervical facet joint blocks. Eur Radiol 2007;17:959-964.
10. Kim KH, Choi SH, Kim TK, et al. Cervical facet joint injections in the neck and shoulder pain. J Korean Med Sci 2005;20:659-662.
11. Heckmann JG, Maihofner C, Lanz S, et al. Transient tetraplegia after cervical facet joint injection for chronic neck pain administered without imaging guidance. Clin Neurol Neurosurg 2006;108:709-711.
12. Pneumaticos SG, Chatziioannou SN, Hipp JA, et al. Low back pain: prediction of short-term outcomes of facet joint injection with bone scintigraphy. Radiology 2006;238:693-698.
13. Mazanec D, Reddy A. Medical management of cervical spondylosis. Neurosurgery 2007;60(Suppl 1):S43-S50.
14. Bronfort G, Haas M, Evans RL, Bouter LM. Efficacy of spinal manipulation and mobilization for low back pain and neck pain: a systematic review and best evidence synthesis. Spine J 2004;4:335-356.
15. Bronfort G, Evans R, Nelson B, et al. A randomized clinical trial of exercise and spinal manipulation for patients with chronic neck pain. Spine 2001;26:788-797.
16. Jordan A, Bendix T, Nielsen H, et al. Intensive training, physiotherapy, or manipulation for patients with chronic neck pain. A prospective, single-blinded, randomized clinical trial. Spine 1998;23:311-318.
17. Skargren EI, Oberg BE, Carlsson PG, Gade M. Cost and effectiveness analysis of chiropractic and physiotherapy treatment for low back and neck pain. Six month follow up. Spine 1997;22:2167-2177.
18. Galiano K, Obwegeser AA, Bodner G, et al. Ultrasound guidance for facet joint injections in the lumbar spine: a computed tomography–controlled feasibility study. Anesth Analg 2005;101:579-583.
19. Manchikanti L, Damron K, Cash K. Therapeutic cervical medial branch blocks in managing chronic neck pain: a preliminary report of a randomized, double-blind, controlled trial. Pain Physician 2006;9:333-346.
20. Boswell MV. Therapeutic cervical medial branch blocks: a changing paradigm in interventional pain management. Pain Physician 2006;9:279-281.
21. Cherkin DC, Sherman KJ, Deyo RA, et al. A review of the evidence for the effectiveness, safety, and cost of acupuncture, massage therapy, and spinal manipulation for back pain. Ann Intern Med 2003;138:898-906.

Cervical Degenerative Disease 3

Avital Fast, MD, and Miriam Segal, MD

Synonyms

Spinal stenosis of cervical region
Intervertebral disc disorder with myelopathy
Cervical spondylosis with myelopathy

ICD-9 Codes

721.1   Cervical spondylosis with myelopathy
722.7   Intervertebral disc disorder with myelopathy
723.0   Spinal stenosis of cervical region

DEFINITION

The term *cervical degenerative disease* encompasses a wide range of pathologic changes affecting all the components of the cervical spine that may lead to axial or radicular pain.

The mechanisms underlying cervical degenerative disease are complex and multifactorial. Genetics, aging, and attrition may all play an important role. It is believed that disc degeneration results in altered, abnormal load distribution, which in turn leads to a cascade of structural changes that affect the various components of the spinal column. This leads to structural changes that may change spinal posture and stability and may compromise neural function. The pathomechanisms underlying axial and radicular pain are still not completely clear. Increased vascularization after discal herniation and the presence of inflammatory mediators such as nitric oxide, prostaglandin E_2, interleukin-6, matrix metalloproteinase, and others play an important role in the pathogenesis of pain.[1]

In the seventh and eighth decades of life, most if not all individuals display diffuse degenerative changes throughout the cervical spine. Only a fraction of these individuals, however, have clinical signs and symptoms. Not uncommonly, individuals who are symptomatic early on become asymptomatic as the degenerative process evolves.

The lowest five cervical vertebrae are connected by five structural elements: the intervertebral disc, the facet joints, and the neurocentral joints (joints of Luschka).[2]

The neurocentral joints are unique to the cervical spine and do not appear anywhere else in the spinal column. These joints, located in the posterolateral aspect of the vertebral bodies, consist of bone projections that articulate with the vertebral body above them (Fig. 3-1). They provide some stability to the very mobile cervical spine and protect the exiting nerve roots from pure lateral disc herniations. Once the disc degenerates, however, these joints may hypertrophy, narrow the intervertebral foramina, and modify their shape, thus compromising the radicular nerves or the dorsal root ganglia. A similar degenerative process may involve the facet joints that are posteriorly located, and they in turn may compress the exiting neural elements from the back. Indeed, the most common cause of cervical radiculopathy is foraminal narrowing due to facet or neurocentral joint hypertrophy.[3] The lower cervical spine, especially C4-5, C5-6, and to a lesser extent C6-7, is the source of pain in most symptomatic individuals. Unlike in the lumbar spine, nucleus pulposus herniation is less frequent and is the cause of radicular pain in only 20% to 25% of cases.[3,4] As the spinal cord occupies a substantial proportion of the cervical spinal canal, posteriorly directed herniations can result in significant cord compression as well as radicular symptoms.

In the general population, the point prevalence for neck pain ranges between 9.5% and 22%, whereas lifetime prevalence may be as high as 66%. The annual incidence is higher in men and peaks around 50 to 54 years of age.[5,6]

SYMPTOMS

The most common symptom, one that drives most of the patients to the physician's office, is pain. In this respect, two large groups of patients can be recognized: patients whose main complaint is limited to axial pain and patients with radicular pain. Patients with axial pain typically complain of stiffness and pain in the cervical spine. The pain is usually more severe in the upright position and relieved only with bed rest. Cervical motion, especially hyperextension and side bending, increases the pain. In patients with pathologic changes involving the upper cervical joints or degeneration of

11

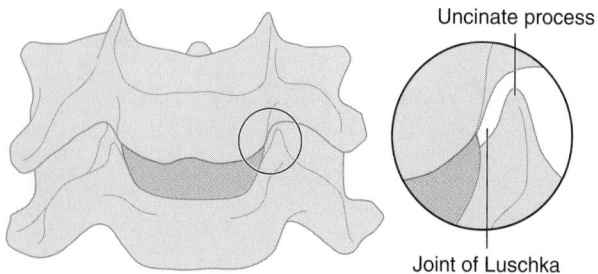

FIGURE 3-1. Schematic representation of the joint of Luschka in the coronal plane. (Reprinted with permission from Fast A, Goldsher D. Navigating the Adult Spine. New York, Demos Medical Publishing, 2007.)

upper cervical discs, the pain may radiate into the head, typically into the occipital region. In patients with lower cervical disease, the pain radiates into the region of the superior trapezius or the interscapular region. On occasion, patients present with atypical symptoms such as jaw pain or chest pain–cervical angina.

Identification of the pain generator and its management are far more challenging in patients with axial pain because imaging studies frequently show multilevel pathologic changes, such as multilevel disc degeneration, facet arthropathy, and uncovertebral joint disease. It is often difficult and quite challenging to identify the exact source of pain. As the facets and the uncovertebral joints, peripheral discs, and ligaments all contain nerve endings, each one or a combination of them could be the source of pain.[4]

Patients with radicular pain have symptoms commensurate with the involved nerve root. The pain usually follows a myotomal distribution and is frequently described as boring, aching, deep-seated pain. The pain is made worse by tilting the head toward the affected side or by hyperextension and side bending. Infrequently, patients find that the pain may be made more tolerable when the hand of the symptomatic side is placed over the top of the head (shoulder abduction release).[7] The sensory symptoms (numbness, tingling, and burning sensation) usually follow the dermatomal distribution. When carpal tunnel syndrome accompanies cervical radiculopathy (double crush syndrome), the sensory changes may be in median nerve distribution. Sclerotomal pain, frequently overlooked or interpreted as trigger points, may be present and commonly resides in the medial or lateral scapular borders.[8,9] On occasion,

patients complain of arm or hand weakness as they may drop things or find difficulty with routine activities of daily living.

PHYSICAL EXAMINATION

Because of severe axial pain, the patient may keep the head and neck immobile as cervical movements may increase the symptoms. Frequently, the only comfortable position is when the patient reclines and the neck is unloaded. Axial pain may increase with cervical extension or side bending. The Spurling sign, whereby simultaneous axial loading and tilting of the head toward the symptomatic side in the upright position are performed, elicits neck and radicular pain. Manual neck distraction may alleviate the symptoms. Tender spots are frequently found over the cervical paraspinal muscles, within the superior trapezius muscles, or in muscles supplied by the compromised root. These spots refer to areas within the muscles that, when stimulated, elicit a sensation of local pain.[9] Tender spots may be of diagnostic significance, especially when they are found unilaterally or in conjunction with other symptoms of cervical radiculopathy.

In patients with radicular pain, depending on the root involved, examination may reveal weakness in myotomal distribution, sensory changes in dermatomal distribution, and reflex changes (Table 3-1). Meticulous physical examination helps identify the compromised root: C5 root compromise will affect shoulder abduction; C6, elbow flexors; C7, elbow extensors; and C8, finger flexors. Finding of concomitant sensory and reflex changes is helpful. Dermatomal arrangement is not fixed and may vary in different patients because of aberrant rootlets or anastomoses between peripheral nerves. Frequently, dermatomes represent only a portion of the root's domain.[10] The dermatomal charts are useful, however, and play a role in the patient's diagnosis. Radicular pain frequently occurs without weakness, reflex, or apparent sensory changes. The most frequently affected roots are C5, C6, and C7.[3,6] In the cervical region, unlike in other regions of the spine, the nerve roots exit the spine above their respective vertebrae; the C5 nerve root exits above C5 vertebra and hence may be compromised by herniation of the C4-5 intervertebral disc. The C8 nerve root exits below the C7 vertebral body; all the subsequent nerves below that level follow the same pattern.

TABLE 3-1 Salient Features of the Most Frequently Affected Roots

	Predominantly Affected Muscles	Sensory Distribution	Reflex Changes
C5	Deltoid, supraspinatus, and infraspinatus	Shoulder and lateral aspect of arm	Supinator reflex
C6	Elbow flexors: biceps brachialis, brachioradialis, and radial extensors of the wrist	Distal lateral forearm, thumb, and index fingers	Biceps reflex
C7	Triceps, wrist flexors	Dorsal aspects of forearm and middle finger	Triceps reflex
C8	Flexor digitorum superficialis and profundus	Ulnar aspects of forearm, hand, and fourth and fifth fingers	No reflex changes

Looking for long tract signs is of paramount importance because their presence points toward cord compression and may modify the treatment plan. The diagnostic accuracy of the physical examination is fairly reliable and may correlate well with imaging studies.[8,11,12]

FUNCTIONAL LIMITATIONS

The functional limitations associated with cervical degenerative disease depend on the extent of the degenerative changes and the neurologic involvement. Not infrequently, patients are asymptomatic, and the only functional limitation noted is loss of cervical range of motion. They tend to hold the neck in a forward stooped posture; the neck is held in forward flexion and cannot achieve extension. When these patients stand against a wall, the back of the head may be inches away from it, and they cannot straighten the cervical spine. These patients may function well but have limited range of motion in all planes and cannot look up. When weakness is present, patients may have functional deficits corresponding with their spinal level of involvement (e.g., patients with C8-T1 involvement may drop things and have difficulties with movements requiring fine motor coordination).

DIAGNOSTIC STUDIES

Radiographs are frequently obtained but are of limited use. Anteroposterior, lateral, oblique, and flexion and extension views should be obtained. The vertebral components are clearly seen in these studies but not the intervertebral discs, spinal cord, or peripheral nerves. The x-ray films clearly show degenerative changes (narrowing intervertebral discs; spurs and calcified or ossified soft tissues). Frequently, there is no good correlation between the symptoms and the extent of degenerative findings on radiographs.[12] Diffuse multilevel changes are frequently observed but are, for the most part, irrelevant to the patient's symptoms. Flexion and extension views are important as they can detect degenerative instability that is responsible for the symptoms and that may not be seen in the static views.[6] Radiographs are not helpful in the early stages of infection and tumors.

Magnetic resonance imaging is the diagnostic modality of choice because it allows visualization of the whole cervical spine without irradiation and enables the clinician to assess the neural structures (cord, roots) as well as the soft tissues (discs, ligaments). Correlation of the imaging studies with the history and clinical examination is of utmost importance because in many individuals, the magnetic resonance imaging studies reveal significant pathologic changes (herniated discs, neural foraminal stenosis) that are totally irrelevant to the patient's complaints and symptoms (Fig. 3-2). Computed tomographic myelography is frequently obtained before surgery and should not be obtained on a routine basis. Patients with axial pain who do not respond to conservative measures can be referred for discography to identify the pain generator. Discography may be the only

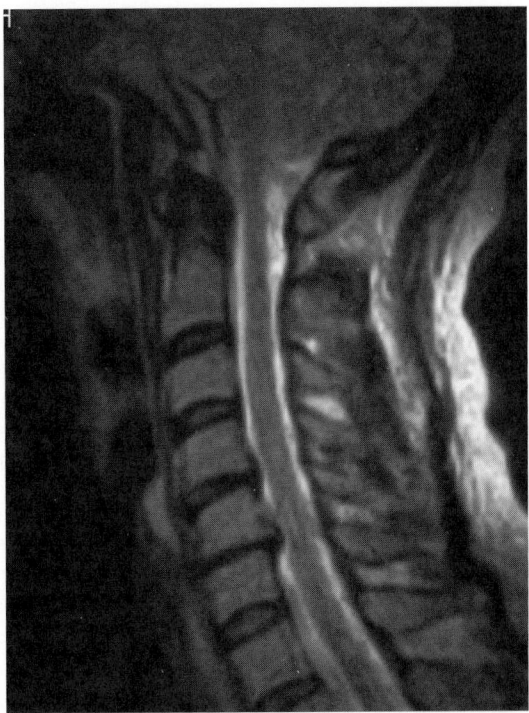

FIGURE 3-2. Sagittal T2-weighted image of the cervical spine showing spinal cord compression at the C3-4 and C4-5 levels. At the C3-4 level, the cord is compressed from the front and from the back. No cerebrospinal fluid is visible in the compressed regions.

Differential Diagnosis[14]

Rotator cuff tendinitis

Rotator cuff tear

Peripheral neuropathies

Carpal tunnel syndrome

Spine tumors

Spinal infection

Brachial plexopathy

Thoracic outlet syndrome

way to identify the disc responsible for the symptoms; however, it remains controversial at present. Electrodiagnostic studies play an important role, especially in the patient with diabetes or whenever peripheral neuropathies are suspected.[13]

TREATMENT

Initial

The management of axial pain without radicular pain is much more challenging than the management of radicular pain. In the case of axial pain, it is often difficult to identify the pain generator and thus to initiate a direct therapeutic response. Anti-inflammatory drugs along with analgesic drugs should be prescribed as a first line of treatment in the initial stages of the disease. Patients with severe radicular pain may be managed with systemic steroids, such as Medrol Dosepak, when they do not respond to other anti-inflammatory drugs. A substantial percentage of patients with spondylotic radicular nontraumatic pain are expected to improve significantly after fluoroscopically guided therapeutic selective nerve root injections.[15,16] Steroids may be beneficial in relieving pain because they reduce inflammation and swelling, thereby facilitating neural nutrient and blood supply, and stabilize neural membranes, thus suppressing ectopic discharges within the affected nerve fibers. They may be administered during the course of a week to 10 days in tapering dose. For severe pain, a starting dose of 70 mg of prednisone decreasing by 10 mg daily may be recommended. Medrol Dosepak (methylprednisolone) is quite handy, as the daily dose is prearranged separately within the package. Steroid administration carries certain risks. These should be considered before steroid administration. Patients with severe burning pain may respond favorably to gabapentin (Neurontin) or pregabalin (Lyrica).

The patient should be instructed to try the shoulder abduction release maneuver as a therapeutic measure (i.e., put the affected hand over the head) with the hope that this might decrease the tension on the affected nerve root and bring some symptomatic relief.[17]

Rehabilitation

Conclusive quality works that clearly define the most efficient rehabilitation approach to patients with neck pain are still lacking.[5] The following paragraph summarizes the more commonly applied methods.

Activity modifications are of paramount importance. It has been demonstrated in vivo that the neural foraminal dimensions vary with flexion and extension. It has been shown that cervical flexion increases foraminal height, width, and cross-sectional area, whereas extension has the opposite effects.[18,19] Because foraminal narrowing plays a major clinical role in patients with cervical radicular pain, patients should be advised to avoid activities in which cervical extension is involved. The patients should be instructed to drink with a straw, to avoid overhead activities, to face the sink while shampooing the hair, to adjust the monitor height, and the like. Temporary immobilization of the cervical spine may bring about some relief. This can be accomplished with a collar when the patient is mobile but should be used only temporarily. Cervical traction, provided it is administered in slight flexion, may be of value in patients with radicular pain. Traction could be administered manually or, preferably, through a mechanized approach. The distraction forces that are applied to the neck can, to some extent, relieve nerve compression by increasing the foraminal height and the intervertebral distance.[20] Traction application in the supine position is preferable because the weight of the head is eliminated and all the traction forces are effectively directed to the cervical spine. No conclusive evidence that proves the therapeutic efficacy of cervical traction exists, however.[21]

Superficial heat should be applied concomitantly with the traction as an adjunct therapy to relax the muscles before and during traction. Isometric neck exercises should be recommended as they may preserve muscle tone and strength without leading to pain. Cervical range of motion exercises are not recommended in patients with acute pain.

Manual medicine (massage, mobilization, manipulation), acupuncture, and electrical stimulation are also widely used. Although these approaches are popular, studies demonstrating their efficacy are still lacking.[22-28]

Procedures

Translaminar and transforaminal (selective nerve root) steroid administration may provide significant and at times long-term relief in patients with radicular pain. Properly selected, up to 60% of patients who are managed with selective nerve root injection may have good to excellent outcome.[3,15] Because there may be a significant risk with these injections (vertebral artery injury), they should be fluoroscopically guided and administered only by physicians with proper training.

Surgery

The main indications for surgery are severe or progressive neurologic deficits and persistent pain that does not respond to conservative measures.

The standard surgical treatment of cervical radiculopathy for many decades has been anterior cervical decompression and fusion. This approach prevailed because in most patients with cervical radiculopathy, the symptoms are caused by osteophytes compressing the nerves within the intervertebral foramina, and laminectomy is not effective in these cases.

The anterior approach permits excellent access to anteriorly impinging structures, such as discs and spondylotic spurs. Some surgeons add instrumentation (i.e., plate) to increase the fusion rate and the postoperative stability.[12] Adequate foraminal decompression can result in early pain relief and enhanced muscle strength. Long term, however, no significant differences have been found between conservatively and surgically treated patients.[24,29]

The negative long-term effects of fusion have only recently been appreciated. Fusion leads to stiffness and lost range of motion, and over the years, it results in next-level degeneration (i.e., accelerated discal degeneration above and below the fused vertebrae). This has led to the development of disc replacement surgery. Whereas the concept of disc replacement is attractive because disc replacement maintains the intervertebral discal height while preserving spinal motion,[30] the indications for this approach and its long-term effects have not yet been determined. Patients with single-level soft disc herniation may be operated on from the back. In these patients, laminotomy with foraminotomy may bring about relief without fusion and its complications while maintaining cervical stability.[12]

POTENTIAL DISEASE COMPLICATIONS

Chronic pain and permanent neurologic deficits may develop in some patients. These may compromise the quality of life and interfere with activities of daily living.

POTENTIAL TREATMENT COMPLICATIONS

Surgical complications include infection, nerve injury, pain, stiffness, pseudarthrosis, and next-level degeneration.

References

1. Peng B, Hao J, Hou S, et al. Possible pathogenesis of painful intervertebral disc degeneration. Spine 2006;31:560-566.
2. Macnab I. Cervical spondylosis. Clin Orthop 1973;109:69-77.
3. Carette S, Fehlings MG. Cervical radiculopathy. N Engl J Med 2005;353:392-399.
4. Bogduk N, Windsor M, Inglis A. The innervation of the cervical intervertebral discs. Spine 1988;13:2-8.
5. Davidson RI, Dunn EJ, Metzmaker JN. The shoulder abduction test in the diagnosis of radicular pain in cervical extradural compressive monoradiculopathies. Spine 1981;6:441-446.
6. Haymaker W, Woodhall B. Peripheral Nerve Injuries. Principles of Diagnosis. Philadelphia, WB Saunders, 1953:47-53.
7. Letchuman R, Gay RE, Shelerud RA, VanOstrand LA. Are tender points associated with cervical radiculopathy? Arch Phys Med Rehabil 2005;86:1333-1337.
8. Slipman CW, Plastaras CT, Palmitier RA, et al. Symptom provocation of fluoroscopically guided cervical nerve root stimulation: are dynatomal maps identical to dermatomal maps? Spine 1998;23:2235-2242.
9. Rao R. Neck pain, cervical radiculopathy, and cervical myelopathy. J Bone Joint Surg Am 2002;84:1872-1881.
10. Wainner RS, Fritz JM, Irrgang JJ, et al. Reliability and diagnostic accuracy of the clinical examination and patient self-report measures for cervical radiculopathy. Spine 2003;28:52-62.
11. Heller JG. The syndrome of degenerative cervical disease. Orthop Clin North Am 1993;23:381-394.
12. Truumees E, Herkowitz HN. Cervical spondylotic myelopathy and radiculopathy. Instr Course Lect 2000;49:339-360.
13. Wainner RS, Gill H. Diagnosis and nonoperative management of cervical radiculopathy. J Orthop Sports Phys Ther 2000;30:728-744.
14. Honet JC, Ellenberg MR. What you always wanted to know about the history and physical examination of neck pain but were afraid to ask. Phys Med Rehabil Clin North Am 2003;14:473-491.
15. Slipman CW, Lipetz JS, Jackson HB, et al. Therapeutic selective nerve root block in the nonsurgical treatment of atraumatic cervical spondylotic radicular pain: a retrospective analysis with independent clinical review. Arch Phys Med Rehabil 2000;81:741-746.
16. Bush K, Hillier S. Outcome of cervical radiculopathy treated with periradicular/epidural corticosteroid injections: a prospective study with independent clinical review. Eur Spine J 1996;5:319-325.
17. Fast A, Parikh S, Marin EL. The shoulder abduction relief sign in cervical radiculopathy. Arch Phys Med Rehabil 1989;70:402-403.
18. Hoving JL, Gross AR, Gasner D, et al. A critical appraisal of review articles on the effectiveness of conservative treatment for neck pain. Spine 2001;26:196-205.
19. Kitagawa T, Fujiwara A, Kobayashi N, et al. Morphologic changes in the cervical neural foramen due to flexion and extension. In vivo imaging study. Spine 2004;29:2821-2825.
20. Craig Humphreys S, Chase J, Patwardhan A, et al. Flexion and traction effect on C5-C6 foraminal space. Arch Phys Med Rehabil 1998;79:1105-1109.
21. van der Heijden GJ, Beurskens AJ, Koes BW, et al. The efficacy of traction for back and neck pain: a systematic, blinded review of randomized clinical trial methods. Phys Ther 1995;75:93-104.
22. Wang WTJ, Olson SL, Campbell AH, et al. Effectiveness of physical therapy for patients with neck pain: an individualized approach using a clinical decision-making algorithm. Am J Phys Med Rehabil 2003;82:203-218.
23. Klaber Moffett JA, Hughes GI, Griffiths P. An investigation of the effects of cervical traction. Part 1. Clinical effectiveness. Clin Rehabil 1990;4:205-211.
24. Persson LCG, Carlsson CA, Carlsson JY. Long-lasting cervical radicular pain managed with surgery, physiotherapy, or a cervical collar. Spine 1997;22:751-758.
25. Taimela S, Takala EP, Asklof T, et al. Active treatment of chronic neck pain: a prospective randomized intervention. Spine 2000;25:1021-1027.
26. Kjellman GV, Skargren EI, Oberg BE. A critical analysis of randomised clinical trials on neck pain and treatment efficacy: a review of the literature. Scand J Rehabil Med 1999;31:139-152.
27. Wolff L, Levine LA. Cervical radiculopathies: conservative approaches to management. Phys Med Rehabil Clin North Am 2002;13:589-608.
28. Weintraub MI. Complementary and alternative methods of treatment of neck pain. Phys Med Rehabil Clin North Am 2003;14:659-674.
29. Fouyas IP, Statham PFX, Sanderock AG. Cochrane review on the role of surgery in cervical spondylotic radiculomyelopathy. Spine 2002;27:736-747.
30. Phillips FM, Garfin SR. Cervical disc replacement. Spine 2005;30:S27-S33.

Cervical Radiculopathy 4

Isaac Cohen, MD, and Cristin Jouve, MD

Synonyms

Cervical disc herniation
Cervical radiculitis
Brachialgia

ICD-9 Codes

722.0 Displacement of cervical intervertebral disc without myelopathy

723.4 Brachial neuritis or radiculitis; cervical radiculitis; radicular syndrome of upper limbs

DEFINITION

Cervical radiculopathy is characterized by signs and symptoms related to cervical nerve root dysfunction. The patient usually presents with neck pain that radiates into the arm. It can be associated with loss of motor function, sensory loss, or reflex changes in the affected nerve root distribution.

There are eight cervical nerve roots, and each cervical nerve root exits above the vertebra of the same numeric designation, except for C8, which exits above the T1 vertebra. The neuroforamina are bordered anteromedially by the uncovertebral joint, posterolaterally by the facet joint, and superiorly and inferiorly by the pedicles of the vertebral bodies above and below.

The most common causes of cervical radiculopathy are cervical disc herniation (most commonly posterolateral) and cervical spondylosis (osteophytic spurs from the vertebral body, uncovertebral joint, facet joint, or a combination) causing nerve root compression[1-3] (Figs. 4-1 and 4-2; see also Chapter 3). C7 is the most commonly affected nerve root, followed by C6, C8, and C5 in descending order of incidence.[4-7] Radiculopathies of the C2 to C4 nerve roots are thought to be uncommon and clinically difficult to distinguish from other sources of pain. The exact pathogenesis of radicular pain is unclear, but it is thought that inflammation, in addition to compression, is necessary for pain to develop.[8-11]

This chapter primarily focuses on cervical radiculopathy arising from extradural compression by disc material or osteophytes.

SYMPTOMS

Patients usually present with neck and predominantly sharp, radiating pain in the upper extremity; the specific distribution depends on the nerve root involved. In general, there is no preceding trauma or inciting event.[4,5] In a majority of patients, neck or scapular pain precedes the onset of radicular symptoms.[6,12,13] Pain radiates in a myotomal pattern, but it also may be felt in the shoulder, interscapular, scapular, suboccipital, and rarely chest wall regions. Numbness and paresthesias follow a dermatomal pattern and most commonly are noted in the distal aspect of the dermatome. Of the subjective complaints, the distribution of hand paresthesias appears to have the greatest localizing value.[7] Cervical hyperextension and lateral bending or rotation ipsilateral to the pain exacerbate symptoms, as do coughing and Valsalva maneuvers. Association of symptoms with unusual exacerbating factors, such as eating or running, is a clue to possible visceral disease.[14] Patients may obtain relief with tilting of the head away from the painful side or elevation of the hand over the head. Patients may note arm weakness or inability to perform certain daily activities, such as pulling, pushing, or grasping. Mild weakness that is demonstrable by careful examination often goes unnoticed by the patient.

A small percentage of patients will present only with weakness without significant pain or sensory complaints. Alternative diagnoses, such as motor neuron disease, myelopathy, myopathy, and chronic rotator cuff tear, should especially be considered for patients with this type of presentation. Clinicians should routinely inquire about symptoms of myelopathy. Bilateral hand numbness and difficulty with fine hand motor skills, such as handling change or small objects, are usually early signs of myelopathy. Poor balance, falls, and bowel or bladder dysfunction are not features of a discrete radiculopathy and should alert the clinician to rule

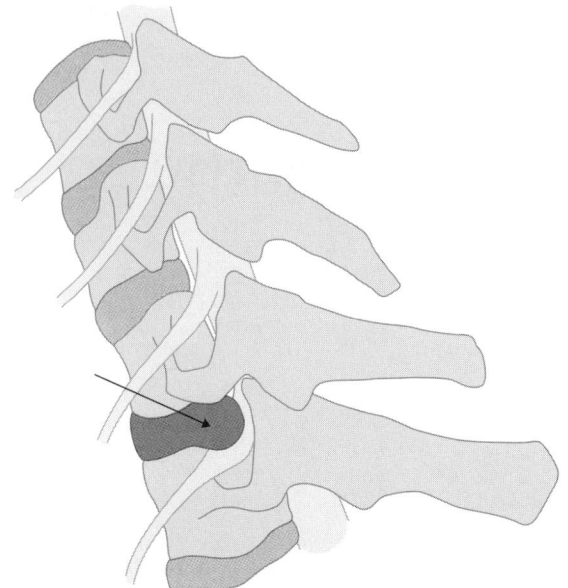

FIGURE 4-1. Discs typically herniate posterolaterally and cause radicular symptoms when they compromise exiting nerve roots.

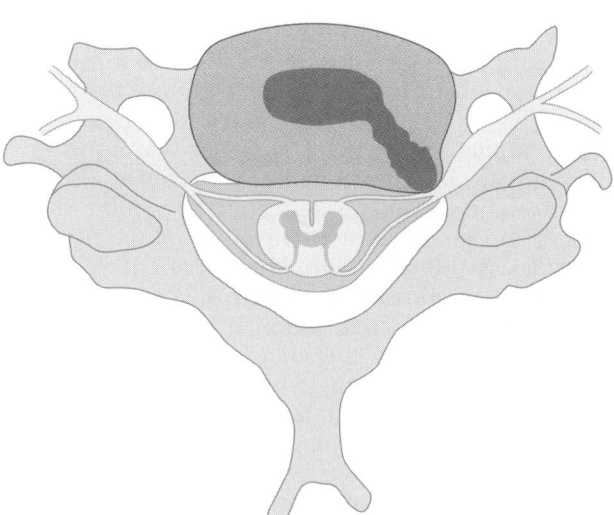

FIGURE 4-2. Axial view of disc herniation illustrated in Figure 4-1.

out spinal cord compression. Cervical myelopathy related to spondylosis is more commonly seen in the elderly.

PHYSICAL EXAMINATION

A useful approach to the patient with neck and arm pain involves categorization of the clinical presentation into axial pain, radiculopathy, myelopathy, or some combination of these. The distinction between radiculopathy and myelopathy is important as it will guide workup and treatment.

The clinician should observe the patient's gait, posture, and muscle bulk in the shoulder girdle and upper extremities. The bone and soft tissue structures of the cervical spine are palpated to assess for deformity or tenderness. Tenderness and muscle spasm are commonly present ipsilaterally. The cervical range of motion is assessed to determine its relation to symptoms, to identify impairments, and to establish a baseline for serial examinations. There is usually a reduction in active cervical range of motion, especially with extension, lateral bending, and rotation toward the symptomatic side, as these cause neuroforaminal narrowing and hence compression of the symptomatic nerve root. The normal cervical range of motion is as follows[15]: flexion, 45 degrees; extension, 55 degrees; lateral bending, 40 degrees; rotation, 70 degrees. A screening test of the shoulder involves asking the patient to abduct the arms overhead as well as to place the hands behind the low back. If an abnormality is noted, one should perform a more detailed assessment of the shoulder. Limited or painful shoulder motion, localized tenderness, and positive impingement signs are more suggestive of shoulder disease.

The main objectives of the neurologic examination are to demonstrate specific nerve root involvement and to rule out myelopathy. The examiner should look for myotomal weakness, diminished or absent muscle stretch reflexes, and dermatomal hypesthesia of the involved nerve root (Table 4-1). Comparison to the contralateral (uninvolved) side is helpful, and the distribution of motor weakness appears to be the most reliable physical examination sign to localize the lesion to a single root level.[7] The examiner may be able to detect subtle weakness by putting the tested muscle at a mechanical disadvantage. The C5-6 myotomes can be examined by testing external shoulder rotation with elbows flexed to 90 degrees and stabilized against the sides of the body. Alternatively, these myotomes can be examined by applying downward resistance against abducted, internally rotated arms. The C6-7 myotomes may be tested by having the patient pronate the hand from the neutral position against resistance while

TABLE 4-1 Diagnosing Cervical Radiculopathy			
Root	**Motor**	**Reflex**	**Sensory**
C5	Deltoid, spinati, biceps	Biceps	Lateral aspect of upper arm
C6	Biceps, brachioradialis, wrist extensors, pronator teres	Biceps, brachioradialis, pronator	Radial distal forearm and thumb, occasionally index finger
C7	Triceps, wrist extensors, pronator teres	Triceps, pronator	Posterior arm, dorsal forearm, middle and index fingers, occasionally index and ring fingers
C8	Intrinsic hand muscles	No reliable reflex is available	Medial forearm, fourth and fifth digits

the elbows are kept flexed to 90 degrees and stabilized against the sides of the body. The C7 myotome can also be examined by applying resistance against a fully flexed elbow and asking the patient to extend the elbow. Myotomal weakness of less than 3/5 is rare, given that all muscle groups in the upper extremity receive innervation from more than one root. This finding should prompt the clinician to consider alternative diagnoses, such as polyradiculopathy, brachial plexopathy, and shoulder disease. Diminished muscle stretch reflexes can localize the level to one of two roots. The pronator reflex may be helpful to distinguish a C6 from a C7 nerve root lesion compared with other reflexes.[16] Dermatomal examination of light touch and pinprick assessment should be performed at the distal aspect of the dermatome. Gait and lower extremity strength should be tested to screen the patient for myelopathy. In addition, upper motor neuron findings are sought: Hoffmann sign, hyperreflexia of the lower extremities, Babinski response, and clonus. There are several provocative and relief maneuvers available to supplement the examination, and these appear to have greater yield for the lower cervical nerve roots (i.e., C6 to C8).[17-19] The Spurling test (Fig. 4-3), as originally described by Spurling and Scoville in 1944, is performed by having the patient tilt the head and neck toward the painful side, with application of pressure on top of the head.[20] Reproduction of the patient's radicular symptoms is considered a positive test result. Currently, the test is performed by combining cervical hyperextension, lateral rotation, and axial compression. Having the patient elevate the hand above the head (shoulder abduction test) and providing gentle manual axial traction with the patient in a supine position (axial manual distraction test) are relief maneuvers that decrease nerve root tension and distract neuroforamina, respectively. These maneuvers do not localize the level of pathologic change. A literature review indicated low sensitivity (40% to 50%), high specificity (greater than 80%), and fair to good interexaminer reliability for the Spurling neck compression test, the neck distraction test, and the shoulder abduction (relief) test.[20]

FUNCTIONAL LIMITATIONS

Limitation of cervical rotation secondary to pain may limit a patient's ability to drive and to perform overhead activities. Patients may experience arm weakness, fatigue, or diminished grip strength. Triceps weakness may go unnoticed by a sedentary patient because gravity can assist in elbow extension. Pain commonly interferes with sleep, work, or social activities. Headaches may also be experienced, probably secondary to muscle spasm and guarding.

DIAGNOSTIC STUDIES

Magnetic resonance imaging is the study of choice for evaluation of cervical radiculopathy because it provides the best definition of the nerve root and herniation of the nucleus pulposus.[2,21] Plain radiographs should be

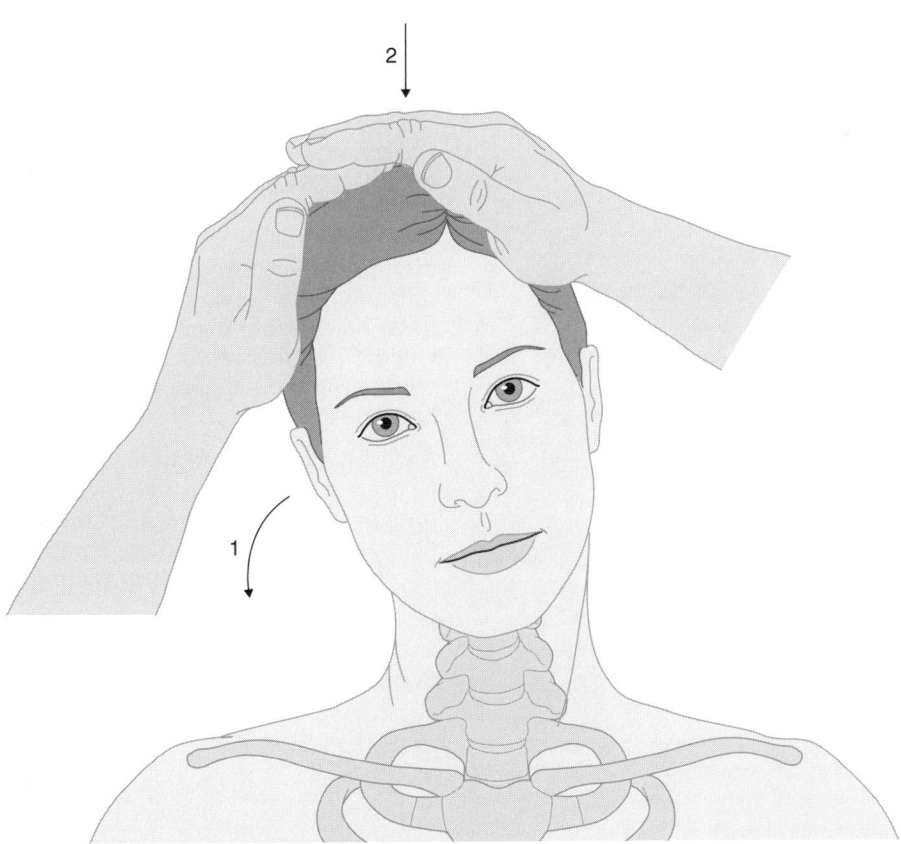

FIGURE 4-3. Spurling test. The patient flexes the head to one side (1), and the examiner presses straight down on the head (2).

performed in patients with a history or suggestion of trauma, infection, inflammatory diseases, or cancer. Computed tomographic examination of the cervical spine can be beneficial to rule out fractures and to obtain further bone definition. All imaging studies require correlation for meaningful interpretation as radiologic abnormalities may be clinically irrelevant.

Electrodiagnostic testing (electromyography and nerve conduction studies) is not necessary if the diagnosis of cervical radiculopathy is apparent by history, physical examination, and imaging studies. It may be required to rule out neurologic conditions that mimic radiculopathy. It may be helpful when the clinical presentation is discordant with the imaging findings or to assess clinical relevancy of nonspecific structural changes.[22] It may also be useful to verify subjective muscle weakness in patients who are pain inhibited or uncooperative with physical examination. The timing of electromyographic studies is important because evidence of denervation in peripheral muscles may not appear until 3 to 4 weeks after the onset of symptoms. The sensitivity of electromyography for cervical radiculopathy generally ranges from 50% to 70%, depending on the "gold standard" that is being used.[23] Electromyography is biased toward assessing for conduction block or axonal loss in motor nerves, and therefore it may not detect mild or pure sensory lesions of the nerve root.

Differential Diagnosis

Neurologic

Cervical myelopathy

Tumor (spinal, Pancoast)

Syringomyelia

Motor neuron disease

Herpes zoster

Brachial plexopathy

Peripheral nerve entrapment (median, ulnar, radial)

Musculoskeletal

Shoulder disease

Cervical spondylosis

Myofascial pain syndrome

Inflammatory spine disease

Infection

Tumor

Tendinitis (epicondylitis, de Quervain)

Other

Cardiac ischemia

TREATMENT

Initial

The initial treatment focuses on education of the patient and control of pain and inflammation. The patient should be informed that most patients (70% to 80%) have good to excellent outcomes with conservative management[24-32] and that most of the pain subsides within several weeks. Nonsteroidal anti-inflammatory drugs may be used to decrease pain and inflammation, and if necessary, a short course of tapering oral corticosteroids may be prescribed. Non-narcotic analgesics may be used for pain. Narcotic analgesics can be prescribed for short periods if this regimen is not sufficient in controlling pain.

Patients should be encouraged to maintain their normal activities of daily living in conjunction with light stretches and application of ice to the neck. Although soft cervical collars are frequently prescribed for short courses, there is risk of cervical soft tissue contracture and disuse weakness.

Rehabilitation

A multitude of treatments have been empirically described for cervical disc herniation; these include heat, cold, massage, mobilization, traction, manipulation, trigger point therapy, acupuncture, and transcutaneous electrical nerve stimulation. However, the paucity of well-designed (randomized, controlled, prospective) studies in the literature makes it difficult to assess their efficacy and whether they alter the long-term outcome.[24-32] Furthermore, there are no published guidelines in the literature for management of cervical radiculopathy.[3]

Supervised physical therapy is generally not necessary in treating cervical radiculopathy if the patient's pain resolves and the patient makes a functional recovery. However, patients who have persistent impairments or disability after resolution of acute radicular pain (e.g., difficulty with cervical range of motion or arm weakness) may benefit from a course of physical therapy involving progressive stretching and strengthening exercises of the cervical paraspinal, shoulder girdle, and low back muscles.[33-35]

A workstation evaluation may be beneficial to facilitate recovery or return to work. The focus should be on improving posture and keeping the head and neck in a neutral position. Ergonomic equipment may include a telephone headset, slanted writing board, document holder, and book stand.

Procedures

The clinician may consider referral for a cervical epidural steroid injection if the aforementioned treatments do not alleviate the patient's pain within 4 to 6 weeks. A clinician who is experienced in this procedure should perform this injection; either an interlaminar or transforaminal technique may be used. The efficacy of cervical epidurals is not known because prospective, randomized, controlled trials are lacking. Uncontrolled studies in the literature have reported good to excellent results in 60% to 76% of patients.[36-42]

It is unclear in the literature how many injections a patient may receive and how often they may be performed. Clinicians usually perform up to three injections in a 6- to 12-month period that are at least several weeks apart to assess the outcome of the previous injection.

Surgery

Indications for surgery are threefold: (1) progressive weakness, (2) myelopathy, and (3) intractable pain despite aggressive conservative management.

Both anterior (anterior discectomy with or without fusion) and posterior (foraminotomy) approaches have been documented in the surgical literature to have good outcomes.[43,44] The approach in a given patient depends on the nature of the anatomic lesion and the preference of the surgeon. A detailed discussion of surgical procedures is beyond the scope of this chapter.

POTENTIAL DISEASE COMPLICATIONS

Possible complications of cervical radiculopathy are persistent or progressive neurologic weakness, residual neck or radicular pain, chronic pain syndrome, disability, and myelopathy (rare, usually associated with spondylosis or large central disc herniation).

POTENTIAL TREATMENT COMPLICATIONS

Nonsteroidal anti-inflammatory drugs may produce gastropathy, hyperkalemia, renal toxicity, hepatic toxicity, exacerbation of asthma, drug-drug interaction, bleeding, and central nervous system effects. The use of steroids (short course) may result in mood changes, fluid retention, facial flushing, hyperglycemia, gastropathy, and suppression of the hypothalamic-pituitary-adrenal axis. The side effects of narcotics are constipation, nausea, vomiting, sedation, impaired mentation or motivation, suppression of endogenous opioid production, tolerance, addiction, biliary spasm, and respiratory depression.

Cervical collars may cause disuse weakness of the cervical muscles, decreased range of motion, and reinforcement of the sick role. Traction and exercise can exacerbate symptoms. Manipulation also may exacerbate symptoms and may result in recurrent disc herniation, worsening weakness, carotid dissection, stroke, and quadriplegia.

Epidural injection may produce vasovagal reactions, facial flushing, temporary exacerbation of symptoms, allergic reaction, hyperglycemia, spinal headache, epidural hematoma, infection, neural damage, and cardiopulmonary arrest. Surgery carries the following risks: infection; neurologic damage to the spinal cord, nerve roots, or peripheral nerves; nonunion of fusion; hardware loosening, migration, or failure; persistent neck and arm pain; and accelerated degeneration of the segment adjacent to fusion.

References

1. Ahlgren BD, Garfin SR. Cervical radiculopathy. Orthop Clin North Am 1996;27:253-263.
2. Malanga GA. The diagnosis and treatment of cervical radiculopathy. Med Sci Sports Exerc 1997;29(Suppl):S236-S245.
3. Carette S, Fehlings M. Cervical radiculopathy. N Engl J Med 2005;353:392-399.
4. Odom GL, Finney W, Woodhall B, et al. Cervical disc lesions. JAMA 1958;166:23-38.
5. Radhakrishan K, Litchy WJ, O'Fallon WM, et al. Epidemiology of cervical radiculopathy: a population-based study from Rochester, Minnesota, 1976 through 1990. Brain 1994;117:325-335.
6. Murphey F, Simmons JCH, Brunson B. Ruptured cervical discs 1939-1972. Clin Neurosurg 1973;20:9-17.
7. Yoss RE, Corbin KB, MacCarty CS, et al. Significance of symptoms and signs in localization of involved root in cervical disc protrusion. Neurology 1957;7:673-683.
8. Boulu P, Benoist M. Recent data on the pathophysiology of nerve root compression and pain. Rev Rhum Engl Ed 2006;63:358-363.
9. Van Zundert J, Harney D, Joosten EA, et al. The role of the dorsal root ganglion in cervical radicular pain: diagnosis, pathophysiology, and rationale for treatment. Reg Anesth Pain Med 2006;31:152-167.
10. Kang JD, Georgescu HI, McIntyre-Larkin L, et al. Herniated cervical intervertebral discs spontaneously produce matrix metalloproteinases, nitric oxide, interleukin-6 and prostaglandin E_2. Spine 1995;20:2373-2378.
11. Kang JD, Stefanovic-Racic M, McIntyre LA, et al. Toward a biochemical understanding of human intervertebral disc degeneration and herniation: contributions of nitric oxide, interleukins, prostaglandin E_2, and matrix metalloproteinases. Spine 1997;22:1065-1073.
12. Spurling RG, Scoville WB. Lateral rupture of the cervical intervertebral discs. A common cause of shoulder and arm pain. Surg Gynecol Obstet 1944;78:350-358.
13. Tanaka Y, Kokubun S, Sato T, et al. Cervical roots as origin of pain in the neck or scapular regions. Spine 2006;31:E568-E573.
14. Honet JC, Ellenberg MR. What you always wanted to know about the history and physical examination of neck pain but were afraid to ask. Phys Med Rehabil Clin North Am 2003;14:473-491.
15. Bates B. A Guide to Physical Examination and History Taking, 5th ed. Philadelphia, JB Lippincott, 1991:472.
16. Malanga GA, Campagnolo DI. Clarification of the pronator reflex. J Phys Med Rehabil 1994;73:338-340.
17. Fast A. The shoulder abduction relief sign in cervical radiculopathy. Arch Phys Med Rehabil 1989;70:402-403.
18. Davidson RI, Dunn EJ, Metzmaker JN. The shoulder abduction test in the diagnosis of radicular pain in cervical extradural compressive monoradiculopathies. Spine 1981;6:441-446.
19. Viikari-Juntura E, Porras M, Laasonen EM. Validity of clinical tests in diagnosis of root compression in cervical disease. Spine 1989;14:253-257.
20. Malanga GA, Landes P, Nadler SF. Provocative tests in cervical spine examination: historical basis and scientific analyses. Pain Physician 2003;6:199-205.
21. Ellenberg MR, Honet JC, Treanor WJ. Cervical radiculopathy. Arch Phys Med Rehabil 1994;75:342-352.
22. Wilbourn AJ, Aminoff MJ. AAEM minimonograph 32: the electrodiagnostic examination in patients with radiculopathies. American Association of Electrodiagnostic Medicine. Muscle Nerve 1998;21:1612-1631.
23. Dillingham TR. Evaluating the patient with suspected radiculopathy. In 2006 Course A. Numbness, Tingling, Pain, and Weakness: A Basic Course in Electrodiagnostic Medicine. Rochester, Minn, American Association of Neuromuscular and Electrodiagnostic Medicine, 2006.
24. Caplan LR, van Gijn J, Reiners K, et al. Management of cervical radiculopathy. Eur Neurol 1995;35:309-320.

25. Goldie I, Landquist A. Evaluation of the effects of different forms of physiotherapy in cervical pain. Scand J Rehabil Med 1970;2-3: 117-121.

26. Heckmann JG, Lang CJ, Zöbelein I, et al. Herniated cervical intervertebral discs with radiculopathy: an outcome study of conservatively or surgically treated patients. J Spinal Disord 1999;12:396-401.

27. Honet JC, Puri K. Cervical radiculitis: treatment and results in 82 patients. Arch Phys Med Rehabil 1976;57:12-16.

28. Martin GM, Corbin KB. An evaluation of conservative treatment for patients with cervical disc syndrome. Arch Phys Med Rehabil 1954;35:87-92.

29. Saal JS, Saal JA, Yurth EF. Nonoperative management of herniated cervical intervertebral disc with radiculopathy. Spine 1996;21: 1877-1883.

30. Sampath P, Bendebba M, Davis JD, et al. Outcome in patients with cervical radiculopathy: prospective, multicenter study with independent clinical review. Spine 1999;24:591-597.

31. Murphy DR, Hurwitz EL, Gregory A, et al. A nonsurgical approach to the management of patients with cervical radiculopathy: a prospective observational cohort study. J Manipulative Physiol Ther 2006;29:279-287.

32. Cleland JA, Whitman JM, Fritz JM, et al. Manual physical therapy, cervical traction and strengthening exercises in patients with cervical radiculopathy: a case series. J Orthop Sports Phys Ther 2005;35:802-811.

33. Rainville J, Sobel JB, Banco RJ, et al. Low back and cervical spine disorders. Orthop Clin North Am 1996;27:729-746.

34. Tan JC, Nordin MD. Role of physical therapy in the treatment of cervical radiculopathy. Orthop Clin North Am 1992;23:435-449.

35. Wolff MW, Levine LA. Cervical radiculopathies: conservative approaches to management. Phys Med Rehabil Clin North Am 2002;13:589-608.

36. Rowlingson JC, Kirschenbaum LP. Epidural analgesic techniques in the management of cervical pain. Anesth Analg 1986;65:938-942.

37. Cicala RS, Thoni K, Angel JJ. Long-term results of cervical epidural steroid injections. Clin J Pain 1989;5:143-145.

38. Stav A, Ovadia L, Sternberg A, et al. Cervical epidural steroid injection for cervicobrachialgia. Acta Anaesthesiol Scand 1993;37:562-566.

39. Bush K, Hillier S. Outcome of cervical radiculopathy treated with periradicular/epidural corticosteroid injections: a prospective study with independent clinical review. Eur Spine J 1996;5:319-325.

40. Berger O, Dousset V, Delmer O, et al. Evaluation of the efficacy of foraminal infusions of corticosteroids guided by computed tomography in the treatment of radicular pain by foraminal injection. J Radiol 1999;80:917-925.

41. Slipman CW, Lipetz JS, Jackson HB, et al. Therapeutic selective nerve root block in the nonsurgical management of atraumatic cervical spondylotic radicular pain: a retrospective analysis with independent clinical review. Arch Phys Med Rehabil 2000;81:741-746.

42. Cyteval C, Thomas E, Decoux E, et al. Cervical radiculopathy: open study on percutaneous periradicular foraminal steroid infiltration performed under CT control in 30 patients. AJNR Am J Neuroradiol 2004;25:441-445.

43. Hacker RJ, Cauthen JC, Gilbert TJ, et al. A prospective randomized multicenter clinical evaluation of an anterior cervical fusion cage. Spine 2000;25:2646-2654.

44. Ahn NU, Ahn UM, Andersson GB, An HS. Operative treatment of the patient with neck pain. Phys Med Rehabil Clin North Am 2003;14:675-692.

Cervical Sprain or Strain 5

Thomas H. Hudgins, MD, Lena Shahban, MD, and Joseph T. Alleva, MD

Synonyms

None

ICD-9 Code

723.1 Cervicalgia

DEFINITION

Cervical sprain or strain typically refers to acute pain arising from injured soft tissues of the neck, including muscles, tendons, and ligaments. The most common event leading to such injuries is motor vehicle collision. The mechanism of injury is complex. During a rear-end motor vehicle collision, the initial head and neck acceleration lags behind vehicular acceleration. Eventually, head and neck acceleration reaches up to $2\frac{1}{2}$ times the maximum car acceleration, which subsequently results in dramatic deceleration at end range of motion of the neck.[1,2] Whereas such injury can also result in fracture, disc, or neurologic injury, cervical strain or sprain, by definition, excludes these entities.

Although these other entities need to be excluded from the differential diagnosis, recent evidence implicates the zygapophyseal joints as a source of neck pain after whiplash injury. Specifically, in a randomized controlled trial in which the medial branches of the cervical dorsal rami were blocked with local anesthetics or treated with saline, it was shown that 60% of patients with whiplash injury had complete neck pain relief after injection of local anesthetic compared with no relief by injection of placebo.[3]

Many factors have been associated with worse outcome in acceleration-deceleration injuries involving motor vehicles. Older women tend to have a worse prognosis than that of younger women and men in general. In addition, poor education and a history of prior neck pain are prognostic factors for worse pain in women. Low family income, a history of prior neck pain, and lack of awareness of head position in the crash are associated with a poor prognosis in men.[4] Additional crash-related factors associated with a worse outcome include occupancy in a truck, being a passenger, colliding with a moving object, and getting hit head-on or perpendicularly.[5] A high intensity of neck pain, a decreased onset of latency of the initial pain, and radicular symptoms are also prognostic of worse outcomes.[6] Because many of these injuries result in initiation of litigation by patients, this too is a poor prognostic indicator.

Other causes include sleeping in awkward positions, lifting or pulling heavy objects, and repetitive motions involving the head and neck.

Estimates exist that 1 million whiplash injuries each year are due to motor vehicle collisions.

SYMPTOMS

The most common presentation of patients with cervical strain or sprain is nonradiating neck pain (Fig. 5-1). Patients will also complain of neck stiffness, fatigue, and worsening of symptoms with cervical range of motion. The pain often extends into the trapezius region or interscapular region. Headache, probably the most common associated symptom, originates in the occiput region and radiates frontally. Increased irritability and sleep disturbances are common. Paresthesias, radiating arm pain, dysphagia, visual symptoms, auditory symptoms, and dizziness may be reported.[6,7] Whereas an isolated cervical sprain or strain injury should be without these symptoms, there is the possibility of concomitant neurologic or bone injury. If these symptoms are present, alternative diagnoses should be suspected. Myelopathic symptoms, which suggest a different diagnosis that is more serious, such as bowel and bladder dysfunction, must be investigated.

PHYSICAL EXAMINATION

The primary finding in a cervical sprain or strain injury is decreased or painful cervical range of motion. This may be accompanied by tenderness of the cervical paraspinal, trapezius, occiput, or anterior cervical (i.e., sternocleidomastoid) muscles (Fig. 5-2).

A thorough neurologic examination should be performed to rule out myelopathic or radicular processes.

23

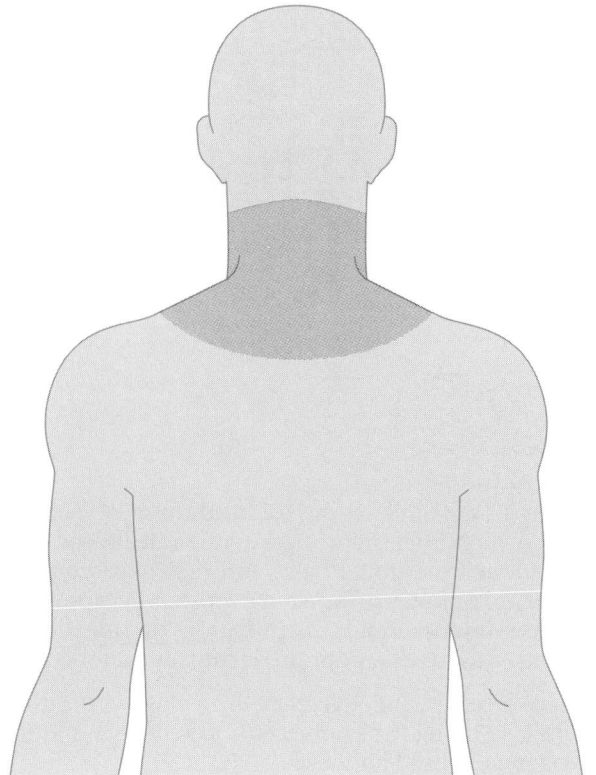

FIGURE 5-1. Typical pain distribution for a patient with an acute cervical sprain or strain injury.

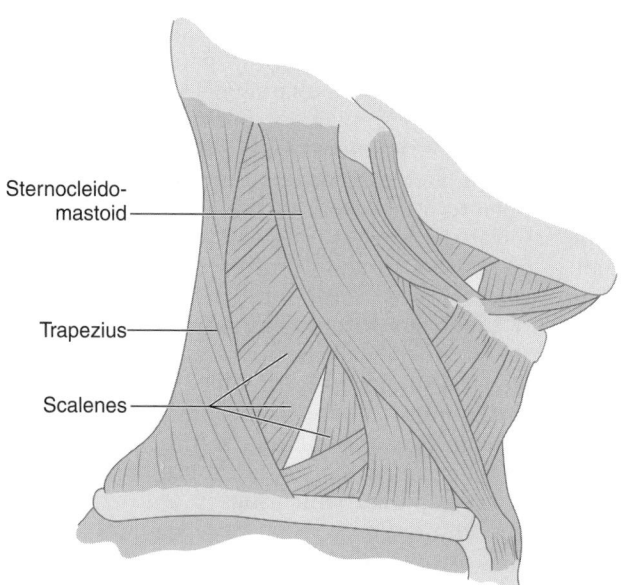

Sternocleido-mastoid

Trapezius

Scalenes

FIGURE 5-2. Muscles commonly involved in a cervical sprain or strain injury.

In an isolated cervical sprain injury, the neurologic examination findings should be normal.

The result of the neurocompression test, in which the patient is asked to rotate and extend the head, thereby reducing the neuroforaminal space, should be negative with cases of cervical sprain or strain.

FUNCTIONAL LIMITATIONS

Restricted range of motion of the cervical spine may contribute to difficulty with daily activities such as driving. Patients often complain of neck fatigue, heaviness, and pain with static cervical positions such as reading and working at the computer. Sleep may be affected as well.

DIAGNOSTIC STUDIES

It is generally accepted that radiographs to exclude fracture should be obtained in patients involved in a traumatic event and who have altered consciousness, are intoxicated, or exhibit cervical tenderness and focal neurologic signs with decreased range of motion on physical examination.[8] Although the clinician may commonly see straightening of the cervical lordosis on the lateral cervical radiograph, this is thought to be related to spasm of the paracervical musculature and bears no other significance (Fig. 5-3).

Studies such as magnetic resonance imaging scans, computed tomographic scans, and electrodiagnostics are typically used to rule out alternative or coexisting entities. All of these studies will have normal findings in cases of cervical sprain or strain.

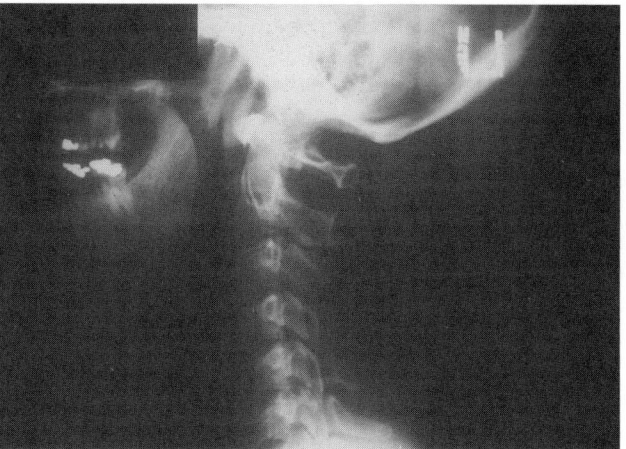

FIGURE 5-3. Cervical spine radiograph showing straightening of the spine and loss of the normal cervical lordosis.

Differential Diagnosis

Occult cervical fracture or dislocation

Cervical discogenic pain

Cervical herniated disc, radiculopathy

Cervical facet syndrome

Cervical spine tumor

Cervical spine infection

TREATMENT

Initial

Initial interventions used in patients with cervical sprain or strain have not been scientifically tested. Education of the patient is critical for a realistic expectation of resolution of symptoms. In most cases, symptoms will resolve within 4 to 6 weeks. In some cases, however, resolution of symptoms may be delayed up to 6 to 12 months.

It is reasonable to recommend rest within the first 24 to 72 hours of injury. The detriments of prolonged bed rest and the use of cervical collars have been clearly described, and these "treatments" may, in fact, promote disability.[9] The short-term use of nonsteroidal anti-inflammatory drugs, muscle relaxants, and analgesic medications on a judicious basis is accepted to promote early return to activity.[10] Muscle relaxants or low-dose tricyclic antidepressants (nortriptyline or amitriptyline, 10 to 50 mg at bedtime) are also used to help restore sleep in the patient for whom this is an issue.

High-dose intravenous methylprednisolone within 8 hours of the whiplash injury has been studied and was shown to be associated with decreased pain at 1 week after injury and fewer total sick days taken at 6 months. However, larger trials are needed to further evaluate the cost-benefit ratio for this treatment.[11]

Rehabilitation

No rehabilitation approach has been proved unequivocally effective, although early mobilization and return to function is the key to successful rehabilitation. Cervical manipulation, massage, and mobilization on a limited basis are geared toward correction of segmental restrictions and restoration of normal range of motion. Such approaches have been shown to be more effective than passive modalities with regard to range of motion and reduction of pain.[12] Therapeutic modalities such as ultrasound and electrical stimulation can be tried for pain control but have no proven efficacy for long-term recovery. In addition, cervical traction done either manually (by a physical therapist) or with a mechanical unit (prescribed for home use) may be tried if there are no contraindications (i.e., fracture). Educational videos that make recommendations about posture, return to activity, exercise, and pain relief methods may help reduce rates of persistent symptoms at 6 months after injury.[13]

Strengthening and stretching exercises for muscles with a tendency for tightness should be used in conjunction with the aforementioned techniques. Muscle imbalances must be addressed, and weak muscle groups such as the scapular stabilizers (middle-lower trapezius, serratus anterior, and levator scapulae) should be strengthened. This is typically done after muscles with a tendency for tightness (upper trapezius, sternocleidomastoid, scalenes, latissimus dorsi, and pectoralis major and minor) are stretched.[14] Cumulative data suggest that such an approach to cervical sprain injuries produces both long- and short-term benefits.[8] The overall treatment goal is to achieve an independent, customized home exercise program so that the patient can become active in his or her treatment.[15] An exercise protocol targeting shoulder and neck muscle strength and endurance was effective in decreasing chronic neck pain and disability in 180 female police officers.

Evaluation of the home or work environment by an occupational therapist can also be of benefit. Specifically, ergonomic alterations, such as the use of a telephone headrest and document holders, may aid in recovery.

Procedures

Trigger point injections are a reasonable adjunct to decrease pain so that patients may participate in physical therapy. The upper trapezius, scalenes, and semispinalis capitis are the most common muscles to develop trigger points after acceleration-deceleration injuries. Other trigger points tend to arise in the splenius capitis, longus capitis, and longus colli after such injuries.[16] Botulinum toxin injections may be useful as well.[17]

Facet injections, epidural injections, and cervical traction may be instituted for conditions such as cervical radiculopathy and facet syndrome, which are often associated with cervical sprains and strains.

Surgery

Surgery is not indicated.

POTENTIAL DISEASE COMPLICATIONS

The main complication from the injury itself is chronic intractable pain leading to permanent loss of cervical range of motion and functional disability.

POTENTIAL TREATMENT COMPLICATIONS

Analgesics and nonsteroidal anti-inflammatory drugs have well-known side effects that most commonly affect the gastric, hepatic, and renal systems. Muscle relaxants and low-dose tricyclic antidepressants can cause sedation. Overly aggressive manipulation or manipulation done when there is a concomitant unidentified injury (i.e., fracture) may result in serious injury. Injections are rarely associated with infection and allergic reactions to the medications used.

References

1. Bogduk N. The anatomy and pathophysiology of whiplash. Clin Biomech 1986;1:92-100.
2. Stovner L. The nosologic status of the whiplash syndrome: a critical review based on methodological approach. Spine 1996;21:2735-2746.
3. Lord SM, Barnsley L, Wallis BJ, Bogduk N. Chronic cervical zygapophysial joint pain after whiplash. A placebo-controlled prevalence study. Spine 1996;21:1737-1744.
4. Holm LW, Carroll LJ, Cassidy JD, Ahlbom A. Factors influencing neck pain intensity in whiplash-associated disorders. Spine 2006;31:E98-E104.

5. Harder S, Veilleux M, Suissa S. The effect of socio-demographic and crash-related factors on the prognosis of whiplash. J Clin Epidemiol 1998;51:377-384.

6. Radanov B, Sturzenegger M. Long-term outcome after whiplash injury. A 2-year follow-up considering features of injury mechanism and somatic, radiologic, and psychosocial findings. Medicine (Baltimore) 1995;1974:281-297.

7. Norris S, Watt I. The prognosis of neck injuries resulting from rear-end vehicle collisions. J Bone Joint Surg Br 1983;65:608-611.

8. Spitzer W, Skovron M, Salmi LR, et al. Scientific monograph of the Quebec Task Force on Whiplash-Associated Disorders: redefining "whiplash" and its management. Spine 1995;20(Suppl):S1-S5.

9. Mealy K, Brennan H, Fenelon GC. Early mobilization of acute whiplash injury. Br Med J (Clin Res Ed) 1986;292:656-657.

10. McKinney L. Early mobilisation and outcome in acute sprains of the neck. BMJ 1989;299:1006-1008.

11. Pettersson K, Toolanen G. High-dose methylprednisolone prevents extensive sick leave after whiplash injury. A prospective, randomized, double-blind study. Spine 1998;23:9844-9889.

12. Rosenfeld M, Gunnarsson R, Borenstein P. Early intervention in whiplash-associated disorder. Spine 2000;25:1782-1787.

13. Brison RJ, Hartling L, Dostaler S, et al. A randomized controlled trial of an educational intervention to prevent the chronic pain of whiplash associated disorders following rear-end motor vehicle collisions. Spine 2005;30:1799-1807.

14. Janda V. Muscles and cervicogenic pain syndromes. In Grant R, ed. Physical Therapy of the Cervical and Thoracic Spine. New York, Churchill Livingstone, 1998:153-166.

15. Nikander R, Mälkiä E, Parkkari J, et al. Dose-response relationship of specific training to reduce chronic neck pain and disability. Med Sci Sports Exerc 2006;38:2068-2074.

16. Simons DG, Travell JG, Simons LS. Travell & Simons' Myofascial Pain and Dysfunction: The Trigger Point Manual, 2nd ed. Upper Half of Body, vol 1. Baltimore, Williams & Wilkins, 1999:278-307, 432-444, 445-471, 504-537.

17. Freund JB, Schwartz M. Treatment of chronic cervical-associated headache with botulinum toxin A: a pilot study. Headache 2000;40:231-236.

Cervical Stenosis 6

Alec L. Meleger, MD

Synonyms

Cervical spondylotic myelopathy
Spinal stenosis
Cervical myelopathy

ICD-9 Code

723.0 Spinal stenosis in cervical region

DEFINITION

Cervical stenosis refers to pathologic narrowing of the spinal canal that can be either congenital or acquired. The congenital type is commonly due to short pedicles that produce an abnormally shallow central spinal canal.[1] The main contributing factors to the development of the acquired type are the degenerative, hypertrophic, age-related changes that affect the intervertebral discs, facet joints, and uncovertebral joints as well as the ligamentum flavum (Fig. 6-1). On radiologic imaging, these degenerative changes are present in 25% to 50% of the population by the age of 50 years and in 75% to 85% by 65 years.[2-4] Some of the other factors that may contribute to pathologic narrowing of the spinal canal include degenerative spondylolisthesis, ossification of posterior longitudinal ligament, and atlantoaxial subluxation as seen in rheumatoid arthritis; rarely, it may be secondary to such extradural pathologic processes as metastatic disease, abscess formation, and trauma.[5]

Spinal cord compression, or cervical myelopathy in symptomatic patients, commonly occurs at the cervical level C5-7, given the relatively increased mobility of those segments and the subsequent development of degenerative "wear and tear." Concomitant compression of the exiting cervical nerve roots is also typically observed in cervical spondylotic disease. Symptom production can occur by constant, mechanical compression of the neural elements or be of an intermittent, dynamic nature as seen with extremes of cervical flexion and extension. Chronic compression can lead to local cord ischemia with subsequent development of cervical myelopathy.[6]

SYMPTOMS

Symptomatic presentation of cervical spinal stenosis can differ from patient to patient, depending on the pathologic process, the anatomic structures, and the cervical levels involved. Intervertebral disc degeneration and zygapophyseal joint arthritis commonly present with axial neck pain. Patients with cervical foraminal stenosis may complain of radicular arm pain as well as of paresthesias, dysesthesias, numbness, and weakness of the upper extremity. On the other hand, patients with cervical central canal stenosis can present with myelopathic symptoms of the upper and lower extremities, neurogenic bladder and bowel, sexual dysfunction, and unsteady and stiff-legged gait as well as weakness, paresthesias, or numbness of the lower extremities. Lower extremity pain is not known to be a clinical symptom unless concomitant lumbar spinal disease is present.

PHYSICAL EXAMINATION

Physical examination findings of the patient with cervical stenosis should be consistent with upper or lower motor neuron signs, depending on the spinal level involved. Lower motor neuron findings are more commonly seen in the upper extremities; these include muscle atrophy, diminished sensation, decreased reflexes, diminished muscle tone, and weakness. Upper extremity myelopathic findings, such as hyperactive reflexes, increased tone, and present Hoffmann sign, can also be observed in cases of upper and mid cervical spinal cord involvement. A Spurling sign (radicular pain on axial loading of an extended head rotated toward the involved extremity) can also be present.

Lower extremity examination is more consistent with upper motor neuron findings in the presence of cervical stenosis with myelopathy. Increased reflexes, Babinski sign, sustained or unsustained clonus, spasticity, weakness, decreased tactile and vibratory sensation, impaired proprioception, and neurogenic bowel and bladder can be seen. Lhermitte sign, an electric-like sensation that the patient reports going down the back when the neck is flexed (Fig. 6-2), can sometimes be elicited.[7] Refer to Chapter 1 for more detail.

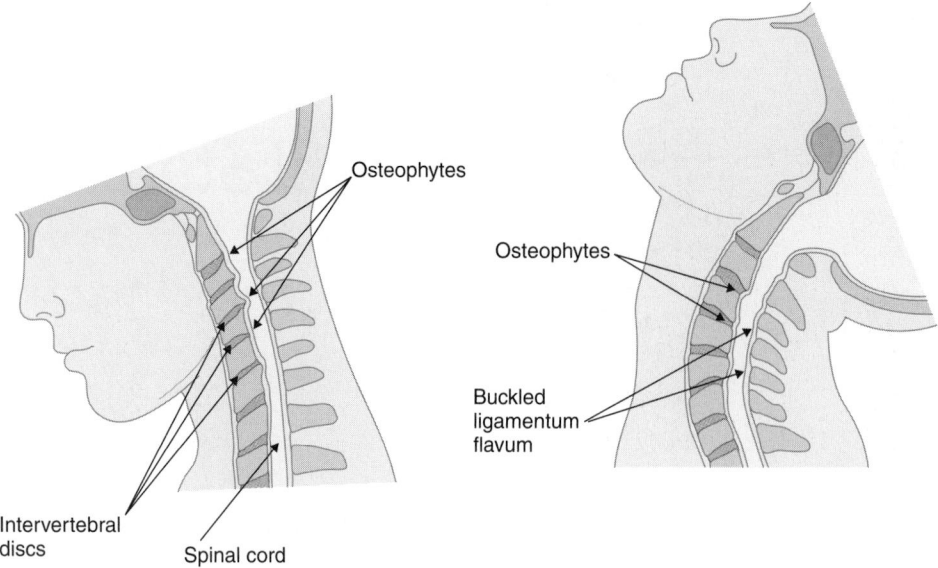

FIGURE 6-1. Cervical stenosis is a narrowing of the spinal canal that may be due to a variety of factors (e.g., congenital narrowing, osteophyte formation, hypertrophy of the ligamentum flavum).

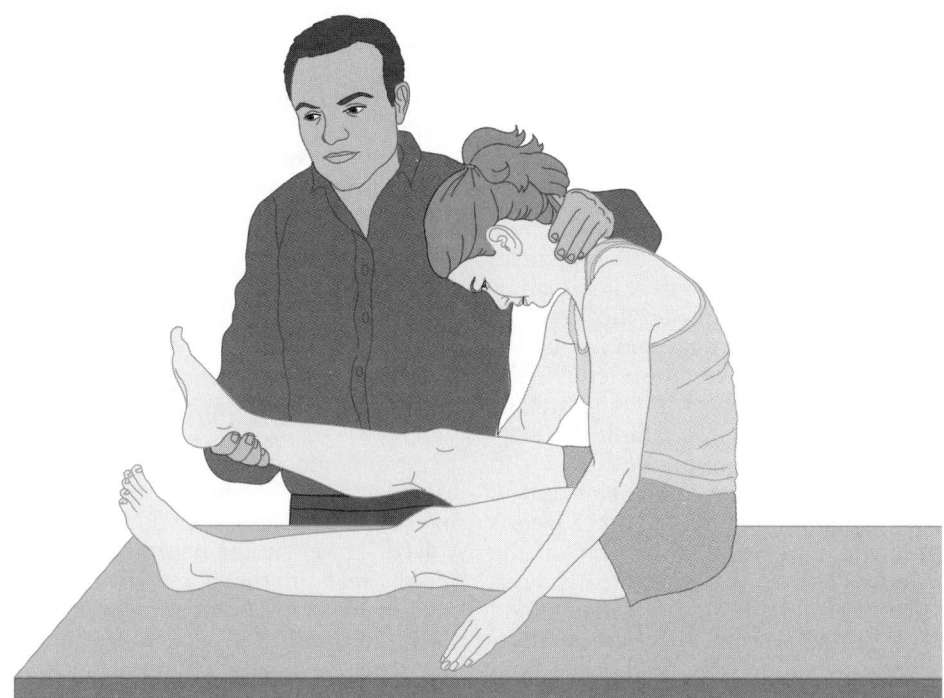

FIGURE 6-2. Lhermitte sign. The examiner flexes the patient's head and hip simultaneously.

FUNCTIONAL LIMITATIONS

The functional limitations depend on the extent of neurologic involvement. A person with mild symptoms can still be completely independent with activities of daily living, mobility, household chores, and work duties. In some cases, pain and weakness can produce various degrees of disability in self-care, such as grooming, bathing, and dressing, as well as in more physically demanding functions, especially in the community setting, such as lifting, carrying, and ambulation. Bowel and bladder incontinence as well as abnormalities of mood and sleep can further lead to social isolation and an increased level of actual and self-perceived disability. In extreme cases, paraplegia and quadriplegia can limit nearly all functional activities.

DIAGNOSTIC STUDIES

Facet and uncovertebral joint arthropathy, intervertebral disc space narrowing, neuroforaminal size reduction, and presence of spondylolisthesis can be evaluated with cervical spine radiographs; if dynamic instability is

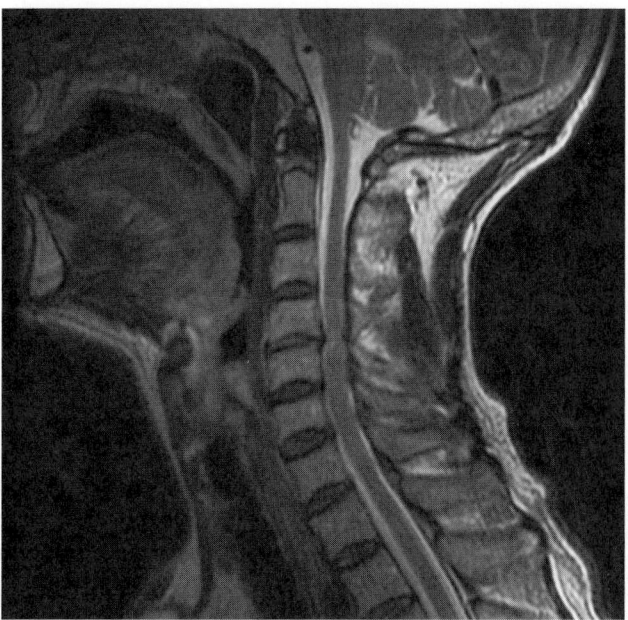

FIGURE 6-3. Severe C4-5 cervical stenosis. Disc-osteophyte complex and hypertrophic ligamentum flavum are producing an indentation of the spinal cord. Notice an intramedullary hyperintensity signal consistent with spinal cord injury.

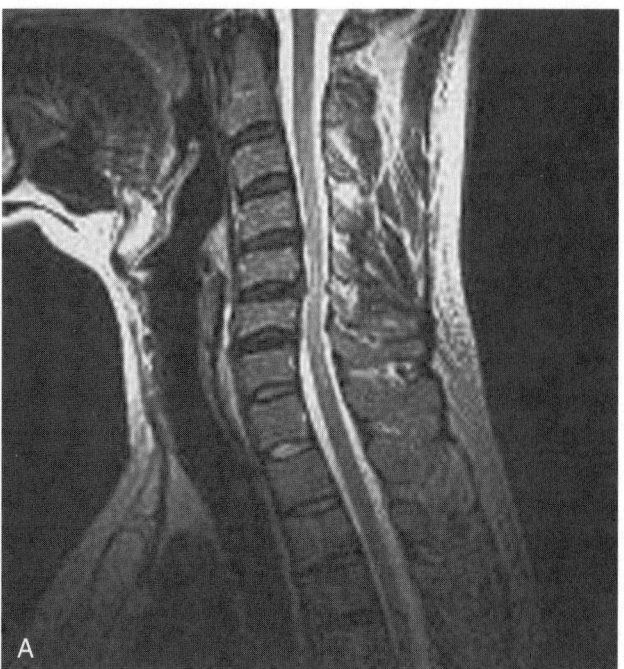

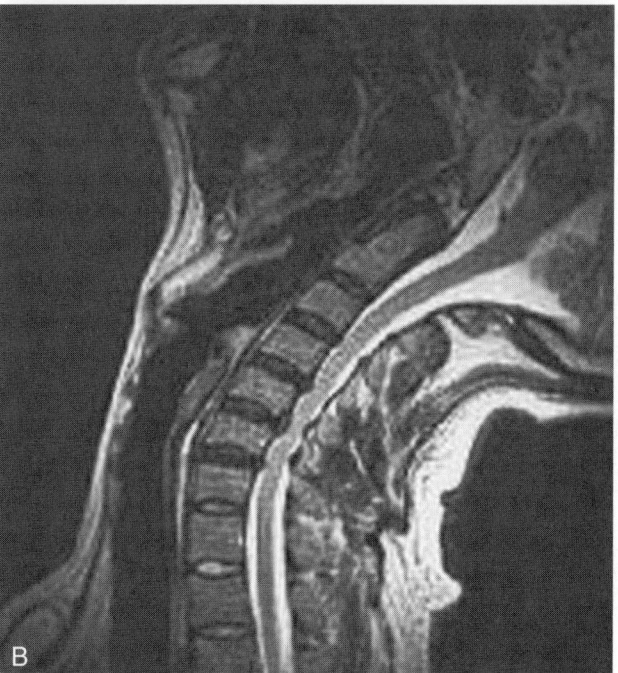

FIGURE 6-4. Sagittal magnetic resonance images of cervical spine with the patient recumbent **(A)** and standing with the neck extended **(B)**.

suspected, standing flexion-extension views are advised. Presence of osseous and soft tissue disease as well as the extent of nerve root and spinal cord compression can be assessed by magnetic resonance imaging (Fig. 6-3). Computed tomographic myelography can provide additional information on the extent of bone disease and the dynamic nature of neural compression during flexion and extension. The new development of upright magnetic resonance imaging may be able to provide the same information on the dynamic behavior of spinal stenosis with less procedural invasiveness[8] (Fig. 6-4). Somatosensory evoked potentials can confirm the presence of myelopathy, and electromyography can confirm peripheral nerve root involvement.[9]

Several radiologic criteria exist to define what constitutes significant stenosis of the cervical spine. According to some sources, an absolute cervical spinal stenosis is present when the sagittal spinal canal diameter is less than 10 mm, and relative spinal stenosis is present when this measurement is 10 to 13 mm.[10,11] The Torg ratio of less than 0.8, which is measured by dividing the sagittal diameter of the spinal canal by the sagittal diameter of the respective vertebral body, predicts the presence of significant spinal stenosis and tries to eliminate any inherent radiographic measurement errors.[12] A more widely accepted approach in evaluating the extent of stenotic pathologic changes is through the use of magnetic resonance imaging, which permits the functional capacity of the surrounding subarachnoid space and the state of the spinal cord itself to be more definitively assessed. The presence of intramedullary signal abnormalities warrants further investigation and a more aggressive treatment approach (see Fig. 6-3).

TREATMENT

Initial

Conservative treatment is generally undertaken in the absence of clinical evidence of cervical myelopathy. If cervical myelopathy is suspected or clearly evident, the patient must be immediately referred for an evaluation by a spine surgical specialist. When a patient is symptomatic with pain but does not have myelopathic symptoms, relative decrease in physical activity for no longer

Differential Diagnosis

Thoracic spinal stenosis

Cervical intramedullary or extramedullary neoplasm

Cervical osteomyelitis with or without epidural abscess

Multiple sclerosis (spinal)

Transverse myelitis

Cerebrovascular accident

Syringomyelia

Spinal cord injury

Arteriovenous malformation

Tabes dorsalis

Progressive multifocal leukoencephalopathy

Tropical spastic paraparesis

Lumbar spinal stenosis

Thoracic outlet syndrome

Idiopathic brachial neuritis

Brachial plexopathy

than 2 or 3 days is initially recommended. For severe cervical or radicular pain, a soft neck collar can be prescribed for a few days with subsequent self-weaning by alternating periods of collar removal.[13]

Self-application of ice or heat for cervical pain and transcutaneous electrical nerve stimulation for radicular symptoms can be of benefit to some patients.

Initial analgesics of choice are acetaminophen and nonsteroidal anti-inflammatory drugs, which may show some effect in cervical as well as in radicular pain when they are taken at regular intervals. More than one family of nonsteroidals should be tried before they are deemed to be ineffective. A short course of opioids and muscle relaxants may benefit those patients with severe pain and strong contraindications to the use of acetaminophen and nonsteroidal anti-inflammatory drugs. For recalcitrant, functionally limiting radicular symptoms, a 7- to 10-day course of oral steroids is recommended. A tapering dose of oral prednisone can be prescribed starting with 60 mg and followed by 10- to 20-mg decrements every 2 or 3 days. Persistent radicular pain can be treated with neuropathic pain medications, such as gabapentin, pregabalin, tricyclic antidepressants, clonazepam, and others.[14]

Education of the patient about the nature of cervical stenosis, its worrisome signs and symptoms (e.g., progressive difficulties with gait, urinary retention or incontinence), injury prevention, and the importance of staying active is of paramount importance. In older patients, fall prevention and fall precautions should be immediately addressed to prevent catastrophic neurologic consequences. In individuals with magnetic resonance imaging evidence of severe cervical stenosis, certain physical activities, such as horseback or motorcycle riding, climbing ladders, and participation in contact sports, should be strongly discouraged. Patients should also be advised to avoid the extremes of cervical extension and flexion, as in swimming the breast stroke, painting a ceiling, or performing legs over head backward stretching.

Rehabilitation

Physical and occupational therapy should focus on keeping patients as active as possible while educating them about activities that might place them at risk for further injury. Continued physical activity, such as walking and the use of a stationary bicycle, is recommended to prevent overall muscle and aerobic deconditioning. Gentle cervical traction may also be tried in the absence of severe stenosis or myelopathic findings. With passing of the acute phase, a program consisting of stretching and isometric neck exercises should be undertaken. Once the pain-free range of motion is achieved, isotonic neck strengthening is initiated.[15] Eventually, patients should be graduated to a home exercise program.

Work site evaluation and institution of certain job restrictions are recommended to prevent repetitive hyperextension or hyperflexion activities. These might include adjustment of computer monitor height, recommendation for a phone headset, and restriction of duties requiring activities above eye level. The use of bifocals should also be addressed because these require frequent head positional changes.

Depression and anxiety can lead to symptom magnification and should be addressed by a mental health provider. Cognitive-behavioral therapy, biofeedback, self-hypnosis, and relaxation techniques must always be considered part of the comprehensive pain management treatment.

Procedures

A trial of interlaminar or transforaminal epidural steroid injections is advocated for acute or subacute radicular symptoms of severe intensity unresponsive to more conservative measures. Care should be taken to avoid the introduction of a spinal needle at the level of stenosis when an interlaminar approach is used. Transforaminal epidural steroid injections should be performed by a well-trained practitioner under continuous fluoroscopic imaging to avoid catastrophic complications. Patients without significant central spinal canal compromise and who continue to suffer with chronic severe radicular symptoms, unresponsive to conservative approaches, may be candidates for a spinal cord stimulator trial and implantation. Arthritic cervical facet joints, which are innervated by medial branch nerves, can be another source of pain. Intra-articular steroid injections can provide up to several months of significant pain relief. If these fail to provide significant analgesic effect, diagnostic medial branch nerve blocks can be performed; if results are found to be positive, radiofrequency nerve ablation should follow.

Surgery

Immediate surgical intervention should be sought with symptoms of progressive weakness, bladder or bowel incontinence, unsteady gait, and upper motor neuron findings. A surgical specialist should also assess intractable pain of 3 months' duration, unresponsive to conservative treatment. Decompressive single-level or multilevel laminectomy, discectomy, foraminotomy, and cervical fusion by use of bone graft or instrumentation are the common surgical procedures. Referral to a surgical specialist should be considered for intractable radicular symptoms.[16,17]

POTENTIAL DISEASE COMPLICATIONS

If left untreated, continued pressure on the exiting cervical nerve roots and the cervical segment of the spinal cord may lead to progressive weakness, loss of sensation, dysfunction of the bladder and bowel, tetraplegia, or paraplegia.

The natural course of cervical spondylotic myelopathy, when it is treated conservatively, demonstrates continued neurologic progression in one third to two thirds of patients.[18,19]

POTENTIAL TREATMENT COMPLICATIONS

Application of aggressive or improper physical or occupational therapy treatments can lead to further injury to the already compromised spinal cord and the exiting nerve roots. Cervical traction may promote signs and symptoms of myelopathy and radiculopathy. Atrophy of cervical musculature can occur with prolonged use of a cervical collar. Aggressive cervical manual technique can cause vertebral artery dissection and severe neurologic sequelae.

Nonsteroidal anti-inflammatory medications carry well-known side effects of gastrointestinal irritation, bleeding, edema, and nephropathy. These medications are to be used cautiously or avoided in patients with a past history of peptic ulcer disease or with decreased renal function. A proton pump inhibitor or misoprostol should be considered for ulcer prophylaxis in individuals at high risk. All of the neuropathic pain medications carry significant side effects; gabapentin possesses the best tolerance. The most common complaints are sedation, dizziness, and gait imbalance. Continued use of opioids can lead to physiologic dependence, tolerance, sedation, constipation, and rarely addiction. Objective evidence of improved function and decreased level of pain is required for their continued use.

Interlaminar epidural steroid injections carry a small risk of dural puncture and subsequent development of a post–dural puncture headache. In the majority of patients, these headaches are self-limited and respond well to bed rest, hydration, and caffeine. Improper placement of needle tip and intravascular injection of particulate steroid can lead to spinal cord injury, stroke, and brain stem infarct. All interventions, percutaneous and surgical, carry a rare risk of spinal infection, compressive hematoma, and nerve and spinal cord injury.

References

1. Epstein JA, Carras R, Hyman RA, Costa S. Cervical myelopathy caused by developmental stenosis of the spinal canal. J Neurosurg 1979;51:362-367.
2. Bohlman HH, Emery SE. The pathophysiology of cervical spondylosis and myelopathy. Spine 1988;13:843-846.
3. Adams CBT, Logue V. Studies in cervical spondylitic myelopathy: I-III. Brain 1971;94:557-594.
4. Connell MD, Wiesel SW. Natural history and pathogenesis of cervical disc disease. Orthop Clin North Am 1992;23:369-380.
5. Ono K, Yonenobu K, Miyamoto S, Okada K. Pathology of ossification of the posterior longitudinal ligament and ligamentum flavum. Clin Orthop Relat Res 1999;359:18-26.
6. Singh A, Crockard HA, Platts A, Stevens J. Clinical and radiological correlates of severity and surgery-related outcome in cervical spondylosis. J Neurosurg 2001;94(Suppl):189-198.
7. Clark CR. Cervical spondylotic myelopathy: history and physical findings. Spine 1988;13:847-849.
8. Jinkins JR, Dworkin JS, Damadian RV. Upright, weight-bearing, dynamic-kinetic MRI of the spine: initial results. Eur Radiol 2005;15:1815-1825.
9. Yiannikas C, Shahani BT, Young RR. Short-latency somatosensory-evoked potentials from radial, median, ulnar, and peroneal nerve stimulation in the assessment of cervical spondylosis. Comparison with conventional electromyography. Arch Neurol 1986;43:1264-1271.
10. Matsuura P, Waters RL, Adkins RH, et al. Comparison of computerized tomography parameters of the cervical spine in normal control subjects and spinal cord–injured patients. J Bone Joint Surg Am 1989;71:183-188.
11. Edwards WC, LaRocca H. The developmental segmental sagittal diameter of the cervical spinal canal in patients with cervical spondylosis. Spine 1983;8:2027.
12. Pavlov H, Torg JS, Robie B, Jahre C. Cervical spinal stenosis: determination with vertebral body ratio method. Radiology 1987;164:771-775.
13. Persson L, Carlsson CA, Carlsson JY. Long lasting cervical radicular pain managed with surgery, physiotherapy, or a cervical collar: a prospective, randomized study. Spine 1997;22:751-758.
14. van Seventer R, Feister HA, Young JP Jr, et al. Efficacy and tolerability of twice-daily pregabalin for treating pain and related sleep interference in postherpetic neuralgia: a 13-week, randomized trial. Curr Med Res Opin 2006;22:375-384.
15. Levoska S, Keinanen-Kiukaanniemi S. Active or passive physiotherapy for occupational cervicobrachial disorders? A comparison of two treatment methods with a 1-year follow up. Arch Phys Med Rehabil 1993;74:425-430.
16. Orr RD, Zdeblick TA. Cervical spondylotic myelopathy: approaches to surgical treatment. Clin Orthop Relat Res 1999;359:58-66.
17. Edwards RJ, Cudlip SA, Moore AJ. Surgical treatment of cervical spondylotic myelopathy in extreme old age. Neurosurgery 1999;45:696.
18. Epstein JA. The surgical management of cervical spinal stenosis, spondylosis and myeloradiculopathy by means of the posterior approach. Spine 1988;13:864-869.
19. Symon L, Lavender P. The surgical treatment of cervical spondylotic myelopathy. Neurology 1967;17:117-127.

Cervicogenic Vertigo   7

Joanne Borg-Stein, MD

Synonyms

Cervicogenic dizziness
Neck pain associated with dizziness

ICD-9 Codes

723.1   Neck pain
780.4   Vertigo
780.4   Dizziness

DEFINITION

Cervicogenic vertigo is the false sense of motion that is due to cervical musculoskeletal dysfunction. The symptoms may be secondary to post-traumatic events with resultant whiplash or postconcussive syndrome. Alternatively, cervicogenic vertigo may be part of a more generalized disorder, such as fibromyalgia or underlying osteoarthritis.

Cervicogenic vertigo is believed to result from convergence of the cervical nerve inputs as well as the cranial nerve input and their close approximation in the upper cervical spinal segments of the spinal cord.[1,2] Dizziness and vertigo, common presenting symptoms, account for 8 million primary care visits to physicians in the United States each year and represent the most common presenting complaint in patients older than 75 years.[3] In fact, 40% to 80% of patients with neck trauma experience vertigo, particularly after whiplash injury. The incidence of symptoms of dizziness and vertigo in whiplash patients has been reported as 20% to 58%.[4]

SYMPTOMS

Patients with cervicogenic vertigo experience a false sense of motion, often whirling or spinning. Some patients experience sensations of floating, bobbing, tilting, or drifting. Others experience nausea, visual motor sensitivity, and ear fullness.[5] The symptoms are often provoked or triggered by neck movement or sustained awkward head positioning.[6-8] Cervical pain or headache may interfere with sleep and functional activities. At times, patients with

coexistent cervical radiculitis may complain of paresthesias in the upper cervical dermatomes.

PHYSICAL EXAMINATION

The essential elements of the physical examination are normal neurologic, ear, and eye examinations for nystagmus. Abnormalities in any of these aspects of the examination indicate a need to exclude other otologic or neurologic conditions, such as Meniere disease, benign paroxysmal positional vertigo, and stroke.[9] A careful cervical examination should be performed, including range of motion testing and palpation of the facet joints to assess mechanical dysfunction. Myofascial trigger points should be sought in the sternocleidomastoid, cervical paraspinal, levator scapulae, upper trapezius, and suboccipital musculature. Patients with cervicogenic headache and disequilibrium have a significantly higher incidence of restricted cervical flexion or extension and painful cervical joint dysfunction and muscle tightness.[10] Palpation in these areas can often reproduce the symptoms experienced as cervicogenic vertigo.[11]

FUNCTIONAL LIMITATIONS

Functional limitations may include difficulty with walking, balance, or equilibrium. As a result, patients may not feel confident with activities such as driving because cervical rotation may induce symptoms. Occupations that require balance and coordination (such as construction) are often limited. Anxiety about the occurrence of disequilibrium may contribute to secondary disability.

DIAGNOSTIC STUDIES

Cervicogenic dizziness is a clinical diagnosis. Testing may include cervical radiographs to rule out cervical osteoarthritis or instability. Cervical magnetic resonance imaging is indicated when cervical spondylosis is suspected, either as a cause of the condition or as an associated diagnosis. Brain magnetic resonance imaging or magnetic resonance angiography may be ordered to exclude vascular lesions or tumor (i.e., acoustic neuroma). A comprehensive neurotologic test battery and consultation are

Differential Diagnosis

Meniere disease

Benign paroxysmal positional vertigo

Labyrinthitis

Vestibular neuronitis

Cardiovascular causes: arrhythmia, carotid stenosis, or postural hypotension

Migraine-associated dizziness

Progressive dysequilibrium of aging

Post-traumatic vertigo

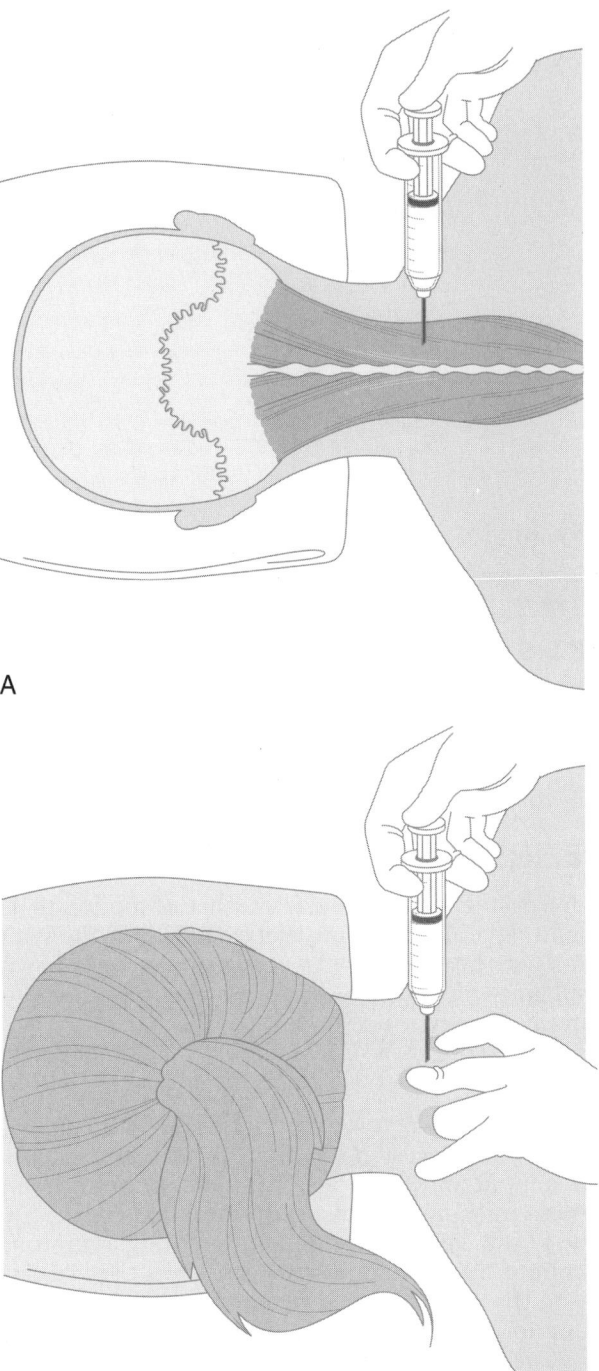

A

B

FIGURE 7-1. A and **B,** Trigger points in the sternocleidomastoid muscle frequently involved in cervicogenic vertigo. (Reprinted with permission from Simons DG, Travell JG, Simons LS. Travell & Simons' Myofascial Pain and Dysfunction: The Trigger Point Manual, 2nd ed. Upper Half of Body, vol 1. Baltimore, Williams & Wilkins, 1999:310.)

preferred if a primary otologic disorder or post-traumatic vertigo is considered.[12]

TREATMENT

Initial

Initial treatment involves reassurance and education of the patient. Nonsteroidal anti-inflammatory drugs are useful to help pain control for those who have underlying cervical osteoarthritis. Muscle relaxants such as cyclobenzaprine, carisoprodol, and low-dose tricyclic antidepressants may be used at bedtime to facilitate sleep and muscle relaxation for myofascial pain. I occasionally prescribe ondansetron (4 to 8 mg every 8 hours as needed) if disequilibrium is accompanied by significant nausea.

Rehabilitation

Rehabilitation is aimed at reducing muscle spasm, increasing cervical range of motion, improving posture, and restoring function. A physical therapist with experience and training in manual therapy, myofascial and trigger point treatment, and therapeutic exercise should evaluate and treat the patient to restore normal cervical function.[13] Occupational therapy can improve posture, ergonomics, and functional daily activities.[14]

Ergonomic accessories, such as telephone earset or headset, may help the patient avoid awkward head and neck postures that contribute to symptoms. Psychological or behavioral medicine consultation and treatment can aid the patient in overcoming the fear, avoidance, and anxiety that often develop.[15]

Procedures

Trigger point injections with local anesthetic (1% lidocaine or 0.25% bupivacaine) are often helpful to decrease cervical muscle pain (Fig. 7-1). The clinician should locate those trigger point areas that reproduce the patient's symptoms. Acupuncture with an emphasis on local treatment of muscle spasm may be an alternative to trigger point injection.[16,17]

Botulinum toxin injection may have a role in the treatment of cervicogenic headache; however, more research is needed in this area.[18] There are no data yet on the treatment of cervicogenic vertigo with botulinum toxin.

Surgery

There is no surgery indicated for treatment of this disorder, unless there is coexistent neurologically significant cervical stenosis or disc herniation.

POTENTIAL DISEASE COMPLICATIONS

The major complications are inactivity, deconditioning, falls, fear of going outside the home, anxiety, and depression. Chronic intractable neck pain and persistent dizziness may persist in spite of treatment.

POTENTIAL TREATMENT COMPLICATIONS

Side effects from nonsteroidal anti-inflammatory drugs may include gastric, renal, hepatic, and hematologic complications. Muscle relaxants and tricyclics may induce fatigue, somnolence, constipation, urinary retention, and other anticholinergic side effects. Local injections may result in local pain, ecchymosis, intravascular injection, or pneumothorax if they are improperly executed.

References

1. Norre M. Cervical vertigo. Acta Otorhinolaryngol Belg 1987;25: 495-499.
2. Revel M, Andre-Deshays C, Mingeut M. Cervicocephalic kinesthetic sensibility in patients with cervical pain. Arch Phys Med Rehabil 1991;72:288-291.
3. Colledge NR, Barr-Hamilton RM, Lewis SJ, et al. Evaluation of investigations to diagnose the cause of dizziness in elderly people: a community based controlled study. BMJ 1996;313:788-793.
4. Wrisley D, Sparto P, Whitney S, Furman J. Cervicogenic dizziness: a review of diagnosis and treatment. J Orthop Sports Phys Ther 2000;30:755-766.
5. Karlberg M, Magnusson M, Malmström EM, et al. Postural and symptomatic improvement after physiotherapy in patients with dizziness of suspected cervical origin. Arch Phys Med Rehabil 1996;77:874-882.
6. Jongkees L. Cervical vertigo. Laryngoscope 1969;79:1473-1484.
7. Praffenrath V, Danekar R, Pollmann W. Cervicogenic headache—the clinical picture, radiological findings, and hypotheses on its pathophysiology. Headache 1987;25:495-499.
8. Sjaastad O, Frediksen T, Praffenrath V. Cervicogenic headache: diagnostic criteria. Headache 1990;30:725-726.
9. Froehling DA, Silverstein MD, Mohr DN, Beatty CW. Does this dizzy patient have a serious form of vertigo? JAMA 1994;271:385-388.
10. Zito G, Jull G, Story I. Clinical tests of musculoskeletal dysfunction in the diagnosis of cervicogenic headache. Manual Therapy 2006;11:118-129.
11. Simons DG, Travell JG, Simons LS. Travell & Simons' Myofascial Pain and Dysfunction: The Trigger Point Manual, 2nd ed. Upper Half of Body, vol 1. Baltimore, Williams & Wilkins, 1999.
12. Ernst A, Basta D, Seidl RO, et al. Management of posttraumatic vertigo. Otolaryngol Head Neck Surg 2005;132:554-558.
13. Reid SA, Rivett DA. Manual therapy treatment of cervicogenic dizziness: a systematic review. Manual Therapy 2005;10:4-13.
14. Karlberg M, Persson L, Magnusson M. Impaired postural control in patients with cervico-brachial pain. Acta Otolaryngol Suppl 1995;520:440-442.
15. Borg-Stein J, Rauch S, Krabak B. Evaluation and management of cervicogenic dizziness. Clin Rev Phys Med Rehabil 2001;13:255-264.
16. deJong P, de Jong M, Cohen B, Jongkees LB. Ataxia and nystagmus induced by injection of local anesthetics in the neck. Ann Neurol 1977;1:240-246.
17. Carlson J, Fahlerantz A, Augustinsson L. Muscle tenderness in tension headaches treated with acupuncture and physiotherapy. Cephalalgia 1990;10:131-141.
18. Sycha T, Kranz G, Auff E, Schnider P. Botulinum toxin in the treatment of rare head and neck pain syndromes: a systematic review of the literature. J Neurol 2004;251(Suppl 1):I19-I30.

Trapezius Strain   8

Isaac Cohen, MD, and Cristin Jouve, MD

Synonyms

Myofascial shoulder pain
Trapezius myositis
Myofasciitis
Tension neckache
Nonarticular rheumatism
Fibrositis
Fibromyalgia
Repetitive stress injury

ICD-9 Codes

729.1   Myalgia and myositis, unspecified
847.0   Neck (sprain or strain); whiplash injury
847.1   Thoracic (sprain or strain)
847.9   Unspecified site of the back (sprain or strain)

DEFINITION

Trapezius strain describes tenderness and pain involving the trapezius muscle due to overstretching or overuse.[1] This condition is also referred to as trapezius myofascial pain and dysfunction.

The numerous causes of trapezius strain include acute causes, such as trauma (e.g., motor vehicle accidents, falls), and chronic causes, such as overload (e.g., repetitive lifting), poor positioning (e.g., tilting the head to the side when using the phone), and skeletal variations (e.g., scoliosis, leg length discrepancy).

The usual expectation is that strains heal within a matter of weeks, forming a scar within the muscle and leaving the patient with no residual pain. However, patients may continue to experience pain beyond this initial time frame. The theory of myofascial pain provides a framework that explains how acute muscle pain can become chronic, even when there is no evidence of persisting tissue damage or injury to the muscle-tendon unit.[2] Tissue overload and fatigue are manifested as trigger points, the pathognomonic sign of myofascial pain. A trigger point has several characteristics: a hyperintense nodule within a taut band of muscle that on palpation produces local and referred pain, a twitch-like response, and even autonomic phenomena. The validity of the myofascial pain concept, however, has been questioned in the scientific literature. Myofascial pain is a clinical diagnosis, yet multiple studies demonstrate low interrater reliability for identification of trigger points.[3-6]

Historically, various terms have been used to describe nonarticular soft tissue pain problems, such as nonarticular rheumatism, myositis, and fibrositis, resulting in confusion.[7] Fibromyalgia is defined as chronic, widespread, axial pain that is bilateral, above and below the waist, and involving at least 11 of 18 characteristic tender points.[8] These patients also present with a host of other complaints, such as fatigue, sleep disturbances, and depression. The relationship between tender points and trigger points is unclear. The term *repetitive strain syndrome* is often used when myofascial pain occurs in an industrial setting, involving repetitive movement or prolonged postures. The term derives from early observations of the epidemic of arm pain and disability that occurred in the mid-1980s in Australia.[9] These diagnoses are discussed in other chapters in this book.

SYMPTOMS

The pain is typically described as a deep aching discomfort, tightness, or spasm in the region of the trapezius muscle. The location of pain is clearly regional and does not follow spinal segmental or peripheral nerve distribution. The patient may be able to identify one or more areas that are tender. The specific areas that are tender and referral patterns depend on which portion of the trapezius is involved (upper, middle, or lower).[2] The pain may radiate to the head, shoulder, arm, or interscapular region. The upper fibers are most commonly involved, referring pain to the posterolateral neck, behind the ear and temple. Middle trapezius fibers refer to the interscapular region. Lower trapezius fibers refer to the interscapular, suprascapular, posterior neck, and mastoid regions. Paresthesias, heaviness, or fatigue may be experienced in the shoulder girdle. Pain can increase with repetitive tasks involving the upper extremity, such as abduction or forward flexion, or with assumption of prolonged postures. Cervical movement such as forward flexion or contralateral side bending may also aggravate the symptoms. The examiner should determine the relationship of symptoms to nonmechanical factors, such as psychological distress, impaired sleep, fatigue, and poor nutrition. These factors may impair a patient's ability to cope with the discomfort.

PHYSICAL EXAMINATION

The goals of physical examination are to rule out concomitant diagnoses and to determine the degree of impairment. Examination begins with observation of posture. Forward head posture, with scapular protraction and compensatory cervical hyperextension, is commonly seen.[10,11] Overdeveloped or shortened anterior shoulder girdle muscles may also be seen in a chronic setting. Cervical motion is assessed in sagittal, coronal, and horizontal planes to establish a baseline for serial examinations, to identify impairment, and to establish relation to symptoms. Active cervical range of motion may be limited by pain. Normal cervical range of motion is as follows: flexion, 45 degrees; extension, 55 degrees; lateral bending, 40 degrees; rotation, 70 degrees.[12] Shoulder range of motion is assessed to screen for shoulder disease, and it should be within normal limits. Palpation of the cervical and shoulder girdle region is performed to identify tender areas and trigger points. Motor, reflex, and sensory examination of the upper extremities is performed, with the expectation of normal neurologic findings with a primary trapezius strain.

FUNCTIONAL LIMITATIONS

Trapezius pain may interfere with activities of daily living and vocational and recreational activities. Activities requiring continuous movement with arms in a forward position, such as typing or playing piano, may exacerbate pain. Driving, which requires lateral rotation, may be impaired. The patient may limit or avoid activities that exacerbate symptoms.

DIAGNOSTIC STUDIES

Trapezius strain is a clinical diagnosis based on history and physical examination. There is no routine laboratory test or imaging study available to confirm the presence of muscle spasm or trigger points. Blood work and imaging and electrodiagnostic studies may be necessary to rule out other conditions.

TREATMENT

Initial

Initial treatment begins with education of the patient. Patients should be reassured that their pain is benign and has a favorable prognosis. The importance of the pain sensation should be de-emphasized, and patients should be encouraged to return to their usual activities as soon as possible.[13,14]

The patient should also be educated about proper positioning and posture. Encourage the patient to identify

Differential Diagnosis

Cervical spondylosis

Cervical herniation

Cervical radiculopathy

Cervical facet syndrome

Peripheral nerve entrapment (e.g., suprascapular, spinal accessory)

Inflammatory disease (e.g., myositis, polymyalgia rheumatica)

Endocrine disorders (e.g., hypothyroidism)

Electrolyte abnormalities

Tumor

and to correct precipitating or perpetuating factors. The impact of stress and poor sleep on symptoms should be explored. Work-related recommendations should be made about the use of a telephone headset or adjustments in seating, armrest, or keyboard height. A patient may be counseled on proper sleeping positions or pillow height; ensure that existing canes are the appropriate lengths. Use of heel lifts may be considered if a significant leg length discrepancy is noted.

Moist heat, such as a hot shower, or ice can be used to reduce spasm and pain. Choice of specific thermal modality is determined by individual preference. Stretching exercises may also be demonstrated to the patient. The upper trapezius fibers can be stretched by placing the ipsilateral arm behind the back and laterally bending the neck to the contralateral side. The middle trapezius fibers can be stretched by clasping the hands together in front of the body and reaching forward. The lower trapezius fibers can be stretched by flexing the neck forward. These stretches should be held for 30 seconds per repetition for a total of three to five repetitions and may be repeated three times daily.

Medications such as nonsteroidal anti-inflammatory drugs may be used on a short-term basis for their analgesic and anti-inflammatory effects. Muscle relaxants, used sparingly and primarily in evening doses, may reduce anxiety and promote sleep. Similarly, low-dose tricyclic antidepressants taken in the evening may be used to relieve pain and assist with sleep.

Cervical collars are generally not indicated as they may promote disability.[15,16]

Rehabilitation

The goals of physical or occupational therapy are to reduce pain and to restore function. Therapeutic exercises directed toward the neck and shoulder girdle region are the cornerstone of treatment. The current literature suggests that early mobilization with active treatment is superior to rest, immobilization, or passive modalities in the population with acute whiplash injury.[14-19] Randomized controlled trials have demonstrated that exercise-based therapy is effective for chronic neck pain.[20-22] However, there is a paucity of well-designed studies documenting the benefit of physical therapy specifically in the population with chronic whiplash injury.

Impairments in posture, range of motion, strength, and endurance are addressed. Stretches are performed, targeting the specific portion of the trapezius that is involved and the anterior neck and chest muscles. The trapezius, cervical extensor, and scapular stabilizer muscles are strengthened with progressive resistive exercises. Postural correction exercises may consist of chin tuck, wall sitting, or wall standing exercises. Modalities such as ice, heat, ultrasound, and massage may therefore be used as optional adjuncts during the first 3 weeks of treatment to modulate pain.[14] Although physiologic effects of various modalities have been demonstrated, their clinical efficacy remains unproven.[23] Patients should be educated about a home exercise program. The therapist may make job-related recommendations or even visit the work site to perform an ergonomic analysis. The patient may bring in photographs of the work site if a visit by the therapist is not feasible.

Procedures

Trigger point injections may be considered for patients who demonstrate trigger points on examination and are not responding to initial measures and therapy (Fig. 8-1). The rationale is to inactivate the trigger point by mechanical disruption. Postinjection care may include application of spray and stretch technique with vapocoolant by the clinician. Patients may be instructed in use of heat or ice to reduce postinjection pain and in temporary activity modification.

Anecdotal experience and uncontrolled studies suggest that trigger point injections are effective in treating myofascial pain.[2,24] A systematic review of needling treatment for myofascial pain concluded that efficacy of trigger point injections beyond placebo has not been supported or refuted in the literature.[25] Comparative studies reveal that injection is therapeutically equivalent to dry needling[26-28] and that the nature of the injected substance makes no difference in the outcome.[29-32]

During the past decade, there has been increasing interest in the injection of botulinum toxin (primarily type A) for treatment of recalcitrant myofascial pain. Initial studies seemed promising, yet several double-blind, randomized, controlled studies refute the efficacy of botulinum toxin for treatment of myofascial pain.[33-35]

Acupuncture may be effective in treating myofascial pain, but this has not been clearly demonstrated in the literature.

Surgery

Surgery is not indicated for treatment of trapezius strain.

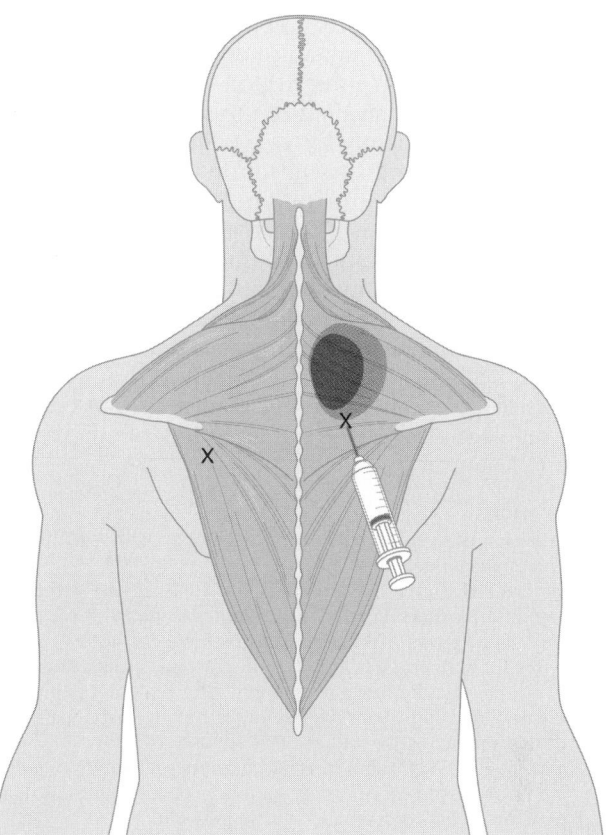

FIGURE 8-1. Ask the patient to point with one finger to the area of most intense pain, then palpate for a taut band. Once it is localized, under sterile conditions, using a 25-gauge or 27-gauge 1½-inch needle, inject approximately 0.1 to 0.3 mL of a local anesthetic (e.g., 1% lidocaine) into the trapezius muscle in several areas of this same site (puncture the skin only once). This should be accompanied by needling of the entire taut band to mechanically break up the abnormal and sensitized tender tissue. It is generally not advisable to inject local steroids into the muscle. This may be repeated in several areas during a single procedure visit. In addition, this procedure may need to be repeated on several occasions, depending on the patient's symptoms and reported relief from the treatment.

POTENTIAL DISEASE COMPLICATIONS

A patient may limit or avoid activities that cause pain. Avoidance behaviors may lead to disuse muscle atrophy and loss of flexibility and endurance. These impairments may produce significant personal and occupational disability. Depression and chronic pain behaviors may complicate this condition and may be disabling in and of themselves.

POTENTIAL TREATMENT COMPLICATIONS

Tylenol may produce hepatic toxicity. Nonsteroidal anti-inflammatory drugs may produce gastropathy, renal toxicity, hepatic toxicity, bleeding, central nervous system effects, exacerbation of asthma, and drug-drug interactions. Muscle relaxants may cause somnolence. Tricyclic antidepressants may cause sedation, dry mouth, constipation, urinary retention, weight gain, orthostatic hypotension, and electroencephalographic abnormalities. Cervical collars may cause disuse weakness of the cervical or shoulder girdle region, decreased range of motion, and reinforcement of the sick role. Aggressive exercise may transiently increase pain in some patients. Patients may become dependent on passive modalities. Local injections may result in local pain (typically lasting for several days), ecchymosis, and syncope. Although rare, hematoma, pneumothorax, infection, or neural injury may complicate either trigger point injection or acupuncture. Botulinum toxin injection may cause influenza-like illness, transient muscle weakness, and dysphagia in addition to local effect from the injection itself. Antibodies to botulinum toxin can develop after repeated injection, resulting in lack of efficacy.

References

1. Anderson DM, ed. Dorland's Pocket Dictionary, 24th ed. Philadelphia, WB Saunders, 1989:562.
2. Simons DG, Travell JG, Simons LS. Travell & Simons' Myofascial Pain and Dysfunction: The Trigger Point Manual, 2nd ed. Upper Half of Body, vol 1. Baltimore, Williams & Wilkins, 1999:278-307.
3. Wolfe F, Simons DG, Fricton J, et al. The fibromyalgia and myofascial pain syndromes: a preliminary study of tender points and trigger points in persons with fibromyalgia, myofascial pain syndrome and no disease. J Rheumatol 1992;19:944-951.
4. Nice D, Riddle D, Lamb R, et al. Inter-tester reliability of judgements of the presence of trigger points in patients with low back pain. Arch Phys Med Rehabil 1992;73:893-898.
5. Njoo K, Van der Does E. The occurrence and inter-rater reliability of myofascial trigger points in the quadratus lumborum and gluteus medius: a prospective study in non-specific low back pain patients and controls in general practice. Pain 1994;58:317-323.
6. Gerwin R, Shannon S, Hong C, et al. Inter-rater reliability in myofascial trigger point examination. Pain 1997;69:65-73.
7. Margoles M. Myofascial pain syndrome: clinical evaluation and management of patients. In Weiner R, ed. Pain Management: A Practical Guide for Clinicians. Boca Raton, St Lucie Press, 1998:191.
8. Bennett R. The fibromyalgia syndrome. In Kelley WN, ed. Textbook of Rheumatology, 5th ed. Philadelphia, WB Saunders, 1997:511-513.
9. Goldenberg D. Fibromyalgia and related syndromes. In Klippel J, Dieppe P, eds. Rheumatology, 2nd ed. London, Mosby, 1998:15.5.
10. Kendall F, McCreary E, Provance P. Muscles, Testing and Function, 4th ed. Baltimore, Williams & Wilkins, 1993:339-342.
11. Hertling D, Kessler R. Management of Common Musculoskeletal Disorders: Physical Therapy Principles and Methods, 3rd ed. Philadelphia, JB Lippincott, 1996:549-550.
12. Bates B. A Guide to Physical Examination and History Taking, 5th ed. Philadelphia, JB Lippincott, 1991:472.
13. Borchegrevink G, Kaasa A, McDonoagh D, et al. Acute treatment of whiplash neck sprain injuries. Spine 1998;23:25-31.
14. Spitzer WO, Skovron ML, Salmi L, et al. Scientific monograph of the Quebec Task Force on Whiplash-Associated Disorders: redefining "whiplash" and its management. Spine 1995;20(Suppl):S1-S73.
15. McKinney L, Dornan J, Ryan M. The role of physiotherapy in the management of acute neck sprains following road-traffic accidents. Arch Emerg Med 1989;6:27-33.
16. Mealy K, Brennan H, Fenelon G. Early mobilization of acute whiplash injuries. BMJ 1986;292:656-657.
17. Jette D, Jette A. Physical therapy and health outcomes in patients with spinal impairments. Phys Ther 1996;76:930-944.
18. Pennie B, Agambar L. Whiplash injuries: a trial of early management. J Bone Joint Surg Br 1990;72:277-279.
19. Rosenfeld M, Gunnarsson R, Borenstein P. Early intervention in whiplash-associated disorders. Spine 2000;25:1782-1787.
20. Kay TM, Gross A, Goldsmith C, et al. Exercises for mechanical neck disorders. Cochrane Database Syst Rev 2005;20:CD004250.
21. Chiu TT, Lam TH, Hedley AJ. A randomized controlled trial on the efficacy of exercise for patients with chronic neck pain. Spine 2005;30: E1-E7.
22. Chiu TT, Hui-Chan CW, Chein G. A randomized clinical trial of TENS and exercise for patients with chronic neck pain. Clin Rehabil 2005;19:850-860.
23. Edelson T. Rehabilitation of whiplash injuries. In Malanga G, Nadler S, eds. Whiplash. Philadelphia, Hanley & Belfus, 2002:289-291.
24. Hong CZ, Hsueh TC. Difference in pain relief after trigger point injections in myofascial pain patients with and without fibromyalgia. Arch Phys Med Rehabil 1996;77:1161-1166.
25. Cummings T, White A. Needling therapies in the management of myofascial trigger point pain: a systematic review. Arch Phys Med Rehabil 2001;82:986-992.
26. Garvey T, Marks M, Wiesel S. A prospective, randomized, double-blind evaluation of trigger-point injection therapy for low back pain. Spine 1989;14:962-964.
27. Hong CZ. Lidocaine injection versus dry needling to myofascial trigger point. The importance of the local twitch response. Am J Phys Med Rehabil 1994;73:256-263.
28. McMillan A, Nolan A, Kelly P. The efficacy of dry needling and procaine in the treatment of myofascial pain in the jaw muscles. J Orofac Pain 1997;11:307-314.
29. Wheeler AH, Goolkasian P, Gretz SS. A randomized, double-blind, prospective pilot study of botulinum toxin injection for refractory, unilateral, cervicothoracic, paraspinal, myofascial pain syndrome. Spine 1998;23:1662-1666.
30. Drewes AM, Andreasen A, Poulsen LH. Injection therapy for treatment of chronic myofascial pain: a double-blind study comparing corticosteroid versus diclofenac injections. J Musculoskel Pain 1993;1:289-294.
31. Tschopp KP, Gysin C. Local injection therapy in 107 patients with myofascial pain syndrome of the head and neck. ORL J Otorhinolaryngol Relat Spec 1996;58:306-310.
32. Garvey TA, Marks MR, Wiesel SW. A prospective, randomized, double-blind evaluation of trigger-point injection therapy for low-back pain. Spine 1989;14:962-964.
33. Ferrante F, Bearn L, Rothrock R, et al. Evidence against trigger point injection technique for the treatment of cervicothoracic myofascial pain with botulinum toxin type A. Anesthesiology 2005;103:377-383.
34. Graboski C, Gray D, Burnham R. Botulinum toxin A versus bupivacaine trigger point injections for the treatment of myofascial pain syndrome: a randomized double blind crossover study. Pain 2005;118:170-175.
35. Querama E, Fuglsang-Frederiksen A, Kasch H, et al. A double-blind, controlled study of botulinum toxin A in chronic myofascial pain. Neurology 2006;67:241-245.

Acromioclavicular Injuries 9

Thomas D. Rizzo, Jr., MD

Synonyms

Acromioclavicular joint injuries
Acromioclavicular pain
Acromioclavicular separation
Separated shoulder
Acromioclavicular osteoarthritis
Atraumatic osteolysis of the distal clavicle

ICD-9 Codes

831.04   Closed dislocation acromioclavicular joint
840.0   Acromioclavicular (joint) (ligament) sprain

DEFINITION

The acromioclavicular joint is a diarthrodial joint found between the lateral end of the clavicle and the medial side of the acromion.[1] The joint is surrounded by a fibrous capsule and stabilized by ligaments. The acromioclavicular ligaments cross the joint. Three ligaments begin at the coracoid process on the scapula and attach to the clavicle (trapezoid and conoid ligaments) or the acromion (coracoacromial ligament). This complex provides passive support and suspension of the scapula from the clavicle while allowing rotation of the clavicle to be transmitted to the scapula.[1,2]

Injuries to the acromioclavicular complex are graded I to VI (Table 9-1). Injuries to the acromioclavicular joint were originally classified as grades 1, 2, and 3 by Tossy.[3] This classification was extended to include more complicated injuries, and grades 4, 5, and 6 were described. The extended grading system uses roman numerals.[4]

The coracoacromial (lateral) ligament is not disrupted in injuries to the acromioclavicular joint. Therefore, the fibrous connection persists between structures of the scapula emanating anteriorly and posteriorly.[5] In rare instances, there is an intra-articular fracture of the distal clavicle in addition to the ligamentous injuries.[6]

There are few demographic data on differences of the disorder based on gender. Problems with the acromioclavicular joint can be associated with trauma and with overhead and throwing activities. Concomitant injuries

can vary on the basis of age; 86% of individuals older than 50 years have rotator cuff tears.[7]

Most patients with grade I or grade II injuries respond to conservative measures and become asymptomatic within 3 weeks.[8]

SYMPTOMS

Patients often provide a history of trauma to the shoulder or in the vicinity of the acromioclavicular joint. Participants in contact or collision sports (e.g., football, downhill skiing) are particularly susceptible. Patients seek care because of pain in the anterior aspect of the shoulder.[2] The pain may radiate into the base of the neck and the trapezius or deltoid muscles or down the arm in a radicular pattern.[2,5,9]

Patients may describe pain brought on by activities of daily living that bring the arm across the chest (e.g., reaching into a jacket pocket) or behind the back (e.g., tucking in a shirt). Pain can also occur with shoulder flexion (reaching overhead) or with adduction of the arm across the chest.

PHYSICAL EXAMINATION

Appropriate examination for suspected acromioclavicular injuries includes an examination of the neck and shoulder joint and girdle to eliminate the possibility of a radiculopathy or referred pain. Patients should have normal neck and neurologic examination findings. The presence of neurologic or vascular injury suggests that a greater degree of trauma has been sustained.[5]

On inspection, there may be a raised area at the acromioclavicular joint. This is caused by depression of the scapula relative to the clavicle or swelling of the joint itself. This area is commonly tender to touch. On active range of motion, the patient may complain of pain or wince near the extreme of shoulder flexion.

Shoulder range of motion is typically within normal limits. Supporting the arm at the elbow and gently directing the arm superiorly may decrease the pain and allow more complete assessment of the patient's

TABLE 9-1 Grades of Acromioclavicular Joint Injuries and Treatments

Grade of Injury	AC Ligament	CC Ligament	Clavicle Displacement	Treatment
I	Sprain	Intact	Mild superior displacement	Conservative
II	Torn	Sprain	Definite superior displacement	Conservative
III	Torn	Torn	25%-100% increase in CC space	Conservative or surgical
IV	Torn	Torn	Posterior displacement	Surgical
V	Torn	Torn	100%-300% increase in CC space	Surgical
VI	Torn	Torn	Subacromial or subcoracoid location	Surgical

AC, acromioclavicular; CC, coracoclavicular.

shoulder range of motion. The pain may become worse as the shoulder is further flexed, whether it is done actively or passively. This is in distinction to impingement syndromes, which often hurt at a particular point in the arc of motion but are painless as the motion proceeds. Pain is typically absent with isometric manual muscle testing of the rotator cuff. Rotator cuff injuries will be painful with activation of the muscles of the rotator cuff. These problems are best identified with the shoulder in a neutral position (i.e., elbow next to the body) because the rotator cuff muscles are in a lengthened position and are easily made symptomatic.

Special tests to identify acromioclavicular joint disease attempt to compress the joint. The most common test is the cross-body adduction test (Fig. 9-1). The shoulder is abducted to 90 degrees and the elbow is flexed to the same degree. The clinician then brings the arm across the patient's body until the elbow approaches the midline (or the patient reports pain).[2]

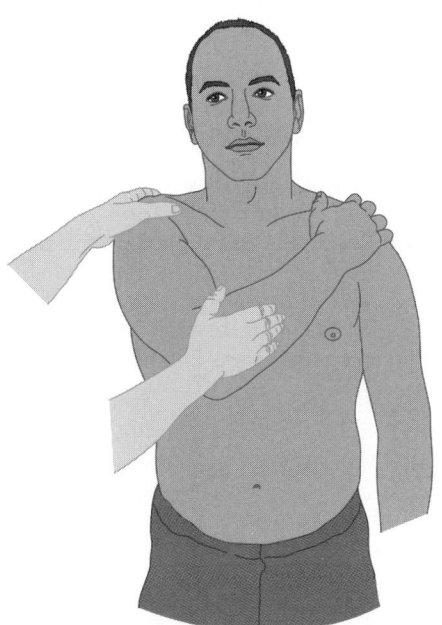

FIGURE 9-1. Cross-body adduction test for a sprain of the acromioclavicular joint.

Other tests help differentiate between impingement syndrome and acromioclavicular joint pain. If the shoulder is passively flexed while it is internally rotated, the greater tuberosity can pinch (impinge) the supraspinatus tendon and subacromial bursa. The same test performed with the shoulder externally rotated will compress the acromioclavicular joint without impinging the subacromial space.[10] In the active compression test, the shoulder is flexed to 90 degrees and then adducted to 10 degrees (Fig. 9-2). The patient first maximally internally rotates the arm and then tries to flex the shoulder against the clinician's resistance. This puts pressure on the acromioclavicular joint and may reproduce pain if disease is present. The test is repeated with the shoulder in full external rotation. This will put stress on the biceps tendon and its labral attachment while excluding the acromioclavicular joint.[11]

In the acromioclavicular resisted extension test, the shoulder is abducted to 90 degrees and adducted across the body to 90 degrees (Fig. 9-3). The examiner resists active shoulder extension. A positive test result reproduces pain in the acromioclavicular joint. A combination of these tests will improve the diagnostic accuracy over isolated tests.[12]

The Paxinos sign, along with bone scan, is purported to have a high degree of diagnostic accuracy in acromioclavicular joint disease.[13] The examiner stands behind the patient and, using the hand contralateral to the affected shoulder, stabilizes the clavicle and pushes the acromion into the clavicle with the thumb. The test response is considered positive if pain occurs or increases in the region of the acromioclavicular joint; the test response is considered negative if there is no change in the pain level (Fig. 9-4).

FUNCTIONAL LIMITATIONS

Reaching up, reaching across the body, and carrying heavy weights are limited because of pain. Patients may have no pain at rest and little or no pain with many activities. Patients may complain of difficulty with putting on a shirt, combing the hair, and carrying a briefcase or grocery bag. Most recreational activities, especially those that incorporate throwing, will be limited as well. Sleep may be affected because of pain.

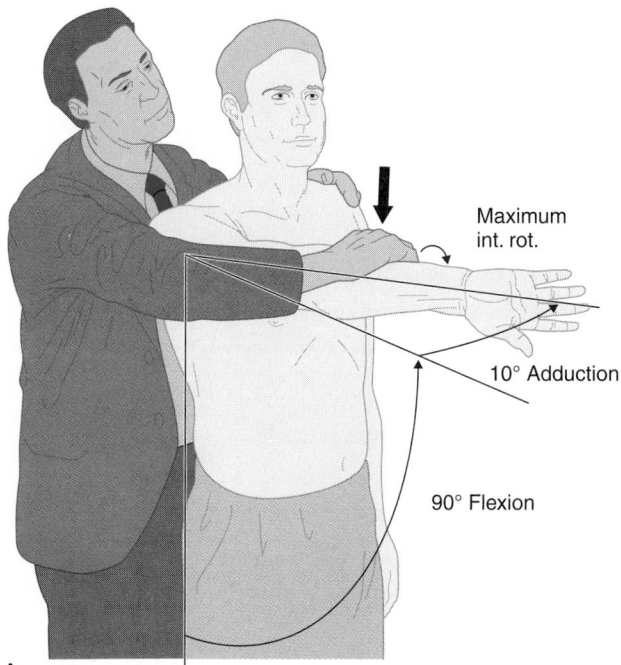

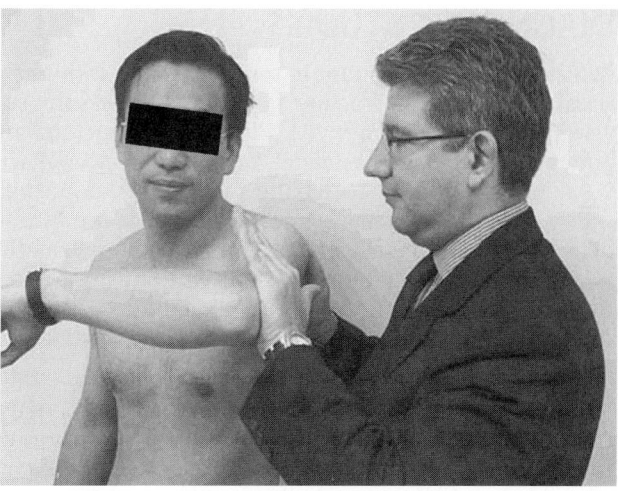

FIGURE 9-3. In the acromioclavicular resisted extension test, the examiner resists active shoulder extension. A positive test result reproduces pain in the acromioclavicular joint. (Reprinted with permission from Chronopoulos E, Kim TK, Park HB, et al. Diagnostic value of physical tests for isolated chronic acromioclavicular lesions. Am J Sports Med 2004;32: 655-661.)

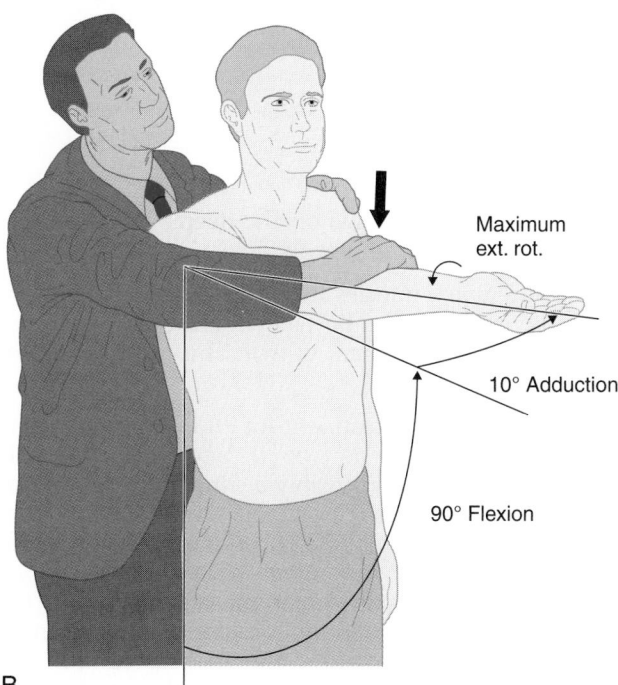

FIGURE 9-2. The active compression test. **A,** The arm is forward flexed and internally rotated maximally. Downward force is applied, and pain indicates acromioclavicular joint disease. **B,** The test is repeated with the arm externally rotated. Pain indicates disease of the biceps tendon and its labral attachment. (Reprinted with permission from O'Brien SJ, Pagnani MJ, Fealy S, et al. The active compression test: a new and effective test for diagnosing labral tears and acromioclavicular joint abnormality. Am J Sports Med 1998;26:610-613.)

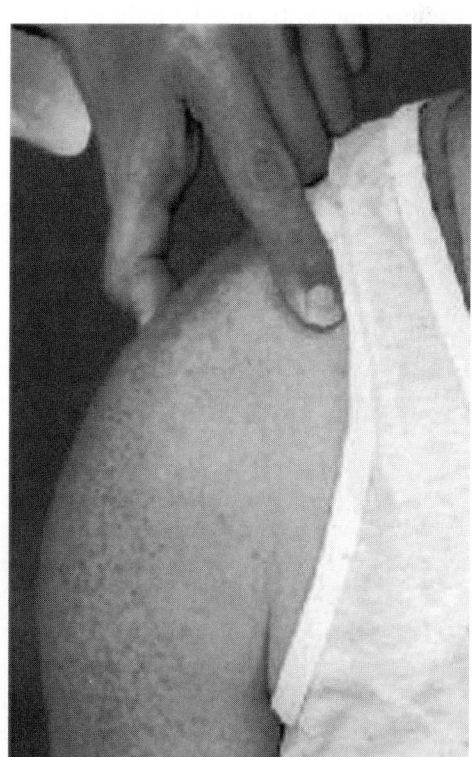

FIGURE 9-4. To elicit Paxinos sign, stand behind the patient and use the hand contralateral to the affected shoulder. (Reprinted with permission from Walton J, Mahajan S, Paxinos A, et al. Diagnostic values of tests for acromioclavicular joint pain. J Bone Joint Surg Am 2004;86:807-812.)

DIAGNOSTIC STUDIES

Radiographs are important in most cases and should be obtained to rule out fracture as well as to assess the severity of the injury (Fig. 9-5). Views should include an anteroposterior view, a lateral Y view, and an axillary view. It is important to let the radiologist know that injury to the acromioclavicular joint, not just the shoulder, is in question. Stress or weighted views are usually not helpful and cause undue pain without improving the accuracy of diagnosis.[2,14] Overpenetration of films may make the interpretation of the acromioclavicular joint and distal clavicle difficult.[5]

A 15-degree cephalad anteroposterior view helps diagnose sprains by decreasing x-ray penetration and showing separation between the acromion and clavicle, whereas the 40-degree cephalic tilt anteroposterior view should be used for suspected fractures of the clavicle. If the fracture is medial to the coracoclavicular ligaments, both an anterior and a posterior 45-degree view should be obtained.[5] Typically, the decision to obtain these views is made by a radiologist.

Certainly, if there are concerns about a fracture or arthrosis and the x-ray images do not provide confirmation, further evaluation with a bone scan[2,5] or magnetic resonance imaging (MRI) may be indicated.[15]

MRI evaluation of symptomatic acromioclavicular joints revealed that 80% had active bone edema in the distal clavicle or acromion or on both sides, but no asymptomatic patients had this finding.[16] MRI will detect the extent of acromioclavicular arthrosis more frequently than conventional radiology will.[17] MRI does not appear to add any further information to the clinical assessment.[18]

Ultrasonography is a reproducible method of evaluating the joint space and joint capsule, but the measurements may vary from those obtained by MRI.[19] The findings on ultrasound evaluation correlate well with the diagnosis obtained by clinical examination and radiographs.[20]

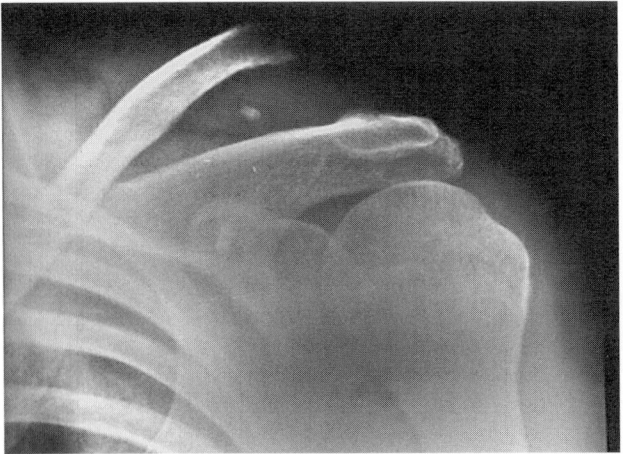

FIGURE 9-5. Grade III acromioclavicular joint dislocation. There is marked superior displacement of the distal clavicle relative to the acromion and coracoid processes. (Reprinted with permission from Katz DS, Math KR, Groskin SA. Radiology Secrets. Philadelphia, Hanley & Belfus, 1998:445.)

Differential Diagnosis

Adhesive capsulitis

Arthritis (e.g., rheumatoid, crystal induced, and septic)[21-23]

Calcific tendinitis

Cervical radiculopathy

Distal osteolysis of the clavicle[2,23]

Fractures of the acromion or distal clavicle[24]

Ganglia and cysts in the acromioclavicular joint[2]

Os acromiale syndrome[23]

Rotator cuff tears[2,6,25]

Shoulder impingement syndrome[26]

Tendinitis of the long head of the biceps[2]

Tears of the glenohumeral labrum[11]

Tumors[2,27]

Referred pain may come from cardiac, pulmonary, and gastrointestinal disease.[2]

TREATMENT

Initial

Initial treatment depends on the degree of injury and the patient's activity and goals.

Type I and type II injuries are exclusively treated nonoperatively, whereas type IV, type V, and type VI injuries require surgery. Treatment of type III injuries is controversial (see Table 9-1).

The initial phase of treatment for all injuries not going to surgery (i.e., type I, type II, and some type III) includes rest, ice, and possibly a sling or brace for 1 to 6 weeks (2 to 3 weeks average). Over-the-counter or prescription non-narcotic analgesics are usually sufficient. Nonsteroidal anti-inflammatory drugs can be used for pain and inflammation. Injections into the joint can also be done in the initial phase of treatment for immediate pain control and to help confirm the diagnosis.

Rest should be relative, that is, the patient should avoid aggravating activities and should not be immobilized if at all possible.

Ice massage can be done over the painful area for 5 to 10 minutes every 2 hours, as needed. An ice pack can be used for 20 minutes at a time and also can be repeated every 2 hours. The usual precautions for the use of ice should be followed.

Type I and type II sprains can be treated with a sling to help support the arm and shoulder. This should be used symptomatically and discontinued for painless activities and when the patient's pain is under control.

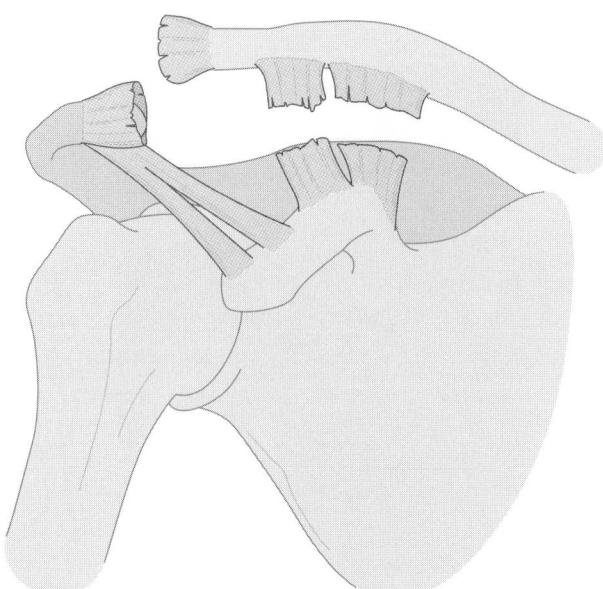

FIGURE 9-6. Grade III acromioclavicular joint sprain. (Reprinted with permission from Mellion MB. Office Sports Medicine, 2nd ed. Philadelphia, Hanley & Belfus, 1996:217.)

Type III injuries have been treated operatively and nonoperatively (Fig. 9-6). The majority of orthopedists favor nonoperative treatment as a rule, even in throwing athletes.[5,14,28-30] One study suggested greater long-term satisfaction in patients who had surgery but showed no difference in range of motion or strength.[31] The majority of patients have no long-term difficulty with nonoperative management. There are also reports of high complication rates with surgery.[5,30] Surgery may be considered in symptomatic individuals with type III injuries and in those who do not respond to conservative measures.

One approach for type III injuries is to treat conservatively with relative rest, support, modalities, medications for symptoms, and gradual return to activity during 6 to 12 weeks. If there is a significant limitation in function, including avocational or sport activities, or if the patient is not progressing as expected, further evaluation is warranted.[5] Unlike with musculotendinous injuries, delayed surgery does not lead to poorer outcomes.

Rehabilitation

Physical or occupational therapy can be ordered to assist with education of the patient, pain control, and, in later stages, gradual range of motion and strengthening exercises. Modalities to control pain can include, in addition to ice, ultrasound or phonophoresis with 10% lidocaine. Alternatively, interferential current can be used. As pain is controlled, motion can be obtained in a pain-free range. Codman and pendulum exercises can progress to active or active-assisted range of motion to restore shoulder flexion and abduction, both individually and in combination. In the initial phase of a rehabilitation program, it is reasonable to avoid painful positions or movements. These include extremes of flexion—even when they are done passively—and adduction across the chest. When the shoulder is pain free and has full range of motion, rehabilitation can progress to gradual strengthening and return to activity. A typical shoulder strengthening rehabilitation program can be used. Light dumbbell exercises with 1 to 5 pounds to strengthen the internal and external rotators or resistance bands can be used initially. This program can be advanced to isolate the shoulder abductors and to incorporate internal and external rotator strengthening at different degrees of shoulder abduction. Further progression depends on the patient's goals and requires incorporation of the scapular stabilizers and training in coordinated movements.

Procedures

Patients with acromioclavicular joint pain due to type I or mild type II injuries can receive injections and return to play or work immediately with little risk of injury as long as they have full functional range of motion and symmetric[2] strength. For diagnostic purposes, a local anesthetic injection may confirm the diagnosis of a type I sprain[2] if the patient has complete pain relief immediately after the injection. Intra-articular injection of a combination of a local anesthetic and a corticosteroid may give immediate and longer acting relief. Injections into the joint can be done for higher grade injuries as well as to give quick symptomatic relief. However, this is not a substitute for relative rest in more seriously injured joints (type II and higher), and 1 week of avoiding provocative maneuvers after the injection is advised.[2]

With the patient sitting or supine with the shoulder propped under a pillow, the acromioclavicular joint is injected under sterile conditions with use of a 25-gauge, $1^{1}/_{2}$-inch disposable needle and a local anesthetic or anesthetic and corticosteroid combination (Fig. 9-7). Typically, a 1- to 3-mL aliquot of solution is injected (e.g., 1 mL of 1% lidocaine mixed with 1 mL of betamethasone). Keep in mind that the acromioclavicular joint is small and close to the surface.

Postinjection care should include local icing for 10 to 15 minutes and instructions to the patient to avoid aggravating activities for at least 1 week.

Surgery

Type IV, type V, and type VI injuries are forms of dislocation of the acromioclavicular joint. These need to be reduced surgically with some form of reconstruction attempted. Early referral is indicated to minimize pain and dysfunction. Because the scapula is no longer suspended from the clavicle, the deltoid and trapezius muscles will become involved in an attempt to hold the scapula in place. These muscles may have been injured directly and therefore are ill-suited to take on the role of suspending the arm. The result is more significant pain and a greater chance for prolonged disability.

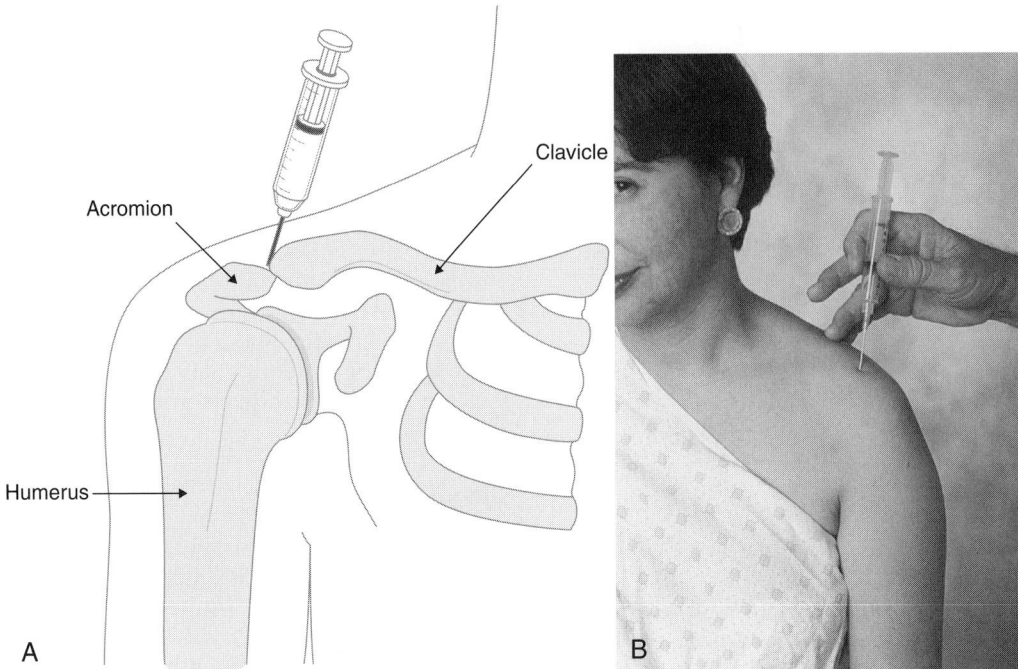

FIGURE 9-7. Internal anatomic **(A)** and approximate surface anatomic **(B)** sites for injection of the acromioclavicular joint. (Reprinted with permission from Lennard TA. Pain Procedures in Clinical Practice, 2nd ed. Philadelphia, Hanley & Belfus, 2000:129.)

If the patient has sustained a fracture, surgery may be necessary, and referral to an orthopedist is appropriate. The severity of the injury depends on whether the fracture is medial to the coracoclavicular ligaments or involves the acromioclavicular joint itself. Fractures medial to the ligaments can result in displacement of the clavicle, and the patient therefore runs the risk of delayed union or nonunion. The displacement can look like a type II or type III sprain. Careful examination of the location and degree of pain should suggest an injury to the clavicle. Regardless, radiographs are indicated to assess the possibility of fracture.

Fractures into the joint are likely to lead to arthrosis in the future. These patients may not need surgery initially—that will be decided by the patient and the orthopedist—but may require a protracted conservative course of symptomatic treatment.

Resection of the distal clavicle, tacking of the acromion to the clavicle, re-creation of the ligaments, and screw fixation of the acromioclavicular joint or of the clavicle to the coracoid process have been used to stabilize the joint. The goal of any surgical procedure is to try to re-create a stable, pain-free joint.[5]

POTENTIAL DISEASE COMPLICATIONS

Patients may be left with a "bump" due to the depression of the acromion relative to the clavicle. This should be expected and is unavoidable without surgery. Acromioclavicular joint pain due to chronic instability is the most common complication.[5,25] Degenerative arthritis can occur because of the injury or instability. This can be treated symptomatically with modalities and injections. One in five patients with a grade I or grade II injury will have

restriction in range of motion, but less than 10% will have symptoms that restrict daily or athletic activity.[32]

If the pain persists, surgery should be considered. In one study, more than 25% of patients with grade I or grade II injuries required surgery 2 years after the injury.[9]

Concomitant disorders of the glenohumeral joint complex can develop along with acromioclavicular arthrosis. These include rotator cuff tears, glenoid labrum tears, glenohumeral arthrosis, and biceps tendon disease.[8]

POTENTIAL TREATMENT COMPLICATIONS

Analgesics and nonsteroidal anti-inflammatory drugs have well-known side effects that most commonly affect the gastric, hepatic, and renal systems. Cyclooxygenase 2 (COX-2) inhibitors may have fewer gastric side effects, but cardiovascular risks should be considered. Injection of the joint with too long a needle may result in injection into the subacromial space. This can cause diagnostic confusion, if not outright injury.[2] Injections can also be associated with infection in rare cases.

Direct complications of surgery can include infection, pain, wound or skin breakdown, and hypertrophic scar.[5,29,33] After surgery, there can be a recurrence of the deformity,[29,31] hardware failure or migration,[6,29,33] or limitation of movement. Pain may persist as a result of insufficient resection, weakness, or joint instability.[2]

Recalcification after acromioclavicular joint resection can be a cause of pain and may require revision of the distal clavicle resection.[33]

References

1. Stecco A, Sgambati E, Brizzi E, et al. Morphometric analysis of the acromioclavicular joint. Ital J Anat Embryol 1997;102: 195-200.
2. Shaffer BS. Painful conditions of the acromioclavicular joint. J Am Acad Orthop Surg 1999;7:176-188.
3. Tossy JD, Mead NC, Sigmond HM. Acromioclavicular separations: useful and practical classification for treatment. Clin Orthop Relat Res 1963;28:111-119.
4. Rockwood CA, Williams GR, Young DC. Acromioclavicular injuries. In Rockwood CA, Green DP, Bucholz RW, eds. Rockwood and Green's Fractures in Adults, 3rd ed, vol 1. Philadelphia, JB Lippincott, 1991:1181-1239.
5. Turnbull JR. Acromioclavicular joint disorders. Med Sci Sports Exerc 1998;30:S26-S32.
6. Berg EE. An intra-articular fracture dislocation of the acromioclavicular joint. Am J Orthop 1998;7:555-559.
7. Brown JN, Roberts SN, Hayes MG, Sales AD. Shoulder pathology associated with symptomatic acromioclavicular joint degeneration. J Shoulder Elbow Surg 2000;9:173-176.
8. Mouhsine E, Garofalo R, Crevoisier X, Farron A. Grade I and II acromioclavicular dislocations: results of conservative treatment. J Shoulder Elbow Surg 2003;12:599-602.
9. Gerber C, Galantay RV, Hersche O. The pattern of pain produced by irritation of the acromioclavicular joint and subacromial space. J Shoulder Elbow Surg 1998;7:352-355.
10. Buchberger DJ. Introduction of a new physical examination procedure for the differentiation of acromioclavicular joint lesions and subacromial impingement. J Manipulative Physiol Ther 1999;22: 316-321.
11. O'Brien SJ, Pagnani MJ, Fealy S, et al. The active compression test: a new and effective test for diagnosing labral tears and acromioclavicular joint abnormality. Am J Sports Med 1998;26:610-613.
12. Chronopoulos E, Kim TK, Park HB, et al. Diagnostic value of physical tests for isolated chronic acromioclavicular lesions. Am J Sports Med 2004;32:655-661.
13. Walton J, Mahajan S, Paxinos A, et al. Diagnostic values of tests for acromioclavicular joint pain. J Bone Joint Surg Am 2004;86: 807-812.
14. Lemos M. Evaluation and treatment of the injured acromioclavicular joint in athletes. Am J Sports Med 1998;26:137-144.
15. Yu JS, Dardani M, Fischer RA. MR observations of posttraumatic osteolysis of the distal clavicle after traumatic separation of the acromioclavicular joint. J Comput Assist Tomogr 2000;24: 159-164.
16. Shubin Stein BE, Ahmad CS, Pfaff CH, et al. A comparison of magnetic resonance imaging findings of the acromioclavicular joint in symptomatic versus asymptomatic patients. J Shoulder Elbow Surg 2006;15:56-59.
17. de Abreu MR, Chung CB, Wesselly M, et al. Acromioclavicular joint osteoarthritis: comparison of findings derived from MR imaging and conventional radiography. Clin Imaging 2005;29:273-277.
18. Jordan LK, Kenter K, Griffiths HL. Relationship between MRI and clinical findings in the acromioclavicular joint. Skeletal Radiol 2002;31:516-521.
19. Heers G, Gotz J, Schachner H, et al. Ultrasound evaluation of the acromioclavicular joint. A comparison with magnetic resonance imaging [in German]. Sportverletz Sportschaden 2005;19:177-181.
20. Iovane A, Midiri M, Galia M, et al. Acute traumatic acromioclavicular joint lesions: role of ultrasound versus conventional radiography. Radiol Med (Torino) 2004;107:367-375.
21. Hammel JM, Kwon N. Septic arthritis of the acromioclavicular joint. J Emerg Med 2005;29:425-427.
22. Kudawara I, Aono M, Ohzono K, Mano M. Synovial chondromatosis of the acromioclavicular joint. Skeletal Radiol 2004;33:600-603.
23. Gordon BH, Chew FS. Isolated acromioclavicular joint pathology in the symptomatic shoulder on magnetic resonance imaging: a pictorial essay. J Comput Assist Tomogr 2004;28:215-222.
24. Richards DP, Howard A. Distal clavicle fracture mimicking type IV acromioclavicular joint injury in the skeletally immature athlete. Clin J Sport Med 2001;11:57-59.
25. Clarke HD, McCann PD. Acromioclavicular injuries. Orthop Clin North Am 2000;31:177-187.
26. Chen AL, Rokito AS, Zuckerman JD. The role of the acromioclavicular joint in impingement syndrome. Clin Sports Med 2003;22:343-357.
27. Echols PG, Omer GE Jr, Crawford MK. Juxta-articular myxoma of the shoulder presenting as a cyst of the acromioclavicular joint: a case report. J Shoulder Elbow Surg 2000;9:157-159.
28. McFarland EG, Blivin SJ, Doehring CB, et al. Treatment of grade III acromioclavicular separations in professional throwing athletes: results of a survey. Am J Orthop 1997;26:771-774.
29. Phillips AM, Smart C, Groom AF. Acromioclavicular dislocation. Conservative or surgical therapy. Clin Orthop Relat Res 1998;353:10-17.
30. Spencer EE Jr. Treatment of grade III acromioclavicular joint injuries: a systematic review. Clin Orthop Relat Res 2007;455:38-44.
31. Press J, Zuckerman JD, Gallagher M, Cuomo F. Treatment of grade III acromioclavicular separations. Bull Hosp Joint Dis 1997; 56:77-83.
32. Shaw MB, McInerney JJ, Dias JJ, Evans PA. Acromioclavicular joint sprains: the post-injury recovery interval. Injury 2003;34:438-442.
33. Rudzki JR, Matava MJ, Paletta GA Jr. Complications of treatment of acromioclavicular and sternoclavicular joint injuries. Clin Sports Med 2003;22:387-405.

Adhesive Capsulitis 10

Brian J. Krabak, MD, MBA, and Norman L. Banks, MD, MS

Synonyms

Frozen shoulder
Periarthritis of the shoulder
Stiff and painful shoulder
Periarticular adhesions
Humeroscapular fibrositis

ICD-9 Code

726.0   Adhesive capsulitis of shoulder

DEFINITION

Primary adhesive capsulitis of the shoulder is an idiopathic, progressive, but self-limited restriction of active and passive range of motion.[1-3] The onset is insidious and progresses through three phases, usually during the course of 1 to 2 years. These phases include the painful phase, the freezing or adhesive phase, and the thawing or resolution phase.[1,4] Adhesive capsulitis occurs in approximately 3% of the general population and approximately 6% of office visits to shoulder specialists (orthopedists and physiatrists) on a yearly basis.[5] The condition preferentially affects women after the age of 50 years, although it is not clear exactly why. In addition, it is associated with numerous secondary causes, including immobilization, diabetes, and hypothyroidism (Table 10-1).

The pathologic process related to adhesive capsulitis involves structures intrinsic to the glenohumeral joint and surrounding it (Fig. 10-1). The pathologic findings of adhesive capsulitis ultimately depend on its stage of development.[1,2,4,6] The painful phase is characterized by synovitis that progresses to capsular thickening (particularly in the anterior and inferior portions of the capsule) with an associated reduction in synovial fluid. As the adhesive phase continues, fibrosis of the capsule is more pronounced, and thickening of the rotator cuff tendons is common. As this phase continues, the glenohumeral joint space becomes contracted and often obliterated.[4,6-8] Pathologic change is more consistent with chronic inflammation with resolution of joint space loss during the final stage.

SYMPTOMS

In the painful phase, pain is progressive, worse nocturnally, and exacerbated by overhead activities. The progressive increase in pain is associated with a reduction in range of motion and decreased use of the affected shoulder. As the adhesive phase ensues, pain is reduced; however, there is a significant reduction in the range of motion in all planes.[1,4] In the latter portion of the adhesive stage, complaints of stiffness with both active and passive range of motion are common. The resolution phase is characterized by a gradual increase in the pain-free range of motion back to normal (Table 10-2).

PHYSICAL EXAMINATION

The findings noted on physical examination reflect the stage of adhesive capsulitis development. During the painful phase of adhesive capsulitis, there is a measurable reduction in *both* passive and active shoulder range of motion. Motion is painful, particularly at the extremes of external rotation and abduction.[1,2,8] This pattern of motion loss is consistent with a capsular pattern of passive range of motion loss, which demonstrates a greater limitation in external rotation and abduction followed by an increasing loss of flexion. These signs are similar to those found in osteoarthritis of the glenohumeral joint, in which there is a similar loss of motion with shoulder pain. However, this presentation is in contrast to findings seen in rotator cuff tears, in which active range of motion is restricted but passive range of motion may approximate normal values. A reduced glenohumeral glide is often noted with adhesive capsulitis, especially with inferior translation. The relationship of glenohumeral joint movements independent of scapulothoracic motion should also be noted. Last, the shoulder is often painful to palpation around the rotator cuff tendons distally.[1,2,8]

Neurologic evaluation is usually normal in adhesive capsulitis, although manual muscle testing may detect weakness secondary to pain. However, concomitant rotator cuff involvement is common and could explain true weakness if it is noted on physical examination. The combination of myotomal weakness, altered dermatomal sensation, reflex asymmetry, and positive

TABLE 10-1 Diseases and Conditions Associated with Secondary Adhesive Capsulitis

Immobilization	Pulmonary tuberculosis	Scleroderma
Diabetes mellitus	Chronic lung disease	Post mastectomy
Thyroid disease	Myocardial infarction	Cervical radiculitis
Rheumatoid arthritis	Cerebrovascular accidents	Peripheral nerve injury
Trauma	Rotator cuff disease	Lung cancer
		Breast cancer

Modified from Siegel LB, Cohen NJ, Gall EP. Adhesive capsulitis: a sticky issue. Am Fam Physician 1999;59:1843-1852.

findings with cervical spine provocative testing is more suggestive of a neurologic cause of shoulder pain.[8]

FUNCTIONAL LIMITATIONS

Patients often experience sleep disruption as a result of pain or inability to sleep on the affected side. Inability to perform activities of daily living (e.g., fastening a bra in the back, putting on a belt, reaching for a wallet in the back pocket, reaching for a seat belt, combing the hair) is common. Work activities may be limited, particularly those that involve overhead activities (e.g., filing above waist level, stocking shelves, lifting boards or other items). Recreational activities (e.g., difficulty serving or

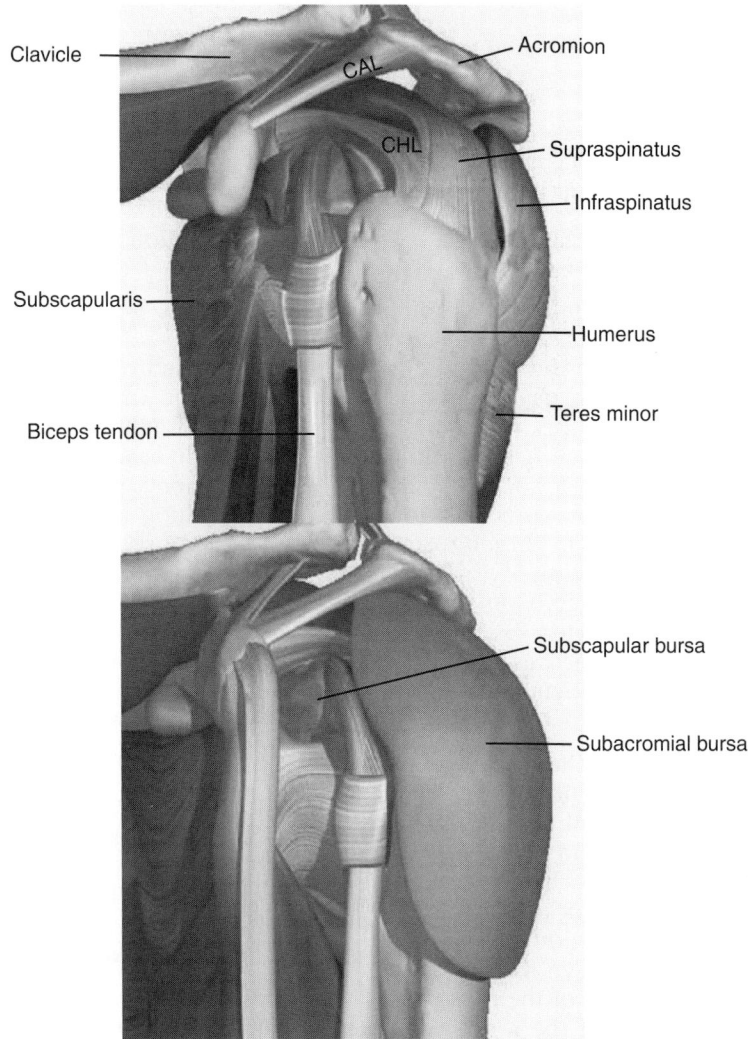

FIGURE 10-1. Relevant anatomy of the glenohumeral joint. Note the rotator cuff tendon insertion sites, biceps tendon, subacromial bursa, and coracoacromial ligament (CAL); the subcoracoid triangle is formed by the coracoid process, coracohumeral ligament (CHL), and joint capsule. (Reprinted with permission from Stubblefield MD, Custodio CM. Upper extremity pain disorders in breast cancer. Arch Phys Med Rehabil 2006;87[Suppl 1]:S96-S99.)

TABLE 10-2 The Three Stages of Adhesive Capsulitis

Painful stage

Pain with movement

Generalized ache that is difficult to pinpoint

Muscle spasm

Increasing pain at night and at rest

Adhesive stage

Less pain

Increasing stiffness and restriction of movement

Decreasing pain at night and at rest

Discomfort felt at extreme ranges of movement

Resolution stage

Decreased pain

Marked restriction with slow, gradual increase in range of motion

Recovery is spontaneous but frequently incomplete

Modified from Siegel LB, Cohen NJ, Gall EP. Adhesive capsulitis: a sticky issue. Am Fam Physician 1999;59:1843-1852.

throwing a ball, inability to do the crawl stroke in swimming) are also affected.

DIAGNOSTIC STUDIES

Because adhesive capsulitis is associated with other comorbidities and a population of patients in whom neoplastic processes are common, routine blood work and radiographs should be performed to rule out secondary causes.[6-10] Radiographs in patients with adhesive capsulitis are generally normal. In advanced stages, joint space narrowing may be noted on arthrograms, as there is a reduced volume of injectable contrast material into the joint (Fig. 10-2). Magnetic resonance imaging may also

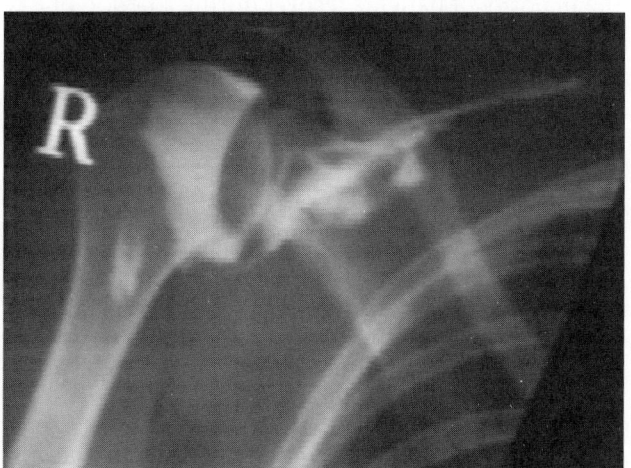

FIGURE 10-2. Arthrogram of shoulder with advanced adhesive capsulitis with a contracted joint space. Note the absence of the axillary recess and the reduced amount of contrast material injected. (Reprinted with permission from Smith LL, Burnet SP, McNeil JD. Musculoskeletal manifestations of diabetes mellitus. Br J Sports Med 2003;37:30-35.)

prove to be a useful diagnostic tool; studies have confirmed findings seen at arthroscopy, including thickening of the coracohumeral ligament and obliteration of the subcoracoid space (Fig. 10-3). If conservative management fails, magnetic resonance imaging and arthrography may be helpful in the confirmation of adhesive capsulitis and evaluation of other causes of shoulder disease consistent with adhesive capsulitis.[10,11]

Differential Diagnosis

Labral disease

Rotator cuff disease

Subacromial bursitis

Osteoarthritis

Acromioclavicular joint disease

Calcific tendinosis

Synovitis

Fractures

Bicipital tendinosis

Cervical radiculopathy (C5, C6)

Peripheral nerve entrapment (suprascapular)

Complex regional pain syndrome

Brachial plexopathies, thoracic outlet syndrome

Neoplastic conditions

Rheumatic conditions

TREATMENT

Initial

The treatment goals depend on the stage of adhesive capsulitis, but the general aim is to decrease pain and inflammation while increasing the shoulder range of motion in all planes.[1,12-14] Initially, pain and inflammation should be managed by use of ice, anti-inflammatories, and activity modifications. Reducing inflammation and pain through the use of nonsteroidal anti-inflammatory drugs is generally advocated; a short trial of oral steroids is another effective option to reduce inflammation. Injections of corticosteroid (with or without lidocaine) into the subacromial space are in many cases useful in breaking pain cycles to allow patients to participate more actively in therapy sessions (particularly in patients with concomitant rotator cuff disease or subacromial bursitis).

Rehabilitation

Restoration of range of motion is of extreme importance in treatment of adhesive capsulitis.[2,6,12,15] Pendulum exercises, overhead stretches, and crossed adduction of the

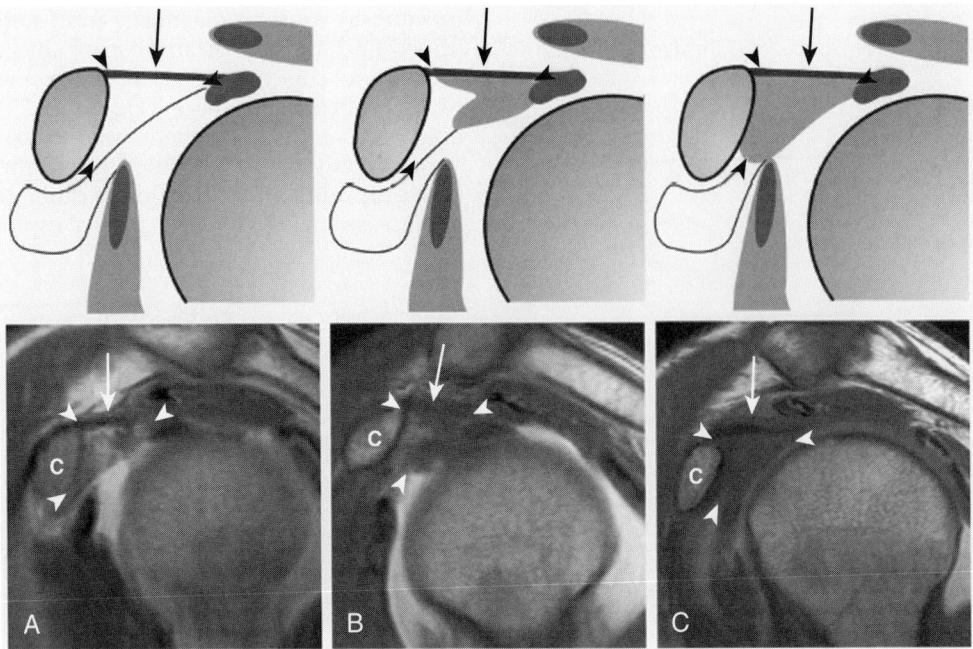

FIGURE 10-3. Note thickening of the coracohumeral ligament *(arrows)* and obliteration of the subcoracoid space *(arrowheads)* on T1-weighted magnetic resonance imaging. C, coracoid space. **A,** Normal shoulder. **B,** Partial obliteration of subcoracoid space. **C,** Complete obliteration of subcoracoid space. (Reprinted with permission from Mengiardi B, Pfirrmann CW, Gerber C, et al. Frozen shoulder: MR arthrographic findings. Radiology 2004;233:486-492.)

affected arm should be taught to patients while they are in the physician's office once adhesive capsulitis is suspected to prevent further loss of function (Fig. 10-4). Physical therapy should be implemented early to improve the pain-free range of motion and to prevent further contraction of the joint capsule.[2,3,15-17] As the patient progresses with physical therapy, a more detailed home exercise program should be implemented. If the patient shows continued progress, exercises should be graduated to strengthening of rotator cuff muscles and periscapular stabilizers. Patients should be encouraged to continue the home exercise program once physical therapy ends to maintain range of motion and to prevent recurrence of adhesive capsulitis.

Procedures

In the treatment of adhesive capsulitis, procedures are often performed in conjunction with physical therapy sessions and primarily involve pain-alleviating modalities. These modalities should include post-therapy icing (especially in the beginning, for inflammation control), pretherapy and home moist heating sessions,[2] transcutaneous electrical nerve stimulation trials, ultrasound, and iontophoresis, depending on the patient's response to therapies. As mentioned, subacromial space injections can be used to break pain cycles. In addition to these injections, suprascapular nerve blocks have also been reported to be helpful in breaking pain cycles associated with adhesive capsulitis.[18,19] Acupuncture has also been shown to be an effective treatment option.[20]

Surgery

The decision to perform surgery is based on failure of conservative management or an unacceptable quality of life. The two commonly used options are glenohumeral injections with saline or lidocaine (to lyse adhesions and to distend the capsule) and manipulation under anesthesia.[21,22] Both are typically followed by immediate physical therapy focusing on improvement of range of motion of the glenohumeral joint. The literature has shown both methods to be effective, and the majority of patients recover during a period of 6 to 8 weeks as opposed to 18 to 24 months noted with conservative management. If both of these options fail, arthroscopic lysis of adhesions may be an effective option.[23-25]

POTENTIAL DISEASE COMPLICATIONS

Most of the complications associated with adhesive capsulitis are related to pain and range of motion loss. Pain is usually transient but can persist for months as the condition runs its clinical course. The loss of range of motion that is seen in adhesive capsulitis is usually regained, but it has been reported that as many as 15% of patients develop permanent loss of full range of motion. This range of motion loss is often not associated with functional deficits.[1] Last, there are also reports of a loss of bone mass and density in the affected shoulder of patients with adhesive capsulitis; however, the significance of this is unclear.[26]

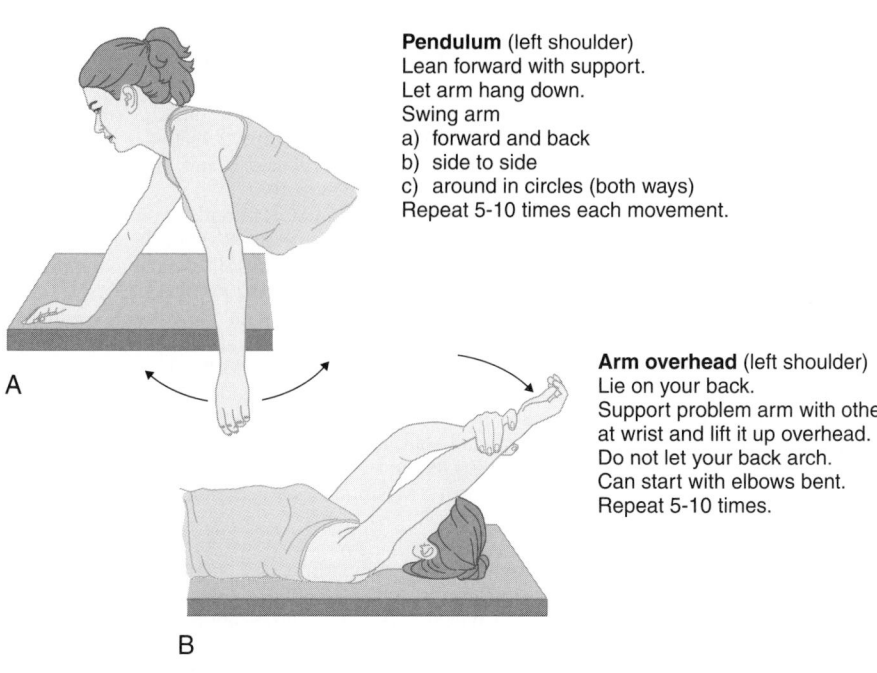

Pendulum (left shoulder)
Lean forward with support.
Let arm hang down.
Swing arm
a) forward and back
b) side to side
c) around in circles (both ways)
Repeat 5-10 times each movement.

A

Arm overhead (left shoulder)
Lie on your back.
Support problem arm with other hand at wrist and lift it up overhead.
Do not let your back arch.
Can start with elbows bent.
Repeat 5-10 times.

B

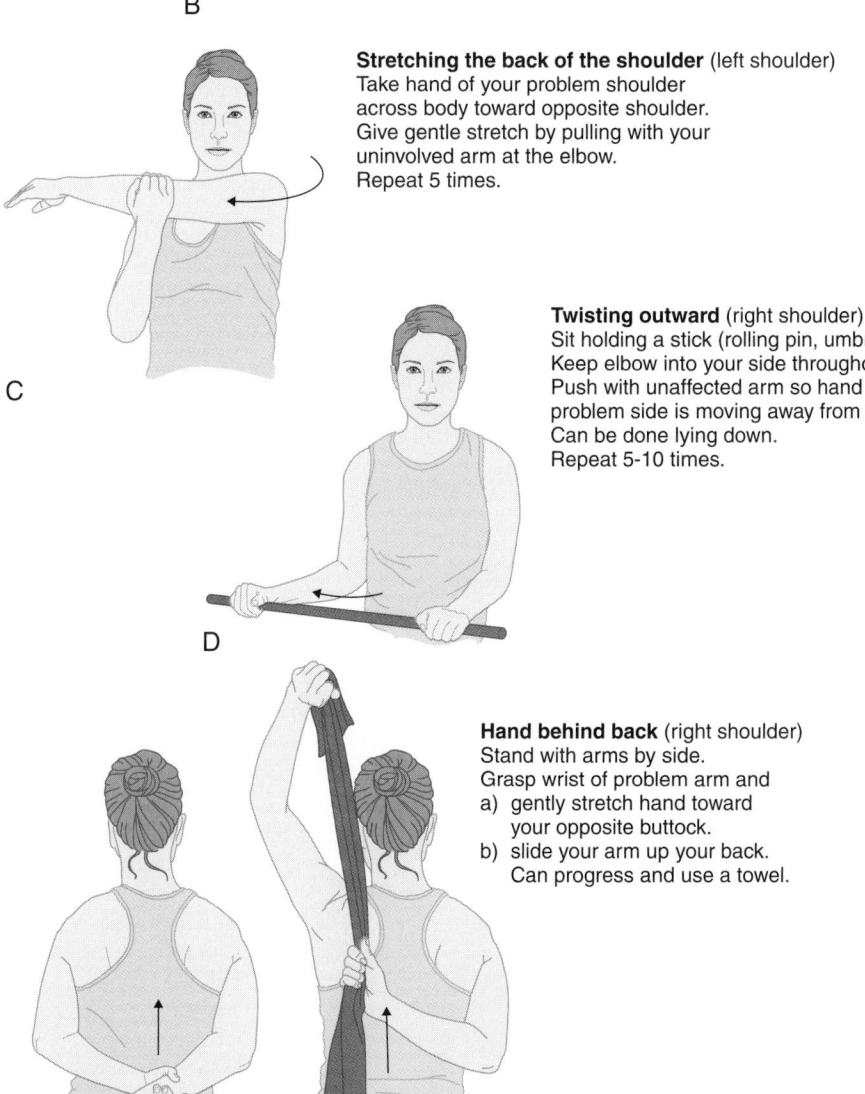

Stretching the back of the shoulder (left shoulder)
Take hand of your problem shoulder across body toward opposite shoulder.
Give gentle stretch by pulling with your uninvolved arm at the elbow.
Repeat 5 times.

C

Twisting outward (right shoulder)
Sit holding a stick (rolling pin, umbrella).
Keep elbow into your side throughout.
Push with unaffected arm so hand of problem side is moving away from midline.
Can be done lying down.
Repeat 5-10 times.

D

FIGURE 10-4. Pendulum and University of Washington (Jackins) exercises for improving range of motion. These exercises should be implemented early. Explanations of the procedures are provided. **A,** Pendulum exercises. **B,** Overhead stretch. **C,** Cross-body reach. **D,** External rotation. **E,** Internal rotation with adduction. (Reprinted with permission from Yeovil Elbow and Shoulder Service. Available at: www.yess.uk.com/patient_information.)

Hand behind back (right shoulder)
Stand with arms by side.
Grasp wrist of problem arm and
a) gently stretch hand toward your opposite buttock.
b) slide your arm up your back.
Can progress and use a towel.

E

POTENTIAL TREATMENT COMPLICATIONS

Treatment complications from conservative management are rare but can include side effects associated with nonsteroidal anti-inflammatory drugs and analgesic medications; these include gastrointestinal bleeds, gastritis, toxic hepatitis, and renal failure.[27] Caution should be used in the treatment of patients with congestive heart failure and hypertension due to fluid retention associated with the use of nonsteroidal anti-inflammatory drugs.[28,29] In patients undergoing suprascapular nerve blocks, care must be taken to prevent intraneural and intravascular injections. There has been one reported case of a patient suffering a pneumothorax during a suprascapular nerve block when a spinal needle was used.[30] A common surgical complication that can occur is a humeral fracture during manipulations under anesthesia.

References

1. Siegel LB, Cohen NJ, Gall EP. Adhesive capsulitis: a sticky issue. Am Fam Physician 1999;59:1843-1852.
2. Nye K, Fallano J, Reid C, DeChaves L. Standard of Care: Adhesive Capsulitis. Physical Therapy Management of the Patient with Adhesive Capsulitis. Boston, Mass, Brigham and Women's Hospital, Department of Rehabilitation Services, 2005:1-7.
3. Rundquist PJ, Anderson DD, Guanche CA, Ludewig PM. Shoulder kinematics in subjects with frozen shoulder. Arch Phys Med Rehabil 2003;84:1473-1479.
4. Miller MD. Review of Orthopedics, 3rd ed. Philadelphia, WB Saunders, 2000:218-225.
5. Vermeulen HM, Rozing PM, Obermann WR, et al. Comparison of high-grade and low-grade mobilization techniques in the management of adhesive capsulitis of the shoulder: randomized controlled trial. Phys Ther 2006;86:355-368.
6. Braddom RL. Handbook of Physical Medicine and Rehabilitation. Philadelphia, WB Saunders, 2004:521-522.
7. Mengiardi B, Pfirrmann CW, Gerber C, et al. Frozen shoulder: MR arthrographic findings. Radiology 2004;233:486-492.
8. McGee DJ. Orthopedic Physical Assessment, 4th ed. Philadelphia, WB Saunders, 2002:296-308.
9. Lee MH, Ahn JM, Muhle C, et al. Adhesive capsulitis of the shoulder: diagnosis using magnetic resonance arthrography, with arthroscopic findings as the standard. J Comput Assist Tomogr 2003;27:901-906.
10. Quan GM, Carr D, Schlicht S, et al. Lessons learnt from the painful shoulder: a case series of malignant shoulder girdle tumours misdiagnosed as frozen shoulder. Int Semin Surg Oncol 2005;2:2.
11. Connell D, Padmanabhan R, Buchbinder R. Adhesive capsulitis: role of MR imaging in differential diagnosis. Eur Radiol 2002;12:2100-2106.
12. Hannafin JA, Chiaia TA. Adhesive capsulitis. A treatment approach. Clin Orthop Relat Res 2000;372:95-109.
13. Warner JJ. Frozen shoulder: diagnosis and management. J Am Acad Orthop Surg 1997;5:130-140.
14. Bell S, Coghlan J, Richardson M. Hydrodilatation in the management of shoulder capsulitis. Australas Radiol 2003;47:247-251.
15. Smith LL, Burnet SP, McNeil JD. Musculoskeletal manifestations of diabetes mellitus. Br J Sports Med 2003;37:30-35.
16. Owens-Burkhard H. Management of the frozen shoulder. In Donatelli R, ed. Physical Therapy of the Shoulder, 2nd ed. New York, Churchill Livingstone, 1991:91-113.
17. Coumo F. Diagnosis, classification, and management of the stiff shoulder. In Iannotti J, Williams G, eds. Disorders of the Shoulder: Diagnosis and Management. Philadelphia, Lippincott Williams & Wilkins, 1999:397-417.
18. Dias R, Cutts S, Massoud S. Frozen shoulder. BMJ 2005;331: 1453-1456.
19. Karatas GK, Meray J. Suprascapular nerve block for pain relief in adhesive capsulitis: comparison of 2 different techniques. Arch Phys Med Rehabil 2002;83:593-597.
20. Sun KO, Chan KC, Lo SL, Fong DY. Acupuncture for frozen shoulder. Hong Kong Med J 2001;7:381-391.
21. Buchbinder R, Green S. Effect of arthrographic shoulder joint distention with saline and corticosteroid for adhesive capsulitis. Br J Sports Med 2004;38:384-385.
22. Kivimaki J, Pohjolainen T. Manipulation under anesthesia for frozen shoulder with and without steroid injection. Arch Phys Med Rehabil 2001;82:1188-1190.
23. Warner JJ, Allen A, Marks PH, Wong P. Arthroscopic release for chronic, refractory adhesive capsulitis of the shoulder. J Bone Joint Surg Am 1996;78:1808-1816.
24. Diwan D, Murrell G. An evaluation of the effects of the extent of capsular release and of postoperative therapy on the temporal outcomes of adhesive capsulitis. Arthroscopy 2005;21:1105-1113.
25. Berghs B. Arthroscopic release of adhesive capsulitis. J Shoulder Elbow Surg 2004;13:180-185.
26. Leppala J, Kannus P, Sievanen H, et al. Adhesive capsulitis of the shoulder (frozen shoulder) produces bone loss in the affected humerus, but long-term bony recovery is good. Bone 1998;22: 691-694.
27. Laine L. Gastrointestinal effects of NSAIDs and coxibs. J Pain Symptom Manage 2003;25(Suppl):S32-S40.
28. Glasser DL, Burroughs SH. Valdecoxib-induced toxic epidermal necrolysis in a patient allergic to sulfa drugs. Pharmacotherapy 2003;23:551-553.
29. Schuster C, Wuthrich B. Anaphylactic drug reaction to celecoxib and sulfamethoxazole: cross reactivity or coincidence? Allergy 2003;58:1072-1075.
30. Marhofer P, Greher M, Kapral S. Ultrasound guidance in regional anaesthesia. Br J Anaesth 2005;94:7-17.

Biceps Tendinitis 11

Brian J. Krabak, MD, MBA, and William Moore, MD

Synonyms

Biceps tendinosis
Bicipital tendinitis

ICD-9 Codes

726.11 Calcifying tendinitis of shoulder
726.12 Bicipital tenosynovitis

DEFINITION

First documented in 1932, biceps tendinitis is a general term used to describe inflammation, pain, or tenderness in the region of the biceps tendon.[1] The actual origin of the pain may be a degenerative process called tendinosis. This usually occurs in "watershed" areas of compromised vascular supply of tendons, but proinflammatory neural mechanisms may also play a role.[2,3]

Primary biceps tendinitis describes isolated inflammation of the tendon as it runs in the intertubercular groove; it typically occurs in the younger, athletic populations.[4,5] The precipitating forces in primary biceps tendinitis are multifactorial and include repetitive overuse, multidirectional shoulder instability, calcifications into the tendon, and direct trauma.[6,7] A flat medial wall of the bicipital groove can predispose to subluxation of the long head tendon, increasing risk for inflammation.[8] A shallow bicipital groove can also promote subluxation.[9] Primary biceps tendinitis is rare. Secondary bicipital tendinitis is typically seen in the older population and more commonly than primary biceps tendinitis.[1,4] Studies have found that up to 95% of patients with bicipital tendinitis have associated rotator cuff disease.[9] A more recent study has noted biceps tendinopathy as a source of anterior shoulder pain after a total shoulder arthroplasty.[10] Focal chondromalacia near the bicipital groove (a biceps tendon "footprint") on arthroscopy is often seen with rotator cuff tears or multidirectional shoulder instability.[11] The presence of the footprint increases the risk for tendinitis.[11]

The majority of shoulder movement occurs about the glenohumeral joint, which is a ball-and-socket joint. This joint has great mobility at the expense of stability, and dynamic effects of muscle strength and function are highly interdependent. Injury to or compromise of a single muscle of the dynamic shoulder stabilizers can adversely affect other muscles and impair function of the entire joint. The biceps is known to help prevent superior translation of the humeral head during shoulder abduction.[4,12]

SYMPTOMS

Biceps tendinitis usually presents with complaints of anterior shoulder pain that is worse with activity. Often, pain will also occur with prolonged rest and subsequent immobility, particularly at night.[13] Attention should be given to onset, duration, and character of the pain. Some individuals present with only complaints of fatigue with shoulder movement in the early stages of tendinitis. History of prior trauma, athletic and occupational endeavors, and systemic diseases should be considered in evaluating the shoulder. The pain can be difficult to separate from impingement or rotator cuff syndrome.[4] Patients with accompanying supraspinatus tendinitis or "impingement syndrome" often complain of a "pinching" sensation with overhead activities and a "toothache" sensation in the lateral proximal arm.[14] A throwing athlete, such as a baseball pitcher, may hear or feel a "snap" if the tendon subluxates in the groove.[1] In bicipital tendinitis, anterior shoulder pain occurs with shoulder flexion and lifting activities that involve elbow flexion.[15]

PHYSICAL EXAMINATION

A physical examination begins with adequate inspection of the shoulder and neck region. Attention is given to prior scars, structural deformities, posture, and muscle bulk. Determination of the exact location of pain can be helpful for diagnosis. Biceps tendinitis commonly presents with palpable tenderness over the bicipital groove (Fig. 11-1). Side-to-side comparisons should be made because the tendon is typically slightly tender to direct palpation. Tenderness over the lateral aspect of the shoulder suggests tendinitis or strain of the deltoid muscle or the underlying bursa. Shoulder range

55

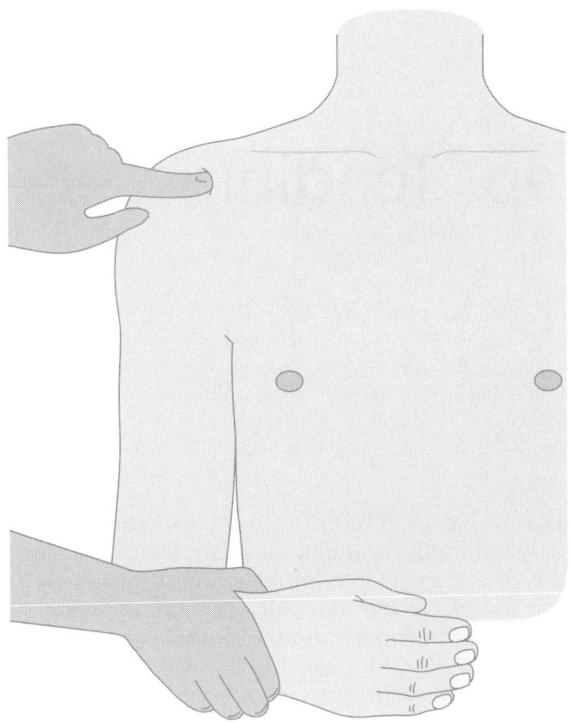

FIGURE 11-1. Palpation of the bicipital groove.

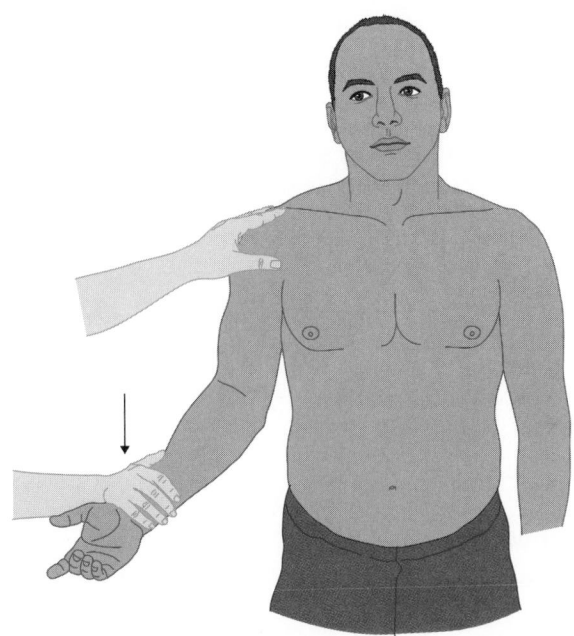

FIGURE 11-2. Demonstration of Speed test for bicipital tendinitis. The examiner provides resistance to forward flexion of the shoulder with the elbow in extension and supination of the forearm. Pain is elicited in the intertubercular groove in a positive test result.

of motion may be limited if the rotator cuff is involved. Motion limitation is not seen in isolated tendinopathies but is often seen in concomitant degenerative joint diseases, impingement syndromes, tendon tears, or adhesive capsulitis. A neurologic examination should be normal, including sensation and deep tendon reflexes. On occasion, strength is limited by pain.

Special tests of the shoulder should be performed routinely. The Speed and Yergason tests (Figs. 11-2 and 11-3) are often used to help evaluate for bicipital tendinitis.[16,17] The Speed test has been shown to be a sensitive but nonspecific indicator of biceps or labral injury.[18] Impingement tests[13] and supraspinatus tests[19] will help assess for any concurrent rotator cuff tendinitis. Other maneuvers to assess for instability (anterior apprehension, anterior-posterior load and shift), labral disease (O'Brien test), and acromioclavicular joint arthritis (Scarf test) should be performed.

FUNCTIONAL LIMITATIONS

Biceps tendinitis may cause patients to limit their activities at home and at work. Limitations may include difficulty with lifting and carrying groceries, garbage bags, and briefcases. Athletics that involve the affected arm, such as swimming, tennis, and throwing sports, may be curtailed. Pain may impair sleep.

DIAGNOSTIC STUDIES

Biceps tendinitis is generally diagnosed on a clinical basis, but imaging studies are helpful for excluding other pathologic processes. Plain radiographs are usu-

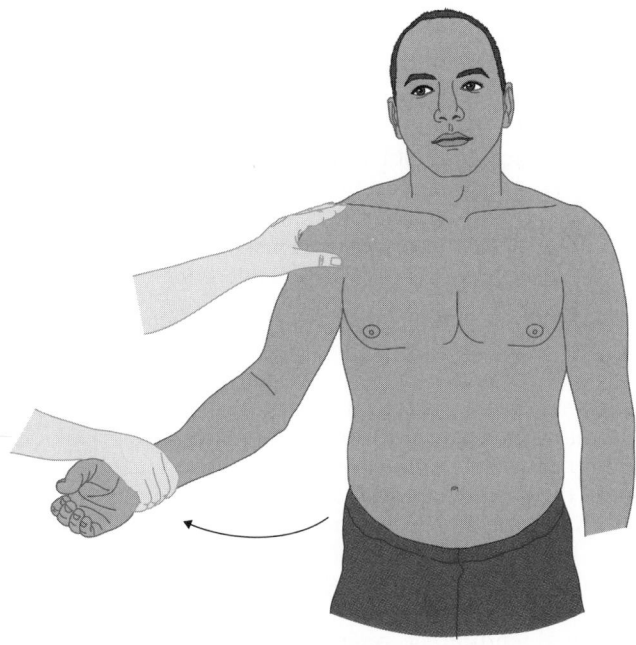

FIGURE 11-3. Demonstration of Yergason test. The examiner provides resistance against supination of the forearm with the elbow flexed at 90 degrees. The test result is considered positive when pain is produced or intensified in the intertubercular groove.

ally normal with biceps tendinitis.[1] However, they can show calcifications in the tendon and degenerative disease of the joint that may predispose to tendinitis. The Fisk view is used in evaluating bicipital tendinitis to assess the size of the intertubercular groove. This helps determine whether there is a relative risk for development of recurrent subluxation of the tendon, which is seen in individuals with short and narrow margins of the intertubercular groove.[20]

Arthrography has been used in the past for rotator cuff disease, but it is generally helpful only in full-thickness tears and has lost favor to magnetic resonance imaging. Magnetic resonance imaging can detect partial-thickness tendon tears, examine muscle substance, evaluate soft tissue abnormalities and labral disease, and assess for masses. In biceps tendinitis, increased signal intensity is seen on T2-weighted images.[21] However, this finding is also seen with partial tears of the tendon.[21] Tendinosis presents with increased tendon thickness and intermediate signal in the surrounding sheath.[22]

Beginning in the early 1980s, ultrasonography has been used by some centers for dynamic assessment of tendon function.[23] A few research articles have found it sensitive for detection of biceps tendinitis and cost-effective, but it can be very operator dependent and has not yet reached widespread acceptance.[23-25] With ultrasound evaluation, the inflamed areas of the tendon have low reflectivity.[21]

Electrodiagnosis is used when concomitant peripheral neuropathies need assessment. Arthroscopy is a useful procedure for the evaluation of intra-articular disease but does not play a role in isolated tendinitis.

TREATMENT

Initial

The hallmark for treatment of biceps tendinitis involves activity modification, anti-inflammatory measures, heat and cold modalities, and a therapeutic exercise program for promoting strength and flexibility of the dynamic shoulder stabilizers.[17] Overhead activities and lifting are to be avoided initially. Workstation assessment and modification can be helpful for laborers. Evaluation of athletic technique and training adaptations are important in athletes. Nonsteroidal anti-inflammatory drugs can assist with decreasing the pain and inflammation. Shoulder stretching helps maintain range of motion and flexibility and is emphasized in all parameters of abduction, adduction, and internal and external rotation.[26] Posterior capsule stretching is also important, particularly with concomitant impingement syndrome.[1] Moist heat can be useful before activity. Ice is helpful after exercise for minimizing pain.

Rehabilitation

Rehabilitation for biceps tendinitis is similar to that for rotator cuff tendinitis (see Chapter 14). Moreover, because biceps tendinitis rarely occurs in isolation, it is important to rehabilitate the patient by accounting for all of the shoulder disease that is present (e.g., instability, impingement). Modalities such as ultrasound can be applied easily to focal tendinitis as a deep heating modality using 1 to 2.5 watts/cm^2. Once full, pain-free active range of motion is achieved, progressive resistance exercises are used to strengthen the dynamic shoulder stabilizers, progressing from static to dynamic exercise as tolerated.[4] Eccentric strengthening may be beneficial for biceps tendinopathy, but more research is needed.[3] Overhead and shoulder abduction activities should be avoided early in treatment because they can exacerbate symptoms.[4] Athletes return to play gradually when pain is minimal or absent. Other modalities, such as iontophoresis and electrical stimulation, have been used, but there are no significant studies supporting their efficacy.

Procedures

Steroid injections are a useful adjunct for biceps tendinitis (Fig. 11-4). Care is taken to avoid injection into the tendon substance itself.

Immediate postinjection care includes icing for 5 to 10 minutes, and the patient may continue to apply ice at home for 15 to 20 minutes, two or three times daily, for several days. The patient should be instructed to avoid heavy lifting or vigorous exercise for 48 to 72 hours after injection. It is advisable not to repeat the injection more than two or three times because of the possibility of weakening the tendon.

These injections serve as an adjunct to diminish pain and inflammation and to facilitate the rehabilitation process. Injections must be used judiciously to avoid weakening of the tendon substance.[27] Depending on the shoulder disease, other injections may also be useful (e.g., subacromial).[28]

Surgery

Surgery is generally not indicated for isolated biceps tendinitis. However, biceps tenodesis in conjunction with acromioplasty in chronic, refractory cases and in those cases associated with rotator cuff impingement

Differential Diagnosis

Rotator cuff tendinitis and tears

Multidirectional instability

Biceps brachii rupture

Acromioclavicular joint sprain

Glenohumeral or acromioclavicular degenerative joint disease

Rheumatoid arthritis

Crystalline arthropathy

Adhesive capsulitis

Cervical spondylosis

Cervical radiculopathy

Brachial plexopathy

Peripheral entrapment neuropathy

Referral from visceral organs

Diaphragmatic referred pain

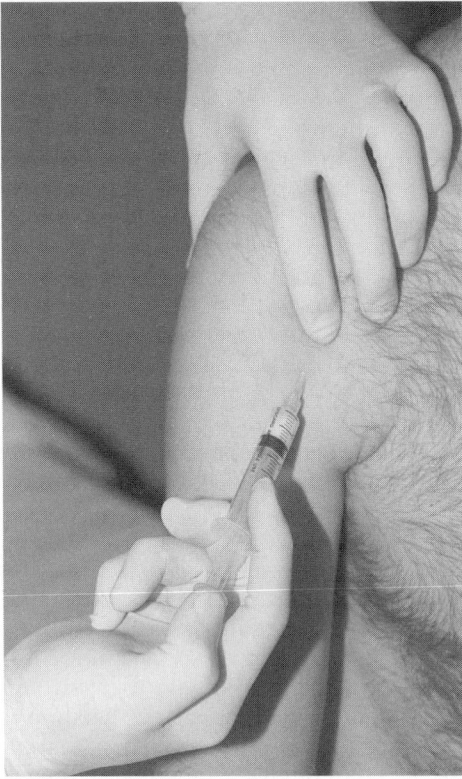

FIGURE 11-4. Injection technique for the long head of the biceps brachii. Under sterile conditions with use of a 25-gauge, 1¹/₂-inch disposable needle and a local anesthetic-corticosteroid combination, the area surrounding the biceps tendon is injected. It is important to bathe the tendon sheath in the preparation rather than to inject the tendon itself. Typically, a 1- to 3-mL aliquot of the mixture is used (e.g., 1 mL of 1% lidocaine mixed with 1 mL of betamethasone). (Reprinted with permission from Lennard TA. Pain Procedures in Clinical Practice, 2nd ed. Philadelphia, Hanley & Belfus, 2000:150.)

has been found to have good results.[1,4] Tenotomy of the long head of the biceps for chronic tendinitis remains controversial, and long-term results are unknown.[1,29]

POTENTIAL DISEASE COMPLICATIONS

Progressive biceps tendinitis and pain can lead to diminished activity and subsequent adhesive capsulitis. Compensatory problems with other tendons can develop because of their interdependence for proper shoulder movement. The development of myofascial pain of the surrounding shoulder girdle muscles is another common complication in shoulder tendinitis.

POTENTIAL TREATMENT COMPLICATIONS

The exercise program should be properly supervised initially to prevent aggravation of tendinitis of other muscle groups. Analgesics and nonsteroidal anti-inflammatory drugs have well-known side effects that most commonly affect the gastric, hepatic, and renal systems. Repeated steroid injections in or near tendons result in compromise of the tendon substance and should be avoided.

References

1. Patton WC, McCluskey GM. Overuse injuries in the upper extremity. Clin Sports Med 2001;20:439-451.
2. Brooks CH, Rewell WJ, Heaely FW. A quantitative histological study of the vascularity of the rotator cuff tendon. J Bone Joint Surg Br 1992;74:151-153.
3. Rees JD, Wilson AM, Wolman RL. Current concepts in the management of tendon disorders. Rheumatology (Oxford) 2006;45:508-521.
4. Paynter KS. Disorders of the long head of the biceps tendon. Phys Med Rehabil Clin North Am 2004;15:511-528.
5. Wang Q. Baseball and softball injuries [review]. Curr Sports Med Rep 2006;5:115-119.
6. Codman EA. Rupture of the supraspinatus tendon and lesions in or about the subacromial bursa. In Codman EA. The Shoulder. Boston, Thomas Todd, 1934:65-177.
7. Wolf WB. Shoulder tendinoses. Clin Sports Med 1992;11:871-890.
8. Pfahler M, Branner S, Refior HJ. The role of the bicipital groove in tendopathy of the long biceps tendon. J Shoulder Elbow Surg 1999;8:419-424.
9. Harwood MI, Smith CT. Superior labrum, anterior-posterior lesions and biceps injuries: diagnostic and treatment considerations. Prim Care Clin Office Pract 2004;31:831-855.
10. Tuckman DV, Dines DM. Long head of the biceps pathology as a cause of anterior shoulder pain after shoulder arthroplasty. J Shoulder Elbow Surg 2006;15:415-418.
11. Sistermann R. The biceps tendon footprint. Acta Orthop 2005;76:237-240.
12. Warner JJ, McMahon PJ. The role of the long head of the biceps brachii in superior stability of the glenohumeral joint. J Bone Joint Surg Am 1995;77:366-372.
13. Neer CS, Foster CR. Impingement lesions. Clin Orthop 1983;173:70-77.
14. Hawkins RJ, Kennedy JC. Impingement syndrome in athletes. Am J Sports Med 1980;May-June;8:151-8.
15. Post M, Benca P. Primary tendinitis of the long head of the biceps. Clin Orthop 1989;246:117-125.
16. Neviaser RJ. Lesions of the biceps and tendonitis of the shoulder. Orthop Clin North Am 1980;11:334-340.
17. Jobe FW, Brodley JP. The diagnosis and nonoperative treatment of shoulder injuries in athletes. Clin Sports Med 1989;8:419-438.
18. Bennett WF. Specificity of the Speed's test: arthroscopic technique for evaluating the biceps tendon at the level of the bicipital groove. Arthroscopy 1998;14:789-796.
19. Jobe FW, Jobe CM. Painful athletic injuries of the shoulder. Clin Orthop 1983;173:117-124.
20. Cone RO, Danzig L, Resnick D, Godman AB. The bicipital groove: radiographic, anatomic and pathologic study. AJR Am J Roentgenol 1983;141:781-788.
21. Campbell RSD, Grainger AJ. Current concepts in imaging of tendinopathy. Clin Radiol 2001;56:253-267.
22. Tirman PF, Smith ED, Stoller DW, Fritz RC. Shoulder imaging in athletes. Semin Musculoskelet Radiol 2004;8:29-40.
23. Moosmayer S, Smith HJ. Diagnostic ultrasound of the shoulder—a method for experts only? Acta Orthop 2005;76:503-508.
24. Middleton WD, Reinus WR, Totty WG. Ultrasonographic evaluation of the rotator cuff and biceps tendon. J Bone Joint Surg Am 1986;68:440-450.
25. Read JW, Perko M. Shoulder ultrasound: diagnostic accuracy for impingement syndrome, rotator cuff tear, and biceps tendon pathology. J Shoulder Elbow Surg 1998;7:264-271.
26. Neviaser RJ. Painful shoulder conditions. Clin Orthop 1983;173:63-69.
27. Fatal PD, Wigins ME. Corticosteroid injections: their use and abuse. J Am Acad Orthop Surg 1994;2:133-140.
28. Larson HM, O'Connor FG, Nirschl RP. Shoulder pain: the role of diagnostic injections. Am Fam Physician 1996;53:1637-1647.
29. Kelly AM, Drakos MC, Fealy S, et al. Arthroscopic release of the long head of the biceps tendon: functional outcome and clinical results. Am J Sports Med 2005;33:208-213.

Biceps Tendon Rupture 12

Michael F. Stretanski, DO

DEFINITION

Biceps tendon rupture is either complete or partial disruption of the tendon of the biceps brachii muscle that can occur proximally or distally. The more common proximal ruptures are frequently seen in older individuals who have had chronic tendinosis of the long head of the biceps tendon associated with concomitant rotator cuff disease and degenerative joint disease of the shoulder[1] (Fig. 12-1). The incidence is 1.2 per 100,000 patients, with a majority on the dominant side of men who smoke and are in the fourth decade of life.[2] Most cases involve the long head of the biceps brachii and present as a partial or complete avulsion from the superior rim of the anterior glenoid labrum.[3]

The distal biceps rupture is relatively uncommon and typically occurs in middle-aged men. This often develops suddenly with stressing of the flexor mechanism of the elbow. Distal biceps rupture usually occurs as a single traumatic event, such as heavy lifting; it is often an avulsion of the tendon from the radial tuberosity, but it can also occur as a midsubstance tendon rupture.[4]

SYMPTOMS

Proximal ruptures are often asymptomatic and are commonly discovered with awareness of distal migration of the biceps brachii muscle mass, or they may occur suddenly by a seemingly trivial event. Often, individuals will note an acute "popping" sensation. Edema and ecchymosis may be seen with tendon rupture but also with other regional pathologic processes. The proximal ruptures are typically less painful but can be preceded by chronic shoulder discomfort.[5]

An acute distal rupture is often associated with pain at the antecubital fossa that is typically aggravated by resisted elbow flexion. The pain is usually sharp initially but improves with time and is often described as a dull ache.[6] Swelling, distal ecchymosis, and proximal migration of the biceps brachii muscle mass accompany this injury with a magnitude dependent on the degree of injury. Patients often present with a cosmetic rather than a functional complaint.

PHYSICAL EXAMINATION

Visual inspection of the biceps brachii, including comparison with the unaffected limb, is usually the first and most critical element in the physical examination of this condition. The Ludington test[7] is a recommended position in which to observe differences in the contour and shape of the biceps (Fig. 12-2). Complete ruptures are relatively easy to diagnose; patients often come in aware of the biceps muscle retraction, whereas partial ruptures exist along a spectrum and can be more difficult. The clinician should also assess for the presence of ecchymosis or swelling as a sign of acute injury. Palpation for point tenderness will often reveal pain at the rupture site. Effort should also be made to determine whether the rupture is complete by palpation of the tendon. Thorough assessment of the shoulder and elbow should be made for range of motion and laxity. The Yergason[8] and Speed[9] tests (see Chapter 11), which are used in the assessment of bicipital tendinitis, are also recommended. Posterior dislocation of the long head of the biceps tendon has been reported[10] and may share some common physical examination findings, but not muscle retraction.

In patients with inconsistent physical examination findings and questionable secondary gain issues, the American Shoulder and Elbow Surgeons subjective shoulder scale has demonstrated acceptable psychometric performance for outcomes assessment in patients with shoulder instability, rotator cuff disease, and glenohumeral arthritis.[11] It is important to examine the entire shoulder and to keep in mind that it is a complex, inherently unstable, well-innervated joint

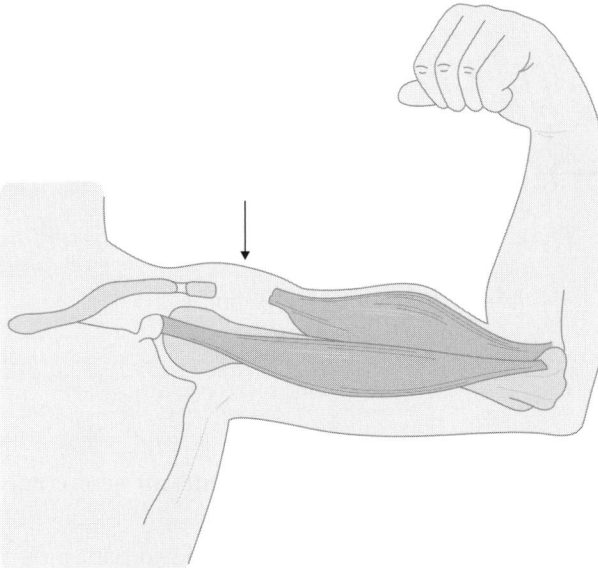

FIGURE 12-1. Proximal biceps tendon rupture.

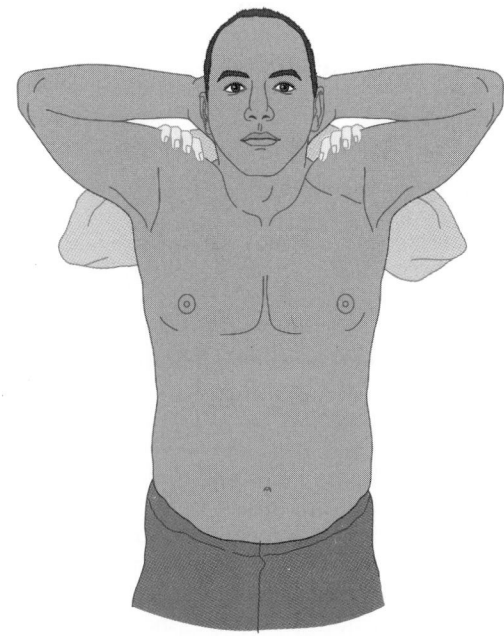

FIGURE 12-2. The Ludington test is performed by having the patient clasp both hands onto or behind the head, allowing the interlocking fingers to support the arms. This action permits maximum relaxation of the biceps tendon in its resting position. The patient then alternately contracts and relaxes the biceps while the clinician palpates the tendon and muscle. In a complete tear, contraction is not felt on the affected side.

that tends to function, and fail, as a unit—therefore, additional lesions that are the true pain generator may be evident. One study[12] looking at shoulder magnetic resonance findings showed no statistical relationship between the level of disability and either biceps tendon rupture or biceps tendinopathy; rather, disability was linked to supraspinatus tendon lesions and bursitis.

A thorough neurologic and vascular examination is performed, and findings should be normal in the absence of concomitant problems. Caution should be used with strength testing to avoid worsening of an incomplete tear.

FUNCTIONAL LIMITATIONS

The functional limitations are generally relatively minimal with proximal biceps rupture,[13] and the patient's concern is commonly centered around cosmetic considerations. More significant weakness of elbow flexion and supination is noted after a distal tendon disruption. Pain can be acutely limiting after both situations but is typically more of a problem in distal rupture. The primary role of the biceps brachii is supination of the forearm. Elbow flexion is functional by the action of the brachialis and brachioradialis. A degree of residual weakness with supination and elbow flexion, particularly after distal tendon rupture, can cause functional impairment for individuals who perform heavy physical labor, such as moving boxes, wood boards, or heavy equipment.[14] Fatigue with repetitive work is also a common complaint with nonsurgically treated distal tendon ruptures.[15] The long head of the biceps is believed to play a role in anterior stability of the shoulder[16,17]; this is an issue for people who perform overhead activities (such as lifting, filing, and painting), powerlifting (in which the last 10% of strength is crucial), and nonsports activities in which the appearance of symmetry is important (such as bodybuilding).

DIAGNOSTIC STUDIES

The diagnosis of biceps brachii rupture is often made on a clinical basis alone. Magnetic resonance imaging is helpful in confirming the diagnosis and assessing the extent of the injury, but it should be performed in the FABS (flexed elbow, abducted shoulder, forearm supinated) position to obtain a true longitudinal view.[18] It is particularly useful in partial ruptures.[19] Magnetic resonance imaging studies can also assess concomitant rotator cuff disease. Diagnostic ultrasonography is a musculoskeletal imaging modality that is gaining popularity in the United States; it may be more cost-effective as a screening tool when clinical index of suspicion is low.[20] Imaging of the entire insertion site as well as of elbow structures should be performed in distal ruptures. Plain radiographs sometimes show hypertrophic bone formation related to chronic degenerative tendon abnormalities as a predisposition to rupture. Radiographs are also performed in acute traumatic cases to rule out fractures. Electrodiagnostic medicine consultation for possible peripheral nerve damage should be considered when appropriate.

TREATMENT

Initial

For most patients, treatment of proximal biceps tears is conservative. Surgery is rarely necessary because there is little loss of function, and the cosmetic deformity is

Differential Diagnosis

Musculocutaneous neuropathy

Rotator cuff disease

Brachial plexopathy

Pectoralis major muscle rupture

Tumor

Hematoma

Dislocated biceps tendon

Cervical radiculopathy

Parsonage-Turner syndrome

generally acceptable without surgical repair.[21] Young athletes or heavy laborers may be the exception; they typically need the lost strength that occurs with loss of the continuity of the biceps tendon. Distal tears are more commonly referred to surgery acutely. However, initial treatment of partial distal ruptures consists of splint immobilization in flexion, which should be continued for 3 weeks. This is followed by a gradual return to normal activities. Analgesics, nonsteroidal anti-inflammatory drugs, and ice may assist with the discomfort and swelling in both proximal and distal ruptures.

Rehabilitation

Nonsurgical treatment includes range of motion exercises of the elbow and shoulder for contracture prevention. Modalities such as iontophoresis and therapeutic ultrasound can be used for pain control. Electrical stimulation should probably be considered to be contraindicated in partial tears and not indicated in complete tears because of the counterphysiologic type II motor unit recruitment, lack of control of power-length relationship, and concern for converting a partial to a complete tear. Gentle strengthening can typically be done after the acute phase (i.e., when there is little swelling or pain) in complete tears that are not going to be repaired because there is little chance of further injury.

Postoperative rehabilitation for distal biceps rupture repairs consists of immobilization of the elbow in 90 degrees of flexion for 7 to 10 days, followed by the use of a hinged flexion-assist splint with a 30-degree extension block for 8 weeks after surgery. Gentle range of motion and progressive resistance exercises are started after that. Unlimited activity is not allowed until 5 months postoperatively.[22]

Procedures

No procedures are performed in the treatment of biceps tendon rupture. Musculocutaneous nerve or upper trunk brachial plexus block may have a role either perioperatively or palliatively in selected cases.

Surgery

Prompt assessment is necessary for complete distal biceps ruptures under consideration for surgical repair because muscle shortening occurs over time. The same is true for proximal ruptures in very active individuals who require maximal upper body strength for their vocation or sport. Optimal surgical outcomes are obtained if treatment occurs within the first 4 weeks after injury. Partial distal ruptures are generally observed nonoperatively until a complete rupture occurs. The partial rupture can scar and remain in continuity.[5] The goal of surgical treatment is to restore strength of supination and flexion. For distal repairs, this is typically performed by a two-incision technique involving reinsertion of the biceps tendon to the radial tuberosity.[23] A single-incision technique with use of suture anchors in the bicipital tuberosity has shown excellent long-term functional results by the Disabilities of the Arm, Shoulder, and Hand (DASH) questionnaire.[24]

POTENTIAL DISEASE COMPLICATIONS

Complications from isolated biceps rupture are relatively rare. Partial tears can become complete tears. Attention should be given to potential contracture formation. Median nerve compression has been reported presumably to be related to an enlarged synovial bursa associated with a partial distal biceps tendon rupture.[25] Compartment syndrome has also been reported in proximal biceps rupture in a patient receiving systemic anticoagulation.[26]

POTENTIAL TREATMENT COMPLICATIONS

Analgesics and nonsteroidal anti-inflammatory drugs have well-known side effects that most commonly affect the gastric, hepatic, and renal systems. Advancement of the extent of the rupture can occur with overly aggressive strengthening measures and passive stretching. The potential for serious surgical complications is most significant with distal rupture because of the important neurovascular structures in that region, including the median and radial nerves and brachial artery and vein.[27] The complication rate increases with the length of time after rupture that surgery is performed. Proximal radial-ulnar synostosis and heterotopic ossification have also been reported as rare postsurgical complications.[22] Stiffness and contractures are possible with or without surgical intervention.

References

1. Neer CS. Impingement lesions. Clin Orthop 1983;173:70-77.
2. Safran MR, Graham SM. Distal biceps tendon ruptures: incidence, demographics and the effect of smoking. Clin Orthop Relat Res 2002;404:275-283.
3. Gilcreest EL. The common syndrome of rupture, dislocation and elongation of the long head of the biceps brachii: an analysis of one hundred cases. Surg Gynecol Obstet 1934;58:322.

4. Le Huec JC, Moinard M, Liquois F, Zipoli B. Distal rupture of the tendon of biceps brachii: evaluation by MRI and the results of repair. J Bone Joint Surg Br 1996;78:767-770.

5. Waugh RI, Hathcock TA, Elliott JL. Ruptures of muscles and tendons: with particular reference of rupture (or elongation of the long tendon) of biceps brachii with report of fifty cases. Surgery 1949;25:370-392.

6. Bourne MH, Morrey BF. Partial rupture of the distal biceps tendon. Clin Orthop Relat Res 1991;271:143-148.

7. Ludington NA. Rupture of the long head of the biceps flexor cubiti muscle. Ann Surg 1923;77:358-363.

8. Yergason RM. Rupture of biceps. J Bone Joint Surg 1931;13:160.

9. Gilcreest EL, Albi P. Unusual lesions of muscles and tendons of the shoulder girdle and upper arm. Surg Gynecol Obstet 1939;68: 903-917.

10. Bauer T, Vuillemin A, Hardy P, Rousselin B. Posterior dislocation of the long head of the biceps tendon: a case report. J Shoulder Elbow Surg 2005;14:557-558.

11. Kocher MS, Horan MP, Briggs KK, et al. Reliability, validity and responsiveness of the American Shoulder and Elbow Surgeons subjective shoulder scale in patients with shoulder instability, rotator cuff disease and glenohumeral arthritis. J Bone Joint Surg Am 2005;87:2006-2011.

12. Krief OP, Huguet D. Shoulder pain and disability: comparison with MR findings. AJR Am J Roentgenol 2006;186:1234-1239.

13. Phillips BB, Canale ST, Sisk TD, et al. Ruptures of the proximal biceps tendon in middle-aged patients. Orthop Rev 1993;22:349-353.

14. Pearl ML, Bessos K, Wong K. Strength deficits related to distal biceps tendon rupture and repair: a case report. Am J Sports Med 1998;26:295-296.

15. Davison BL, Engber WD, Tigert LJ. Long term evaluation of repaired distal biceps brachii tendon ruptures. Clin Orthop Relat Res 1996;333:188-191.

16. Rodosky MW, Harner CD, Fu FH. The role of the long head of the biceps muscle and superior glenoid labrum in anterior stability of the shoulder. Am J Sports Med 1994;22:121-130.

17. Warner JJ, McMahon PJ. The role of the long head of the biceps brachii in superior stability of the glenohumeral joint. J Bone Joint Surg Am 1995;77:366-372.

18. Chew ML, Giuffrè BM. Disorders of the distal biceps brachii tendon. Radiographics 2005;25:1227-1237.

19. Erickson SJ, Fitzgerald SW, Quinn SF, et al. Long bicipital tendon of the shoulder: normal anatomy and pathologic findings on MR imaging. AJR Am J Roentgenol 1992;158:1091-1096.

20. Belli P, Costantini M, Mirk P, et al. Sonographic diagnosis of distal biceps tendon rupture: a prospective study of 25 cases. J Ultrasound Med 2001;20:587-595.

21. Hawkins RJ, Kennedy JC. Impingement syndrome in athletes. Am J Sports Med 1980;8:151-158.

22. Ramsey ML. Distal biceps tendon injuries: diagnosis and management. J Am Acad Orthop Surg 1999;7:199-207.

23. Boyd HD, Anderson LD. A method for reinsertion of the distal biceps brachii tendon. J Bone Joint Surg Am 1961;43:1041-1043.

24. McKee MD, Hirji R, Schemitsch EH, et al. Patient-oriented functional outcome after repair of distal biceps tendon ruptures using a single-incision technique. J Shoulder Elbow Surg 2005;14:302-306.

25. Foxworthy M, Kinninmonth AWG. Median nerve compression in the proximal forearm as a complication of partial rupture of the distal biceps brachii tendon. J Hand Surg Br 1992;17:515-517.

26. Richards AM, Moss AL. Biceps rupture in a patient on long-term anticoagulation leading to compartment syndrome and nerve palsies. J Hand Surg Br 1997;22:411-412.

27. Rantanen J, Orava S. Rupture of the distal biceps tendon. A report of 19 patients treated with anatomic reinsertion, and a meta-analysis of 147 cases found in the literature. Am J Sports Med 1999;27:128-132.

Glenohumeral Instability 13

William Micheo, MD, and Edwardo Ramos, MD

Synonyms
Dislocation
Subluxation
Recurrent dislocation
Multidirectional instability

ICD-9 Codes

718.81   Instability of shoulder joint
831.00   Closed dislocation of shoulder, unspecified

DEFINITIONS

Shoulder instability represents a spectrum of disorders ranging from shoulder subluxation, in which the humeral head partially slips out of the glenoid fossa, to shoulder dislocation, which is a complete displacement out of the glenoid. It is classified as anterior, posterior, or multidirectional and on the basis of its frequency, etiology, direction, and degree.[1] Instability can result from macrotrauma, such as shoulder dislocation, or repetitive microtrauma associated with throwing, and it can occur without trauma in individuals with generalized ligamentous laxity.

The glenohumeral joint has a high degree of mobility at the expense of stability. Static and dynamic restraints combine to maintain the shoulder in place with overhead activity. Muscle action, particularly of the rotator cuff and scapular stabilizers, is important in maintaining joint congruity in midranges of motion. Static stabilizers such as the glenohumeral ligaments, joint capsule, and glenoid labrum are important for stability in the extremes of motion.[2]

Damage to the shoulder capsule, the glenohumeral ligaments, and the inferior labrum results from acute dislocation. Repeated capsular stretch, rotator cuff, and superior labral injuries are associated with anterior instability in athletes who participate in overhead sports; a loose patulous capsule is the primary pathologic change with multidirectional instability, and patients may present with bilateral symptoms.[3,4] Shoulder instability affects, in particular, young individuals, females, and athletes, but it may also affect sedentary individuals.[5,6]

In the case of traumatic instability, the individual usually falls on the outstretched, externally rotated, and abducted arm with a resulting anterior dislocation. A blow to the posterior aspect of the externally rotated and abducted arm can also result in anterior dislocation. Posterior dislocation usually results from a fall on the forward flexed and adducted arm or by a direct blow in the posterior direction when the arm is above the shoulder.[2]

Recurrent shoulder instability after a traumatic dislocation is common, particularly when the initial event happens at a young age. In these individuals, it may occur repeatedly in association with overhead activity, and it may even happen at night in those with severe symptoms.[6] The patients may initially require visits to the emergency department or reduction of recurrent dislocation by a team physician; but as the condition becomes more chronic, some may be able to reduce their own dislocations.

Patients with neurologic problems such as stroke, brachial plexus injury, and poliomyelitis may present with shoulder girdle muscle weakness, scapular dysfunction, and resultant shoulder instability.

SYMPTOMS

With atraumatic instability or subluxation, it may be difficult to identify an initial precipitating event. Usually, symptoms result from repetitive activity that places great demands on the dynamic and static stabilizers of the glenohumeral joint, leading to increased translation of the humeral head in racket sports, swimming, or work-related tasks. Pain is the initial symptom, usually associated with impingement of the rotator cuff under the coracoacromial arch. Patients may also report that the shoulder slips out of the joint or that the arm goes "dead," and they may report weakness associated with overhead activity.[7]

Patients with neurologic injury present with pain with motion and shoulder subluxation as well as scapular and shoulder girdle muscle weakness.

PHYSICAL EXAMINATION

The shoulder is inspected for the presence of deformity, atrophy of surrounding muscles, asymmetry, and scapular winging. Individuals are observed from the anterior, lateral, and posterior positions. Palpation of soft tissue and bone is systematically addressed and includes the rotator cuff, biceps tendon, and subacromial region.

Passive and active range of motion is evaluated. Differences between passive and active motion may be secondary to pain, weakness, or neurologic damage. Repeated throwing may lead to an increase in measured external rotation accompanied by a reduction in internal rotation; tennis players may present with an isolated glenohumeral internal rotation deficit.[8]

Manual strength testing is performed to identify weakness of specific muscles of the rotator cuff and the scapular stabilizers. The supraspinatus muscle can be tested in the scapular plane with internal rotation or external rotation of the shoulder. The external rotators can be tested with the arm at the side of the body; the subscapularis muscle can be tested by the lift-off test, in which the palm of the hand is lifted away from the lower back (Fig.13-1). The scapular stabilizers, such as the serratus anterior and the rhomboid muscles, can be tested in isolation or by doing wall pushups.[9] Sensory and motor examination of the shoulder girdle is performed to rule out nerve injuries.

Testing the shoulder in the position of 90 degrees of forward flexion with internal rotation, or in extreme forward flexion with the forearm supinated, can assess for rotator cuff impingement and may reproduce symptoms of pain[10] (Fig. 13-2). Glenohumeral translation testing for ligamentous laxity or symptomatic instability should be documented. Apprehension testing can be performed with the patient sitting, standing, or in the supine position. The shoulder is stressed anteriorly in the position of 90 degrees of abduction and external rotation to reproduce the feeling that the shoulder is coming out of the joint (Fig. 13-3). A relocation maneuver that reduces the symptoms of instability also aids in the diagnosis but appears to be less specific than apprehension testing[11] (Fig. 13-4). The causation of posterior shoulder pain (rather than symptoms of instability) with apprehension testing may be associated with internal impingement of the rotator cuff and posterior superior labrum.

Other tests include the load and shift maneuver with the arm at the side to document humeral head translation in anterior and posterior directions; the sulcus sign to document inferior humeral head laxity; and the active compression test described by O'Brien and colleagues in which a downward force is applied to the forward flexed, adducted, and internally rotated shoulder to reproduce pain associated with superior labral tears or acromioclavicular joint disease.[8,12-15]

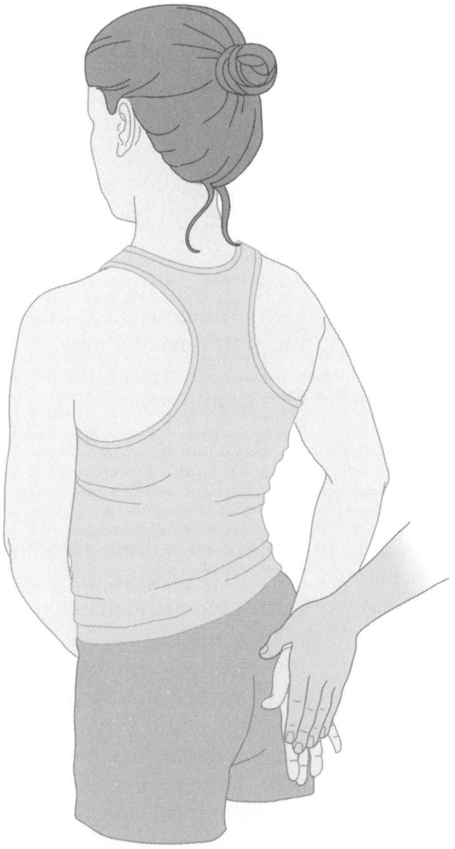

FIGURE 13-1. In the lift-off test of the subscapularis, the patient places the arm on the lower back area and attempts to forcefully internally rotate against the examiner's hand. It is important to document first that the patient has enough passive motion to allow the shoulder to be internally rotated away from the lower back area.

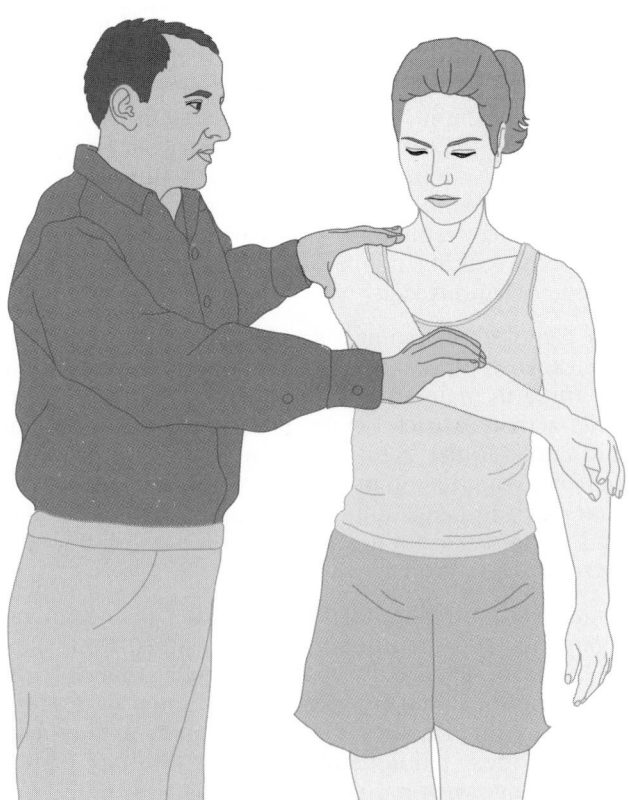

FIGURE 13-2. Impingement test for impingement against the coracoacromial arch.

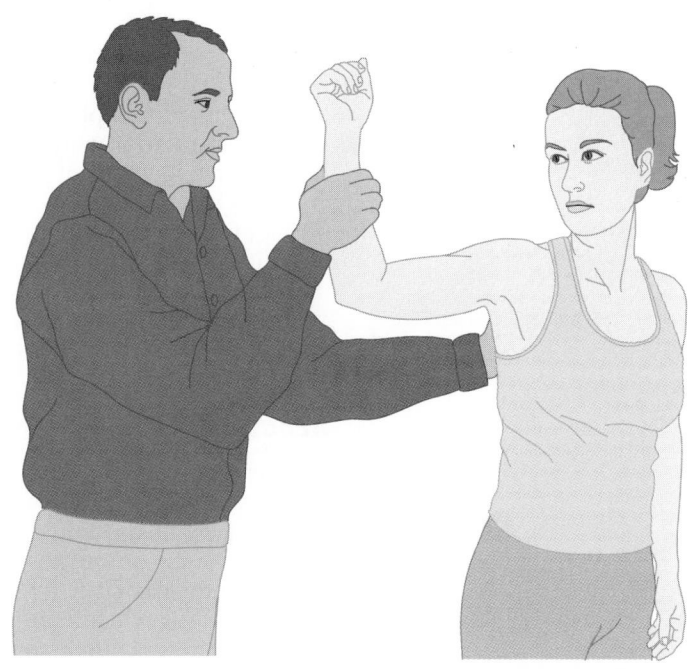

FIGURE 13-3. In the apprehension test, the arm is abducted to approximately 90 degrees and progressively externally rotated while the patient's response is noted. A positive response is elicited by the patient's having a sensation that the shoulder will slip out of the joint.

FUNCTIONAL LIMITATIONS

Limitations include reduced motion, muscle weakness, and pain that interferes with activities of daily living, such as reaching into cupboards and brushing hair. Athletes, particularly those participating in throwing sports, may experience a decrease in the velocity of their pitches, and tennis players may lose control of their serve. Occupational limitations may include inability to reach or to lift weight above the level of the head or pain with rotation of the arm in a production line. Recurrent instability often leads to avoidance of activities that require abduction and external rotation because of reproduction of symptoms.

DIAGNOSTIC STUDIES

The standard radiographs that are obtained to evaluate the patient with shoulder symptoms include anteroposterior views in external and internal rotation, outlet view, axillary lateral view, and Stryker notch view. These allow an assessment of the greater tuberosity and the shape of the acromion and reveal irregularity of the glenoid or posterior humeral head.

Special tests that can also be ordered include arthrography, computed tomographic arthrography, and magnetic resonance imaging. These should be ordered in looking for rotator cuff or labral abnormalities in the patient who has not responded to treatment. Magnetic resonance imaging has become the current standard technique for evaluation of rotator cuff and labral disease. Gadolinium contrast enhancement and modification of the position of the arm for the test appear to increase the sensitivity of magnetic resonance imaging in identifying the specific location of capsular or labral

pathologic changes associated with recurrent instability and dislocation.[15-18] Diagnostic arthroscopy can be used in some cases but is generally not necessary.

TREATMENT

Initial

Acute management of glenohumeral instability is nonoperative in the majority of cases. This includes relative rest, ice, and analgesic or anti-inflammatory medication. Goals at this stage are pain reduction, protection from further injury, and initiation of an early rehabilitation program.

If the injury was observed (as often occurs in athletes) and no evidence of neurologic or vascular damage is evident on clinical examination, reduction may be attempted with traction in forward flexion and slight abduction,

Differential Diagnosis

Glenohumeral joint instability

    Post-traumatic

    Atraumatic

    Multidirectional

Rotator cuff tendinitis or tendinosis

Rotator cuff tear

Glenoid labral tear

Suprascapular neuropathy

immobilization in a sling, in which the arm is positioned in internal rotation, followed by an exercise program and gradual return to activity. Several studies have suggested that placement of the arm in a position of external rotation may be more appropriate because of better realignment of anatomic structures.[19,20] However, this issue still merits further study because there is a lack of randomized controlled studies demonstrating a significant reduction in redislocation rates or a difference in return to activity levels in comparing the positions of immobilization after reduction or the duration of the postreduction immobilization period.[21]

Rehabilitation

The rehabilitation of glenohumeral instability should begin as soon as the injury occurs. The goals of nonsurgical management are reduction of pain, restoration of full motion, correction of muscle strength deficits, achievement of muscle balance, and return to full activity free of symptoms. The rehabilitation program consists of acute, recovery, and functional phases[22,23] (Table 13-1).

Acute Phase (1 to 2 weeks)

This phase should focus on treatment of tissue injury and clinical signs and symptoms. The goal in this stage is to allow tissue healing while reducing pain and inflammation. Reestablishment of nonpainful active range of motion, prevention of shoulder girdle muscle atrophy, reduction of scapular dysfunction, and maintenance of general fitness are addressed.

Recovery Phase (2 to 6 weeks)

This phase focuses on obtaining normal passive and active glenohumeral range of motion, restoring posterior capsule flexibility, improving scapular and rotator cuff muscle strength, and achieving normal core muscle strength and balance. This phase can be started as soon as pain is controlled and the patient can participate in an exercise program without exacerbation of symptoms. Young individuals with symptomatic instability need to progress slowly to the position of shoulder abduction and external rotation. Athletes can progress rapidly through the program and emphasize exercises in functional ranges of motion. Older patients with goals of returning to activities of daily living may require slower progression, particularly if they have significant pain, muscle inhibition, and weakness. Biomechanical and functional deficits including abnormalities in the throwing motion should also be addressed.

Functional Phase (6 weeks to 6 months)

This phase focuses on increasing power and endurance of the upper extremities while improving neuromuscular control because a normal sensorimotor system is key in returning to optimal shoulder function.[24] Rehabilitation at this stage works on the entire kinematic chain to address specific functional deficits.

After the completion of the rehabilitation program, prehabilitation strategies with goals of preventing recurrent injury should be instituted for individuals who

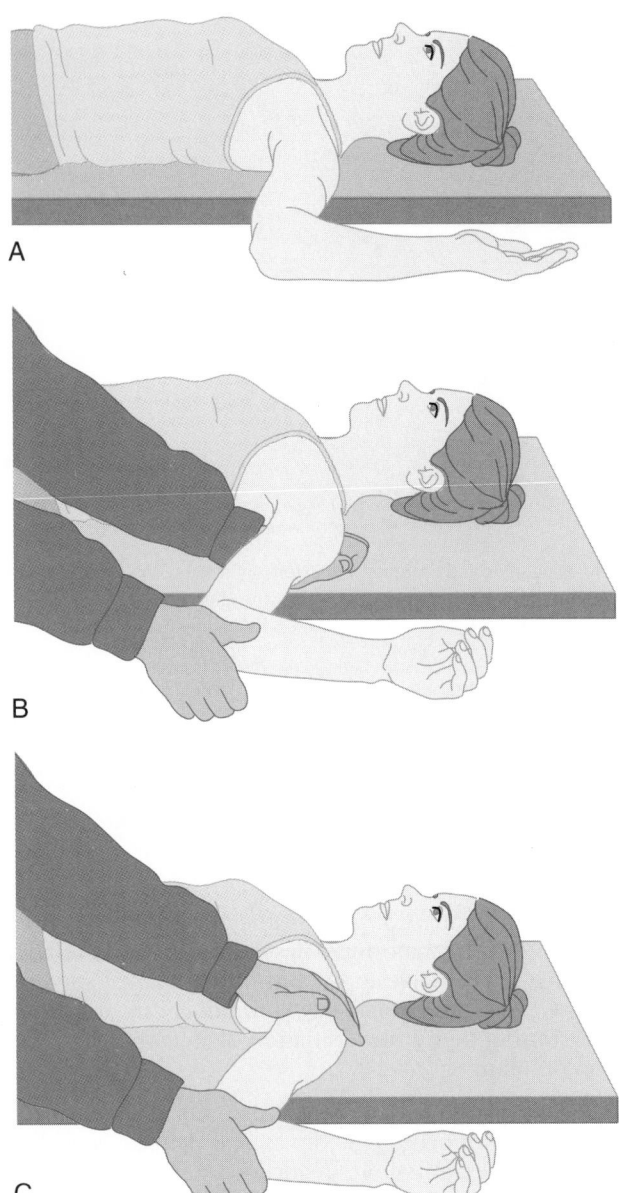

FIGURE 13-4. A, Apprehension relocation test in supine position with arm in 90 degrees of abduction and maximal external rotation. **B,** Reduction of symptoms of apprehension with posteriorly directed force on proximal humerus. **C,** Increased symptoms of apprehension or pain with anterior force applied on proximal humerus.

followed by gentle internal rotation. If this fails, the patient should be transported away from the playing area; reduction may be attempted by placing the patient prone, sedating the individual, and allowing the injured arm to hang from the bed with a 5- to 10-pound weight attached to the wrist.[2] If fracture or posterior dislocation is suspected, the patient should undergo radiologic evaluation before a reduction is attempted. After the reduction, radiologic studies should be repeated.

When acute shoulder dislocations are treated nonoperatively, they are usually managed with variable periods of

TABLE 13-1 Glenohumeral Instability Rehabilitation

	Acute Phase	Recovery Phase	Functional Phase
Therapeutic intervention	Active rest Cryotherapy Electrical stimulation Protected motion Isometric and closed chain exercise to shoulder and scapular muscles General conditioning Nonsteroidal anti-inflammatory drugs	Modalities: superficial heat, ultrasound, electrical stimulation Range of motion exercises, flexibility exercises for posterior capsule Scapular control: closed chain exercises, proprioceptive neuromuscular facilitation patterns Dynamic upper extremity strengthening exercise: isolated rotator cuff exercises Sports-specific exercises: surgical tubing, multiplanar joint exercises, core and lower extremity Gradual return to training	Power and endurance in upper extremities: diagonal and multiplanar motions with tubing, light weights, medicine balls, plyometrics Increased multiple-plane neuromuscular control Maintenance: general flexibility training, strengthening, power and endurance exercise program Sports-specific progression
Criteria for advancement	Pain reduction Recovery of pain-free motion Strength of the shoulder muscles to 4/5	Full nonpainful motion Normal scapular stabilizers and rotator cuff strength Correction of posterior capsule inflexibility Symptom-free progression in a sports-specific program	Normal clinical examination Normal shoulder mechanics Normal kinematic chain integration Completed sports-specific program Normal throwing motion

participate in sports, recreational activities, or work-related tasks in which high demands on the shoulder joint are expected. A training program that combines flexibility and strengthening exercises with neuromuscular as well as proprioceptive training should be ongoing. Patients with multidirectional instability need to work specifically on strengthening of the scapular stabilizers and balancing the force couples between the rotator cuff and the deltoid muscle.

Procedures

If the individual persists with some symptoms of pain secondary to rotator cuff irritation despite an appropriate rehabilitation program, a subacromial injection could be considered (Figs.13-5 and 13-6). The patient at that time should be reevaluated for identification of residual functional and biomechanical deficits that need to be addressed in combination with the injection. Under sterile conditions, with use of a 23- to 25-gauge, 1½-inch disposable needle, inject an anesthetic-corticosteroid preparation by an anterior, posterior, or lateral approach. Typically, 3 to 8 mL is injected (e.g., 4 mL of 1% lidocaine and 2 mL of 40 mg/mL triamcinolone). Alternatively, the lidocaine may be injected first, followed by the corticosteroid. Postinjection care includes local ice for 5 to 10 minutes. The patient is instructed to ice the shoulder for 15 to 20 minutes three or four times daily for the next few days and to avoid aggressive overhead activities for the following week.

Surgery

The treatment of an acute initial shoulder dislocation has traditionally consisted of a period of immobilization followed by rehabilitation and a gradual return to full activity. However, because of high rates of recurrent instability after conservative treatment in the active athletic population and, in particular, throwers, early surgical intervention is gaining acceptance.[25] Open repair of Bankart lesions has been the standard surgical intervention after traumatic instability, and it is still reported by some authors as the preferred method because of predictable results in regard to recurrence of dislocation and return to activity.[26] Early arthroscopic repair of the inferior labral defect associated with acute shoulder dislocation is becoming widespread because of an apparent reduction in postoperative morbidity that may allow the athlete an early return to function.[27,28]

In the individual with recurrent instability, surgical treatment may need to address abnormalities in the shoulder capsule, glenoid labrum, and rotator cuff. Surgical interventions include capsular procedures, such as the capsular shift and thermal capsulorrhaphy, and labral as well as rotator cuff procedures, such as débridement and repair.[29,30]

In many instances, these procedures need to be combined for optimal results in the patient, followed by an accelerated rehabilitation program with guidelines similar to those for the patient treated nonoperatively.[31]

POTENTIAL DISEASE COMPLICATIONS

Complications include recurrent instability with overhead activity, pain of the shoulder region, nerve damage, and weakness of the rotator cuff and scapular muscles. These tend to occur more commonly in patients with multidirectional atraumatic instability. Loss of function may include inability to lift overhead and loss of throwing velocity and accuracy. Recurrent episodes of instability in the older individual may also be related to the development of rotator cuff tears.[32]

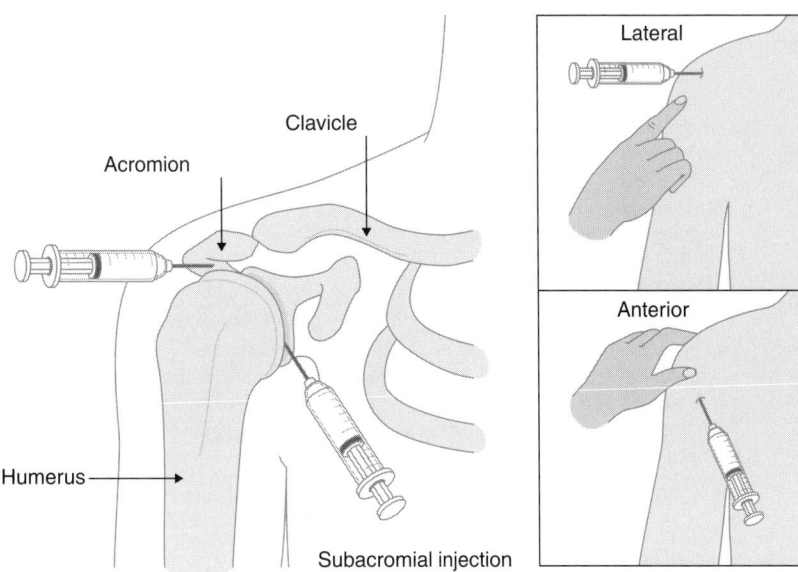

FIGURE 13-5. Approximate surface anatomy *(insets)* and internal anatomic sites for injection of the glenohumeral joint laterally and anteriorly. See also Figure 13-6. (Reprinted with permission from Lennard TA. Physiatric Procedures. Philadelphia, Hanley & Belfus, 1995.)

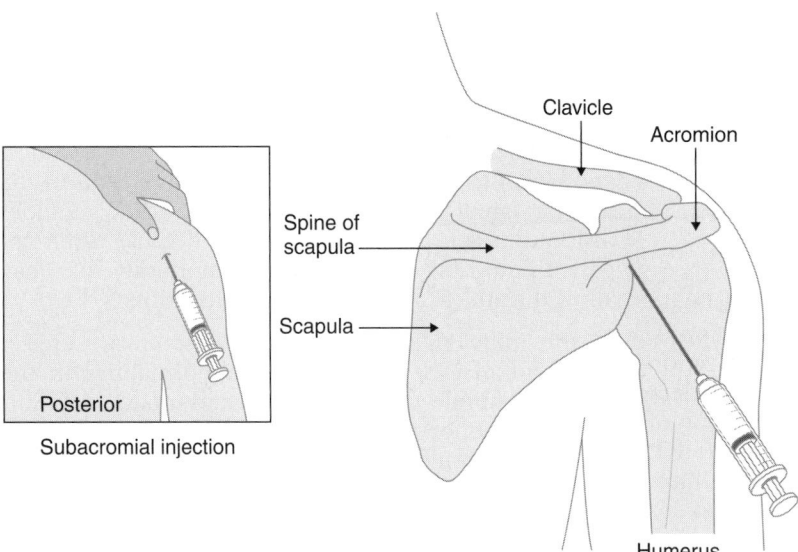

FIGURE 13-6. Posterior injection of the glenohumeral joint. (Reprinted with permission from Lennard TA. Physiatric Procedures. Philadelphia, Hanley & Belfus, 1995.)

POTENTIAL TREATMENT COMPLICATIONS

Complications of treatment include loss of motion, failure of surgical repair with recurrent instability, and inability to return to previous level of function. Failure of conservative treatment may be associated with incomplete rehabilitation or poor technique.

Recurrent dislocation after surgical treatment can be related to not addressing all the sites of pathologic change at the time of the operation.[33,34] Analgesics and non-steroidal anti-inflammatory drugs have well-known side effects that most commonly affect the gastric, hepatic, cardiovascular, and renal systems.

References

1. Speer KP. Anatomy and pathomechanics of shoulder instability. Clin Sports Med 1995;14:751-760.
2. Bahr R, Craig E, Engerbretsen L. The clinical presentation of shoulder instability including on-field management. Clin Sports Med 1995;14:761-776.
3. Takase K, Yamamoto K. Intraarticular lesions in traumatic anterior shoulder instability. Acta Orthop 2005;76:854-857.

4. Cordasco FA. Understanding multidirectional instability of the shoulder. J Athl Train 2000;35:278-285.

5. Loud KJ, Micheli LJ. Common athletic injuries in adolescent girls. Curr Opin Pediatr 2001;13:317-322.

6. Wasserlauf BL, Paletta GA Jr. Shoulder disorders in the skeletally immature throwing athlete. Orthop Clin North Am 2003;34:427-437.

7. Satterwhite YE. Evaluation and management of recurrent anterior shoulder instability. J Athl Train 2000;35:273-277.

8. Laurencin CT, O'Brien SJ. Anterior shoulder instability: anatomy, pathophysiology, and conservative management. In Andrews JR, Zarims B, Wilk K, eds. Injuries in Baseball. Philadelphia, Lippincott-Raven, 1998:189-197.

9. Myers JB, Laudner KG, Pasquale MR, et al. Glenohumeral range of motion deficits and posterior shoulder tightness in throwers with pathologic internal impingement. Am J Sports Med 2006;34:385-391.

10. Bowen JE, Malanga GA, Tutankhamen P, et al. Physical examination of the shoulder. In Malanga GA, Nadler SF, eds. Musculoskeletal Physical Examination: An Evidence-Based Approach. Philadelphia, Elsevier, 2006:59-118.

11. Pappas GP, Blemker SS, Beaulieu CF, et al. In vivo anatomy of the Neer and Hawkins sign positions for shoulder impingement. J Shoulder Elbow Surg 2006;15:40-49.

12. Farber AJ, Castillo R, Clough M, et al. Clinical assessment of three common tests for traumatic anterior shoulder instability. J Bone Joint Surg Am 2006;88:1467-1474.

13. Clarnette RC, Miniaci A. clinical exam of the shoulder. Med Sci Sports Exerc 1998;30(Suppl):1-6.

14. Meister K. Injuries to the shoulder in the throwing athlete. Part one: biomechanics/pathophysiology/classification of injury. Am J Sports Med 2000;28:265-275.

15. O'Brien SJ, Pagnani MJ, Fealy S, et al. The active compression test: a new and effective test for diagnosing labral tear and acromioclavicular joint abnormality. Am J Sports Med 1998;26:610-613.

16. Meister K. Injuries to the shoulder in the throwing athlete. Part two: evaluation/treatment. Am J Sports Med 2000;28:587-601.

17. Liu SH, Henry MH, Nuccion S, et al. Diagnosis of labral tears. A comparison between magnetic resonance imaging and clinical examinations. Am J Sports Med 1996;24:149-154.

18. Moosikasuwan JB, Miller TT, Dines DM. Imaging of the painful shoulder in throwing athletes. Clin Sports Med 2006;25:433-443.

19. Song HT, Huh YM, Kim S, et al. Antero-inferior labral lesions of recurrent shoulder dislocation evaluated by MR arthrography in an adduction internal rotation (ADIR) position. J Magn Reson Imaging 2006;23:29-35.

20. De Baere T, Delloye C. First-time traumatic anterior dislocation of the shoulder in young adults: the position of the arm during immobilization revisited. Acta Orthop Belg 2005;71:516-520.

21. Funk L, Smith M. Best evidence report. How to immobilize after shoulder dislocation? Emerg Med J 2005;22:814-815.

22. Handoll HH, Hanchard NC, Goodchild L, et al. Conservative management following closed reduction of traumatic anterior dislocation of the shoulder. Cochrane Database Syst Rev 2006;1:CD004962.

23. Cavallo RJ, Speer KP. Shoulder: instability and impingement in throwing athletes. Med Sci Sports Exerc 1998;30(Suppl):18-25.

24. Kibler WB, Livingston B, Bruce R. Current concepts in shoulder rehabilitation. Adv Oper Orthop 1995;3:249-300.

25. Myers JB, Lephart SM. The role of the sensorimotor system in the athletic shoulder. J Athl Train 2000;35:351-363.

26. Nelson BJ, Arciero RA. Arthroscopic management of glenohumeral instability. Am J Sports Med 2000;28:602-614.

27. Mohtadi NG, Bitar IJ, Sasyniuk TM, et al. Arthroscopic versus open repair for traumatic anterior shoulder instability: a meta-analysis. Arthroscopy 2005;21:652-658.

28. Carreira DS, Mazzocca AD, Oryhon J, et al. A prospective outcome evaluation of arthroscopic Bankart repairs: minimum 2 years follow-up. Am J Sports Med 2006;34:771-777.

29. Fabbriciani C, Milano G, Demontis A, et al. Arthroscopic versus open treatment of Bankart lesions of the shoulder: a prospective randomised study. Arthroscopy 2004;20:456-462.

30. Ticker JB, Warner JJP. Selective capsular shift technique for anterior and anterior-inferior glenohumeral instability. Clin Sports Med 2000;19:1-17.

31. Marquard B, Potzl W, Witt KA, et al. A modified capsular shift for atraumatic anterior-inferior shoulder instability. Am J Sports Med 2005;33:1011-1015.

32. Kim SH, Ha KI, Jung MW, et al. Accelerated rehabilitation after arthroscopic Bankart repair for selected cases: a prospective randomized clinical trial. Arthroscopy 2003;19:722-731.

33. Porcellini G, Paladini P, Campi F, et al. Shoulder instability and related rotator cuff tears: arthroscopic findings and treatment in patients aged 40 to 60 years. Arthroscopy 2006;22:270-276.

34. Tauber M, Resch H, Forstner R, et al. Reasons for failure after surgical repair of anterior shoulder instability. J Shoulder Elbow Surg 2004;13:279-285.

Rotator Cuff Tendinitis 14

Jay E. Bowen, DO, and Gerard A. Malanga, MD

DEFINITION

Rotator cuff tendinitis is a common phenomenon affecting both athletes and nonathletes. The muscles that compose the rotator cuff—the supraspinatus, infraspinatus, subscapularis, and teres minor—may become inflamed or impinged by the acromion, coracoacromial ligament, acromioclavicular joint, and coracoid process. Fibroblastic hyperplasia (tendinosis) may play a role as well. The supraspinatus tendon is the most commonly involved.

Rotator cuff tendinitis may result from a variety of factors. The tendon or its musculotendinous junction can be "squeezed" along its course from a relatively narrowed space. Tendinosis can be a result of degeneration from the aging process or from underlying subtle instability of the humeral head.

In chronic rotator cuff tendinitis, the muscles of the rotator cuff and surrounding scapulothoracic stabilizers may become weak by disuse. Under these conditions, the muscles can fatigue early, resulting in altered biomechanics. The humeral head moves excessively off the center of the glenoid, usually superiorly. From this abnormal motion, impingement of the rotator cuff occurs, causing inflammation of the tendon. With the passage of time, modifications of the acromion occur, resulting in osteophyte formation or "hooking" of the acromion (Fig. 14-1). With repeated superior migration and acromial changes, degeneration of the musculotendinous junction can lead to tearing of the rotator cuff (see Chapter 15). This is what many refer to as impingement or impingement syndrome. This particularly occurs during forward flexion when the anterior portion of the acromion impinges on the supraspinatus tendon.

With prolonged pain, adhesive capsulitis can develop from the lack of active motion (see Chapter 10).

SYMPTOMS

Patients normally present with pain in the posterolateral shoulder region and, often, deltoid muscle pain, which is referred from the shoulder. The pain is described as dull and achy and often occurs at night. Complaints occur with activities above the shoulder level, usually when the arm is abducted more than 90 degrees. Pain is also noted in movements involving eccentric contractions and from sleeping on the affected side. Rotator cuff tendinitis is common in persons with overhead activity requirements (e.g., swimmers, painters).

PHYSICAL EXAMINATION

The shoulder examination is approached systematically in every patient. It includes inspection, palpation, range of motion, muscle strength, and performance of special tests of the shoulder as clinically indicated.

The examination begins with observation of the patient during the history portion of the evaluation. The shoulder should be carefully inspected from the anterior, lateral, and posterior positions. Because shoulder pain is usually unilateral, comparison with the contralateral shoulder is often useful. Atrophy of the supraspinatus and infraspinatus muscles can be seen in massive rotator cuff tears as well as in entrapments of the suprascapular nerve. Scapular winging is rare in rotator cuff injuries; however, abnormalities of scapulothoracic motion are often present and should be addressed as part of the treatment plan.

Tenderness is often localized to the greater tuberosity, subacromial bursa, or long head of the biceps.

Total active and passive range of motion in all planes and scapulohumeral rhythm should be evaluated. Maximal total elevation occurs in the plane of the scapula, which lies approximately 30 degrees forward of the coronal plane. Patients with rotator cuff tears tend to have altered scapulothoracic motion during active shoulder elevation. Decreased active elevation with normal passive range of

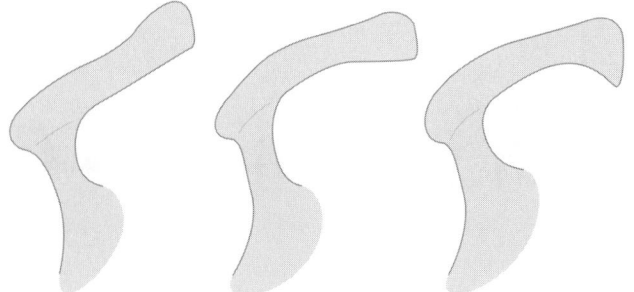

FIGURE 14-1. Types of acromial shape (lateral view).

motion is usually seen in rotator cuff tears secondary to pain and weakness. When both active and passive range of motion are similarly decreased, this usually suggests the onset of adhesive capsulitis. Glenohumeral internal rotation is assessed most accurately by abduction of the shoulder to 90 degrees and manual fixation of the scapula. From this point, the elbow is flexed to 90 degrees and the humerus is internally rotated. The impingement syndrome associated with rotator cuff injuries tends to cause pain with elevation between 60 and 120 degrees (painful arc), when the rotator cuff tendons are compressed against the anterior acromion and coracoacromial ligament.

Muscle strength testing should be done to isolate the relevant individual muscles. The anterior cuff (subscapularis) can be assessed by the lift-off test (see Chapter 13, Fig. 13-1), which is performed with the arm internally rotated behind the back. Lifting of the hand away from the back against resistance tests the strength of the subscapularis muscle. The posterior cuff (infraspinatus and teres minor) can be tested with the arm at the side and the elbow flexed to 90 degrees. Significant weakness in external rotation will be seen in large tears of the rotator cuff. The supraspinatus muscle is specifically tested by abduction of the patient's arm to 90 degrees, horizontal adduction to 20 to 30 degrees, and internal rotation of the arm to the thumbs down position. Testing of the scapula rotators, the trapezius, and the serratus anterior is also important. The serratus anterior can be tested by having the patient lean against a wall; winging of the scapula as the patient pushes against the wall indicates weakness.

Drop Arm Test

The clinician abducts the patient's shoulder to 90 degrees and then asks the patient to slowly lower the arm to the side in the same arc of movement. The test result is positive if the patient is unable to return the arm to the side slowly or has severe pain when attempting to do so. A positive result indicates a tear of the rotator cuff.

Impingement Sign

The shoulder is forcibly forward flexed with the humerus internally rotated, causing a jamming of the greater tuberosity against the anterior inferior surface of the acromion. Pain with this maneuver reflects a posi-

tive test result and indicates an overuse injury to the supraspinatus muscle and possibly to the biceps tendon (see Chapter 13, Fig. 13-2).

Apprehension Test

The arm is abducted 90 degrees and then fully externally rotated while an anteriorly directed force is placed on the posterior humeral head from behind. The patient will become apprehensive and resist further motion if chronic anterior instability is present (see Chapter 13, Fig. 13-3).

Relocation Test

Perform the apprehension test with the patient supine and the shoulder at the edge of the table (Fig. 14-2). A posteriorly directed force on the proximal humerus will cause resolution of the patient's symptoms of apprehension, which is another indicator of anterior instability (see Chapter 13, Fig. 13-4).

FUNCTIONAL LIMITATIONS

Patients with rotator cuff tendinitis complain of pain with overhead activities (e.g., throwing a baseball, painting a ceiling), greatest above 90 degrees of abduction. Pain may also occur with internal and external rotation and may affect daily self-care activities. Women typically have difficulty hooking the bra in back. Work activities such as filing, hammering overhead, and lifting can be affected. The patient can be awoken by pain in the shoulder, which impairs sleep.

DIAGNOSTIC STUDIES

In the event of trauma to the shoulder and complaints consistent with rotator cuff tendinitis, the clinician should obtain radiographs to avoid missing an occult fracture. The anteroposterior view with internal and external rotation is sufficient for screening. If dislocation is suspected, further views should be obtained, including West Point axillary, true anteroposterior, and Y views.

Magnetic resonance imaging is the study of choice when a patient is not progressing with conservative management or to rule out an alternative pathologic process (e.g., rotator cuff tear). In tendinitis, magnetic resonance imaging will demonstrate an increased signal within the substance of the tendon. Diagnostic arthroscopy is used in some cases but is generally not necessary.

Electrodiagnostic studies can be ordered to exclude alternative diagnoses as well (e.g., cervical radiculopathy).

Subacromial anesthetic injections (see Chapter 13, Figs. 13-5 and 13-6) have been discussed as diagnostic tools to assist in the confirmation of rotator cuff tendinitis. This procedure is not as important for diagnosis of tendinitis as it is for ruling out a tear. If the patient cannot provide good effort to abduction during the physical examination, the clinician can inject the anesthetic into the subacromial space. After the injection, if there is

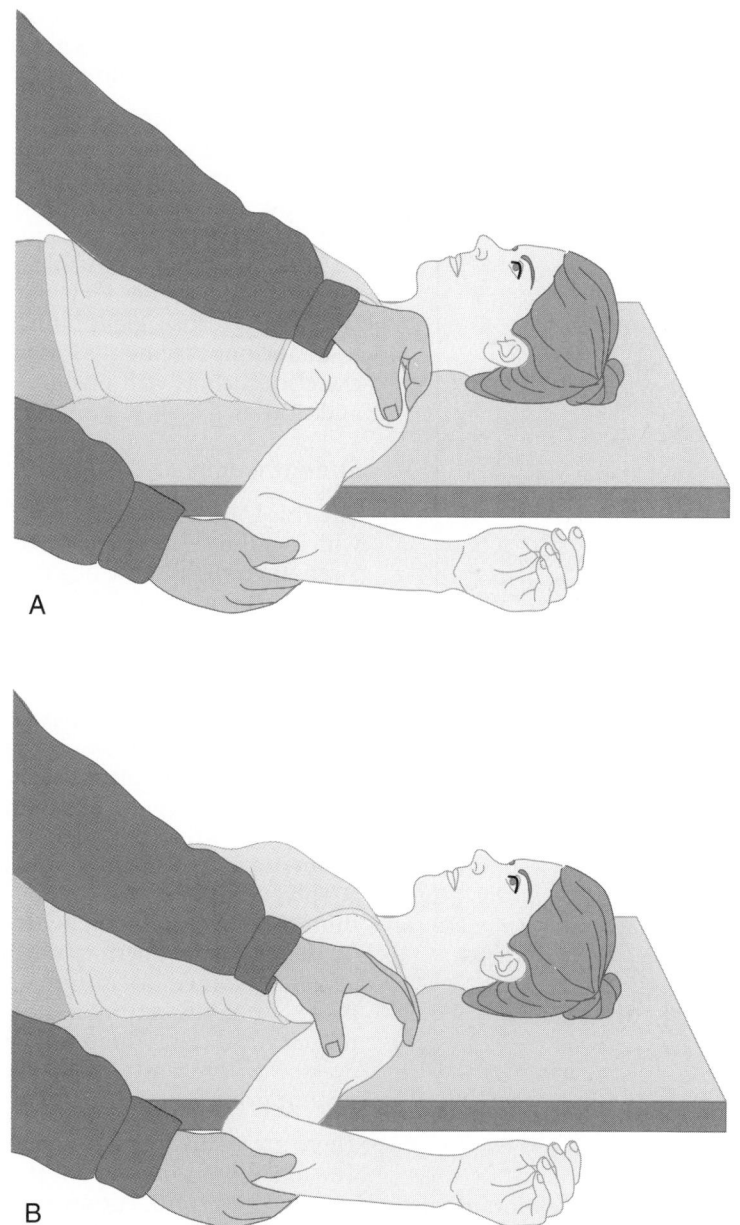

FIGURE 14-2. Relocation test. **A,** In certain shoulders, pain limits abduction and maximum external rotation. **B,** By the application of pressure on the anterior shoulder, the discomfort is eliminated and greater external rotation is noted.

significant reduction in the pain level and the patient can provide adequate and nearly maximal abduction, tendinitis is more likely than a rotator cuff tear.

TREATMENT

Initial

There are five basic phases of treatment (Table 14-1). These phases may overlap and can be progressed as rapidly as tolerated, but each should be performed to speed recovery and to prevent reinjury.

Initially, pain control and inflammation reduction are required to allow progression of healing and the initiation of an active rehabilitation program. This can be accom-

plished with a combination of relative rest from aggravating activities, icing (20 minutes three or four times a day), and electrical stimulation. Acetaminophen may help with pain control. Nonsteroidal anti-inflammatory drugs may be used to help control pain and inflammation.

Having the patient sleep with a pillow between the trunk and arm will decrease the tension on the supraspinatus tendon and prevent compromise of blood flow in its watershed region.

Rehabilitation

Physical therapy may also help with pain management. Initially, ultrasound to the posterior capsule followed by gentle, passive, prolonged stretch may be needed.

Differential Diagnosis

Rotator cuff tear

Glenolabral tear

Muscle strain

Subacromial bursitis

Bicipital tendinitis

Myofascial pain

Fracture

Acromioclavicular sprain

Tumor

Myofascial or vascular thoracic outlet syndrome

Cervical radiculopathy

Traumatic or atraumatic brachial plexus disease (e.g., Parsonage-Turner [acute brachial neuritis])

Suprascapular neuropathy

Thoracic outlet syndrome

TABLE 14-1 Treatment Phases for Rotator Cuff Tendinitis

Pain control and reduction of inflammation

Restoration of normal shoulder motion, both scapulothoracic and glenohumeral

Normalization of strength and dynamic muscle control

Proprioception and dynamic joint stabilization

Sport- or task-specific training

The use of ultrasound should be closely monitored to avoid heating of an inflamed tendon, which will worsen the situation.

Restoration of Shoulder Range of Motion

After the pain has been managed, restoration of shoulder motion can be initiated. The focus of treatment in this early stage is on improvement of range, flexibility of the posterior capsular, and postural biomechanics and restoration of normal scapular motion. Codman pendulum exercises, wall walking, stick or towel exercises, and a physical therapy program are useful in attaining full pain-free range. It is important to address any posterior capsular tightness because it can cause anterior and superior humeral head migration, resulting in impingement. A tight posterior capsule and the imbalance it causes force the humeral head anterior, producing shearing of the anterior labrum and causing additional injury. Stretching of the posterior capsule is a difficult task to isolate. The horizontal adduction that is usually performed tends to stretch the scapular stabilizers, not the posterior capsule.

However, stretching of the posterior capsule is possible if care is taken to fix and to stabilize the scapula, preventing stretching of the scapulothoracic stabilizers.

Postural biomechanics are important because with poor posture (e.g., excessive thoracic kyphosis and protracted shoulders), there is increased acromial space narrowing, resulting in greater risk for rotator cuff impingement. Restoration of normal scapular motion is also essential because the scapula is the platform on which the glenohumeral joint rotates.[1,2] Thus, an unstable scapula can secondarily cause glenohumeral joint instability and resultant impingement. Scapular stabilization includes exercises such as wall pushups and biofeedback (visual and tactile).

Strengthening

The third phase of treatment is muscle strengthening, which should be performed in a pain-free range. Strengthening should begin with the scapulothoracic stabilizers and the use of shoulder shrugs, rowing, and pushups, which will isolate these muscles and help return smooth motion, allowing normal rhythm between the scapula and the glenohumeral joint. This will also provide a firm base of support on which the arm can move. Attention is then turned to strengthening of the rotator cuff muscles. Positioning of the arm at 45 and 90 degrees of abduction for exercises prevents the "wringing out" phenomenon that hyperadduction can cause by stressing the tenuous blood supply to the tendon of the exercising muscle. The thumbs down position with the arm in more than 90 degrees of abduction and internal rotation should also be avoided to minimize subacromial impingement. After the scapular stabilizers and rotator cuff muscles are rehabilitated, the prime movers are addressed to prevent further injury and to facilitate return to prior function.

There are many ways by which to strengthen muscles. The rehabilitation program should start with static exercises and co-contractions, progress to concentric exercises, and be completed with eccentric exercises. A therapy prescription should include the number of repetitions, the number of sets, and the intensity at which the specific exercise should be performed. When strength is restored, a maintenance program should be continued for fitness and prevention of reinjury. Local muscle endurance should also be trained.

Proprioception

The fourth phase is proprioceptive training. This is important to retrain the neurologic control of the strengthened muscles, providing improved dynamic interaction and coupled execution of tasks for harmonious movement of the shoulder and arm. Tasks should begin with closed kinetic chain exercises to provide joint stabilizing forces. As the muscles are reeducated, exercises can progress to open chain activities that may be used in specific sports or tasks. In addition, proprioceptive neuromuscular facilitation is designed to stimulate muscle-tendon stretch receptors for reeducation.

Task or Sport Specific

The last phase of rehabilitation is to return to task- or sport-specific activities. This is an advanced form of training for the muscles to relearn prior activities. This is important and should be supervised so the task is performed correctly and to eliminate the possibility of reinjury or injury in another part of the kinetic chain from improper technique. The rehabilitation begins at a cognitive level but must be repeated so that it transitions to unconscious motor programming.

Procedures

A subacromial injection of anesthetic can be beneficial in differentiating a rotator cuff tear from tendinitis. Patients with pain that limits the validity of their strength testing may be able to provide almost full resistance to abduction and external rotation after the injection, suggesting rotator cuff tendinitis. On the other hand, if there is continued weakness, one must consider a rotator cuff tear.

Many clinicians include a corticosteroid with the anesthetic to avoid the need for a second injection. This procedure can be both diagnostic and therapeutic. If one makes the diagnosis of rotator cuff tendinitis, the corticosteroid injection will decrease the inflammation and allow accelerated rehabilitation.

Refer to the injection procedure in Chapter 13.

Surgery

Surgery should be considered if the patient fails to improve with a progressive nonoperative therapy program of 3 to 6 months. Surgical procedures may include subacromial decompression arthroscopically or, less commonly, open. At that time, the surgeon may débride the tendon and explore for other pathologic changes.

POTENTIAL DISEASE COMPLICATIONS

The greatest risk in not treating rotator cuff tendinitis is rupture or tear of a tendon or the development of a labral tear. As previously discussed, with prolonged impairment in motion and strength and subtle instability, hooking of the acromion can develop. Adhesive capsulitis may develop with chronic pain and decreased shoulder movement as well.

POTENTIAL TREATMENT COMPLICATIONS

There are minimal possible complications from nonoperative treatment of rotator cuff tendinitis. Because nonsteroidal anti-inflammatory drugs are used frequently, one must remain vigilant to their potential side effects (e.g., gastritis, ulcers, renal impairment, bronchospasm). Injections may cause rupture of the diseased tendon.

References

1. Andrews JR. Diagnosis and treatment of chronic painful shoulder: review of nonsurgical interventions. Arthoscopy 2005;21: 333-347.
2. Rees JD, Wilson AM, Wolman RL. Current concepts in the management of tendon disorders. Rheumatology (Oxford) 2006;45: 508-521.
3. Gross J, Fetto J, Rosen E. Musculoskeletal Examination. Massachusetts, Blackwell Science, 1996.
4. Smith L, Weiss E, Lehmkuh L. Brunnstrom's Clinical Kinesiology, 5th ed. Philadelphia, FA Davis, 1996.
5. Cailliet R. Shoulder Pain, 3rd ed. Philadelphia, FA Davis, 1991:42-46.
6. Malanga GA, Bowen JE, Nadler SF, Lee A. Nonoperative management of shoulder injuries. J Back Musculoskeletal Rehab 1999;12:179-189.
7. Hawkins RJ. Basic science and clinical application in the athlete's shoulder. Clin Sports Med 1991;10:955-971.
8. Poppen NK, Walker PS. Normal and abnormal motion of the shoulder. J Bone Joint Surg Am 1976;58:195-201.
9. Kibler WB. Role of the scapula in the overhead throwing motion. Contemp Orthop 1991;22:525-532.
10. DeLateur BI. Exercise for strength and endurance. In Basmajian JV, ed. Therapeutic Exercise, 4th ed. Baltimore, Williams & Wilkins, 1984.
11. Steindler A. Kinesiology of Human Body under Normal and Pathological Conditions. Springfield, Ill, Charles C Thomas, 1995.
12. Howell SM, Galinat BJ. The glenoid-labral socket—a constrained articular surface. Clin Orthop 1989;243:122-125.
13. Steinbeck J, Liljenqvist U, Jerosch J. The anatomy of the glenohumeral ligamentous complex and its contribution to anterior shoulder stability. J Shoulder Elbow Surg 1998;7:122-126.
14. Inman VT, Saunders JB, Abbott LC. Observations of the function of the shoulder. J Bone Joint Surg 1944;26:1-30.
15. Saha AK. Dynamic stability of the glenohumeral joint. Acta Orthop Scand 1971;42:491.
16. Wuelker N, Korell M, Thren K. Dynamic glenohumeral joint stability. J Shoulder Elbow Surg 1998;7:43-52.
17. Ozaki J, Fujimoto S, Nakagawa Y, et al. Tears of the rotator cuff of the shoulder associated with pathologic changes in the acromion: a study in cadavers. J Bone Joint Surg Br 1988;70:1224-1230.
18. Codman EA. The Shoulder: Rupture of The Supraspinatus Tendon and Other Lesions in or About the Subacromial Bursa. Boston, Thomas Todd, 1934.
19. Rathbun JB, Macnab I. The microvascular pattern of the rotator cuff of the shoulder. J Bone Joint Surg Br 1970;52:540.
20. Lohr JF, Uhthoff HK. The microvascular pattern of the supraspinatus tendon. Clin Orthop Relat Res 1990;254:35-38.
21. Swiontkowski M, Iannotti JP, Esterhai JL, et al. Intraoperative assessment of rotator cuff vascularity using laser Doppler flowmetry. Presented at the 56th annual meeting of the American Academy of Orthopaedic Surgeons; Las Vegas, Nev; Feb 10, 1989.
22. Biglianni LU, Morrison D, April EW. The morphology of the acromion and its relationship to rotator cuff tears. Orthop Trans 1986;10:228.
23. Neer CS. Anterior acromioplasty for the chronic impingement syndrome in the shoulder: a preliminary report. J Bone Joint Surg Am 1972;54:41-50.
24. Flatow E, Soslowsky L, Ticker J, et al. Excursion of the rotator cuff under the acromion: patterns of subacromial contact. Am J Sports Med 1994;22:779-787.
25. Brems JJ. Management of atraumatic instability: techniques and results. Instructional Course Lecture 179. American Academy of Orthopaedic Surgeons annual meeting; Atlanta, Ga; Feb 26, 1996.
26. Yoneda B, Welsh R. Conservative treatment of shoulder dislocation in young males. J Bone Joint Surg Br 1982;64:254-255.
27. Burkhead WZ Jr, Rockwood CA Jr. Treatment of instability of the shoulder with an exercise program. J Bone Joint Surg Am 1992;74:890-896.
28. Rockwood CA, Matsen FA. The Shoulder. Philadelphia, WB Saunders, 1990.

29. Nicholas JA, Hershman EB. The Upper Extremity in Sports Medicine. St. Louis, Mosby, 1990.

30. Reid DC. Sports Injury Assessment and Rehabilitation. New York, Churchill Livingstone, 1992.

31. Simonet WT, Cofield RH. Prognosis in anterior shoulder dislocation. Am J Sports Med 1984;12:19-24.

32. Plancher KD, Litchfield R, Hawkins RJ. Rehabilitation of the shoulder in tennis players. Clin Sports Med 1995;14: 116-118.

33. Dines DM, Levinson M. The conservative management of the unstable shoulder including rehabilitation. Clin Sports Med 1995;14:799-813.

34. Harryman DT, Sidles JA, Clark JM, et al. Translation of the humeral head on the glenoid with passive glenohumeral motion. J Bone Joint Surg Am 1990;72:1334-1343.

35. Kibler WB, Chandler TJ. Functional scapular instability in throwing athletes. Presented at the 15th annual meeting of the American Orthopaedic Society for Sports Medicine; Traverse City, Mich; June 19-22, 1989.

36. Borsa PA, Lephart SM, Kocher MS, Lephart SP. Functional assessment and rehabilitation of shoulder proprioception for the glenohumeral instability. J Sports Rehab 1994;3:84-104.

37. Janda DH, Loubert P. A preventive program focusing on the glenohumeral joint. Clin Sports Med 1991;10:955-971.

38. Kabat H. Proprioception facilitation in therapeutic exercise. In Kendall HD, ed. Therapeutic Exercises. Baltimore, Waverly Press, 1965:327-343.

39. Malanga GA, Jenp Y, Growney E, An K. EMG analysis of shoulder positioning in testing and strengthening the supraspinatus. Med Sci Sports Exerc 1996;28:661-664.

40. Jenp Y, Malanga GA, Growney E, An K. Activation of the rotator cuff in generating isometric shoulder rotation torque. Am J Sports Med 1996;24:477-485.

41. Wang JC, Shapiro MS. Changes in acromial morphology with age. J Shoulder Elbow Surg 1997;6:55-59.

42. Cordasco FA, Wolfe IN, Wootten ME, Bigliani LU. An electromyographic analysis of the shoulder during a medicine ball rehabilitation program. Am J Sports Med 1996;24:386-392.

43. Blasier RB, Carpenter JE, Huston LJ. Shoulder proprioception: effect of joint laxity, joint position, and direction of motion. Orthop Rev 1994;23:45-50.

44. Basmajian J. Muscles Alive: Their Functions Revealed by Electromyography, 5th ed. Philadelphia, Williams & Wilkins, 1985.

45. Andrews JR. Diagnosis and treatment of chronic painful shoulder: review of nonsurgical interventions. Arthroscopy 2005;21:333-347.

46. Rees JD, Wilson AM, Wolman RL. Current concepts in the management of tendon disorders. Rheumatology (Oxford) 2006;45: 508-521.

Rotator Cuff Tear 15

Gerard A. Malanga, MD, and Jay E. Bowen, DO

Synonyms

Shoulder tear
Torn shoulder

ICD-9 Codes

726.10   Rotator cuff syndrome
727.61   Nontraumatic complete rupture of rotator cuff
840.4   Rotator cuff sprain

DEFINITION

The rotator cuff has three main functions in the shoulder. It compresses the humeral head into the fossa, increases joint contact pressure, and centers the humeral head on the glenoid. Three types of tears can occur to the rotator cuff. A full-thickness tear can be massive and cause immediate functional impairments. Another type of tear, a partial-thickness tear, can be broken down into a tear on the superior surface into the subacromial space or a tear on the inferior surface on the articular side. As a result of a rotator cuff tear, the humeral head will be displaced superiorly during abduction because of the unopposed action of the deltoid. These tears can be either traumatic or degenerative[1-7] (Figs. 15-1 to 15-3).

Traumatic tears occur in the younger population of athletes and laborers, whereas degenerative tears occur in older individuals. One reason that rotator cuff tears are more common in men is because there are more male heavy laborers. The incidence of degenerative tears is increased for both sexes older than 35 years and for those with chronic impingement syndrome, repetitive microtrauma, tendon degeneration, and hypovascularity.[4,6,8]

SYMPTOMS

Symptoms are similar to those of rotator cuff tendinitis. Pain is referred to the lateral triceps and sometimes more globally in the shoulder. There is often coexisting inflammation, and the pain quality is dull and achy. Weakness occurs because of the pain, which is caused by the impaired motion or the tear itself. Persons have difficulty with overhead activities. Patients may report pain at night in a side-lying position.

PHYSICAL EXAMINATION

Examination is essentially the same as for rotator cuff tendinitis. The most common physical findings of a tear are supraspinatus weakness, external rotator weakness, and impingement. The arm drop test may demonstrate greater weakness than expected from an inflamed, intact tendon, although one can be easily fooled. As with rotator cuff tendinitis, an anesthetic injection into the subacromial space may help discern tear. Even though the pain may be improved or resolved from the injection, resisted abduction will be just as weak because the torn tendon cannot withstand the stress.[9]

Remember to examine the cervical spine to avoid missing underlying pathologic changes. A rotator cuff tear develops in some individuals as a result of a radiculopathy or other nerve impairment. The dysfunction of the shoulder from a radiculopathy or suprascapular neuropathy results in weakness of the rotator cuff or the scapular stabilizers. This dysrhythmia causes impingement of the tendons with other structures and eventually leads to fraying and tearing.[10-12]

FUNCTIONAL LIMITATIONS

The greatest limitation that patients complain of is performing overhead activities.[2,7,13-15]

Patients with rotator cuff tendinitis complain of difficulty with overhead activities (e.g., throwing a baseball, painting a ceiling), greatest above 90 degrees of abduction, secondary to pain or weakness. Internal and external rotation may be compromised and may affect daily self-care activities. Women typically have difficulty hooking the bra in back. Work activities, such as filing, hammering overhead, and lifting, will be affected. The patient can be awaken by pain in the shoulder, which impairs his or her sleep.

Posterior view

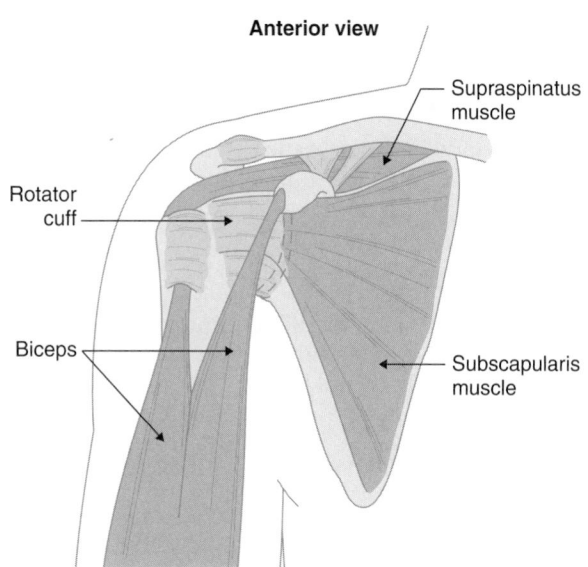

Anterior view

FIGURE 15-1. Muscles of the rotator cuff, posterior *(top)* and anterior *(bottom)* views. (Reprinted with permission from Snider RK. Essentials of Musculoskeletal Care. Rosemont, Ill, American Academy of Orthopaedic Surgeons, 1997.)

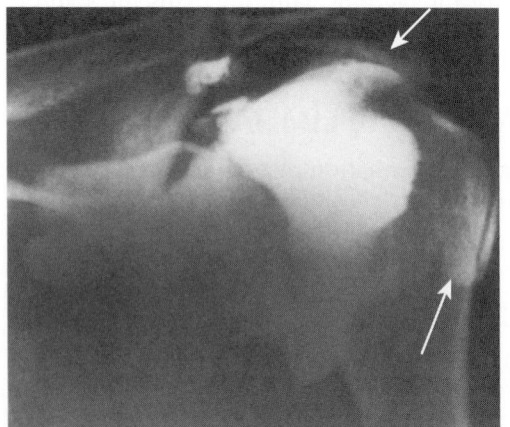

FIGURE 15-2. Rotator cuff tear with extension of contrast material into the subacromial *(short arrow)* and subdeltoid *(long arrow)* bursae. (Reprinted with permission from West SG. Rheumatology Secrets. Philadelphia, Hanley & Belfus, 1997:373.)

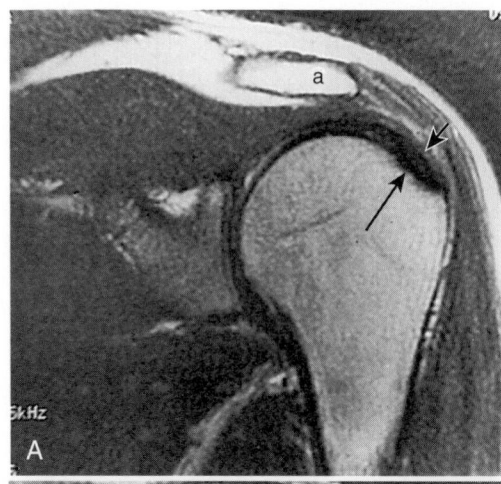

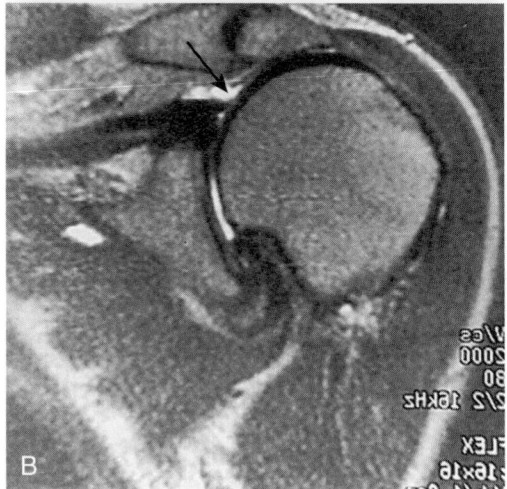

FIGURE 15-3. A, Normal shoulder MRI. The supraspinatus tendon is uniformly low signal and continuous *(arrows).* The space between the humeral head and the acromion (a) is maintained. **B,** Chronic rotator cuff tear. The supraspinatus tendon is completely torn and retracted to the level of the glenohumeral joint *(arrow),* where it is surrounded by fluid. Note the high-riding humeral head, close to the acromion. This is due to the atrophy of the cuff muscles associated with chronic tendon tears.

DIAGNOSTIC STUDIES

The diagnosis of a rotator cuff tear depends mostly on the history and physical examination. However, imaging studies may be used to confirm the clinician's diagnosis and to eliminate other possible pathologic processes.

Radiographs are often obtained to rule out any osseous problem. A tear can be inferred if there is evidence of humeral head upward migration or sclerotic changes at the greater tuberosity where the tendons insert. Radiographs are helpful with active 90-degree abduction showing a decreased acromiohumeral distance secondary to absence of the supraspinatus and unopposed action of the deltoid.

Magnetic resonance imaging (MRI) of the shoulder is the "gold standard."[16] Computed tomographic scans show osseous structures better but are less effective at demonstrating a soft tissue injury. By evaluation of the amount of retraction, the clinician is also better able to predict the course of recovery.

As in the evaluation of a person with rotator cuff tendinitis, an anesthetic injection can be performed to differentiate a tear from tendinitis.

Shoulder arthrography is performed less often since the advent of MRI. Arthrography involves injection of contrast material into the glenohumeral joint followed by plain radiography. Dye should remain contained in the joint space. If it extravasates, this signifies a tear. Partial-thickness rotator cuff tears can be missed, especially tears on the superior surface. Some centers have been combining gadolinium dye injections with MRI. This is used mostly to identify a labral tear, not a rotator cuff tear.

Ultrasound imaging can also be used in the diagnosis of full-thickness rotator cuff tears.[17] Ultrasonography is becoming more popular in the United States, and it can be a very helpful study when it is performed in centers with clinicians who have experience in musculoskeletal ultrasound imaging. It is now believed that ultrasonography is as accurate as MRI in the diagnosis of supraspinatus tendon tears. Full-thickness tears appear hypoechoic or anechoic where fluid has replaced the area of torn tendon. Manual compression will be able to displace the fluid. In an area of torn tendon without fluid, compression will show the "sagging peribursal fat" sign.[4,6,8,9,12,13,18,19]

Diagnostic arthroscopy is done in some instances but is not generally necessary.

Differential Diagnosis

Non-neurologic
Rotator cuff tendinitis

Glenolabral tear

Acromioclavicular sprain

Occult fracture

Osteoarthritis

Rheumatoid arthritis

Adhesive capsulitis

Myofascial pain syndrome

Myofascial thoracic outlet syndrome

Neurologic
Cervical radiculopathy

Brachial plexopathy

Suprascapular neuropathy

Neurogenic (true) thoracic outlet syndrome

TREATMENT

Initial

Initial treatment of a rotator cuff tear is similar to that of rotator cuff tendinitis as previously discussed (see Chapter 14). However, if the symptoms do not respond to a rehabilitation program, the clinician should consider surgical consultation earlier in the course of injury.

Rehabilitation

Because of the interrelationship of instability and impingement previously discussed, there is a great deal of overlap in the rehabilitation of these shoulder problems. Treatment must be individualized and based on the restoration of optimal *function*, not merely based on surgical correction of anatomic changes. Supervised physical therapy is the mainstay of treatment and is successful in most patients.

The basic phases of rehabilitation include the following[12]: pain control and reduction of inflammation; restoration of normal shoulder motion, both scapulothoracic and glenohumeral; normalization of strength and dynamic joint stabilization; proprioception and dynamic joint stabilization; and sport-specific training. The rehabilitation phases may overlap and can be progressed as rapidly as tolerated, but all should be performed to speed recovery and to prevent reinjury.

Pain Control and Reduction of Inflammation

Initially, pain control and inflammation reduction are required to allow progression of healing and the initiation of an active rehabilitation program. These can be accomplished with a combination of relative rest, icing (20 minutes, three or four times a day), electrical stimulation, and acetaminophen or a nonsteroidal anti-inflammatory drug. The next section's rehabilitation program can be added as tolerated by the patient. Having the patient sleep with a pillow between the trunk and the arm will decrease the tension on the supraspinatus tendon and prevent compromise of blood flow in its watershed region.

Restoration of Shoulder Range of Motion

As with all musculoskeletal disorders, the entire body must be taken into consideration. Abnormalities in the kinetic chain can also affect the shoulder. If there are restrictions or limitations in range of motion or strength, the forces will be transmitted to other portions of the kinetic chain, resulting in an overload of those tissues and possibly injury.

After the pain has been managed, restoration of motion can be initiated. The use of Codman pendulum exercises, wall walking, stick or towel exercises, or a physical therapy program is beneficial in attaining full pain-free range. It is important to address any posterior capsular tightness because this can cause anterior and superior humeral head migration, resulting in impingement. A tight posterior capsule and the imbalance it causes force the humeral head anteriorly, producing shearing of the anterior labrum and causing an additional injury. Stretching of the posterior capsule is a difficult task. The horizontal adduction that is usually performed tends to stretch the scapular stabilizers rather than the posterior capsule. If care is taken to fix and to stabilize the scapula and therefore to prevent the stretching of the scapulo-thoracic stabilizers, stretching of the posterior capsule can be achieved. The focus of treatment in this early stage should be on improving range and flexibility of the posterior capsule, improving postural biomechanics, and restoring normal scapular motion.

Initially, ultrasound to the posterior capsule followed by gentle, passive prolonged stretch may be needed. The use of ultrasound should be closely monitored to prevent heating of an inflamed tendon, which will worsen the injury.

Postural biomechanics are important because with poor posture (e.g., excessive thoracic kyphosis and protracted shoulders), there is increased outlet narrowing, resulting in greater risk for rotator cuff impingement. Restoration of normal scapular motion is also essential because the scapula is the platform on which the glenohumeral joint rotates.[20,21] Thus, an unstable scapula can secondarily cause glenohumeral joint instability and resultant impingement. Scapular stabilization includes exercises such as wall pushups and biofeedback (visual and tactile).

Strengthening

The third phase of treatment is strengthening, and it should be performed in a pain-free range. Strengthening should begin with the scapulothoracic stabilizers and the use of shoulder shrugs, rowing, and pushups, which will isolate these muscles and help return smooth motion, allowing normal rhythm between the scapula and the glenohumeral joint. This will also provide a firm base of support on which the arm can move. Attention should then be turned toward strengthening of the rotator cuff muscles. Positioning of the arm at 45 and 90 degrees of abduction for exercises prevents the "wringing out" phenomenon that hyperadduction can cause by stressing the tenuous blood supply to the tendon of the exercising muscle. The "thumbs-down" position with the arm in greater than 90 degrees of abduction and internal rotation should also be avoided to minimize subacromial impingement. After the scapular stabilizers and rotator cuff muscles are rehabilitated, the prime movers should be addressed to prevent further injury and to facilitate return to prior function.

There are many ways by which to strengthen muscles. The rehabilitation program should start with static contractions and co-contractions, progress to concentric exercises, and be completed with eccentric exercises and endurance training. The BodyBlade can be used for co-contraction in multiple planes and positions for rhythmic stabilization. There are many techniques to strengthen muscles, including static and dynamic exercises. A therapy prescription should include the number of repetitions, the number of sets of repetitions, and the intensity at which the specific exercise should be performed. When

strength is restored, a maintenance program should be continued for fitness and prevention of reinjury.

Proprioception

The fourth phase is proprioceptive training. This is important to retrain the neurologic control of the strengthened muscles in providing improved dynamic interaction and coupled execution of tasks for harmonious movement of the shoulder and arm. Tasks should begin with closed kinetic chain exercises to provide joint stabilizing forces. As the muscles are reeducated, exercises can progress to open chain activities that may be used in specific sports or tasks. Exercises such as those using the Body-Blade or plyometrics will also address proprioception. In addition, proprioceptive neuromuscular facilitation is designed to stimulate muscle-tendon stretch receptors for reeducation. Kabat[22] has described shoulder proprioceptive neuromuscular facilitation techniques in detail.

Task or Sport Specific

The last phase of rehabilitation is to return to task- or sport-specific activities. This is an advanced form of training for the muscles to relearn prior activities. This is important and should be supervised so that the task performed is correct and to eliminate the possibility of reinjury or injury in another part of the kinetic chain from improper technique. The rehabilitation begins at a cognitive level but must be practiced so that it ultimately becomes part of unconscious motor programming.

Procedures

Subacromial injections of anesthetic and corticosteroid may be both diagnostic and therapeutic (see Chapter 14).

Surgery

If the patient's condition has not progressed with a conservative rehabilitation after 2 to 3 months, a surgical consultation should be considered. If the patient is unable to perform all the activities he or she demands (vocationally and avocationally) after 6 months of treatment and independent exercise performance, a surgical consultation should be obtained. If the patient is a high-level athlete or worker, earlier consultation may be appropriate. The population of younger patients is more amenable to surgical intervention.[6,8]

If surgery is contemplated, repair, débridement, decompression, or a combination of these may be considered. A concomitant injury should be considered, such as a labral tear. The detail of these surgical procedures is beyond the scope of this text.

POTENTIAL DISEASE COMPLICATIONS

Partial rotator cuff tears can progress to full-thickness tears, especially if untreated. Rehabilitation attempts to restore biomechanics close to normal to prevent excessive wear on the tendon, which can cause further degeneration. Chronic untreated rotator cuff tears can lead to shoulder arthropathy.[6,11]

POTENTIAL TREATMENT COMPLICATIONS

Analgesics and nonsteroidal anti-inflammatory drugs have well-known side effects that most commonly affect the gastric, hepatic, and renal systems. There are minimal disadvantages to coordinating a rehabilitation program that may improve the patient's symptoms to a level at which the patient is satisfied and functional. However, an overly aggressive program can progress a partial tear to a complete tear. As for surgery, in general, the potential problems include bleeding, infection, worsening of the complaints, and nerve injury.

References

1. Biglianni LU, Morrison D, April EW. The morphology of the acromion and its relationship to rotator cuff tears. Orthop Trans 1986;10:228.
2. Codman EA. The Shoulder: Rupture of the Supraspinatus Tendon and Other Lesions in or About the Subacromial Bursa. Boston, Thomas Todd, 1934.
3. Flatow E, Soslowsky L, Ticker J, et al. Excursion of the rotator cuff under the acromion: patterns of subacromial contact. Am J Sports Med 1994;22:779-787.
4. Hawkins RJ. Basic science and clinical application in the athlete's shoulder. Clin Sports Med 1991;10:693-971.
5. Neer CS. Anterior acromioplasty for the chronic impingement syndrome in the shoulder. A preliminary report. J Bone Joint Surg Am 1972;54:41-50.
6. Rockwood CA, Matsen FA. The Shoulder. Philadelphia, WB Saunders, 2004:795-871.
7. Ozaki J, Fujimoto S, Nakagawa Y, et al. Tears of the rotator cuff of the shoulder associated with pathologic changes in the acromion: a study in cadavers. J Bone Joint Surg Am 1988;70:1224-1230.
8. Reid DC. Sports Injury Assessment and Rehabilitation. New York, Churchill Livingstone, 1992.
9. Gross J, Fetto J, Rosen E. Musculoskeletal Examination. Boston, Blackwell Science, 1996.
10. Basmajian J. Muscles Alive: Their Functions Revealed by Electromyography, 5th ed. Philadelphia, Williams & Wilkins, 1985.
11. Kibler WB. Role of the scapula in the overhead throwing motion. Contemp Orthop 1991;22:525-532.
12. Malanga GA, Bowen JE, Nadler SF, Lee A. Nonoperative management of shoulder injuries. J Back Musculoskelet Rehab 1999;12:179-189.
13. Dines DM, Levinson M. The conservative management of the unstable shoulder including rehabilitation. Clin Sports Med 1995;14:799-813.
14. Harryman DT, Sidles JA, Clark JM, et al. Translation of the humeral head on the glenoid with passive glenohumeral motion. J Bone Joint Surg Am 1990;72:1334-1343.
15. Steinbeck J, Liljenqvist U, Jerosch J. The anatomy of the glenohumeral ligamentous complex and its contribution to anterior shoulder stability. J Shoulder Elbow Surg 1998;7:122-126.
16. Chaipat L, Palmer WE. Shoulder magnetic resonance imaging. Clin Sports Med 2006;25:371-386.
17. Moosikasuwan JB, Miller TT, Burke BJ. Rotator cuff tears: clinical, radiographic, and US findings. Radiographics 2005;25:1591-1607.
18. Cailliet R. Shoulder Pain, 3rd ed. Philadelphia, FA Davis, 1991:42-46.
19. Nicholas JA, Hershman EB. The Upper Extremity in Sports Medicine, 2nd ed. St. Louis, Mosby, 1996:209-222.
20. Kibler WB, Chandler TJ. Functional scapular instability in throwing athletes. Presented at the 15th annual meeting of the American Orthopaedic Society for Sports Medicine; Traverse City, Mich; June 19-22, 1989.
21. Nuber GW, Jobe FW, Perry J, et al. Fine wire electromyography analysis of the shoulder during swimming. Am J Sports Med 1985;13:216-222.
22. Kabat H. Proprioception facilitation in therapeutic exercise. In Kendall HD, ed. Therapeutic Exercises. Baltimore, Waverly Press, 1965:327-343.

Scapular Winging 16

Peter M. McIntosh, MD

Synonyms

Scapulothoracic winging
Long thoracic nerve palsy
Spinal accessory nerve palsy
Scapula alata
Alar scapula
Rucksack palsy

ICD-9 Codes

352.4   Spinal accessory nerve disorder
353.3   Neuropathy long thoracic
353.5   Neuralgic amyotrophy
354.9   Mononeuritis of upper limb, unspecified
723.4   Cervical radiculopathy NOS
724.4   Long thoracic nerve entrapment
728.87   Muscle weakness NOS

DEFINITION

Scapular winging refers to prominence of the vertebral (medial) border of the scapula.[1] The inferomedial border can also be rotated or displaced away from the chest wall. This well-defined medical sign was first described by Velpeau[2] in 1837. It is associated with a wide array of medical conditions or injuries that typically result in dysfunction of the scapular stabilizers and rotators and, ultimately, glenohumeral and scapulothoracic biomechanics.

Fiddian and King[1] classified scapular winging as either static or dynamic after examination of 25 patients with 23 different causes of scapular winging. Static winging is attributable to a fixed deformity in the shoulder girdle, spine, or ribs; it is characteristically present with the patient's arms at the sides. Dynamic winging is ascribed to a neuromuscular disorder; it is produced by active or resisted movement and is usually absent at rest. Scapular winging has also been classified anatomically according to whether the etiology of the lesion is related to nerve, muscle, bone, or joint disease (Table 16-1).

The scapula is a triangular bone that is completely surrounded by muscles and attaches to the clavicle by the coracoclavicular ligaments and acromioclavicular joint capsule. Motion of the scapula along the chest wall occurs through the action of the muscle groups that originate or insert on the scapula and proximal humerus. These muscles include the rhomboids (major and minor), trapezius, serratus anterior, levator scapulae, and pectoralis minor. The rotator cuff and deltoid muscles are involved with glenohumeral motion. Innervation of these muscle groups includes all the roots of the brachial plexus and several peripheral nerves. Scapular winging may be caused by brachial plexus injuries but most often is related to a peripheral nerve injury (see Table 16-1).

Injury to the long thoracic and spinal accessory nerves with weakness of the serratus anterior and trapezius muscles, respectively, is most commonly associated with scapular winging. The serratus anterior muscle originates on the outer surface and superior border of the upper eight or nine ribs and inserts on the costal surface of the medial border of the scapula. It abducts the scapula and rotates it so the glenoid cavity faces cranially and holds the medial border of the scapula against the thorax.

The serratus anterior muscle is innervated by the pure motor long thoracic nerve, which arises from the ventral rami of the fifth, sixth, and seventh cervical roots. The nerve passes through the scalenus medius muscle, beneath the brachial plexus and the clavicle, and over the first rib. It then runs superficially along the lateral aspect of the chest wall to supply all the digitations of the serratus anterior muscles.[34] Because of its long and superficial course, the long thoracic nerve is susceptible to both traumatic and nontraumatic injuries (Fig. 16-1).

The trapezius muscle consists of upper, middle, and lower fibers. The upper fibers originate from the external occipital protuberance, superior nuchal line, nuchal ligament, and spinous process of the seventh cervical vertebra and insert on the lateral clavicle and acromion. The middle fibers arise from the spinous process of the first through fifth thoracic vertebrae and insert on the superior lip of the scapular spine. The lower fibers originate from the spinous process of the sixth through twelfth thoracic vertebrae and insert on the apex of the scapular spine. They are innervated by the pure motor spinal accessory nerve (cranial nerve XI) and afferent

83

TABLE 16-1 Etiology of Scapular Winging

Characteristic	Nerve	Muscle	Bone	Joint
Site of lesion	LTN SAN DSN[3] C5-7 nerve root lesion[4,5] Brachial plexus lesion[6]	SA T R	Scapula Clavicle Spine Ribs	GHJ ACJ
Traumatic	Acute, repetitive, or chronic compression of LTN, SAN, DSN Trauma or traction injury to LTN, nerve roots, brachial plexus[7] Whiplash injury[8]	Direct muscle injury to SA, T, R[3,9,10] Avulsion of SA, T, R[11] RTC disease Sports-related injury[12-16]	Nonunion Malunion Fractures of scapula,[17] clavicle, acromion	Glenoid fracture ACJ dislocation Shoulder instability
Congenital, hereditary	Cerebral palsy	Congenital contracture of infraspinatus muscle[18] Agenesis of SA, T, R Duchenne muscular dystrophy FSHD[19-21] Fibrous bands (deltoid)	Scoliosis Craniocleidodysostosis Ollier disease Sprengel deformity	Arthrogryposis multiplex congenita Congenital posterior shoulder dislocation
Degenerative, inflammatory	SLE[22] Neuritis Amyotrophic brachial neuralgia[3]	Toxin exposure Infection Myositis		Abduction-internal rotation contracture[23] from AVN of humeral head Arthropathy
Iatrogenic	Epidural or general anesthesia[24] Radical neck dissection[25] Lymph node biopsy First rib resection[26] Radical mastectomy Posterolateral thoracotomy incision Axillary node dissection	Postinjection fibrosis (deltoid) Division of SA		
Miscellaneous	Vaginal delivery[27] Cervical syringomyelia[28]	Chiropractic manipulation Electrocution[29]	Scapulothoracic bursa Enchondroma Subscapular osteochondroma[30-32] Exostoses of rib or scapula[33]	Voluntary posterior shoulder subluxation

ACJ, acromioclavicular joint; AVN, avascular necrosis; DSN, dorsal scapular nerve; FSHD, facioscapulohumeral muscular dystrophy; GHJ, glenohumeral joint; LTN, long thoracic nerve; R, rhomboid muscles; RTC, rotator cuff muscles; SA, serratus anterior muscle; SAN, spinal accessory nerve; SLE, systemic lupus erythematosus; T, trapezius muscle.
With permission from Fiddian NJ, King RJ. The winged scapula. Clin Orthop Relat Res 1984;185:228-236.

fibers from the second through fourth cervical spinal nerves. The root fibers unite to form a common trunk that ascends to enter the intracranial cavity through the foramen magnum. It exits with the vagus nerve through the jugular foramen, pierces the sternocleidomastoid muscle, and descends obliquely across the floor of the posterior triangle of the neck to the trapezius muscle.[34] In the posterior triangle, the nerve lies superficially, covered only by fascia and skin, and is susceptible to injury. Cadaver studies have shown considerable variations in the course and distribution of the spinal accessory nerve in the posterior triangle and in the nerve's relationship to the borders of the sternocleidomastoid and trapezius muscles.[35] The trapezius muscle adducts the scapula (middle fibers), rotates the glenoid cavity upward (upper and lower fibers), and elevates and depresses the scapula. Overall, the trapezius muscles maintain efficient shoulder function by both supporting the shoulder and stabilizing the scapulae (Fig. 16-2).

A rare cause of scapular winging is dorsal scapular nerve palsy. The dorsal scapular nerve is a pure motor nerve from the fifth cervical spinal nerve that supplies the rhomboid and levator scapulae muscles. It arises above the upper trunk of the brachial plexus and passes through the middle scalene muscle on its way to the levator scapulae and rhomboids. The rhomboids (major and minor) adduct and elevate the scapula and rotate it so the glenoid cavity faces caudally.

The levator scapulae muscles originate on the transverse process of the first four cervical vertebrae and insert on the medial borders of the scapulae between the superior angle and the root of the spine. They elevate the scapulae and assist in rotation of the glenoid cavity caudally. They are innervated by the dorsal scapular nerve (emanating from the fifth cervical spinal nerve) and the cervical plexus (emanating from the third and fourth cervical spinal nerves) (Fig. 16-3).

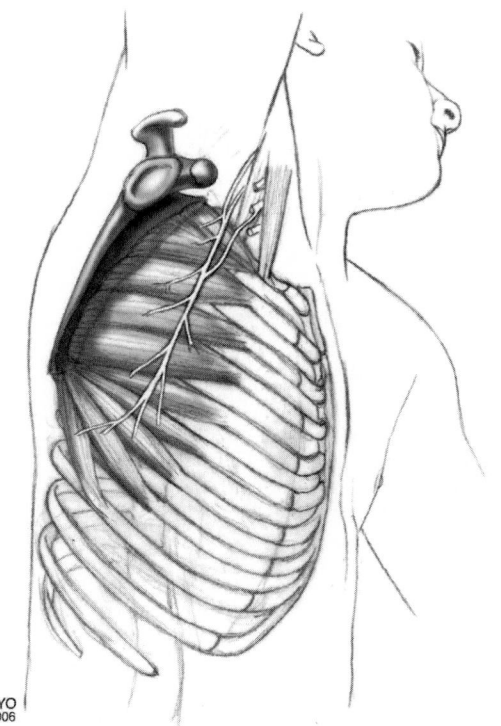

FIGURE 16-1. Anterolateral view of the right upper chest and shoulder showing the course of the long thoracic nerve and innervation of the serratus anterior muscles. Note the superficial location of the long thoracic nerve. (Reprinted with permission of Mayo Foundation for Medical Education and Research. © Mayo Foundation, 2007.)

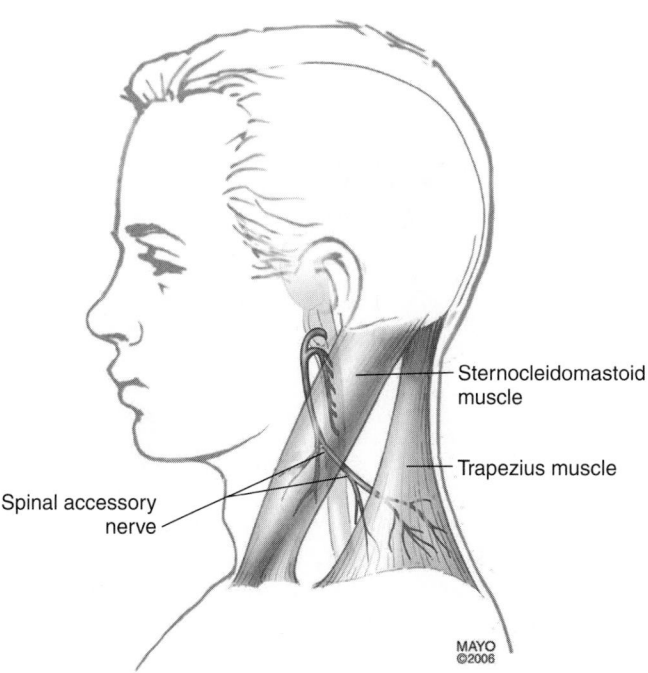

FIGURE 16-2. Lateral view of the neck showing the course of the spinal accessory nerve and innervation of the trapezius muscle. (Reprinted with permission of Mayo Foundation for Medical Education and Research. © Mayo Foundation, 2007.)

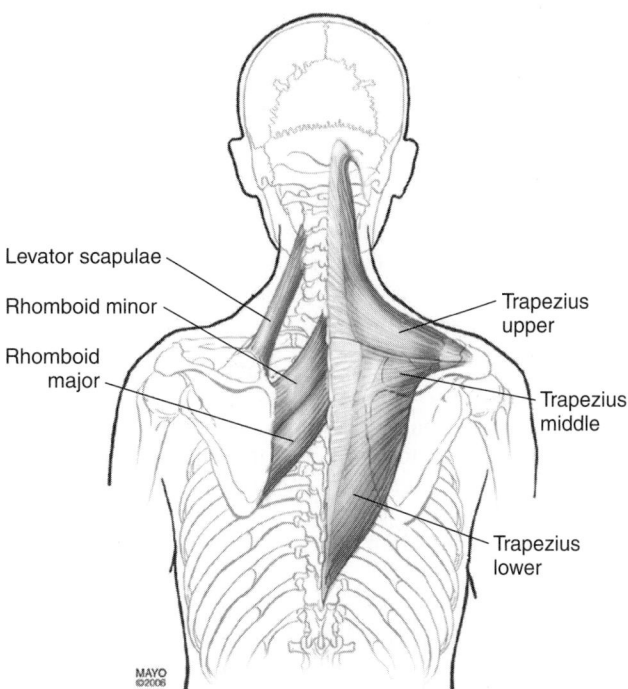

FIGURE 16-3. View of upper back showing origins and insertions of rhomboid, levator scapulae, and trapezius muscles. (Reprinted with permission of Mayo Foundation for Medical Education and Research. © Mayo Foundation, 2007.)

SYMPTOMS

A patient's presenting symptoms depend on the type and chronicity of the injury. Most patients, however, complain of upper back or shoulder pain, muscle fatigue, and weakness with use of the shoulder. The diagnosis of scapular winging is made clinically. A pain profile should be obtained, including onset and duration of pain, location, severity, and quality as well as exacerbating and relieving factors, not only to provide baseline information but also to help develop a differential diagnosis. The patient should also be questioned about hand dominance because the dominant shoulder is usually more muscular but sits lower than the non-dominant shoulder. Knowledge of the patient's age, occupation and hobbies, and current and previous level of functioning may also contribute to the diagnosis and treatment plan. The mechanism of injury in patients with traumatic palsy is important, as are associated findings including muscle spasm, paresthesia, and muscle wasting or weakness.[36,37] The scapular winging of long thoracic neuropathy and serratus anterior muscle weakness must be distinguished from that of a spinal accessory neuropathy and trapezius muscle weakness. Serratus anterior muscle dysfunction is the most common cause of scapular winging. Typically, patients complain of a dull aching pain in the shoulder and periscapular region. The periscapular pain may be related to spasm from unopposed contraction of the other scapular stabilizers in the presence of serratus anterior muscle weakness. There may be "clicking" or "popping" noise emanating from the periscapular area when the patient moves, which is made worse with stressful upper extremity activities.[36] Because the serratus anterior muscle rotates the scapula forward as the arm is abducted or forward flexed above the shoulder level, these movements are affected. Shoulder fatigue and weakness are related to loss of scapular rotation and stabilization.

A cosmetic deformity may occur in the upper back as a result of the winged scapula. It may be apparent at rest but usually is more obvious on raising of the arm. Patients may find it difficult to sit for prolonged periods with the back resting against a hard surface, such as driving for long periods.

With trapezius muscle weakness, the affected shoulder is depressed, and the inferior scapular border rotates laterally, which makes prolonged use of the arm painful and tiresome. Patients often complain of a dull ache around the shoulder girdle and difficulty with overhead activities and heavy lifting, especially with shoulder abduction greater than 90 degrees.[37]

PHYSICAL EXAMINATION

The patient should be suitably undressed so that the examiner can observe, both front and back, the normal bone and soft tissue contours of both shoulders and scapulae for symmetry and their relationship to the thorax. The patient's overall posture is assessed, as are the presence of muscle spasm and trapezius or rhomboid muscle atrophy. Scapulothoracic motion is examined with both passive and active range of motion activities of the shoulder.[38]

With long thoracic neuropathy and serratus anterior muscle weakness, the cardinal sign is winging of the scapula, in which the vertebral border of the scapula moves away from the posterior chest wall and the inferior angle is rotated toward midline.[38] This scapular winging may be visible with the patient standing normally, but if the weakness is mild, it may be visible only when the patient extends the arm and pushes against a wall in a pushup position (Fig. 16-4).

Spinal accessory neuropathy and trapezius muscle weakness are usually accompanied by an asymmetric neckline with noticeable shoulder droop when the patient's arms are unsupported at the sides. On the affected side, deepening of the supraclavicular fossa is evident and shoulder shrug is difficult. With shoulder elevation, the scapula is displaced laterally, rotating downward and outward. There is usually difficulty with shoulder abduction above 90 degrees, more so than with forward flexion. Weakness with attempted shoulder elevation against resistance is characteristic. Normal muscle testing can elicit weakness in the trapezius muscle (Fig. 16-5).[37]

With weakness of the rhomboids, winging of the scapula is minimal. The wing is best demonstrated by slowly lowering the arms from a forward elevated position. Atrophy of the rhomboids may be present. The scapula is displaced downward and laterally.[39]

A complete neurologic and musculoskeletal examination, with manual muscle strength testing and sensory and

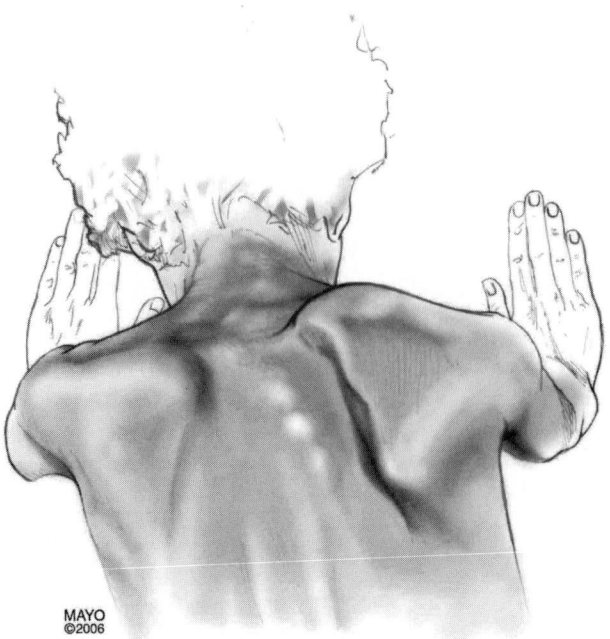

FIGURE 16-4. Winging of the right scapula with forward flexion of the extended arms due to injury of the long thoracic nerve. Note the upward displacement of the scapula with prominence of the vertebral border and medial displacement of the inferior angle. (Reprinted with permission of Mayo Foundation for Medical Education and Research. © Mayo Foundation, 2007.)

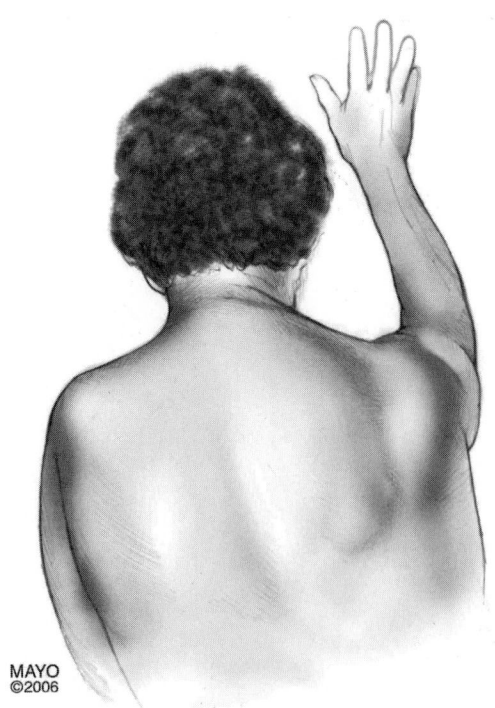

FIGURE 16-5. Right trapezius palsy. The neckline is asymmetric, the shoulder droops, the scapula is translated laterally, and the glenoid labrum is rotated downward. (Reprinted with permission of Mayo Foundation for Medical Education and Research. © Mayo Foundation, 2007.)

reflex testing, should be completed to rule out underlying neuromuscular disease processes. In addition, thorough examination of the neck and shoulder with provocative maneuvers should be completed to rule out additional musculoskeletal sources of scapular winging.

FUNCTIONAL LIMITATIONS

Functional limitations depend not only on the cause of the scapular winging but also on the severity of weakness and pain. Difficulty with activities of daily living may be evident as a result of pain, weakness, and altered scapulothoracic and glenohumeral motion. Especially affected are activities that require arm elevation above the level of the shoulder (e.g., brushing hair or teeth or shaving). Recreational and vocational activities such as golf, tennis, and volleyball that entail working or reaching overhead may be affected. Chronic shoulder pain and dysfunction can lead to depression and anxiety, irritability, concentration difficulties, lack of sleep, and chronic fatigue. Overuse of the shoulder and scapular stabilizer muscles can lead to myofascial pain syndromes.

DIAGNOSTIC STUDIES

Plain radiography of the shoulder, cervical spine, chest, and scapulae is recommended as part of the initial evaluation for scapular winging, especially if the cause is not obvious. Plain radiography can help rule out other causes of scapular winging, such as subscapular osteochondroma, avulsion fracture of the scapula, or other primary shoulder and cervical spine disease. With radiographs of the scapula, oblique views are recommended because osteochondroma may be hidden on anteroposterior views.[40,41]

Computed tomography and magnetic resonance imaging are usually not necessary unless the coexistence of other disease processes is suspected. The patient's presentation and examination findings are pivotal in deciding whether advanced imaging is necessary.

Electrodiagnostic studies, namely, electromyography and nerve conduction studies, are valuable tools clinically to aid in the evaluation of scapular winging. They can assist in localizing injury and disease of peripheral nerves or muscles related to scapular function. These studies can help evaluate patients with abnormal scapulothoracic motion but in whom it cannot be clearly established clinically whether the weakness lies in a particular muscle or in the actions of other muscles acting on the scapula.

Serial electromyographic and nerve conduction studies have been used to follow recovery in patients with isolated long thoracic or spinal accessory nerve palsies and to help in decisions of whether to undertake nerve exploration or muscle transfer.[36,37] However, caution has been advised in the use of needle electromyographic findings to predict the prognosis and to guide the timing of surgical repair.[42] Long thoracic and spinal accessory neuropathies may be associated with a good prognosis, irrespective of needle electromyographic findings.

Differential Diagnosis [43]

Rotator cuff disease

Shoulder impingement syndromes

Glenohumeral instability (especially posterior instability)

Acromioclavicular joint disease

Shoulder arthritis

Adhesive capsulitis

Bicipital tendinitis

Cervical radiculopathy (especially C5-7)

Suprascapular nerve entrapment

Myofascial pain syndromes

Scoliosis (associated rib deformities can cause asymptomatic scapular winging on convex side of curve)[41]

Sprengel deformity (congenital deformity of shoulder with high-riding and downward-rotated scapula, often confused with scapular winging)[41]

Fracture or malunion of clavicle and acromion

Tumors of shoulder girdle, lung, or spine

TREATMENT

In most patients, scapular winging is a result of neurapraxic injuries. Fortunately, these types of injuries usually resolve spontaneously within 6 to 9 months after traumatic injury and within 2 years after nontraumatic injuries. In one study,[42] traumatic long thoracic and spinal accessory nerve injuries were associated with a poor prognosis compared with nontraumatic neuropathies. Once the diagnosis is made, conservative treatment should be initiated. Some clinicians have recommended a trial of conservative treatment for at least 12 to 24 months to allow adequate time for nerve recovery.[36-38,41]

Initial

Pain control may be achieved early with use of an analgesic or an anti-inflammatory medication. Activity modification is recommended. The patient should avoid precipitating activities and strenuous use of the involved extremity. Physical modalities, such as ice massage, superficial moist heat, and ultrasound, can be applied to help with pain control. Ice massage may additionally help control swelling and relieve associated muscle spasm.

Immobilization should be a part of the initial management to prevent overstretching of the weakened muscle. This can be accomplished with the use of a sling to rest the arm initially.[38]

Long-term use of scapular winging shoulder braces to maintain the position of the scapula against the thorax is controversial. Various shoulder braces and orthotics have been used with mixed results. Some authors[14,44] recommend against use of shoulder braces because they are cumbersome, poorly tolerated, and ineffective. Others have advocated their use to protect against muscle overstretching and scapulothoracic overuse.[45-47]

Rehabilitation

Specific treatment varies, depending on the etiology of the scapular winging. In general, range of motion exercises should be initiated early to prevent contractures or adhesive capsulitis, especially if the affected extremity is immobilized.

A stretching and strengthening exercise program can be undertaken after pain control is achieved. Stretching the scapular stabilizers and shoulder capsules without overstretching the weakened muscle is important and should be supervised by a physical therapist. The scapular stabilizer, cervical muscles, and rotator cuff muscle should be strengthened, especially the affected muscle groups. Neuromuscular electrical stimulation may be used to prevent muscle atrophy. Functional glenohumeral and scapulothoracic muscle patterns must be relearned. Progression to an independent structured home exercise program is recommended, but the patient should first be able to perform the exercises appropriately under supervision of a physical therapist.

Procedures

Localized injections are not routinely administered for isolated scapular winging. Injection therapy may be indicated for other coexisting shoulder disease to help with pain control.

Surgery

Conservative treatment has been recommended for a prolonged period (12 to 24 months) to allow adequate time for recovery before surgical options are considered.[36-38,41] Surgery should be considered for patients who do not recover in this time. In patients with penetrating trauma in which the nerve may have been injured, spontaneous recovery is less likely, and early nerve exploration with neurolysis, direct nerve repair, or nerve grafting may be indicated.

Surgery may also be indicated if scapular winging appears to have been caused by a surgically treatable lesion (e.g., a subscapular osteochondroma) and the patient is symptomatic or has a cosmetic disfigurement. In general, surgical options are many but can be divided into two categories: static stabilization procedures and dynamic muscle transfers.

Static stabilization procedures involve scapulothoracic fusion and scapulothoracic arthrodesis in which the scapula is fused to the thorax. These procedures may be effective in cases of generalized weakness (e.g., facioscapulo-humeral muscular dystrophy) when the patient has disabling pain and functional loss and no transferable mus-cles.[19,48,49] They can relieve shoulder fatigue and pain and allow functional abduction and flexion of the upper extremity.[20,21] Static stabilization procedures have fallen out of favor for scapular winging related to isolated muscle weakness because the results deteriorate over time with recurrence of winging. The usual incidence of complications associated with some of these procedures is high.[49]

Dynamic muscle transfers have shown better results for correction of scapular winging and restoration of function. Several different muscles have been used in various muscle transfer techniques to provide dynamic control of the scapula and to improve scapulothoracic and glenohumeral motion. Transfer of the sternal head of the pectoralis major muscle to the inferior angle of the scapula with fascia lata autograft reinforcement is the preferred method of treatment for scapular winging related to long thoracic nerve injury.[44,47] The surgical procedure of choice for scapular winging related to chronic trapezius muscle dysfunction involves the lateral transfer of the insertions of the levator scapulae and the rhomboid major and minor muscles. This procedure enables the muscles to support the shoulder girdle and to stabilize the scapula.[37]

POTENTIAL DISEASE COMPLICATIONS

Disease complications are usually related to scapulothoracic dysfunction as a result of scapular winging. This can contribute to glenohumeral instability and subsequent shoulder range of motion and functional deficits, as well as chronic periscapular, upper back, and shoulder pain. Secondary impingement syndromes can result from the muscle dysfunction. Adhesive capsulitis can occur from loss of shoulder mobility and function. Cosmetic deformity is a common result of scapular winging, especially if there is a combined serratus anterior and trapezius muscle weakness.

POTENTIAL TREATMENT COMPLICATIONS

Pharmacotherapy can lead to treatment complications. Nonsteroidal anti-inflammatory drugs have well-documented adverse effects that most commonly involve the gastrointestinal system. Analgesics may have adverse effects that predominantly involve the hepatorenal system. These complications can be minimized by having a working knowledge of the patient's ongoing medical problems, current medications, and potential drug interactions.

Local injections may cause allergic reactions, infection at the injection site, and, rarely, sepsis. Tendon rupture is a potential complication if inadvertent injection into a tendon occurs.

Surgical complications are numerous and include a large, cosmetically unpleasant incision over the shoulder and upper back, postoperative musculoskeletal deformities (e.g., scoliosis), infection, pulmonary complications (e.g., pneumothorax and hemothorax), hardware failure, pseudoarthrosis, recurrent winging, and persistent pain.

References

1. Fiddian NJ, King RJ. The winged scapula. Clin Orthop Relat Res 1984;185:228-236.
2. Velpeau AALM. Luxations de l'epaule. Arch Gen Med 1837;14: 269-305.
3. Burdett-Smith P. Experience of scapula winging in an accident and emergency department. Br J Clin Pract 1990;44:643-644.
4. Cast IP, Jamjoom AH. C7 radiculopathy: importance of scapular winging in clinical diagnosis. J Neurol Neurosurg Psychiatry 1987;50:506.
5. Makin GJ, Brown WF, Ebers GC. C7 radiculopathy: importance of scapular winging in clinical diagnosis. J Neurol Neurosurg Psychiatry 1986;49:640-644.
6. Parsonage MJ, Turner JWA. Neuralgic amyotrophy: the shoulder-girdle syndrome. Lancet 1948;251:973-978.
7. Oakes MJ, Sherwood DL. An isolated long thoracic nerve injury in a Navy Airman. Mil Med 2004;169:713-715.
8. Bodack MP, Tunkel RS, Marini SG, et al. Spinal accessory nerve palsy as a cause of pain after whiplash injury: case report. J Pain Symptom Manage 1998;15:321-328.
9. Sanitate S, Jurist KA. Medical scapular winging in a patient with normal electromyograms. Orthopedics 1995;18:292-293.
10. Lee SG, Kim JH, Lee SY, et al. Winged scapula caused by rhomboideus and trapezius muscles rupture associated with repetitive minor trauma: a case report. J Korean Med Sci 2006;21:581-584.
11. Hayes JM, Zehr DJ. Traumatic muscle avulsion causing winging of the scapula: a case report. J Bone Joint Surg Am 1981;63:495-497.
12. Gregg JR, Labosky D, Harty M, et al. Serratus anterior paralysis in the young athlete. J Bone Joint Surg Am 1979;61:825-832.
13. Packer GJ, McLatchie GR, Bowden W. Scapula winging in a sports injury clinic. Br J Sports Med 1993;27:90-91.
14. Schultz JS, Leonard JA Jr. Long thoracic neuropathy from athletic activity. Arch Phys Med Rehabil 1992;73:87-90.
15. Sherman SC, O'Connor M. An unusual cause of shoulder pain: winged scapula. J Emerg Med 2005;28:329-331.
16. van Tuijl JH, Schmid A, van Kranen-Mastenbroek VH, et al. Isolated spinal accessory neuropathy in an adolescent: a case study. Eur J Paediatr Neurol 2006;10:83-85. Epub 2006 Mar 10.
17. Bowen TR, Miller F. Greenstick fracture of the scapula: a cause of scapular winging. J Orthop Trauma 2006;20:147-149.
18. Kitano K, Tada K, Oka S. Congenital contracture of the infraspinous muscle: a case report. Arch Orthop Trauma Surg 1988;107:54-57.
19. Diab M, Darras BT, Shapiro F. Scapulothoracic fusion for facioscapulohumeral muscular dystrophy. J Bone Joint Surg Am 2005;87:2267-2275.
20. Rhee YG, Ha JH. Long-term results of scapulothoracic arthrodesis of facioscapulohumeral muscular dystrophy. J Shoulder Elbow Surg 2006;15:445-450.
21. Ziaee MA, Abolghasemian M, Majd ME. Scapulothoracic arthrodesis for winged scapula due to facioscapulohumeral dystrophy (a new technique). Am J Orthop 2006;35:311-315.
22. Delmonte S, Massone C, Parodi A, et al. Acquired winged scapula in a patient with systemic lupus erythematosus. Clin Exp Rheumatol 1998;16:82-83.
23. Simotas AC, Tsairis P. Adhesive capsulitis of the glenohumeral joint with an unusual neuropathic presentation: a case report. Am J Phys Med Rehabil 1999;78:577-581.
24. Hubbert CH. Winged scapula associated with epidural anesthesia. Anesth Analg 1988;67:418-419.
25. Witt RL, Gillis T, Pratt R Jr. Spinal accessory nerve monitoring with clinical outcome measures. Ear Nose Throat J 2006;85:540-544.
26. Wood VE, Frykman GK. Winging of the scapula as a complication of first rib resection: a report of six cases. Clin Orthop Relat Res 1980;149:160-163.
27. Debeer P, Devlieger R, Brys P, et al. Scapular winging after vaginal delivery. BJOG 2004;111:758-759.
28. Niedermaier N, Meinck HM, Hartmann M. Cervical syringomyelia at the C7-C8 level presenting with bilateral scapular winging. J Neurol Neurosurg Psychiatry 2000;68:394-395.
29. Marmor L, Bechtol CO. Paralysis of the serratus anterior due to electric shock relieved by transplantation of the pectoralis major muscle: a case report. J Bone Joint Surg Am 1963;45:156-160.
30. Cooley LH, Torg JS. "Pseudowinging" of the scapula secondary to subscapular osteochondroma. Clin Orthop Relat Res 1982;162:119-124.
31. Cuomo F, Blank K, Zuckerman JD, Present DA. Scapular osteochondroma presenting with exostosis bursata. Bull Hosp Jt Dis 1993;52:55-58.
32. Danielsson LG, el-Haddad I. Winged scapula due to osteochondroma: report of 3 children. Acta Orthop Scand 1989;60:728-729.
33. Parsons TA. The snapping scapula and subscapular exostoses. J Bone Joint Surg Br 1973;55:345-349.
34. Hollinshead WH. Anatomy for Surgeons. Hagerstown, Md, Harper & Row, 1982:259-340.
35. Symes A, Ellis H. Variations in the surface anatomy of the spinal accessory nerve in the posterior triangle. Surg Radiol Anat 2005;27:404-408. Epub 2005 Aug 23.
36. Wiater JM, Flatow EL. Long thoracic nerve injury. Clin Orthop Relat Res 1999;368:17-27.
37. Wiater JM, Bigliani LU. Spinal accessory nerve injury. Clin Orthop Relat Res 1999;368:5-16.
38. Kuhn JE, Hawkins RJ. Evaluation and treatment of scapular disorders. In Warner JJP, Iannotti JP, Gerber C, eds. Complex and revision problems in shoulder surgery. Philadelphia, Lippincott-Raven, 1997:357-376.
39. Saeed MA, Gatens PF Jr, Singh S. Winging of the scapula. Am Fam Physician 1981;24:139-143.
40. Banerjee A. X-rays as a diagnostic aid in winged scapula. Arch Emerg Med 1993;10:261-263.
41. Duralde XA. Evaluation and treatment of the winged scapula. J South Orthop Assoc 1995;4:38-52.
42. Friedenberg SM, Zimprich T, Harper CM. The natural history of long thoracic and spinal accessory neuropathies. Muscle Nerve 2002;25:535-539.
43. Belville RG, Seupaul RA. Winged scapula in the emergency department: a case report and review. J Emerg Med 2005;29:279-282.
44. Warner JJ, Navarro RA. Serratus anterior dysfunction: recognition and treatment. Clin Orthop Relat Res 1998;349:139-148.
45. Marin R. Scapula winger's brace: a case series on the management of long thoracic nerve palsy. Arch Phys Med Rehabil 1998;79: 1226-1230.
46. Zeier FG. The treatment of winged-scapula. Clin Orthop Relat Res 1973;91:128-133.
47. Iceton J, Harris WR. Treatment of winged scapula by pectoralis major transfer. J Bone Joint Surg Br 1987;69:108-110.
48. Jeon IH, Neumann L, Wallace WA. Scapulothoracic fusion for painful winging of the scapula in nondystrophic patients. J Shoulder Elbow Surg 2005;14:400-406.
49. Krishnan SG, Hawkins RJ, Michelotti JD, et al. Scapulothoracic arthrodesis: indications, technique, and results. Clin Orthop Relat Res 2005;435:126-133.

Shoulder Arthritis 17

Michael F. Stretanski, DO

Synonyms

Glenohumeral arthritis
Osteoarthritis
Arthritic frozen shoulder

ICD-9 Codes

715.11   Primary osteoarthritis, shoulder
715.21   Secondary osteoarthritis, shoulder (rotator cuff
         arthropathy)
716.11   Traumatic arthropathy, shoulder
716.91   Arthropathy, unspecified, shoulder

DEFINITION

Osteoarthritis of the glenohumeral joint occurs when there is loss of articular cartilage that results in narrowing of the joint space (Fig. 17-1). Synovitis and osteocartilaginous loose bodies are commonly associated with glenohumeral arthritis. Pathologic distortion of the articular surfaces of the humeral head and glenoid can be due to increasing age, overuse, heredity, alcoholism, trauma, or disease of bone. This condition is most commonly seen beyond the fifth decade and is more common in men. Long-standing complete rotator cuff tears, multidirectional instability from any cause, lymphoma[1] (chronic lymphocytic lymphoma or immunocytoma), or prior capsulorrhaphy for anterior instability[2] can predispose one to glenohumeral arthritis. Acute septic arthritis should not be heedlessly ruled out in the face of severe osteoarthritis.[3] The medical history should include any history of fracture, dislocation, rotator cuff tear, repetitive motion, metabolic disorder, chronic glucocorticoid administration, or prior shoulder surgery.

SYMPTOMS

Symptoms include constant shoulder pain intensified by activity and partially relieved with rest. Pain is usually noted with all shoulder movements. Major restriction of shoulder motion and disuse weakness or pain inhibitory weakness are common and potentially progressive. Adhesive capsulitis may result. The pain is typically restricted to the area of the shoulder and may be felt around the deltoid region but not typically into the forearm. The pain is generally characterized as dull and aching but may become sharp at the extremes of range of motion. Shoulder pain is typically worse when supine and in attempting to sleep on the arthritic side. Neurologic symptoms such as numbness and paresthesias should be absent. Pain may interfere with sleep and may be worse in the morning or while supine.

PHYSICAL EXAMINATION

Restriction of shoulder range of motion is a major clinical component, especially loss of external rotation and abduction. Both active and passive range of motion is affected in shoulder arthritis, compared with only active motion in rotator cuff tears (passive range is normal in rotator cuff injuries unless adhesive capsulitis is present). Pain increases when the extremes of the restricted motion are reached, and crepitus is common with movement. Tenderness may be present over the anterior rotator cuff and over the posterior joint line. If acromioclavicular joint osteoarthritis is an accompanying problem, the acromioclavicular joint may be tender. There may be wasting of the muscles surrounding the shoulder because of disuse atrophy. Sensation and deep tendon reflexes should be normal. Electrodiagnostic medicine consultation will help rule out idiopathic brachial plexopathy (Parsonage-Turner syndrome), cervical radiculopathy, and isolated suprascapular, dorsal scapular, or axillary neuropathy. In patients with inconsistent physical examination findings and questionable secondary gain issues, the American Shoulder and Elbow Surgeons subjective shoulder scale has demonstrated acceptable psychometric performance for outcomes assessment in patients with shoulder instability, rotator cuff disease, and glenohumeral arthritis.[4]

FUNCTIONAL LIMITATIONS

Any activities that require upper extremity strength, endurance, and flexibility can be affected. Most commonly, activities that require reaching overhead in external rotation are limited. These include activities of daily

91

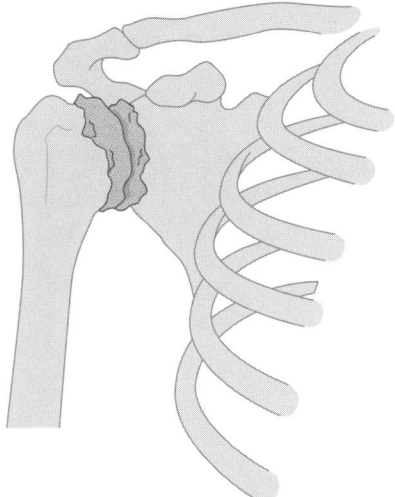

FIGURE 17-1. Osteoarthritis of the shoulder.

living (such as brushing hair or teeth, donning or doffing upper torso clothes) and activities such as overarm throwing or reaching for items overhead. If pain is severe and constant, sleep may be interrupted, sleep-wake cycle disruption may occur, and situational reactive depression is not uncommon.

DIAGNOSTIC STUDIES

Routine shoulder radiographs with four views (anteroposterior internal and external rotation, axillary, and scapular Y) are generally sufficient for evaluating loss of articular cartilage and glenohumeral joint space narrowing (Fig. 17-2). Varying degrees may be seen of flattening of the humeral head, marginal osteophytes, calcific tendinitis, subchondral cysts in the humeral head and glenoid, sclerotic bone, bone erosion, and humeral head migration. Specifically, if there is a chronic rotator cuff tear that is contributing to the destruction of the articular cartilage, the humeral head will be seen pressing against the undersurface of the acromion. Associated acromioclavicular joint arthritis can be seen on the anteroposterior view.

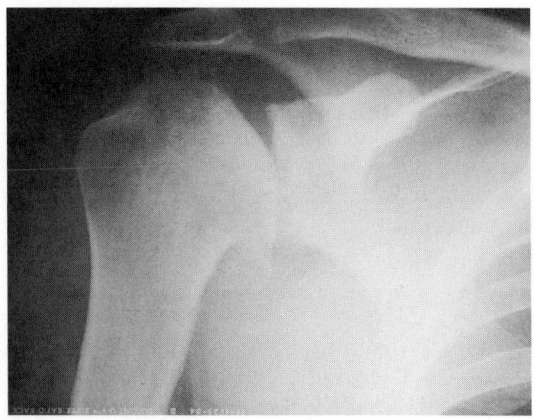

FIGURE 17-2. Radiograph typical of glenohumeral osteoarthritis.

Conventional magnetic resonance imaging is the "gold standard" to assess soft tissues for rotator cuff tear; but when more sensitive evaluation of the labrum, capsule, articular cartilage, and glenohumeral ligaments is required or when a partial-thickness rotator cuff tear is suspected, magnetic resonance arthrography with intra-articular administration of contrast material may be required to visualize these subtle findings.[5] Paralabral cysts (extraneural ganglia), which can result with posterior labrocapsular complex tears and cause suprascapular nerve compression, may be visualized on magnetic resonance imaging.[6] Electrodiagnostic medicine consultation should be obtained for needle electromyography of the suprascapularis and subscapularis muscles in such cases. Computed tomography may have a unique role in finding the glenohumeral arthritis risk factor of posterior humeral head subluxation relative to the glenoid in the absence of posterior glenoid erosion,[7] and magnetic resonance imaging to assess the rotator cuff may be indicated.

A rise in popularity of diagnostic ultrasonography in musculoskeletal medicine is undeniable. The modality may play a role in full-thickness rotator cuff tear diagnosis in experienced hands, but significant interrater reliability has been called into question.[8,9] This fact and this diagnostic tool contribute little to the current glenohumeral joint body of knowledge. Additionally, I suggest that any woman with shoulder pain recalcitrant to seemingly appropriate treatment be considered for mammography.

Differential Diagnosis

Rotator cuff disease

Synovitis

Cervical osteoarthritis

Shoulder instability

Rheumatoid arthritis

Cervical radiculopathy

Labral degeneration and tear

Pseudogout

Charcot joint

Biceps tendon abnormalities

Infection

Fracture of the humerus

Adhesive capsulitis

Parsonage-Turner syndrome

Neoplasms

Leukemic arthritis

Avascular necrosis

TREATMENT

Initial

Shoulder arthritis is a chronic issue, but acute exacerbations in pain can be managed conservatively. Nonsteroidal anti-inflammatory drugs or analgesic medications can help with pain and enable rehabilitation. Capsaicin cream, lidocaine patches, ice, or moist heat may be used topically as needed. Gentle stretching exercises help keep the range of motion and prevent secondary adhesive capsulitis.

Rehabilitation

The shoulder is a complicated structure composed of several joints with both static and dynamic stabilizers that tend to function, and fail, as a concerted unit. A well-designed rehabilitation program must take this into account and treat glenohumeral arthritis within this context. The rehabilitative efforts are dedicated to the restoration of strength, endurance, and flexibility of the shoulder musculature. Supervised physical or occupational therapy should focus on the upper thoracic, neck, and scapular muscle groups but address the entire upper extremity kinetic chain, including the rotator cuff, arm, forearm, wrist, and hand. Patients benefit from aquatic therapy and can easily be taught exercises and then transitioned to an independent pool exercise program that they can continue long term. In cases of severe rheumatoid arthritis, joint-sparing isometric exercises may prevent atrophy and maintain strength of dynamic stabilizers of the shoulder without placing undue stress on the remaining articular surfaces. The consensus[10] on glenohumeral involvement in rheumatoid arthritis is that narrowing of the joint space is a turning point that indicates a risk of rapid joint destruction, and surgical interventions should be considered before musculoskeletal sequelae are too severe to enable adequate recovery.

The success of flexibility return will be determined by the extent of mechanical bone blockade, which in turn is determined by the magnitude of glenohumeral incongruous distortion, loose bodies, and osteophyte formation. Pain control can be assisted with modalities such as ultrasound and iontophoresis. Electrical stimulation may have a limited role in posterior shoulder strengthening in patients with poor posture and "rounded shoulders" on examination, but it should not take the place of volitional contraction and not be used routinely across arthritic joints for obvious reasons of enabling passive dependence and counterphysiologic type II motor unit recruitment. The rehabilitation medicine specialist may also have a role along the continuum of care of the shoulder patient. In caring for arthroplasty patients, the Neer protocol for postoperative total shoulder arthroplasty rehabilitation is widely used and based on tradition and the basic science of soft tissue and bone healing.[11]

Procedures

If therapies fail or are impossible because of pain, the patient has several treatment options. Periarticular injections may offer some help to control pain of associated problems, such as subacromial bursitis and rotator cuff tendinitis or tendinosis. Intra-articular glenohumeral joint injections may also afford some pain relief, particularly in the early stages. The accuracy of intra-articular injections not fluoroscopically guided is less than perfect at 80%; the anterior approach is slightly more accurate than the posterior approach at 50%.[12] However, injections have not been shown to alter the underlying arthritis pathoanatomy (Fig. 17-3). Great care should be taken in anticoagulated patients. Viscosupplementation (hylan G-F 20) is not approved by the Food and Drug Administration for the glenohumeral joint but may have a role in mild osteoarthritis.

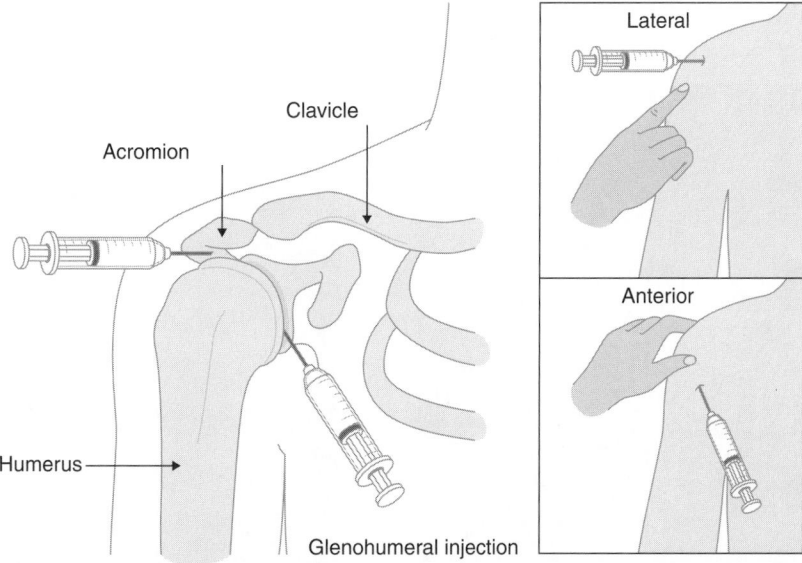

FIGURE 17-3. Approximate surface anatomy *(insets)* and internal anatomic sites for injection of the glenohumeral joint laterally and anteriorly. (Reprinted with permission from Lennard TA. Physiatric Procedures in Clinical Practice. Philadelphia, Hanley & Belfus, 1995:17.)

The initial setup can be identical for either intra-articular glenohumeral or subacromial injection. With the patient seated with the arm either in the lap or hanging down by the side, the internal rotation and gravity pull of the arm will open the space, leading to the glenohumeral joint or subacromial space. Several approaches have been described. Most commonly for a subacromial injection, the skin entry point is 1 cm inferior to the acromion, and the needle is tracked anteriorly at a lateral to medial 45-degree angle in the axial plane and slightly superior (under the acromion). A 5- to 10-mL mixture of a local anesthetic-corticosteroid combination (e.g., 1 mL of 1% lidocaine mixed with 3 mL of betamethasone [Celestone], 6 mg/mL) is then injected. The injectate should flow with minimal resistance into this potential space. If resistance is encountered, the needle should be repositioned to avoid intratendinous injection and increased risk of tendon rupture. For glenohumeral injection, a more inferior and medial approach is used (Fig. 17-4).

Postinjection care includes icing of the shoulder for 5 to 10 minutes immediately and then for 15 to 20 minutes two or three times a day during the next 24 to 48 hours. Patients are cautioned to avoid aggressive activities for the first few days after the injection. If the adhesive capsulitis component is specifically being treated, a suprascapular nerve block with 5 to 10 mL of 0.25% bupivacaine (Marcaine) can be performed immediately before therapy, with an appropriately trained therapist aware of the safe handling of such an anesthetized joint. I typically employ a combined suprascapular and subacromial approach in these cases.

Surgery

If unacceptable symptoms persist despite conservative treatment, the patient may decide to reduce his or her activity level to minimize pain or proceed with one of a number of surgical interventions. It is important to inform the patient that regardless of the treatment approach, with osteoarthritis, a return to normal shoulder function, by either rehabilitation or surgery, is not possible. Pain control and some increased function are usually achievable, however.

Surgical options include débridement of the glenohumeral joint by either open or arthroscopic techniques and joint replacement.[13] If reasonable congruity between the humeral head and glenoid is present, good improvement in pain control and some functional improvement can be anticipated with débridement, even in the presence of severe chondromalacia. The glenoid may be amenable to arthroscopic resurfacing with a meniscal allograft.[14] Other arthroscopic techniques are successful, provided mechanical blockading osteophytes and loose bodies are removed (Fig. 17-5).[15] Hemiarthroplasty may be indicated in the absence of advanced glenohumeral disease if the glenoid can at least be converted to a smooth concentric surface.[16] Hemiarthroplasty has also been suggested as the procedure of choice in moderate to severe glenohumeral arthritis and irreparable rotator cuff tears.[17] If major incongruity is present between the humeral head and glenoid, total shoulder arthroplasty may be indicated.[18] There is some suggestion of better long-term outcomes when biceps tenodesis is performed concomitantly with shoulder arthroplasty.[19] Whereas it may seem counterintuitive, proprioception actually improves after total shoulder arthroplasty over prearthroplasty measurements.[20] This is important from the standpoint of activities of daily life in osteoarthritic patients. Most shoulders, however, can be aided arthroscopically with appropriate technique, which often necessitates a second posterior portal and a highly experienced shoulder arthroscopist.[15] Although a greater risk of more advanced glenohumeral arthritis is associated with arthroscopic procedures that result in limited external rotation,[21] arthrodesis may be required for irreversible and nonreconstructible massive rotator cuff tears, tumor, and deltoid muscle denervation as well as for detachment of the deltoid from its origin or to stabilize the glenohumeral joint after many failed attempts at shoulder reconstruction.[22] Arthrodesis for failed prosthetic arthroplasty or tumor resection presents additional challenges and additional risk of the aforementioned complications. A newer procedure, thermal capsulorrhaphy, has come in and out of favor;

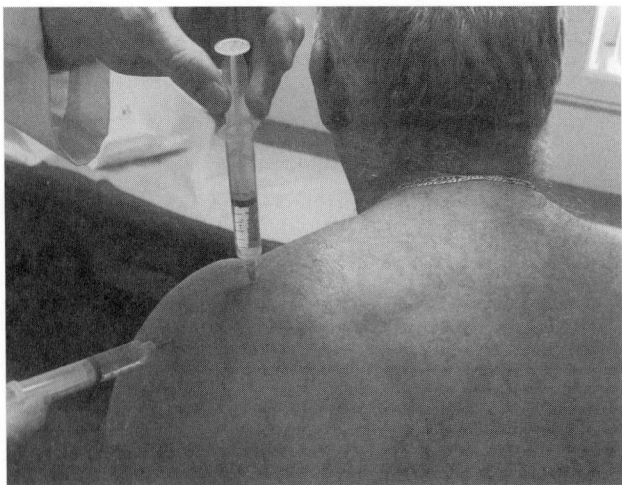

FIGURE 17-4. Combined subacromial and suprascapular injection. The site is marked for intra-articular glenohumeral injection.

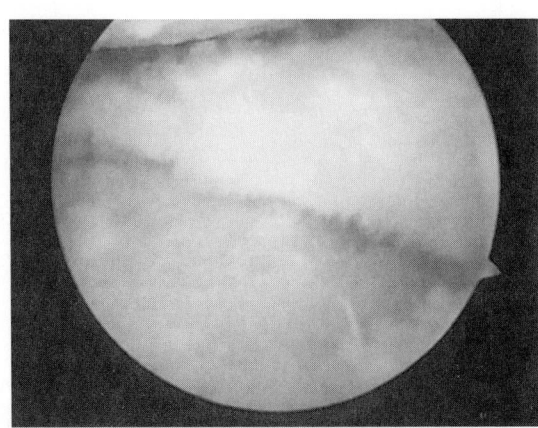

FIGURE 17-5. Arthroscopic surgical view of osteoarthritis.

it is usually used more in high-functioning athletes for isolated posterior instability without labral detachment, rather than in isolated glenohumeral osteoarthritis.[23]

POTENTIAL DISEASE COMPLICATIONS

Disease complications include chronic intractable pain and loss of shoulder range of motion. These result in diminished functional ability to use the arm, disuse weakness, difficulty with sleep, inability to perform work and recreational activities, and reactive depression.

POTENTIAL TREATMENT COMPLICATIONS

Analgesics and nonsteroidal anti-inflammatory drugs have well-known side effects that most commonly affect the gastric, hepatic, and renal systems. Infection, hemarthrosis, and allergic reaction to the medications are rare side effects of injections. In particular, there may be an association between subdeltoid septic bursitis and concomitant systemic isotretinoin (Accutane).[24] Fluid retention or transient hyperglycemia may be seen with a single exogenous glucocorticoid injection. Arthroscopic complications are not common, but the usual possibilities, including neurovascular issues, have been reported. Arthrodesis complications include nonunion, malposition, pain associated with prominent hardware, and periarticular fractures. Arthrodesis after cancer reconstruction has a higher risk of complication.[22]

References

1. Braune C, Rittmeister M, Engels K, Kerschbaumer F. Non-Hodgkin lymphoma (immunocytoma) of low malignancy and arthritis of the glenohumeral joint [in German]. Z Orthop Ihre Grenzgeb 2002;140:199-202.
2. Green A, Norris TR. Shoulder arthroplasty for advanced glenohumeral arthritis after anterior instability repair. J Shoulder Elbow Surg 2001;10:539-545.
3. Martinez OA, Gracia SP, Pueo E, Chopo JM. Septic arthritis as an initial manifestation of bacterial endocarditis caused by *Staphylococcus aureus*. An Med Interna 2006;23:184-186.
4. Kocher MS, Horan MP, Briggs KK, et al. Reliability, validity and responsiveness of the American Shoulder and Elbow Surgeons subjective shoulder scale in patients with shoulder instability, rotator cuff disease and glenohumeral arthritis. J Bone Joint Surg Am 2005;87;2006-2011.
5. Chaipat L, Palmer WE. Shoulder magnetic resonance imaging. Clin Sports Med 2006;25:371-386.
6. Spinner RJ, Amrami KK, Kliot M, et al. Suprascapular intraneural ganglia and glenohumeral joint connections. J Neurosurg 2006;104:551-557.
7. Walch G, Ascani C, Boulahia A, et al. Static posterior subluxation of the humeral head: an unrecognized entity responsible for glenohumeral osteoarthritis in the young adult. J Shoulder Elbow Surg 2002;11:309-314.
8. Naredo E, Miller I, Moragues C, et al. Interobserver reliability in musculoskeletal ultrasonography: results from a "Teach the Teachers" rheumatologist course. Ann Rheum Dis 2006;65:14-19.
9. O'Connor PJ, Rankine J, Gibbon WW, et al. Interobserver variation in sonography of the painful shoulder. J Clin Ultrasound 2005;33:53-56.
10. Thomas T, Nol E, Goupille P, et al. The rheumatoid shoulder: current consensus on diagnosis and treatment. Joint Bone Spine 2006;73:139-143.
11. Wilcox RB, Arslanian LE, Millett P. Rehabilitation following total shoulder arthroplasty. J Orthop Sports Phys Ther 2005;35:821-836.
12. Sethi PM, El Attrache N. Accuracy of intra-articular injection of the glenohumeral joint: a cadaveric study. Orthopedics 2006;29:149-152.
13. Williams GR, Iannotti JP. Biomechanics of the glenohumeral joint: influence on shoulder arthroplasty. In Iannotti J, Williams G, eds. Disorders of the Shoulder: Diagnosis and Management. Philadelphia, Lippincott Williams & Wilkins, 1999.
14. Pennington WT, Bartz BA. Arthroscopic glenoid resurfacing with meniscal allograft: a minimally invasive alternative for treating glenohumeral arthritis. Arthroscopy 2005;21:1517-1520.
15. Nirschl RP. Arthroscopy in the treatment of glenohumeral osteoarthritis. Presented to the Brazilian Congress of Upper Extremity Surgeons; Belo Horizonte, Brazil; Sept 29, 2000.
16. Wirth MA, Tapscott RS, Southworth C, Rockwood CA. Treatment of glenohumeral arthritis with a hemiarthroplasty: a minimum of five-year follow-up outcome study. J Bone Joint Surg Am 2006;88:964-973.
17. Laudicina L, D'Ambrosia R. Management of irreparable rotator cuff tears and glenohumeral arthritis. Orthopaedics 2005;28:382-388.
18. Schenk T, Iannotti JP. Prosthetic arthroplasty for glenohumeral arthritis with an intact or repairable rotator cuff: indications, techniques, and results. In Iannotti J, Williams G, eds. Disorders of the Shoulder: Diagnosis and Management. Philadelphia, Lippincott Williams & Wilkins, 1999.
19. Fama G, Edwards TB, Boulahia A, et al. The role of concomitant biceps tenodesis in shoulder arthroplasty for primary osteoarthritis: results of a multicentric study. Orthopedics 2004;27:401-405.
20. Cuoma F, Birdzell MG, Zuckerman JD. The effect of degenerative arthritis and prosthetic arthroplasty on shoulder proprioception. J Shoulder Elbow Surg 2005;14:345-348.
21. Brophy RH, Marx RG. Osteoarthritis following shoulder instability. Clin Sports Med 2005;24:47-56.
22. Safran O, Iannotti JP. Arthrodesis of the shoulder. J Am Acad Orthop Surg 2006;14:145-153.
23. Bisson LJ. Thermal capsulorrhaphy for isolated posterior instability of the glenohumeral joint without labral detachment. Am J Sports Med 2005;33:1898-1904.
24. Drezner JA, Sennett BJ. Subacromial/subdeltoid septic bursitis associated with isotretinoin therapy and corticosteroid injection. J Am Board Fam Pract 2004;17:299-302.

Elbow Arthritis 18

Charles Cassidy, MD, and Chien Chow, MD

DEFINITION

In the simplest of terms, arthritis of the elbow reflects a loss of articular cartilage in the ulnotrochlear and radiocapitellar articulations. Destruction of the articulating surfaces and bone loss or, alternatively, excess bone formation in the form of osteophytes can be present. Joint contractures are common. Joint instability can result from inflammatory or traumatic injury to the bone architecture, capsule, and ligaments. The spectrum of disease ranges from intermittent pain or loss of motion with minimal changes detectable on radiographs to the more advanced stages of arthritis with a limited, painful arc of motion and radiographic demonstration of osteophyte formation, cysts, and loss of joint space. Ultimately, these destructive processes may result in complete ankylosis or total instability of the elbow.

The major causes of elbow arthritis are the inflammatory arthropathies, of which rheumatoid arthritis is the predominant disease. Arthritis of the elbow eventually develops in approximately 20% to 50% of patients with rheumatoid arthritis.[1] Involvement of the elbow in juvenile rheumatoid arthritis is not uncommon. Other inflammatory conditions affecting the elbow joint include systemic lupus erythematosus, the seronegative spondyloarthropathies (ankylosing spondylitis, psoriatic arthritis, Reiter syndrome, and enteropathic arthritis), and crystalline arthritis (gout and pseudogout). Post-traumatic arthritis may result from intra-articular fractures of the elbow. Osteonecrosis of the capitellum or trochlea, leading to arthritis, has also been described.[2,3] Primary osteoarthritis of the elbow

is a rare condition, responsible for less than 5% of elbow arthritis.[4] Interestingly, the incidence is significantly higher in the Alaskan Eskimo and Japanese populations.[5] Primary elbow arthritis usually affects the dominant arm of men in their 50s. Repetitive, strenuous arm use appears to be a risk factor; primary elbow arthritis has been reported in heavy laborers, weightlifters, and throwing athletes. Synovial chondromatosis is another rare cause of elbow arthritis.[3]

SYMPTOMS

The symptoms of elbow arthritis reflect, in part, the underlying etiology and severity of the disease process. Regardless of the etiology, however, the inability to fully straighten (extend) the elbow is a nearly universal complaint of patients with elbow arthritis. Associated symptoms of cubital tunnel syndrome (ulnar neuropathy at the elbow) include numbness in the ring and small fingers, loss of hand dexterity, and aching pain along the ulnar aspect of the forearm. Cubital tunnel syndrome is neither uncommon nor unexpected, given the proximity of the ulnar nerve to the elbow joint (see Chapter 23).

Patients with early rheumatoid involvement complain of a swollen, painful joint with morning stiffness. Progressive loss of motion or instability is seen in later stages. Compression of the posterior interosseous nerve by rheumatoid synovitis can occasionally produce the inability to extend the fingers.

Patients with crystalline arthritis of the elbow may complain of severe pain, swelling, and limited motion; an expedient evaluation is warranted to rule out a septic elbow in such cases.

Post-traumatic or idiopathic arthritis of the elbow, in contrast, usually manifests with painful loss of motion without the significant effusions, warmth, or constant pain associated with an inflamed synovium. These patients usually complain of pain at the extremes of motion secondary to osteophyte impingement, and they typically have more trouble extending the elbow than flexing it. Pain throughout the arc of motion implies advanced arthritis.

The final stages of arthritis, irrespective of cause, can include complaints of severe pain and decreased motion that hinder activities of daily living as well as the cosmetic deformity of the flexed elbow posture.

PHYSICAL EXAMINATION

Physical examination findings vary according to the cause and stage of the elbow arthritis. A flexion contracture is almost always present. The range of motion should be monitored at the initial examination and at subsequent follow-up examinations.

Normal adult elbow range of motion in extension-flexion is from 0 degrees to about 150 degrees; pronation averages 75 degrees, and supination averages 85 degrees. A functional range of motion is considered to be 30 degrees to 130 degrees, with 50 degrees of both pronation and supination.[6]

All other joints should be assessed as well. Strength should be normal but may be impaired in long-standing elbow arthritis because of disuse or, in more acute cases, pain. Weakness may also be noted in the presence of associated neuropathies. In the absence of associated neuropathies, deep tendon reflexes and sensation should be normal.

Associated ulnar nerve irritation can produce a sensitive nerve with the presence of Tinel sign over the cubital tunnel, diminished sensation in the small finger and ulnar half of the ring finger, and weakness of the intrinsic muscles (see Chapter 23). Numbness provoked by acute flexion of the elbow for 30 to 60 seconds is a positive elbow flexion test result.

Effusions, synovial thickenings, and erythema are commonly noted in the inflammatory arthropathies during acute flares. Loss of motion in flexion and extension, as well as in pronation and supination, can be present because the synovitis affects all articulating surfaces in the elbow. Pain, limited motion, and crepitus worsen as the disease progresses. On occasion, rheumatoid destruction of the elbow will produce instability, which may be perceived by the patient as weakness or mechanical symptoms. Examination of such elbows will demonstrate laxity to varus and valgus stress; posterior instability may also be seen.

In contrast, progressive primary or post-traumatic arthritis of the elbow results in stiffness. The loss of extension is usually worse than the loss of flexion. Pain is present with forced extension or flexion. Crepitus may be palpable throughout the arc of flexion-extension or with forearm rotation.

FUNCTIONAL LIMITATIONS

The elbow functions to position the hand in space. Significant loss of extension can hinder an individual's ability to interact with the environment, making activities that require nearly full extension, like carrying groceries or briefcases, painful. Significant loss of flexion can interfere with activities of daily living such as eating, shaving, and washing. A normal shoulder can compen-

TABLE 18-1	Radiographic Classification of Rheumatoid Arthritis[7]
I	Synovitis with a normal-appearing joint
II	Loss of joint space but maintenance of the subchondral architecture
IIIa	Alteration of the subchondral architecture
IIIb	Alteration of the architecture with deformity
IV	Gross deformity

sate well for a lack of pronation, whereas a normal shoulder, wrist, and cervical spine can compensate, albeit awkwardly, for a lack of elbow flexion. There is no simple solution for a significant lack of elbow extension; the body must be moved closer to the desired object. Compensatory mechanisms are often impaired in patients with rheumatoid arthritis, magnifying the impact of the elbow arthritis on function.

DIAGNOSTIC STUDIES

Anteroposterior, lateral, and oblique radiographic views of the elbow are usually sufficient for diagnosis of elbow arthritis. The radiographs should be inspected for joint space narrowing, osteophyte and cyst formation, and bone destruction. For the rheumatoid patient, the Mayo Clinic radiographic classification of rheumatoid involvement is useful (Table 18-1).[7] Dramatic loss of bone is evident as the disease progresses (Fig. 18-1). This pattern of destruction is not seen, however, in the post-traumatic or idiopathic patient. Radiographic features in these patients include spurs or osteophytes on the coronoid and olecranon, loose bodies, and narrowing of the coronoid and olecranon fossae (Fig. 18-2).

Magnetic resonance arthrography or computed tomographic arthrography may help localize suspected loose bodies. Magnetic resonance imaging is most valuable for confirmation of suspected osteonecrosis.

The diagnosis of rheumatoid arthritis will have already been made in the majority of patients who present with rheumatoid elbow involvement. When isolated inflammatory arthritis of the elbow is suspected, appropriate serologic studies may include analysis of rheumatoid factor, antinuclear antibody, HLA-B27, and erythrocyte sedimentation rate. Elbow aspiration may be needed to rule out a crystalline or infectious cause in patients who present with a warm, stiff, swollen, and painful joint with no history of trauma or inflammatory arthritis.

TREATMENT

Initial

Treatment of elbow arthritis depends on the diagnosis, degree of involvement, functional limitations, and pain. When the elbow is one of a number of joints actively involved with inflammatory arthritis, the obvious treatment

Differential Diagnosis

Medial or lateral epicondylitis

Median nerve compression

Elbow instability

Radial tunnel syndrome

Septic arthritis

Cervical radiculopathy

Acute fracture

Elbow contracture

Cubital tunnel syndrome

is systemic. Disease-modifying agents have had a dramatic effect in relieving symptoms and retarding the progression of arthritis for many of these patients. For systemic disease, a rheumatology consultation can be beneficial.

The initial local treatment of an acutely inflamed elbow joint includes rest. A simple sling places the elbow in a relatively comfortable position. The patient should be encouraged to remove the sling for gentle range of motion exercises of the elbow and shoulder several times daily. Icing of the elbow for 15 minutes several times a day for the first few days may be beneficial.

Nonoperative treatment of primary osteoarthritis of the elbow primarily consists of rest, activity modification, and nonsteroidal anti-inflammatory drugs. Oral analgesics may help with pain control. Topical treatments such as capsaicin can be tried as well.

Patients who have associated cubital tunnel symptoms are instructed to avoid direct pressure over the elbow and to avoid prolonged elbow flexion. A static night splint that maintains the elbow in about 30 degrees of flexion may help alleviate cubital tunnel symptoms (see Chapter 23).

Rehabilitation

Once the acute inflammation has subsided, physical or occupational therapy may be instituted to regain elbow motion and strength and to educate the patient in activity modification and pain control measures.

Therapy should focus on improving range of motion and strength throughout the upper body with a goal of improving function regardless of the degree of elbow arthritis. Adaptive equipment, such as reachers, can be recommended. Ergonomic workstation equipment may also be useful (e.g., voice-activated computer software, forearm rests).

Modalities such as ultrasound and iontophoresis may help with pain control.

Nighttime static, static-progressive, or dynamic extension splinting may be indicated to relieve significant elbow contractures. Braces may be effective in the setting of instability. The goal of therapy is *functional* rather than full elbow motion.

In primary osteoarthritis of the elbow, corrective splinting is not indicated because bone impingement is usually present. Similarly, therapy may actually aggravate the symptoms and should be ordered judiciously.

Rehabilitation is critical to the success of surgical procedures around the elbow. The rheumatoid patient commonly has multiple joint problems that must not be neglected during treatment of the elbow. The shoulder is at particular risk for stiffness. A good operation, a motivated patient, and a knowledgeable and skillful therapist are necessary to optimize postoperative results. Postoperative rehabilitation depends on the procedure and the

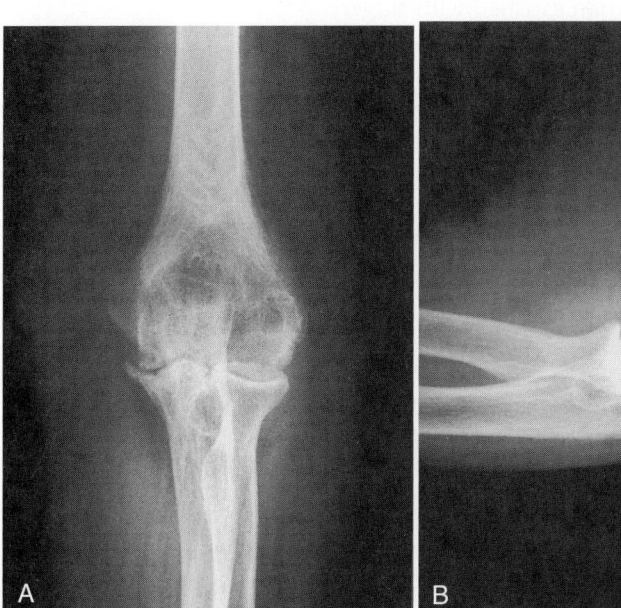

FIGURE 18-1. Rheumatoid arthritis. Anteroposterior (**A**) and lateral (**B**) elbow radiographs of a 40-year-old woman with long-standing elbow pain. Osteopenia and symmetric joint space narrowing are present. The lateral radiograph demonstrates early bone loss in the ulna. This is categorized as stage IIIa.

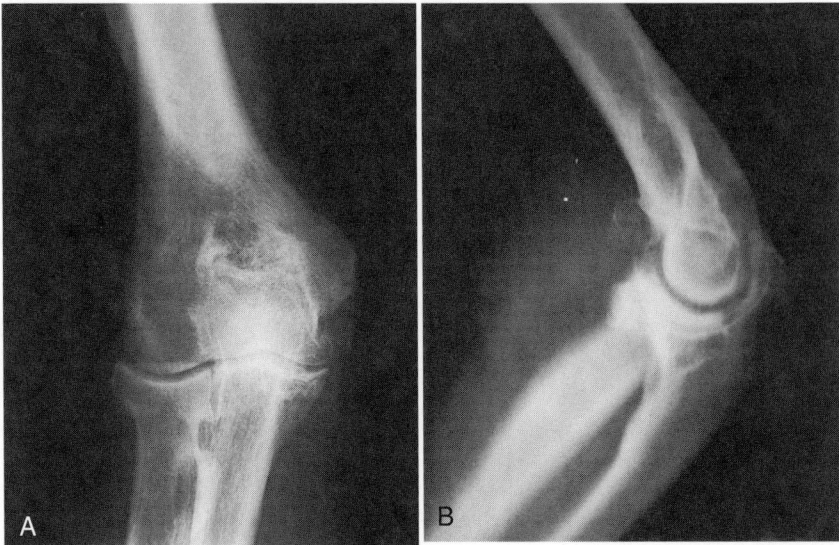

FIGURE 18-2. Primary degenerative elbow arthritis. Anteroposterior **(A)** and lateral **(B)** elbow radiographs of a 52-year-old man with dominant right elbow pain at the extremes of motion. **A,** Joint space narrowing and obliteration of the coronoid fossa. **B,** Coronoid and olecranon spurs and a large anterior loose body are evident.

surgeon's preference. However, in general, physical or occupational therapy should be recommended to restore range of motion and strength.

Procedures

For recalcitrant symptoms, intra-articular steroid injections are effective in relieving the pain associated with synovitis (Fig. 18-3).

The elbow joint is best accessed through the "soft spot," the center of the triangle formed by the lateral epicondyle, the tip of the olecranon, and the radial head. The patient is placed with the elbow between 50 degrees and 90 degrees of flexion. For the posterolateral approach, the lateral epicondyle and the posterior olecranon are palpated. Under sterile conditions, with use of a 25-gauge, 1½-inch needle, 3 to 4 mL of an anesthetic-corticosteroid mixture (e.g., 1 mL of 80 mg/mL methylprednisolone and 3 mL of 1% lidocaine) is injected. The needle is directed proximally toward the head of the radius and medially into the elbow joint. No resistance should be noted as the needle enters the joint. If an effusion is present, aspiration may be done before the anesthetic-corticosteroid mixture is injected.

For the posterior approach, the olecranon fossa is palpated just proximal to the tip of the olecranon. The needle is then inserted above the superior aspect of and lateral to the olecranon. Again, it should enter the joint without resistance.

Postinjection care may include icing of the elbow for 10 to 20 minutes after the injection and then two or three times daily thereafter. The patient should be informed that the pain may worsen for the first 24 to 36 hours and that the medication may take 1 week to work.

In general, repeated injections are not recommended. Although the intra-articular steroids are effective in treating synovitis, they also temporarily inhibit chondrocyte synthesis, an effect that could potentially accelerate arthritis.

Surgery

Patients whose treatment has failed after 3 to 6 months of adequate medical therapy are potential candidates for surgery. Refractory pain is the best indication for surgery. In assessment of the surgical candidate with primary elbow arthritis, it is important to listen carefully to the patient's complaints. Many patients are dissatisfied with the simple fact that they cannot fully straighten the elbow. Such patients will usually be less than satisfied with surgery.

Intermittent locking or catching suggestive of a loose body is often best treated with arthroscopy. Pain at the extremes of motion is consistent with olecranon and coronoid osteophyte impingement. An ulnohumeral arthroplasty, or surgical débridement of the elbow joint, may be recommended. Traditionally, open surgical techniques have been performed to remove impinging osteophytes. More recent arthroscopic advances have permitted this débridement to be performed in a less invasive manner, with potentially less morbidity. However, arthroscopic treatment of elbow contractures is a technically demanding procedure.[8] Ulnohumeral arthroplasty is successful at achieving its principal goal—pain relief at the extremes of motion. However, it is only marginally successful at actually improving motion, with an average improvement in extension of 7 to 12 degrees and an average improvement in flexion of 8 to 17 degrees in four reported series.[4,9-11] Overall, 85% of patients in these series were satisfied with the results. As expected, the results deteriorate with time as the arthritis progresses.

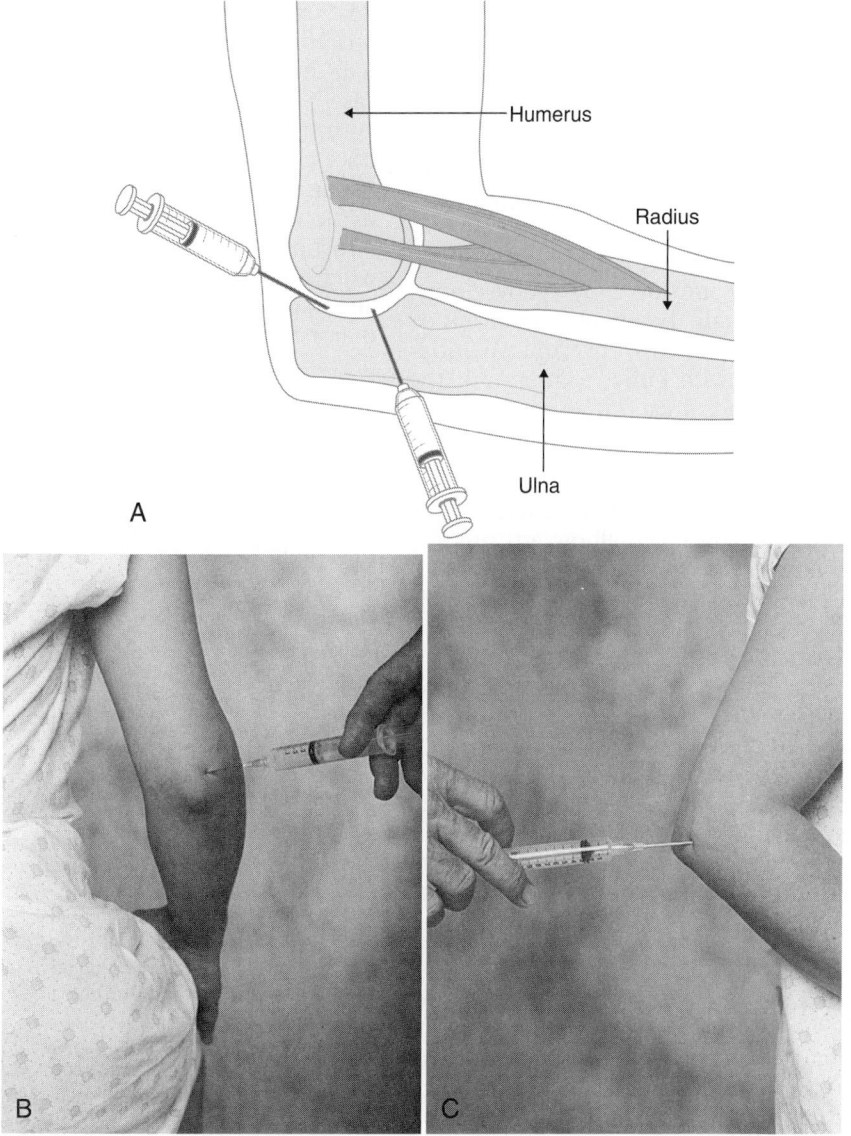

FIGURE 18-3. Internal anatomic (**A**) and approximate surface anatomic (**B,** lateral; **C,** posterior) sites for injection of the elbow laterally and posteriorly. (Reprinted with permission from Lennard TA. Pain Procedures in Clinical Practice, 2nd ed. Philadelphia, Hanley & Belfus, 2000.)

Less commonly, patients with primary arthritis complain of pain throughout the arc of motion. Their radiographs will probably demonstrate advanced arthritis with severe joint space narrowing. Simple removal of the osteophytes is not likely to be successful. Total elbow arthroplasty would seem to be a reasonable option. However, unlike their rheumatoid counterparts, most of these patients are otherwise healthy, vigorous people who would regularly stress their joint replacement. For this reason, total elbow arthroplasty in this setting is best reserved for the sedentary patient older than 65 years.[12]

For the younger patient with advanced primary arthritis, a distraction interposition arthroplasty is recommended.[3,14,15] This procedure involves a radical débridement of the joint followed by a resurfacing of the joint surfaces with an interposition material, such as autologous fascia lata or allograft Achilles tendon. A hinged external fixator is then applied, which will protect the healing interposition material while simultaneously maintaining elbow stability and permitting motion. In the one relatively large series of distraction interposition arthroplasty,[15] pain relief was satisfactory in 69% of patients at an average of 5 years postoperatively. An advantage of interposition arthroplasty is the potential for conversion to total elbow arthroplasty, ideally after the age of 60 years,[16] but this procedure certainly does not produce a normal elbow.

Other nonimplant surgical options include elbow arthrodesis and resection arthroplasty. There is no ideal position for an elbow fusion. The elbow looks more cosmetically appealing when it is relatively straight. However, this position is relatively useless. Consequently, elbow arthrodesis is performed rarely, usually in the setting of intractable infection. Resection arthroplasty is an option for a failed total elbow arthroplasty.

This procedure permits some elbow motion, although the elbow tends to be very unstable.

For the rheumatoid patient with elbow arthritis, elbow synovectomy and débridement provide predictable short-term pain relief.[17] Interestingly, the results do not necessarily correlate with the severity of the arthritis. The results do, however, deteriorate somewhat over time, drifting down from 90% success at 3 years to 70% success by 10 years as the synovitis recurs.[18-20] Elbow motion is not necessarily improved by synovectomy; only 40% of patients obtain better motion. A study comparing arthroscopic and open synovectomy demonstrated equivalent results with either technique if the preoperative arc of flexion is greater than 90 degrees.[19] For stiff rheumatoid elbows, arthroscopic synovectomy performed better than the open method did.

Total elbow arthroplasty is a reliable procedure for the rheumatoid patient with advanced elbow arthritis.[21,22] The Mayo Clinic has reported excellent results with a semiconstrained prosthesis,[23] with pain relief in 92% of patients and an average arc of motion of 26 to 130 degrees, with 64 degrees of pronation and 62 degrees of supination. An outcomes study demonstrated good satisfaction of the patients, although the majority of patients continued to have some functional impairments, presumably due, in part, to rheumatoid involvement in other joints.[24] In spite of the excellent clinical results, the patient should be made aware that the complication rate for total elbow arthroplasty is significantly higher than that for the more conventional hip and knee replacements.

POTENTIAL DISEASE COMPLICATIONS

End-stage rheumatoid arthritis of the elbow can produce either severe stiffness or instability. Advanced primary arthritis invariably produces stiffness. Either outcome results in pain and limited function of the involved extremity. In addition, entrapment or traction neuritis of the ulnar nerve is not uncommon. Compressive injury to the posterior interosseous nerve from rheumatoid synovial hyperplasia has also been reported.

POTENTIAL TREATMENT COMPLICATIONS

The systemic complications of the disease-modifying agents used in treatment of rheumatoid arthritis are numerous and are beyond the scope of this chapter (see Chapters 30 and 37). Analgesics and nonsteroidal anti-inflammatory drugs have well-known side effects that most commonly affect the gastric, hepatic, and renal systems. Intra-articular steroid injections introduce the risk of iatrogenic infection and may produce transient chondrocyte damage.

Potential surgical complications include infection, wound problems, neurovascular injury, stiffness, recurrent synovitis, triceps disruption, periprosthetic lucency, fracture, and iatrogenic instability. In the primary and post-traumatic osteoarthritic elbow, motion-improving procedures such as ulnohumeral arthroplasty do not halt the inevitable radiographic progression of the disease. Similarly, synovectomy of the rheumatoid elbow, even if it is successful in alleviating pain and synovitis, does not reliably prevent further joint destruction. Preoperative ulnar nerve symptoms can occasionally be made worse by surgery, and simultaneous ulnar nerve transposition should be considered in such patients when the preoperative range of motion is limited.[11] In an analysis of 473 consecutive elbow arthroscopies, major and temporary minor complications occurred in 0.8% and 11% of patients, respectively.[8] The most significant risk factors for development of temporary nerve palsies were rheumatoid arthritis and contracture.

With total elbow arthroplasty, wound healing problems, infection, triceps insufficiency, and implant loosening are the principal complications, occurring in approximately 5% to 7% of patients. As a result, most surgeons place lifelong restrictions on high-impact loading (no golf, no lifting of more than 10 pounds) to minimize the need for revision surgery.

References

1. Porter BB, Park N, Richardson C, Vainio K. Rheumatoid arthritis of the elbow: the results of synovectomy. J Bone Joint Surg Br 1974;56:427-437.
2. Le TB, Mont MA, Jones LC, et al. Atraumatic osteonecrosis of the adult elbow. Clin Orthop 2000;373:141-145.
3. Gramstad GD, Galatz LM. Management of elbow osteoarthritis. J Bone Joint Surg Am 2006;88:421-430.
4. Morrey BF. Primary degenerative arthritis of the elbow: treatment by ulnohumeral arthroplasty. J Bone Joint Surg Br 1992;74:409-413.
5. Ortner DJ. Description and classification of degenerative bone changes in the distal joint surface of the humerus. Am J Phys Anthropol 1968;28:139-155.
6. Morrey BF, Askew L, An KN, et al. A biomechanical study of normal functional elbow motion. J Bone Joint Surg Am 1981;63:872-877.
7. Morrey BF, Adams RA. Semi-constrained arthroplasty for the treatment of rheumatoid arthritis of the elbow. J Bone Joint Surg Am 1992;74:479-490.
8. Kelly EW, Morrey BF, O'Driscoll SW. Complications of elbow arthroscopy. J Bone Joint Surg Am 2001;83:25-34.
9. Oka Y. Debridement arthroplasty for osteoarthrosis of the elbow. Acta Orthop Scand 2000;71:185-190.
10. Wada T, Isogai S, Ishii S, Yamashita T. Debridement arthroplasty for primary osteoarthritis of the elbow. J Bone Joint Surg Am 2004;86:233-241.
11. Antuña SA, Morrey BF, Adams RA, O'Driscoll SW. Ulnohumeral arthroplasty for primary degenerative arthritis of the elbow. J Bone Joint Surg Am 2002;84:2168-2173.
12. Moro JK, King GJ. Total elbow arthroplasty in the treatment of posttraumatic conditions of the elbow. Clin Orthop Relat Res 2000;370:102-114.
13. Gramstad GD, King GJ, O'Driscoll SW, Yamagushi K. Elbow arthroplasty using a convertible implant. Tech Hand Up Extrem Surg 2005;9:153-163.
14. Wright PE, Froimson AI, Morrey BF. Interposition arthroplasty of the elbow. In Morrey BF, ed. The Elbow and Its Disorders, 3rd ed. Philadelphia, WB Saunders, 2000:718-730.
15. Cheng SL, Morrey BF. Treatment of the mobile, painful, arthritic elbow by distraction interposition arthroplasty. J Bone Joint Surg Br 2000;82:223-228.

16. Blaine TA, Adams R, Morrey BF. Total elbow arthroplasty after interposition arthroplasty for elbow arthritis. J Bone Joint Surg Am 2005;87:286-292.

17. Ferlic DC, Patchett CE, Clayton ML, Freeman AC. Elbow synovectomy in rheumatoid arthritis. Clin Orthop 1987;220:119-125.

18. Alexiades MM, Stanwyck TS, Figgie MP, Inglis AE. Minimum ten-year follow-up of elbow synovectomy for rheumatoid arthritis. Orthop Trans 1990;14:255.

19. Tanaka N, Sakahashi H, Hirose K, et al. Arthroscopic and open synovectomy of the elbow in rheumatoid arthritis. J Bone Joint Surg Am 2006;88:521-525.

20. Horiuchi K, Momohara S, Tomatsu T, et al. Arthroscopic synovectomy of the elbow in rheumatoid arthritis. J Bone Joint Surg Am 2002;84:342-347.

21. Hargreaves D, Emery R. Total elbow replacement in the treatment of rheumatoid disease. Clin Orthop Relat Res 1999;366:61-71.

22. Ferlic DC. Total elbow arthroplasty for treatment of elbow arthritis. J Shoulder Elbow Surg 1999;8:367-378.

23. Gill DR, Morrey BF. The Coonrad-Morrey total elbow arthroplasty in patients with rheumatoid arthritis: a 10- to 15-year follow-up study. J Bone Joint Surg Am 1998;80:1327-1335.

24. Angst F, John M, Pap G, et al. Comprehensive assessment of clinical outcome and quality of life after total elbow arthroplasty. Arthritis Rheum 2005;53:73-82.

Epicondylitis 19

Lyn D. Weiss, MD, and Jay M. Weiss, MD

Synonyms

Tendinosis[1]
Lateral epicondylitis
Medial epicondylitis
Tennis elbow
Pitcher's elbow
Golfer's elbow

ICD-9 Codes

726.31   Medial epicondylitis
726.32   Lateral epicondylitis

DEFINITION

Epicondylitis is a general term used to describe inflammation, pain, or tenderness in the region of the medial or lateral epicondyle of the humerus. The actual nidus of pain and pathologic change has been debated. Lateral epicondylitis implies an inflammatory lesion with degeneration at the origin of the extensor muscles (the lateral epicondyle of the humerus). The extensor carpi radialis brevis is the muscle primarily affected. Other muscles that can contribute to the condition are the extensor carpi radialis longus and the extensor digitorum communis. In medial epicondylitis, the flexor muscle group is affected (flexor carpi radialis, flexor carpi ulnaris, flexor digitorum superficialis, and palmaris longus).

Although the term *epicondylitis* implies an inflammatory process, inflammatory cells are not identified histologically. Instead, the condition may be secondary to failure of the musculotendinous attachment with resultant fibroplasia,[2] termed tendinosis. Other postulated primary lesions include angiofibroblastic tendinosis, periostitis, and enthesitis.[3] In children, medial elbow pain may result from repetitive stress on the apophysis of the medial epicondyle ossification center (little leaguer's elbow).[4] Overall, the focus of injury appears to be the muscle origin. Symptoms may be related to failure of the repair process.[5]

Repetitive stress has been implicated as a factor in this condition.[6] Poor throwing mechanics and excessive throwing have been implicated in little leaguer's elbow. Overuse from a tennis backhand (especially a one-handed backhand with poor technique) can frequently lead to lateral epicondylitis (hence, the term *tennis elbow* is frequently used synonymously with lateral epicondylitis, regardless of its etiology). Repetitive wrist flexion as in the trailing arm in a golf swing can cause a medial epicondylitis (hence, the term *golfer's elbow* is frequently used for medial epicondylitis, also regardless of etiology).

SYMPTOMS

Patients usually report pain in the area just distal to the lateral epicondyle (lateral epicondylitis) or the medial epicondyle (medial epicondylitis). The patient may complain of pain radiating proximally or distally. Patients may also complain of pain with wrist or hand movement, such as gripping a doorknob, carrying a briefcase, or shaking hands. Patients occasionally report swelling as well.

PHYSICAL EXAMINATION

On examination, the hallmark of epicondylitis is tenderness over the extensor muscle origin (lateral epicondylitis) or flexor muscle origin (medial epicondylitis). The origin of the extensor or flexor muscles can be located one fingerbreadth below the lateral or medial epicondyle, respectively. With lateral epicondylitis, pain is increased with resisted wrist extension, especially with the elbow extended, the forearm pronated, the wrist radially deviated, and the hand in a fist. The middle finger test can also be used to assess for lateral epicondylitis. Here, the proximal interphalangeal joint of the long finger is resisted in extension, and pain is elicited over the lateral epicondyle. Swelling is occasionally present. With medial epicondylitis, pain is increased with resisted wrist flexion. In cases of recalcitrant lateral epicondylitis, the diagnosis of radial nerve entrapment should be considered. The radial nerve can become entrapped just distal to the lateral epicondyle where the nerve pierces the intermuscular septum (between the brachialis and brachioradialis muscles). There may be localized tenderness

105

along the course of the radial nerve around the radial head. Motor and sensory findings are usually absent.

FUNCTIONAL LIMITATIONS

The patient may complain of an inability to lift or to carry objects on the affected side secondary to increased pain. Typing, using a computer mouse, or working on a keyboard may re-create the pain. Even handshaking or squeezing may be painful in both lateral and medial epicondylitis. Athletic activities may cause pain, especially with an acute increase in repetition, poor technique, and equipment changes (frequently with a new racket or stringing).

DIAGNOSTIC STUDIES

The diagnosis is usually made on clinical grounds. Magnetic resonance imaging, which is particularly useful for soft tissue definition, can be used to assess for tendinitis, tendinosis, degeneration, partial tears or complete tears, and detachment of the common flexor or common extensor tendons at the medial or lateral epicondyles, respectively.[7] Magnetic resonance imaging is rarely needed, however, except in recalcitrant epicondylitis, and it will not alter the treatment significantly in the early stages. The medial and lateral collateral ligament complexes can be evaluated for tears as well as for chronic degeneration and scarring. Arthrography may be beneficial if capsular defects and associated ligament injuries are suspected. Barring evidence of trauma, early radiographs are of little help in this condition but may be useful in cases of resistant tendinitis and to rule out occult fractures, arthritis, and/or osteochondral loose body.

Differential Diagnosis

Posterior interosseous nerve syndrome

Bone infection or tumors

Median or ulnar neuropathy around the elbow

Osteoarthritis

Acute calcification around the lateral epicondyle[8]

Osteochondral loose body

Anconeus compartment syndrome[9]

Triceps tendinitis

Degenerative arthrosis[10]

Elbow synovitis

Lateral ligament instability[11]

Radial head fracture

Bursitis

Collateral ligament tears

Hypertrophic synovial plica[12]

TREATMENT

Initial

Initial treatment consists of relative rest, avoidance of repetitive motions involving the wrist, activity modification to avoid stress on the epicondyles, anti-inflammatory medications, and thermal modalities such as heat and ice for acute pain. Patients who develop lateral epicondylitis from tennis should modify their stroke (especially improving the backhand stroke to ensure that the forearm is in midpronation and the trunk is leaning forward) and their equipment, usually by reducing string tension and enlarging the grip size.[6] Frequently, a two-handed backhand will relieve the stress sufficiently. Patients who develop medial epicondylitis from golf should consider modifying their swing to avoid excessive force on wrist flexor muscles. Biomechanical modifications may help reduce symptoms if the medial epicondylitis is thought to be due to poor pitching technique.

In addition, a forearm band (counterforce brace) worn distal to the flexor or extensor muscle group origin can be beneficial. The theory behind this device is that it will dissipate forces over a larger area of tissue than the medial or lateral attachment site. Alternatively, the use of wrist immobilization splints may be helpful. A splint set in neutral can be helpful for either medial or lateral epicondylitis by relieving the tension on the flexors and extensors of the wrist and fingers. A splint set in 30 to 40 degrees of wrist extension (for lateral epicondylitis only) will relieve the tension on the extensors, including the extensor carpi radialis brevis muscle as well as other wrist and finger extensors.[13,14] Dynamic extension bracing has also been proposed.[15]

Rehabilitation

Rehabilitation may include physical or occupational therapy. Therapy should include two phases. The first phase is directed at decreasing pain (ultrasound, electrical stimulation, phonophoresis, heat, ice, massage) and decreasing disability (education, reduction of repetitive stress, and preservation of motion). When the patient is pain free, a gradual program is implemented to improve strength and endurance of wrist extensors (for lateral epicondylitis) or wrist flexors (for medial epicondylitis) and stretching. This program must be carefully monitored to permit strengthening of the muscles and work hardening of the tissues, without itself causing an overuse situation. The patient should start with static exercises and advance to progressive resistive exercises. Thera-Band, light weights, and manual (self) resistance exercises can be used.

Work or activity restrictions or modifications may be required for a time.

Procedures

Injection of corticosteroid, usually with a local anesthetic, into the area of maximum tenderness (approximately 1 to 5 cm distal to the lateral epicondyle) has been shown to be effective in treatment of lateral epicondylitis (Fig. 19-1).[16] To confirm the diagnosis, a trial of lidocaine alone may be given. An immediate improvement in grip strength should be noted after injection. Postinjection treatment includes icing of the affected area both immediately (for 5 to 10 minutes) and thereafter (a reasonable regimen is 20 minutes two or three times per day for 2 weeks) and wearing of a wrist splint (particularly for activities that involve wrist movement). The wrist splint should be set in slight extension for lateral epicondylitis and neutral for medial epicondylitis. Exacerbating activities are to be avoided.

Injection of botulinum toxin into the extensor digitorum communis muscles to the third and fourth digits has been reported to be beneficial in treating chronic treatment-resistant lateral epicondylitis.[17,18]

Injections for medial epicondylitis must be used cautiously because of the risk of injury to the ulnar nerve (either by direct injection or by tissue changes that may promote nerve injury). There are studies that support acupuncture as an effective modality in the short-term relief of lateral epicondylitis.[19-21]

Surgery

Surgery may be indicated in those patients with continued severe symptoms who do not respond to conservative management. For lateral epicondylitis, surgery is aimed at excision and revitalization of the pathologic tissue in the extensor carpi radialis brevis and release of the muscle origin.[22] Pinning may be done if the elbow joint is unstable.[4]

POTENTIAL DISEASE COMPLICATIONS

Possible long-term complications of untreated epicondylitis include chronic pain, loss of function, and possible elbow contracture. Medial epicondylitis may lead to reversible impairment (neurapraxia) of the ulnar

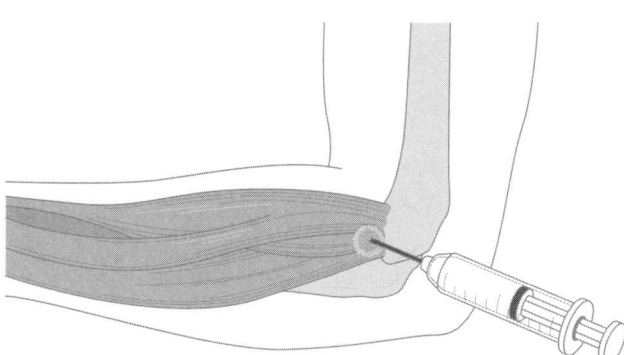

FIGURE 19-1. Under sterile conditions, with use of a 27-gauge needle and 1 to 2 mL of a local anesthetic combined with 1 to 2 mL of a corticosteroid preparation, inject the solution approximately 1 to 5 cm distal to the lateral epicondyle. The injected materials should flow smoothly. Resistance generally indicates that the solution is being injected directly into the tendon, and this should be avoided.

nerve.[23] In general, epicondylitis is more easily and successfully treated in the acute phase.

POTENTIAL TREATMENT COMPLICATIONS

Analgesics and nonsteroidal anti-inflammatory drugs have well-known side effects that most commonly affect the gastric, hepatic, and renal systems. Local steroid injections may increase the risk for disruption of tissue planes, create high-pressure tissue necrosis, rupture tendons,[1] damage nerves, promote skin depigmentation or atrophy, or cause infection.[24]

References

 1. Kraushaar BS, Nirschl RP. Tendinosis of the elbow (tennis elbow): clinical features and findings of histological, immunohistochemical, and electron microscopy studies. J Bone Joint Surg Am 1999;81:259-278.
 2. Nirschl RP, Pettrone FA. Tennis elbow. J Bone Joint Surg Am 1979;61:832-839.
 3. Nirschl RP. Elbow tendinosis/tennis elbow. Clin Sports Med 1992;11:851-870.
 4. Brown D, Freeman E, Cuccurullo S. Elbow disorders. In Cuccurullo S, ed. Physical Medicine and Rehabilitation Board Review. New York, Demos, 2004:163-173.
 5. Putnam MD, Cohen M. Painful conditions around the elbow. Orthop Clin North Am 1999;30:109-118.
 6. Cassvan A, Weiss LD, Weiss JM, et al. Cumulative Trauma Disorders. Boston, Butterworth-Heinemann, 1997:123-125.
 7. Braddom RL. Physical Medicine and Rehabilitation. Philadelphia, WB Saunders, 1996:222.
 8. Hughes E. Acute deposition of calcium near the elbow. J Bone Joint Surg Br 1950;32:30-34.
 9. Abrahamsson S, Sollerman C, Soderberg T, et al. Lateral elbow pain caused by anconeus compartment syndrome. Acta Orthop Scand 1987;58:589-591.
10. Brems JJ. Degenerative joint disease of the elbow. In Nicholas JA, Hershman EB, eds. The Upper Extremity in Sports Medicine. St. Louis, Mosby, 1995:331-335.
11. Morrey BF. Anatomy of the elbow joint. In Morrey BF, ed. The Elbow and Its Disorders, 2nd ed. Philadelphia, WB Saunders, 1993:16.
12. Kim DH, Gambardella RA, El attrache NS, et al. Arthroscopic treatment of posterolateral elbow impingement from lateral synovial plicae in throwing athletes and golfers. Am J Sports Med 2006;34:438-444. Epub 2005 Dec 19.
13. Plancher KD. The athletic elbow and wrist, part I. Diagnosis and conservative treatment. Clin Sports Med 1995;15:433-435.
14. Derebery VJ, Devenport JN, Giang GM, Fogarty WT. The effects of splinting on outcomes for epicondylitis. Arch Phys Med Rehabil 2005;86:1081-1088.
15. Faes M, van den Akker B, de Lint JA, et al. Dynamic extensor brace for lateral epicondylitis. Clin Orthop Relat Res 2006;442:149-157.
16. Hay EH, Paterson SM, Lewis M, et al. Pragmatic randomized controlled trial of local corticosteroid injection and naproxen for treatment of lateral epicondylitis of elbow in primary care. BMJ 1999;319:964-968.
17. Morre HH, Keizer SB, van Os JJ. Treatment of chronic tennis elbow with botulinum toxin. Lancet 1997;349:1746.
18. Wong SM, Jui AC, Tong PY, et al. Treatment of lateral epicondylitis with botulinum toxin: a randomized, double-blind, placebo-controlled trial. Ann Intern Med 2005;143:793-797.
19. Trinh KV, Phillips SD, Ho E, Damsma K. Acupuncture for the alleviation of lateral epicondyle pain: a systematic review. Rheumatology (Oxford) 2004;43:1085-1090.

20. Fink M, Wolkenstein E, Luennemann M, et al. Chronic epicondylitis: effects of real and sham acupuncture treatment: a randomised controlled patient- and examiner-blinded long-term trial. Forsch Komplementarmed Klass Naturheilkd 2002;9:210-215.

21. Fink M, Wolkenstein E, Karst M, Gehrke A. Acupuncture in chronic epicondylitis: a randomized controlled trial. Rheumatology (Oxford) 2002;41:205-209.

22. Organ SW, Nirschl RP, Kraushaar BS, Guidi EJ. Salvage surgery for lateral tennis elbow. Am J Sports Med 1997;25:746-750.

23. Barry NN, McGuire JL. Overuse syndromes in adult athletes. Rheum Dis Clin North Am 1996;22:515-530.

24. Nichols AW. Complications associated with the use of corticosteroids in the treatment of athletic injuries [review]. Clin J Sport Med 2005;15:370-375.

Median Neuropathy 20

Francisco H. Santiago, MD, and Ramon Vallarino, Jr., MD

Synonyms

Pronator teres syndrome
Pronator syndrome
Anterior interosseous syndrome
Kiloh-Nevin syndrome

ICD-9 Code

354.1   Other lesion of median nerve (median nerve neuritis)

DEFINITION

There are three general areas in which the median nerve can become entrapped around the elbow and forearm. Because this chapter mainly deals with entrapment below the elbow and above the wrist, the most proximal and least frequent entrapment is not discussed but merely mentioned. Elbow median nerve entrapment is the compression of the nerve by a dense band of connective tissue called the ligament of Struthers, an aberrant ligament found immediately above the elbow. The topics discussed in this chapter are compression of the median nerve at or immediately below the elbow, where the pronator teres muscle usually compresses it, and compression distally of a branch of the median nerve—the anterior interosseous nerve.

Pronator Teres Syndrome

Pronator teres syndrome[1,3] is a symptom complex that is produced where the median nerve crosses the elbow and becomes entrapped as it passes first beneath the lacertus fibrosus—a thick fascial band extending from the biceps tendon to the forearm fascia—then between the two heads (superficial and deep) of the pronator teres muscle and under the edge of the flexor digitorum sublimis (Fig. 20-1). Compression may be related to a local process such as pronator teres hypertrophy, tenosynovitis, muscle hemorrhage, fascial tear, postoperative scarring, or anomalous median artery. The median nerve may also be injured by occupational strain, such as carrying a grocery bag, guitar playing, or insertion of a catheter.[1,3-10]

Anterior Interosseous Syndrome

The anterior interosseous nerve arises from the median nerve 5 to 8 cm distal to the lateral epicondyle.[1,2,4] Slightly distal to its course through the pronator teres muscle, the median nerve gives off the anterior interosseous nerve, a purely motor branch (Fig. 20-2). It contains no fibers of superficial sensation but does supply deep pain and proprioception to some deep tissues, including the wrist joint. This nerve may be damaged by direct trauma, forearm fractures, humeral fracture, injection into or blood drawing from the cubital vein, supracondylar fracture, and fibrous bands related to the flexor digitorum sublimis and flexor digitorum profundus muscles. In some patients, it is a component of brachial amyotrophy of the shoulder girdle (proximal fascicular lesion) or related to cytomegalovirus infection or a bronchogenic carcinoma metastasis. The nerve may be partially involved, but in a fully established syndrome, three muscles are weak: flexor pollicis longus, flexor digitorum profundus to the second and sometimes the third digits, and pronator quadratus.[1,2,4,10-15]

SYMPTOMS

Pronator Teres Syndrome

In an acute compression, with unmistakable symptoms, the diagnosis is relatively simple to establish.[2,3] In many cases of intermittent, mild, or partial compression, the signs and symptoms are vague and nondescript. The most common symptom is mild to moderate aching pain in the proximal forearm, sometimes described as tiredness and heaviness. Use of the arm may cause a mild or dull aching pain to become deep or sharp. Repetitive elbow motions are likely to provoke symptoms. As the pain intensifies, it may radiate proximally to the elbow or even to the shoulder. Paresthesias in the distribution of the median nerve may be reported, but they are generally not as severe or well localized as the complaints in carpal tunnel syndrome. When numbness is a prominent symptom, the complaints may mimic carpal tunnel syndrome. However, unlike carpal tunnel syndrome, pronator teres syndrome rarely has nocturnal exacerbation and the symptoms are not exacerbated by a change of wrist position.

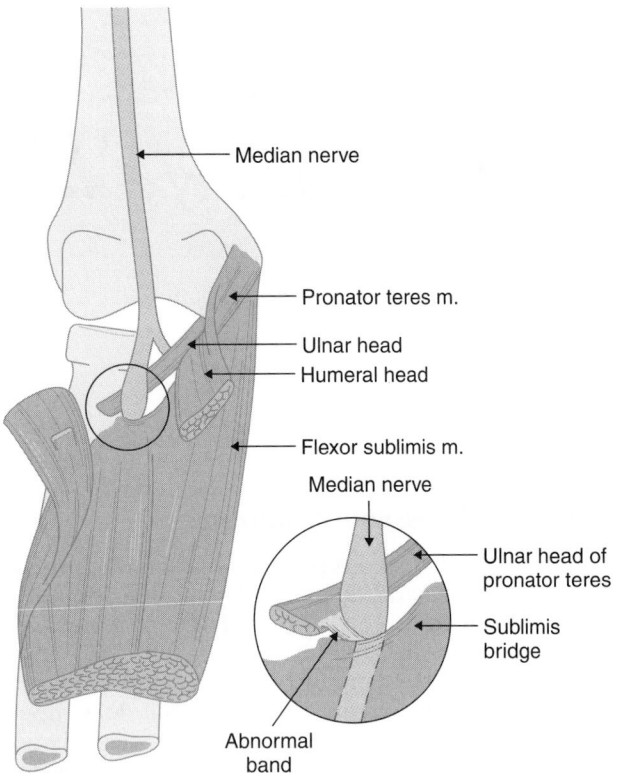

FIGURE 20-1. The median nerve is shown descending beneath the sublimis bridge after traversing the space between the two heads of the pronator teres. The nerve is compressed at the sublimis bridge. (Reprinted with permission from Kopell HP, Thompson WAL. Pronator syndrome: a confirmed case and its diagnosis. N Engl J Med 1958;259: 713-715.)

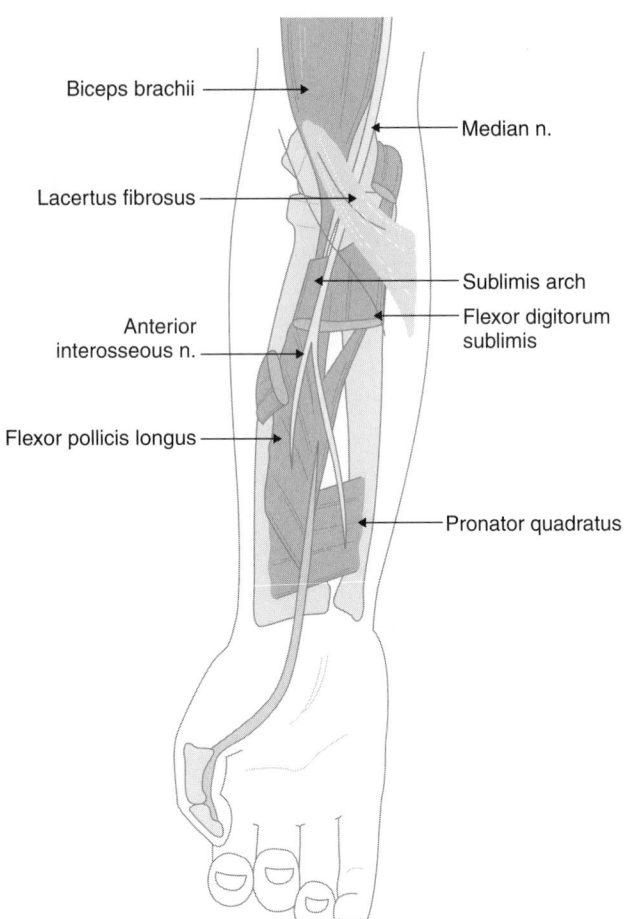

FIGURE 20-2. Course of the median nerve and its anterior interosseous branch.

Anterior Interosseous Syndrome

The onset of anterior interosseous syndrome can be related to exertion, or it may be spontaneous. In classic cases of spontaneous anterior interosseous nerve paralysis, there is acute pain in the proximal forearm or arm lasting for hours or days. There may be a history of local trauma or heavy muscle exertion at the onset of pain. As mentioned, the patient may complain of weakness of the forearm muscles innervated by the anterior interosseous nerve. Theoretically, there should be no sensory complaints.[4]

PHYSICAL EXAMINATION

Pronator Teres Syndrome

Findings may be ill-defined and difficult to substantiate in pronator teres syndrome.[2,3] The most important physical finding is tenderness over the proximal forearm. Pressure over the pronator teres muscle produces discomfort and may produce a radiating pain and digital numbness. The symptomatic pronator teres muscle may be firm to palpation compared with the other side. The contour of the forearm may be depressed, caused by the thickening of the lacertus fibrosus. Distinctive findings are weakness of both the intrinsic muscles of the hand supplied by the median

nerve and the muscles proximal to the wrist and in the forearm with tenderness, Tinel sign over the point of entrapment, and absence of Phalen sign. Pain may be elicited by pronation of the forearm, elbow flexion, or even contraction of the superficial flexor of the second digit. Sensory examination findings are usually poorly defined but may involve not only the median nerve distribution of the digits but also the thenar region of the palm because of involvement of the palmar cutaneous branch of the median nerve. Deep tendon reflexes and cervical examination findings should be normal.[5,10-16]

Anterior Interosseous Syndrome

To test the muscles that the anterior interosseous nerve innervates,[2,3] the clinician braces the metacarpophalangeal joint of the index finger and the patient is asked to flex only the distal phalanx. This isolates the action of the flexor digitorum profundus on the terminal phalanx and eliminates the action of the flexor digitorum superficialis. There is no terminal phalanx flexion if the anterior interosseous nerve is injured.

Another useful test is to ask the patient to make the "OK" sign.[17] In anterior interosseous syndrome, the distal interphalangeal joint cannot be flexed, and this

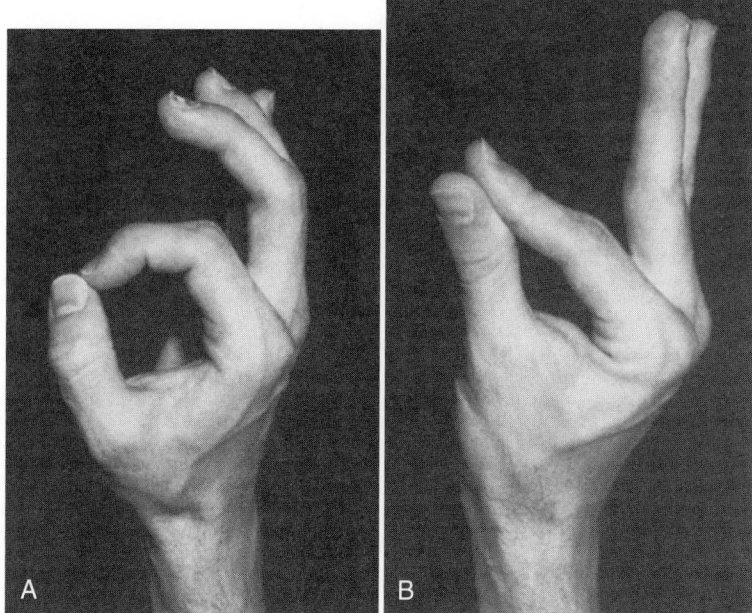

FIGURE 20-3. The anterior interosseous nerve innervates the flexor pollicis longus as well as the flexor digitorum profundus to the index and long fingers. **A,** It is responsible for flexion of the thumb interphalangeal joint and the index finger distal interphalangeal joint. **B,** An injury to the median nerve high in the forearm or to the anterior interosseous branch of the median nerve results in inability to forcefully flex these joints. (From Concannon MJ. Common Hand Problems in Primary Care. Philadelphia, Hanley & Belfus, 1999:137, with permission.)

results in the index finger's remaining relatively straight during this test (Fig. 20-3). The patient is asked to forcefully approximate the finger pulps of the first and second digits. The patient with weakness of the flexor pollicis longus and digitorum profundus muscles cannot touch with the pulp of the fingers, but rather the entire volar surfaces of the digits are in contact. This is due to the paralysis of the flexor pollicis longus and flexor digitorum profundus of the second digit. The pronator quadratus is difficult to isolate clinically, but an attempt can be made by flexing the forearm and asking the patient to resist supination. Sensation and deep tendon reflexes should be normal.[5,10-16]

FUNCTIONAL LIMITATIONS

Pronator Teres Syndrome

In pronator teres syndrome, there is clumsiness, loss of dexterity, and a feeling of weakness in the hand. This may lead to functional limitations both at home and at work. Repetitive elbow motions, such as hammering, cleaning fish, serving tennis balls, and rowing, are most likely to provoke symptoms.

Anterior Interosseous Syndrome

As weakness develops in anterior interosseous syndrome, there is loss of dexterity and pinching motion with difficulty picking up small objects with the first two digits. Activities of daily living, such as buttoning shirts and tying shoelaces, can be impaired. Patients may have difficulty with typing, handwriting, cooking, and so on.

DIAGNOSTIC STUDIES

Pronator Teres Syndrome

Electrodiagnostic testing (nerve conduction studies and electromyography) is the "gold standard" for confirming pronator teres syndrome.[1,17] Nerve conduction studies may be abnormal in the median nerve distribution; however, the diagnosis may be best established by electromyographic studies demonstrating membrane instability (including increased insertional activity, fibrillation and positive sharp waves at rest, wide and high amplitude polyphasics on minimal contraction, and decreased recruitment pattern on maximal contraction) of the median nerve muscles below and above the wrist in the forearm, but with *sparing of the pronator teres.*[17,18] Imaging studies (e.g., radiography, computed tomography, sonography, and magnetic resonance imaging) are used to exclude alternative diagnoses.[19-24]

Anterior Interosseous Syndrome

Electrodiagnostic studies may also help establish the diagnosis of anterior interosseous syndrome.[3] In general, routine motor and sensory studies are normal. The most appropriate technique is surface electrode recording from the pronator quadratus muscle with median nerve stimulation at the antecubital fossa. On electromyography, findings of membrane instability are restricted to the flexor pollicis longus, flexor digitorum profundus (of the second and third digits), and pronator quadratus.[7,18]

Again, imaging studies are useful in excluding other diagnoses.[19-22]

Differential Diagnosis

Pronator Teres Syndrome

Carpal tunnel syndrome

Cervical radiculopathy, particularly lesions affecting C6 or C7

Thoracic outlet syndrome with involvement of the medial cord

Elbow arthritis

Epicondylitis

Anterior Interosseous Syndrome

Paralytic brachial plexus neuritis

Entrapment or rupture of the tendon of the flexor pollicis longus

Rupture of the flexor pollicis longus and flexor digitorum profundus

TREATMENT

Initial

Pronator Teres Syndrome

Treatment is initially conservative, with rest and avoidance of the offending repetitive trauma.[2,4] Nonsteroidal anti-inflammatory drugs may help with pain and inflammation. Analgesics may be used for pain. Low-dose tricyclic antidepressants may be used for pain and to help with sleep. Antiseizure medications are also often used for neuropathic pain (e.g., carbamazepine, gabapentin).

Anterior Interosseous Syndrome

Treatment of the anterior interosseous syndrome depends on the cause.[2,3] Penetrating wounds require immediate exploration and repair. Impending Volkmann contracture demands immediate decompression. In spontaneous cases associated with specific occupations, a trial of nonoperative therapy is indicated. If spontaneous improvement does not occur by 6 to 8 weeks, consideration should be given to surgical exploration. Conservative management includes avoiding the activity that exacerbates the symptoms. Pharmacologic treatment is similar to that for pronator teres syndrome.

Rehabilitation

Pronator Teres Syndrome

A splint that can put the thumb in an abducted, opposed position, such as a C bar or a thumb post-static orthosis, can be used (Fig. 20-4).[6,7,9] Taping of the index and middle fingers in a buddy splint to stabilize the lack of distal interphalangeal flexion may be helpful.[9]

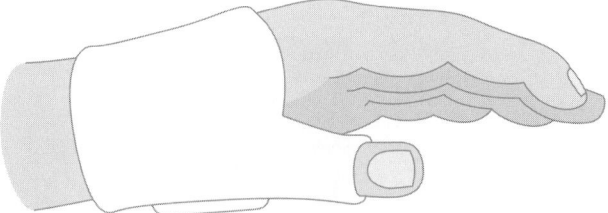

FIGURE 20-4. A typical splint used in pronator teres syndrome.

Rehabilitation may include modalities such as ultrasound, electrical stimulation, iontophoresis, and phonophoresis. The patient can be instructed in ice massage as well. Once the acute symptoms have subsided, physical or occupational therapy can focus on exercises to improve forearm flexibility, muscle strength responsible for thumb abduction, opposition, and wrist radial flexion.

Anterior Interosseous Syndrome

Resting the arm by immobilization in a splint may be tried (Fig. 20-5).[25] If the symptoms subside, conservative physical or occupational therapy, including physical modalities as previously described and exercises to improve strength and function of the pronator quadratus, flexor digitorum profundus, and flexor pollicis longus, can be initiated.[9]

Procedures

In both anterior interosseous and pronator teres syndromes, a median nerve block may be attempted[26] (Figs. 20-6 and 20-7).

Surgery

Pronator Teres Syndrome

If symptoms fail to resolve, surgical release of the pronator teres muscle and any constricting bands (ligament of Struthers and lacertus fibrosus) should be considered with direct exploration of the area. An S-shaped incision is typically used to extensively expose the entire median nerve from the forearm to the hand.[27]

Anterior Interosseous Syndrome

If spontaneous improvement does not occur by 6 to 8 weeks, consideration should be given to surgical exploration. The surgical technique for exploration is exposure

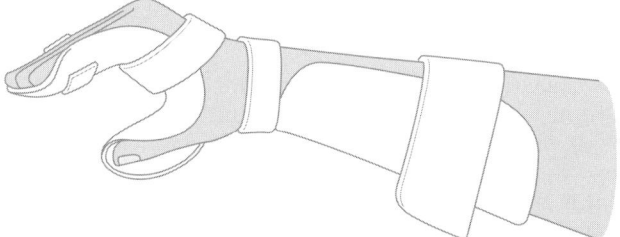

FIGURE 20-5. A typical splint used in anterior interosseous syndrome.

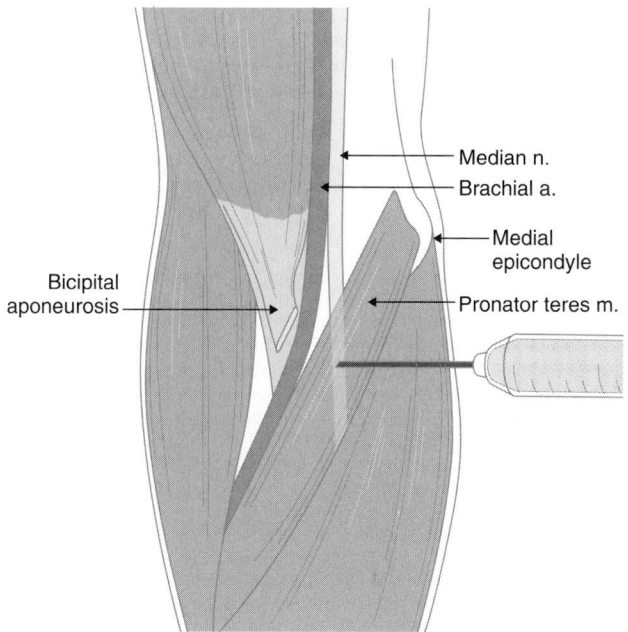

FIGURE 20-6. Pronator teres nerve block. At the elbow crease, make a mark at the midpoint between the medial epicondyle and the biceps tendon. Then, under sterile conditions, insert a 25-gauge, 1¹/₂ -inch disposable needle into the pronator teres muscle approximately 2 cm below the mark or at the point of maximal tenderness in the muscle. Confirmation of needle placement can be made by a nerve stimulator. Then, inject 3 to 5 mL of a corticosteroid-anesthetic solution (e.g., 2 mL of methylprednisolone [40 mg/mL] combined with 2 mL of 1% lidocaine). Postinjection care may include icing for 10 to 15 minutes and splinting of the wrist and forearm in a functional position for a few days. Also, the patient should be cautioned to avoid aggressive use of the arm for at least 1 to 2 weeks. (Reprinted with permission from Lennard TA. Pain Procedures in Clinical Practice, 2nd ed. Philadelphia, Hanley & Belfus, 2000:98.)

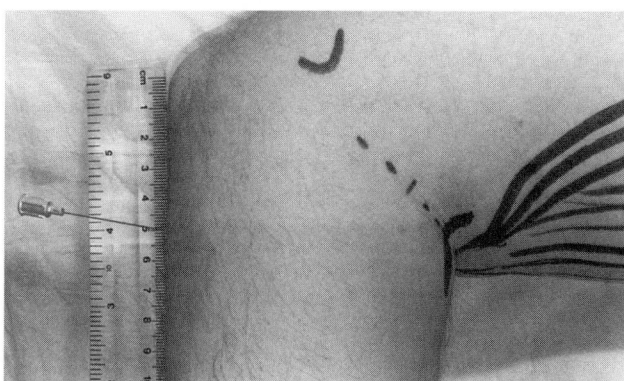

FIGURE 20-7. Anterior interosseous nerve block. The anterior interosseous nerve can be blocked by either an anterior or a posterior approach. For the posterior approach, the posterior elbow is exposed and the forearm is placed in neutral. Under sterile conditions with use of a 2-inch, 25-gauge disposable needle, inject 3 to 5 mL of a corticosteroid-anesthetic solution (e.g., 2 mL of methylprednisolone [40 mg/mL] combined with 2 mL of 1% lidocaine) approximately 5 cm distal to the tip of the olecranon. The needle should penetrate about 3.5 to 5 cm toward the biceps tendon insertion at the radius. A nerve stimulator is necessary to ensure proper placement. Postinjection care is similar to that of the pronator teres nerve block. (Reprinted with permission from Lennard TA. Pain Procedures in Clinical Practice, 2nd ed. Philadelphia, Hanley & Belfus, 2000:99.)

of the median nerve directly beneath the pronator teres or separation of this muscle from the flexor carpi radialis, identification of the anterior interosseous nerve, and release of the offending structures.

If surgical decompression was performed and failed to resolve the weakness, tendon transfers may be considered after a more proximal fascicular lesion is ruled out.[27]

POTENTIAL DISEASE COMPLICATIONS

Pronator Teres Syndrome

Disease-related complications, if the condition is left unresolved, include permanent loss of the use of the pinch grasp, lack of wrist flexion, and incessant pain.

Anterior Interosseous Syndrome

If it is allowed to persist, this syndrome will cause inability to perform the pinch grasp, resulting in the functional deficits mentioned before.

POTENTIAL TREATMENT COMPLICATIONS

Use of anti-inflammatory medications such as nonsteroidal anti-inflammatory drugs can induce gastric, renal, and hepatic side effects. Local steroid injections can induce skin depigmentation, local atrophy, or infection. Surgical complications include infection, bleeding, and injury to surrounding structures.

References

1. Liveson J. Peripheral Neurology—Case Studies in Electrodiagnosis, 2nd ed. Philadelphia, FA Davis, 1991:23-26.
2. Dawson D, Hallett M, Millender L. Entrapment Neuropathies, 3rd ed. Boston, Little, Brown, 1999:98-109.
3. Shapiro BE, Preston DC. Entrapment and compressive neuropathies. Med Clin North Am 2003;87:663-696.
4. Lee MJ, La Stayo PC. Pronator syndrome and other nerve compressions that mimic carpal tunnel syndrome. J Orthop Sports Phys Ther 2004;34:601-609.
5. Bilecenoglu B, Uz A, Karalezli N. Possible anatomic structures causing entrapment neuropathies of the median nerve: an anatomic study. Acta Orthop Belg 2005;71:169-176.
6. Puhaindran ME, Wong HP. A case of anterior interosseous nerve syndrome after peripherally inserted central catheter (PICC) line insertion. Singapore Med J 2003;44:653-655.
7. Rieck B. Incomplete anterior interosseous syndrome in a guitar player [in German]. Handchir Mikrochir Plast Chir 2005;37:418-422.
8. Lederman RJ. Neuromuscular and musculoskeletal problems in instrumental music. Muscle Nerve 2003;27:549-561.
9. Burke SL, Higgins J, Saunders R, et al. Hand and Upper Extremity Rehabilitation: A Practical Guide, 3rd ed. St. Louis, Elsevier Churchill Livingstone, 2006:87-95.
10. Bromberg MB, Smith AG, eds. Handbook of Peripheral Neuropathy. Boca Raton, Taylor & Francis, 2005:476-478.
11. Stewart J, Jablecki C, Medina N. XVI-Mononeuropathies, 49-median nerve. In Brown W, Boulton C, Aminoff J, eds. Neuromuscular Function and Disease, Basic Clinical and Electrodiagnostic Aspects. Philadelphia, WB Saunders, 2002:873.
12. Spinner RJ, Amadio PC. Compressive neuropathies of the upper extremities. Clin Plast Surg 2003;30:158-159.

13. Proximal median neuropathy. In Campbell WW, ed. DeJong's the Neurologic Examination, 6th ed. Philadelphia, Lippincott Williams & Wilkins, 2005:553-554.

14. Prescott D, Shapiro B. 18-Proximal Median Neuropathy Electromyography and Neuromuscular Disorders: Clinical Electrophysiologic Correlations, 2nd ed. Philadelphia, Elsevier, 2005: 281-290.

15. Dyck PJ, Thomas PK. Peripheral Neuropathy, vol 2. Philadelphia, Elsevier Saunders, 2005:1453-1454.

16. Mackinnon SE. Pathophysiology of nerve compression. Hand Clin 2002;18:231-241.

17. Dumitru D. Electrodiagnostic Medicine. Philadelphia, Hanley & Belfus, 1994:864-867.

18. Wilbourne AS. Electrodiagnostic examination with peripheral nerve injuries. Clin Plast Surg 2003;30:150-151.

19. Kimura J. Electrodiagnosis in Diseases of Nerve and Muscle: Principles and Practice, 3rd ed. New York, Oxford University Press, 2001:14-15, 719-723.

20. Martinoli C, Bianchi S, Pugliese F, et al. Sonography of entrapment neuropathies in the upper limb (wrist excluded). J Clin Ultrasound 2004;32:438-450.

21. Peer S, Bodner G, eds. High-Resolution Sonography of the Peripheral Nervous System. New York, Springer, 2003.

22. Andreisik G, Crook DW, Burg D, et al. Peripheral neuropathies of the median, radial, and ulnar nerves: MR imaging features. Radiographics 2006;26:1267-1287.

23. Kim S, Choi JY, Huh YM, et al. Role of magnetic resonance imaging in entrapment and compressive neuropathy—what, where, and how to see the peripheral nerves on the musculoskeletal magnetic resonance image: part 2. Upper extremity. Eur Radiol 2007;17:509-522. Epub 2006 Mar 30.

24. Braddom R. Physical Medicine and Rehabilitation. Philadelphia, WB Saunders, 1996:328-329.

25. Hunter J, Mackin E, Callahan A, eds. Rehabilitation of the Hand and Upper Extremity, 5th ed. St. Louis, Mosby-Year Book, 2002.

26 Trombly C, ed. Occupational Therapy for Physical Dysfunction, 4th ed. Philadelphia, Lippincott Williams & Wilkins, 1997:556-558.

27. Lennard T. Physiatric Procedures in Clinical Practice. Philadelphia, Hanley & Belfus, 1995:140-142.

Olecranon Bursitis **21**

Charles Cassidy, MD, and Sarah S. Banerjee, MD

Synonyms

Miner's elbow
Student's elbow
Draftsman's elbow
Dialysis elbow
Elbow bursitis

ICD-9 Code

726.23   Olecranon bursitis

DEFINITION

Olecranon bursitis is a swelling of the subcutaneous, synovium-lined sac that overlies the olecranon process. The bursa functions to cushion the tip of the olecranon and to reduce friction between the olecranon and the overlying skin during elbow motion. Because of the paucity of soft tissue covering the elbow, the olecranon bursa is susceptible to injury.

The causes of olecranon bursitis can be classified as traumatic, inflammatory, septic, and idiopathic.[1] Traumatic bursitis may result from a single, direct blow to the elbow or from repetitive stress. Football players, particularly those who play on artificial turf, are at risk for development of acute bursitis. More commonly, repeated minor trauma from direct pressure on the elbow or elbow motion is responsible for the problem. Trauma is thought to stimulate increased vascularity, resulting in bursal fluid production and fibrin coating of the bursal wall.[2] Persons engaged in certain occupations or certain activities are susceptible to olecranon bursitis, including auto mechanics, gardeners, plumbers, carpet layers, students, gymnasts, wrestlers, and dart throwers. Interestingly, approximately 7% of hemodialysis patients develop olecranon bursitis.[3] Repeated, prolonged positioning of the elbow and anticoagulation appear to be contributing factors.

Inflammatory causes include diseases that affect the bursa primarily, such as rheumatoid arthritis, gout, and chondrocalcinosis. Olecranon bursitis is commonly seen in rheumatoid patients, in whom the bursa may actually communicate with the affected elbow joint. Crystal-induced olecranon bursitis may be difficult to differentiate from septic bursitis.

Septic olecranon bursitis represents 20% of olecranon bursitis.[4] The source is most often transcutaneous, and about half have identifiable breaks in the skin. When culture samples are positive, the bursal fluid usually contains *Staphylococcus aureus*.[5] Sepsis is unusual. Both underlying bursal disease (gout, rheumatoid arthritis, chondrocalcinosis) and systemic conditions such as diabetes mellitus, uremia, alcoholism, intravenous drug use, and steroid therapy are considered predisposing factors. There appears to be a seasonal trend, with a peak of staphylococcal septic bursitis during the summer months.[6]

In approximately 25% of cases, no identifiable cause of the olecranon bursitis is found. Presumably, repetitive, minor irritation is responsible for the bursal swelling.

SYMPTOMS

Painless swelling is the chief complaint in noninflammatory, aseptic olecranon bursitis. When patients are symptomatic, they usually have discomfort when the elbow is flexed beyond 90 degrees and have trouble resting on the elbow. Moderate to severe pain is the predominant complaint of patients with septic or crystal-induced olecranon bursitis. These patients may also have fever, malaise, and limited elbow motion.

PHYSICAL EXAMINATION

The physical examination varies somewhat, depending on the underlying condition. With noninflammatory aseptic bursitis, a nontender fluctuant mass is present over the tip of the elbow (Fig. 21-1). Elbow motion is usually full and painless. With chronic bursitis, the fluctuance may be replaced with a thickened bursa (Fig. 21-2).

The distinction between crystal-induced and septic bursitis may be subtle. Both conditions may produce tender fluctuance, induration, swelling, warmth, and local erythema. Elbow flexion may be somewhat limited, although not as limited as with septic arthritis of the elbow joint.

115

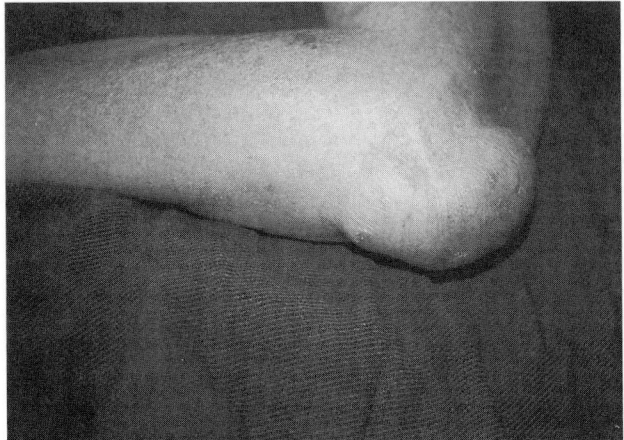

FIGURE 21-1. Atraumatic olecranon bursitis in a 55-year-old woman. A large fluctuant mass is present.

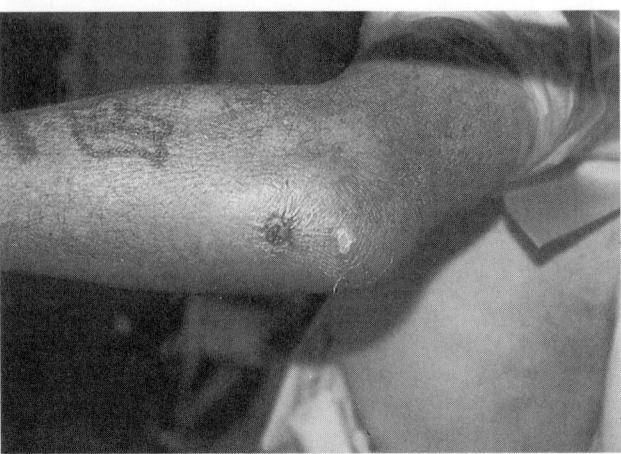

FIGURE 21-3. Septic olecranon bursitis. Cellulitis is present over a wide area. The white scab at the tip of the elbow represents the site of the penetrating injury. Distally, the draining area of granulation tissue developed at the site of needle aspiration. Aspiration of the bursa should be done by use of a long needle inserted well away from the fluctuant area.

Fever and a break in the skin over the elbow are important clues to an underlying septic process (Fig. 21-3). Cellulitis extending distally along the forearm is also more likely to be due to an infection.

In inflammatory cases, pain inhibition may produce mild weakness of elbow flexion and extension. Sensation and distal pulses are unaffected. Examination findings of other joints should also be normal.

FUNCTIONAL LIMITATIONS

Functional limitations depend on the underlying diagnosis. Traumatic olecranon bursitis usually causes minimal functional limitation. Patients may note some mild discomfort with direct pressure over the tip of the elbow (e.g., when sitting at a desk or resting the arm on the armrest of a chair or in the car). With crystal-induced and septic bursitis, pain is the predominant issue. Patients may have trouble sleeping and have difficulty with most activities of daily living that involve the affected extremity (e.g., dressing, grooming, cleaning, shopping, and carrying packages).

DIAGNOSTIC STUDIES

The diagnosis of aseptic, noninflammatory olecranon bursitis is usually straightforward, based on a characteristic appearance on physical examination. In this setting, additional studies are not usually necessary. However, plain radiographs may demonstrate an olecranon spur in about one third of cases (Fig. 21-4). Because this is an extra-articular process, a joint effusion is not present.

If crystal-induced or septic bursitis is suspected, aspiration of the bursal fluid is usually indicated. The fluid should be sent for cell count, Gram stain and culture, and crystal analysis. Acute, traumatic bursal fluid typically has a serosanguineous appearance, containing fewer than 1000 white blood cells per high-power field, with a predominance of monocytes. Infected bursal fluid usually contains an increased white blood cell count, with a high percentage of polymorphonuclear cells. The Gram stain is positive in only 50% of septic

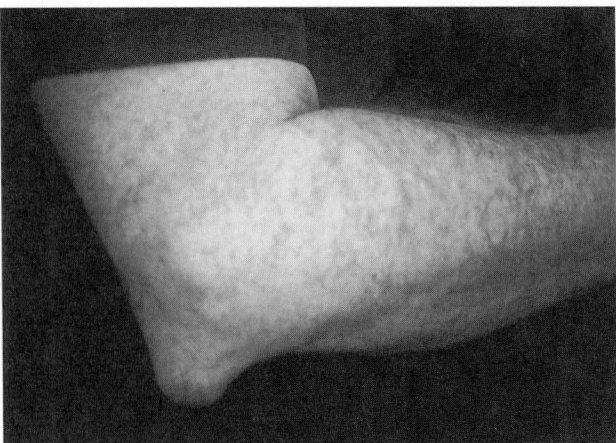

FIGURE 21-2. Chronic gouty olecranon bursitis. The prominence at the tip of the elbow is firm with thinning of the overlying skin.

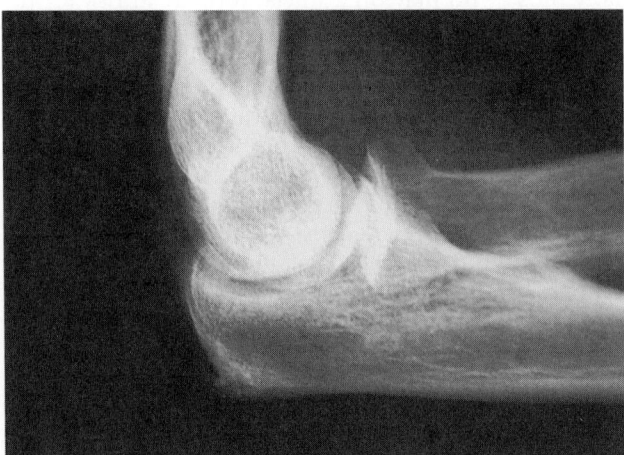

FIGURE 21-4. Lateral radiograph of the elbow in a patient with chronic olecranon bursitis. Note the olecranon spur.

cases. Even in the setting of infection, the fluid should be examined under a polarizing microscope because simultaneous infectious and crystal-induced arthritis can occur.[7]

A complete blood cell count and determination of serum uric acid level may provide supportive information in confusing cases, although a normal serum white blood cell count does not preclude septic bursitis.

Magnetic resonance imaging may be of some value to distinguish septic from nonseptic olecranon bursitis, although there is considerable overlap of findings.[8] Absence of bursal and soft tissue enhancement is consistent with nonseptic olecranon bursitis. Olecranon marrow edema is suggestive but not diagnostic of septic olecranon bursitis. The use of magnetic resonance imaging may also help clarify the diagnosis of unusual masses around the elbow.

TREATMENT

Initial

Treatment of traumatic olecranon bursitis begins with prevention of further injury to the involved elbow. An elastic elbow pad provides compression and protects the bursa. The patient should be counseled in ways of protecting the elbow at work and during recreation. Nonsteroidal anti-inflammatory drugs are usually prescribed. Traumatic, noninflammatory bursitis usually resolves with this treatment.[9] On occasion, when the bursa is very large, aspiration of the bloody fluid will be a first-line treatment. This is followed by application of a compressive wrap and splint for several days.

In suspected cases of septic olecranon bursitis, it is important to palpate for fluctuance. If a fluid collection is appreciated, the bursa should be aspirated (see the section on procedures). When cellulitis over the tip of the elbow is present without an obvious collection, empirical treatment with antibiotic therapy to cover penicillin-resistant S. aureus, the most common offender, is recommended. (Less common organisms include group A streptococcus and Staphylococcus epidermidis.) The decision whether to use oral or intravenous antibiotics depends on the appearance of the elbow, the signs of systemic illness, and the general health of the patient. The elbow should be splinted in a semiflexed position (approximately 60 degrees) without pressure on the

olecranon. Nonsteroidal anti-inflammatory drugs may be prescribed unless they are contraindicated for empirical treatment of gout and pseudogout. When final culture results return, the antibiotic therapy is adjusted appropriately. Outpatient cases are observed closely, with any changes in the size of the bursa and the quality of the overlying skin noted; oral antibiotic therapy should continue for at least 10 days.

Patients with extensive infection or underlying bursal disease, systemic disease, or immunosuppression and outpatients refractory to oral treatment should be treated with an intravenous cephalosporin. In one study, the average duration of intravenous therapy was 4.4 days if symptoms had been present for less than 1 week and 9.2 days if symptoms had been present for longer than 1 week.[10] The conversion to oral antibiotics should occur only after consistent improvement is seen in the appearance of the patient and the elbow. Serial aspirations may also constitute part of the therapy; alternatively, some clinicians use a suction irrigation system placed into the bursa. We recommend surgical consultation if the bursitis has failed to improve within several days of appropriate management.

Rehabilitation

Because the process is extra-articular, permanent elbow stiffness is not usually a problem. Physical or occupational therapy for gentle range of motion may be indicated once the olecranon wound has clearly healed. Extreme flexion should be avoided early on because this position puts tension on the already compromised skin. If prolonged immobilization is necessary to permit the soft tissues to heal, therapy may include range of motion and strengthening of the arm and forearm.

Patients who have traumatic or recurrent olecranon bursitis should be counseled in ways to modify their home and work activities to eliminate irritation to the bursa. This might include the use of ergonomic equipment such as forearm rests (also called data arms) that do not contact the elbow. In some instances, vocational retraining may be indicated.

Procedures

Needle aspiration is therapeutic as well as diagnostic and usually reduces symptoms (Fig. 21-5). It can be performed for patients with traumatic bursitis if they have symptoms compromising their regular activities and should be done (as previously described) for patients in whom inflammatory or septic causes are suspected.

The elbow is prepared in a sterile fashion. The skin is infiltrated locally with 1% lidocaine (Xylocaine). To minimize the risk of persistent drainage after aspiration, it is recommended to insert a long 18-gauge needle at a point well proximal to the tip of the elbow. The bursa should be drained as completely as possible. The fluid should be sent for Gram stain, culture and sensitivity, cell count, and crystal analysis.

Differential Diagnosis

Rheumatoid nodule

Lipoma

Tophus

Elbow synovitis

Olecranon spur

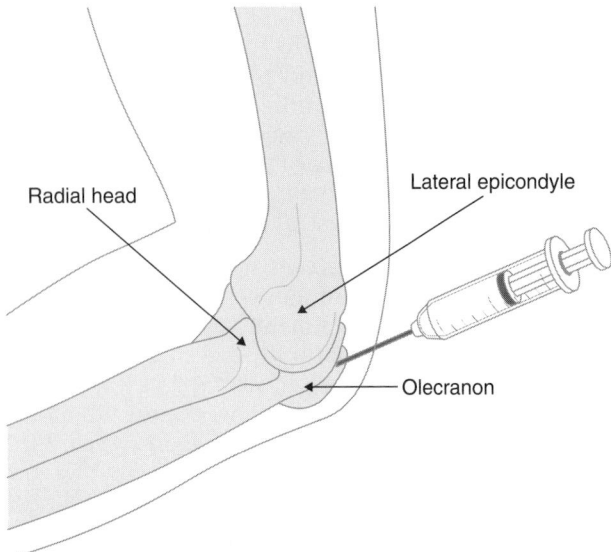

FIGURE 21-5. Approach for olecranon aspiration and injection.

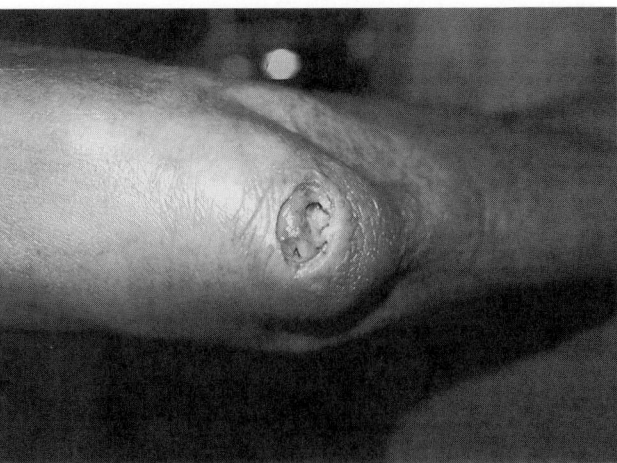

FIGURE 21-6. Untreated septic bursitis with a large olecranon ulcer. The periosteum of the olecranon is visible in the wound. This problem is difficult to manage and often requires flap coverage.

Postinjection care includes local icing for 10 to 20 minutes. A sterile compressive dressing is then applied, followed by an anterior plaster splint that maintains the elbow in 60 degrees of flexion.

Corticosteroid injections into the bursa have been shown to hasten the resolution of traumatic and crystal-induced olecranon bursitis.[11] However, the risk of complications is high, including infection, skin atrophy, and chronic local pain. Consequently, the routine use of steroid injections for olecranon bursitis is not recommended.

Surgery

Surgery is rarely indicated for traumatic olecranon bursitis. Chronic drainage of bursal fluid is the most common indication for surgery.[1] Bursectomy is conventionally done through an open technique, although a recently developed arthroscopic method has shown some promise. Surgery is usually curative for both traumatic and septic bursitis. However, the success rates are very different for patients with rheumatoid arthritis—surgery provides successful relief for 5 years in only 40% of patients with rheumatoid arthritis versus 94% of nonrheumatoid patients.[12]

After surgery, suction drains are often placed for several days. Splinting of the elbow at 60 degrees of flexion or greater for 2 weeks is thought to help prevent recurrence.

POTENTIAL DISEASE COMPLICATIONS

Septic bursitis poses the greatest threat with regard to disease complications. If it is neglected, the infection may thin the overlying skin and eventually erode through it (Fig. 21-6). This complication is quite difficult to manage, often requiring extensive débridement and flap coverage. Persistent infection can also result in osteomyelitis of the olecranon process. Immunocompromised patients are at risk for sepsis from olecranon bursitis. Necrotizing fasciitis originating from a septic olecranon bursitis, although rare, may prove to be fatal.

POTENTIAL TREATMENT COMPLICATIONS

Analgesics and nonsteroidal anti-inflammatory drugs have well-known side effects that most commonly affect the gastric, hepatic, and renal systems. Persistent drainage from a synovial fistula is an uncommon complication of aspiration of the olecranon bursa; however, this problem is serious enough to discourage the routine aspiration of olecranon bursal fluid in noninflammatory conditions. Complications of steroid injection, as described earlier, can be serious. In addition, wound problems are the major complication associated with surgical treatment of olecranon bursitis. Because of the superficial location of the olecranon and the tenuous blood supply of the overlying skin, wound healing can be difficult. Malnourished and chronically ill patients are especially at risk for surgical complications.

References

1. Morrey BF. Bursitis. In Morrey BF, ed. The Elbow and Its Disorders, 3rd ed. Philadelphia, WB Saunders, 2000:901-908.
2. Canoso JJ. Idiopathic or traumatic olecranon bursitis. Clinical features and bursal fluid analysis. Arthritis Rheum 1977;20:1213-1216.
3. Irby R, Edwards WM, Gatter RJ. Articular complications of hemotransplantation and chronic renal hemodialysis. Rheumatology 1975;2:91-99.
4. Jaffe L, Fetto JF. Olecranon bursitis. Contemp Orthop 1984;8:51-56.
5. Zimmerman B III, Mikolich DJ, Ho G Jr. Septic bursitis. Semin Arthritis Rheum 1995;24:391-410.
6. Cea-Pereiro JC, Garcia-Meijide J, Mera-Varela A, Gomez-Reino JJ. A comparison between septic bursitis caused by *Staphylococcus aureus* and those caused by other organisms. Clin Rheumatol 2001;20:10-14.

7. Gerster JC, Lagier R, Boivin G. Olecranon bursitis related to calcium pyrophosphate dihydrate deposition disease. Arthritis Rheum 1982;25:989-996.

8. Floemer F, Morrison WB, Bongartz G, Ledermann HP. MRI characteristics of olecranon bursitis. AJR Am J Roentgenol 2004;183:29-34.

9. Smith DL, McAfee JH, Lucas LM, et al. Treatment of nonseptic olecranon bursitis. A controlled, blinded prospective trial. Arch Intern Med 1989;149:2527-2530.

10. Ho G, Su EY. Antibiotic therapy of septic bursitis. Arthritis Rheum 1981;24:905-911.

11. Weinstein PS, Canso JJ, Wohlgethan JR. Long-term follow-up of corticosteroid injection for traumatic olecranon bursitis. Ann Rheum Dis 1984;43:44-46.

12. Stewart NJ, Manzanares JB, Morrey BF. Surgical treatment of aseptic olecranon bursitis. J Shoulder Elbow Surg 1997;6:49-54.

Radial Neuropathy 22

Lyn D. Weiss, MD, and Thomas E. Pobre, MD

Synonyms

Radial nerve palsy
Radial nerve compression
Wristdrop neuropathy
Finger or thumb extensor paralysis
Saturday night palsy
Supinator syndrome
Radial tunnel syndrome
Cheiralgia paresthetica

ICD-9 Code

354.3   Lesion of the radial nerve

DEFINITION

The radial nerve originates from the C5 to T1 roots. These nerve fibers travel along the upper, middle, and lower trunks. They continue as the posterior cord and terminate as the radial nerve.

The radial nerve is prone to entrapment in the axilla (crutch palsy), the upper arm (spiral groove), the forearm (posterior interosseous nerve), and the wrist (cheiralgia paresthetica). Radial neuropathies can result from direct nerve trauma, compressive neuropathies, neuritis, or complex humerus fractures.[1]

In the proximal arm, the radial nerve gives off three sensory branches (posterior cutaneous nerve of the arm, lower lateral cutaneous nerve of the arm, and posterior cutaneous nerve of the forearm). The radial nerve supplies a motor branch to the triceps and anconeus before wrapping around the humerus in the spiral groove, a common site of radial nerve injury. The nerve then supplies motor branches to the brachioradialis, the long head of the extensor carpi radialis, and the supinator. Just distal to the lateral epicondyle, the radial nerve divides into the posterior interosseous nerve (a motor nerve) and the superficial sensory nerve (a sensory nerve). The posterior interosseous nerve supplies the supinator muscle and then travels under the arcade of Frohse (another potential site of compression) before coursing distally to supply the extensor digitorum com-

munis, extensor digiti minimi, extensor carpi ulnaris, abductor pollicis longus, extensor pollicis longus, extensor pollicis brevis, and extensor indicis proprius. The superficial sensory nerve supplies sensations to the dorsum of the hand, excluding the fifth and medial aspect of the fourth digit, which is supplied by the ulnar nerve (Fig. 22-1).

SYMPTOMS

Symptoms of radial neuropathy depend on the site of nerve entrapment[2] (Table 22-1). A Tinel sign may be present at the site of compression. In the axilla, the entire radial nerve can be affected. This may be seen in crutch palsy if the patient is improperly using crutches in the axilla instead of distal to the axilla. With this type of injury, the median, axillary, or suprascapular nerves may also be affected. All radially innervated muscles (including the triceps) as well as sensation in the posterior arm, forearm, and dorsum of the hand may be affected.

The radial nerve is especially prone to injury in the spiral groove (also known as Saturday night palsy or honeymooner's palsy). Symptoms include weakness of all radially innervated muscles except the triceps and sensory changes in the posterior arm and hand. In the forearm, the radial nerve is susceptible to injury as it passes through the supinator muscle and the arcade of Frohse. Because the superficial radial sensory nerve branches before this area of impingement, sensation will be spared. The patient will complain of weakness in the wrist and finger extensors. On occasion, the superficial radial sensory nerve is entrapped at the wrist, usually as a result of lacerations at the wrist or a wristwatch that is too tight. In this situation, the symptoms will be sensory, involving the dorsum of the hand.

PHYSICAL EXAMINATION

The findings on physical examination depend on where the injury is along the anatomic course of the nerve. Injury in the axilla will lead to weakness in elbow extension, wrist extension, and finger extension. There is usually radial deviation of the wrist with extension, as the flexor carpi radialis (which is innervated by the median nerve) is

121

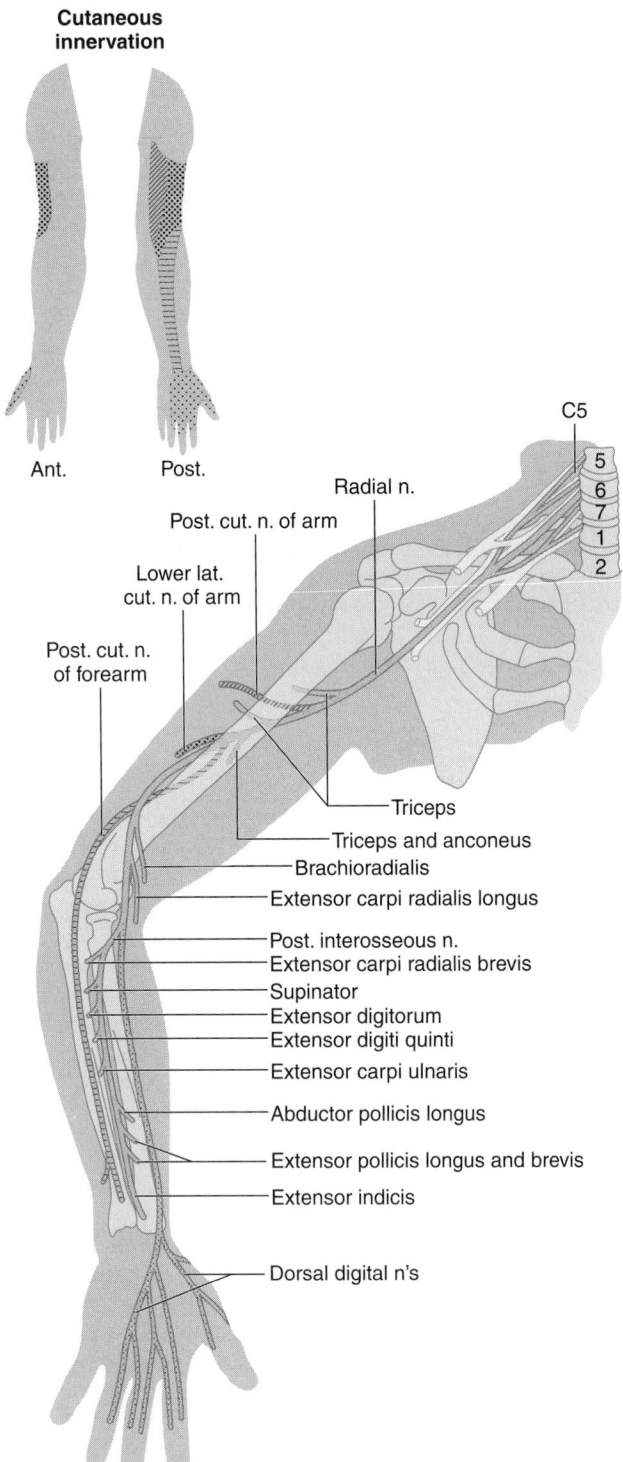

Cutaneous innervation

Ant.   Post.

C5

5
6
7
1
2

Radial n.

Post. cut. n. of arm

Lower lat. cut. n. of arm

Post. cut. n. of forearm

Triceps

Triceps and anconeus

Brachioradialis

Extensor carpi radialis longus

Post. interosseous n.

Extensor carpi radialis brevis

Supinator

Extensor digitorum

Extensor digiti quinti

Extensor carpi ulnaris

Abductor pollicis longus

Extensor pollicis longus and brevis

Extensor indicis

Dorsal digital n's

FIGURE 22-1. Neural branching of the radial nerve. Its origin in the axilla to the termination of its motor and sensory branches is shown. The inset demonstrates the cutaneous distribution of the various sensory branches of the radial nerve. (Reprinted with permission from Haymaker W, Woodhall B. Peripheral Nerve Injuries. Philadelphia, WB Saunders, 1953:265.)

not affected. The entire sensory distribution of the radial nerve will be affected. If the injury is in the spiral groove, the examination findings will be the same, except that *triceps function will be spared*. Radial neuropathy in the forearm will usually result in sparing of sensory functions. If the nerve is entrapped in the supinator muscle, supinator strength should be normal. This is because the branch to innervate the supinator muscle is given off proximal to the muscle. The patient will have radial deviation with wrist extension and weakness of finger extensors. Injury to the superficial radial sensory nerve will result in paresthesias or dysesthesias over the radial sensory distribution in the hand.

FUNCTIONAL LIMITATIONS

Functional limitation also depends on the level of the lesion. In high radial nerve palsy, wrist and finger extension are impaired. However, the inability to stabilize the wrist in extension leads to the main functional limitation. The loss of the power of the wrist and finger extensors destroys the essential reciprocal tenodesis action vital to the normal grasp and release pattern of the hand and results in ineffective finger flexion function. Activities such as gripping or holding objects will therefore be impaired. The sensory loss associated with radial nerve palsy is of lesser functional consequence compared with that of median or ulnar nerve lesions. Sensory loss is limited to the dorsoradial aspect of the hand, and this leaves the more functionally important palmar surface intact. Pain from posterior interosseous nerve entrapment can be disabling enough to limit the function of the involved extremity.

DIAGNOSTIC STUDIES

Electrodiagnostic testing (electromyography and nerve conduction studies) is usually the most useful test to assess for radial neuropathies. This test can be used to diagnose, to localize, to prognosticate, and to rule out other nerve injuries. Radiography and magnetic resonance imaging can be used to rule out a mass (ganglion or tumor)[3] or fracture[4,5] as the reason for the radial neuropathy.

TREATMENT

Initial

Radial neuropathies from compression can be managed conservatively in nearly all cases. Elimination of offending factors, such as improper use of crutches, and avoidance of provocative activities are the first steps in the treatment of radial neuropathy. Medications, including tricyclic agents, anticonvulsants, antiarrhythmics, topical solutions, clonidine, and opioids, can be considered for pain management. Nonpharmaceutical treatments, including transcutaneous electrical nerve stimulation and acupuncture, may be considered as adjuvants to medication.[10]

TABLE 22-1 Extensor Tendon Compartments—Wrist

Muscles	Insertion	Evaluation
Abductor pollicis longus	Dorsal base of thumb metacarpal	Bring thumb out to side
Extensor pollicis brevis	Proximal phalanx of the thumb	
Extensor carpi radialis longus	Dorsal base of index and middle metacarpals	Dorsiflex the wrist with the hand in a fist and
Extensor carpi radialis brevis		apply resistance radially
Extensor pollicis longus	Distal phalanx of the thumb	Hand flat on table
		Lift only thumb
Extensor digitorum communis	Extensor hood and base of proximal	Extend fingers with wrist in neutral
Extensor indicis proprius	phalanges of the ulnar four digits	Extend index finger
Extensor digiti minimi	Proximal phalanx of the little finger	Straighten little finger with other fingers in fist
Extensor carpi ulnaris	Dorsal base of the fifth metacarpal	Wrist extension with ulnar deviation

From American Society for Surgery of the Hand. The Hand: Examination and Diagnosis. New York, Churchill Livingstone, 1983.

Differential Diagnosis

Cervical radiculopathy (C6, C7)

Brachial neuritis

Posterior cord brachial plexopathy

Upper or middle trunk brachial plexopathy

Extensor tendon rupture

Epicondylitis

de Quervain tenosynovitis

Wristdrop secondary to lead polyneuropathy

Posterior interosseous nerve mononeuropathy

Peripheral neuropathy

Axillary nerve injury

Tumor

Chondroma[6]

Hematoma

Carpal tunnel syndrome

Upper extremity extensor compartment syndrome

Ulnar neuropathy

Entrapment neuropathy due to chronic injection-induced triceps fibrosis[7]

Superficial radial neuropathy caused by intravenous injection[8]

Neuropathy after vascular access cannulation for hemodialysis[9]

Rehabilitation

The main goals of rehabilitation are prevention of joint contractures, shortening of the flexor tendons, and over-stretching of the extensors while waiting for nerve recovery. These goals can be achieved by range of motion exercises, passive stretching, and proper splinting. Functional splinting can make relatively normal use of the hand possible. Dynamic splints use elastic to passively extend the finger at the metacarpophalangeal joints with the wrist immobilized in slight dorsiflexion. This provides stability to the wrist joint, passive extension of the digits by the elastic band, and active flexion of the fingers. A splint designed at the Hand Rehabilitation Center in Chapel Hill, North Carolina, uses a static nylon cord rather than a dynamic rubber band to suspend the proximal phalanges. The design simulates the tenodesis action of normal grasp and release pattern of the hand.

Postsurgical release of compression should be immediately followed by range of motion exercises and a nerve gliding program to prevent adhesions. Overly aggressive strengthening should be avoided during reinnervation. In tendon transfers, preoperative strengthening of the muscle to be transferred and postoperative muscle re-education are vital to the success of the procedure.

Procedures

Local anesthetic blocks or injections of hydrocortisone can be used[11] but are rarely necessary. Lateral epicondylitis may mimic posterior interosseous nerve entrapment at the elbow. When lateral epicondylitis does not respond to conservative treatment, including injections of the lateral epicondyle, a diagnostic and therapeutic radial nerve injection at the elbow may be indicated.[12]

Surgery

Surgical decompression may be required for patients who do not respond to conservative treatment or patients with severe nerve injury. Radial tunnel release has been advocated for compression neuropathies of the posterior interosseous nerve, but the results have been questionable.[13] Surgical intervention for anastomosis may be indicated in cases of complete radial injury (neurotmesis). Tendon transfers may be considered in these instances if the surgery is not performed or is not successful.[14,15] Care must be exercised to avoid the radial sensory branch during operations involving the wrist.[11]

POTENTIAL DISEASE COMPLICATIONS

Patients with incomplete recovery may suffer significant functional loss in the upper extremity. Like any patient with nerve injury, they are at risk for development of complex regional pain syndrome (reflex sympathetic dystrophy).[16] Contractures and chronic pain may develop as well.

POTENTIAL TREATMENT COMPLICATIONS

There are inherent risks with any surgery, including failure to correct the problem, infection, additional deformity, and death. Any injection or surgery involving the wrist should avoid the superficial radial sensory nerve as this could cause additional paresthesias or dysesthesias.

References

1. Lowe JB 3rd, Sen SK, Mackinnon SE. Current approach to radial nerve paralysis. Plast Reconstr Surg 2002;110:1099-1113.
2. Silver J. Radial neuropathy. In Weiss L, Silver J, Weiss J, eds. Easy EMG. New York, Butterworth-Heinemann, 2004:135-139.
3. Bordalo-Rodrigues M, Rosenberg ZS. MR imaging of entrapment neuropathies at the elbow [review]. Magn Reson Imaging Clin North Am 2004;12:247-263, vi.
4. Ring D, Chin K, Jupiter JB. Radial nerve palsy associated with high-energy humeral shaft fractures. J Hand Surg Am 2004;29: 144-147.
5. Larsen LB, Barfred T. Radial nerve palsy after simple fracture of the humerus. Scand J Plast Reconstr Surg Hand Surg 2000;34: 363-366.
6. De Smet L. Posterior interosseous neuropathy due to compression by a soft tissue chondroma of the elbow. Acta Neurol Belg 2005;105:86-88.
7. Midroni G, Moulton R. Radial entrapment neuropathy due to chronic injection-induced triceps fibrosis. Muscle Nerve 2001;24:134-137.
8. Sheu JJ, Yuan RY. Superficial radial neuropathy caused by intravenous injection. Acta Neurol Belg 1999;99:138-139.
9. Kalita J, Misra UK, Sharma RK, Rai P. Femoral and radial neuropathy following vascular access cannulation for hemodialysis. Nephron 1995;69:362.
10. Weiss L, Weiss J, Johns J, et al. Neuromuscular rehabilitation and electrodiagnosis: peripheral neuropathy. Arch Phys Med Rehabil 2005;86:(Suppl 1):511-517.
11. Braidwood AS. Superficial radial neuropathy. J Bone Joint Surg Br 1975;57:380-383.
12. Weiss L, Silver J, Lennard T, Weiss J. Easy Injection. Philadelphia, Elsevier, 2007.
13. De Smet L, Van Raebroeckx T, Van Ransbeeck H. Radial tunnel release and tennis elbow: disappointing results. Acta Orthop Belg 1999;65:510-513.
14. Kozin SH. Tendon transfers for radial and median nerve palsies [review]. J Hand Ther 2005;18:208-215.
15. Herbison G. Treatment of peripheral neuropathies. Plenary Session. Neuropathy: From Genes to Function. Philadelphia, American Association of Electrodiagnostic Medicine, 2000.
16. Wasner G, Backonja MM, Baron R. Traumatic neuralgias: Complex regional pain syndrome (reflex sympathetic dystrophy and causalgia): Clinical characteristics, pathophysiological mechanism and therapy. Neurology Clin 1998;16:851-868.

Ulnar Neuropathy (Elbow) 23

Lyn D. Weiss, MD, and Jay M. Weiss, MD

Synonyms

Cubital tunnel syndrome
Tardy ulnar palsy
Ulnar neuritis
Compression of the ulnar nerve

ICD-9 Code

354.2 Lesion of ulnar nerve

DEFINITION

The ulnar nerve is derived predominantly from the nerve roots of C8 and T1 with a small contribution from C7. The C8 and T1 fibers form the lower trunk of the brachial plexus. The ulnar nerve is the continuation of the medial cord of the brachial plexus at the level of the axilla.

Ulnar neuropathy at the elbow is the second most common entrapment neuropathy. Only carpal tunnel syndrome (median neuropathy at the wrist) is more frequent. The ulnar nerve is susceptible to compression at the elbow for several reasons. First, the nerve has a superficial anatomic location at the elbow. Hitting the "funny bone" (ulnar nerve at the elbow) creates an unpleasant sensation that most people have experienced. If the ulnar nerve is susceptible to subluxation, further injury may result. Second, the nerve is prone to repeated trauma from leaning on the elbow or repetitively flexing and extending the elbow. Poorly healing fractures at the elbow may damage this nerve. Finally, and perhaps most important, the ulnar nerve can become entrapped at the arcade of Struthers, in the cubital tunnel (ulnar collateral ligament and aponeurosis between the two heads of the flexor carpi ulnaris; Fig. 23-1), or within the flexor carpi ulnaris muscle. The nerve lengthens and becomes taut with elbow flexion. In addition, there is decreased space in the cubital tunnel in this position. The volume of the cubital tunnel is maximal in extension and can decrease by 50% with elbow flexion.[1] The nerve may also become compromised after a distal humerus fracture, either as a direct result of the fracture or because of an altered carrying angle of the elbow and decreased elbow extension (tardy ulnar palsy). Repetitive or incorrect throwing can lead to damage of the ulnar nerve at the elbow.[2] Biomechanical risk factors (repetitive holding of a tool in one position), obesity, and other associated upper extremity work-related musculoskeletal disorders (especially medial epicondylitis and other nerve entrapment disorders) have also been associated with the development of ulnar neuropathy at the elbow.[3]

SYMPTOMS

If the ulnar nerve is entrapped at the elbow, both the dorsal ulnar cutaneous nerve (which arises just proximal to the wrist) and the palmar cutaneous branch of the ulnar nerve will be affected. Patients will therefore complain of numbness or paresthesias in the dorsal and volar aspects of the fifth and ulnar side of the fourth digits. Hand intrinsic muscle weakness may be apparent. In cases of severe ulnar neuropathy, clawing of the fourth and fifth digits (with attempted hand opening) and atrophy of the intrinsic muscles may be noted. Symptoms may be exacerbated by elbow flexion. Pain may be noted and may radiate proximally or distally.

PHYSICAL EXAMINATION

The ulnar nerve may be palpable in the posterior condylar groove (posterior to the medial epicondyle) with elbow flexion and extension. A Tinel sign may be present at the elbow; however, it should be considered significant only if the Tinel sign is absent on the nonaffected side. The ulnar nerve may be felt subluxing with flexion and extension of the elbow. Sensory deficits may be noted in the fifth and ulnar half of the fourth digits. Atrophy of the intrinsic hand muscles and hand weakness may be noted as well (although this is generally seen in more advanced cases). Wartenberg sign (abduction of the fourth and fifth digits) may occur. The patient should be tested for Froment sign. Here, a patient is asked to grasp a piece of paper between the thumb and radial side of the second digit. The examiner tries to pull the paper out of the patient's hand. If the patient has injury to the adductor pollicis muscle

125

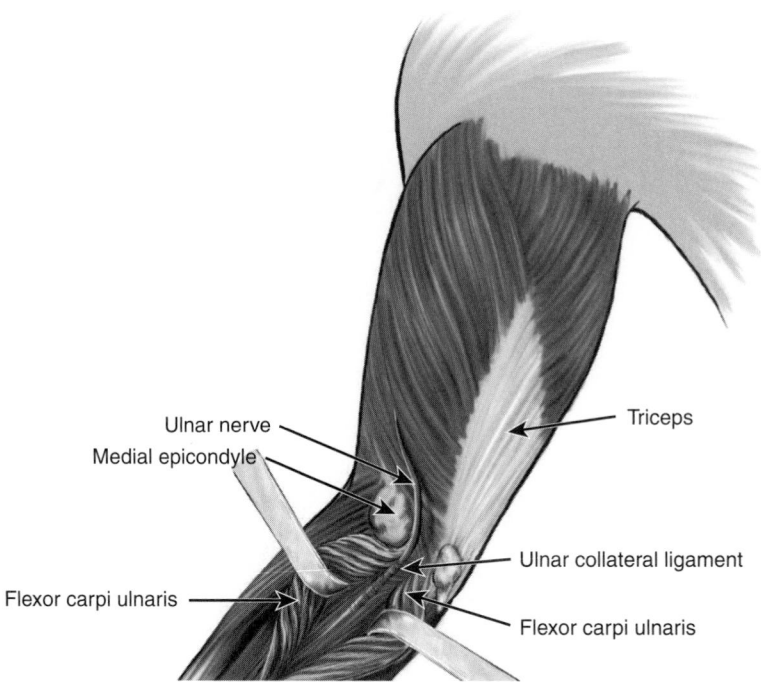

FIGURE 23-1. The cubital tunnel. (Reprinted with permission from Bernstein J, ed. Musculoskeletal Medicine. Rosemont, III, American Academy of Orthopaedic Surgeons, 2003:238.)

(ulnar innervated), the patient will try to compensate by using the median-innervated flexor pollicis longus muscle (Fig. 23-2).

FUNCTIONAL LIMITATIONS

The patient with ulnar neuropathy at the elbow may have poor hand function and complain of dropping things or clumsiness. There may be difficulty with activities of daily living, such as dressing, holding a pen, or using keys.

DIAGNOSTIC STUDIES

Electrodiagnostic studies can help identify, localize, and gauge the severity of an ulnar nerve lesion at the elbow. The findings of abnormal spontaneous potentials (fibrillations and positive sharp waves) in ulnarly innervated muscles on needle electromyographic study indicate axonal damage and portend a worse prognosis than with injury to the myelin only. Slowing of the ulnar nerve across the elbow or conduction block (a drop in compound motor action potential amplitude across the elbow) indicates myelin injury. These studies can also identify other areas of nerve compression that may accompany ulnar neuropathy at the elbow. Radiographs of the elbow with cubital tunnel views can be obtained if fractures, spurs, arthritis, and trauma are suspected. In rare cases, magnetic resonance imaging[4] with arthrography may be used to assess for tears in the ulnar collateral ligament or soft tissue disease.

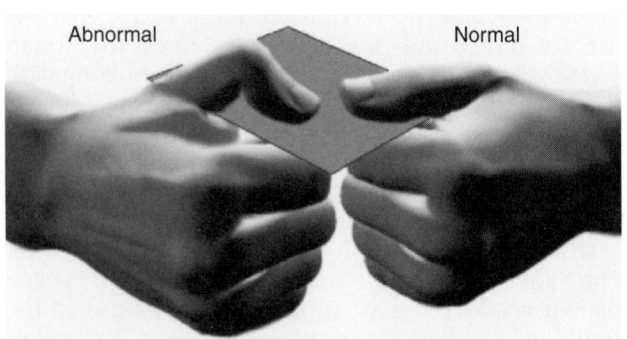

FIGURE 23-2. Froment sign. (Reprinted with permission from Weiss L, Silver J, Weiss J, eds. Easy EMG. New York, Butterworth-Heinemann, 2004.)

Differential Diagnosis

Ulnar neuropathy at a location other than the elbow

C8-T1 radiculopathy

Brachial plexopathy (usually lower trunk)

Thoracic outlet syndrome

Elbow fracture

Elbow dislocation

Medial epicondylitis

Carpal tunnel syndrome

TREATMENT

Initial

Treatment initially involves relative rest and protecting the elbow. Nonsteroidal anti-inflammatory drugs may be prescribed. Elbow pads or night splinting in mild flexion may be beneficial. Treatment should be directed at avoidance of aggravating biomechanical factors, such as leaning on the elbows, prolonged or repetitive elbow flexion, and repetitive valgus stress in throwing.

Rehabilitation

Successful rehabilitation of ulnar neuropathy at the elbow includes identification and correction of biomechanical factors. This may include workstation modifications to decrease the amount of elbow flexion, substitution of headphones for telephone handsets, and use of forearm rests. Often, an elbow pad can be beneficial; the pad protects the ulnar nerve and keeps the elbow in relative extension. A rehabilitation program should include strengthening of forearm pronator and flexor muscles. Flexibility exercises should be instituted to maintain range of motion and to prevent muscle tightness. Advanced strengthening, including eccentric and dynamic joint stabilization exercises, can be added.[5,6]

Procedures

Procedures are not typically performed to treat ulnar neuropathy at the elbow.

Surgery

If conservative management has failed or if significant damage to the ulnar nerve is evident, surgery may be considered.[7-9] The type of surgery depends on the area of ulnar nerve injury and may involve release of the cubital tunnel, ulnar nerve transposition,[10] decompression of the ulnar nerve,[11] subtotal medial epicondylectomy,[12,13] or ulnar collateral ligament repair.

POTENTIAL DISEASE COMPLICATIONS

If ulnar neuropathy at the elbow is left untreated, complications may include hand weakness, poor coordination, intrinsic muscle atrophy, sensory loss, and pain. In addition, flexion contractures and valgus deformity may develop at the elbow.[5]

POTENTIAL TREATMENT COMPLICATIONS

The results of surgery depend on the extent of ulnar nerve compression, accuracy of identifying the site of compression, type of procedure, thoroughness of compression release, comorbid factors, degree of prior intrinsic muscle loss, and previous sensory loss.[5,14-18] Nonsteroidal anti-inflammatory drugs may cause gastric, hepatic, or renal complications.

References

1. Weiss L. Ulnar neuropathy. In Weiss L, Silver J, Weiss J, eds. Easy EMG. New York, Butterworth-Heinemann, 2004:127-134.
2. Aoki M, Takasaki H, Muraki T, et al. Strain on the ulnar nerve at the elbow and wrist during throwing motion. J Bone Joint Surg Am 2005;87:2508-2514.
3. Descatha A, Leclerc A, Chastang JF, Roquelaure Y; Study Group on Repetitive Work. Incidence of ulnar nerve entrapment at the elbow in repetitive work. Scand J Work Environ Health 2004;30:234-240.
4. Timmerman L, Schwartz M, Andrew J. Preoperative evaluation of the ulnar collateral ligament by magnetic resonance imaging and computed tomography arthrography: evaluation of 25 baseball players with surgical confirmation. Am J Sports Med 1994;22:26-32.
5. Stokes W. Ulnar neuropathy (elbow). In Frontera W, Silver J, eds. Essentials of Physical Medicine and Rehabilitation. Philadelphia, Hanley & Belfus, 2002:139-142.
6. Wilk K, Chmielewski T. Rehabilitation of the elbow. In Canavan P, ed. Rehabilitation in Sports Medicine. Stamford, Conn, Appleton & Lange, 1998:237-256.
7. Asamoto S, Boker DK, Jodicke A. Surgical treatment for ulnar nerve entrapment at the elbow. Neurol Med Chir (Tokyo) 2005;45:240-244; discussion 244-245.
8. Nathan PA, Istvan JA, Meadows KD. Intermediate and long-term outcomes following simple decompression of the ulnar nerve at the elbow. Chir Main 2005;24:29-34.
9. Beekman R, Wokke JH, Schoemaker MC, et al. Ulnar neuropathy at the elbow: follow-up and prognostic factors determining outcome. Neurology 2004;63:1675-1680.
10. Matei CI, Logigian EL, Shefner JM. Evaluation of patients with recurrent symptoms after ulnar nerve transposition. Muscle Nerve 2004;30:493-496.
11. Nabhan A, Ahlhelm F, Kelm J, et al. Simple decompression or subcutaneous anterior transposition of the ulnar nerve for cubital tunnel syndrome. J Hand Surg Br 2005;30:521-524.
12. Anglen J. Distal humerus fractures. J Am Acad Orthop Surg 2005;13:291-297.
13. Popa M, Dubert T. Treatment of cubital tunnel syndrome by frontal partial medial epicondylectomy. A retrospective series of 55 cases. J Hand Surg Br 2004;29:563-567.
14. Dellon A. Review of treatment for ulnar nerve entrapment at the elbow. J Hand Surg Am 1989;14:688-700.
15. Jobe F, Fanton G: Nerve injuries. In Morrey B, ed. The Elbow and Its Disorders. Philadelphia, WB Saunders, 1985:497.
16. Efstathopoulos DG, Themistocleous GS, Papagelopoulos PJ, et al. Outcome of partial medial epicondylectomy for cubital tunnel syndrome. Clin Orthop Relat Res 2006;444:134-139.
17. Davis GA, Bulluss KJ. Submuscular transposition of the ulnar nerve: review of safety, efficacy and correlation with neurophysiological outcome. J Clin Neurosci 2005;12:524-528.
18. Gervasio O, Gambardella G, Zaccone C, Branca D. Simple decompression versus anterior submuscular transposition of the ulnar nerve in severe cubital tunnel syndrome: a prospective randomized study. Neurosurgery 2005;56:108-117.

de Quervain Tenosynovitis **24**

Carina J. O'Neill, DO

Synonyms

Washerwoman's sprain[1]
Stenosing tenosynovitis[2]
Tenovaginitis[3,4]
Tendinosis[5]
Tendinitis[6]
Peritendinitis[6]

ICD-9 Codes

727.0   Synovitis and tenosynovitis
727.04   de Quervain tenosynovitis
727.05   Other tenosynovitis of hand and wrist

DEFINITION

Tenosynovitis is defined as inflammation of a tendon and its enveloping sheath.[7] de Quervain tenosynovitis is classically defined as a stenosing tenosynovitis of the synovial sheath of tendons of abductor pollicis longus and extensor pollicis brevis in the first compartment of the wrist due to repetitive use[2] (Fig. 24-1). Fritz de Quervain first described this condition in 1895.[3] Histologic studies have found that this disorder is characterized by degeneration and thickening of the tendon sheath and that it is not an active inflammatory condition.[8]

de Quervain described thickening of the tendon sheath compartment at the distal radial end of the extensor pollicis brevis and abductor longus.[3] Extensor triggering, which is manifested by locking in extension, is rare but has also been reported in de Quervain disease with prevalence of 1.3%.[1]

Overexertion related to household chores and recreational activities including piano playing, sewing, knitting, typing, bowling, golfing, and fly-fishing have been reported to cause de Quervain tenosynovitis. Workers involved with fast repetitive manipulations such as pinching, grasping, pulling, or pushing are also at risk.[6]

For a majority of cases, the onset of de Quervain tenosynovitis is gradual and not associated with a history of acute trauma, although several authors have noted traumatic etiology, such as falling on the tip of the thumb.[6]

de Quervain tenosynovitis primarily affects women (gender ratio approximately 10:1) between the ages of 35 and 55 years. There is no predilection for right versus left side, and no racial differences have been observed.[6]

SYMPTOMS

Patients may complain of pain in the lateral wrist during grasp and thumb extension.[3] They may also describe pain with palpation over the lateral wrist.[9] Symptoms are often persistent for several weeks or months, and there is often a history of chronic overuse of the wrist and the hand.[10] Pain is the most prominent symptom quality, but some patients report stiffness or neuralgia-like complaints; however, true paresthesia in the distribution of the superficial radial nerve is uncommon.[6]

PHYSICAL EXAMINATION

On examination, the findings of local tenderness and moderate swelling around the radial styloid are likely to be present.[10] A positive Finkelstein test result can confirm the diagnosis.[11] The Finkelstein test is performed by grasping the patient's thumb and quickly abducting the hand in ulnar deviation[4] (Fig. 24-2). Reproduction of pain is a positive test result. A similar test, described by Eichhoff in 1927, provides ulnar deviation while the patient is flexing the thumb and curling fingers around it. Pain should disappear the moment the thumb is again extended, even if the ulnar abduction is maintained.[3] The Eichhoff test is sometimes erroneously called the Finkelstein test. The Brunelli test maintains the wrist in radial deviation while forcibly abducting the thumb.[3] Pain over the radial styloid from these provocative stretch maneuvers differentiates de Quervain tenosynovitis from arthritis of the first metacarpal.[9] Strength, particularly grip and pinch strength, may be decreased from pain or disuse secondary to pain.[12] Strength and sensation are expected to be normal in de Quervain tenosynovitis. A comprehensive examination of the neck and entire upper extremity should be performed before conduction of the wrist examination to rule out radiating pain from a more proximal problem, such as a herniated cervical disc.[9]

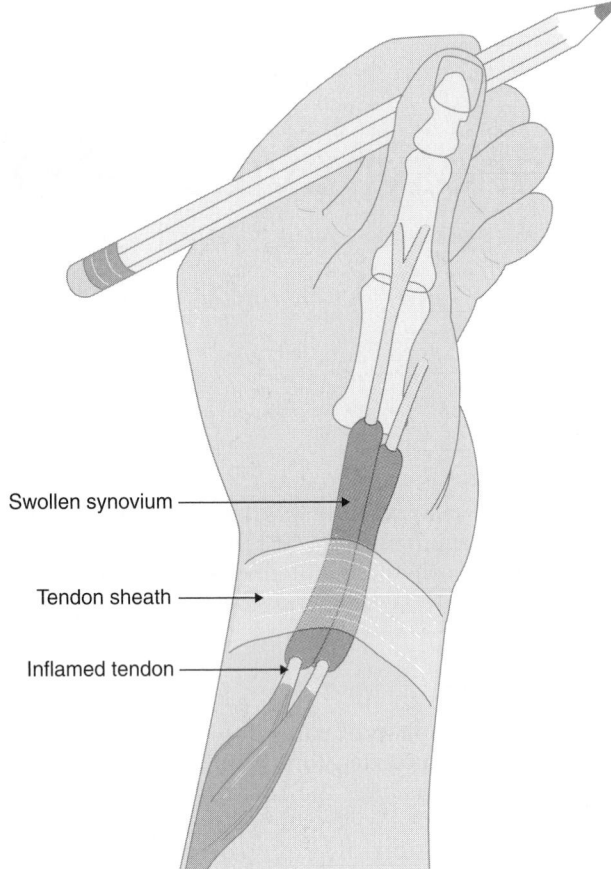

Swollen synovium

Tendon sheath

Inflamed tendon

FIGURE 24-1. de Quervain tenosynovitis of the first extensor compartment.

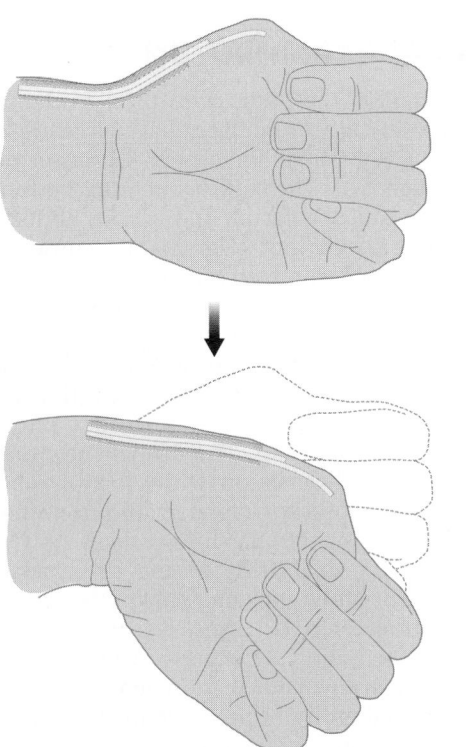

FIGURE 24-2. The result of the Finkelstein test is positive when the patient has pain with full thumb flexion and ulnar deviation of the wrist.

FUNCTIONAL LIMITATIONS

Mechanically, functional impairment is believed to be caused by impaired gliding of the abductor pollicis longus or extensor pollicis brevis tendon due to a narrowed fibro-osseous canal.[6] Functional impairment of the thumb is a result of mechanical impingement or pain. Activities of daily living, such as difficulty with dressing, can be affected; fastening of buttons often causes significant pain. In addition, household chores can be limited secondary to pain. Limits in recreational activities, such as bowling, fly-fishing, sewing, and knitting, are also seen in de Quervain tenosynovitis. Workers with repetitive motions such as pushing or pulling in a factory setting are at risk for development of the condition, and therefore pain from the condition can have a significant economic inpact.[6]

DIAGNOSTIC STUDIES

Tenosynovitis of the wrist is a clinical diagnosis, but some authors recommend obtaining a wrist radiograph to rule out other potential causes of wrist pain.[6] Some clinicians report that relief of symptoms after injection of a local anesthetic into the first dorsal compartment is often helpful as a diagnostic tool.[6] When clinical findings are nondiagnostic, a bone scan can help confirm a diagnosis.[2] On ultrasound examination, tenosynovitis is characterized by hypoechoic fluid distending the tendon sheath with inflammatory changes within the tendon.[13]

TREATMENT

Initial

It is unclear whether conservative treatments are effective in de Quervain tenosynovitis. The current literature is limited to effectiveness of ice, nonsteroidal anti-inflammatory drugs (NSAIDs), heat, splints, strapping,

Differential Diagnosis

Carpal joint arthritis

Triscaphoid arthritis

Rheumatoid arthritis

Intersection syndrome

Radial nerve injury

Ganglion cyst

Cervical radiculopathy

Scaphoid fracture

Carpal tunnel syndrome

Radioscaphoid arthritis

Kienböck disease

Extensor pollicis longus tenosynovitis

rest, and massage. In the research available, these techniques seem to be ineffective in treatment of de Quervain tenosynovitis[6]; however, no randomized controlled study has been performed. One study compared splinting with rest and NSAID therapy. Only 14% of patients who were splinted were cured versus 0% with rest and NSAIDs.[14]

Rehabilitation

Goals of therapy are to reduce pain and to improve function of the affected hand. Classically, therapy includes physical modalities such as ice, heat, transcutaneous electrical nerve stimulation, ultrasound, and iontophoresis.[8] In addition, friction massage and active exercises have been employed.[8] A thumb spica splint has been used for immobilization as well.[15] A thumb spica splint is believed to be an effective way to manage symptoms because it inhibits gliding of the tendon through the abnormal fibro-osseous canal.[6] Research has been limited to the effectiveness of therapy in reduction of symptoms of de Quervain tenosynovitis. One small, randomized study demonstrated that patients with mild symptoms are more likely to improve with therapy and NSAIDs alone versus the majority of patients with moderate to severe symptoms not responding to therapy.[15] Although steroid injection is the mainstay for treatment of de Quervain tenosynovitis, because of the benign profile of therapy, it is reasonable to consider these less invasive approaches (such as ice, thumb spica splinting, and NSAIDs) when this disorder is first treated.[16]

Procedure

Injection of local anesthetics and corticosteroids, with or without immobilization, became popular in the 1950s.[6] It is currently the most frequent treatment modality for patients with de Quervain tenosynovitis. Injection into the first extensor compartment can relieve symptoms (see Fig. 24-2). One study described an 83% cure rate with injection.[14] Interestingly, the same study compared injection with thumb splint immobilization, in which there was only a 61% cure rate. Care must be taken not to inject directly into a tendon.[17]

Surgery

Before 1950, surgery was considered the treatment of choice for de Quervain tenosynovitis. Now, with the success of injections, it is reserved for those whose injection therapy fails.[18] Surgery involves incision of the skin, slitting or removal of a strip of the tendon sheath, closure of the skin, and application of a compression bandage that is removed in a week. The patient returns to normal activities after 2 to 3 weeks. On average, surgical success rates range from 83% to 92%.[6]

POTENTIAL DISEASE COMPLICATIONS

de Quervain tenosynovitis has been described as a vicious circle. It is postulated that increased friction is the likely pathogenetic mechanism. Because of friction, the tendon sheath becomes edematous, which can further increase friction. This can eventually lead to fibrosis of the tendon.[6] The condition is characterized not by inflammation[6] but by thickening of the tendon sheath and most notably by the accumulation of mucopolysaccharide, an indicator of myxoid degeneration. These changes are pathognomonic of the condition and are not seen in control tendon sheaths. The term *stenosing tenovaginitis* is a misnomer; de Quervain disease is a result of intrinsic, degenerative mechanisms rather than of extrinsic, inflammatory ones.[19]

POTENTIAL TREATMENT COMPLICATIONS

NSAIDs have well-known side effects that most commonly affect the gastric, hepatic, and renal systems. The most common immediate adverse reaction reported with injection was immediate pain at the injection site (35%), followed by immediate inflammatory flare reaction (10%), temporary radial nerve paresthesia (4%), and vasovagal reaction (4%); 31% had late adverse reactions ranging from minimal skin color lightening to subcutaneous fat atrophy.[6] In this study, no postinjection infection, bleeding, or tendon rupture was seen; however, this could be possible with any injection. With any type of steroid injection, there is a risk of bleeding. Repeated steroid injections have the potential to weaken the tendon and may cause a tendon rupture. Surgical treatment complications include radial nerve injury, incomplete retinacular release, and tendon subluxation.[18]

References

1. Alberton GM, High WA, Shin AY, Bishop AT. Extensor triggering in de Quervain's stenosing tenosynovitis. J Hand Surg Am 1999;24:1311-1314.
2. Leslie WD. The scintigraphic appearance of de Quervain tenosynovitis. Clin Nucl Med 2006;31:602-604.
3. Ahuja NK, Chung KC. Fritz de Quervain, MD (1868-1940): stenosing tendovaginitis at the radial styloid process. J Hand Surg Am 2004;29:1164-1170.
4. Finkelstein H. Stenosing tendovaginitis at the radial styloid process. J Bone Joint Surg 1930;12:509-540.
5. Ashe MC, McCauley T, Khan KM. Tendinopathies in the upper extremity: a paradigm shift. J Hand Ther 2004;17:329-334.
6. Moore JS. De Quervain's tenosynovitis: stenosing tenosynovitis of the first dorsal compartment. J Occup Environ Med 1997;39:990-1002.
7. http://medical-dictionary.thefreedictionary.com/tenosynovitis.
8. Walker MJ. Manual physical therapy examination and intervention of a patient with radial wrist pain: a case report. J Orthop Sports Phys Ther 1994;34:761-769.
9. Forman TA, Forman SK, Rose NE. A clinical approach to diagnosing wrist pain. Am Fam Physician 2005;72:1753-1758.
10. Abe Y, Tsue K, Nagai E, et al. Extensor pollicis longus tenosynovitis mimicking de Quervain's disease because of its course through the first extensor compartment: a report of 2 cases. J Hand Surg Am 2004;29:225-229.
11. Alexander RD, Catalano LW, Barron OA, Glickel SZ. The extensor pollicis brevis entrapment test in the treatment of de Quervain's disease. J Hand Surg Am 2002;27:813-816.

12. Fournier K, Bourbonnais D, Bravo G, et al. Reliability and validity of pinch and thumb strength measurements in de Quervain's disease. J Hand Ther 2006;19:2-10.

13. Torriani M, Kattapuram SV. Musculoskeletal ultrasound: an alternative imaging modality for sports-related injuries. Top Magn Reson Imaging 2003;14:103-111.

14. Richie CA, Briner WW. Corticosteroid injection for treatment of de Quervain's tenosynovitis: a pooled quantitative literature evaluation. J Am Board Fam Pract 2003;16:102-106.

15. Lane LB, Boretz RS, Stuchin SA. Treatment of de Quervain's disease: role of conservative management. J Hand Surg Br 2001;26:258-260.

16. Slawson D. Best treatment for de Quervain's tenosynovitis uncertain. Am Fam Physician 2003;68:533.

17. Tallia AF, Cardone DA. Diagnostic and therapeutic injection of the wrist and hand region. Am Fam Physician 2003;67:745-750.

18. Kent TT, Eidelman D, Thomson JG. Patient satisfaction and outcome of surgery for de Quervain's tenosynovitis. J Hand Surg Am 1999;24:1071-1077.

19. Clark MT, Lyall HA, Grant JW, et al. The histopathology of de Quervain's disease. J Hand Surg Br 1998;23:732-734.

Dupuytren Contracture 25

Michael F. Stretanski, DO

Synonym

Dupuytren disease

ICD-9 Code

728.6   Dupuytren contracture

DEFINITION

Dupuytren disease is a nonmalignant fibroproliferative disease causing progressive and permanent contracture of the palmar fascia; subsequent flexion contracture usually begins with the fourth and fifth digits on the ulnar side of the hand (Fig. 25-1). The eponym Cooper contracture has been suggested for Astley Cooper, who first described the disease in 1822 and lectured and wrote extensively on it. A nodule in the palm is the primary lesion in Dupuytren contracture. It is a firm, soft tissue mass fixed to both the skin and the deeper fascia. It is characterized histologically by dense, noninflammatory, chaotic cellular tissue and appears on the anterior aspect of the palmar aponeurosis.

The key cell response for tissue contraction in Dupuytren disease is thought to be the fibroblast and its differentiation into a myofibroblast.[1] This idiopathic activation happens in response to the fibrogenic cytokines interleukin-1, prostaglandin F_2, prostaglandin E_2, platelet-derived growth factor, connective tissue–derived growth factor, and, most important, transforming growth factor-β and fibroblast growth factor 2. As the nodule extends slowly, it induces shortening and tension on the longitudinal fascial bands of the palmar aponeurosis, resulting in cords of hypertrophied tissue. It is unique among ailments of the hand, and one could conceive of it as a focal autoimmune—collagen vascular phenomenon. Dupuytren disease is believed to begin in the overlying dermis.[2] Unlike the nodule, the cord is strikingly different histologically; it contains few or no myofibroblasts and few fibroblasts in a dense collagen matrix with less vascularity. Skin changes can be the earliest signs of Dupuytren disease, including thickening of the palmar skin and underlying subcutaneous tissue. Rippling of the skin can occur before the development of a digital flexion deformity.[3]

A controversy exists as to whether there is a relationship between Dupuytren disease and repetitive "microtrauma."[4] This suggestion has not held up under scrutiny, and it is now believed that microruptures are related to the contracture rather than a primary cause of it.[5] Cessation of manual labor, like immobilization, can lead to acceleration of the disease, which has been noted in laborers after retirement.[6] However, one self-reported study seems to suggest that there may be an association with rock climbing in men.[7]

Dupuytren disease is known to have a genetic predisposition and is believed to be inherited as an autosomal dominant trait with variable penetrance.[8] Family history is often unreliable; many individuals are unaware that they have family members who have the diagnosis. Dupuytren disease has been termed Viking disease[9] because it has a high prevalence in areas that were populated by the Vikings and where the Vikings eventually migrated. It is rare in nonwhite populations. Dupuytren disease occurs more commonly in the elderly but tends to be associated with greater functional compromise in younger patients. Women are affected half as often as men are.[10] There is no relationship to handedness; however, affected individuals tend to complain more frequently about the dominant hand. Other associations with the condition include diabetes mellitus[11] (specifically with an increased risk from diet-controlled diabetes to sulfonylureas to metformin to insulin requiring), alcohol consumption,[12] cigarette smoking,[12,13] human immunodeficiency virus infection,[14] and antecedent Colles fracture. Conflicting reports exist for an association with epilepsy, but antiepileptic drugs do not present an increased risk.[11,15]

There are secondary findings in Dupuytren disease that are rarely seen but when present suggest a strong Dupuytren diathesis (genetic penetrance of the disease). These findings include knuckle pads (Garrod nodes), plantar fascial disease, and contracture of the penile fascial envelope (Peyronie disease). The contractile tissue in all of these conditions resembles the pathologic findings of Dupuytren disease in the palm,[16] and alterations in the expression of certain gene families, fibroblast to myofibroblast differentiation among others, are similar.[17] However, these associated conditions are found in only

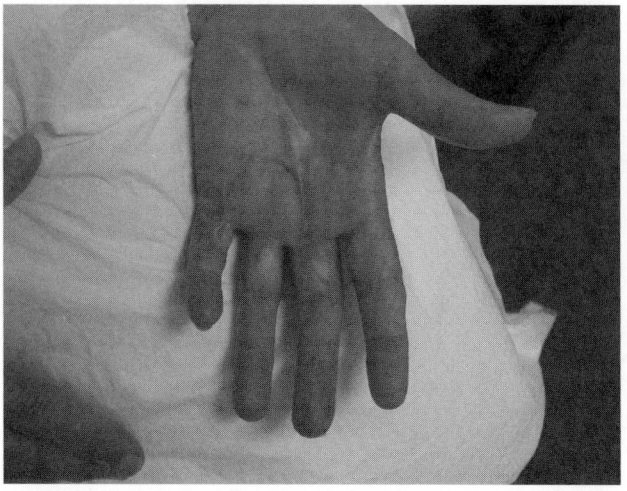

FIGURE 25-1. Typical appearance of ulnar palmar surface after surgical release; notice scarring and incomplete extension.

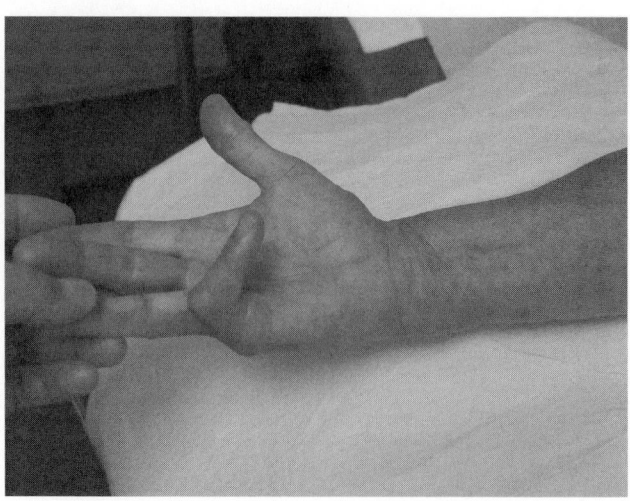

FIGURE 25-2. Dupuytren contracture of the ring finger.

an estimated 1% or less of patients with Dupuytren disease.[18] All patients with the disease have a diathesis. The association with these conditions, as well as onset at an early age and family history, suggests that the diathesis is strong. Recognition of a strong diathesis is important for planning an appropriate rehabilitation protocol, including long-term follow-up and awareness of possible poor prognosis and likelihood of recurrence with surgical treatment.

SYMPTOMS

Dupuytren disease typically has a painless onset and progression. Decreased range of motion, loss of dexterity, and getting the hand "caught" when trying to place it in one's pant-pocket are common presenting symptoms. Pain can be a result of concomitant injuries to the hand and fingers that can precede the development or worsening of Dupuytren disease. Abrasions or ecchymosis to the distal interphalangeal and proximal interphalangeal joints of the affected digits may be seen and may be the reason for the initial consultation. The progression of the condition is generally considered to be a result of immobility after an injury in a predisposed individual rather than of the injury itself.

PHYSICAL EXAMINATION

The most common first sign of Dupuytren disease is a lump in the palm close to the distal palmar crease and in the axis of the ray of the fourth digit (ring finger) (Fig. 25-2). It can also present in the digit, generally over the proximal phalanx. The thumb and index finger are the least affected of the five digits. The nodule can be tender to palpation. In most cases, the skin is closely adherent to the nodule, and movement with tendon excursion often suggests other conditions, such as stenosing tenosynovitis. The condition is more readily apparent when it presents in a more advanced stage with palmar nodule, cord, and digital flexion contracture. Conditions as-

sociated with this disease include fat pads at the knuckles as well as evidence of the disease in the plantar fascia. "Swan-neck" deformity as a dorsal variant of Dupuytren disease has been suggested.[19] The examination should evaluate the entire upper limb for associated adhesive capsulitis. Determination of hemoglobin A_{1c} or thyroid-stimulating hormone values and autoimmune workup may be appropriate. Neurosensory examination findings, muscle stretch reflexes, and shoulder muscle bulk should be normal with normal manual motor testing.

FUNCTIONAL LIMITATIONS

The majority of individuals with this condition have little functional limitation. With more advanced contracture, properly opening the palm while grasping can become difficult, making gripping activities such as activities of daily living, opening cans, buttoning shirts, or placing keys in automotive ignitions troublesome.

DIAGNOSTIC STUDIES

The diagnosis of Dupuytren disease is generally made on a clinical basis. Biopsy is considered when a palmar soft tissue mass cannot be reliably differentiated from sarcoma. The suspicion for this is higher in a younger individual with no strong evidence of Dupuytren disease because sarcoma is more likely in younger age groups. Unfortunately, histologic differentiation is not always easy because a Dupuytren nodule can appear cellular with mitotic figures and closely resemble an aggressive sarcoma.

TREATMENT

Initial

Appropriate identification of the purpose of the encounter with the patient is important. Clinical manifestations of Dupuytren disease exist along a spectrum, and at the time of consultation, they may not be painful

Differential Diagnosis

Fibromas

Lipomas

Epithelioid sarcoma

Giant cell tumors

Neurofibromas

Tendon nodules of stenosing tenosynovitis

Inclusion cysts

Dorsal Dupuytren disease

Retinacular ganglions at the A1 pulley

Non-Dupuytren palmar fascial disease

Tophi

Cooper contracture (eponym)

or functionally limiting. Many patients who seek consultation for Dupuytren disease are merely looking for reassurance that they do not have a malignant neoplasm and are satisfied to learn that the contracture is not a sign of a more ominous disease.

Conventional noninvasive treatment has generally been of little or no value in the prevention of contracture or recurrence in Dupuytren disease. This includes the use of steroid injections, splinting, ultrasound, and nonsteroidal anti-inflammatory medications. Radiotherapy, topical dimethyl sulfoxide, colchicine, and interferon have also been proposed but lack data demonstrating long-term efficacy. Topical 5-fluorouracil,[20] topical imiquimod (Aldara),[21] and oral simvastatin[22] seem to target the underlying fibroblastic process and are slightly more promising, but long-term outcome studies do not exist. Traumatic rupture has never gained acceptance as a method of correcting flexion contracture; however, anecdotal reports of individuals correcting their deformity in such a fashion exist.[23] Recurrence in true Dupuytren disease would be expected. Continuous passive traction has been proposed by some for severely flexed digit contractures[24]; however, this is used as a preoperative adjunctive procedure and not done in isolation.

Ergonomic assessment and equipment modification can be of use in some instances with laborers who are functionally limited by contracture. Tobacco abuse or excessive alcohol consumption should be addressed if applicable.

Rehabilitation

Rehabilitation efforts are minimal preoperatively and focus on adaptive equipment recommendations for work and home (e.g., large-handled tools for gripping). Splinting may be done by therapists with prefabricated or custom designs, but there is no controlled evidence that this delays contracture and does not affect the

underlying pathohistologic changes. Continuous passive traction has been proposed by some for severely flexed digit contractures[25]; however, this is used as a preoperative adjunctive procedure and not done in isolation.

Postoperative rehabilitation is needed to facilitate a satisfactory outcome. The length of the rehabilitation generally reflects the invasiveness of the surgical procedure; limited fasciotomies often involve a period of 4 to 6 weeks, whereas more extensive surgery may necessitate a formal rehabilitation process of up to 3 to 6 months. Stretching, splinting in palmar extension, and continuous passive traction in some individuals are used early postoperatively. Strengthening and functional activities are added later after incision healing. Again, splinting may be an option to prevent recurrence, and adaptive equipment recommendations can help with resumption of functions that involve gripping or repetitive hand use.

Procedures

Closed needle fasciotomy has been used[25] but is prone to complications, including infection, nerve injury, and skin breakdown as well as recurrence.

Enzymatic fasciotomy with collagenase has more recently shown promise for nonsurgical relief of contracture. Purified collagenase is derived from *Clostridium histolyticum*. This treatment has been used in the past for débridement of burns and skin ulcers as well as for Peyronie disease.[26] In vitro studies have shown efficacy,[27] and current clinical studies are ongoing.

Steroid injection into the palmar nodule can be a useful adjunct to flatten the nodule. Concern for potential adverse effect on the underlying flexor tendons has prevented widespread use. Injection of collagenase into the central cord is gaining popularity. Care must be taken to avoid injection into the underlying flexor tendons.[28]

Surgery

Appropriate selection is critical for patients considering surgical treatment. The potential for recurrence and worsening after surgery is high in patients with a strong diathesis. Recurrence is defined as the development of nodules and contracture in the area of previous surgery. Extension is the development of lesions outside of the surgical area where there had previously been no disease. All patients should be made aware that surgery is not curative of this disease and that recurrence and extension are likely at some time. Extensive recurrence is more likely if surgery is performed during the proliferative phase of the condition.

Nevertheless, many individuals have improved hand function after surgical treatment, compared with their preoperative status, for years on follow-up.[29] The goals of surgical treatment, when it is indicated, are to improve function, to reduce deformity, and to prevent recurrence. Surgical indication is generally thought to include digital flexion contracture of the proximal interphalangeal and metacarpophalangeal joints and web space contracture. Metacarpophalangeal joint contractures are often fully correctable; however, proximal interphalangeal joint contractures often have residual deformity.[30]

Multiple surgical procedures have been described for the treatment of Dupuytren contracture. These include variations of subcutaneous fasciotomy, fasciectomy, and skin grafting. A controlled randomized trial between the two most common approaches found no statistical difference at 2 years.[31] Fewer complications are seen with limited fasciectomy, and this is often the procedure of choice for higher risk patients, for whom temporary relief is a therapeutic goal. A diseased cord arising from the abductor digiti minimi is noted to be present in approximately 25% of cases,[32] and it should be released at the time of surgery if it is present. Full-thickness skin grafting has been shown to prevent recurrence and is considered in patients with a strong diathesis who have functionally limiting contracture.

POTENTIAL DISEASE COMPLICATIONS

In some individuals, the condition can become functionally limiting because of severe contracture. The thumb and index finger tend to be less affected than the other digits. Secondary contracture of the proximal interphalangeal joints can also develop in long-standing deformity. Vascular compromise is rare and more often part of complex regional pain syndrome after surgery. It appears that there is an advantage with axillary block or intravenous regional anesthesia with clonidine over lidocaine alone or general anesthesia in preventing complex regional pain syndrome in patients undergoing Dupuytren surgery.[33]

POTENTIAL TREATMENT COMPLICATIONS

Recurrence of the disease after surgery is common (approximately 31%).[34] This is probably because surgery does not alter the underlying histopathologic process. Loss of flexion into the palm is particularly disturbing to patients. The presence of thickly calloused hands can result in increased postoperative swelling, leading to longer postoperative follow-up. "Flare reaction"[35] is a postoperative complication that occurs 3 to 4 weeks after surgery and is characterized by redness, swelling, pain, and stiffness. This occurs in 5% to 10% of patients.[36] Complication rates are higher with greater disease severity, in particular proximal interphalangeal joint flexion contracture of 60 degrees or more.[34] Amputation and ray resections are reported complications more common in surgery for recurrences.[37] Although women with the disease less frequently meet operative criteria, they are thought to have a higher incidence of complex regional pain syndrome postoperatively.[38] Other potential surgical complications are digital hematoma, granulation, scar contracture, inadvertent division of a digital nerve or artery, infection, and graft failure in full-thickness grafting procedures. A potential complication of injection therapy is injury to nearby structures, including the digital artery, nerve, and flexor tendons.

References

1. Cordova A, Tripoli M, Corradino B, et al. Dupuytren's contracture: an update of biomolecular aspects and therapeutic perspectives. J Hand Surg Br 2005;30:557-562.
2. Hueston JT. Digital Wolfe grafts in recurrent Dupuytren's contracture. Plast Reconstr Surg 1962;29:342.
3. McFarlane RM. Patterns of the diseased fascia in the fingers in Dupuytren's contracture. Plast Reconstr Surg 1974;54:31-44.
4. Skoog T. The pathogenesis and etiology of Dupuytren's contracture. Plast Reconstr Surg 1963;31:258.
5. Early P. Population studies in Dupuytren's contracture. J Bone Joint Surg Br 1962;44:602-613.
6. Liss GM, Stock SR. Can Dupuytren's contracture be work-related? Review of the literature. Am J Indust Med 1996;29:521-532.
7. Logan AJ, Mason G, Dias J, Makwana N. Can rock climbing lead to Dupuytren's disease? Br J Sports Med 2005;39:639-644.
8. Ling RSM. The genetic factors in Dupuytren's disease. J Bone Joint Surg Br 1963;45:709.
9. Hueston J. Dupuytren's contracture and occupation. J Hand Surg Am 1987;12:657.
10. Yost J, Winters T, Fett HC. Dupuytren's contracture: a statistical study. Am J Surg 1955;90:568-572.
11. Geoghegan JM, Forbes J, Clark DI, et al. Dupuytren's disease risk factors. J Hand Surg Br 2004;29:423-426.
12. Godtfredson NS, Lucht H, Prescott E, et al. A prospective study linked both alcohol and tobacco to Dupuytren's disease. J Clin Epidemiol 2004;57:858-863.
13. An JS, Southworth SR, Jackson T, et al. Cigarette smoking and Dupuytren's contracture of the hand. J Hand Surg Am 1994;19:442.
14. Bower M, Nelson M, Gazzard BG. Dupuytren's contractures in patients infected with HIV. Br Med J 1990;300:165.
15. Lund M. Dupuytren's contracture and epilepsy. Acta Psychiatr Neurol 1941;16:465-492.
16. Hueston JT. Some observations on knuckle pads. J Hand Surg Br 1984;9:75.
17. Qian A, Meals RA, Rajfer J, Gonzalez-Cadavid NF. Comparison of gene expression profiles between Peyronie's disease and Dupuytren's contracture. Urology 2004;64:399-404.
18. Cavolo DJ, Sherwood GF. Dupuytren's disease of the plantar fascia. J Foot 1982;21:12.
19. Boyce DE, Tonkin MA. Dorsal Dupuytren's disease causing a swan-neck deformity. J Hand Surg Br 2004;29:636-637.
20. Bulstrode NW, Mudera V, McGrouther DA. 5-Fluorouracil selectively inhibits collagen synthesis. Plast Reconstr Surg 2005;116:209-221.
21. Namazi H. Imiquimod: a potential weapon against Dupuytren contracture. Med Hypotheses 2006;66:991-992.
22. Namazi H, Emami MJ. Simvastatin may be useful in therapy of Dupuytren contracture. Med Hypotheses 2006;66:683-684.
23. Sirotakova M, Elliot D. A historical record of traumatic rupture of Dupuytren's contracture. J Hand Surg Br 1997;22:198-201.
24. Citron N, Mesina J. The use of skeletal traction in the treatment of severe primary Dupuytren's disease. J Bone Joint Surg Br 1998;80:126-129.
25. Badois F, Lermusiaux J, Masse C, et al. Nonsurgical treatment of Dupuytren's disease using needle fasciotomy. Rev Rhum Engl Ed 1993;60:692-697.
26. Gelbard M, James K, Riach P, et al. Collagenase versus placebo in the treatment of Peyronie's disease: a double-blind study. J Urol 1993;149:56-58.
27. Starkweather KD, Lattuga S, Hurst LC, et al. Collagenase in the treatment of Dupuytren's disease: an in vitro study. J Hand Surg Am 1996;21:490-495.

28. Badalamente M, Hurst L. Enzyme injection as a nonoperative treatment for Dupuytren's disease. Drug Delivery 1996;3:33-40.

29. Forgon M, Farkas G. Results of surgical treatment of Dupuytren's contracture. Handchir Mikrochir Plast Chir 1988;20:279-284.

30. Riolo J, Young VL, Ueda K, Pidgeon L. Dupuytren's contracture. South Med J 1991;84:983-996.

31. Citron ND, Nunez V. Recurrence after surgery of Dupuytren's disease: a randomized trial of two skin incisions. J Hand Surg Br 2005;30:563-566.

32. Meathrel KE, Thoma A. Abductor digiti minimi involvement in Dupuytren's contracture of the small finger. J Hand Surg Am 2004;29:510-513.

33. Reuben SS, Pristas R, Dixon D, et al. The incidence of complex regional pain syndrome after fasciectomy for Dupuytren's contracture: a prospective observational study of four anesthestic techniques. Anesth Analg 2006;102:499-503.

34. Bulstrode NW, Jemec B, Smith PJ. The complications of Dupuytren's contracture surgery. J Hand Surg Br 2005;30:1021-1025.

35. Howard LD Jr. Dupuytren's contracture: a guide for management. Clin Orthop 1959;15:118.

36. McFarlane RM. The current status of Dupuytren's disease. J Hand Surg Br 1983;8:703.

37. Del Frari B, Estermann D, Piza-Katzer H. Dupuytren's contracture—surgery of recurrences. Handchir Mikrochir Plast Chir 2005;37:309-315.

38. Zemel NP, Balcomb TV, Stark HH, et al. Dupuytren's disease in women: evaluation of long-term results after operation. J Hand Surg Am 1987;12:1012.

Extensor Tendon Injuries **26**

Jeffrey S. Brault, DO, PT, and Gregory L. Umphrey, MD

Synonyms

Mallet finger
Extensor hood injury
Central slip injury
Extensor sheath injury
Boutonnière deformity
Buttonhole deformity

ICD-9 Codes

727.63   Hand extensor injury
736.1   Mallet finger
736.21   Boutonnière deformity

DEFINITION

Extensor tendon injuries are injuries to the extensor mechanism of the digits. They include the finger and the thumb extensors and abductors. Extensor tendon injuries are more common than flexor tendon injuries because of their superficial position. As a result, the extensor tendons are prone to laceration, abrasion, crushing, burns, and bite wounds.[1] Demographic data defining age, gender, and occupation for the development of extensor tendon injury are not well documented. However, in our clinical experience, extensor tendon injuries commonly occur from lacerations and fist to mouth injuries.

Extensor tendon injuries result in the inability to extend the finger because of transection of the tendon itself, extensor lag, joint stiffness, and poor pain control.[2,3] There are eight zones to the extensor mechanism where injury can result in differing pathomechanics[4] (Fig. 26-1).

SYMPTOMS

Patients typically lose the ability to fully extend the involved finger (Fig. 26-2). This lack of motion may be confined to a single joint or the entire digit. Pain in surrounding regions often accompanies the loss of motion because of abnormal tissue stresses. Diminished sensation may be present if there is concomitant injury to the digital nerves.

PHYSICAL EXAMINATION

Physical examination begins with observation of the resting hand position. If the extensor tendon is completely disrupted, the unsupported finger will assume a flexed posture. Range of motion, both active and passive, is evaluated for each finger joint. Grip strength is commonly measured by use of a hand-held dynamometer. Individual finger extension strength can be recorded by manual muscle testing or finger dynamometry. Sensation should be checked because of the proximity of the extensor mechanism to the digital nerves. The radial and ulnar sides of the digit should be checked to assess light touch, pinprick, and two-point discrimination.

FUNCTIONAL LIMITATIONS

The positioning of the hand in preparation for grip or pinch is occasionally more important and limiting than the inability to grasp. Functional limitations therefore are manifested as the inability to produce finger extension in preparation for grip or pinch. As a result, writing and manipulation of small objects can be problematic. Patients may also have difficulty reaching into confined areas such as pockets because of a flexed digit with the limited ability to extend.

DIAGNOSTIC STUDIES

Anteroposterior and lateral radiographs of the involved hand and fingers are obtained when there is a possibility of bone or soft tissue injury, such as fracture of a metacarpal from a bite wound, foreign body retention from glass or metal, or air in the soft tissues or joint space secondary to penetration of a foreign object. Ultrasonography is an inexpensive alternative to magnetic resonance imaging for the detection of foreign bodies and identification of traumatic lesions of tendons. However, ultrasonography and magnetic resonance imaging are generally not necessary but can be used to confirm clinical suspicion of a chronic extensor tendon injury.

139

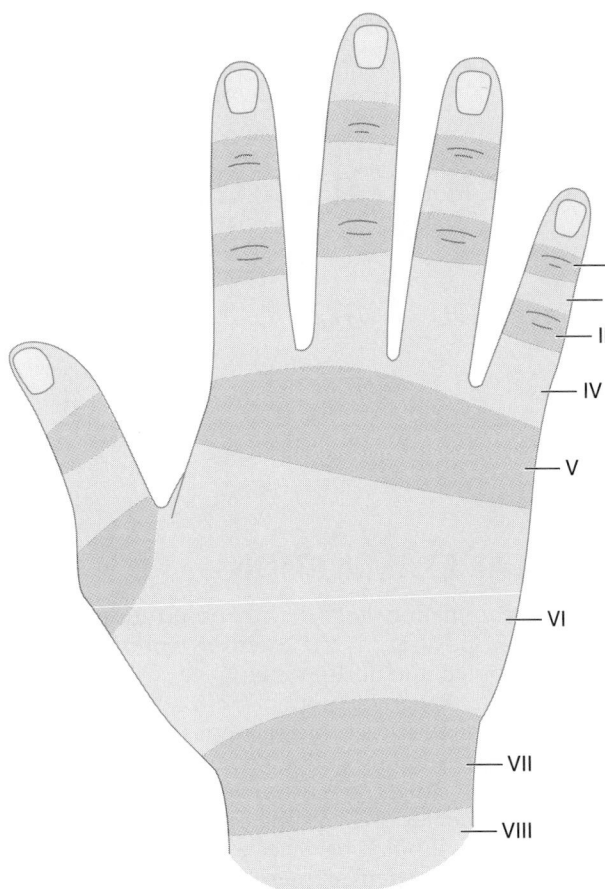

FIGURE 26-1. Zones of extensor tendons. Odd numbers overlie the respective joints, and even numbers overlie areas of intermediate tendon regions.

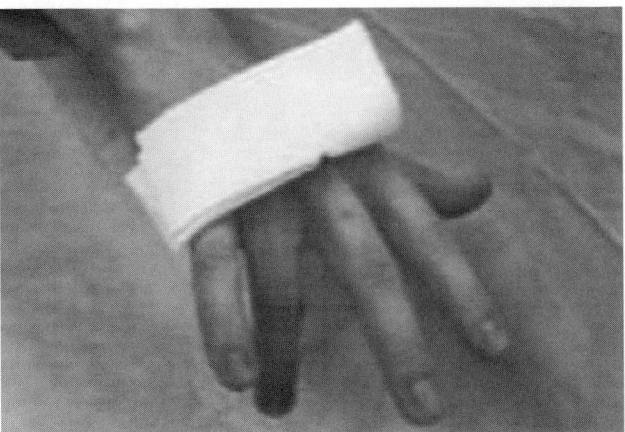

FIGURE 26-2. Extensor tendon disruption of the ring finger resulting in an inability to extend the ring finger. (Modified from Daniels JM II, Zook EG, Lynch JM. Hand and wrist injuries: part I. Nonemergent evaluation. Am Fam Physician 2004;69:1941-1948.)

Differential Diagnosis

Fracture dislocation

Joint dislocation

Peripheral nerve injury

Osteoarthritis

Rheumatoid arthritis

Trigger finger (stenosing tenosynovitis)

TREATMENT

Initial

The treatment protocols for extensor tendon injuries vary by zone, mechanism, and time elapsed since the injury. If the disruption of the extensor mechanism is due to a laceration, crush injury, burn, or bite, surgical referral is warranted. In open injuries, if repair is not immediate, appropriate antibiotics should be initiated, and irrigation and primary coverage of the injured tendon by skin suturing should be performed to protect the tendon and to decrease the potential of infection. The surgeon who will be performing the definitive repair should be contacted before this, however.[5] Conservative splinting can be attempted for closed zone I and zone II extensor tendon injuries.

Rehabilitation

Conservative treatment and splinting have been recommended for zone I and zone II injuries. Conservative treatment of injuries involving zones III through VIII has limited success in restoring normal range of motion and function. Acute injuries in these zones usually require surgical repair, and chronic injuries often require surgical review.

Zone I (Mallet Deformity)

Disruption of continuity of the extensor tendon over the distal interphalangeal (DIP) joint produces the characteristic flexion deformity of the DIP joint.[6] Injury in this region is the result of a traumatic event, such as sudden forced hyperflexion of an extended DIP joint with tendinous disruption or avulsion fracture at the site of insertion. The digits most commonly involved are the long, ring, and small fingers of the dominant hand.[7] When it is left untreated for a prolonged time, hyperextension of the proximal interphalangeal (PIP) joint (swan-neck deformity) may develop because of proximal retraction of the central band.[6]

In a closed injury, the most common method of treatment is 6 weeks of continuous immobilization of the DIP joint in full extension or slight hyperextension (0 to 15 degrees).[8,9,10] The DIP joint should not be immobilized in excessive hyperextension because of compromise of the vascular supply to the dorsal skin.[7] Stack splints are commonly used to achieve extension at the DIP joint. The splint should be worn continuously, except during hygiene. When the splint is removed, the DIP joint should be maintained in extension. If no extensor lag is identified after 7 weeks, range of motion exercises consisting of 10 repetitions hourly of passive, pain-free motion of the DIP joint can be initiated. The splint should be worn during exercise and at night. Splinting may be discontinued and exercises progressed to active extension after 8 weeks. In chronic mallet deformities, in which no treatment is initiated for 3 weeks after injury, splinting is recommended for 8 weeks before beginning of range of motion exercises (Table 26-1).[9]

Zone II

Injuries in zone II are often due to a laceration or crush injury. Treatment involves routine wound care and splinting for 7 to 10 days, followed by active motion if less than 50% of the tendon width is cut. If more than 50% of the tendon is cut, it should be repaired primarily, followed by 6 weeks of splinting.[6]

Zone III (Boutonnière Deformity)

Zone III injuries usually result from direct forceful flexion of an extended PIP joint, laceration, or bite. If the lateral bands slip volarly, a boutonnière deformity results. The boutonnière deformity develops gradually and usually appears 10 to 14 days after the initial injury. Diagnosis is best made after splinting of the finger straight for a few days and reexamination of the finger after swelling subsides. Absent or weak active extension of the PIP joint is a positive finding.[6]

Closed injuries are initially treated with 4 to 6 weeks of splinting of the PIP joint in extension with the metacarpophalangeal (MCP) and wrist joints left free. The splint is reapplied for recurrence of deformity.[6]

Displaced closed avulsion fractures at the base of the middle phalanx, axial and lateral instability of the PIP joint with loss of joint motion, and failed nonoperative treatment are indications for surgical intervention.[6] In addition, acute open injuries require primary surgical repair.

Postoperative rehabilitation has changed in recent years with the implementation of early protected motion.[8-11] Postoperatively, the finger is immobilized in a PIP joint gutter splint. This splint is removed hourly to perform guarded active motion exercises, which may consist of using two exercise braces that provide optimal gliding of the extensor mechanism (Table 26-2).

Zone IV

Injuries in zone IV usually spare the lateral bands. However, there is often considerable adhesion with resultant loss of motion that develops because of the intricate relationship of the tendon and bone in this area. Rehabilitation and splinting techniques are similar to those in zone III (see Table 26-2).

Zone V

Zone V is located over the MCP joints. This is the most common area of extensor tendon injuries resulting from bites, lacerations, or joint dislocation.[1] The injury more often occurs with the joint in flexion, so the tendon injury will actually be proximal to the dermal injury.[6] Acute open injuries are surgically repaired after thorough irrigation if they are not the result of a human bite or fist to mouth injury.

TABLE 26-1 Zone I and Zone II Injuries

	Splint	Exercises	Wound and Skin Care
Acute DIP joint injuries, mallet deformity (less than 3 weeks)			
0-5 weeks	Continuous DIP joint extension (stack)	Active flexion and extension of PIP and MCP joints (hourly)	Remove splint daily to check for skin integrity and hygiene (maintain DIP joint in extension)
6 weeks	Worn between exercises and at night	Active flexion and extension of DIP joint (hourly)	Remove splint daily to check for skin integrity and hygiene (maintain DIP joint in extension)
7 weeks	Worn between exercises and at night	Passive flexion and extension of DIP joint (hourly)	Remove splint daily to check for skin integrity and hygiene (maintain DIP joint in extension)
8 weeks	If no extensor lag, may gradually wean splint	Continue with active and passive DIP joint exercises	Remove splint daily to check for skin integrity and hygiene (maintain DIP joint in extension)
Chronic DIP joint injuries, mallet deformity (more than 3 weeks)			
0-7 weeks	Continuous DIP joint extension (stack)	Active flexion and extension of PIP and MCP joints (hourly)	Remove splint daily to check for skin integrity and hygiene (maintain DIP joint in extension)
8 weeks	Worn between exercises and at night	Active flexion and extension of DIP joint (hourly)	Remove splint daily to check for skin integrity and hygiene (maintain DIP joint in extension)
9 weeks	Worn between exercises and at night	Passive flexion and extension of DIP joint (hourly)	Remove splint daily to check for skin integrity and hygiene (maintain DIP joint in extension)
10 weeks	If no extensor lag, may gradually wean splint	Continue with active and passive DIP joint exercises	Remove splint daily to check for skin integrity and hygiene (maintain DIP joint in extension)

Reprinted with permission from Brault J. Rehabilitation of extensor tendon injuries. Oper Tech Plast Reconstr Surg 2000;7:25-30.

TABLE 26-2 Zone III and Zone IV Injuries (Immediate Motion)

	Splint	Exercises	Wound and Skin Care
Start 24-48 hours	DIP joint and PIP joint neutral splint	Exercise hourly with two splints	Daily removal of splint for wound cleaning Edema control with compressive wrap
0-2 weeks		Splint 1: allows 30 degrees of PIP joint and 25 degrees of DIP joint range of motion Splint 2: PIP joint in neutral, DIP joint	Daily removal of splint for wound cleaning Edema control with compressive wrap
2-3 weeks	If no extensor lag noted	Splint 1: increase PIP joint in flexion to 40 degrees Splint 2: continue	Daily removal of splint for wound cleaning Edema control with compressive wrap
4-5 weeks	If no extensor lag noted	Splint 1: increase PIP joint in flexion to 40 degrees Splint 2: continue	Daily removal of splint for wound cleaning Edema control with compressive wrap
6 weeks	If no extensor lag noted, discontinue use of splints	Allow full active PIP joint and DIP joint flexion	Daily removal of splint for wound cleaning Edema control with compressive wrap

Reprinted with permission from Brault J. Rehabilitation of extensor tendon injuries. Oper Tech Plast Reconstr Surg 2000;7:25-30.

Many authors have recently recommended that dynamic splinting be initiated in the first week.[8,9,12,13] This is accomplished with a dorsal dynamic extension splint that has stop beads on the suspension line, which limits flexion (Fig. 26-3A). Patients are instructed to perform active flexion of the fingers hourly (Fig. 26-3B). The rubber band suspension provides passive extension. Therapy is initiated early by a skilled therapist by positioning the wrist in 20 degrees of flexion and passively flexing the MCP joint to 30 degrees. This provides for safe protected gliding of the extensor mechanism. At postoperative week 7, progressive strengthening exercises can be initiated. At week 9, all bracing may be discontinued if no extensor lag is present (Table 26-3).

When the wound is associated with a human bite, it is extensively inspected and débrided; culture specimens are obtained, and the wound is irrigated and left open. Broad-spectrum antibiotics are initiated. The hand is splinted with the wrist in approximately 45 degrees of extension and the MCP joint in 15 to 20 degrees of flexion. The wound typically heals within 5 to 10 days, and secondary repair is rarely needed.[6]

Zone VI

Zone VI is located over the metacarpals. Injuries to this area have a clinical picture similar to that of zone V injuries and are treated as such (see Table 26-3).[9,12,13]

Zone VII

Zone VII lies at the level of the wrist. Tendons in this region course through a fibro-osseous tunnel and are covered by the extensor retinaculum. Complete laceration of the tendons in this region is rare. Tendon retraction can be a significant problem in this region, and primary repair is warranted, with preservation of a portion of the retinaculum to prevent extensor bowstringing.[6] Rehabilitation is similar to that in zone V (see Table 26-3).

Zone VIII

Zone VIII lies at the level of the distal forearm. Multiple tendons may be injured in this area, making it difficult to identify individual tendons. Restoration of independent wrist and thumb extension should be given priority.[6] Injuries in this location often require tendon retrieval for complete lacerations, and surgical intervention is warranted.

Postoperative rehabilitation consists of static immobilization of the wrist in 45 degrees of extension with the MCP joints in 15 to 20 degrees of flexion. Splinting is generally

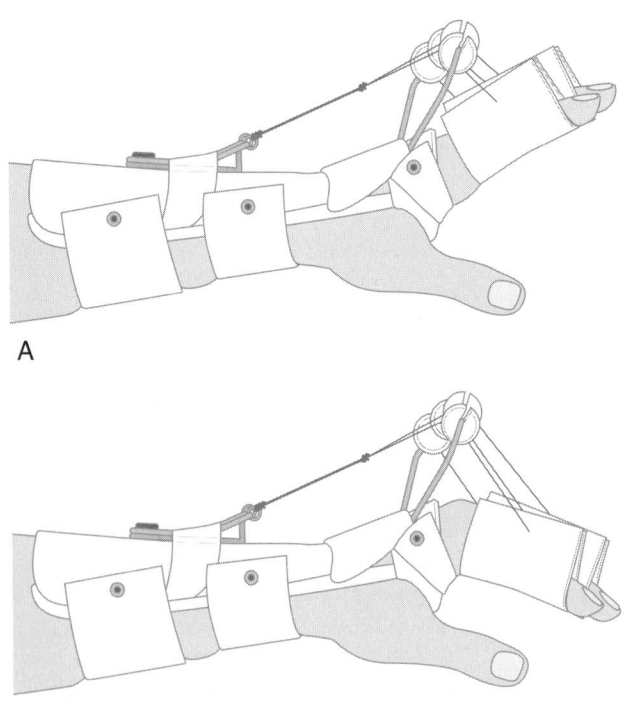

A

B

FIGURE 26-3. A, Splint allows 30 to 40 degrees of active MCP joint flexion with passive return to neutral. **B,** Flexion is limited by stop beads on the outrigger strings.

TABLE 26-3 Zone V, Zone VI, and Zone VII Injuries

	Splint	Exercises	Wound and Skin Care
Start 24-48 hours	Dorsal dynamic extension splint (see Fig. 26-3) Night splint: MCP joint	Exercise hourly in extension splint: allows 30-40 degrees of MCP joint flexion With skilled therapist: wrist at 20 degrees, passive MCP joint flexion to 30 degrees; patient performs active extension (daily to 3 three times a week)	Daily removal of splint for wound cleaning Edema control with 0-3 compressive wrap
4 weeks	Continue with dynamic day splint, static night splint	Increase active range of motion to 50-60 degrees	Daily removal of splint for wound cleaning Edema control with 0-3 compressive wrap
5 weeks	Discontinue dynamic extension splint MCP joint block splint worn at night and between exercises	Increase active range of motion exercises to full motion	Daily removal of splint for wound cleaning Edema control with 0-3 compressive wrap
6 weeks	MCP joint block splint	Passive flexion exercises of MCP and IP joints (buddy tape)	Daily removal of splint for wound cleaning Edema control with 0-3 compressive wrap
7 weeks	MCP joint block splint	Progressive extension exercises, with mild resistance	Daily removal of splint for wound cleaning Edema control with 0-3 compressive wrap
9 weeks	If no extensor lag, discontinue all splints	Continue with active and passive DIP joint exercises	Daily removal of splint for wound cleaning Edema control with 0-3 compressive wrap

Reprinted with permission from Brault J. Rehabilitation of extensor tendon injuries. Oper Tech Plast Reconstr Surg 2000;7:25-30.

maintained for 4 to 5 weeks. However, early controlled motion with a dynamic extensor splint may help decrease adhesions and subsequent contractures. Dynamic motion of the MCP joints may be started at 2 weeks.

Procedures

Surgical repair is the mainstay for treatment of most extensor tendon injuries. Injections are typically not appropriate for the management of these conditions.

Surgery

Zone I and zone II injuries are typically treated nonoperatively, unless there is laceration of the terminal extensor slip (zone II injury), which may then require surgical repair. Surgical correction of zone I and zone II injuries usually results from failed conservative bracing, usually in a younger patient. In addition, patients may elect to have the terminal extensor tendon repaired or the DIP joint fused for cosmetic reasons. In older individuals with fixed deformities and painful arthritic conditions that limit function, joint arthrodesis is a reasonable approach.

Surgical intervention in zones III through VIII is usually primary repair of the injured extensor tendon mechanism. If primary repair is not possible, tendon grafting has been described.[4]

POTENTIAL DISEASE COMPLICATIONS

Extensor tendon injury can result in permanent loss of finger extension, primarily due to adhesion formation or joint contracture. Painful degeneration of the affected joints can occur if normal motion is not restored.

POTENTIAL TREATMENT COMPLICATIONS

Analgesics and nonsteroidal anti-inflammatory drugs have well-known side effects that most commonly affect the gastric, hepatic, renal, and cardiovascular systems. Acute tendon ruptures as a result of aggressive therapy necessitate reoperation, which may include tendon grafting. Therapy programs that are not aggressive enough often result in reduced range of motion and strength. Surgical complications include infection, adhesion formation, and advanced joint degeneration.

References

1. Hart R, Uehara D, Kutz J. Extensor tendon injuries of the hand. Emerg Med Clin North Am 1993;11:637-649.
2. Evans R, Burkhalter W. A study of the dynamic anatomy of extensor tendons and implications for treatment. J Hand Surg Am 1986;11:774-779.
3. Newport M, Blair W, Steyers C. Long-term results of extensor tendon repair. J Hand Surg Am 1990;15:961-966.
4. Kleinert H, Verdan C. Report of the committee on tendon injuries. J Hand Surg Am 1983;8:794-798.
5. Daniels JM II, Zook EG, Lynch JM. Hand and wrist injuries: part II. Emergent evaluation. Am Fam Physician 2004;69:1949-1956.
6. Rockwell WB, Butler PN, Byrne BA. Extensor tendon: anatomy, injury, and reconstruction. Plast Reconstr Surg 2000;106:1592-1603.
7. Bendre AA, Hartigan BJ, Kalainov DM. Mallet finger. J Am Acad Orthop Surg 2005;13:336-344.
8. Evans R. An update on extensor tendon management. In Hunter J, Mackin E, Callahan A, eds. Rehabilitation of the Hand: Surgery and Therapy, vol 1, 4th ed. St. Louis, Mosby, 1995:656-606.

9. Minamikawa Y. Extensor repair and rehabilitation. In Peimer C, ed. Surgery of the Hand and Upper Extremity, vol 1. New York, McGraw-Hill, 1996:1163-1188.

10. Rosenthal E. The extensor tendon: anatomy and management. In Hunter J, Mackin E, Callahan A, eds. Rehabilitation of the Hand: Surgery and Therapy, vol 1, 4th ed. St. Louis, Mosby, 1995: 519-564.

11. Evans RB. Early short arc motion for the repaired central slip. J Hand Surg Am 1994;19:991-997.

12. Brault J. Rehabilitation of extensor tendon injuries. Oper Tech Plast Reconstr Surg 2000;7:25-30.

13. Thomas D. Postoperative management of extensor tendon repairs in zones V, VI, VII. J Hand Ther 1996;9:309-314.

Flexor Tendon Injuries 27

Jeffrey S. Brault, DO, PT, and Gregory L. Umphrey, MD

Synonyms

Flexor tendon injury, laceration, or rupture
Jersey or sweater finger

ICD-9 Codes

727.64   Rupture of flexor tendons of hand and wrist, nontraumatic
842.1   Sprains and strains of the wrist and hand, unspecified site
848.9   Lacerated tendon (not specific to the hand)

DEFINITION

The flexor tendons of the hand are vulnerable to laceration and rupture. These injuries are most commonly seen in individuals who work around moving equipment, use knives, or wash glass dishes; in people with rheumatoid arthritis; and in athletes (jersey finger).[1] The flexor digitorum profundus (FDP) of the ring finger is the most commonly involved.[2] Incomplete injuries to the flexor tendon are easily missed on physical examination and can progress to full ruptures.

Regions of potential tendon injury are divided into five zones (Fig. 27-1).[3] Zone I is from the tendon insertion at the base of the distal phalanx to the midportion of the middle phalanx. Laceration or injury in this zone results in disruption of the FDP tendon and the inability to flex the distal interphalangeal (DIP) joint. Zone II extends from the midportion of the middle phalanx to the distal palmar crease. This zone is known as no man's land because of the poor functional results after tendon repair.[4,5] Tendon injury in this zone usually involves both FDP and flexor digitorum superficialis (FDS) tendons and results in inability to flex the DIP and proximal interphalangeal (PIP) joints. Zone III is located from the distal palmar crease to the distal portion of the transverse carpal ligament. This zone includes the intrinsic hand muscles and vascular arches. Zone IV overlies the transverse carpal ligament in the area of the carpal tunnel. In this zone, injuries usually involve multiple FDP and FDS tendons. Zone V extends from the wrist crease to the level of the musculotendinous junction of the flexor tendons. Injuries in this region most often result from self-inflicted laceration (suicide attempts).

The flexor tendons are held close to the bone in zone I and zone II by a complex series of pulleys and vincula. These structures are frequently injured with the tendons.[1]

SYMPTOMS

Inability to flex the affected joint may be the presenting complaint. Sensation of the involved finger is often affected because of the proximity of the flexor tendons to the neurovascular bundle.

PHYSICAL EXAMINATION

It is important to obtain a detailed history to outline the mechanism of injury. Evaluation begins with observation of the resting hand position. If the flexor tendon is completely severed, the unsupported finger will assume an extended position (Fig. 27-2).[1,6] Active flexion of all finger joints needs to be assessed. If active finger flexion is not observed because of pain, tenodesis can be employed to determine whether the tendon is intact. The wrist is passively extended, and all fingers should assume a relatively flexed posture. If the flexor tendons are disrupted, the finger will remain in a relatively extended posture.

Flexion strength of each digit should be evaluated by manual muscle testing or finger dynamometry. Strength is evaluated by having the patient individually flex first the DIP joint and then the PIP joint against applied resistance. It is possible to have a complete laceration of the flexor tendons with preservation of peritendinous structures and active motion. In these cases, however, flexion will be weak.[7]

For individual function of the FDP tendon to be checked, the patient is asked to flex the fingertip at the DIP joint while the PIP joint is maintained in extension. If there is injury to the FDP tendon, the patient will be unable to flex the DIP joint.

It is difficult to diagnose solitary injuries of the FDS tendon because of the FDP tendon's ability to perform

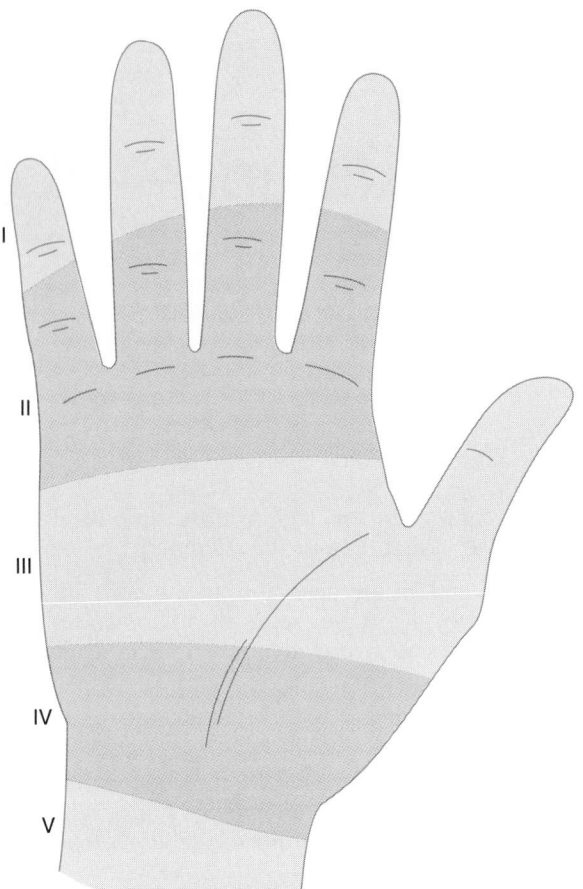

FIGURE 27-1. Zones of flexor tendons.

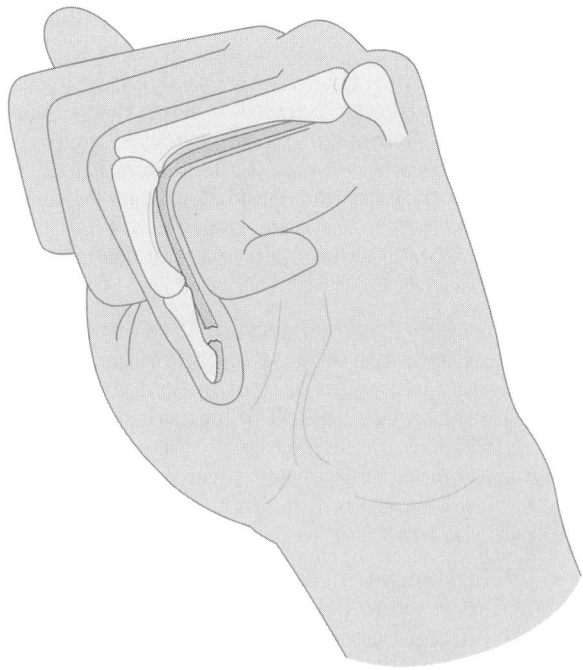

FIGURE 27-2. Jersey finger. The flexor profundus tendon is detached by a forced hyperextension of the DIP joint. (Reprinted with permission from Mellion MB. Office Sports Medicine, 2nd ed. Philadelphia, Hanley & Belfus, 1996.)

flexion of all finger joints through intertendinous connections. For the integrity of the FDS tendon to be isolated, all the fingers are held straight, placing the FDP tendon in a biomechanically disadvantaged position. The patient actively attempts to flex the finger to be tested while the other fingers are held in relative extension. If the patient is unable to move the finger, injury most likely has occurred to the FDS tendon. This test is reliable only for the middle, ring, and small fingers.

Sensation of the finger should be evaluated because open tendon injuries often are accompanied by injuries of the nearby digital nerves. Two-point discrimination should be assessed before injection of local anesthetic for wound care.[1]

FUNCTIONAL LIMITATIONS

Functional limitations include difficulty with power grasp if the ulnarly sided tendons are involved, and precision grasp problems if the radially sided tendons are involved. The patient may present with inability to button shirts, to pinch small objects, or to firmly grasp objects.

DIAGNOSTIC STUDIES

Radiographic evaluation includes anteroposterior and lateral views of the involved fingers. These assist in identification of joint dislocation, articular disruption, avulsion, long bone fractures, and potential for retained foreign bodies. Ultrasonography and magnetic resonance imaging are used to identify partially lacerated or ruptured tendons.

TREATMENT

Initial

Surgical intervention is almost always required for flexor tendon injuries.[1,7] Protection of the affected finger in a bulky dressing and meticulous wound care are recommended before surgical correction.

Cleaning and repair of superficial wounds should be performed if surgical referral is delayed. Optimally, surgical correction of the flexor tendon injury occurs within the first 12 to 24 hours. Delayed primary repair is performed in the first 10 days. If primary repair is not performed because of infection, secondary repair can be

---

Differential Diagnosis

Partial tendon laceration

Anterior interosseous nerve injury

Trigger finger (stenosing tenosynovitis)

Median nerve injury

performed up to 4 weeks. If repair is not performed within 4 weeks, the tendon usually is retracted within the sheath, making surgical repair difficult.[7]

Newer surgical repair and suture techniques have improved the strength of repaired flexor tendons, providing for earlier rehabilitation.[7-9]

Analgesics and nonsteroidal anti-inflammatory drugs are frequently used for pain control.

Rehabilitation

Postoperative rehabilitation of repaired tendons has changed greatly in the past two decades through initiation of early protected motion.[10-13] Historically, the repaired fingers were placed in an immobilization splint for up to 2 months. This often led to adhesion formation and ultimately the loss of motion and function.[12]

The currently accepted rehabilitation schemes for repaired flexor tendons are essentially the same for all zones (Table 27-1). Immediately postoperatively, the hand is placed in a protective dorsal splint with 20 to 30 degrees of wrist flexion. All metacarpophalangeal (MCP) joints are placed in 50 to 70 degrees of flexion.[13] A dorsal hood extends to the fingertip level, allowing PIP joint and DIP joint extension to 0 degrees. All of the fingers are held in flexion by dynamic traction applied by rubber bands originating from the proximal forearm with a pulley at the palm and attachment to the fingernails (Fig. 27-3A).

The patient is typically seen by the therapist 24 to 48 hours after surgical repair. Dressings are changed, edema control measures are initiated, and rehabilitation goals are discussed.[12,13]

The patient is instructed to actively extend the fingers against the rubber band traction to the dorsal block, 10 repetitions hourly, to prevent flexion contractures (see Fig. 27-3B). The rubber band traction passively returns the fingers to a flexed position. At night, the traction is removed and the fingers are strapped to the dorsal hood with the PIP and DIP joints in extension.

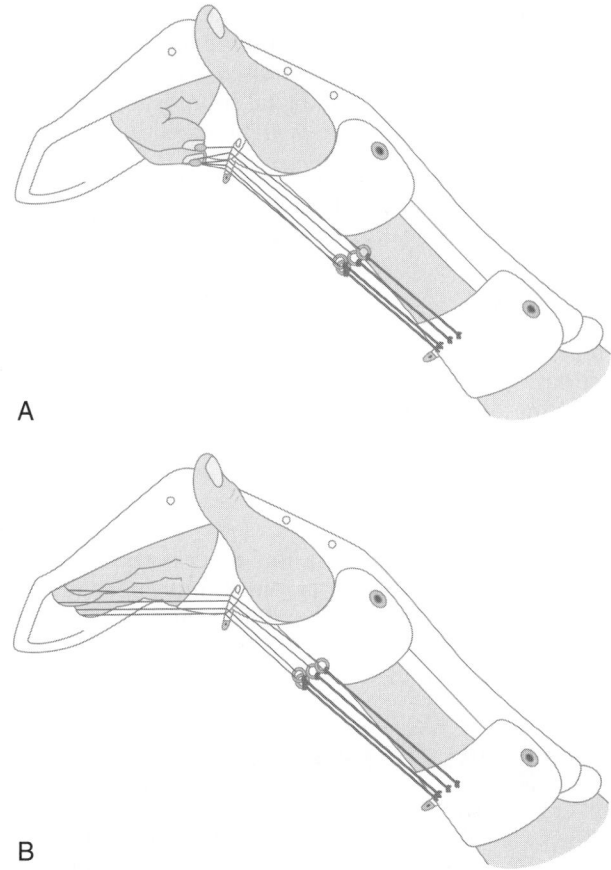

A

B

FIGURE 27-3. A, Dorsal dynamic protection splint; fingers in resting position. **B,** Dorsal dynamic protection splint; active extension exercises.

The rehabilitation program may involve immediate short arc motion.[12-15] Under the supervision of a skilled therapist, the injured digit is placed in moderate flexion with the wrist in 30 to 40 degrees of extension, the MCP joints in 80 degrees of flexion, the PIP joints in 75 degrees of flexion, and the DIP joints in 30 to 40 degrees of flexion. The patient is then instructed to actively hold this position for 10 seconds. On completion of the static

TABLE 27-1 Flexor Tendon Injuries (Immediate Motion)

	Splint	Exercises	Wound and Skin Care
Postoperatively to 21 days	Postoperative dynamic flexion splint with dorsal hood (see Fig. 27-3) Wrist flexion at 20-30 degrees MCP joint, 50-70 degrees; PIP and DIP joints, 0 degrees of extension	Patient actively extends each finger 10 times hourly (start postoperative day 2) Under the direction of a hand therapist, wrist flexion is used to produce less tension on the flexor tendon during passive exercises Initiate supervised active flexion exercises (postoperative day 14)	Daily removal of splint for wound cleaning Edema control with compressive wrap
21-35 days	Progressive reduction in use of splint	Patient may begin to perform active flexion exercises without therapist	Continue with wound care and edema control as needed.
35 days	Discontinue splint	Progress to increased active and passive flexion exercises; grip strengthening	Continue with wound care and edema control as needed.

Modified from Lund A. Flexor tendon rehabilitation: a basic guide. Oper Tech Plast Reconstr Surg 2000;7:20-24; Evans R. Early active motion after flexor tendon repair. In Berger RA, Weiss APC. Hand Surgery. Lippincott Williams & Wilkins, 2003:710-735; Groth GN. Current practice patterns of flexor tendon rehabilitation. J Hand Ther 2005;18:169-174.

contraction, the therapist passively flexes the wrist. This allows natural tenodesis to extend the fingers. At day 21, the patient can initiate unsupervised active flexion exercises. At 35 days, the dorsal digital splint is removed and active tendon gliding exercises are initiated.[12,15,16]

Modalities such as ultrasound, contrast or paraffin baths, whirlpool, and fluidized therapy may be used to promote wound healing and range of motion.

Procedures

Procedures are generally not indicated in flexor tendon injuries. Corticosteroid injections can be performed if stenosing tenosynovitis (triggering) develops at the flexor pulleys.

Surgery

Optimally, repair of the flexion tendon should occur within the first 48 hours after injury. Improper handling of tissues during repair can result in hematoma, damage to the pulley integrity, and damage to the vincula—the vascular supply of the tendons.

POTENTIAL DISEASE COMPLICATIONS

Injury to the flexor tendon mechanism can result in permanent loss of finger flexion. Partial tendon damage can easily be missed and result in either weakness or complete rupture.

POTENTIAL TREATMENT COMPLICATIONS

Analgesics and nonsteroidal anti-inflammatory drugs have well-known side effects that most commonly affect the gastric, hepatic, and renal systems. Postsurgical complications include adhesion formation and tendon rupture. Postsurgical tendon rupture is usually the result of aggressive motion, by either the patient or therapist, that results in failure of the repair. Reoperation is often required, which results in the greater propensity for adhesion formation. Adhesion formation and the loss of motion and strength complicate surgical repair, particularly in zone II.[4,5]

Many other factors affect healing of the tendon and postoperative rehabilitation. Factors such as advanced age, poor circulation, tobacco and caffeine use, and generalized poor health can contribute to impaired healing. Scar formation can result in adhesion formation and decreased movement. Poor motivation and compliance with the therapy program result in less than optimal recovery.

References

1. Mass DP. Early repairs of flexor tendon injuries. In Berger RA, Weiss APC. Hand Surgery. Philadelphia, Lippincott Williams & Wilkins, 2003:679-698.
2. Amadio P. Epidemiology of hand and wrist injuries in sports. Hand Clin 1990;6:429-453.
3. Kleinert H, Schepel S, Gill T. Flexor tendon injuries. Surg Clin North Am 1981;61:267-286.
4. Chow J, Thomas L, Dovelle S, et al. A combined regimen of controlled motion following flexor tendon repair in "no man's land." Plast Reconstr Surg 1987;79:447-453.
5. Hister GD, Kleinert HE, Kutz JE, Atasoy E. Primary flexor tendon repair followed by immediate controlled mobilization. J Hand Surg Am 1977;2(6):441-451.
6. Idler R, Manktelow R, Lucus G, et al. The Hand: Examination and Diagnosis, 3rd ed. New York, Churchill Livingstone, 1990:59-62.
7. Strickland J. Flexor tendons—acute injuries. In Green D, Hotchkiss R, Peterson W, eds. Green's Operative Hand Surgery, 4 ed. Philadelphia, Churchill Livingstone, 1999:1851-1897.
8. Miller L, Mas DP. A comparison of four repair techniques for Camper's chiasma flexor digitorum superficialis lacerations: tested in an in vitro model. J Hand Surg Am 2000;25:1122-1126.
9. Angeles JG, Heminger H, Mass DP. Comparative biomechanical performances of 4-strand core suture repairs for zone II flexor tendon lacerations. J Hand Surg Am 2002;27:508-517.
10. Strickland J. Biologic rationale, clinical application and result of early motion following flexor tendon repair. J Hand Ther 1989;2:71-83.
11. Pettengill KM. The evolution of early mobilization of the repaired flexor tendon. J Hand Ther 2005;18:157-168.
12. Evans R. Early active motion after flexor tendon repair. In Berger RA, Weiss APC. Hand Surgery. Lippincott Williams & Wilkins, 2003:710-735.
13. Groth GN. Current practice patterns of flexor tendon rehabilitation. J Hand Ther 2005;18:169-174.
14. Evans R. Immediate active short arc motion following tendon repair. In Hunter J, Schneider L, Mackin E, eds. Tendon and Nerve Surgery in the Hand—A Third Decade. St. Louis, Mosby, 1997:362-393.
15. Lund A. Flexor tendon rehabilitation: a basic guide. Oper Tech Plast Reconstr Surg 2000;7:20-24.
16. Werntz J, Chesher S, Breiderbach W, et al. A new dynamic splint and postoperative treatment of flexor tendon injury. J Hand Surg Am 1989;14:559-566.

Hand and Wrist Ganglia 28

Charles Cassidy, MD, and Victor Chung, BS

Synonyms

Carpal cyst
Synovial cyst
Mucous cyst
Intraosseous cyst

ICD-9 Codes

727.41 Ganglion of joint
727.42 Ganglion of tendon sheath

DEFINITION

Hand and wrist ganglia account for 50% to 70% of all hand masses. The ganglion is a benign, mucin-filled cyst found in relation to a joint, ligament, or tendon. It is typically filled from the joint through a tortuous duct or "stalk" that functions as a valve directing the flow of fluid. The mucin itself contains high concentrations of hyaluronic acid as well as glucosamine, albumin, and globulin.[1] When it is used to describe ganglia, the term *synovial cyst* is actually a misnomer because ganglion cysts do not contain synovial fluid and are not true cysts lined by epithelium but rather by flat cells. The etiology of ganglia remains a mystery, although many believe that ligamentous degeneration or trauma plays an important role.[1,2]

By far, the most common location for a ganglion is the dorsal wrist (Fig. 28-1), with the pedicle arising from the scapholunate ligament in virtually all cases. Only 20% of ganglia are found on the volar wrist (Fig. 28-2). This type may originate from either the radioscaphoid or scaphotrapezial joint. Alternatively, ganglia can occur near the joints of the finger. One subtype of hand-wrist ganglia is the "occult" cyst, which is not palpable on physical examination.

Ganglion cysts occur more commonly in women, usually between the ages of 20 and 30 years. However, they can develop in either sex at any age. Ganglia of childhood usually resolve spontaneously during the course of 1 year.[3] The most commonly seen ganglion of the elderly, the mucous cyst, arises from an arthritic distal interphalangeal joint (Fig. 28-3).

Other common types of ganglia in the hand include the retinacular cyst (flexor tendon sheath ganglion; Fig. 28-4), proximal interphalangeal joint ganglion, and first extensor compartment cyst associated with de Quervain tenosynovitis. Less common ganglia include cysts within the extensor tendons or carpal bones (intraosseous) and those associated with a second or third carpometacarpal boss (arthritic spur). Rarely, ganglia within the carpal tunnel or Guyon canal can produce carpal tunnel syndrome or ulnar neuropathy.

As noted, the cause of ganglion cyst formation is not known, but there may be a link to light, repetitive activity, demonstrated by an increased incidence in typists, musicians, and draftsmen. Interestingly, there is no increased risk in heavy laborers, who bear a greater load on their wrists. Wrist instability has also been discussed as both a possible cause and an effect of the disease. Overall, there is a history of trauma in 10% to 30% of people presenting with the disease.[2]

SYMPTOMS

Patients with a wrist ganglion usually present with a painless wrist or hand mass of variable duration. The cyst may fluctuate in size or disappear altogether for a time. Pain and weakness of grip are occasional presenting symptoms; however, an underlying concern about the appearance or seriousness of the problem is usually the reason for seeking medical attention. The pain, when present, is most often described as aching and aggravated by certain motions. With dorsal wrist ganglia, patients often complain of discomfort as the wrist is forcefully extended (e.g., when pushing up from a chair). Interestingly, dorsal wrist pain may be the principal complaint of patients with an occult dorsal wrist ganglion, which is not readily visible. The wrist pain usually subsides as the mass enlarges.

With a retinacular cyst, patients usually complain of slight discomfort when gripping, for example, a racket handle or shopping cart. Patients whose complaints of pain are primarily related to de Quervain tenosynovitis (see Chapter 24) may notice a bump over the radial styloid area. Pain with grip is also a complaint of patients

149

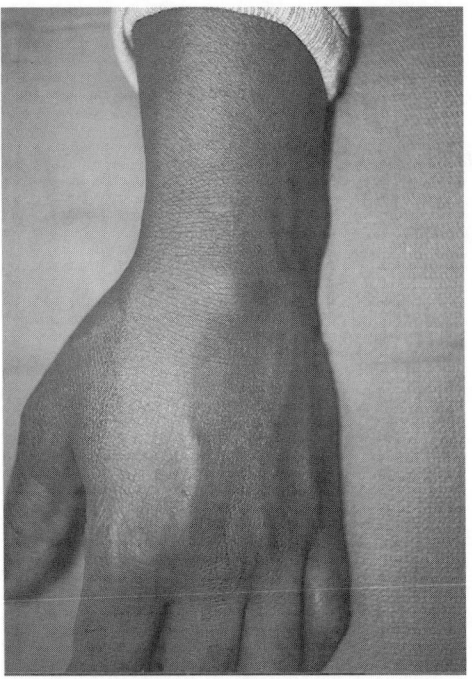

FIGURE 28-1. Dorsal wrist ganglion. The mass is typically found overlying the scapholunate area in the center of the wrist.

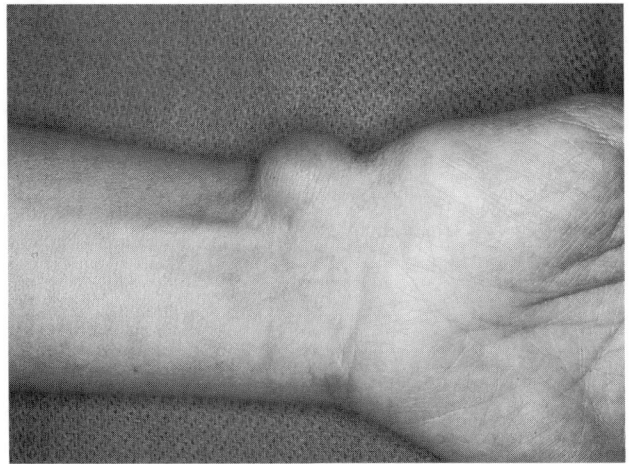

FIGURE 28-2. Clinical appearance of a volar wrist ganglion.

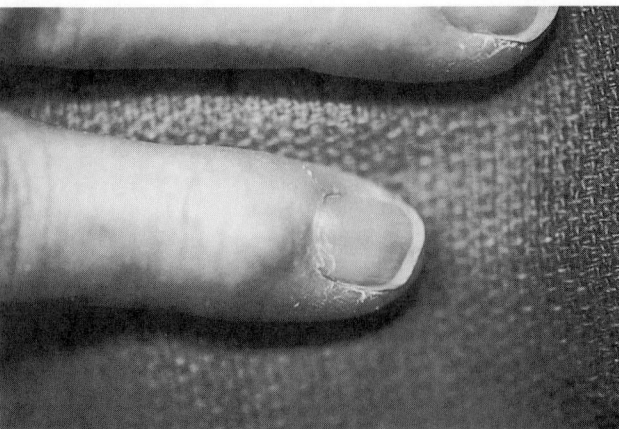

FIGURE 28-3. Mucous cyst. This ganglion originates from the distal interphalangeal joint. Pressure on the nail matrix by the cyst may produce flattening of the nail plate, as is seen here.

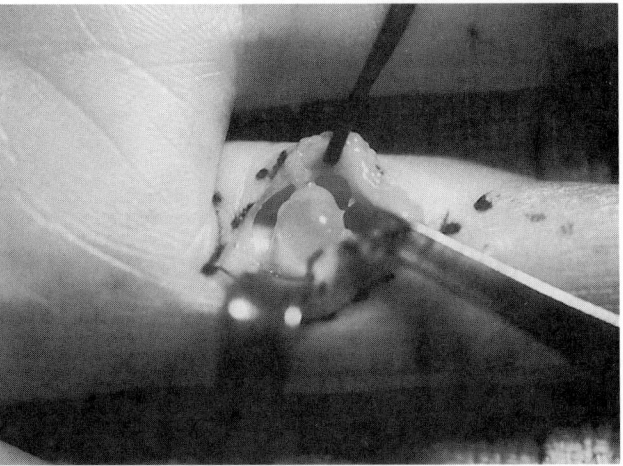

FIGURE 28-4. Retinacular cyst. This ganglion originates from the flexor tendon sheath.

with a carpometacarpal boss. Mucous cysts can drain spontaneously and can also produce nail deformity, either of which may be a presenting complaint. Symptoms identical to those of carpal tunnel syndrome will be noted by patients with a carpal tunnel ganglion. A ganglion in Guyon canal will produce hand weakness (due to loss of intrinsic function) and may produce numbness in the ring and small fingers.

PHYSICAL EXAMINATION

Ganglia are typically solitary cysts, although they are often found to be multiloculated on surgical exploration. They are usually mobile a few millimeters in all directions on physical examination. The mass may be slightly tender. When the cyst is large, transillumination (placing a penlight directly onto the skin overlying the mass) will help differentiate it from a solid tumor.

The classic location for a dorsal wrist ganglion is ulnar to the extensor pollicis longus, between the third and fourth tendon compartments, or directly over the scapholunate ligament.[1] However, these ganglia may have a long pedicle that courses through various tendon compartments and exits at different locations on the dorsal wrist or even the volar wrist. When the ganglion is small, it may be apparent only with wrist flexion. Wrist extension and grip strength may be slightly diminished. Dorsal wrist pain and tenderness with no obvious mass or instability should suggest an occult ganglion.

Volar ganglia occur most commonly at the wrist flexion crease on the radial side of the flexor carpi radialis tendon but may extend into the palm or proximally, or even dorsally, into the carpal tunnel. They can involve the radial artery, complicating their surgical removal. They may seem to be pulsatile, although careful inspection will demonstrate that the radial artery is draped over the mass.

Retinacular cysts are usually not visible but are palpable as pea-sized masses, typically located at the volar aspect of the digit at the palmar digital crease. They are adherent to the flexor tendon sheath and do not move with finger flexion. Alternatively, intratendinous ganglia are distinguished by the fact that they move with finger motion.

Mucous cysts are located over the distal interphalangeal joint, and the overlying skin may be quite thin. They are occasionally mistaken for warts. Spontaneous drainage and even septic distal interphalangeal joint arthritis are not uncommon. Nail plate deformity is an associated finding. Proximal interphalangeal joint ganglia are located on the dorsum of the digit, slightly off midline. Ganglia associated with carpometacarpal bosses produce tender prominences on the dorsum of the hand distal to the typical location for a wrist ganglion.

An important sign to look for on physical examination, especially in planning for surgery, is compression of the median or ulnar nerve or of the radial artery. An Allen test should be performed before surgery to evaluate radial and ulnar artery patency, particularly in the case of a volar cyst (Fig. 28-5).

FUNCTIONAL LIMITATIONS

Physical limitations due to ganglion cysts are rare. With dorsal wrist ganglia, fatigue and weakness are occasional findings. Patients may have difficulty with weight bearing on the affected extremity with the wrist extended (e.g., when pushing up from a chair).

DIAGNOSTIC STUDIES

The diagnosis of a ganglion cyst is usually straightforward, and ancillary studies are often unnecessary. With wrist ganglia, plain radiographs of the wrist are usually obtained preoperatively to evaluate the carpal relationships and to exclude the possibility of an intraosseous ganglion. With a mucous cyst, radiographs of the affected digit will usually demonstrate a distal interphalangeal joint osteophyte. Ultrasonography or magnetic resonance imaging may be useful in identifying deep cysts in cases of vague dorsal wrist pain. Specifically, magnetic resonance imaging is indicated to rule out Kienböck disease in patients with dorsal wrist pain and no obvious ganglion or wrist instability. Cyst aspiration is the single best confirmatory study. Aspiration characteristically yields a viscous, clear to yellowish fluid with the appearance and consistency of apple jelly. On occasion, the fluid will be blood tinged.

Differential Diagnosis

Lipoma

Carpal boss

Extensor tenosynovitis

Scapholunate ligament injury or sprain

Giant cell tumor of tendon sheath

Kienböck disease (avascular necrosis of the lunate)

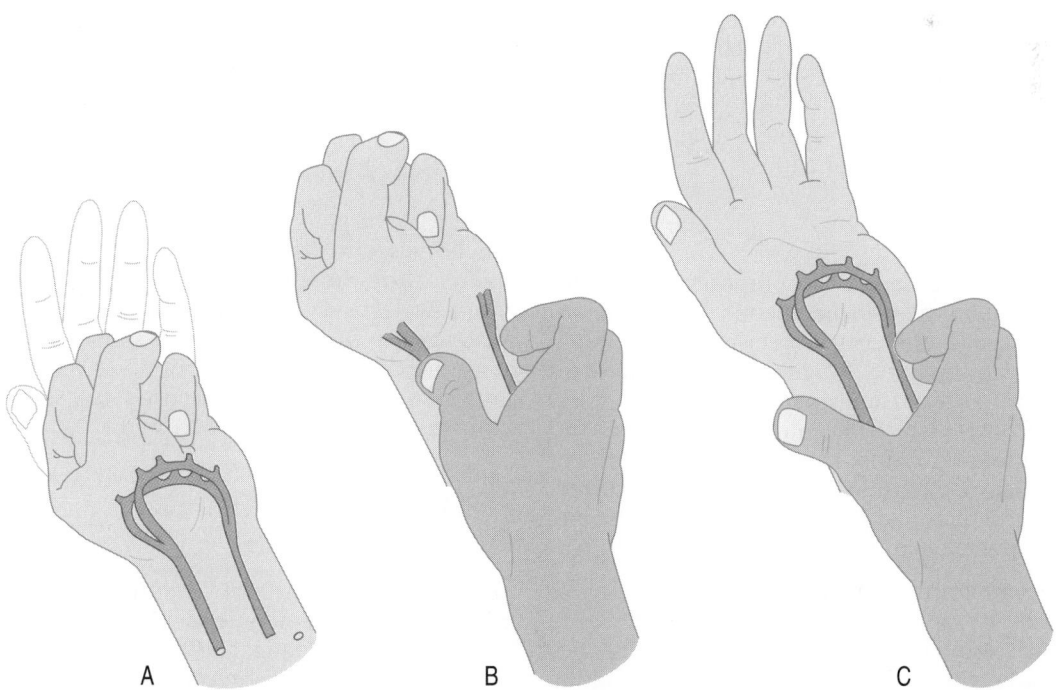

FIGURE 28-5. The Allen test is performed by asking the patient to open and close the hand several times as quickly as possible and then to make a tight fist (**A**). The examiner then compresses the radial and ulnar arteries as the hand is opened (**B**). One artery is tested by releasing the pressure over the artery to see whether the hand flushes (**C**). The other artery is tested in a similar fashion, and the opposite hand is tested for comparison.

TREATMENT

Initial

Reassurance is the single most important initial treatment. Many patients are satisfied to know that they do not have a serious illness. It is important to tell patients that the cyst often fluctuates in size and occasionally disappears on its own. Undoubtedly, observation is the most appropriate treatment of ganglia in children, as long as the diagnosis is certain. In adults, splinting is an appropriate initial treatment of cysts associated with discomfort. A cock-up wrist splint is prescribed for carpometacarpal and dorsal and volar wrist ganglia, whereas a radial gutter splint is prescribed for ganglia associated with de Quervain tenosynovitis. Traditional methods of crushing the cyst with a coin or a Bible, even though occasionally successful, are not recommended. Anecdotally, daily massage of mucous cysts by patients may be successful in resolving them as long as the overlying skin is healthy. Analgesics or nonsteroidal anti-inflammatory drugs may be used on a limited basis for discomfort but do little to treat the disorder.

Rehabilitation

Rehabilitation has a role primarily in the postsurgical setting. The usual course of treatment after dorsal ganglion excision involves 7 to 14 days of immobilization in slight wrist flexion to minimize loss of wrist *flexion* secondary to scarring. Frequent, active range of motion of the wrist should be started after splint removal, and the patient should be able to return to relatively normal activity approximately 3 weeks after surgery.[1] Most patients are able to carry out their own rehabilitation at home. Formal therapy can be ordered if patients have difficulty returning to normal functioning. Therapy may include modalities for pain control, active-assisted and passive range of motion exercises, and strengthening exercises. Therapists may also evaluate return to work issues, including adaptive equipment that may assist patients in their daily work functions.

Procedures

Aspiration of the cyst serves two purposes: it confirms the diagnosis, and it may be therapeutic. Unfortunately, the recurrence rate after ganglion aspiration is high. One study[4] demonstrated long-term success rates of 27% and 43% for dorsal and volar wrist ganglia, respectively, treated with aspiration, multiple puncture, and 3 weeks of immobilization. Importantly, cysts present for longer than 6 months almost uniformly recurred. The results for aspiration of retinacular cysts were somewhat better, averaging 69% successful.

However, a significant number of patients may elect to proceed with cyst aspiration despite the high likelihood of recurrence. Aspiration of volar wrist ganglia may cause displacement of the cyst and envelop the radial artery. Aspiration of proximal interphalangeal joint ganglia may be successful in eliminating the cyst.[5] Aspiration of mucous cysts is not recommended.

Steroids have *not* been shown to add any therapeutic benefit to ganglia aspiration.

Surgery

Many patients opt for surgical excision of the cyst, often for primarily cosmetic reasons. Surgery should be advised when the diagnosis is unclear. To minimize the likelihood of recurrence, the surgeon should not only remove the cyst but trace the stalk to its origin within the joint. For wrist ganglia, the surgeon often finds that the visible mass grossly underestimates its actual size and extent. Because these procedures require opening of the wrist joint, they cannot be performed with the use of local anesthesia. With proper technique, recurrence rates should be less than 5%. Volar ganglia are more difficult to access and more often variable in their shape and location, making for more complicated surgery. A prospective cohort study of volar wrist ganglion treatment by observation, aspiration, or surgery concluded that at 5 years, there were no significant differences in the recurrence rates with any of the treatments; 42% of the excised ganglia recurred, whereas 51% of the untreated ganglia had resolved spontaneously.[6] Clearly, it is important that the risks and benefits of surgical treatment of ganglion cysts be carefully discussed with the patient.

Arthroscopic resection of dorsal wrist ganglia has been advocated recently to be a safe and reliable procedure, with recurrence rates of less than 5%.[7] A small case series of arthroscopic débridement of volar wrist ganglia has demonstrated excellent results as well.[8]

The surgical management of mucous cysts must include excision of the cyst stalk as well as the offending osteophyte, which originates from either the dorsal base of the distal phalanx or the head of the middle phalanx. The nail deformity should resolve during several months.[9]

POTENTIAL DISEASE COMPLICATIONS

Chronic wrist pain as the result of an untreated wrist ganglion is rare. The cosmetic deformity, however, is obvious. The most important complication associated with a neglected cyst is septic arthritis of the distal interphalangeal joint resulting from spontaneous drainage of a mucous cyst. For that reason, we recommend mucous cyst excision when the overlying skin is thin or spontaneous drainage has occurred.

POTENTIAL TREATMENT COMPLICATIONS

Analgesics and nonsteroidal anti-inflammatory drugs have well-known side effects that most commonly affect the gastric, hepatic, and renal systems. The patient must understand that surgery will replace a bump with a scar. Slight limitation of wrist flexion after dorsal ganglion excision is not uncommon. Another risk is iatrogenic injury to the scapholunate ligament, extensor tendon, and cutaneous nerve. Recurrence is another possibility.

Surgery performed on the *volar* wrist carries a greater risk of injury to artery and nerve. The structures most at risk are the palmar cutaneous branch of the median nerve and the terminal branches of the lateral antebrachial cutaneous nerve as well as the radial artery, which is often intertwined with the cyst. Perhaps because of the more intricate nature of its surgical removal, the volar cyst is associated with a higher rate of recurrence after surgery.

References

1. Athanasian EA. Bone and soft tissue tumors. In Green DP, Hotchkiss RN, Pederson WC, et al, eds. Green's Operative Hand Surgery, 5th ed. Philadelphia, Churchill Livingstone, 2005.
2. Peimer C, ed. Surgery of the Hand and Upper Extremity, vol 1. New York, McGraw-Hill, 1996: 837-852.
3. Wang AA, Hutchinson DT. Longitudinal observation of pediatric hand and wrist ganglia. J Hand Surg Am 2001;26:599-602.
4. Richman JA, Gelberman RH, Engber WD, et al. Ganglions of the wrist and digits: results of treatment by aspiration and cyst wall puncture. J Hand Surg Am 1987;12:1041-1043.
5. Cheng CA, Rockwell WB. Ganglions of the proximal interphalangeal joint. Am J Orthop 1999;28:458-460.
6. Dias J, Buch K. Palmar wrist ganglion: does intervention improve outcome? A prospective study of the natural history and patient-reported treatment outcomes. J Hand Surg Br 2003;28:172-176.
7. Rizzo M, Berger RA, Steinmann SP, Bishop AT. Arthroscopic resection in the management of dorsal wrist ganglions: results with a minimum 2-year follow-up period. J Hand Surg Am 2004;29: 59-62.
8. Ho PC, Lo WN, Hung LK. Arthroscopic resection of volar ganglion of the wrist: a new technique. Arthroscopy 2003;19:218-221.
9. Kasdan ML, Stallings SP, Leis VM, Wolens D. Outcome of surgically treated mucous cysts of the hand. J Hand Surg Am 1994;19: 504-507.

Hand Osteoarthritis 29

David Ring, MD, PhD

Synonyms

Arthritis
Degenerative arthritis
Osteoarthritis
Degenerative joint disease
Joint destruction

ICD-9 Codes

715.14   Osteoarthritis, primary, localized to the hand
715.24   Osteoarthritis, secondary, localized to the hand
716.14   Traumatic arthropathy of the hand

DEFINITION

Osteoarthritis of the hand is a degenerative condition of hyaline cartilage in diarthrodial joints. It is distinct from inflammatory arthropathies, such as rheumatoid arthritis, in which the primary component is an inflammatory or systemic pathophysiologic process. Idiopathic osteoarthritis excludes post-traumatic arthritis or arthritic conditions resulting from pyrophosphate deposition disease, infection, or other known causes. It is associated with aging, but variations in onset and severity seem genetically determined. In particular, the early onset of osteoarthritis of the distal interphalangeal and trapeziometacarpal joints is genetically mediated separate from osteoarthritis at other joints; in other words, a 50-year-old person with severe hand arthritis is not at risk for early hip arthritis. The prevalence of osteoarthritis of the hand increases with age and is more common in men than in women until menopause. In individuals older than 65 years, osteoarthritis of the hand has been estimated to be as high as 78% in men and 99% in women.[1] The distal interphalangeal and proximal interphalangeal joints and the base of the thumb are the most affected joints.

SYMPTOMS

Patients typically report pain, stiffness, and dysfunction. Symptoms follow a waxing and waning course as the disease gradually and inevitably progresses. The correlation between radiographic findings and complaints of pain or disability is limited, most likely as a reflection of the psychosocial factors that mediate the difference between disease and illness and between impairment and disability.

PHYSICAL EXAMINATION

Osteoarthritis is insidious. Although it takes decades to wear out a joint, patients often notice an acute onset of symptoms that can make it difficult for them to believe their problem is a chronic degenerative condition. The hallmarks of physical examination are deformity, restriction of motion, pain, and crepitation. The correlation between symptoms (illness behavior) and signs (objective impairment and disease) is poor and likely to be mediated primarily by psychosocial factors (effective coping skills and psychological distress). A careful examination of all of the joints notes any deformity, effusions, erythema, limitations in range of motion, and swelling. A more thorough musculoskeletal examination is also important and should specifically note any weakness due to muscle disuse or other causes. The neurologic examination should be normal.

Interphalangeal Joints

Osteoarthritis of the distal interphalangeal joint is characterized by enlargement of the distal joint by osteophytes, forming the so-called Heberden node (Fig. 29-1). Angulatory and rotatory deformities of the terminal phalanx can develop (Fig. 29-2). Ganglion (or mucous) cysts are associated with osteoarthritis of the distal (and less commonly the proximal) interphalangeal joints. The pressure of these cysts on the germinal matrix can cause a groove in the fingernail. The proximal interphalangeal joint is less commonly involved than the distal joint. The enlargement and deformity at the proximal interphalangeal joint is referred to as a Bouchard node.

Metacarpophalangeal Joints

It is relatively uncommon for the metacarpophalangeal joints to be involved in primary idiopathic osteoarthritis. The presentation at this joint is usually characterized by complaints of pain and stiffness rather than deformity.

155

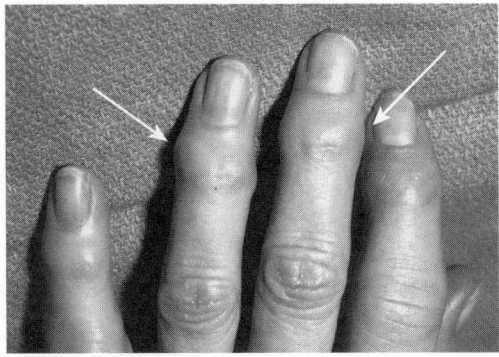

FIGURE 29-1. Patients with degenerative joint disease of the hands can present with Heberden nodes *(arrows)*. These nodules represent osteophytes at the distal interphalangeal joint. (Reprinted with permission from Concannon MJ. Common Hand Problems in Primary Care. Philadelphia, Hanley & Belfus, 1999.)

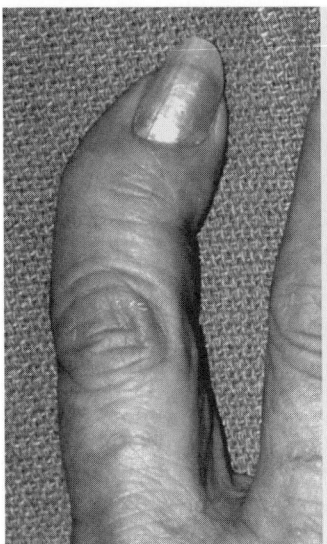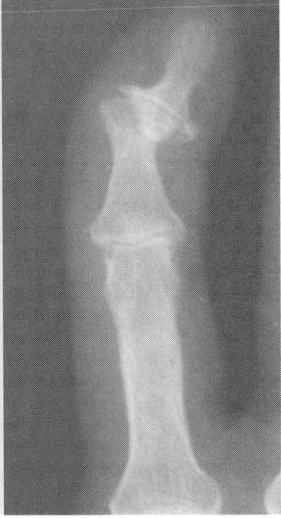

FIGURE 29-2. Severe osteoarthritis at the distal interphalangeal joint of the fifth finger. Osteophyte formation, joint destruction, and angulation are demonstrated. (Reprinted with permission from Concannon MJ. Common Hand Problems in Primary Care. Philadelphia, Hanley & Belfus, 1999.)

Trapeziometacarpal Joint

Arthritis of the trapeziometacarpal joint is associated with aging. Among women aged 80 years and older, 94% have radiographic signs of arthritis; two thirds of these have severe joint destruction.[2] Men develop arthritis more slowly than women do, but by the age of 80 years, 85% have arthritis. The process progresses from subluxation and slight narrowing of the joint to osteophyte formation, deformity, and destruction of the joint.[3] As the disease progresses, the base of the metacarpal subluxates radially, there is an adduction contracture of the metacarpal toward the palm, and laxity and hyperextension of the metacarpophalangeal joint develop in compensation. Axial compression and rotation and shear (the compression test) will produce crepitation and reproduce symptoms. Both active and passive movement is restricted. Grip and pinch strength gradually diminish. It is useful to screen for carpal tunnel

syndrome and trigger thumb, both of which are common in this age group.

FUNCTIONAL LIMITATIONS

The classic forms of reported disability are activities that require a forceful grasp, such as opening a tight jar, turning a key, or opening a doorknob. Whereas fine motor tasks are often impaired by osteoarthritis, complaints of disability are far less common; perhaps because the disease is so gradual, most patients adapt.

DIAGNOSTIC STUDIES

Radiographs are rarely necessary to establish a diagnosis or to guide treatment; their chief use is for ruling out other pathologic processes and increasing the patient's understanding and acceptance of the disease process. Characteristic findings are joint space narrowing, subchondral sclerosis, osteophyte formation, and degenerative cyst formation in the subchondral bone. Eaton and Littler classified trapeziometacarpal arthritis into four radiographic stages.[4] In stage I, the articular contours are normal with no subluxation or joint debris. The joint space may be widened if an effusion is present. In stage II, there is slight narrowing of the thumb trapezial metacarpal joint, but the joint space and articular contours are preserved. Joint debris is less than 2 mm and may be present. In stage III, there is significant trapezial metacarpal joint destruction with sclerotic resistive changes and subchondral bone with osteophytes larger than 2 mm. Stage IV is characterized by pantrapezial arthritis in which both the trapezial metacarpal and scaphoid trapezial joints are affected.

TREATMENT

Initial

There are no proven disease-modifying treatments of osteoarthritis. All treatments take the form of either palliation (management) or salvage (e.g., arthrodesis or arthroplasty). Because osteoarthritis is so common (as people age, they all have some evidence of osteoarthritis to some degree), and at least annoying if not disabling,

---

Differential Diagnosis

Post-traumatic arthritis

Inflammatory arthritis (e.g., Lyme disease, gout, rheumatoid arthritis, psoriatic arthritis)

Calcium pyrophosphate deposition disease

Septic arthritis

Systemic lupus erythematosus

Scleroderma

there is extensive marketing that suggests the disease can be modified, but there is no proof of this assertion. There is also no proof that exercise or activity accelerates osteoarthritis. Exercise and activity can improve muscle strength, proprioception, and range of motion. Physicians should be cautious about advising activity restriction because it can directly create disability in a patient who associates pain with joint damage. Activity restriction is a personal choice determined by desired comfort level; it is entirely appropriate to remain active in spite of painful, degenerated joints.

Non-narcotic analgesics (acetaminophen and non-steroidal anti-inflammatory medications) are useful for pain relief and safe enough for routine use in most patients. Some patients find ice, heat, or topical creams useful. Splints that immobilize arthritic joints (for instance, a hand-based thumb spica with the interphalangeal joint free for trapeziometacarpal arthritis) can provide symptomatic relief, but it must be made clear to the patient that they will not cure the disease or prevent progression by wearing them and that splint wear is optional. The interphalangeal joints are rarely splinted because of the associated functional limitations as well as infrequent requests by patients. Intra-articular injections of corticosteroids or hyaluronate[5] inconsistently provide temporary relief, but patients need to understand that these injections cannot cure the disease and that they must either find effective coping mechanisms or elect salvage reconstructive surgery.

Rehabilitation

Patients can be taught alternative ways to perform tasks that are hindered by arthritis (Table 29-1). For instance, they can get a device that helps them open jars and a larger grip for pens and pencils; they can change their doorknobs to levers. Prefabricated and custom hand-based thumb spica splints can diminish the pain of trapeziometacarpal arthritis and may be most useful during certain tasks. Therapeutic modalities such as paraffin baths may be beneficial for some people.

Contrast baths and ice massage are economical modalities that can bring some relief.

Procedures

Injections

At best, an intra-articular injection of corticosteroids or hyaluronate will provide a few months of relief.[6] Serious complications such as infection are rare. The worst aspect of an injection is the disappointment felt by patients when their hoped-for miracle cure is not forthcoming, or—perhaps even worse—when the helpful injection (be it placebo or otherwise) wears off after a few weeks to months. When the role of injections is accurately described, patients rarely request them. Injections hurt and have some risks; most patients would like to avoid them unless they are going to provide some lasting relief or meaningful disease modification. The number of corticosteroid injections at a single site is limited by the potential for skin discoloration, subcutaneous atrophy, and capillary fragility. I will not give more than three lifetime injections in the same area (Fig. 29-3).

Under sterile conditions, with use of a 25- to 27-gauge needle and a mixture of local anesthetic (e.g., 0.5 to 1 mL of 1% lidocaine) and corticosteroid (e.g., 0.5 to 1 mL of triamcinolone), the joint is injected. Small joints of the hand will not accommodate large volumes, so the total amount of fluid injected should typically be in the range of 1 to 2 mL. It is helpful to distract the joint by pulling on the finger.

Surgery

Osteoarthritis of the hand is a part of human existence that all of us will experience if we are lucky to live long enough. It is probably safe to assume that most patients adapt well to their arthritis, have effective coping skills, and never bring the arthritis to the attention of a physician. Among those who do bring the problem to a physician's attention, most are satisfied with an explanation of the disease process, the reassurance that

TABLE 29-1 Basic Principles of Arthritis Management	
Understand pain	The pain does not reflect ongoing harm; it is the result of the existing, permanent disease process. Any rest or activity restriction is voluntary and intended to diminish pain. Patients should be encouraged to continue in painful activities that they value without feeling guilty, neglectful, or irresponsible.
Activity modification	Patients can be taught alternative, less painful, and easier ways to accomplish daily tasks that do not rely on painful joints. Jar openers, pen grips, and door levers rather than knobs can be useful modifications.
Maintain strength and range of motion	Patients are encouraged to continue both daily activities and sports and exercise as a means for preserving active range of motion and muscle conditioning. Daily activities may be supplemented with active range of motion exercises targeted for specific joints.
Use stronger muscles and larger joints	Other adaptive techniques include instruction in how to limit stress on the smaller joints and weaker muscles of the hand. In addition, the patient can be taught to carry items close to the body or to cradle them in the entire arm to distribute loads, rather than relying on smaller muscles and joints of the hand to bear the entire load.
Use adaptive equipment or splints	The patient is provided with information on specific adaptive devices that are helpful in reducing or eliminating positions of deformity or stress on the smaller joints. Splints can be useful for limiting pain with specific activities.

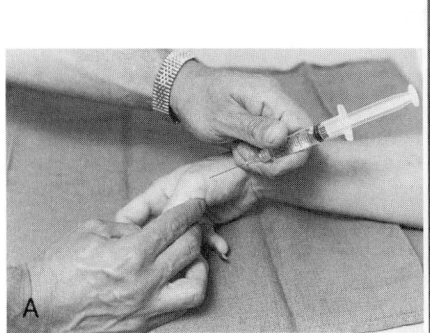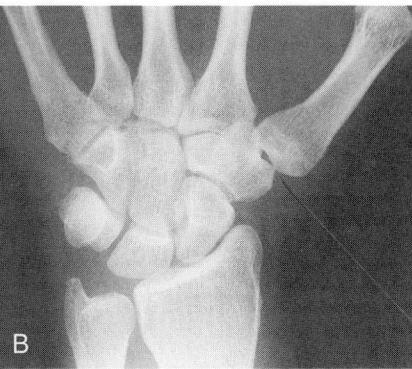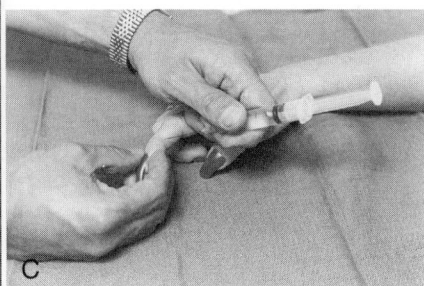

FIGURE 29-3. A, Needle placement into the carpometacarpal joint. **B,** Anteroposterior radiograph of the hand demonstrating needle placement into the first carpometacarpal joint. **C,** Needle placement into the interphalangeal joint. (Reprinted with permission from Lennard TA. Pain Procedures in Clinical Practice, 2nd ed. Philadelphia, Hanley & Belfus, 2000.)

it is normal and inevitable, an understanding that the disease cannot be modified, and suggestions for management and palliation. Although surgery provides fairly predictable pain relief, very few patients request operative treatment to reconstruct or to salvage the arthritic joint.

Distal Interphalangeal Joint

Infected mucous cysts are typically effectively treated with oral antibiotics (cephalexin or the equivalent to treat *Staphylococcus aureus* infection). Operative treatment is necessary only for long-standing cases with potential osteomyelitis. Because the joint is already severely damaged, there is no need to be concerned about joint damage from the infection.

Aspiration of mucous cysts is rarely curative. Patients sometimes elect aspiration to reduce the size of a very large cyst or to improve skin cover when it has become thin and translucent. The recurrence rate is also high after surgery. Patients must choose between leaving the cyst alone and making an attempt to resolve it with surgery, being mindful of the discomfort, inconvenience, and risks of surgery as well as the high recurrence rate. Arthrodesis of the distal interphalangeal joint is the only reliable cure for a mucous cyst, but it is rarely performed for this purpose.

Patients usually request arthrodesis when there is substantial ulnar or radial deviation of the distal interphalangeal joint. It is more cosmetic than functional. Patients rarely request distal interphalangeal joint arthrodesis for pain.

Proximal Interphalangeal Joint

It is extremely uncommon to operate on idiopathic osteoarthritis of the proximal interphalangeal joint, probably a reflection of the relatively low incidence and severity of osteoarthritis at this joint compared with the distal interphalangeal joint and effective coping with an insidious, slowly progressive disease. Arthrodesis and arthroplasty (of nonborder digits with either silicone rubber or, experimentally, pyrocarbon implants) are both options at this joint and are usually considered for

post-traumatic arthritis, and the indication is usually pain relief.

Arthrodesis is more predictable. Arthroplasty is used only in patients who are motivated to retain some mobility at the sacrifice of pain relief and stability.[7]

Trapeziometacarpal Joint

The trapeziometacarpal joint is the most common upper extremity site of surgical reconstruction for osteoarthritis. Operative treatment consists of the salvage procedures arthrodesis and resection arthroplasty.[8,9] Arthrodesis is less used because of the need for protection, the risk of nonunion, and the inability to place the hand flat on the table that is often bothersome to patients. Some surgeons favor arthrodesis in younger patients who use the hand for strength, but this recommendation is not evidence based.

Reconstruction of the palmar oblique ligament without resection of the trapezium and extension osteotomy of the metacarpal are controversial treatments for a painful trapeziometacarpal joint in a relatively young patient with limited radiographic signs of arthritis. Neither procedure is known to affect the natural history of the disease, and until it is demonstrated to be better than sham surgery, it should be considered to be strongly subject to the placebo or meaning effect in my opinion.[8] Patients with laxity related to a connective tissue disorder are not helped by ligament reconstruction; their only option is arthrodesis, and it is elective.

There are many variations of resection arthroplasty.[10-12] The sources of variation include the following: the amount of trapezium resected; whether the palmar oblique ligament is reconstructed and what technique and tendon are used; what, if anything, is placed in the space created by trapeziectomy (rolled up tendon, prosthesis, or other commercial spacers); operative approach (volar, direct radial, arthroscopic); pinning of the joint; and tendons used or included in the reconstruction. The result is that there are probably as many surgeries as surgeons. Simple trapeziectomy has been shown to be as effective as more sophisticated techniques in some prospective randomized trials,[13,14] but many hand surgeons—who tend to be concerned about persistent pain and are rather detail oriented—find this simple resection arthroplasty relatively unappealing. I favor simple trapeziectomy for its simplicity, safety, and quicker recovery,[13] and my patients have been pleased with the results.

POTENTIAL DISEASE COMPLICATIONS

Hand osteoarthritis is a chronic, progressive disease that is a nuisance and not a danger. The only potential complications are associated with treatments.

POTENTIAL TREATMENT COMPLICATIONS

Nonsteroidal anti-inflammatory drugs have well-known side effects that most commonly affect the gastric, hepatic, and renal systems. The newer nonsteroidal anti-inflammatory drugs (e.g., cyclooxygenase 2 inhibitors) have been associated with cardiovascular risks.[15]

The primary risks associated with injections are infection and an allergic reaction to the medication used, but both are extremely rare. Some patients develop a hematoma or complain of substantial pain after an injection.

Potential surgical complications include wound infection, silicone implant synovitis, and dissolution or extrusion of tendon interpositional spacers or implants. The major source of dissatisfaction after surgery is persistent pain, and its sources are controversial.

Complications of arthrodesis procedures include nonunion, infection, implant breakage, and extrusion.

References

1. Chaisson CE, Zhang Y, McAlindon TE, et al. Radiographic hand osteoarthritis incidents, patterns, and influence of preexisting disease in a population base sample. J Rheumatol 1997;24:1337-1343.
2. Sodha S, Ring D, Zurakowski D, Jupiter JB. Prevalence of osteoarthrosis of the trapeziometacarpal joint. J Bone Joint Surg Am 2005;87:2614-2618.
3. Burton RI. Basal joint arthrosis of the thumb. Orthop Clin North Am 1973;4:331-348.
4. Eaton RG, Littler JW. A study of the basal joint of the thumb. Treatment of its disabilities by fusion. J Bone Joint Surg Am 1969;51:661-668.
5. Towheed TE, Anastassiades TP. Glucosamine therapy for osteoarthritis. J Rheumatol 1999;26:2294-2297.
6. Stahl S, Karsh-Zafrir I, Ratzon N, Rosenberg N. Comparison of intraarticular injection of depot corticosteroid and hyaluronic acid for treatment of degenerative trapeziometacarpal joints. J Clin Rheumatol 2005;11:299-302.
7. Dovelle S, Heeter PK. Hand Injuries: A Rehabilitation Perspective in Orthopedic Assessment and Treatment of the Geriatric Patient. St. Louis, Mosby, 1993:205.
8. Lynn HH, Wyrick JD, Stern PJ. Proximal interphalangeal joint silicone replacement arthroplasty: clinical results using an interior approach. J Hand Surg Am 1995;20:123-132.
9. Burton RI, Pellegrini VD Jr. Surgical management of basal joint arthritis of the thumb. Part 2. Ligament reconstruction with tendon interposition arthroplasty. J Hand Surg Am 1986;11:324-332.
10. Eaton RG, Littler JW. A study of the basal joint of the thumb. J Bone Joint Surg Am 1969;51:661-668.
11. Thompson JS. Complications and salvage of trapezial metacarpal arthroplasties. Instr Course Lect 1989;38:3-13.
12. Calandruccio JH, Jobe MT. Arthroplasty of the thumb carpometacarpal joint. Semin Arthroplasty 1997;8:135-147.
13. Taylor EJ, Desari K, D'Arcy JC, Bonnici AV. A comparison of fusion, trapeziectomy and Silastic replacement for the treatment of osteoarthritis of the trapeziometacarpal joint. J Hand Surg Br 2005;30:45-49.
14. Davis TR, Brady O, Dias JJ. Excision of the trapezium for osteoarthritis of the trapeziometacarpal joint: a study of the benefit of ligament reconstruction or tendon interposition. J Hand Surg Am 2004;29:1069-1077.
15. McGettigan P, Henry D. Cardiovascular risk and inhibition of cyclooxygenase: a systematic review of the observational studies of selective and nonselective inhibitors of cyclooxygenase 2. JAMA 2006;296:1633-1644.
16. Foliart EE. Swanson silicone finger joint implants. A review of the literature regarding long-term complications. J Hand Surg Am 1995;20:445-449.

Hand Rheumatoid Arthritis 30

David Ring, MD, PhD, and Jonathan Kay, MD

Synonyms

Rheumatoid arthritis
Rheumatism
Inflammatory arthritis

ICD-9 Code

714.0   Rheumatoid arthritis

DEFINITION

Rheumatoid arthritis is a systemic inflammatory disorder of unknown etiology. It is a progressive condition that results in deformity and dysfunction when synovial inflammation erodes cartilage, bone, and soft tissues. However, the widespread early use of methotrexate during the past 25 years has transformed rheumatoid arthritis into a much less devastating disease.[1] The recent availability of targeted biologic therapies, such as the tumor necrosis factor (TNF) antagonists, has further improved the outcome of rheumatoid arthritis.[2] Surgery is becoming much less common and more straightforward in patients with rheumatoid arthritis.

SYMPTOMS

Presenting symptoms in the hand include joint pain in the fingers as well as stiffness and swelling, typically involving the proximal interphalangeal and metacarpophalangeal joints but sparing the distal interphalangeal joints. Stiffness usually is most pronounced in the morning. If it is left untreated, rheumatoid arthritis may result in progressive deformity and disability.

PHYSICAL EXAMINATION

The evaluation of a rheumatoid arthritic hand should include the following: joint pain and inflammation; joint stability; limitations in active and passive range of motion for grip and pinch strength deficits; limitations in hand dexterity; and degree of disability with respect to self-care, vocational activities, and recreational activities.

Early in the course of disease, involved joints are usually stiff, painful, and swollen as synovitis predominates. In some patients, the first sign of rheumatoid arthritis may be extensor tenosynovitis on the dorsum of the hand and wrist. Chronic synovitis may destroy capsuloligamentous and tendinous structures, creating laxity and deformity. In rheumatoid arthritis, in contrast to the arthritis of systemic lupus erythematosus, this soft tissue damage is usually accompanied by destruction of bone with periarticular erosions evident on plain radiographs.

Typical hand deformities associated with advanced rheumatoid arthritis include boutonnière deformity (flexion deformity of the proximal interphalangeal joint and extension deformity of the distal interphalangeal joint) and swan-neck deformity (hyperextension of the proximal interphalangeal joint with flexion of the distal interphalangeal joint). It is not uncommon to see varying patterns on the fingers of one hand (Fig. 30-1).

Inability to extend the index through small fingers may be due to the following: deformity and subluxation or dislocation of the index through small finger metacarpophalangeal joints; ulnar translocation of the extensor tendons due to laxity and destruction of the radial sagittal bands; extensor tendon ruptures due to a combination of dorsal tenosynovitis and distal radioulnar joint deformity or abrasions; or posterior interosseous nerve compression by elbow synovitis. Ulnar drift of the fingers usually accompanies each of these deformities.

Rupture of the extensor tendons usually proceeds in a sequence from ulnar to radial, referred to as the Vaughn-Jackson syndrome.[3] Mannerfelt syndrome is the equivalent on the volar side, progressing from the thumb to the index and long fingers, producing tendon ruptures as a result of synovitis and scaphotrapezial trapezoid irregularity.[4]

Synovitis in the wrist results in volar and ulnarward subluxation and supination of the hand in relation to the forearm. This wrist deformity can exacerbate the Vaughn-Jackson syndrome and ulnar drift.

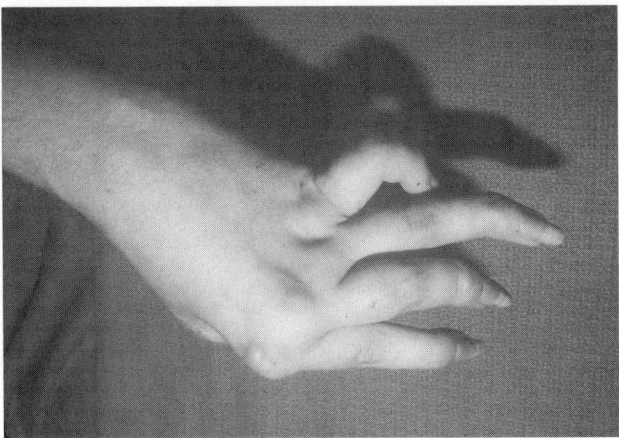

FIGURE 30-1. Rheumatoid hand. Note the multiple presentations in one hand: ulnar drift at the metacarpophalangeal joints, swan-neck deformities of the third and fourth fingers, boutonnière deformity of the fifth finger, volar subluxation at the metacarpophalangeal joint, and radial rotation of the metacarpals.

FUNCTIONAL LIMITATIONS

Surgery is considered when correction of a deformity will improve function. Rheumatoid deformities progress slowly, and patients often adapt well. In some cases, realignment or stabilization of one joint or finger will actually decrease function because it will interfere with an adaptive mechanism. For this reason, surgery for rheumatoid deformity must carefully match the functional desires and goals of the patient with the risks and benefits of operative intervention. Many severe deformities are left untreated when patients have adapted well.

DIAGNOSTIC STUDIES

The diagnosis of rheumatoid arthritis is based predominantly on its clinical presentation. Laboratory testing is used to monitor disease activity and toxicity of drug therapy. Acute-phase reactants, such as C-reactive protein and erythrocyte sedimentation rate, may be elevated in the setting of active joint inflammation. The majority of patients with rheumatoid arthritis have circulating rheumatoid factor or antibodies to cyclic citrullinated peptides. The presence of one of these serologic markers suggests a more aggressive and destructive disease course.

Diffuse periarticular osteopenia is the earliest radiographic sign of rheumatoid arthritis. Joint space narrowing and periarticular erosions may be observed in more than half of patients with rheumatoid arthritis during the first 2 years of disease.[5] If left untreated, joints involved by rheumatoid arthritis may be destroyed by chronic synovitis.

Diagnostic ultrasonography has recently been used to detect early erosions and joint swelling in patients with rheumatoid arthritis.[6] Magnetic resonance imaging of the hand may reveal synovitis and erosions early in the course of rheumatoid arthritis. However, the plain radiograph remains the "gold standard" for diagnostic imaging of rheumatoid arthritis.

Differential Diagnosis

Septic arthritis

Psoriatic arthritis

Systemic lupus erythematosus

Gout

Lyme disease

Calcium pyrophosphate dihydrate deposition disease (pseudogout)

TREATMENT

Initial

Nonsteroidal anti-inflammatory drugs decrease pain and inflammation by inhibiting prostaglandin synthesis; they do not inhibit synovial proliferation and thus do not slow the progression of bone erosion and joint destruction. Low-dose corticosteroids also reduce symptoms of joint inflammation; but unlike nonsteroidal anti-inflammatory drugs, low-dose corticosteroids retard the progression of joint destruction. However, the widespread use of corticosteroids is limited by their many deleterious side effects, including osteoporosis, osteonecrosis of bone, cataracts, cushingoid features, and hyperglycemia.

During the past 25 years, the widespread and early use of low-dose weekly methotrexate has transformed rheumatoid arthritis into a much less destructive disease than it had been previously. Leflunomide also may be used to suppress synovial proliferation and joint destruction.[7] Other slow-acting antirheumatic drugs that have been used to treat rheumatoid arthritis include antimalarial drugs such as hydroxychloroquine, sulfasalazine, intramuscular and oral gold, D-penicillamine, immunosuppressive agents (azathioprine and cyclophosphamide), and cyclosporine.

During the past decade, targeted biologic therapies have been introduced to treat rheumatoid arthritis and other inflammatory diseases. TNF antagonists, such as etanercept, infliximab, and adalimumab, result in the rapid and marked improvement of signs and symptoms of joint inflammation and dramatically slow the rate of joint destruction.[8-10] Abatacept (an inhibitor of T-cell costimulation) and rituximab (a monoclonal anti–B-cell antibody) have recently been approved by the U.S. Food and Drug Administration for treatment of patients with rheumatoid arthritis who have been inadequately responsive to TNF antagonists. Each of these agents is most effective when it is used in combination with methotrexate.[11,12]

Rehabilitation

Rehabilitation of the rheumatoid hand involves resting of the involved joints, modification of activities that stress the joints, joint protection and work simplification instructions (refer to Table 29-1), splinting regimens, heat modalities followed by gentle active range of motion exercise, and resistive exercise (see also Chapter 29).

Flexor and Extensor Tendon Reconstruction Postoperative Rehabilitation

The rehabilitation protocol after flexor and extensor tendon reconstruction varies according to the injury, operative technique, and preferences of the surgeon. Most surgeons protect repairs with cast or splint immobilization for 4 to 6 weeks. Active and active-assisted motion is then encouraged.

Metacarpophalangeal Joint Postoperative Rehabilitation

There is also substantial variation in the preferences of surgeons for rehabilitation after metacarpophalangeal arthroplasty; however, continuous passive motion and dynamic splinting have not proved better than a month of cast immobilization with active-assisted motion exercises thereafter.[13]

Interphalangeal Joint Postoperative Rehabilitation

Interphalangeal joint arthrodesis is usually performed with internal fixation that allows the patient to be splint free and to work on active motion of the metacarpophalangeal joints immediately. Rehabilitation after implant arthroplasty of the proximal interphalangeal joint varies according to operative exposure. Patients treated through a volar exposure begin active exercises within a few days, but patients in whom the extensor tendon or a collateral ligament was taken down and repaired during surgery are immobilized for about 4 weeks initially.

Procedures

Injection of intra-articular steroids may halt progression of the synovitis in a given joint. A good rule of thumb is no more than three injections spaced at least 3 months apart (refer to Chapter 29 for procedure details).

Surgery

Indications for surgery include pain relief and functional restoration; however, one of the most striking benefits—and the source of patients' satisfaction—from hand surgery in rheumatoid arthritis is improvement in the appearance of the hand.[14] The goals may be different when both hands have severe deformities. One may be addressed in a way that enhances fine motor skills, whereas the other is prepared for gross functional tasks requiring strength.

Some have advocated advancement from proximal to distal in rheumatoid hand reconstruction, arguing that if the hand cannot be placed in useful positions in space, postoperative rehabilitation will be hindered. Wrist deformity affects hand deformity and is usually corrected first or simultaneously.[15]

Extensor Tendon Surgery

Patients with extensor tenosynovitis (see also Chapter 26) present with a painless dorsal wrist mass distal to the retinaculum of the wrist. Tenosynovectomy is indicated to establish diagnosis and to prevent tendon rupture, which is uncommon after this surgery. Treatment of tendon rupture involves transfer of the distal end of the ruptured tendon to an adjacent tendon. In the event of multiple tendon ruptures, tendon transfer from the volar side may be indicated. When both wrist extensor tendons are ruptured on the radial side, arthrodesis is required.[16]

Flexor Tendon Surgery

Flexor tenosynovitis (see also Chapter 27) can contribute to a rheumatoid patient's complaints of weak grasp, morning stiffness, volar swelling, and median nerve compression. A tenosynovitis may be diffuse or create discrete nodules that can limit tendon excursion. At the wrist, tenosynovial biopsy is indicated for median nerve compression, painful tenosynovial mass, or tendon rupture. The tendon most commonly ruptured is the flexor pollicis longus. A tendon bridge graft, a two-stage flexor graft, or a tendon transfer can be performed to reconstruct the rupture. A ruptured profundus tendon is sutured to an adjacent intact tendon. The presence of one tendon rupture is an indication to promptly perform surgery to prevent further tendon damage.

The palm is the most common location of flexor tenosynovitis. Indications for flexor tenosynovectomy in the palm include pain with use, triggering, tendon rupture, and passive flexion of the fingers that is greater than active flexion. For tendon rupture within a digit, a distal interphalangeal joint fusion should be considered. When both tendons are ruptured in the digit, consideration should be given to a staged tendon graft or fusion of both the proximal interphalangeal and the distal interphalangeal joints.

Metacarpophalangeal Joint Surgery

The most common deformities of the metacarpophalangeal joint are palmar dislocation of the proximal phalanx and ulnar deviation of the fingers. As the inflammatory process disrupts the digit stabilizers, anatomic forces during use of the hand propel the digits into ulnar deviation. Metacarpophalangeal synovectomy is indicated for the painful, persistent metacarpophalangeal joint synovitis that has not responded to medical treatment and demonstrates minimal cartilage destruction on inspection or radiographically. Silicone implant arthroplasty is indicated in patients with diminished range of motion, marked flexion contractures, poor functional position, severe ulnar drift, and loss of function. Long-term studies have shown mild loss of motion over time and some recurrent deformity in patients whose disease course is progressive, but in general, the results are excellent.[17]

Interphalangeal Joint Surgery

There are two types of proximal interphalangeal joint deformities, the boutonnière deformity and the swan-neck deformity. Surgical intervention, such as flexor sublimis tenodesis or oblique retinacular ligament reconstruction, is designed to prevent hyperextension. On occasion, there is a mallet of the distal interphalangeal joint that can be corrected by partial extension. In later disease, intrinsic tightness requires release. In late swan-neck deformity with loss of proximal interphalangeal movement, implant arthroplasty of the proximal interphalangeal joint as well as sufficient soft tissue immobilization and release to achieve movement in flexion once again is required. In late deformities, especially in the index and middle fingers, arthrodesis may be required. Implant arthroplasties are recommended for the proximal interphalangeal joints of the ring and small fingers.

In early boutonnière deformity, proximal interphalangeal joint synovectomy may be accompanied by postoperative splinting or joint injection. In distal extensor compromise, tenotomy can gain distal interphalangeal joint flexion. In late disease, fixed flexion contracture with inability to passively extend the proximal interphalangeal joint may be present. Restoration of the extensor tendon function by itself will be unsuccessful. Treatment options are proximal interphalangeal arthrodesis or arthroplasty with a Silastic implant. Long-term results reveal significant loss of range of motion of the proximal interphalangeal joint, but the deformity and pain level are markedly improved.

The thumb presents with two types of deformities. One is the boutonnière deformity with flexion of the metacarpophalangeal joint and extension of the interphalangeal joint. The other is the swan-neck deformity with abduction subluxation of the base of the thumb metacarpal, hyperextension of the metacarpophalangeal joint, and flexion deformity of the interphalangeal joint of the thumb. This once again is caused by synovitis, and synovectomy and tendon reconstruction in early deformity may be helpful. For more severe swan-neck deformity, carpometacarpal arthrodesis or arthroplasty may be necessary. There are many more complex deformities that can be discussed, but they are beyond the scope of this chapter.

POTENTIAL DISEASE COMPLICATIONS

Complications of rheumatoid disease in the hand include severe loss of function with complete joint destruction, severe flexion and ulnar deviation deformities of the digits, and severe swan-neck and boutonnière deformities. Chronic intractable pain is also a common complication of the disease.

POTENTIAL TREATMENT COMPLICATIONS

Complications of treatment include infection, hardware breakage, nonunion, Silastic implant breakage, silicone synovitis, and progression of deformity. All of these eventually lead to loss of function of the hand.

Nonsteroidal anti-inflammatory drugs have associated toxicities that most commonly affect the gastric, hepatic, renal, and cardiovascular systems. Methotrexate may cause liver, hematologic, and, less frequently, lung toxicity. Thus, all patients receiving low-dose weekly methotrexate therapy should have complete blood count and liver function monitoring at least every 8 weeks.[18]

The efficacy of targeted biologic therapies is tempered by potential toxicities. Because TNF antagonist therapy increases the risk for reactivation of latent tuberculosis, all patients for whom TNF antagonist therapy is considered should undergo PPD testing. If the PPD test result is reactive, treatment of latent tuberculosis should be initiated before treatment is begun with a TNF antagonist. Also, because the severity of bacterial infections may be increased in patients receiving TNF antagonist therapy, all patients taking these medications should be warned to seek immediate medical attention if signs or symptoms of infection develop.[2]

References

1. Kremer JM. Safety, efficacy, and mortality in a long-term cohort of patients with rheumatoid arthritis taking methotrexate: followup after a mean of 13.3 years. Arthritis Rheum 1997;40:984-985.
2. Furst DE, Breedveld FC, Kalden JR, et al. Updated consensus statement on biological agents for the treatment of rheumatic diseases, 2006. Ann Rheum Dis 2006;65(Suppl 3):iii2-15.
3. Vaughan-Jackson OJ. Attrition ruptures of tendons in the rheumatoid hand [abstract]. J Bone Joint Surg Am 1958;40:1431.
4. Mannerfelt LG, Norman O. Attrition ruptures of flexor tendons in rheumatoid arthritis caused by bony spurs in the carpal tunnel. A clinical and radiological study. J Bone Joint Surg Br 1969;51:270-277.
5. Wolfe F, Sharp JT. Radiographic outcome of recent-onset rheumatoid arthritis: a 19-year study of radiographic progression. Arthritis Rheum 1998;41:1571-1582.
6. Ostergaard M, Szkudlarek M. Ultrasonography: a valid method for assessing rheumatoid arthritis? Arthritis Rheum 2005;52:681-686.
7. O'Dell JR. Therapeutic strategies for rheumatoid arthritis. N Engl J Med 2004;350:2591-2602.
8. Keystone EC, Kavanaugh AF, Sharp JT, et al. Radiographic, clinical, and functional outcomes of treatment with adalimumab (a human anti-tumor necrosis factor monoclonal antibody) in patients with active rheumatoid arthritis receiving concomitant methotrexate therapy: a randomized, placebo-controlled, 52-week trial. Arthritis Rheum 2004;50:1400-1411.
9. Klareskog L, van der Heijde D, de Jager JP, et al. Therapeutic effect of the combination of etanercept and methotrexate compared with each treatment alone in patients with rheumatoid arthritis: double-blind randomised controlled trial. Lancet 2004;363:675-681.
10. Lipsky PE, van der Heijde DM, St. Clair EW, et al. Infliximab and methotrexate in the treatment of rheumatoid arthritis. Anti-Tumor Necrosis Factor Trial in Rheumatoid Arthritis with Concomitant Therapy Study Group. N Engl J Med 2000;343:1594-1602.
11. Emery P, Fleischmann R, Filipowicz-Sosnowska A, et al. The efficacy and safety of rituximab in patients with active rheumatoid arthritis despite methotrexate treatment: results of a phase IIB randomized, double-blind, placebo-controlled, dose-ranging trial. Arthritis Rheum 2006;54:1390-1400.
12. Kremer JM, Genant HK, Moreland LW, et al. Effects of abatacept in patients with methotrexate-resistant active rheumatoid arthritis: a randomized trial. Ann Intern Med 2006;144:865-876.
13. Ring D, Simmons BP, Hayes M. Continuous passive motion following metacarpophalangeal joint arthroplasty. J Hand Surg Am 1998;23:505-511.

14. Mandl LA, Galvin DH, Bosch JP, et al. Metacarpophalangeal arthroplasty in rheumatoid arthritis: what determines satisfaction with surgery? J Rheumatol 2002;29:2488-2491.

15. Millender LH, Phillips C. Combined wrist arthrodesis and metacarpophalangeal joint arthroplasty in rheumatoid arthritis. Orthopedics 1978;1:43-48.

16. Millender LH, Nalebuff EA. Arthrodesis of the rheumatoid wrist. An evaluation of sixty patients and a description of a different surgical technique. J Bone Joint Surg Am 1973;55:1026-1034.

17. Goldfarb CA, Stern PJ. Metacarpophalangeal joint arthroplasty in rheumatoid arthritis. A long-term assessment. J Bone Joint Surg Am 2003;85:1869-1878.

18. Kremer JM, Alarcon GS, Lightfoot RW Jr, et al. Methotrexate for rheumatoid arthritis. Suggested guidelines for monitoring liver toxicity. American College of Rheumatology. Arthritis Rheum 1994;37:316-328.

Kienböck Disease 31

Charles Cassidy, MD, and Vivek M. Shah, MD

DEFINITION

Kienböck disease is defined as avascular necrosis of the lunate, unrelated to acute fracture, often leading to fragmentation and collapse. Although the precise etiology and natural history of this disorder remain unknown, interruption of the blood supply to the lunate is undoubtedly a part of the process. Trauma has been implicated as a cause.[1-3] This disease occurs most often in the dominant hand of men in the age group of 20 to 40 years. Many of these patients are manual laborers who report a history of a major or repetitive minor injury. Associations have also been made between Kienböck disease and corticosteroid use, cerebral palsy, systemic lupus erythematosus, sickle cell disease, gout, and streptococcal infection.

An important radiographic observation has been made regarding the radius-ulna relationship at the wrist and the development of Kienböck disease.[4] In these patients, the ulna is generally shorter than the radius, a finding termed ulnar negative (or minus) variance. Normally, the lunate rests on both the radius and the triangular fibrocartilage complex covering the ulnar head. It has been speculated that when the ulna is significantly shorter than the radius, a shearing effect occurs in the lunate, which can make it more susceptible to injury.

SYMPTOMS

Presenting symptoms include chronic wrist pain, decreased range of motion, and weakness.[5] The pain is usually deep within the wrist, although the patient often points to the dorsum of the wrist, and is aggravated by activity. Some patients complain of a pressure-like pain that may awaken them. A history of recent trauma is often provided; however, many patients report having had long-standing mild wrist pain preceding the recent injury. Symptoms may often be present for months or years before the patient seeks medical attention.

PHYSICAL EXAMINATION

Mild dorsal wrist swelling and tenderness in the mid-dorsal aspect of the wrist may be present. Wrist flexion and extension are limited. Forearm rotation is usually preserved. Grip strength is often considerably less on the affected side.

FUNCTIONAL LIMITATIONS

Functional limitations include difficulty with heavy lifting, gripping, and activities involving the extremes of wrist motion. Many heavy laborers are unable to perform the essential tasks required of their occupation.

DIAGNOSTIC STUDIES

The initial diagnostic imaging for suspected Kienböck disease includes standard wrist radiographs. Early in the disease process, the radiographs may be normal. With time, a characteristic pattern of deterioration occurs, beginning with sclerosis of the lunate, followed by fragmentation, collapse, and finally arthritis[6,7] (Fig. 31-1). A radiographic staging system for Kienböck disease, proposed by Lichtman, is helpful in describing the extent of the disease and guiding treatment[1] (Table 31-1).

For clinical suspicion of Kienböck disease with normal radiographs, a technetium bone scan or magnetic resonance imaging (MRI) may be helpful. In fact, MRI has probably supplanted plain radiography for the detection and evaluation of the early stages of Kienböck disease when there has been no trabecular bone

167

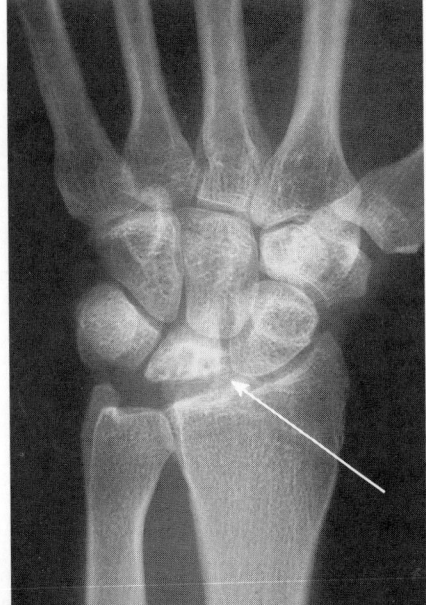

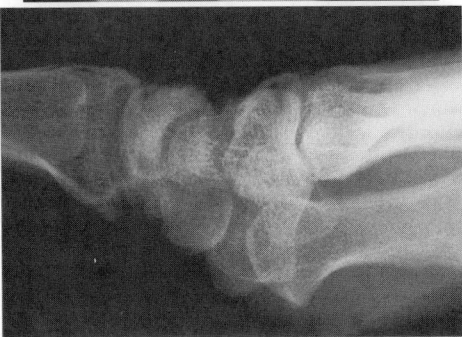

FIGURE 31-1. Advanced Kienböck disease. Cystic and sclerotic changes are present within the collapsed lunate *(arrow)*.

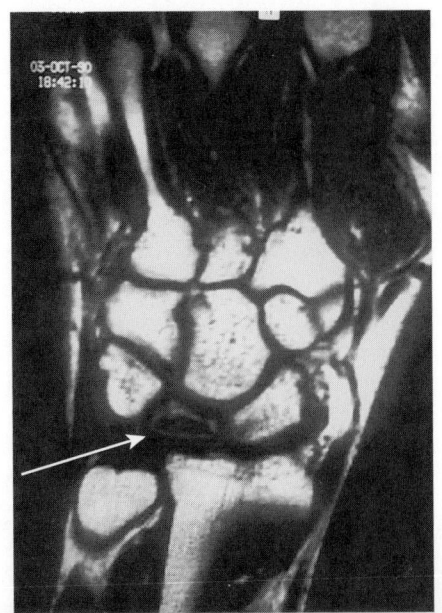

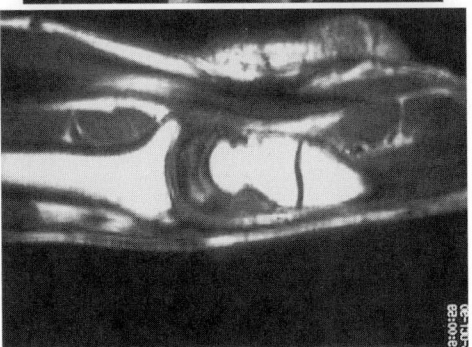

FIGURE 31-2. MRI in Kienböck disease. T1-weighted images demonstrate diffuse low signal within the lunate *(arrow)*.

TABLE 31-1 Stages of Kienböck Disease

Stage I	Normal radiographs or linear fracture
Stage II	Lunate sclerosis, one or more fracture lines with possible early collapse on the radial border
Stage III	Lunate collapse
IIIA	Normal carpal alignment and height
IIIB	Fixed scaphoid rotation (ring sign), carpal height decreased, capitate migrates proximally
Stage IV	Severe lunate collapse with intra-articular degenerative changes at the midcarpal joint, radiocarpal joint, or both

Differential Diagnosis

Wrist sprain

Scapholunate ligament tear

Osteoarthritis

Ganglion

Inflammatory arthritis (e.g., rheumatoid arthritis)

Preiser disease (avascular necrosis of the scaphoid)

Tendinitis

Scaphoid fracture

destruction. Characteristic signal changes include decreased signal on T1-weighted and increased signal on T2-weighted images (Fig. 31-2). Computed tomography is more effective than MRI in assessing for fracture of the lunate, but it provides limited information about its vascularity (Figs. 31-3 and 31-4).

TREATMENT

Initial

Given the limited information about the etiology and natural history of this uncommon disease, it is not surprising that the treatment has not been standardized.

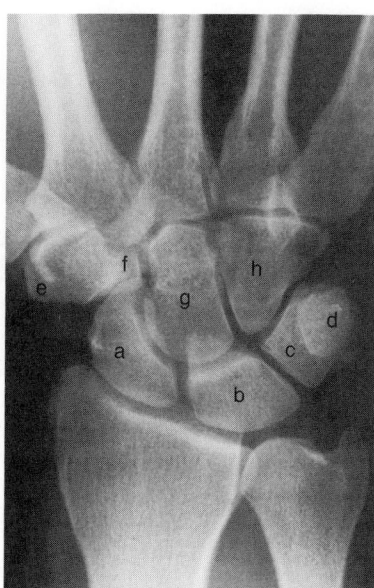

FIGURE 31-3. Posteroanterior view of the wrist demonstrating the proximal and distal carpal rows. a, scaphoid; b, lunate; c, triquetrum; d, pisiform; e, trapezium; f, trapezoid; g, capitate; and h, hamate. (Reprinted with permission from Jebson PJL, Kasdan ML, eds. Hand Secrets. Philadelphia, Hanley & Belfus, 1998:220.)

Without surgery, progressive radiographic collapse and radiographic arthritis almost invariably occur.[5] However, symptoms correlate only weakly with the radiographic appearance, and many patients maintain good long-term function.[8] The goals of surgery ideally would be to relieve the pain and to halt the progression of the disease. Surgical interventions appear to be relatively effective in achieving the first goal but have not as yet reliably altered the radiographic deterioration of the lunate. Consequently, treatment options range from simple splints to external fixation and from radial shortening to vascularized grafts to fusions. Factors taken into consideration in assigning treatment include stage of the disease; ulnar variance; and age, occupation, pain, and functional impairment of the patient.[9] In general, young, active patients should be treated more conservatively before moving to major procedures that compromise wrist function and range of motion.

Many clinicians prefer to begin with symptomatic treatment. Depending on the situation, this may involve a splint and activity modification or a short arm cast. However, an appropriate length of immobilization has not been established. Some clinicians have attempted this treatment for as long as 1 year, but most clinicians prescribe a cast for 6 to 12 weeks. The immobilization probably helps the pain associated with synovitis and with wrist activity and motion; however, it does nothing to alter the vascularity of the bone or the shear stresses across the lunate. The patient should be informed that the radiographs will, in all likelihood, demonstrate worsening of the disease over time.

Pain can be treated with analgesics, including nonsteroidal anti-inflammatory drugs. Narcotic medications are generally not recommended because of the chronicity of this condition.

Rehabilitation

Rehabilitation does not play a major role early in conservative treatment. Once the pain has subsided, gentle range of motion and strengthening may be initiated. Therapy is important for the postoperative patient, particularly if an intra-articular procedure has been performed or an external fixator has been applied. The wrist is typically immobilized postoperatively until the vascularized graft or fusion has healed (about 6 weeks). At that point, occupational or physical therapy can effectively begin with gentle range of motion exercises, gradually progressing to strengthening exercises.

Procedures

Intra-articular steroids are of no proven benefit in the management of Kienböck disease.

Surgery

Some authors believe that the majority of patients treated nonoperatively do well,[6] whereas others believe that surgery is indicated for the majority of patients with Kienböck disease.[10-12] The surgical treatment options for this disease may be divided into stress reduction (unloading), revascularization, lunate replacement, and salvage procedures.[9] Radial shortening of 2 to 3 mm is currently the most popular procedure for early-stage Kienböck disease in the setting of ulnar minus variant.[10,13] The goal is to make the radius and ulna lengths the same and thus to reduce shear forces on the lunate. Other unloading procedures include limited wrist fusion and external fixation.[14] Revascularization procedures have shown promise in the management of avascular necrosis of the lunate.[15,16] The most popular of the pedicled bone grafts, based on the extensor compartmental arteries of the wrist, is transplanted from the distal radius into the lunate. In one series with relatively short-term follow-up, significant pain relief was observed in 92% of patients, and actual lunate revascularization was seen in 60% on follow-up MRI.[15] An intriguing method of indirect revascularization of the lunate has been proposed by Illarramendi and colleagues,[17] who perform a metaphyseal decompression of the radius and ulna, without violating the wrist joint. In their series, 16 of 20 patients were pain free at an average of 10 years postoperatively.

When the lunate has collapsed to the point that it is not reconstructable, salvage procedures such as proximal row carpectomy and partial or total wrist arthrodesis are considered. Obviously, these procedures sacrifice motion in an effort to provide pain relief. The results of the various procedures are dependent, to some extent, on the stage of the disease. Wrist arthroscopy may be of some benefit in determining the extent of the disease and in selecting the appropriate salvage procedure.[18] Regardless of the specific type of salvage procedure, most authors report 70% to 100% satisfaction of patients. Advanced arthritis (stage IV) is generally best treated with a total wrist arthrodesis.

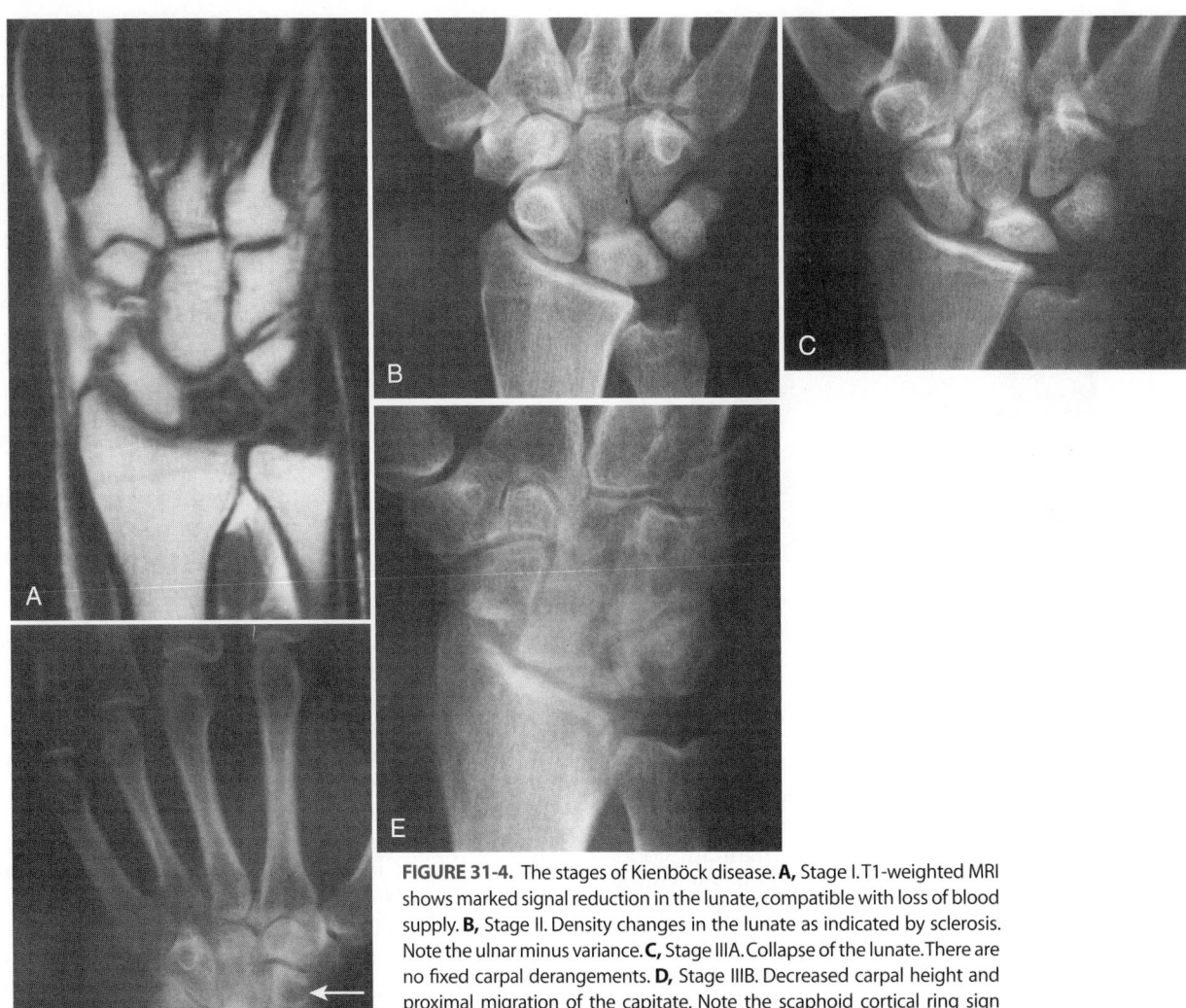

FIGURE 31-4. The stages of Kienböck disease. **A,** Stage I. T1-weighted MRI shows marked signal reduction in the lunate, compatible with loss of blood supply. **B,** Stage II. Density changes in the lunate as indicated by sclerosis. Note the ulnar minus variance. **C,** Stage IIIA. Collapse of the lunate. There are no fixed carpal derangements. **D,** Stage IIIB. Decreased carpal height and proximal migration of the capitate. Note the scaphoid cortical ring sign *(arrow).* **E,** Stage IV. Generalized degenerative changes in the carpus. (Reprinted with permission from Weinzweig J, ed. Plastic Surgery Secrets. Philadelphia, Hanley & Belfus, 1999:605-606.)

POTENTIAL DISEASE COMPLICATIONS

Without surgery, progressive radiographic collapse of the lunate and arthritis of the wrist invariably occur.

POTENTIAL TREATMENT COMPLICATIONS

Analgesics and nonsteroidal anti-inflammatory drugs have well-known side effects that most commonly affect the gastric, hepatic, and renal systems. Infection is uncommon after hand surgery. Complications such as nerve injury, painful hardware, and stiffness of the wrist and digits are inherent in hand surgery. A radial shortening osteotomy or partial wrist fusion may fail to heal (nonunion). Secondary wrist arthritis can develop after partial wrist fusions or proximal row carpectomy. Grip strength virtually never returns to normal. Finally, and most im-

portant, whether surgery favorably alters the natural history of this rare condition remains unproven.

References

1. Fredericks TK, Fernandez JE, Pirela-Cruz MA. Kienböck's disease. I. Anatomy and etiology. Int J Occup Med Environ Health 1997;10:11-17.
2. Fredericks TK, Fernandez JE, Pirela-Cruz MA. Kienböck's disease. II. Risk factors, diagnosis, and ergonomic interventions. Int J Occup Med Environ Health 1997;10:147-157.
3. Watson HK, Guidera PM. Aetiology of Kienböck's disease. J Hand Surg Br 1997;22:5-7.
4. Hulten O. Über anatomische Variationen der Handgelenkknochen. Acta Radiol 1928;9:155-168.
5. Beckenbaugh RD, Shives TS, Dobyns JH, Linscheid RL. Kienböck's disease: the natural history of Kienböck's disease and considerations of lunate fractures. Clin Orthop 1980;149:98-106.
6. Stahl F. On lunatomalacia (Kienböck's disease): clinical and roentgenological study, especially on its pathogenesis and late results of immobilization treatment. Acta Chir Scand Suppl 1947;126:1-133.

7. Lichtman DM, Mack GR, MacDonald RI, et al. Kienböck's disease: the role of silicon replacement arthroplasty. J Bone Joint Surg Am 1977;59:899-908.
8. Mirabello SC, Rosenthal DI, Smith RJ. Correlation of clinical and radiographic findings in Kienböck's disease. J Hand Surg Am 1987;12:1049-1054.
9. Ruby LK, Cassidy C. Fractures and dislocations of the carpus. In Browner BD, Jupiter JB, Levine A, Trefton P, eds. Skeletal Trauma: Fractures, Dislocations, and Ligamentous Injuries, 3rd ed. Philadelphia, Saunders, 2008.
10. Salmon J, Stanley JK, Trail IA. Kienböck's disease: conservative management versus radial shortening. J Bone Joint Surg Br 2000;82:820-823.
11. Mikkelsen SS, Gelineck J. Poor function after nonoperative treatment of Kienböck's disease. Acta Orthop Scand 1987;58:241-243.
12. Delaere O, Dury M, Molderez A, Foucher G. Conservative versus operative treatment for Kienböck's disease. J Hand Surg Br 1998;23:33-36.
13. Almquist EE. Kienböck's disease. Hand Clin North Am 1987;3:141-148.
14. Zelouf DS, Ruby LK. External fixation and cancellous bone grafting for Kienböck's disease. J Hand Surg Am 1996;21:743-753.
15. Moran SL, Cooney WP, Berger RA, et al. The use of the 4 + 5 extensor compartmental vascularized bone graft for the treatment of Kienböck's disease. J Hand Surg Am 2005;30:50-58.
16. Daecke W, Lorenz S, Wieloch P, et al. Vascularized os pisiform for reinforcement of the lunate in Kienböck's disease: an average of 12 years of follow-up study. J Hand Surg Am 2005;30:915-922.
17. Illarramendi AA, Schulz C, De Carli P. The surgical treatment of Kienböck's disease by radius and ulna metaphyseal core decompression. J Hand Surg Am 2001;26:252-260.
18. Bain GI, Begg M. Arthroscopic assessment and classification of Kienböck's disease. Tech Hand Up Extrem Surg 2006;10:8-13.

Median Neuropathy (Carpal Tunnel Syndrome) 32

Meijuan Zhao, MD, and David Burke, MD, MA

Synonyms

Median nerve entrapment at the wrist or carpal tunnel syndrome
Median nerve compression

ICD-9 Code

354.0   Carpal tunnel syndrome

DEFINITION

Carpal tunnel syndrome (CTS), an entrapment neuropathy of the median nerve at the wrist, is the most common compression neuropathy of the upper extremity. This syndrome produces paresthesias, numbness, pain, subjective swelling, and, in advanced cases, muscle atrophy and weakness of the areas innervated by the median nerve. The condition is often bilateral, although the dominant hand tends to be more severely affected.

CTS is thought to result from a compression of the median nerve as it passes through the carpal tunnel. The clinical presentation is variable. Whereas there is some variation as to what should be included in this definition, CTS is most often thought to involve sensory changes in the radial $3\frac{1}{2}$ digits of the hand with burning, tingling, numbness, and a subjective sense of swelling. Those affected often first note symptoms at night. In the later stages, complaints include motor weakness in the thenar eminence.

It is helpful to think of the carpal tunnel as a structure with four sides, three of which are defined by the carpal bones and the fourth, the "top" of the tunnel, by the transverse carpal ligament (Figs. 32-1 and 32-2). Passing through the tunnel are the median nerve and nine tendons with their synovial sheaths; these include the flexor pollicis longus, the four flexor digitorum superficialis, and the four flexor digitorum profundus tendons. None of the sides of the tunnel yields well to expansion of the fluid or structures within. Because of this, swelling will increase pressure within the tunnel and may result in compression of the median nerve. CTS occurs more commonly in women than in men, with a population prevalence of 5.8% in women and 0.6% in men[1]; it is most common in middle-aged persons between the ages of 30 and 60 years. The older adults may have objective clinical and electrophysiologic evidence of a more severe median nerve entrapment.[2] One survey of employees who were frequent computer users found that their frequency of CTS was similar to that in the general population.[3] It has been reported that computer use does not pose a severe occupational hazard for development of symptoms of CTS.[4]

SYMPTOMS

The classic symptoms of CTS include numbness and paresthesias in the radial $3\frac{1}{2}$ fingers (Fig. 32-3). A typical early complaint is awakening in the night with numbness or pain in the fingers. Symptoms during the day are often brought out by activities placing the wrist in substantial flexion or extension or requiring repetitive motion of the structures that traverse the carpal tunnel. Numbness and pain in the hand may also include volar wrist pain and aching at the forearm. The patient may describe the symptoms as being positional, with symptoms relieved by the shaking of a hand, often referred to as the flick sign. Patients may complain of a sense of swelling in the hands, often noting that they have difficulty wearing jewelry or watches, with this sensation fluctuating throughout the day or week.[5] Some patients also report dry skin and cold hands. In the later stages of CTS, the numbness may become constant and motor disturbances more apparent, with complaints of weakness manifested by a functional decrease of strength. Patients may then report dropping objects.

PHYSICAL EXAMINATION

Careful observation of the hands, comparing the affected side with the unaffected side and comparing the thenar and hypothenar eminences of the same hand, may reveal an increasing asymmetry. Weakness of the thenar intrinsic muscles of the hand can be tested with a dynamometer or clinically by testing abduction of the thumb against resistance. A two-point sensory discrimination task is thought to be the most sensitive of the bedside examination techniques. This involves a comparison of the two-point discriminating sensory ability of the median

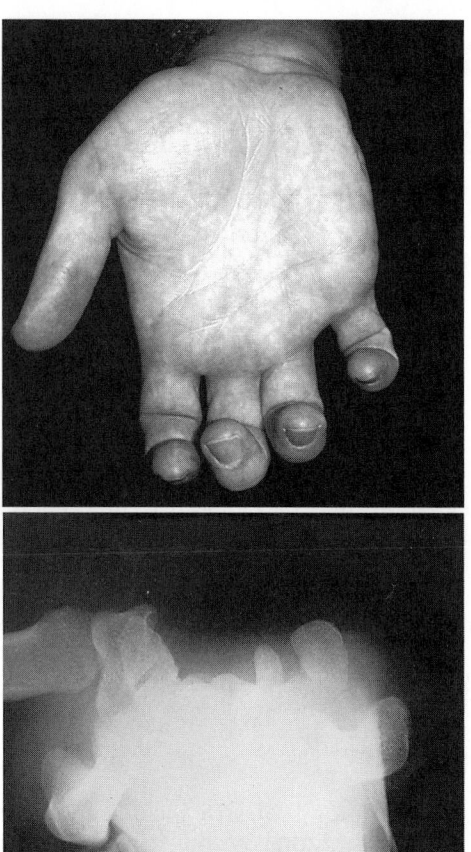

FIGURE 32-1. Radiographic demonstration of the carpal tunnel (for orientation, the hand is in the same position in the radiograph). The carpal tunnel is formed radially, ulnarly, and dorsally by the carpal bones. (Reprinted with permission from Concannon M. Common Hand Problems in Primary Care. Philadelphia, Hanley & Belfus, 1999:134.)

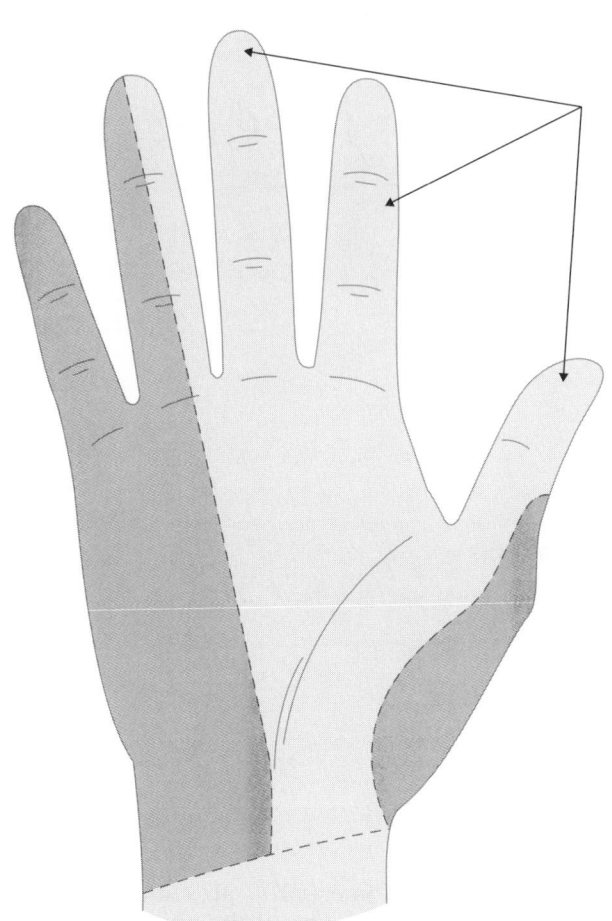

FIGURE 32-3. Patients with carpal tunnel syndrome complain of numbness or paresthesia within the median nerve distribution (*gray area, arrows*). (Reprinted with permission from Concannon M. Common Hand Problems in Primary Care. Philadelphia, Hanley & Belfus, 1999:135.)

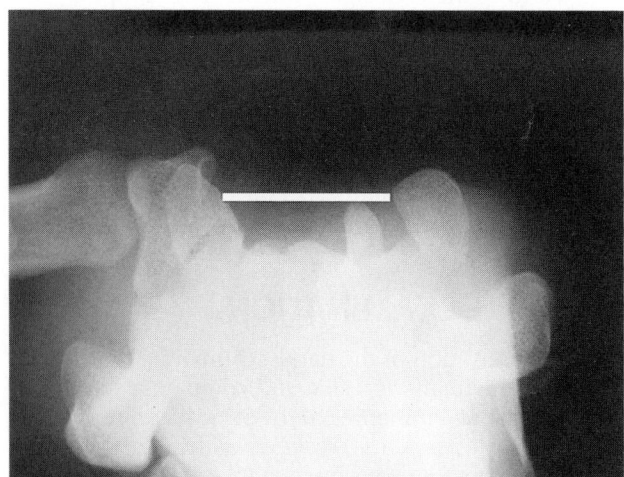

FIGURE 32-2. The volar carpal ligament (*line*) forms the roof of the carpal tunnel. This thick, fibrous structure does not yield to expansion, and increased pressure within the carpal tunnel can cause impingement of the median nerve. (Reprinted with permission from Concannon M. Common Hand Problems in Primary Care. Philadelphia, Hanley & Belfus, 1999:134.)

with that of the ulnar nerve distribution of the hand. The more common special tests include the Phalen, the Tinel, and the nerve compression tests. The Phalen test involves a forced flexion at the wrist to 90 degrees for a period of 1 minute; a positive test result reproduces the symptoms of CTS (Fig. 32-4). The reverse Phalen maneuver is the same test completed with forced extension. The Tinel test involves tapping sharply over the volar aspect of the wrist just distal to the distal wrist crease. The test result is positive when a sensory disturbance radiates down the region of the distribution of the median nerve. The nerve compression test involves the placement of two thumbs over the roof of the carpal tunnel, with pressure maintained for 1 minute. The test result is positive if symptoms are reproduced in the area of the distribution of the median nerve. A review showed an overall estimate of 68% sensitivity and 73% specificity for the Phalen test, 50% sensitivity and 77% specificity for the Tinel test, and 64% sensitivity and 83% specificity for the carpal compression test. Two-point discrimination and testing of atrophy or strength of the abductor pollicis brevis proved to be specific but not very sensitive.[6]

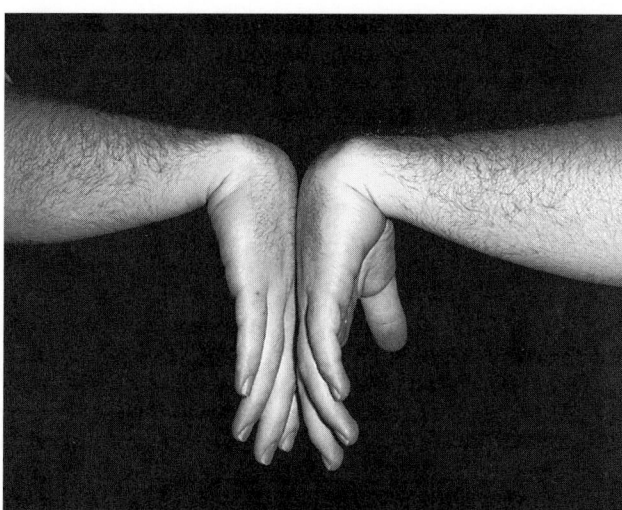

FIGURE 32-4. Phalen test. Patients maximally flex both wrists and hold the position for 1 to 2 minutes. If symptoms of numbness or paresthesia within the median nerve distribution are reproduced, the test result is positive. (Reprinted with permission from Concannon M. Common Hand Problems in Primary Care. Philadelphia, Hanley & Belfus, 1999:136.)

Differential Diagnosis

Cervical radiculopathy in C5 to T1 distribution

Brachial plexopathy

Proximal median neuropathy

Ulnar or radial neuropathy

Generalized neuropathy

Arthritis of carpal-metacarpal joint of thumb

de Quervain tenosynovitis

Tendinitis of the flexor carpi radialis

Raynaud phenomenon

Hand-arm vibration syndrome

Arthritis of the wrist

Gout

FUNCTIONAL LIMITATIONS

Functional limitations of CTS often include difficulty with sleep due to frequent awakenings by the symptoms. Because certain sustained or repetitive motions are difficult, tasks that often become more difficult include driving a car and sustained computer keyboard use at work. The later symptom of weakness in the thenar eminence may result in difficulty maintaining grip. Profound CTS may result in functional limitations such as the inability to tie one's shoes, to button shirts, and to put a key in a lock.

DIAGNOSTIC STUDIES

Whereas CTS is a syndrome rather than a singular finding, it is often suggested that the "gold standard" test of CTS is electrodiagnostic testing. Electromyography and nerve conduction studies can confirm the diagnosis, determine the severity (if any) of nerve damage, guide and measure the effect of treatment, and rule out other conditions such as radiculopathy and brachial plexopathy. Ultrasound studies, which reveal an enlarged median nerve, may assist with the diagnosis.[7]

Others have advocated the injection of corticosteroids or bupivacaine into the carpal tunnel. If the injection is accompanied by a relief of symptoms, it provides diagnostic evidence of CTS.[8]

A wrist radiograph may be helpful if a fracture or degenerative joint disease is suspected.

Blood tests should be ordered if underlying rheumatologic disease or endocrine disturbance is suspected. These include fasting blood glucose concentration, erythrocyte sedimentation rate, thyroid function, and rheumatoid factor.

TREATMENT

Initial

Once the diagnosis is established, treatment should begin with conservative management. Nighttime wrist splinting in a neutral position may help reduce or completely relieve CTS symptoms. Full-time use, if tolerable, has been shown to provide greater improvement of symptoms and electrophysiologic measures. Compliance with full-time use is more difficult.[9] The majority of patients will achieve maximal symptom relief through splinting within 2 to 3 weeks. The optimal length of time for splint placement before it is decided to proceed with more invasive techniques is not completely clear.[10] Nonsteroidal anti-inflammatory drugs are frequently prescribed as an adjunct to wrist splinting. However, some studies have demonstrated that nonsteroidal anti-inflammatory drugs are often no more effective than placebo in relieving the symptoms of CTS.[11,12] The use of oral steroids (prednisone in doses of 20 mg daily for the first week and 10 mg daily for the second week,[13] or prednisolone at 25 mg daily for 10 days[14]) has proved to be of some benefit, although not as impressive as the results noted through injection.[14] Frequent periods of rest of the wrist should be prescribed, especially when vocational activities involve sustained positioning or repetitive and forceful flexion or extension of the wrist. Ice after periods of use may be effective for symptom relief. Positioning of the body while a task is being performed should be reviewed to relieve unnecessary strain as necessary motions are performed.

Rehabilitation

Rehabilitation must address the issue of overuse, which exacerbates the symptoms of CTS in many individuals. As with all overuse symptoms, occupational therapists can be helpful in instructing patients in relative rest and improved ergonomics. During these periods of rest, flexion and extension stretching of the wrist and forearm may be useful, with the patient using the unaffected hand. Although many therapists advocate strengthening as part of a treatment program, aggressive strengthening exercises should be avoided until symptom relief is nearly complete.

Because overuse syndromes involve a degree of edema, icing after long periods of use has been advocated to reduce the pain and swelling. In addition, it is important that patients be instructed in a program of general physical conditioning; generalized deconditioning exacerbates the symptoms of CTS.[15]

Procedures

The patient can also be treated with corticosteroid injections into the carpal tunnel. A number of authors have suggested various injection techniques to avoid direct injury to the median nerve.[16-19]

For injection into the carpal tunnel (Fig. 32-5), 1 mL of steroid (triamcinolone, 40 mg/mL) can be injected under sterile conditions. For delivery, one should use a ⅝-inch, 27-gauge needle, placing the needle proximal to the distal wrist crease and ulnar to the palmaris longus tendon. The needle should be directed dorsally and angled at 30 degrees to a depth of about ⅝ inch (the length of the needle) or contact with a flexor tendon. Slowly inject 1 mL of the corticosteroid. Anesthetics are not typically used in this injection unless for diagnostic verification. In individuals lacking a palmaris longus tendon (about 2% to 20% of the population), the needle can be placed midpoint between the ulna and radial styloid process. The injection will increase the volume of fluid within the carpal tunnel and thus may exacerbate the discomfort for a few hours; relief is expected within the 24 to 48 hours after injection.

Surgery

Carpal tunnel release surgery should be considered in patients with symptoms that do not respond to conservative measures and for whom electrodiagnostic testing clearly confirms median neuropathy at the wrist. Surgery is also indicated when there are signs of atrophy or muscle weakness. The overall efficacy of the operative procedure is good, and it has been reported that open carpal tunnel release results in a better symptomatic and neurophysiologic outcome compared with steroid injection in patients with idiopathic CTS during a 20-week period.[20] The open release of the transverse carpal ligament represents the standard procedure and can be performed by dividing the transverse carpal ligament through a small open wrist incision. The endoscopic techniques were introduced in the late 1980s to be minimally invasive and to prevent the palmar scarring. Both methods have equal efficacy in relieving symptoms of CTS. A Cochrane collaboration review concluded that with the possible exception of quicker recovery after endoscopic surgery, there is no significant difference in outcome.[21] However, others report that endoscopic surgery is associated with less postoperative pain than open surgery but has no advantage regarding the length of work absence, with 28 days of absence in both groups.[22]

POTENTIAL DISEASE COMPLICATIONS

As with any insult to a peripheral nerve, untreated CTS may result in chronic sensory disturbance or motor impairment in the area serviced by the median nerve. It is important that the clinician be wary of this and not allow the nerve disturbance to progress to permanent nerve damage.

POTENTIAL TREATMENT COMPLICATIONS

Although oral analgesics may be important for symptomatic relief early in the stages of CTS, gastric, renal, and hepatic complications of nonsteroidal anti-inflammatory drugs should be monitored. Complications from local corticosteroid injections include infection, bleeding, skin depigmentation, skin atrophy, potential for tendon rupture, and potential for injury to the median nerve at the time of injection.

Surgical complications have been noted to be few in the literature. These include accidental transection of the median nerve, with permanent loss of function distal to the transection. In addition, some have suggested that arthroscopic surgery might damage the Berrettini branch of the median nerve, a sensory branch.[23] Whereas

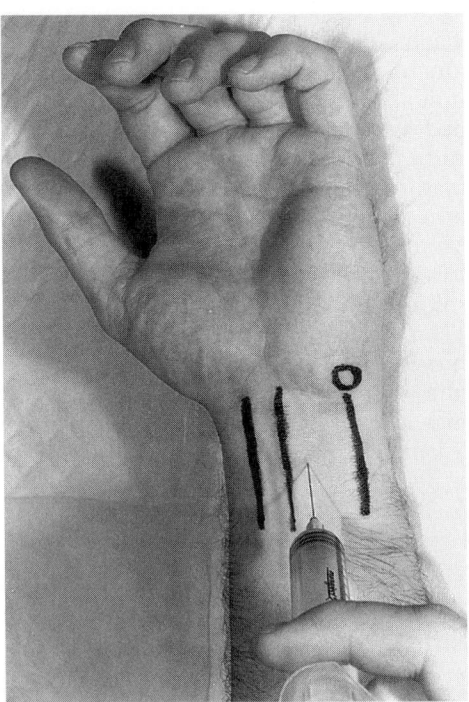

FIGURE 32-5. Preferred method for ulna bursa injection. Needle puncture is just ulnar to the palmaris longus tendon. The circle is over the pisiform bone. (Reprinted with permission from Lennard TA. Pain Procedures in Clinical Practice, 2nd ed. Philadelphia, Hanley & Belfus, 2000:100.)

complications of surgical intervention are thought to be relatively infrequent, a number have been reported. The most common complication of surgical intervention is the incomplete sectioning of the transverse carpal ligament. Other potential complications include injury to the median nerve, palmar cutaneous branch, recurrent motor branch, and superficial palmar arch; hypertrophied or thickened scar due to inappropriate incision; tendon adhesions because of wound hematoma; recurrence because of repair of the ligament; bowstringing of flexor tendons; malposition of the median nerve; inappropriate separation of the nerve fibers from surrounding scars; and reflex sympathetic dystrophy.[24-26]

References

1. de Krom MC, Knipschild PG, Kester AD, et al. Carpal tunnel syndrome, prevalence in the general population. J Clin Epidemiol 1992;45:373-376.
2. Blumenthal S, Herskovitz S, Verghese J. Carpal tunnel syndrome in older adults. Muscle Nerve 2006;34:78-83.
3. Stevens JC, Witt JC, Smith BE, et al. The frequency of carpal tunnel syndrome in computer users at a medical facility. Neurology 2001;56:1568-1570.
4. Andersen JH, Thomsen JF, Overgaard E, et al. Computer use and carpal tunnel syndrome: a 1-year follow-up study. JAMA 2003;289:2963-2969.
5. Burke DT, Burke MAM, Bell R, et al. Subjective swelling: a new sign for carpal tunnel syndrome. Am J Phys Med Rehabil 1999;78:504-508.
6. MacDermid JC, Wessel J. Clinical diagnosis of carpal tunnel syndrome: a systematic review. J Hand Ther 2004;17:309-319.
7. Wiesler ER, Chloros GD, Cartwright MS, et al. The use of diagnostic ultrasound in carpal tunnel syndrome. J Hand Surg Am 2006;31:726-732.
8. Phalen GS. The carpal tunnel syndrome—clinical evaluation of 598 hands. Clin Orthop 1972;83:29-40.
9. Walker WC, Metzler M, Cifu DX, et al. Neutral wrist splinting in carpal tunnel syndrome: a comparison of night-only versus full-time wear instruction. Arch Phys Med Rehabil 2000;81:424-429.
10. Burke DT, Burke MM, Stewart GW, et al. Splinting for carpal tunnel syndrome: in search of the optimal angle. Arch Phys Med Rehabil 1994;75:1241-1244.
11. Gerritsen AA, de Krom MC, Struijs MA, et al. Conservative treatment options for carpal tunnel syndrome: a systematic review of randomized controlled trials. J Neurol 2002;249:272-280.
12. O'Connor D, Marshall S, Massy-Westropp N. Non-surgical treatment (other than steroid injection) for carpal tunnel syndrome. Cochrane Database Syst Rev 2003;1:CD003219.
13. Herskovitz S, Berger AR. Low-dose, short-term oral prednisone in the treatment of carpal tunnel syndrome. Neurology 1995;45:1923-1925.
14. Wong SM, Hui AC, Tang A. Local vs systemic corticosteroids in the treatment of carpal tunnel syndrome. Neurology 2001;56:1565-1567.
15. Nathan PA. Keniston RC. Carpal tunnel syndrome and its relation to general physical condition. Hand Clin 1993;9:253-261.
16. Cyriax JH. The wrist and hand. In Cyriax J, Cyriax P. Illustrated Manual of Orthopaedic Medicine. London, Butterworths, 1983:65.
17. Frederick HA, Carter PR, Littler T. Injection injuries to the median and ulnar nerves at the wrist. J Hand Surg Am 1992;17:645-647.
18. Kay NR, Marshall PD. A safe, reliable method of carpal tunnel injection. J Hand Surg Am 1992;17:1160-1161.
19. Racasan O, Dubert T. The safest location for steroid injection in the treatment of carpal tunnel syndrome. J Hand Surg Br 2005;30:412-414.
20. Hui AC, Wong S, Leung CH, et al. A randomized controlled trial of surgery vs steroid injection for carpal tunnel syndrome. Neurology 2005;64:2074-2078.
21. Scholten RJPM, Gerritsen AAM, Uitdehaag BMJ, et al. Surgical treatment options for carpal tunnel syndrome. Cochrane Database Syst Rev 2004;1:CD003905.
22. Atroshi I, Larsson GU, Ornstein E, et al. Outcomes of endoscopic surgery compared with open surgery for carpal tunnel syndrome among employed patients: randomised controlled trial. BMJ 2006;332:1473. Epub 2006 Jun 15.
23. Stancic MF, Micovic V, Potocnjak M. The anatomy of the Berrettini branch: implications for carpal tunnel release. J Neurosurg 1999;91:1027-1030.
24. Langloh ND, Linscheid RL. Recurrent and unrelieved carpal-tunnel syndrome. Clin Orthop Relat Res 1972;83:41-47.
25. McDonald RI, Lichtman VM, Hanlon JJ, et al. Complications of surgical release for carpal tunnel syndrome. J Hand Surg Am 1978;3:70-76.
26. Kessler FB. Complications of the management of carpal tunnel syndrome. Hand Clin 1986;2:401-406.

Trigger Finger 33

Julie K. Silver, MD

Synonyms

Stenosing tenosynovitis
Digital flexor tenosynovitis
Locked finger
Tendinitis

ICD-9 Code

727.03   Trigger finger

DEFINITION

Trigger finger is defined as the snapping, triggering, or locking of a finger as it is flexed and extended. This is due to a localized inflammation or a nodular swelling of the flexor tendon sheath that does not allow the tendon to glide normally back and forth under a pulley. Trigger finger is believed to arise from high pressures at the proximal edge of the A1 pulley when there is a discrepancy in the diameter of the flexor tendon and its sheath at the level of the metacarpal head[1] (Fig. 33-1). The thumb and the middle and ring fingers of the dominant hand of middle-aged women are most commonly affected.[2] It is often encountered in patients with diabetes and rheumatoid arthritis.[3,4] The relationship of trigger finger to repetitive trauma has been cited frequently in the literature[4-6]; however, the exact mechanism of this correlation is still open for debate.[7] Rarely, it is due to acute trauma or space-occupying lesions.[8-10]

SYMPTOMS

Patients typically complain of pain in the proximal interphalangeal joint of the finger, rather than in the true anatomic location of the problem—at the metacarpophalangeal joint. Some individuals may report swelling or stiffness in the fingers, particularly in the morning. Patients may also have intermittent locking in flexion or extension of the digit, which is overcome with forceful voluntary effort or passive assistance. Involvement of multiple fingers can be seen in patients with rheumatoid arthritis or diabetes.[3,4] In one study, the perioperative symptoms differed for trigger thumbs versus trigger fingers.[11]

In this study, patients complained of pain with motion with trigger thumb; with trigger finger, they complained primarily of triggering and loss of range of motion.

PHYSICAL EXAMINATION

The essential element in the physical examination is the localization of the disorder at the level of the metacarpophalangeal joint. There is palpable tenderness and sometimes a tender nodule over the volar aspect of the metacarpal head. Swelling of the finger may also be noted. Opening and closing of the hand actively produces a painful clicking as the inflamed tendon passes through a constricted sheath. Passive extension of the distal interphalangeal or proximal interphalangeal joint while the metacarpophalangeal joint is kept flexed may be painless and done without triggering.[2] With chronic triggering, the patient may develop interphalangeal joint flexion contractures.[2] Therefore, it is important to determine whether there is normal passive range of motion in the metacarpophalangeal and interphalangeal joints. Neurologic examination, including muscle strength, sensation, and reflexes, should be normal, with the exception of severe cases associated with disuse weakness or atrophy. Comorbidities can affect the neurologic examination findings as well (e.g., someone with diabetic neuropathy may have impaired sensation).

FUNCTIONAL LIMITATIONS

Functional limitations include difficulty with grasping and fine manipulation of objects due to pain, locking, or both. Fine motor problems may include difficulty with inserting a key into a lock, typing, or buttoning a shirt. Gross motor skills may include limitations in gripping a steering wheel or in grasping tools at home or at work.

DIAGNOSTIC STUDIES

This is a clinical diagnosis. Patients without a history of injury or inflammatory arthritis do not need routine radiographs.[12] Magnetic resonance imaging can confirm tenosynovitis of the flexor sheath, but this offers minimal advantage over clinical diagnosis.[13]

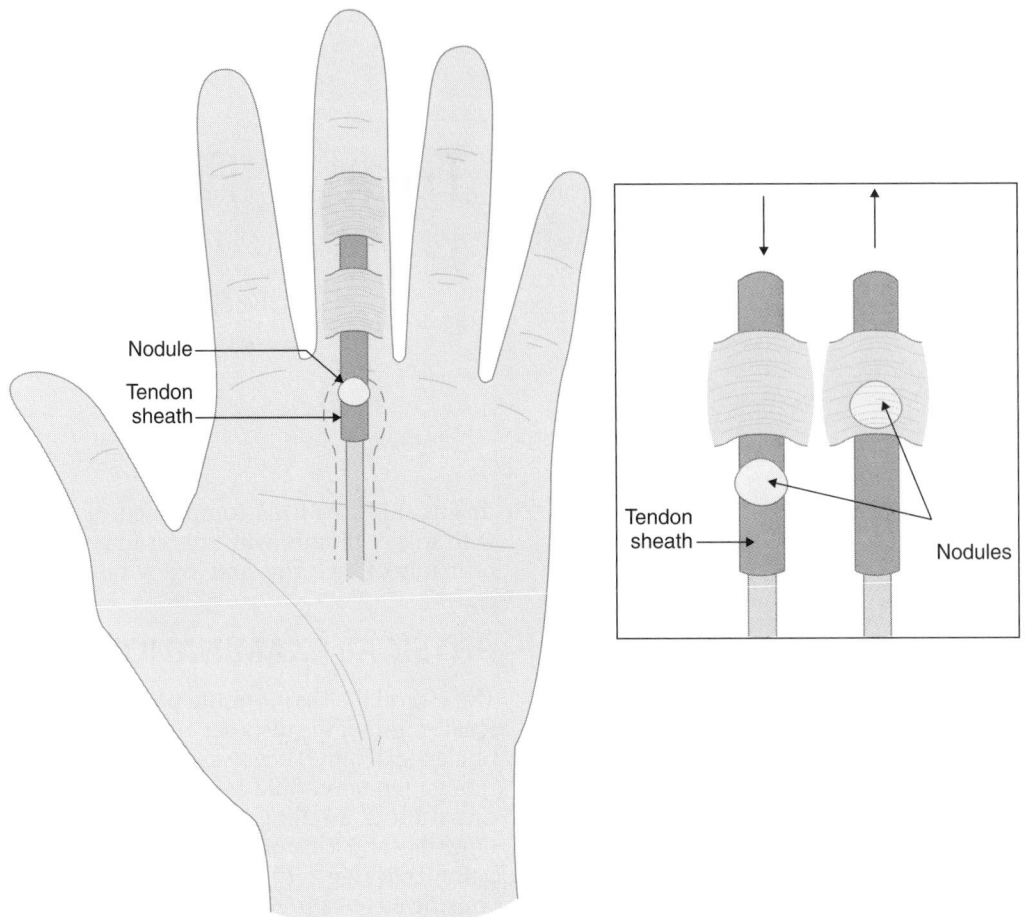

FIGURE 33-1. The flexor tendon nodule catches under the annular ligament and produces the snapping or triggering sensation.

Differential Diagnosis

Anomalous muscle belly in the palm

Dupuytren disease

Ganglion of the tendon sheath

Tumor of the tendon sheath

Rheumatoid arthritis

TREATMENT

Initial

The goal of treatment is to restore the normal gliding of the tendon through the pulley system. This can often be achieved with conservative treatment. Typically, the first line of treatment is a local steroid injection, particularly in nondiabetic patients.[14] The determination of whether to inject first or to try noninvasive measures is often based on the severity of the patient's symptoms (more severe symptoms generally respond better to injections), the level of activity of the patient (e.g., someone who needs to return to work as quickly as possible), and the patient's and clinician's preferences.

Noninvasive measures generally involve splinting of the metacarpophalangeal joint at 10 to 15 degrees of flexion with the proximal interphalangeal and distal interphalangeal joints free, for up to 6 weeks continuously.[15] This has been reported to be quite effective, although less so in the thumbs.[16] Also, splinting provides a reliable and functional means of treating work-related trigger finger without loss of time from work.[17] Additional conservative treatment includes icing of the palm (20 minutes two or three times per day in the absence of vascular disease), nonsteroidal anti-inflammatory drugs, and avoidance of exacerbating activities such as typing and repetitive gripping. Wearing padded gloves provides protection and may help decrease inflammation by avoiding direct trauma.

Rehabilitation

Rehabilitation may include treatment with an occupational or physical therapist experienced in the treatment of hand problems. Supervised therapy is generally not necessary but may be useful in the following

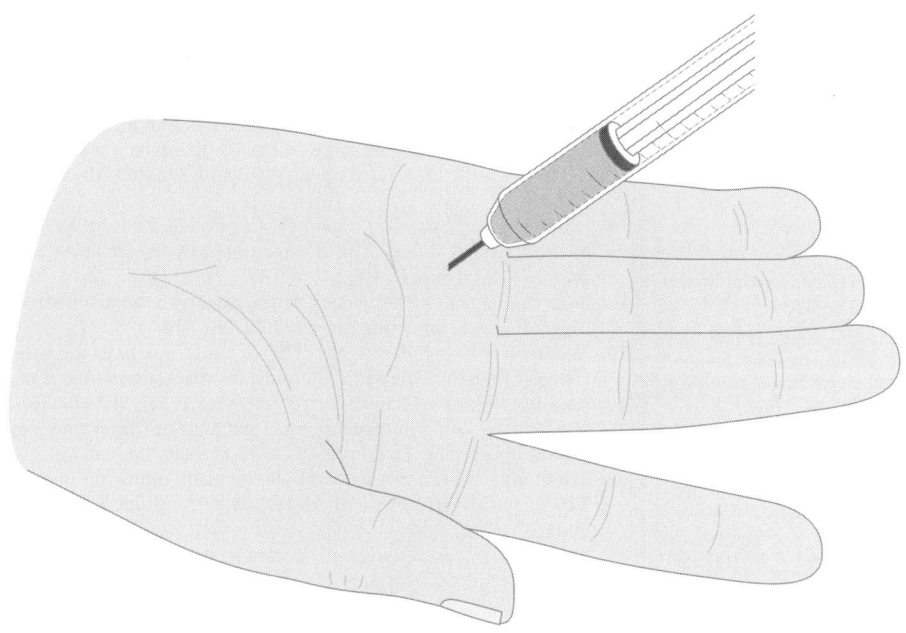

FIGURE 33-2. Under sterile conditions with use of a 27-gauge, $5/8$-inch needle, a 2- to 3-mL aliquot of a local anesthetic and steroid mixture (e.g., 1 mL of 1% lidocaine mixed with 1 mL [40 mg] of methylprednisolone) is injected into the palm at the level of the distal palmar crease, which directly overlies the tendon. Before cleaning of the area to be injected, palpate for the nodule to localize exactly where the injection should be placed.

scenarios: when a patient has lost significant strength, range of motion, or function from not using the hand, from prolonged splinting, or postoperatively; when modalities such as ultrasound and iontophoresis are recommended to reduce inflammation; and when a customized splint is deemed to be necessary.

Therapy should focus on increasing function and decreasing inflammation and pain. This can be done by techniques such as ice massage, contrast baths, ultrasound, and iontophoresis with local steroid use. For someone with a very large or small hand or other anatomic variations (e.g., arthritic joints), a custom splint may fit better and allow him or her to function at work more easily than with a prefabricated splint. Range of motion and strength can be improved through supervised therapy either before surgery or postoperatively.

Procedures

A local corticosteroid injection combined with local anesthetic (Fig. 33-2) can be used as an alternative or in addition to other management.[18,19] Postinjection care includes immediate icing of the palm for 5 to 10 minutes and then two or three times a day for 15 to 20 minutes for the next few days. A splint can be worn after injection for a few days; it will help protect the injected area and allow the medication to take effect. The patient should be cautioned that it is normal to experience some postinjection pain for the first 24 to 48 hours. In addition, the patient should be advised to avoid activities with the affected hand as much as possible for 1 week after the injection.

The injections are usually beneficial and frequently curative.[20,21] In one study, satisfactory results were obtained in 95% of digits injected with triamcinolone.[22] However, the injection may need to be repeated up to three times. This procedure is less effective with involvement of

multiple digits (such as in patients with diabetes or rheumatoid arthritis) or when the condition has persisted longer than 4 months.[21]

Surgery

Although steroid injections should be tried for most trigger finger cases before surgery is considered, surgical intervention is highly successful for conservative treatment failures and should be considered for patients desiring quick and definitive relief from this disability.[23] Individuals with diabetes and rheumatoid arthritis are more likely to require surgery.[3,24] There are two general types of surgery for this condition: the standard operative release of the A1 pulley and the percutaneous A1 pulley release procedure. In one study using a percutaneous trigger finger release technique, the success rate was 94% for "good" or "excellent" results.[25] Both surgical procedures are generally effective and carry a relatively low risk of complications.[23,26]

POTENTIAL DISEASE COMPLICATIONS

Disease-related complications include permanent loss of range of motion from development of a contracture in the affected finger, most commonly at the proximal interphalangeal joint.[2] In rare instances, chronic intractable pain may develop despite treatment.

POTENTIAL TREATMENT COMPLICATIONS

Treatment-related complications from nonsteroidal anti-inflammatory drugs are well known and include gastric, renal, and hepatic side effects. Complications from local corticosteroid injections include skin depigmentation, dermatitis, subcutaneous fat atrophy, tendon rupture, digital sensory nerve injury, and infection.[22,27] Individuals with rheumatoid arthritis are more likely to have tendon rupture[28]; therefore, repeated injections are not recommended in these cases. Possible surgical complications include infection, nerve injury, and flexor tendon bowstringing.[29-31]

References

1. Akhtar S, Bradley MJ, Quinton DN, Burke FD. Management and referral for trigger finger/thumb. BMJ 2005;331:30-33.
2. Lapidus PW. Stenosing tenovaginitis. Surg Clin North Am 1953;33:1317-1347.
3. Stahl S, Kanter Y, Karnielli E. Outcome of trigger finger treatment in diabetes. J Diabetes Complications 1997;11:287-290.
4. Gray RG, Gottlieb NL. Hand flexor tenosynovitis in rheumatoid arthritis. Prevalence, distribution, and associated rheumatic features. Arthritis Rheum 1977;20:1003-1008.
5. Bonnici AV, Spencer JD. A survey of "trigger finger" in adults. J Hand Surg Br 1988;13:202-203.
6. Verdon ME. Overuse syndromes of the hand and wrist [review]. Prim Care 1996;23:305-319.
7. Trezies AJ, Lyons AR, Fielding, K, Davis TR. Is occupation an etiological factor in the development of trigger finger? J Hand Surg Br 1998;23:539-540.
8. Tohyama M. Trigger finger caused by an old partial flexor tendon laceration: a case report. Hand Surg 2005;10:105-108.
9. Lee SJ, Pho RWH. Report of an unusual case of trigger finger secondary to phalangeal exostosis. Hand Surg 2005;10:135-138.
10. Fujiwara M. A case of trigger finger following partial laceration of flexor digitorum superficialis and review of the literature. Arch Orthop Trauma Surg 2005;125:430-432.
11. Moriya K, Uchiyama T, Kawaji Y. Comparison of the surgical outcomes for trigger finger and trigger thumb: preliminary results. Hand Surg 2005;10:83-86.
12. Katzman BM, Steinberg DR, Bozentka DJ, et al. Utility of obtaining radiographs in patients with trigger finger. Am J Orthop 1999;28:703-705.
13. Gottlieb NL. Digital flexor tenosynovitis: diagnosis and clinical significance. J Rheumatol 1991;18:954-955.
14. Nimigan AS, Ross DC, Gan BS. Steroid injections in the management of trigger fingers. Am J Phys Med Rehabil 2005;85:36-43.
15. Ryzewicz M, Wolf JM. Trigger digits: principles, management, and complications. J Hand Surg Am 2006;31:135-146.
16. Patel MR, Bassini L. Trigger fingers and thumb: when to splint, inject, or operate. J Hand Surg Am 1992;17:110-113.
17. Rodgers JA, McCarthy JA, Tiedeman JJ. Functional distal interphalangeal joint splinting for trigger finger in laborers: a review and cadaver investigation. Orthopedics 1998;21:305-309; discussion 309-310.
18. Lambert MA, Morton RJ, Sloan JP. Controlled study of the use of local steroid injection in the treatment of trigger finger and thumb. J Hand Surg Br 1992;17:69-70.
19. Benson LS, Ptaszek AJ. Injection versus surgery in the treatment of trigger finger. J Hand Surg Am 1997;22:138-144.
20. Anderson B, Kaye S. Treatment of flexor tenosynovitis of the hand ("trigger finger") with corticosteroids. A prospective study of the response to local injection. Arch Intern Med 1991;151:153-156.
21. Newport ML, Lane LB, Stuchin SA. Treatment of trigger finger by steroid injection. J Hand Surg Am 1990;15:748-750.
22. Sawaizumi T, Nanno M, Ito H. Intrasheath triamcinolone injection for the treatment of trigger digits in adults. Hand Surg 2005;10:37-42.
23. Turowski GA, Zdankiewicz PD, Thomson JG. The results of surgical treatment of trigger finger. J Hand Surg Am 1997;22:145-149.
24. Stirrat CR. Treatment of tenosynovitis in rheumatoid arthritis [review]. Hand Clin 1989;5:169-175.
25. Ragoowansi R, Acornley A, Khoo CT. Percutaneous trigger finger release: the "lift cut" technique. Br J Plast Surg 2005;58:817-821.
26. Luan TR, Chang MC, Lin CF, et al. Percutaneous A_1 pulley release for trigger digits. Zhonghua Yi Xue Za Zhi (Taipei) 1999;62:33-39.
27. Fitzgerald BT, Hofmeister EP, Fan RA, Thompson MA. Delayed flexor digitorum superficialis and profundus ruptures in a trigger finger after a steroid injection: a case report. J Hand Surg Am 2005;30:479-482.
28. Ertel AN. Flexor tendon ruptures in rheumatoid arthritis [review]. Hand Clin 1989;5:177-190.
29. Thorpe AP. Results of surgery for trigger finger. J Hand Surg Br 1988;13:199-201.
30. Heithoff SJ, Millender LH, Helman J. Bowstringing as a complication of trigger finger release. J Hand Surg Am 1988;13:567-570.
31. Carrozzella J, Stern PJ, Von Kuster LC. Transection of radial digital nerve of the thumb during trigger release. J Hand Surg Am 1989;14(pt 1):198-200

Ulnar Collateral Ligament Sprain 34

Sheila Dugan, MD

DEFINITION

The ulnar collateral ligament (UCL) complex includes the ulnar proper collateral ligament and the ulnar accessory collateral ligament.[1] These ligaments are located deep to the adductor aponeurosis of the thumb and stabilize the first metacarpophalangeal (MCP) joint. Tears can occur if a valgus force is applied to an abducted first MCP joint.[2] A lesion of the UCL is commonly called skier's thumb.

Acute injuries can occur when the strap on a ski pole forcibly abducts the thumb. In the United States, estimates for skiing injuries are three or four per 1000 skier-hours; thumb injuries account for about 10% of skiing injuries.[3] A study of downhill skiing found that thumb injuries accounted for 17% of skiing injuries, second only to knee injuries.[4] Three fourths of the thumb injuries were UCL sprains. UCL injury in football players may be related to falls or blocking. Other sports involving ball handling or equipment with repetitive abduction forces to the thumb, like basketball or lacrosse, can cause injury to the UCL.

UCL injuries may be accompanied by avulsion fractures. Complete tears can fold back proximally when they are ruptured distally and become interposed between the adductor aponeurosis.[1] This injury is known as the Stener lesion and has been described as a complication of complete UCL tears, with a frequency ranging from 33% to 80%.[5]

Chronic ligamentous laxity is more common in occupational conditions associated with repetitive stresses to the thumb. The term *gamekeeper's thumb* was coined in the mid-1950s to describe an occupational injury of Scottish gamekeepers.[6] The term is also used for acute injuries to the UCL.

SYMPTOMS

Patients report pain and instability of the thumb joint. In the acute injury setting, patients can often recall the instant of injury. If the UCL is ruptured, patients report swelling and hematoma formation; pain may be minimal with complete tears. When pain is present, it can cause thumb weakness and reduced function. Numbness and paresthesias are not typical findings.

PHYSICAL EXAMINATION

The physical examination begins with the uninvolved thumb, noting the individual's normal range of motion and stability. Palpate to determine the point of maximal tenderness, assessing for distal tenderness; if the ligament is torn, it tears distally off the proximal phalanx. Initially, the examiner may be able to detect a knot at the site of ligament disruption. Laxity of the UCL is the key finding on examination. Ligament injuries are graded as follows: grade 1 sprains, local injury without loss of integrity; grade 2 sprains, local injury with partial loss of integrity, but end-feel is present; and grade 3 sprains, complete tear with loss of integrity and end-feel (Fig. 34-1). Passive abduction can be painful, especially in acute grade 1 and grade 2 sprains.

The UCL should be tested with the first MCP joint in extension and flexion to evaluate all bands. The excursion is compared with the uninjured side. Testing for disruption of the ulnar proper collateral ligament is done with the thumb flexed to 90 degrees.[1] With the thumb in extension, a false-negative finding may result. The stability of the joint will not be impaired even if the ulnar proper collateral ligament is torn because of the taut ulnar accessory ligament in extension.

A displaced fracture is a contraindication to stress testing. The fracture presents with swelling or discoloration on the ulnar side of the first MCP joint and tenderness

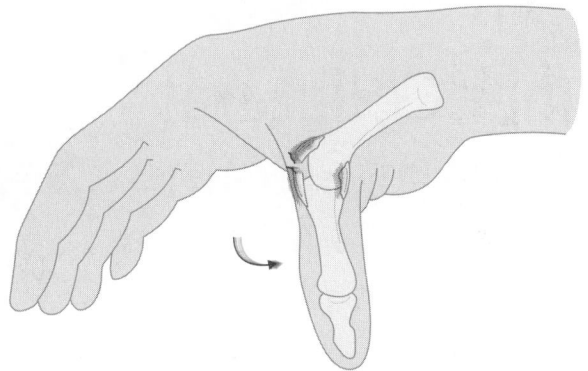

FIGURE 34-1. Skier's thumb. The ulnar collateral ligament to the metacarpophalangeal joint is disrupted by an abduction force. (Reprinted with permission from Mellion MB. Office Sports Medicine, 2nd ed. Philadelphia, Hanley & Belfus, 1996:228.)

Ultrasonography has been used as a less expensive means of diagnosing UCL tears, but controversy exists as to whether it is useful or fraught with pitfalls.[9,11-13]

> ### Differential Diagnosis
>
> Radial collateral ligament sprain or rupture
>
> First MCP joint dislocation with or without volar plate injury
>
> Thumb fracture-dislocation (Bennett fracture)

along the base of the proximal phalanx. Some authors recommend that conventional radiographs be obtained before stressing of the UCL to determine whether a large undisplaced fracture is present because stress testing could cause displacement.[7] More than 3 mm of volar subluxation of the proximal phalanx indicates gross instability. The patient may be unable to pinch.

Pain may limit the complete examination and lead to underestimation of injury extent. Infiltration of local anesthetic around the injury site can reduce discomfort and improve the accuracy of the examination.[8]

FUNCTIONAL LIMITATIONS

Individuals describe difficulty with pinching activities (e.g., turning a key in a lock). Injuries affecting the dominant hand can have an impact on many fine motor manipulations, such as buttoning or retrieving objects from one's pocket. Injuries affecting the nondominant hand can impair bilateral hand activities requiring stabilization of small objects. Sports performance can be reduced with dominant hand injuries, and skiing, ball handling, or equipment use may be contraindicated in the acute stage of injury or on the basis of the extent of injury. In the setting of high-level or professional sports competition, the clinical decision to allow an athlete to compete with appropriate splinting or casting is based on severity of symptoms, with the caveat that the potential for worsening of the injury exists.

DIAGNOSTIC STUDIES

Whereas clinical examination is the mainstay of diagnosis, imaging studies are useful in the setting of uncertain diagnosis.[9] A plain radiograph is essential to rule out an avulsion fracture of the base of the ulnar side of the proximal phalanx. A stress film with the thumb in abduction is occasionally useful and should be compared with the uninjured side. UCL rupture presents with an angle greater than 35 degrees. Magnetic resonance imaging has greater than 90% sensitivity and specificity for UCL tears but is expensive and not always required.[10]

TREATMENT

Initial

Pain and edema are managed with ice, nonsteroidal anti-inflammatory drugs, and rest. Initial treatment of a first-degree (grade 1) UCL sprain is taping for activity. Initial treatment of an incomplete (grade 2) UCL sprain involves immobilization in a thumb spica cast for 3 to 6 weeks with the thumb slightly abducted. Injuries involving nondisplaced or small avulsion fractures associated with an incomplete UCL tear can also be managed nonsurgically and may require a longer course of immobilization. The cast may be extended to include the wrist for greater stability.[14] An alpine splint allows interphalangeal flexion while prohibiting abduction and extension of the first MCP joint.[15] A study of 63 cases of nonoperative and postsurgical patients compared short arm plaster cast immobilization with functional splinting that prevented ulnar and radial deviation of the thumb; there was no difference between the two groups in regard to stability, thumb range of motion or strength, and length of sick leave after an average follow-up of 15 months.[16] Even slightly displaced avulsion fractures without complete UCL rupture tended to do well with immobilization in a study of 30 patients; those with larger bone fragments and larger initial rotation of the fragment were more likely to have residual symptoms.[17]

Grade 3 injuries require surgical repair unless surgery is contraindicated for other reasons. Prompt referral for surgical consultation is recommended to maximize ligament positioning for reattachment. Failure to refer promptly or misdiagnosis of a complete tear can result in a less favorable outcome, including a Stener lesion.[5]

Rehabilitation

Physical or occupational therapy is important in the rehabilitation management of UCL sprains. Therapists who have completed special training and are certified hand therapists (often called CHTs) can be great resources. Range of motion of the unaffected joints of the arm, especially the interphalangeal joint of the thumb, must be maintained. In the setting of a grade 1 sprain, after a short course of relative rest and taping, therapy may be required to restore strength to the preinjury level. In grade 2 sprains, a volar splint replaces the cast after 3 to 6 weeks. Splints may be custom molded by the therapist. They can be removed for daily active range of motion exercises. Passive range of motion and isometric strength training are initiated once pain at rest has resolved, and the patient is progressed to concentric exercise after about 8 weeks for nonsurgical lesions and 10 to 12 weeks for postsurgical lesions. Prophylactic taping is appropriate for transitioning back to sports-specific activity (Fig. 34-2). Postsurgical rehabilitation is less aggressive with avoidance of strengthening, especially a power pinch, for 8 weeks postoperatively.[18] Protected early postoperative range of motion is indicated.[19] Full activity after grade 2 tears with or without nondisplaced avulsion fractures begins at 10 to 12 weeks compared with 12 to 16 weeks for surgically repaired injuries.[20]

Procedures

There are no specific nonsurgical procedures performed for this injury.

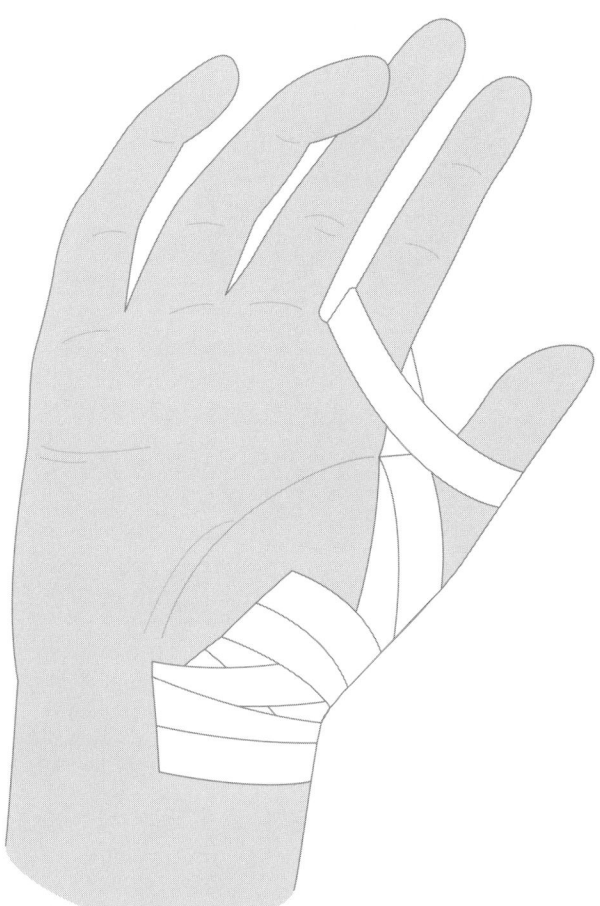

FIGURE 34-2. Taping technique to protect the ulnar collateral ligament.

Surgery

Early direct repair is required in the setting of a ruptured UCL (grade 3) injury. Grade 2 and grade 3 injuries resulting in severe instability, displaced fractures, or intra-articular fragments are also surgical candidates. Surgery is indicated in the setting of gross instability.[21] Tension wiring is used to fixate avulsions; open reduction may be required for large displaced avulsion defects. Surgical approaches that improve stability are the focus of new techniques.[22,23] However, postoperative immobilization is being reconsidered. A cadaver study concluded that a controlled active motion therapy protocol after suture anchor repair of a ruptured UCL is safe from a biomechanical point of view.[24] Reconstruction may be necessary for a chronic tear, including bone-retinaculum-bone reconstruction.[25]

POTENTIAL DISEASE COMPLICATIONS

Disease complications include chronic laxity with associated functional limitations, pain, and inability to pinch[26]; premature arthritis and persistent pain in the first MCP joint; and decreased range of motion of the thumb.

POTENTIAL TREATMENT COMPLICATIONS

Analgesics and nonsteroidal anti-inflammatory drugs have well-known side effects that most commonly affect the gastric, renal, and hepatic systems. Prolonged splinting can lead to loss of range of motion of the joint and weakness and atrophy of the surrounding joints, depending on the extent of the injury and the length of time spent in a splint. Surgical risks include nonunion of avulsed fragments and the typical infrequent surgical complications, such as infection and bleeding. Surgery can result in persistent numbness on the ulnar aspect of the thumb.

References

1. Stener B. Displacement of the ruptured ulnar collateral ligament of the metacarpophalangeal joint of the thumb. A clinical and anatomical study. J Bone Joint Surg Br 1962;44:869-879.
2. McCue FC, Hussamy OD, Gieck JH. Hand and wrist injuries. In Zachazewski JE, Magee DJ, Quillen WS, eds. Athletic Injuries and Rehabilitation. Philadelphia, WB Saunders, 1996:589-599.
3. Schneider T. Snow skiing injuries. Aust Fam Physician 2003;32:499-502.
4. Enqkvist O, Balkfors B, Lindsjo U. Thumb injuries in downhill skiing. Int J Sports Med 1982;3:50-55.
5. Louis DS, Huebner JJ, Hankin FM. Rupture and displacement of the ulnar collateral ligament of the metacarpophalangeal joint of the thumb. Preoperative diagnosis. J Bone Joint Surg Am 1986;68:1320-1326.
6. Campbell CS. Gamekeeper's thumb. J Bone Joint Surg Br 1955;37:148-149.
7. Kibler WB, Press JM. Rehabilitation of the wrist and hand. In Kibler WB, Herring SA, Press JM, eds. Functional Rehabilitation of Sports and Musculoskeletal Injuries. Gaithersburg, Md., Aspen, 1998:186-187.
8. Cooper JG, Johnstone AJ, Hider P, Ardagh MW. Local anaesthetic infiltration increases the accuracy of assessment of ulnar collateral ligament injuries. Emerg Med Australas 2005;17:132-136.

9. Koslowsky TC, Mader K, Gausepohl T, et al. Ultrasonographic stress test of the metacarpophalangeal joint of the thumb. Clin Orthop Relat Res 2004;427:115-119.

10. Plancher KD, Ho CP, Cofield SS, et al. Role of MR imaging in the management of "skier's thumb" injuries. Magn Reson Imaging Clin North Am 1999;7:73-84.

11. Hergan K, Mittler C, Oser W. Pitfalls in sonography of the gamekeeper's thumb. Eur Radiol 1997;7:65-69.

12. Susic D, Hansen BR, Hansen TB. Ultrasonography may be misleading in the diagnosis of ruptured and dislocated ulnar collateral ligaments of the thumb. Scand J Plast Reconstr Surg Hand Surg 1999;33:319-320

13. Schnur DP, DeLone FX, McClellan RM, et al. Ultrasound: a powerful tool in the diagnosis of ulnar collateral ligament injuries of the thumb. Ann Plast Surg 2002;49:19-22.

14. Reid DC, ed. Sports Injury Assessment and Rehabilitation. New York, Churchill Livingstone, 1992:1089-1092.

15. Moutet F, Guinard D, Corcella D. Ligament injuries of the first metacarpophalangeal joint. In Bruser P, Gilbert A, eds. Finger Bone and Joint Injuries. London, Martin Dunitz, 1999:207-211.

16. Kuz JE, Husband JB, Tokar N, McPherson SA. Outcome of avulsion fractures of the ulnar base of the proximal phalanx of the thumb treated nonsurgically. J Hand Surg Am 1999;24:275-282.

17. Sollerman C, Abrahamsson SO, Lundborg G, Adalbert K. Functional splinting versus plaster cast for ruptures of the ulnar collateral ligament of the thumb. A prospective randomized study of 63 cases. Acta Orthop Scand 1991;62:524-526.

18. Neviaser RJ. Collateral ligament injuries of the thumb metacarpophalangeal joint. In Strickland JW, Rettig AC, eds. Hand Injuries in Athletes. Philadelphia, WB Saunders, 1992:95-105.

19. Firoozbakhsh K, Yi IS, Moneim MS, et al. A study of ulnar collateral ligament of the thumb metacarpophalangeal joint. Clin Orthop Relat Res 2002;403:240-247.

20. Brown AP. Ulnar collateral ligament injury of the thumb. In Clark GL, Wilgis EF, Aiello B, et al, eds. Hand Rehabilitation: A Practical Guide, 2nd ed. New York, Churchill Livingstone, 1997:369-375.

21. Jackson M, McQueen MM. Gamekeeper's thumb: a quantitative evaluation of acute surgical repair. Injury 1994;25:21-23.

22. Lee SK, Kubiak EN, Liporace FA, et al. Fixation of tendon grafts for collateral ligament reconstructions: a cadaveric biomechanical study. J Hand Surg Am 2005;30:1051-1055.

23. Lee SK, Kubiak EN, Lawler E, et al. Thumb metacarpophalangeal ulnar collateral ligament injuries: a biomechanical simulation study of four static reconstructions. J Hand Surg Am 2005;30:1056-1060.

24. Harley BJ, Werner FW, Green JK. A biomechanical modeling of injury, repair, and rehabilitation of ulnar collateral ligament injuries of the thumb. J Hand Surg Am 2004;29:915-920.

25. Guelmi K, Thebaud A, Werther JR, et al. Bone-retinaculum-bone reconstruction for chronic posttraumatic instability of the metacarpophalangeal joint of the thumb. J Hand Surg Am 2003;28:685-695.

26. Smith RJ. Post-traumatic instability of the metacarpophalangeal joint of the thumb. J Bone Joint Surg Am 1977;59:14-21.

Ulnar Neuropathy (Wrist) 35

Ramon Vallarino, Jr., MD, and Francisco H. Santiago, MD

Synonym

Guyon canal entrapment

ICD-9 Code

354.2 Lesion of ulnar nerve

DEFINITION

Entrapment neuropathy of the ulnar nerve can be encountered at the wrist in a canal formed by the pisiform and the hamate and its hook (the pisohamate hiatus). These are connected by an aponeurosis that forms the ceiling of Guyon canal (Fig. 35-1). This canal generally contains the ulnar nerve and the ulnar artery and vein. The following three types of lesions can be encountered[1]:

Type I affects the trunk of the ulnar nerve proximally in Guyon canal and involves both the motor and sensory fibers. This is the most commonly seen lesion.

Type II affects only the deep (motor) branch distally in Guyon canal and may spare the abductor digiti quinti, depending on the location of its branching. A further classification is type IIa (still pure motor), in which all the hypothenar muscles are spared because of a lesion distal to their neurologic branching.

Type III affects only the superficial branch of the ulnar nerve, which provides sensation to the volar aspect of the fourth and fifth fingers and the hypothenar eminence. There is sparing of all motor function, although the palmaris brevis is affected in some cases. This is the least common lesion encountered.

This injury is commonly seen in bicycle riders and people who use a cane improperly, as they place excessive weight on the proximal hypothenar area at the canal of Guyon and therefore are predisposed to distal ulnar nerve traumatic injury, especially affecting the deep ulnar motor branch (type II).[2,3] Entrapment at Guyon canal has also been associated with prolonged, repetitive occupational use of tools, such as pliers and screwdrivers.[2]

Other rare causes have been reported in the literature. These include fracture of the hook of the hamate, gan-glion cyst formation, tortuous or thrombosed ulnar artery aneurysm (hypothenar hammer syndrome), osteoarthritis or osteochondromatosis of the pisotriquetral joint, anomalous variation of abductor digiti minimi, schwannomas, aberrant fibrous band, and idiopathic.[4-7]

SYMPTOMS

Signs and symptoms can vary greatly and depend on which part of the ulnar nerve and its terminal branches are affected and where along the Guyon canal itself (Table 35-1). It is of great importance to be able to differentiate entrapment of the ulnar nerve at the wrist from entrapment at the elbow, which occurs far more commonly. The two clinical findings that confirm the diagnosis of Guyon canal entrapment instead of ulnar entrapment at the elbow are (1) sparing of the dorsal ulnar cutaneous sensory distribution in the hand and (2) sparing of function of the flexor carpi ulnaris and the two medial heads of the flexor digitorum profundus (Figs. 35-2 and 35-3). Otherwise, the symptoms in both conditions are generally similar and may include hand intrinsic muscle weakness and atrophy, numbness in the fourth and fifth fingers, hand pain, and sometimes severely decreased function.

PHYSICAL EXAMINATION

Careful examination of the hand and a thorough knowledge of the anatomy of motor and sensory distribution of ulnar nerve innervation are required to determine the location of the lesion. Except for the five muscles innervated by the median nerve (abductor pollicis brevis, opponens pollicis, flexor pollicis brevis superficial head, and first two lumbricals), the ulnar nerve supplies every other intrinsic muscle in the hand. Classically, there is notable atrophy of the first web space due to denervation of the first dorsal interosseous muscle (Fig. 35-4). In lesions involving the motor branches, there will be weakness and eventually atrophy of the interossei, the adductor pollicis, the fourth and fifth lumbricals, and the flexor pollicis brevis deep head. The palmaris brevis, abductor digiti quinti, opponens digiti quinti, and flexor digiti quinti may be involved or spared, depending on the

187

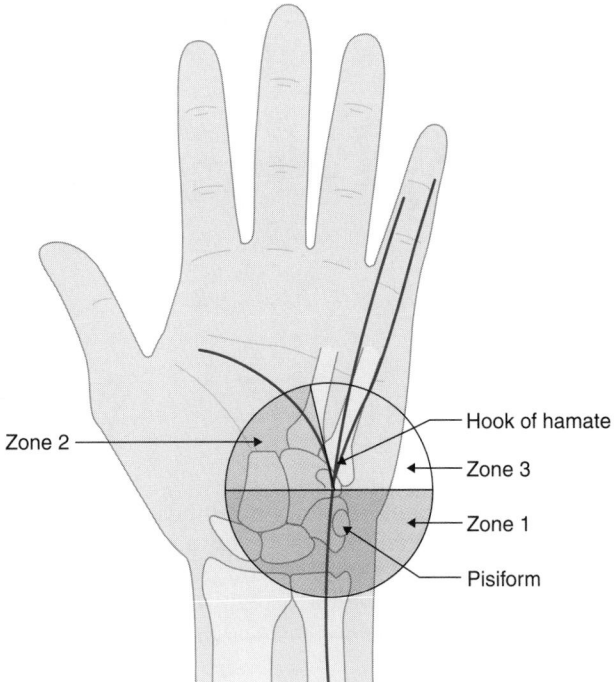

Zone 2
Hook of hamate
Zone 3
Zone 1
Pisiform

FIGURE 35-1. Distal ulnar tunnel (Guyon canal) showing the three zones of entrapment. Lesions in zone 1 give motor and sensory symptoms, lesions in zone 2 cause motor deficits, and lesions in zone 3 create sensory deficits.

lesion. Sensory examination in all but type II reveals decreased sensation of the volar aspect of the hypothenar eminence and the fourth and fifth fingers (with splitting of the fourth in most). There is always sparing of the sensation of the dorsum of the hand medially as it is innervated by the dorsal ulnar cutaneous branch of the ulnar nerve, which branches off the forearm proximal to Guyon canal.[1] The ulnar claw (hyperextension of the fourth and fifth metacarpophalangeal joints with flexion of the interphalangeal joints) seen in more proximal lesions may be more pronounced, probably because of preserved function of the two medial heads of the flexor digitorum profundus, which create a flexion moment

that is unopposed by the weakened interossei and lumbricals.[1,8] The flexor carpi ulnaris has normal strength. All the signs of intrinsic hand muscle weakness that are seen in more proximal ulnar nerve lesions, such as the Froment paper sign, are also found in Guyon canal entrapment, affecting the motor nerve fibers (Fig. 35-5).[9] Grip strength is invariably reduced in these patients when the motor branches of the ulnar nerve are affected.[10]

FUNCTIONAL LIMITATIONS

Functional loss can vary from isolated decreased sensation in the affected region to severe weakness and pain with impaired hand movement and dexterity. As can be anticipated, lesions affecting motor nerve fibers are functionally more severe than those affecting only sensory nerve fibers. The patient may have trouble holding objects and performing many activities of daily living, such as occupation, daily household chores, grooming, and dressing. Vocationally, individuals may not be able to perform the basic requirements of their jobs (e.g., operating a computer or cash register, carpentry work). This can be functionally devastating.

DIAGNOSTIC STUDIES

The cause of the clinical lesion suspected after careful history and physical examination can be investigated with the use of imaging techniques. Plain radiographs could reveal a fracture of the hamate or other carpal bones as well as of the metacarpals and the distal radius, especially if there has been a traumatic injury. Magnetic resonance imaging and computed tomography (multislice spiral computed tomographic angiography, multidetector computed tomography) can be helpful if a fracture, a tortuous ulnar artery, or a ganglion cyst is suspected.[11,12] As technology and accuracy of ultrasound equipment have advanced, there are now reports of the use of conventional and color duplex sonography to diagnose conditions such as thrombosed aneurysm of the ulnar artery.[11,13]

TABLE 35-1 Volar Forearm and Hand: Ulnar Nerve	
Muscle	**Action**
Flexor carpi ulnaris	Flexes wrist, ulnarly deviates
Flexor digitorum profundus	Flexes distal interphalangeal joint (fourth and fifth)
Abductor digiti quinti*	Analogous to dorsal interosseous
Flexor digiti quinti*†	Analogous to dorsal interosseous
Opponens digiti quinti*†	Flexes and supinates fifth metacarpal
Volar interossei*	Adducts fingers, weak flexion metacarpophalangeal
Dorsal interossei*†	Abduct fingers, weak flexion metacarpophalangeal
Lumbricals (ring and fifth)*†	Coordinate movement of fingers; extend interphalangeal joints; flex metacarpophalangeal joints
Adductor pollicis*	Adducts thumb toward index finger
Lumbricals (ring, small)*	Coordinate movement of fingers; extend interphalangeal joints; flex metacarpophalangeal joints

*Hand intrinsic muscles.
†Hypothenar mass.

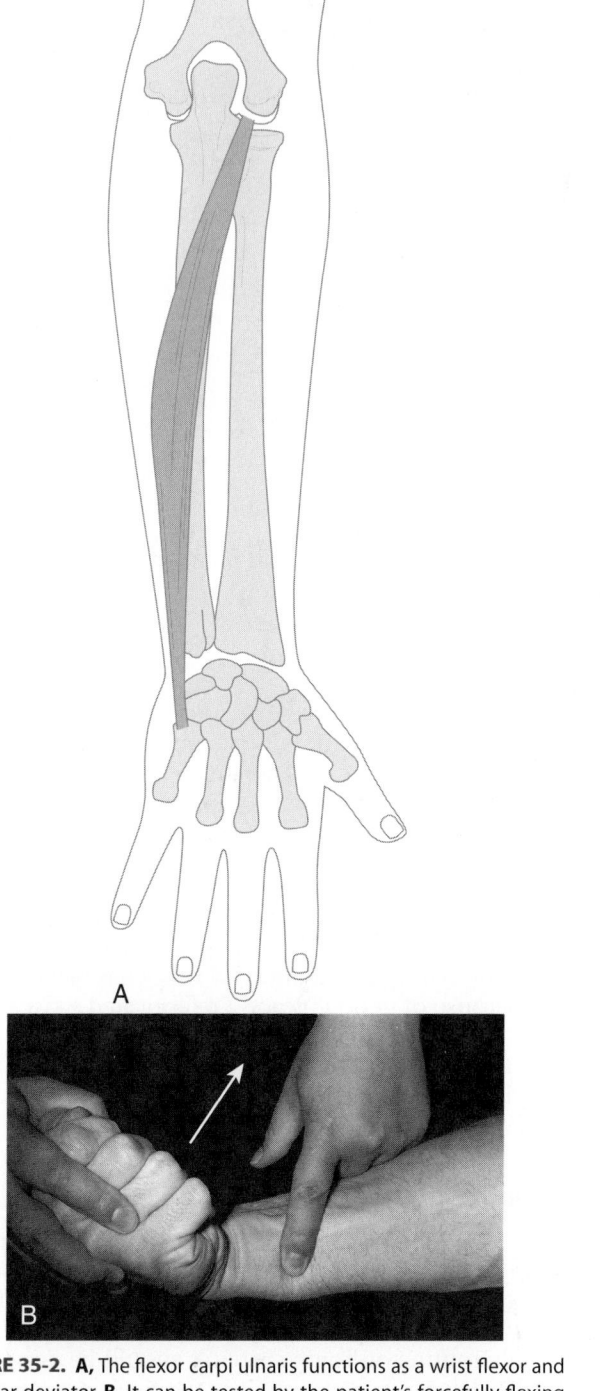

A

B

FIGURE 35-2. A, The flexor carpi ulnaris functions as a wrist flexor and an ulnar deviator. **B,** It can be tested by the patient's forcefully flexing *(arrow)* and ulnarly deviating the wrist. The clinician palpates the tendon while the patient performs this maneuver. (Reprinted with permission from Concannon MD: Common Hand Problems in Primary Care. Philadelphia, Hanley & Belfus, 1999.)

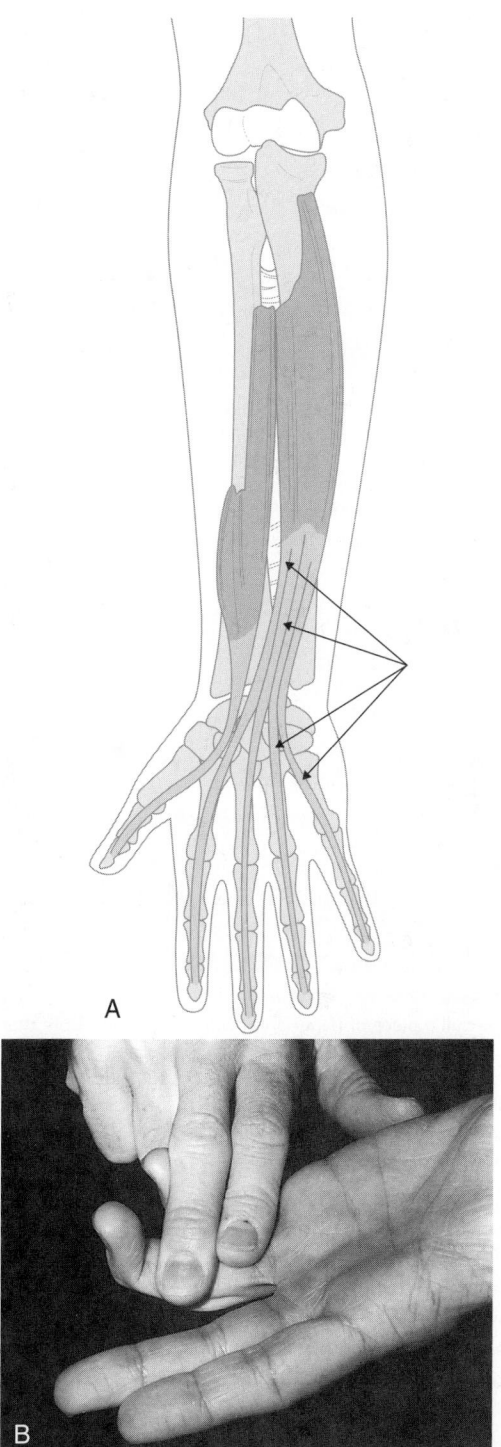

A

B

FIGURE 35-3. A, Flexor digitorum profundi *(arrows)*. **B,** These tendons can be tested by the patient's flexing the distal phalanx while the clinician blocks the middle phalanx from flexing. (Reprinted with permission from Concannon MD: Common Hand Problems in Primary Care. Philadelphia, Hanley & Belfus, 1999.)

Nerve conduction study and electromyography are helpful in confirming the diagnosis and the classification as well as in determining the severity of the lesion and the prognosis for functional recovery. As a rule, the dorsal ulnar cutaneous sensory nerve action potential is normal compared with the unaffected side.[14] Abnormalities in both sensory and motor conduction studies are seen in type I. The ulnar sensory nerve action potential recorded from the fifth finger is normal in type II, and an isolated abnormality is encountered in type III. The compound muscle action potential of the abductor digiti quinti is normal in types IIa and III. For this reason, it is important

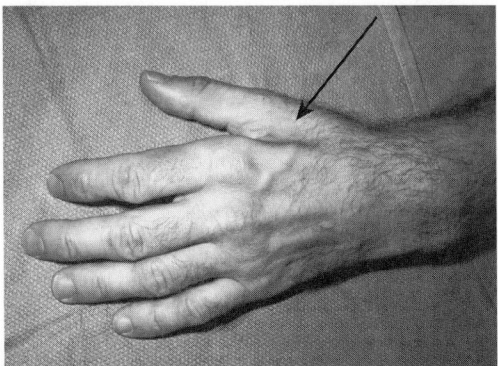

FIGURE 35-4. It is not unusual for patients with ulnar neuropathy to present with signs of muscle atrophy. It is most noticeable at the first web space, where atrophy of the first dorsal interosseous muscle leaves a hollow between the thumb and the index rays *(arrow)*. (Reprinted with permission from Concannon MD. Common Hand Problems in Primary Care. Philadelphia, Hanley & Belfus, 1999.)

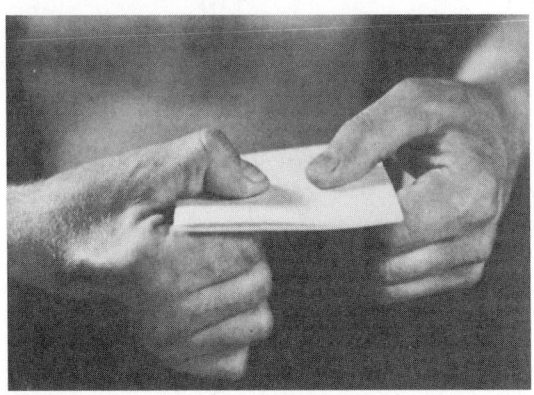

FIGURE 35-5. Ulnar nerve lesion. A patient with an ulnar nerve lesion is asked to pull a piece of paper apart with both hands. Note that the affected side (right hand) uses the flexor pollicis longus muscle to prevent the paper from slipping out of the hand, thus substituting for the adductor pollicis muscle and generating the Froment sign. (Reprinted with permission from Haymaker W, Woodhall B. Peripheral Nerve Injuries. Philadelphia, WB Saunders, 1953.)

to perform motor studies recording from more distal muscles, such as the first dorsal interosseous.[15] Motor conduction studies should include stimulation across the elbow to rule out a lesion there, as it is far more common. Furthermore, ulnar nerve stimulation at the palm, after the traditional stimulation at the wrist and across the elbow, can be useful in sorting out the location of the compression and which fascicles are affected.[16] Care must be taken not to overstimulate because median nerve–innervated muscles are very close (i.e., lumbricals 1 and 2), and their volume-conducted compound muscle action potentials could confuse the diagnosis. A "neurographic" palmaris brevis sign has been described in type II ulnar neuropathy at the wrist.[17] This consists of a positive wave preceding the delayed abductor digiti minimi motor response, presumably caused by volume-conducted depolarization of a spared palmaris brevis muscle. Needle electromyography helps in documenting axonal loss, determining severity of the lesion to allow prognosis for recovery, and more precisely localizing a lesion for an accurate classification. The flexor carpi ulnaris and the ulnar

Differential Diagnosis[18]

Ulnar neuropathy at the elbow (or elsewhere)

Thoracic outlet syndrome (generally lower trunk or medial cord)

Cervical radiculopathy at C8-T1

Motor neuron disease

Superior sulcus tumor (affecting the medial cord of the plexus)

Camptodactyly (an unusual developmental condition with a claw deformity)

heads of the flexor digitorum profundus should be completely spared in a lesion at Guyon canal.[14]

TREATMENT

Initial

Initial treatment involves rest and avoidance of trauma (especially if occupational or repetitive causes are suspected). Ergonomic and postural adjustments can be effective in these cases. The use of nonsteroidal anti-inflammatory drugs in cases in which an inflammatory component is suspected can also be beneficial. Analgesics may help control pain. Low-dose tricyclic antidepressants may be used both for pain and to help with sleep. More recently, the use of antiepileptic medications for neuropathic pain syndromes has been increasing because of good efficacy. Prefabricated wrist splints may be beneficial and are often prescribed for night use. For individuals who continue their sport or work activities, padded, shock-absorbent gloves may be useful (e.g., for cyclists, jackhammer users).

Rehabilitation

A program of physical or occupational therapy performed by a skilled hand therapist can help obtain functional range of motion and strength of the interossei and lumbrical muscles. Instruction of the patient in a daily routine of home exercises should be done early in the diagnosis. Static splinting (often done as a custom orthosis) with an ulnar gutter will ensure rest of the affected area. In more severe cases, the use of static or dynamic orthotic devices may be considered to improve the patient's functional level. Weakness in the ulnar claw deformity can be corrected to improve grasp with the use of a dorsal metacarpophalangeal block (lumbrical bar) to the fourth and fifth fingers with a soft strap over the palmar aspect.[19]

A work site evaluation may be beneficial as well. Ergonomic adaptations can prove helpful to individuals with ulnar nerve entrapment at the wrist (e.g., switching to a foot computer mouse or voice-activated computer software).

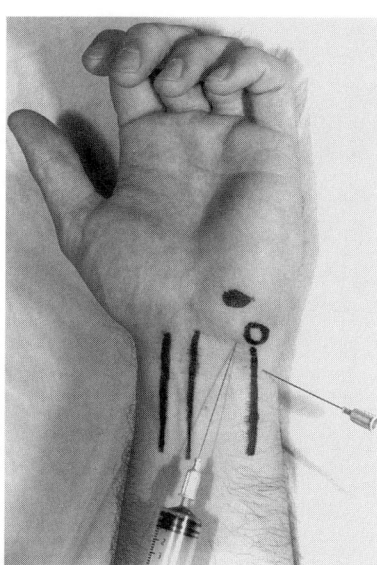

FIGURE 35-6. Approaches for two ulnar nerve blocks. The needle with syringe attached demonstrates the puncture for block at Guyon canal. The circle is over the pisiform bone, and the solid mark is over the hook of the hamate. The second needle demonstrates the puncture site for an ulnar nerve block at the wrist, ulnar approach. (Reprinted with permission from Lennard TA. Pain Procedures in Clinical Practice, 2nd ed. Philadelphia, Hanley & Belfus, 2000:104.)

Procedures

Injections into Guyon canal may be tried if a compressive entrapment neuropathy is suspected and generally provide symptomatic relief (Fig. 35-6).[2]

Under sterile conditions, with use of a 25-gauge, 1½-inch disposable needle, a mixture of corticosteroid and 1% or 2% lidocaine totaling no more than 1 mL is injected into the distal wrist crease to the radial side of the pisiform bone; the needle is angled sharply distally so that its tip lies just ulnar to the palpable hook of the hamate.[2,20] Postinjection care includes ensuring hemostasis immediately after the procedure, local icing for 5 to 10 minutes, and instructions to the patient to rest the affected limb during the next 48 hours.

Surgery

Surgery is recommended when there is a fracture of the hook of the hamate or of the pisiform or a tortuous ulnar artery that causes neurologic compromise. Ganglion cyst and pisohamate arthritis are also indications for surgical treatment. Surgery in general involves exploration, excision of the hook of hamate or pisiform (if fractured), repair of the ulnar artery as necessary, decompression, and neurolysis of the ulnar nerve.[2,4] Experience and a sound knowledge of the possible anatomic variations (i.e., muscles, fibrous bands) and the arborization patterns of the ulnar artery in Guyon canal are of great importance in promoting a positive outcome when surgery is medically necessary.[6,21]

POTENTIAL DISEASE COMPLICATIONS

The severity and type of lesion of the ulnar nerve at the wrist will ultimately determine the complications. Severe motor axon loss will cause profound weakness and atrophy of ulnar-innervated muscles in the hand and render the patient unable to perform even simple tasks because of lack of vital grip strength. Some patients also develop chronic pain in the affected hand, which can be severely debilitating, perhaps inciting a complex regional pain syndrome, and it can predispose them to further problems such as depression and drug dependency.

POTENTIAL TREATMENT COMPLICATIONS

The use of nonsteroidal anti-inflammatory drugs should be carefully monitored because there are potential side effects, including gastrointestinal distress and cardiac, renal, and hepatic disease. Low-dose tricyclic antidepressants are generally well tolerated but may cause fatigue, so they are usually prescribed for use in the evening. Injection complications include injury to a blood vessel or nerve, infection, and allergic reaction to the medication used. Complications after surgery include infection, wound dehiscence, recurrence, and, rarely, complex regional pain syndrome.

References

1. Dumitru D. Electrodiagnostic Medicine. Philadelphia, Hanley & Belfus, 1995:887-891.
2. Dawson D, Hallet M, Millender L. Entrapment Neuropathies, 2nd ed. Boston, Little, Brown, 1990:193-195.
3. Akuthota V, Plastaras C, Lindberg K, et al. The effect of long-distance bicycling on ulnar and median nerves: an electrodiagnostic evaluation of cyclist palsy. Am J Sports Med 2005;33:1224-1230.
4. Murata K, Shih JT, Tsai TM. Causes of ulnar tunnel syndrome: a retrospective study of 31 subjects. J Hand Surg Am 2003;28:647-651.
5. Harvie P, Patel N, Ostlere SJ. Prevalence of epidemiological variation of anomalous muscles at Guyon's canal. J Hand Surg Br 2004;29:26-29.
6. Bozkurt MC, Tajil SM, Ozcakal L, et al. Anatomical variations as potential risk factors for ulnar tunnel syndrome: a cadaveric study. Clin Anat 2005;18:274-280.
7. Jose RM, Bragg T, Srivata S. Ulnar nerve compression in Guyon's canal in the presence of a tortuous ulnar artery. J Hand Surg Br 2006;31:200-202.
8. Liveson JA, Spielholz NI. Peripheral Neurology: Case Studies in Electrodiagnosis. Philadelphia, FA Davis, 1991:162-165.
9. Haymaker W, Woodhall B. Peripheral Nerve Injuries. Philadelphia, WB Saunders, 1953.
10. Snider RK. Essentials of Musculoskeletal Care. Rosemont, Ill, American Academy of Orthopaedic Surgeons, 1997:260-262.
11. Coulier B, Goffin D, Malbecq S, Mairy Y. Colour duplex sonographic and multislice spiral CT angiographic diagnosis of ulnar artery aneurysm in hypothenar hammer syndrome. Journal Belge de Radiologie 2003;86:211-214.
12. Blum AG, Zabel JP, Kohlman R, et al. Pathologic conditions of the hypothenar eminence: evaluation with multidetector CT and MR imaging. Radiographics 2006;26:1021-1044.
13. Peeters EY, Nieboer KH, Osteaux MM. Sonography of the normal ulnar nerve at Guyon's canal and of the common peroneal nerve dorsal to the fibular head. J Clin Ultrasound 2004;32:375-380.

14. Kim DJ, Kalantri A, Guha S, Wainapel SF. Dorsal cutaneous nerve conduction: diagnostic aid in ulnar neuropathy. Arch Neurol 1981;38:321-322.

15. Witmer B, DiBenedetto M, Kang CG. An improved approach to the evaluation of the deep branch of the ulnar nerve. Electromyogr Clin Neurophysiol 2002;42:485-493.

16. Wee AS. Ulnar nerve stimulation at the palm in diagnosing ulnar nerve entrapment. Electromyogr Clin Neurophysiol 2005;45:47-51.

17. Morini A, Della Sala WS, Bianchini G, et al. "Neurographic" palmaris brevis sign in type II degrees ulnar neuropathy at the wrist. Clin Neurophysiol 2005;116:43-48.

18. Patil JJP. Entrapment neuropathy. In O'Young BJ, Young MA, Stiens SA, eds. Physical Medicine and Rehabilitation Secrets, 2nd ed. Philadelphia, Hanley & Belfus, 2002:144-150.

19. Irani KD. Upper limb orthoses. In Braddom RL, ed. Physical Medicine and Rehabilitation. Philadelphia, WB Saunders, 1996: 328-330.

20. Mauldin CC, Brooks DW. Arm, forearm, and hand blocks. In Lennard TA, ed. Physiatric Procedures. Philadelphia, Hanley & Belfus, 1995:145-146.

21. Murata K, Tamaj M, Gupta A. Anatomic study of arborization patterns of the ulnar artery in Guyon's canal. J Hand Surg Am 2006;31:258-263.

Wrist Osteoarthritis 36

José M. Nolla, MD, and Chaitanya S. Mudgal, MD, MS (Orth), MCh (Orth)

Synonyms

Degenerative arthritis of the wrist
Osteoarthritis of the wrist
Post-traumatic arthritis of the wrist
SLAC wrist
SNAC wrist

ICD-9 Codes

715.1	Osteoarthrosis, localized, primary, wrist
715.2	Osteoarthrosis, localized, secondary, wrist
716.1	Traumatic arthropathy, wrist
718.83	Other joint derangement, not elsewhere classified, wrist
719.03	Joint effusion, wrist
719.13	Pain in joint, wrist
842.01	Wrist sprain

DEFINITION

Osteoarthritis of the wrist refers to the painful degeneration of the articular surfaces that make up the wrist due to noninflammatory arthritides. It commonly affects the joints between the distal radius and the proximal row of carpal bones. Symptoms include pain, swelling, stiffness, and crepitation. Radiographs will reveal different degrees of joint space narrowing, cyst formation, subchondral sclerosis, and osteophyte formation.

The most common etiology of wrist osteoarthritis is post-traumatic, as can be seen after distal radius fractures, carpal fractures, and carpal instability.[1] Rare conditions that may cause it include idiopathic osteonecrosis of the lunate (Kienböck disease) and the scaphoid (Preiser disease). As opposed to idiopathic osteoarthritis of the thumb carpometacarpal joint, which is seen in more than 90% of women older than 80 years,[2] idiopathic osteoarthritis of the wrist is rare.

Distal radius fractures that have healed inappropriately (malunited) can also be the cause (Fig. 36-1). In considering malunited fractures of the distal radius, abnormal parameters that have been shown to be associated with wrist arthritis include the following: on an anteroposterior radiograph, an intra-articular step-off of more than 2 mm and radial shortening of more than 5 mm; and on the lateral radiograph, a dorsal angulation of more than 10 degrees.[3-5]

Carpal fractures that fail to heal, particularly of the scaphoid, can also be the cause of arthritis.[6] This bone is predisposed to nonunions biologically because of its fragile vascular supply and biomechanically on account of the shear forces it encounters.[7,8] Other factors associated with nonunions include fracture displacement, fracture location, and delay in initiation of treatment.[9,10] Features of a scaphoid nonunion that appear to be associated with arthritis are the displacement of the cartilaginous surfaces and the loss of carpal stability.[11,12] Both of these lead to abnormal loading of the cartilage and consequently to ensuing arthritis. This pattern of arthritis is known as scaphoid nonunion advanced collapse (SNAC) (Fig. 36-2).

Carpal instability can also result in uneven loading of the articular surfaces and subsequent arthritis[13] (Figs. 36-3 and 36-4). The most common form of carpal instability is scapholunate dissociation.[14] It consists of a disruption of the interosseous ligament between the scaphoid and lunate. The resultant abnormal biomechanics lead to abnormal loading and subsequent arthritis, a pattern known as scapholunate advanced collapse[1] (SLAC).

SYMPTOMS

Wrist pain is the presenting symptom in the overwhelming majority of patients. For the most part, this pain is of insidious onset, although many patients will recall a particular event that brought it to their attention. It is diffusely located across the dorsum of the wrist. It may be activity related and may bear little correlation to radiographic findings. Patients may also report inability to do their daily activities because of weakness, but on further questioning, this weakness is often secondary to pain.

Another presenting symptom is stiffness, particularly in flexion and extension of the wrist. Pronation and supination are usually not affected, unless the arthritic process is extensive and also involves the distal radioulnar

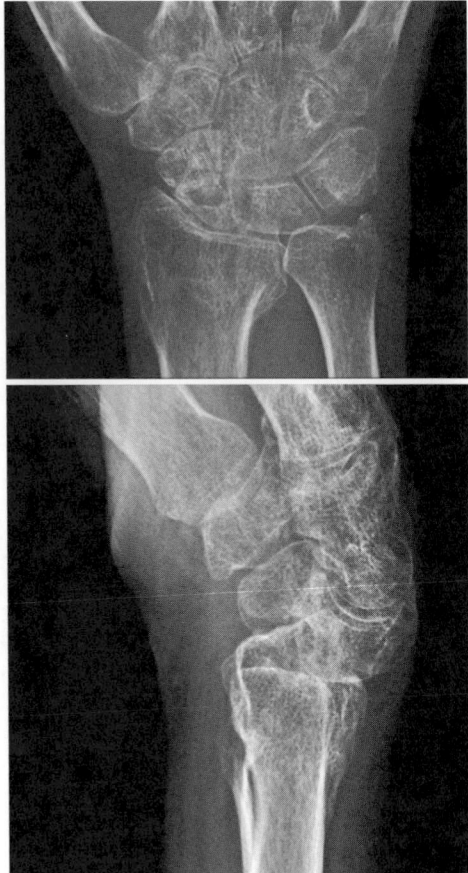

FIGURE 36-1. Wrist osteoarthritis secondary to a malunited wrist frac-ture. Note the dorsal angulation of the distal articular surface and the reduced joint space. This patient also had significant osteopenia second-ary to pain-induced lack of use.

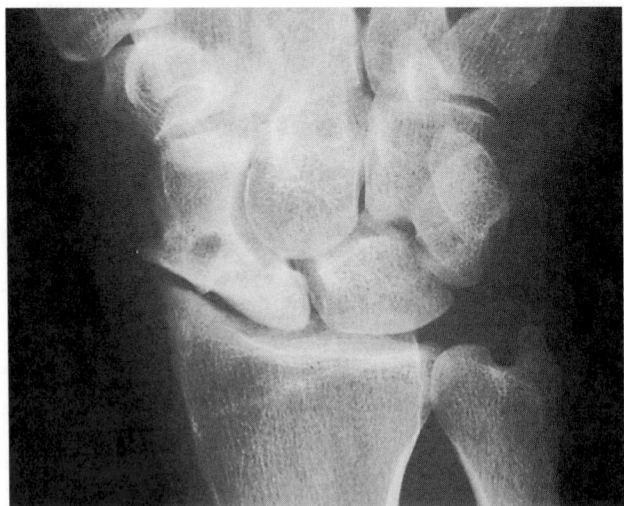

FIGURE 36-2. Osteoarthritic change of a wrist with a scaphoid nonunion (SNAC), stage 2. Notable features include the "beaked" appearance of the radial styloid, cystic change along with a nonunion in the scaphoid, and "kissing" osteophytes on adjoining surfaces of the radius and scaphoid.

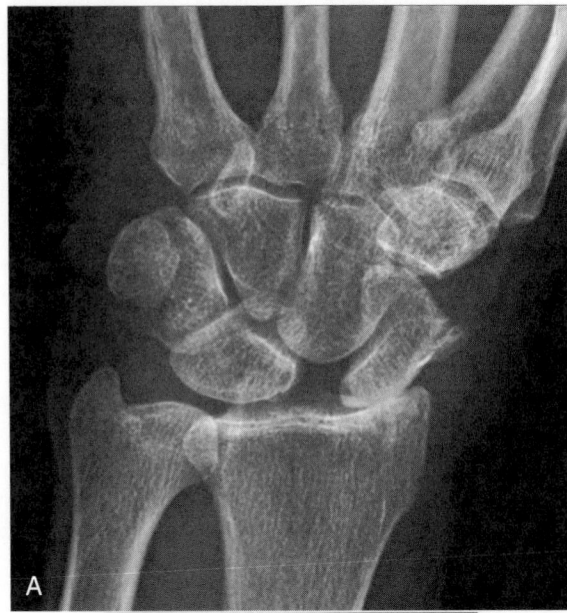

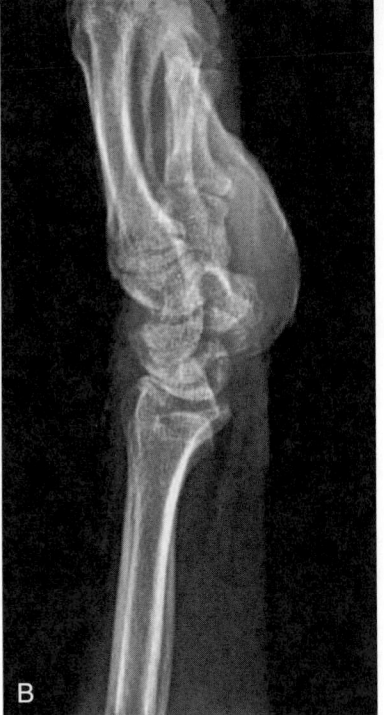

FIGURE 36-3. **A** and **B,** Wrist osteoarthritis secondary to scapholunate advanced collapse (SLAC), stage 2. Note the increased scapholunate space and the sclerosis of the radioscaphoid joint. Early osteophytes are clearly seen on the radial border of the scaphoid. The lateral view shows dorsal osteophytes as well as the dorsally angled lunate.

joint. Motion may also be associated with a clicking sensation or with audible crepitation.

Complaints about cosmetic deformity are also common, particularly after distal radius fractures that have healed with an inappropriate alignment. Swelling is also com-monly noted. This swelling is essentially a representa-tion of the malunited fracture, but in patients with ad-vanced arthritis irrespective of the etiology, it may represent synovial hypertrophy or osteophyte formation.

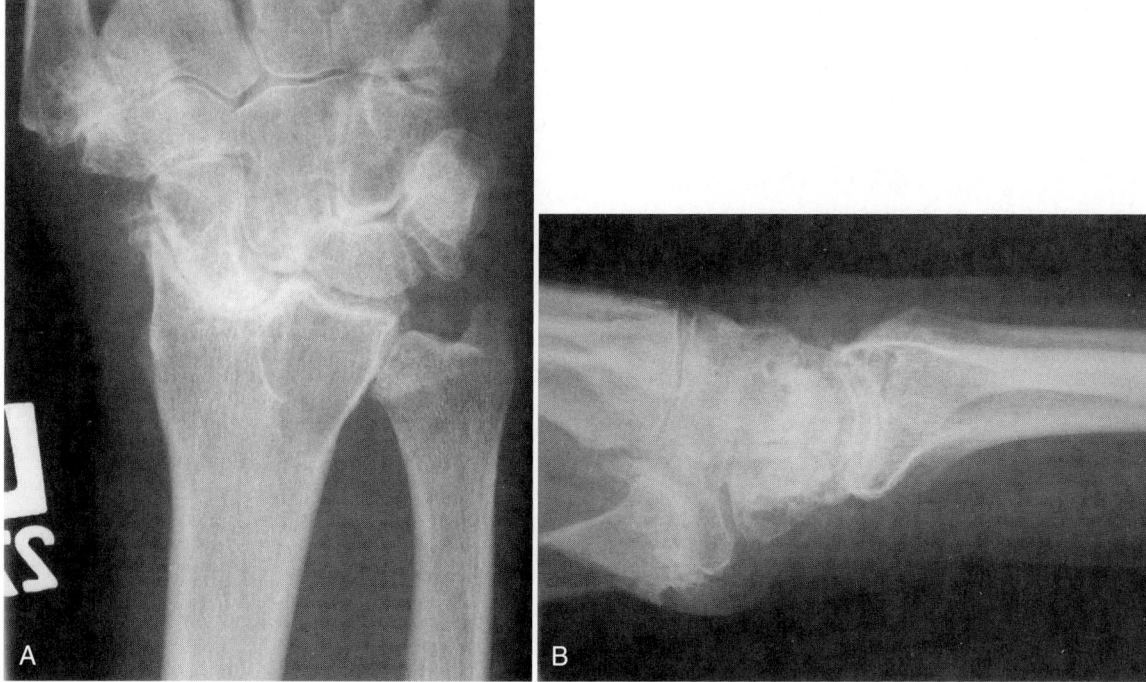

FIGURE 36-4. A and **B,** Advanced wrist osteoarthritis secondary to SLAC (stage 3). Note the increased scapholunate space, the sclerosis in the radioscaphoid and lunocapitate joints, and the proximal migration of the capitate. Most notable in both views is the complete loss of normal wrist alignment.

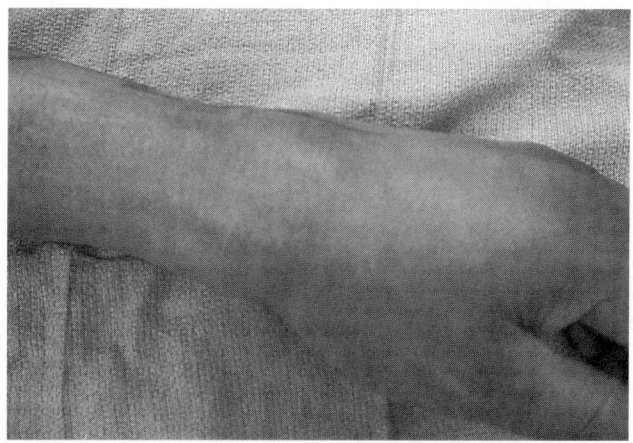

FIGURE 36-5. Clinical appearance of an osteoarthritic wrist that in this particular instance was secondary to a scaphoid nonunion. The diffuse radiodorsal swelling indicates some degree of synovitis.

In this situation, the swelling tends to be located in the dorsoradial region of the wrist (Fig. 36-5).

PHYSICAL EXAMINATION

Examination of the wrist includes a thorough examination of the entire upper limb. Comparison with the opposite side is useful to determine the degree of motion loss, if any. In wrist osteoarthritis, the most obvious finding may be loss of motion. Normal range of motion includes approximately 80 degrees of flexion, 60 degrees of extension, 20 degrees of radial deviation, and 40 degrees of ulnar deviation.[15]

The wrist is palpated for evidence of cysts or tenderness. Tenderness just distal to Lister tubercle may be a sign of pathologic change at the scapholunate joint, including scapholunate dissociation, Kienböck disease, or synovitis of the radiocarpal joint. Tenderness at the anatomic snuffbox may indicate a scaphoid fracture or nonunion, and in early SNAC, wrists may be the site of radioscaphoid degeneration. In the presence of pancarpal arthritis, the tenderness is usually diffuse.

Provocative maneuvers should also be performed to check for signs of carpal instability. The scaphoid shift test of Watson tests for scapholunate instability.[16] In this test, the examiner places a thumb volarly on the patient's scaphoid tubercle, and the rest of the fingers wrap around the wrist to lie dorsally over the proximal pole of the scaphoid. As the wrist is taken from ulnar deviation to radial deviation, the thumb will apply pressure on the scaphoid tubercle and force the scaphoid to sublux out of its fossa dorsally in ligamentously lax patients as well as in those with frank scapholunate instability. Once pressure from the thumb is released, the scaphoid will then shift back into its fossa. This finding is best demonstrated in those who are ligamentously lax or those with recent injuries. Patients who have chronic injuries often develop sufficient fibrosis to prevent subluxation of the scaphoid out of its fossa. However, they often still have pain that is reproduced with the maneuver. Comparison with the unaffected side is essential, especially if the patient has evidence of generalized ligamentous laxity.

The strength of the abductor pollicis brevis is tested by asking the patient to palmar abduct the thumb against resistance, and it should be compared with the opposite side. Similarly, the strength of the first dorsal interosseus should be checked by asking the patient to radially deviate the index finger against resistance. These tests evaluate for motor deficits of the median nerve and ulnar nerve, respectively. Sensation should also be compared with the opposite side. Whereas static two-point discrimination is an excellent way to test sensation in the office, a more precise evaluation of early sensory deficits can be performed by graduated Semmes-Weinstein monofilaments. Frequently, this test requires a referral to occupational therapists who perform it.

FUNCTIONAL LIMITATIONS

The majority of the limitations in wrist arthritis arise from a lack of motion. A range of motion from 10 degrees of flexion to 15 degrees of extension is required for activities involving personal care.[17] The loss of motion mainly affects activities of daily living such as washing one's back, fastening a brassiere, and writing. Eating, drinking, and using a telephone require 35 degrees of extension. However, learned compensatory maneuvers can allow most activities of daily living to be accomplished with as little as 5 degrees of flexion and 6 degrees of extension.[18]

DIAGNOSTIC STUDIES

The initial evaluation of the arthritic wrist includes standard posteroanterior, lateral, and pronated oblique radiographs. In the posteroanterior view, any evidence of arthritis between the radius and proximal row of carpal bones or between the proximal and distal rows should be noted. Radiographic features that indicate an arthritic process include reduction or loss of joint space, osteophyte formation, cyst formation in periarticular regions, and loss of normal bone alignment (see Figs. 36-2 to 36-4).

Injury to the scapholunate ligament is evidenced by a space between the scaphoid and the lunate greater than 2 mm and a cortical ring sign of the scaphoid.[14] Sclerosis or collapse of the lunate is consistent with Kienböck disease.[19] The lateral view can reveal signs of carpal instability, such as a dorsally or palmarly oriented lunate. An angle between the scaphoid and the lunate in excess of 60 degrees is also consistent with scapholunate dissociation. The oblique view will often demonstrate the site of a scaphoid nonunion. Although it may be possible to make a diagnosis of scapholunate dissociation on plain radiographs, some patients can often have bilateral scapholunate distances and angles in excess of normal limits. It is therefore critical to obtain contralateral radiographs before a diagnosis of scapholunate injury is made.

Patterns of arthritic progression in SLAC and SNAC wrists have been classified into three stages. In a SLAC wrist, stage 1 involves arthritis between the radial styloid and the distal pole of the scaphoid; stage 2 results in reduction or loss of joint space between the radius and the proximal pole of the scaphoid (see Fig. 36-3), and stage 3 indicates

capitolunate degeneration with proximal migration of the capitate between the scaphoid and lunate (see Fig. 36-4). In a SNAC wrist, stage 1 and stage 3 are similar to those in a SLAC wrist. However, in stage 2, there is degenerative change between the distal pole of the scaphoid and capitate (see Fig. 36-2).

Other imaging modalities are not necessary for the diagnosis of osteoarthritis. Computed tomography is sometimes used to evaluate the alignment of the scaphoid fragments in cases of nonunion and the amount of collapse of the lunate in Kienböck disease. Magnetic resonance imaging is occasionally used to evaluate the vascularity of the scaphoid proximal pole and lunate in scaphoid nonunions and Kienböck disease, respectively.[19,20] Wrist arthroscopy offers the optimal ability to assess the condition of the articular cartilage; however, this assessment can be made from plain radiographs or at the time of surgical reconstruction of the wrist.

Differential Diagnosis

Acute fracture

Septic arthritis

Crystalline arthritis

Carpal tunnel syndrome

Rheumatoid arthritis

de Quervain tenosynovitis

TREATMENT

Initial

Osteoarthritis of the wrist is a condition that has usually been present for a significant amount of time. However, it is not uncommon for symptoms to be of a short duration, and they can often be manifested after seemingly trivial trauma. It is important for the physician to establish good rapport with the patient during several visits so that the pathophysiologic changes of the process can be emphasized to the patient. This becomes even more important in situations involving workers' compensation or litigation or both. It is also important for the patient to understand that the condition cannot be reversed and that the symptoms are likely to be cyclic. Patients must understand that over time, the condition may worsen radiographically; however, it is impossible to predict the rate of progression or severity of symptoms that might ensue.

Many patients present with symptoms of wrist osteoarthritis that are not severe enough to be limiting but enough to be noticed. These patients are often looking for reassurance about their condition. If they are able to do all the activities that they want to do, intervention is not needed. They should not refrain from doing their activities in fear that they may accelerate the condition; there is no scientific evidence to substantiate this concern. This approach offers the least amount of risk to the patient.

Other patients may prefer to have some symptom reduction, particularly during episodes of acute worsening, despite some inconvenience or small risks. An over-the-counter wrist splint with a volar metal stabilizing bar (cock-up splint) can be a small inconvenience; however, by virtue of immobilizing the wrist, it can provide great symptom relief during daily activities. This metal bar can be contoured to place the wrist in the neutral position rather than in extension, as most splints of this nature tend to do. The neutral position appears to be better tolerated by patients and affords better compliance with splint wear. Nonsteroidal anti-inflammatory drugs can also provide significant pain relief, particularly during periods of acute exacerbation of symptoms. A long-term use of nonsteroidal anti-inflammatory drugs is not indicated. Periodic application of ice, especially during periods of acute symptom exacerbation, can be of help. On occasion, in patients with radioscaphoid arthritis (SNAC), inclusion of the thumb in a custom-made orthoplast splint may provide better pain relief.

Rehabilitation

Once the acute inflammation phase has passed, most patients are able to resume most activities. Some may complain of persistent lack of motion or strength. These patients may benefit from a home exercise program for range of motion and strengthening directed by an occupational therapist. Modalities such as fluidized therapy may help with range of motion. Static progressive splinting is usually not recommended to improve range of motion because there is often a bone block to motion. It is always important to understand that therapy itself may worsen symptoms, especially passive stretching exercises. Active range of motion and active-assisted range of motion exercises are better tolerated by patients, and some patients may be better off without any formal rehabilitation.

Procedures

Nonsurgical procedures, including corticosteroid injections, may be indicated for wrist osteoarthritis, although they appear to have a greater use in crystalline and inflammatory arthritides. Hyaluronan injections for osteoarthritis have been studied in other joints, including the thumb carpometacarpal joint, with beneficial results; however, their use in the wrist is still considered experimental.[21] Typically, all injections around the wrist should be done by aseptic technique with a 25-gauge, 1½-inch needle and a mixture of a nonprecipitating, water-soluble steroid preparation that is injected along with 2 mL of 1% lidocaine.

The radiocarpal joint can be injected from the dorsal aspect approximately 1 cm distal to Lister tubercle, with the needle angled proximally about 10 degrees to account for the slight volar tilt of the distal radius articular surface. This is done with the wrist in the neutral position. Gentle longitudinal traction by an assistant can help widen the joint space, which may be reduced on account of the disease. An alternative radiocarpal injection site is the ulnar wrist, just palmar to the extensor carpi ulnaris tendon at the level of the ulnar styloid process. With strict aseptic technique, a 25-gauge, 1½-inch needle is inserted into the ulnocarpal space, just distal to the ulnar styloid, just dorsal or volar to the easily palpable tendon of the extensor carpi ulnaris. The needle must be angled proximally by 20 to 30 degrees to enter the space between the ulnar carpus and the head of the ulna. It is important to ascertain that the injectate flows freely. Any resistance indicates a need to reposition the needle appropriately. Alternatively, the injection may be performed by fluoroscopic guidance with the help of a mini image intensifier, if one is available in the office.

If a midcarpal injection is required, this is done through the dorsal aspect, under fluoroscopic guidance, with injection into the space at the center of the lunate-triquetrum-hamate-capitate region.

Surgery

The goal of surgery in an osteoarthritic wrist is pain relief. Surgical procedures for osteoarthritis can be divided into motion-sparing procedures and fusions (arthrodesis). However, even motion-sparing procedures often result in significant loss of motion. This is very important in patients who have almost no motion preoperatively. These patients will not benefit from motion-sparing procedures and are better served with total wrist fusions. The decision to proceed with surgery should not be made until nonsurgical means have been tried for an adequate time, which usually amounts to a period of 3 to 6 months. In some patients who are going to have a total wrist fusion, before a decision is made about surgery, it is useful to apply a well-molded fiberglass short arm cast for 2 weeks to accustom the patient to the lack of wrist motion.

Motion-sparing procedures include proximal row carpectomy and limited intercarpal fusions with scaphoid excision. The excision of the scaphoid is essential because 95% of wrist arthritis involves the scaphoid.[1] Proximal row carpectomy involves removal of the scaphoid, lunate, and triquetrum. The capitate then articulates with the radius through the lunate fossa (Fig. 36-6). Wrist stability is maintained by preserving the volar wrist ligaments. As a prerequisite for this procedure, the lunate fossa of the radius and the articular surface over the head of the capitate must be healthy and free of degenerative change (Fig. 36-7). The main advantage of this procedure is that it does not involve any fusions. After a short period of postoperative casting, patients are allowed to start moving the wrist as early as 3 weeks after surgery. Most people are able to attain a flexion-extension arc of 60 to 80 degrees and 60% to 80% of the grip strength of the uninvolved side[22,23] (Fig. 36-8). This

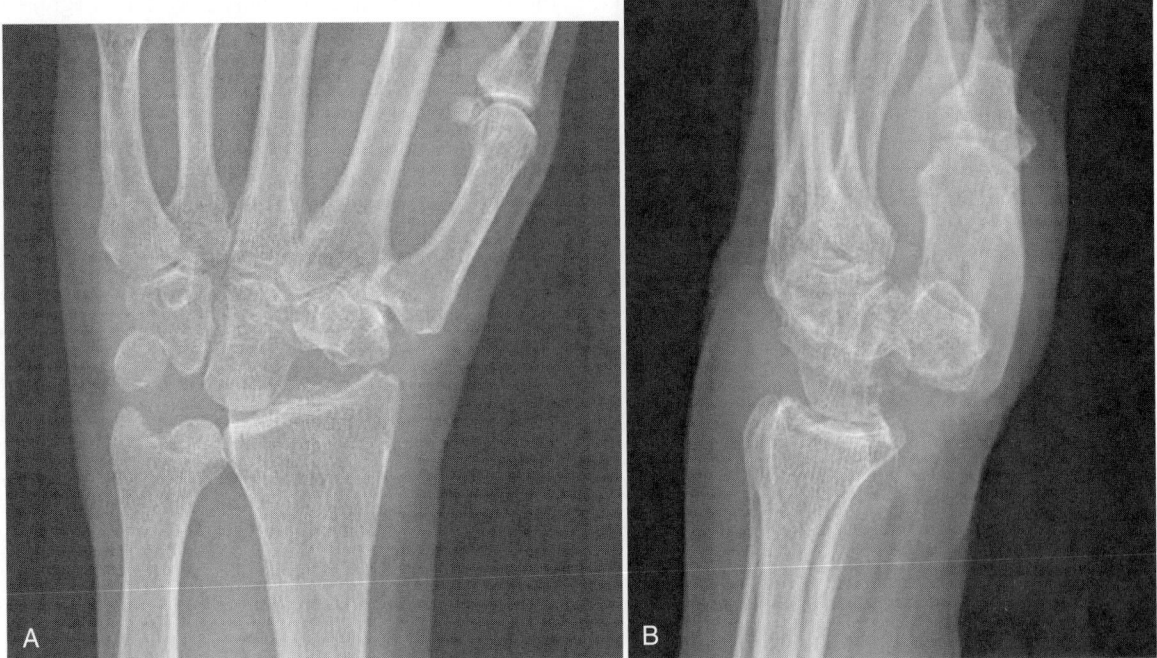

FIGURE 36-6. A and **B,** Plain radiographs of the patient seen in Figure 36-3 after she underwent a proximal row carpectomy. A terminal radial sty-loidectomy has also been performed to reduce impingement of the trapezium on the tip of the radius. Note how well the capitate articulates with the lunate fossa of the distal radius.

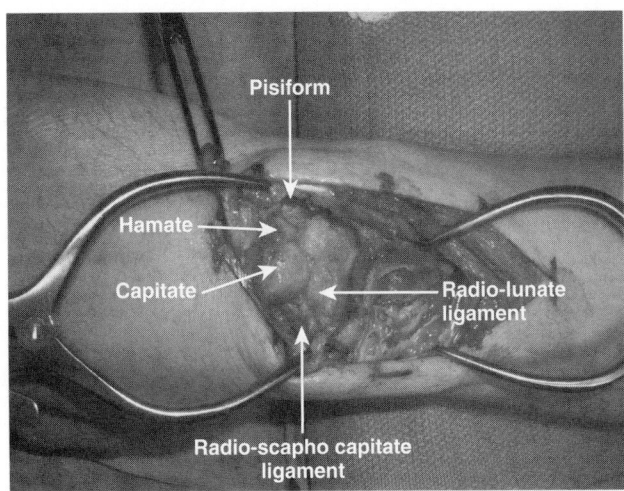

FIGURE 36-7. An intraoperative photograph of the patient seen in Figures 36-3 and 36-6, during a proximal row carpectomy, to show healthy articular cartilage over the head of the capitate.

procedure is appropriate for the early stages of SLAC and SNAC arthritis.

The most common limited intercarpal fusion is known as the four-corner or four-bone fusion. It involves creating a fusion mass between the lunate, triquetrum, capitate, and hamate. The scaphoid is excised. The prerequisite for this procedure is an intact joint between the radius and the lunate. A theoretical advantage of this procedure over a proximal row carpectomy is that it maintains carpal height, leading to a better grip strength

(Fig. 36-9). However, this has not been shown to be the case in larger studies comparing these two procedures. The flexion-extension arc of wrist motion is also not significantly different between these two procedures.[23] Theoretical disadvantages of a four-corner fusion include protracted immobilization until fusion is confirmed (usually 8 weeks) and the possibility of needing a secondary operative procedure to remove hardware (Fig. 36-10). This procedure is also appropriate for the early stages of SLAC and SNAC arthrosis.

Patients with severe arthrosis that involves not only the radiocarpal joint but also the joint between the proximal and distal carpal rows (midcarpal joint) are better served with total wrist fusion. This procedure is also beneficial in patients who present preoperatively with minimal or no wrist motion. It involves a fusion between the radius, proximal row, and distal row of carpal bones. The wrist is protected with a splint for 4 to 6 weeks. Most patients are able to attain a grip strength that is 60% to 80% of the opposite side.[24] A successful fusion abolishes the flexion-extension arc of wrist motion and, more important, can be effective in obtaining pain relief. However, the lost motion makes it difficult for patients to position the hand in tight spaces and can affect perineal care.[25] In these patients, the loss of motion does not appear to have an adverse functional impact because most of these patients have significant reduction of motion at the time of presentation. The pain relief provided by this procedure, however, can have a positive impact on functional outcome to a significant degree. Pronation and supination are unaffected. This procedure is appropriate for the advanced stages of SLAC and SNAC arthritis (Fig. 36-11).

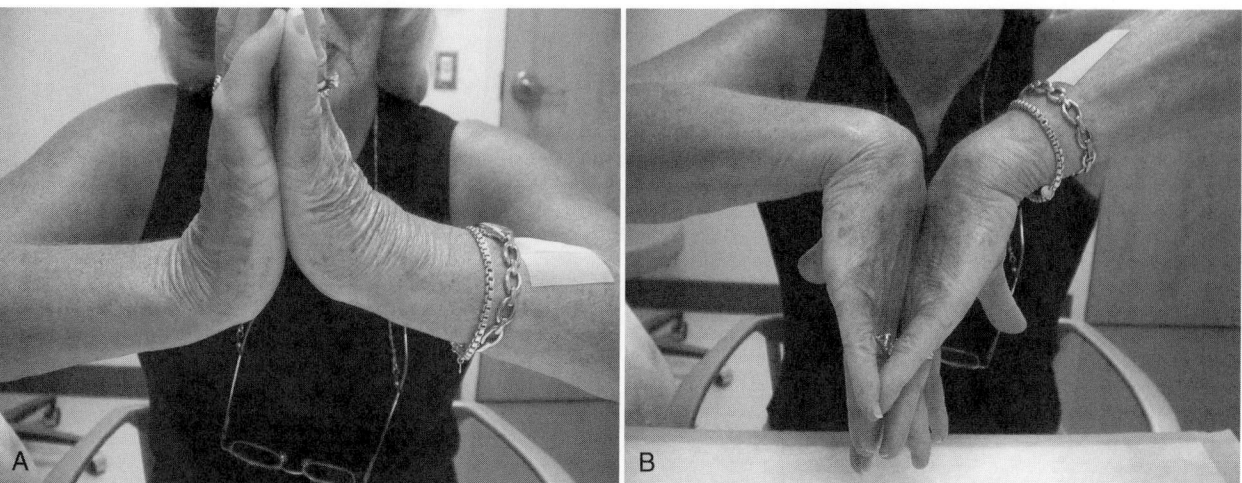

FIGURE 36-8. **A** and **B,** Postoperative function 6 months after a proximal row carpectomy. The patient has recovered nearly a 100-degree arc of motion and has no pain.

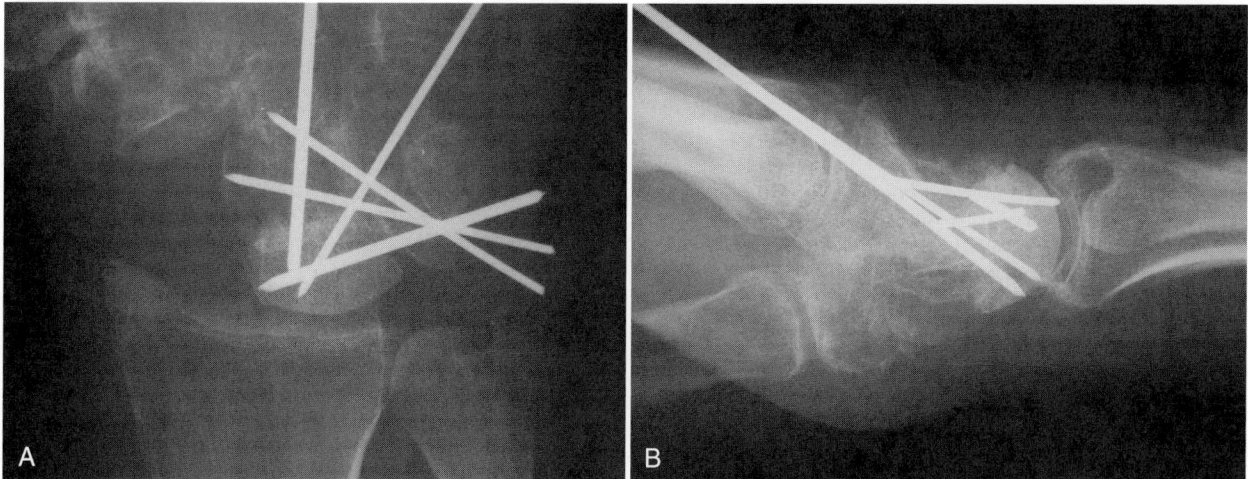

FIGURE 36-9. **A** and **B,** Postoperative radiographs after scaphoid excision and four-bone fusion have been performed.

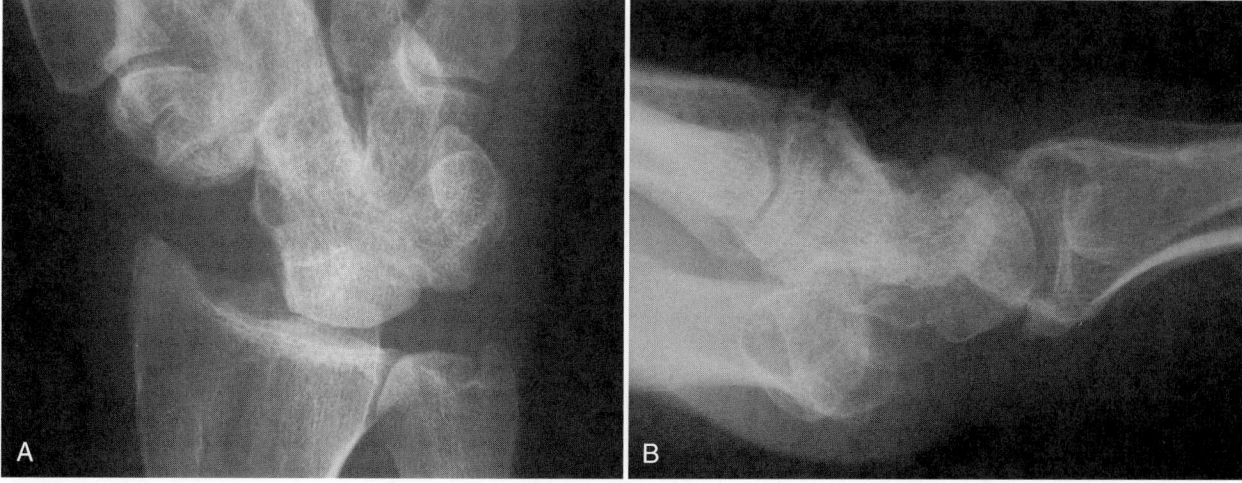

FIGURE 36-10. **A** and **B,** A mature four-bone fusion after a secondary procedure to remove the pins seen in Figure 36-9. To avoid the second operative procedure, some may elect to leave the pins percutaneous and to remove them during an office visit.

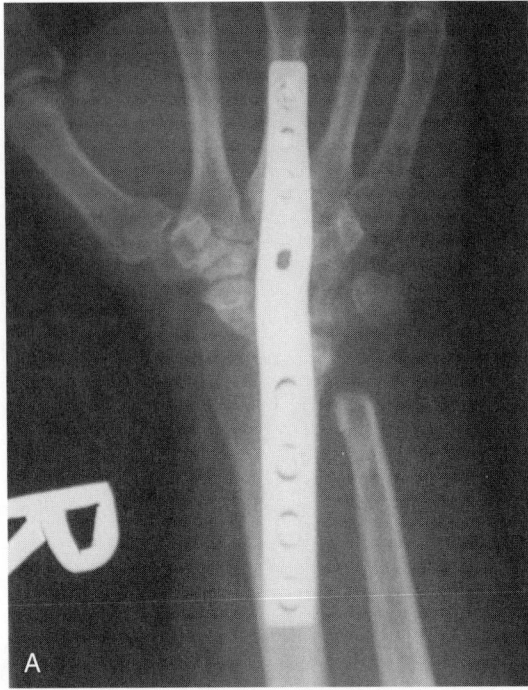

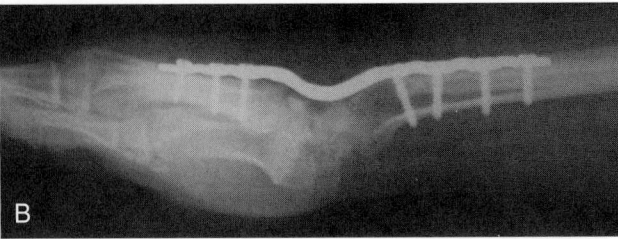

FIGURE 36-11. A and **B,** A total wrist arthrodesis with a contoured plate and screws. In the anteroposterior radiograph, it is evident that the wrist is in mild ulnar deviation; in the lateral radiograph, the wrist appears to be in mild dorsiflexion. This is the optimal position for hand function in such patients. The patient also underwent excision of the distal ulna.

POTENTIAL DISEASE COMPLICATIONS

Wrist osteoarthritis that progresses to advanced stages results in severely painful limitation of motion. Patients are unable to do their activities of daily living because any load across the arthritic wrist joint results in pain. The pain and stiffness can also inhibit the ability of the patient to position the hand in space. Rarely, osteophytes occurring over the dorsal aspect of the distal radius and the distal radioulnar joint can cause attritional ruptures of extensor tendons.

POTENTIAL TREATMENT COMPLICATIONS

Nonsteroidal anti-inflammatory medicines carry risks to the cardiovascular, gastric, renal, and hepatic systems. For these reasons, these medications are typically used for short periods. Surgery exposes the patient to significant risks from anesthesia, infection, nerve injury, and tendon injury. Fusions carry the risk of nonunion and malunion as well as that of hardware complications, such as prominence of the hardware, tendon irritation, and metal sensitivity. Motion-sparing procedures can eventually lead to further degenerative disease (Fig. 36-12) and in the presence of symptoms may require further surgery, which most commonly consists of a total wrist fusion.

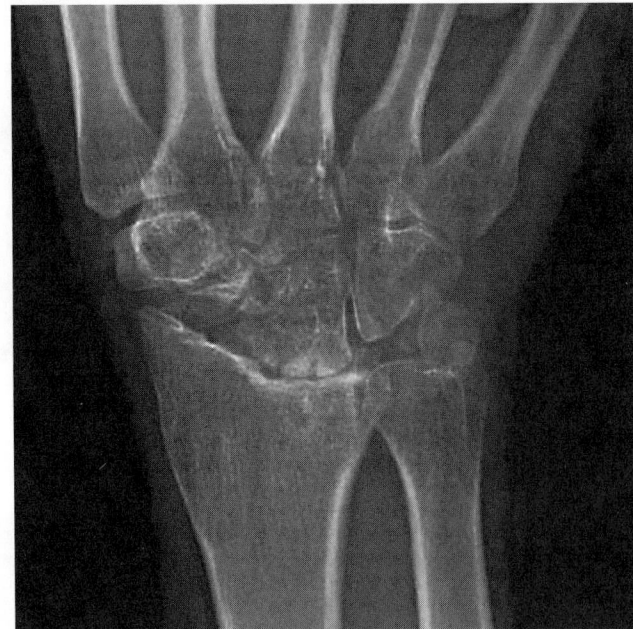

FIGURE 36-12. Advanced degenerative disease in a patient who underwent a proximal row carpectomy a few years before. Despite the radiographic appearance, the patient reported only mild pain.

References

1. Watson HK, Ballet FL. The SLAC wrist: scapholunate advanced collapse pattern of degenerative arthritis. J Hand Surg Am 1984;9:358-365.
2. Sodha S, Ring D, Zurakowski D, Jupiter JB. Prevalence of osteoarthrosis of the trapeziometacarpal joint. J Bone Joint Surg Am 2005;87:2614-2618.
3. Knirk JL, Jupiter JB. Intra-articular fractures of the distal end of the radius in young adults. J Bone Joint Surg Am 1986;68:647-659.
4. Aro HT, Koivunen T. Minor axial shortening of the radius affects outcome of Colles' fracture treatment. J Hand Surg Am 1991;16:392-398.
5. Gliatis JD, Plessas SJ, Davis TR. Outcome of distal radial fractures in young adults. J Hand Surg Br 2000;25:535-543.
6. Ruby LK, Stinson J, Belsky MR. The natural history of scaphoid non-union. A review of fifty-five cases. J Bone Joint Surg Am 1985;67:428-432.
7. Gelberman RH, Menon J. The vascularity of the scaphoid bone. J Hand Surg Am 1980;5:508-513.
8. Slade JF 3rd, Dodds SD. Minimally invasive management of scaphoid nonunions. Clin Orthop Relat Res 2006;445:108-119.
9. Cooney WP, Linscheid RL, Dobyns JH. Scaphoid fractures. Problems associated with nonunion and avascular necrosis. Orthop Clin North Am 1984;15:381-391.
10. Osterman AL, Mikulics M. Scaphoid nonunion. Hand Clin 1988;4:437-455.
11. Lindstrom G, Nystrom A. Incidence of post-traumatic arthrosis after primary healing of scaphoid fractures: a clinical and radiological study. J Hand Surg Br 1990;15:11-13.
12. Mack GR, Bosse MJ, Gelberman RH, Yu E. The natural history of scaphoid non-union. J Bone Joint Surg Am 1984;66:504-509.
13. O'Meeghan CJ, Stuart W, Mamo V, et al. The natural history of an untreated isolated scapholunate interosseous ligament injury. J Hand Surg Br 2003;28:307-310.
14. Walsh JJ, Berger RA, Cooney WP. Current status of scapholunate interosseous ligament injuries. J Am Acad Orthop Surg 2002;10:32-42.
15. Ryu J, Cooney WP III, Askew LJ, et al. Functional ranges of motion of the wrist joint. J Hand Surg Am 1991;16:409-419.
16. Watson HK, Weinzweig J. Physical examination of the wrist. Hand Clin 1997;13:17-34.
17. Brumfield RH, Champoux JA. A biomechanical study of normal functional wrist motion. Clin Orthop Relat Res 1984;187:23-25.
18. Nissen KL. Symposium on cerebral palsy (orthopaedic section). Proc R Soc Med 1951;44:87-90.
19. Allan CH, Joshi A, Lichtman DM. Kienböck's disease: diagnosis and treatment. J Am Acad Orthop Surg 2001;9:128-136.
20. Simonian PT, Trumble TE. Scaphoid nonunion. J Am Acad Orthop Surg 1994;2:185-191.
21. Fuchs S, Monikes R, Wohlmeiner A, Heyse T. Intra-articular hyaluronic acid compared with corticoid injections for the treatment of rhizarthrosis. Osteoarthritis Cartilage 2006;14:82-88.
22. Imbriglia JE, Broudy AS, Hagberg WC, McKernan D. Proximal row carpectomy: clinical evaluation. J Hand Surg Am 1990;15:426-430.
23. Cohen MS, Kozin SH. Degenerative arthritis of the wrist: proximal row carpectomy versus scaphoid excision and four-corner arthrodesis. J Hand Surg Am 2001;26:94-104.
24. Bolano LE, Green DP. Wrist arthrodesis in post-traumatic arthritis: a comparison of two methods. J Hand Surg Am 1993;18:786-791.
25. Weiss AC, Wiedeman G Jr, Quenzer D, et al. Upper extremity function after wrist arthrodesis. J Hand Surg Am 1995;20:813-817.

Wrist Rheumatoid Arthritis 37

Brian T. Fitzgerald, MD, and Chaitanya S. Mudgal, MD, MS (Orth), MCh (Orth)

Synonyms

Rheumatoid wrist
Synovitis of the wrist
Tenosynovitis of the wrist
Rheumatoid synovial hypertrophy

ICD-9 Codes

714.0   Rheumatoid arthritis
718.93 Joint derangement, wrist
719.43 Joint pain, wrist
727.00 Synovitis, wrist
727.05 Tenosynovitis
736.00 Joint deformity

DEFINITION

Rheumatoid arthritis is a systemic autoimmune disorder involving the synovial joint lining and is characterized by chronic symmetric erosive synovitis. It has been estimated that 1% to 2% of the world's population is affected by this disorder. Women are affected more frequently, and the ratio of gender involvement is 2.5:1. The wrist is among the most commonly involved peripheral joints; more than 65% of patients have some symptoms within 2 years of diagnosis, and more than 90% have symptoms by 10 years.[1-3] The wrist articulation can be divided into three compartments, all of which are synovium lined and therefore involved in rheumatoid arthritis: the radiocarpal, midcarpal, and distal radioulnar joints. If medical control of the disease is inadequate, significant damage to joint cartilage and tendons can occur and also may be accompanied by nerve compression syndromes.

Three specific processes are involved in the pathophysiologic development of rheumatoid disease: cartilage degradation, synovial proliferation or expansion, and ligamentous laxity.[4] The cascade of events that lead to articular cartilage damage is thought to begin when platelets, leukocytes, and fibrin clots injure the lumina of synovial endothelial cells. The specific trigger for this endothelial damage is theorized to be the expression of vascular and intercellular adhesion molecules, which promotes the migration of inflammatory cells into the synovium.[5] The result is thickening and proliferation of the synovium, chemotactic attraction of polymorphonuclear cells, and release by the polymorphonuclear cells of lysosomal enzymes and free oxygen radicals. These enzymes destroy joint cartilage and the synovial proliferation causes changes in tendons of both an ischemic and inflammatory nature, which make them susceptible to weakening and eventual rupture.

Expansion of the synovium leading to symmetric erosive joint changes is the sine qua non of rheumatoid disease.[4] Areas of the wrist that display vascular penetration into bone or contain significant synovial folds, such as the radial attachment of the radioscaphocapitate ligament (the most radial of the volar radiocarpal ligaments), the waist of the scaphoid, and the base of the ulnar styloid (prestyloid recess), are the most common sites of progressive synovitis. The results of chronic erosive changes in these areas are bone spicules that can abrade and weaken tendons passing in their immediate vicinity, ultimately causing rupture and functional deterioration. The extensor tendons to the small finger and ring finger and the flexor tendon of the thumb are the most commonly involved. At the wrist, the extensor tendons are enclosed in a sheath of synovium, which makes them susceptible to the damaging changes of synovial hypertrophy that is commonly seen in rheumatoid arthritis.

Both cartilage loss from degradation and synovial proliferation contribute to ligamentous laxity by causing stretching of the normally stout volar radioscaphocapitate ligament, which is an important stabilizer of the carpus in relation to the distal radius. Laxity around the wrist leads to the classic rheumatoid deformities of carpal supination and ulnar translocation. In addition to ulnar translocation of the carpus, laxity of the volar radioscaphocapitate ligament leads to loss of the ligamentous support to the waist of the scaphoid. The scaphoid responds by adopting a flexed posture, and this is accompanied by radial deviation of the hand at the radiocarpal articulation in addition to the ulnar translocation. When the bony carpus supinates, the distal radius subluxates palmarly and the ulna is left relatively prominent on the dorsal aspect of the wrist, a condition sometimes referred to as the caput ulnae syndrome.[6,7] This bone prominence and expanding synovitis in the distal radioulnar joint can cause injury to the extensor tendons in the area. The secondary effect of carpal supination is subluxation of the extensor carpi ulnaris tendon in a volar direction, to the point that it no longer functions effectively as a wrist extensor. The bony architecture of the wrist is affected secondarily, in that the inflammatory cascade also stimulates bone-resorbing osteoclasts, which cause subchondral and periarticular osteopenia.

SYMPTOMS

Three distinct areas of the wrist can be the source of symptoms from rheumatoid disease: the extensor tendons, the distal radioulnar joint, and the radiocarpal joint. However, symptoms can originate as far proximal as the cervical spine or involve the shoulder and the elbow.

Joint-related symptoms in early disease include swelling and pain, with morning stiffness as a classic characteristic. Symmetric involvement of the wrists is commonly present. Loss of motion in the early stages usually results from synovial hypertrophy and pain. Progressive loss of motion is seen with disease progression and represents articular destruction. The prominence of the ulnar head at the distal radioulnar joint can be painful because of inflammation within the joint, and it can be a source of decreased forearm rotation (Figs. 37-1 and 37-2).

Symptoms of median nerve compression and dysfunction creating altered or absent sensation primarily in the radially sided digits and night pain and paresthesias in the hand can be associated with rheumatoid arthritis as well. This is primarily due to hypertrophy of the tenosynovium around the flexor tendons within the confined space of the carpal canal, with resulting compression of the median nerve.

Tenosynovitis of the tendons traversing the dorsal wrist can often present as a painless swelling. Patients with advanced rheumatoid disease in the wrist or those unresponsive to medical management may present with loss of extension of the digits at the metacarpophalangeal joints or with inability to flex the thumb at the interphalangeal articulation. These findings result from extensor digitorum communis tendon ruptures over the dorsal aspect of the wrist or a rupture of the flexor pollicis longus. Deformity of the wrist and hand is often the most concerning factor for patients and is attributable to the progressive carpal rotation and translocation discussed earlier, coupled with the extensor tendon imbalance accentuated at the metacarpophalangeal joints of the hand, which causes ulnar drift of the digits.

Radial deviation at the radiocarpal joint combined with ulnar translocation of the carpus leads to radially directed digits. This, in turn, accentuates the pull of the long extensors that approach the metacarpophalangeal joints from an ulnar direction. Thus, a compensatory ulnar deviation occurs at the metacarpophalangeal joints, and it can often be the presenting symptom in undiagnosed or untreated patients.

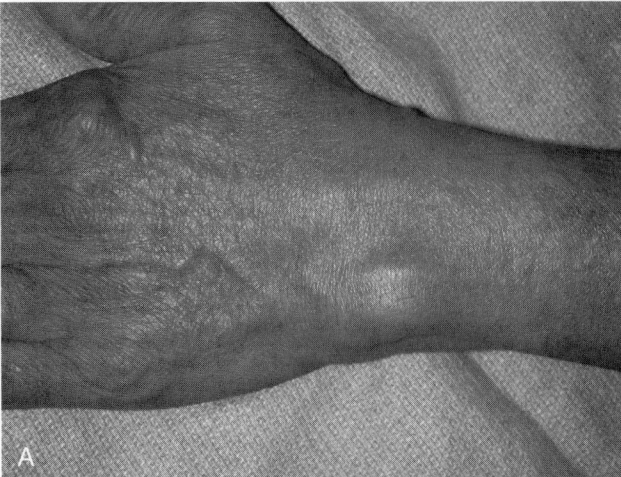

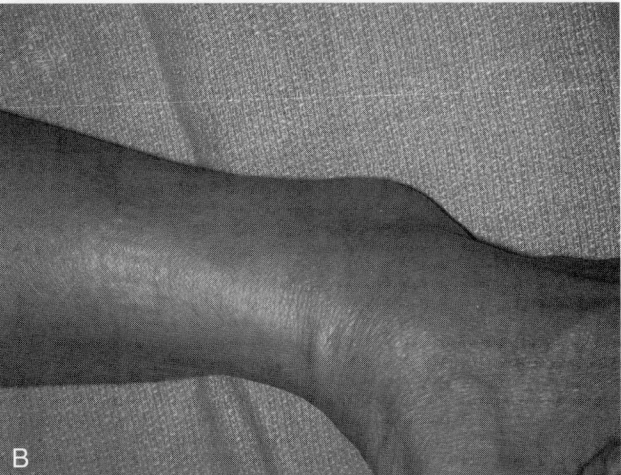

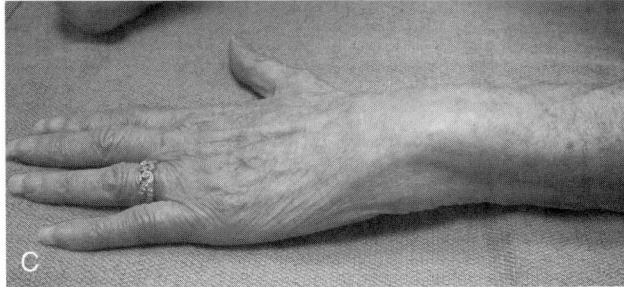

FIGURE 37-1. A, Appearance of the wrist in early rheumatoid arthritis. Note the swelling around the ulnar head. **B,** The synovial hypertrophy around the head of the ulna and distal radioulnar joint is appreciated in profile. There is also an early radial deviation of the hand at the wrist. **C,** The prominence of the ulnar head is compounded by the subluxation and supination of the carpus, creating an appearance of an abrupt change in contour from the wrist to the hand.

Later stages of the disease usually are manifested with complaints of severe pain, decreased motion, significant cosmetic concerns, and difficulties in performing activities of daily living.

PHYSICAL EXAMINATION

Keeping in mind the three primary locations of rheumatoid involvement in the wrist, careful physical examination can help identify the sources of pain and

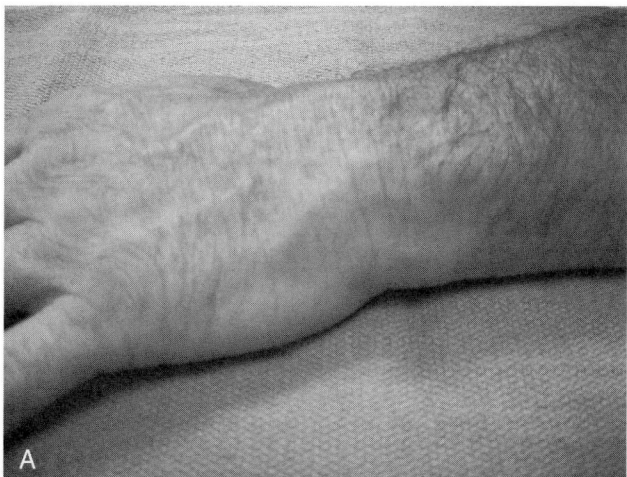

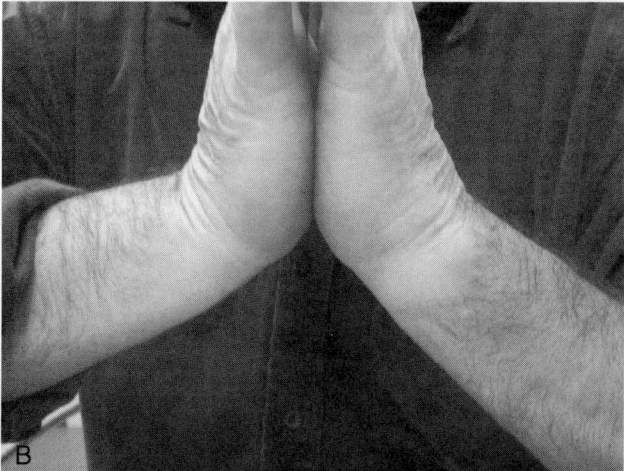

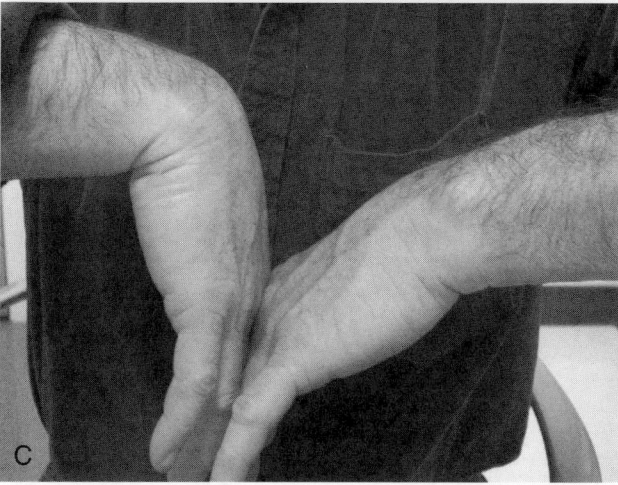

FIGURE 37-2. A, Synovitis around the distal end of the ulna may be manifested with swelling just volar to the ulnar styloid, as in this patient. **B** and **C,** Loss of motion in early rheumatoid disease of the wrist, as in this patient, is often a manifestation of the synovitis and pain associated with it rather than a true joint destruction.

processes. An inflamed synovial membrane surrounding the radiocarpal joint is usually tender to palpation, but there can be surprisingly little swelling on examination if it is confined only to the dorsal capsule. Swelling that is related to the joint usually does not display movement with passive motion of the digits. Tenosynovitis, however, is typically painless and nontender and moves with tendon excursion as the digits are moved.

Distal radioulnar joint involvement is confirmed with tenderness to palpation, pain, crepitation, limitation of forearm rotation, and prominence of the ulnar head, indicating subluxation or dislocation. If the ulnar border of the hand and carpus are in straight alignment with the ulna, it is indicative of radial deviation and carpal supination. As mentioned previously, this is often accompanied by an ulnar drift of the digits at the metacarpophalangeal joints.

It is important to examine the function and integrity of the tendons to the digits, primarily the extensor tendons and flexor pollicis longus tendon, to identify any attritional ruptures that may be present. Rupture of the extensor tendons to the ring and small fingers has been termed the Vaughn-Jackson syndrome,[8] and flexor pollicis longus rupture has been termed the Mannerfelt syndrome.[9]

Examination for provocative signs of carpal tunnel syndrome includes eliciting of Tinel sign over the carpal canal, reproduction or worsening of numbness in the digits with compression over the proximal edge of the canal at the distal wrist crease (Durkan test), or performance of the Phalen test. A careful neurologic examination may detect decreased light touch sensibility in the thumb, index, middle, and radial aspects of the ring finger if there is advanced median nerve dysfunction.

If there is significant synovitis of the radiocapitellar joint proximally, there can be posterior interosseous nerve dysfunction as well. This is manifested during the wrist and hand examination as the inability to extend the thumb and digits and, to some extent, the wrist. This finding, however, needs to be differentiated from tendon rupture or subluxation at the level of the metacarpophalangeal joints. Strength testing may be diminished because of pain from synovitis or the inability to contract a muscle secondary to tendon rupture.

Examination of the shoulder and elbow should be included to identify functional difficulties from these joints that may require treatment before the wrist is addressed.

FUNCTIONAL LIMITATIONS

The most common functional limitations expressed by patients with advanced rheumatoid disease of the wrist are decreased muscle strength, decreased range of motion of both the wrist and forearm, deformity, and pain. Normal joints proximal and distal to an

dysfunction and plan a course of treatment. Swelling around the ulnar styloid and loss of wrist extension secondary to extensor carpi ulnaris subluxation indicate early wrist involvement. Dorsal wrist swelling is commonly present and can be due to radiocarpal synovitis, tenosynovitis, or a combination of the two abnormal joint can usually allow a great deal of compensatory function.

Rheumatoid patients, however, often have shoulder, elbow, and hand involvement and an abnormal wrist, which leads to significant limitations in activities of daily living. The inability to extend one or more digits secondary to extensor tendon rupture, tendon subluxation, or nerve palsy is difficult to compensate for, and splinting can be cumbersome. Because the distal radioulnar joint is important in allowing functional forearm rotation and in helping to position the hand in space, advanced synovitis of this joint causing pain and fixed deformity can have a severe impact on a patient's daily functional activity. Functional difficulties that are commonly experienced by these patients include activities of lifting, carrying, and sustained or repetitive grasp. Whereas a loss of pronation may be compensated for by shoulder abduction and internal rotation, supination loss is very difficult to compensate. This can lead to difficulty in opening doors and turning keys. Simple acts such as receiving change during shopping can be compromised by reduced supination. Furthermore, in patients with shoulder involvement, the freedom of compensatory motion at the shoulder can be severely limited, compounding the functional limitations imposed on the patient's function by limitation of forearm rotation.

DIAGNOSTIC STUDIES

Plain radiographs of the wrist that include posterioranterior, lateral, and oblique views allow thorough examination of the radiocarpal, midcarpal, and distal radioulnar joints. Specifically, a supinated oblique view[10] should be closely inspected for early changes consistent with rheumatoid synovitis. The earliest of these changes are symmetric soft tissue swelling and juxta-articular osteoporosis. Radiographic staging can be performed as well[11] (Table 37-1).

Although a majority of patients may have had a diagnosis of rheumatoid arthritis already made, radiographic examination occasionally detects the earliest signs of the disease by changes in areas of the wrist

where there is a concentration of synovitis. These changes include erosions at the base of the ulnar styloid, the sigmoid notch of the distal radius, and the midwaist of the scaphoid and isolated joint space narrowing of the capitolunate joint seen on the posteroanterior view (Figs. 37-3 and 37-4). Ulnar translocation of the lunate can also be seen on this view. The lateral radiograph can show small bone spikes protruding palmarly, usually from the scaphoid. Late radiographic changes include pancompartmental loss of joint spaces and large subchondral erosions[12] (Fig. 37-5). Although radiographic findings may not always correlate well with clinical findings, the information gained from plain radiographs can be important in influencing which procedures will be of most benefit in patients

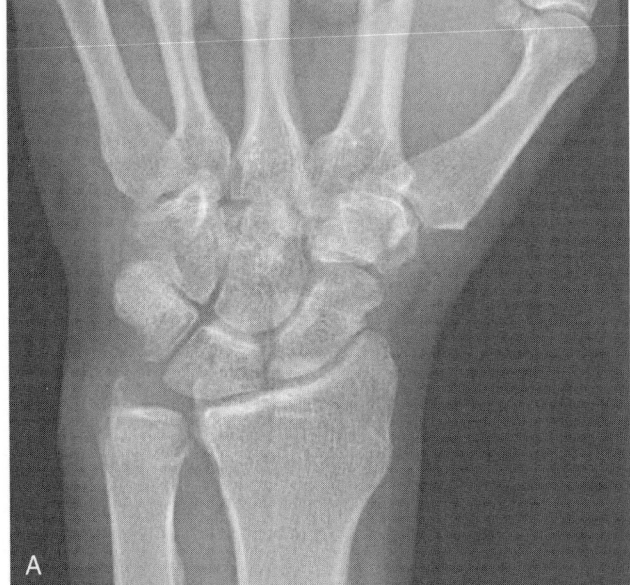

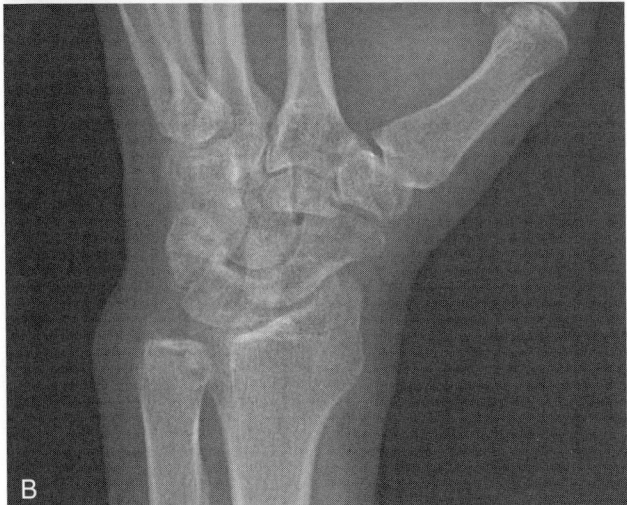

FIGURE 37-3. **A** and **B,** Radiographs (of the patient in Figure 37-2) in early rheumatoid disease of the wrist show bone erosions in areas of synovitis, such as around the ulnar styloid and distal radioulnar joint. There are also early erosive changes in the scapholunate articulation. The soft tissue swelling and deformity around the distal ulna are easily appreciated. These radiographs represent Larsen stage 2 disease.

TABLE 37-1 Larsen Radiographic Staging of Rheumatoid Arthritis	
Larsen Score	**Radiographic Status**
0	No changes, normal joint
1	Periarticular swelling, osteoporosis, slight narrowing
2	Erosion and mild joint space narrowing
3	Moderate destructive joint space narrowing
4	End-stage destruction, preservation of articular surface
5	Mutilating disease, destruction of normal articular surfaces

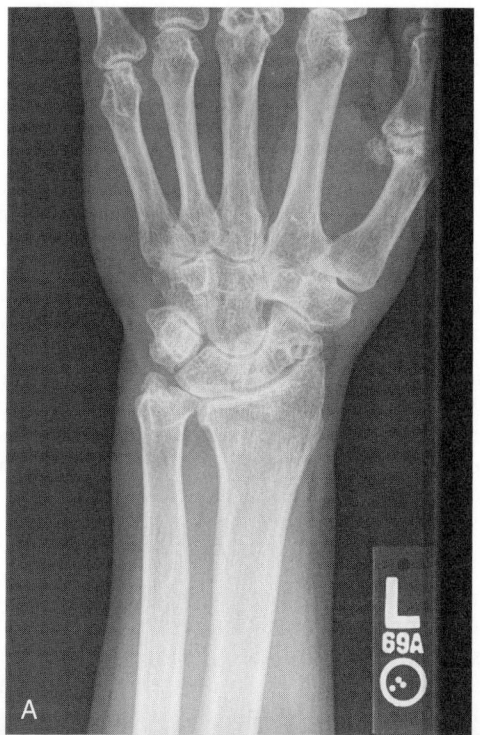

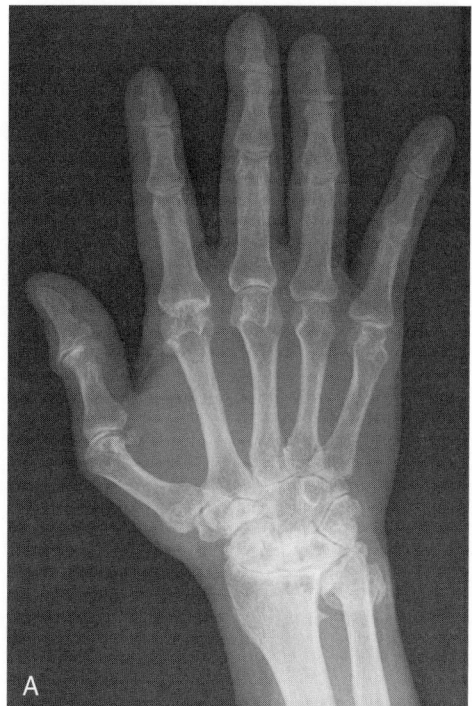

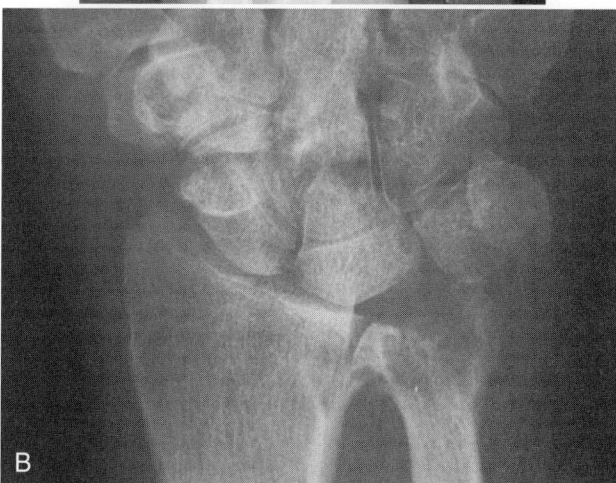

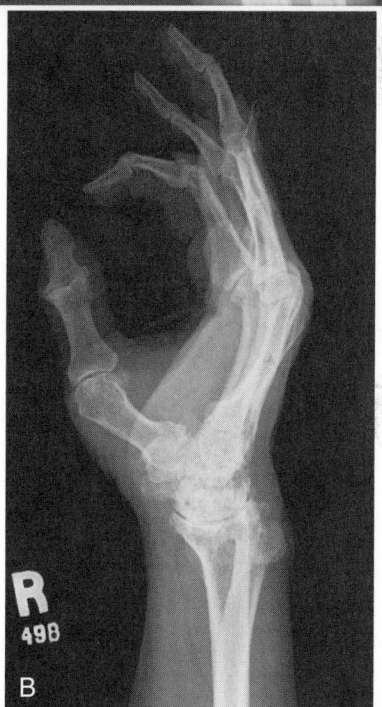

FIGURE 37-4. **A,** As the disease advances, cystic changes in the radioscaphoid articulation, reduction in joint space, and osteophyte formation are clearly seen in this radiograph of stage 3 disease. **B,** Radiographic appearance in stage 3 of persistent synovitis around the ulnar head and distal radioulnar joint, which leads to destruction of the ulnar head and osteophyte formation, both of which can contribute to extensor tendon attrition and rupture. There is ulnar translocation of the carpus best appreciated by the ulnar displacement of the lunate.

FIGURE 37-5. **A** and **B,** In advanced disease (stage 4), there is complete loss of joint space affecting the entire wrist, profuse osteophyte formation best appreciated in the lateral view, and deformation and dorsal dislocation of the ulnar head.

Differential Diagnosis

Post-traumatic arthritis

Chronic scapholunate advanced collapse

Septic arthritis

Wrist instability

Carpal tunnel syndrome

Gout

with poor medical disease control. Significant joint subluxation, bone loss, relative ulnar length, and ulnar translocation can help determine which procedure best serves a patient.

Advanced imaging techniques such as magnetic resonance imaging and computed tomography are not usually helpful in evaluation or planning for surgery. Electrodiagnostic studies are recommended if neurologic symptoms are present.

In patients in whom rheumatoid arthritis is suspected clinically, appropriate diagnostic serologic tests may include rheumatoid factor, antinuclear antibody, HLA-B27, sedimentation rate, and anticitrulline antibody assay. These tests are performed in conjunction with a consultation by a rheumatologist or an internist experienced in the care of rheumatoid disease.

TREATMENT

Initial

The monitored use of disease-modifying agents has dramatically improved control of the disease, especially with early, aggressive treatment. Management of local disease depends on several factors, such as severity of disease, functional limitations, pain, and cosmetic deformity. The patient's education, nutrition, and psychological health should be maximized.

Acutely painful, inflamed wrists are best managed with rest and immobilization and oral anti-inflammatory agents. Splints available over-the-counter are occasionally ill-suited to this population of patients because the material cannot mold to the altered anatomic contours. In such cases, a custom-made, forearm-based, volar resting splint that holds the wrist in the neutral position will provide support and comfort and is likely to be worn with greater compliance. Topical agents such as capsaicin cream may be efficacious in some instances. Steroid injections into the wrist can be useful to control local synovitis and pain.

Patients with associated carpal tunnel syndrome should be issued a wrist splint primarily for nighttime use. Steroid injection into the carpal canal is an option, but the risks of possible attritional tendon rupture need to

be discussed with the patient. Thorough knowledge of local anatomy is essential before an injection into the carpal tunnel is attempted. More important, alteration of local anatomy (and therefore altered location of the median nerve) must be considered very carefully before a carpal tunnel injection.

Rehabilitation

Occupational therapy can offer patients potential pain control measures, activity modification education, custom splinting, and range of motion exercises. A home exercise program can be developed to improve function and strength if the disease is also under adequate medical control.

Splinting, primarily of the resting, static form, is used to alleviate pain by selective immobilization and support, primarily in the acute phase of disease. Splints also serve to stabilize joints that are subjected to subluxation forces and to improve grip when it is impaired by pain.

In patients affected with local tenosynovitis of the extensor aspect and unwilling to have an injection, a trial of iontophoresis may prove beneficial. In patients with large amounts of subcutaneous adipose tissue, iontophoresis may be of limited efficacy in joints or periarticular structures. Studies on the effects of hot and cold in patients with rheumatoid arthritis show benefits in pain, joint stiffness, and strength but do not prove the superiority of one modality over the other.[13] Paraffin baths and moist heat packs are used to improve joint motion and pain, allowing improved activity tolerance. The results with paraffin baths are superior when they are combined with exercise programs.[13] Contrast baths may help in reducing diffuse edema but are less commonly used in rheumatoid arthritis. Hydrotherapy can be an adjunct to many treatment programs, primarily for the purpose of decreasing muscle tension and reducing pain.

Physical therapy may be of benefit if multiple joints are affected and symptomatic. Improvement of shoulder and elbow function is important because it is difficult to position a hand in space with a painful, stiff joint proximal to it.

Potentially the most critical role of therapy is in the postoperative period. It is then that patients particularly require monitored splinting, improvement in range of motion and strength, edema control, and monitoring of progress.

Procedures

Intra-articular cortisone injections are effective in alleviating wrist pain due to synovitis. Typically, all injections around the wrist should be done by aseptic technique with a 25-gauge, $1\frac{1}{2}$-inch needle and a mixture of a nonprecipitating, water-soluble steroid preparation, which is injected along with 2 mL of 1% lidocaine.

The radiocarpal joint can be injected from the dorsal aspect approximately 1 cm distal to Lister tubercle, with the needle angled proximally about 10 degrees to account for the slight volar tilt of the distal radius articular surface. This is done with the wrist in the neutral position. Gentle longitudinal traction by an assistant can help widen the joint space, which may be reduced on account of the disease.

An alternative radiocarpal injection site is the ulnar wrist, just dorsal or volar to the easily palpable extensor carpi ulnaris tendon at the level of the ulnar styloid process. The needle must be angled proximally by 20 to 30 degrees to enter the space between the ulnar carpus and the head of the ulna. It is important to ascertain that the injectate flows freely. Any resistance indicates a need to reposition the needle appropriately. Alternatively, the injection may be performed by fluoroscopic guidance with the help of a mini image intensifier, if one is available in the office.

If a midcarpal injection is required, this is done through the dorsal aspect, under fluoroscopic guidance, with injection into the space at the center of the lunate-triquetrum-hamate-capitate region.

Injections into the carpal tunnel are usually performed at the level of the distal wrist crease with the needle introduced just ulnar to the palmaris longus, which in most patients is just palmar to the median nerve and therefore protects it at this level. In patients who do not display clinical evidence of a palmaris longus, we do not recommend carpal tunnel injections.

Patients must be counseled about the postinjection period. It is not uncommon for patients to experience some increase in local discomfort for 24 to 36 hours after the injection. Use of the splint is recommended during this time, and icing of the area may also be of benefit. In our experience, most steroid injections take a few days to have a therapeutic effect. As is the case with any joint, repeated injections should be minimized if there is no radiographic sign of advanced cartilage wear because of the deleterious effect that corticosteroids can have on articular cartilage by transient inhibition of chondrocyte synthesis. However, in advanced disease, when joint surgery in inevitable, there is no contraindication to repeat injections that have proved beneficial to a patient.

Surgery

The indications for operative treatment of the rheumatoid wrist include one or more of the following: disabling pain and chronic synovitis not relieved by a minimum of 4 to 6 months of adequate medical and nonoperative measures; deformity and instability that limit hand function; tendon rupture; and nerve compression. Deformity alone is rarely an indication for surgery. It is not uncommon to see patients with significant deformities demonstrate excellent function with the use of compensatory maneuvers in the absence of pain. Corrective surgery in these patients is ill-advised.

Surgical procedures can be divided into those involving bone and those involving soft tissue. On occasion, a bone procedure will be combined with a soft tissue procedure in the same setting.

Synovectomy involves the removal of the inflamed, thickened joint lining from the radiocarpal and distal radioulnar joints and is best performed for the painful joint that demonstrates little or no radiographic evidence of joint destruction. Tenosynovectomy involves débridement of the tissue around involved tendons in the hope of avoiding future attritional tendon ruptures. Patients best suited for these procedures have relatively good medical disease control, no fixed joint deformity, and minimal radiographic changes.

If tendon rupture has already occurred, most commonly over the distal ulna, the procedure of choice is some form of tendon transfer, usually combined with resection of the ulnar head (Darrach procedure). Repair is not indicated or possible in most cases because of the poor tissue quality and extensive loss of tendon tissue in the zone of rupture. Depending on the number of tendons ruptured, it is possible to transfer the ruptured distal tendon into a neighboring healthier tendon or to transfer a more distant tendon, such as the extensor indicis proprius or superficial flexor tendon, into the affected tendon. The distal end of a ruptured extensor tendon may also be sutured to its unaffected neighboring extensor, in some cases.

Bone procedures can include resection arthroplasty, resurfacing arthroplasty, and limited or complete wrist fusions. Resection arthroplasty, such as the Darrach procedure, in which the distal ulna is resected, is based on the concept that removal of a prominent region of bone that causes tendon rupture and limits motion will improve both pain and motion of the wrist. There are some modifications to this technique involving removal of a portion of the distal ulna versus the entire head, as well as the option to interpose tissue into the distal radioulnar joint to serve as a spacer.[14] Outcomes with this type of surgery have shown 75% to 84% grip strength improvement and 75% to 85% satisfaction of patients and pain relief.[15,16]

Resurfacing total wrist arthroplasty requires the resection of a portion of the distal radius and carpus and insertion of metallic implants with a polyethylene spacer. It is generally restricted to patients with low functional demands who have bilateral rheumatoid wrist disease and require some motion in one wrist if the other is fused. It is most effective in patients who have good bone stock, relatively good alignment, and intact extensor tendons. The complication rate with contemporary designs is 20% to 25% and usually involves implant failure or loosening.[17,18] However, some studies have shown that with a 5- to 10-year follow-up after surgery, pain relief is maintained in 80% to 85% of patients, and these patients also retain 50 to 60 degrees of combined wrist flexion and extension.[17-19] Improvements in arthroplasty technique and implant design may offer improved outcomes in the future.

Fusion, or arthrodesis, procedures to eliminate pain due to significantly degenerative joints are well described.[20-25] However, depending on the nature of the fusion, these lead to a partial or complete loss of wrist motion. Limited fusions are described for the distal radioulnar joint (Sauvé-Kapandji) and radiolunate joint (Chamay). The potential benefit of limited fusions is some sparing of wrist motion, which can occur through the articulations that remain unfused, and this sparing of some motion can be critical to overall function in this group of patients. The Sauvé-Kapandji procedure involves fusion of the distal radioulnar joint and allows some forearm rotation through an osteotomy of the ulna just proximal to the fusion. This osteotomy is essentially a resection of a small segment of bone proximal to the fused distal radioulnar joint to construct a "false joint" or pseudarthrosis, through which the patient may be able to rotate the forearm. Excellent pain relief has been demonstrated in rheumatoid patients with this procedure.[26,27] A fusion of the radiolunate joint still allows some wrist motion to occur through the midcarpal and distal radioulnar joints.

Total wrist fusion is a reliable, safe, and well-established procedure for relieving pain and providing a stable wrist that improves hand function.[20,21,23] Success rates of 65% to 85% have been shown in terms of eliminating or significantly improving wrist pain.[23] For advanced wrist rheumatoid disease, it has become the most common bone procedure. Fusion can be accomplished either with a contoured dorsal plate fixed to the wrist by screws or with one or more large intraosseous pins placed across the wrist (Fig. 37-6). The intraosseous pins are usually placed through the second or third metacarpal or through both, across the wrist into the medullary canal of the radius. Ideally, the wrist is fused in slight extension to allow improved grip strength. High rates of fusion and a 15% rate of symptomatic hardware removal have been described.[22]

If significant median nerve compression exists, an extended open carpal tunnel release with flexor tenosynovectomy is typically performed through a palmar incision.

POTENTIAL DISEASE COMPLICATIONS

Rheumatoid arthritis is a chronic, progressive disease that can cause significant upper extremity disability at many locations by stiffness or instability from the shoulder to the hand. If wrist involvement becomes advanced, this contributes to problems with motion, pain, stiffness, and nerve compression. Extensor and flexor tendon rupture is a common scenario in rheumatoid disease and can complicate management. During the course of their disease, the majority of patients with rheumatoid disease will lose some functional capacity, and about half will develop disabling disease that requires significant physical dependence on adaptive measures for performance of the activities of daily living. Occupational therapists and social workers play roles in obtaining and using aids and appliances, such as special grips and alterations of household appliances, to maximize the patient's function.

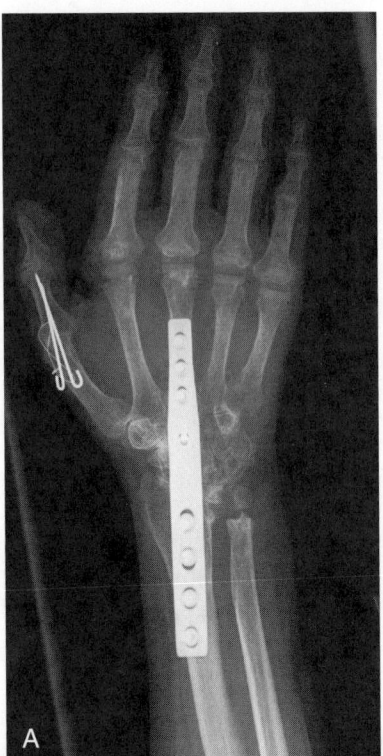

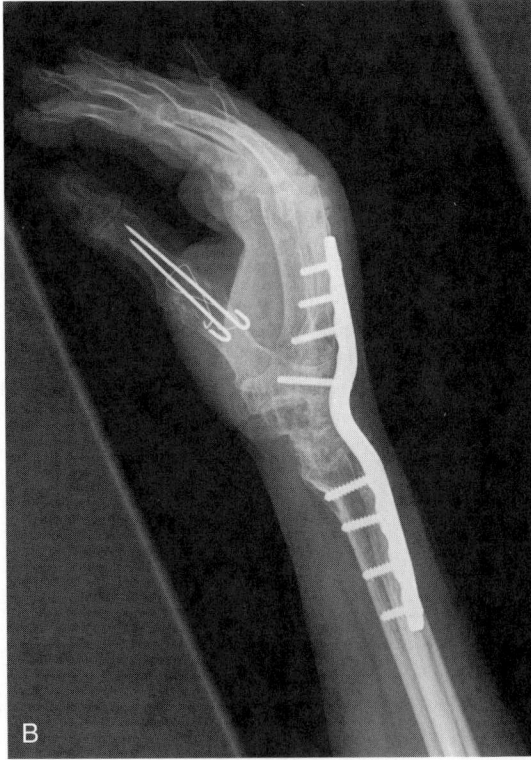

FIGURE 37-6. A and **B,** Radiographs depicting a total wrist arthrodesis with use of a contoured plate and screws. Note that the distal end of the ulna has also been excised (Darrach procedure). The polyarthritic nature of the disease process is emphasized by the metacarpophalangeal joint arthroplasties in the fingers and a metacarpophalangeal arthrodesis of the thumb.

POTENTIAL TREATMENT COMPLICATIONS

Systemic complications from the medical treatment of rheumatoid arthritis with current disease-modifying agents are beyond the scope of this chapter. Analgesics and nonsteroidal anti-inflammatory medications have well-known side effects that can affect the cardiac, gastric, renal, and hepatic systems. Intra-articular corticosteroid injections involve a very small risk of infection as well as cumulative cartilage injury from repeated exposure to steroid.

Surgical complications can result from wound healing problems, infection, neurovascular injury, recurrent synovitis, recurrent tendon rupture, persistent joint instability, and implant loosening or failure. To some extent, the frequency of complications may be reduced by meticulous surgical technique and judicious management of medications affecting wound healing and immunity, such as methotrexate and systemic steroids.

References

1. Hämäläinen M, Kammonen M, Lehtimäki M, et al. Epidemiology of wrist involvement in rheumatoid arthritis. Rheumatology 1992;17:1-7.
2. Lee SK, Hausman MR. Management of the distal radioulnar joint in rheumatoid arthritis. Hand Clin 2005;21:577-589.
3. Papp SR, Athwal GS, Pichora DR. The rheumatoid wrist. J Am Acad Orthop Surg 2006;14:65-77.
4. Shapiro JS. The wrist in rheumatoid arthritis. Hand Clin 1996;12:477-495.
5. Williams DG. Autoantibodies in rheumatoid arthritis. In Klippel JH, Dieppe PA, eds. Rheumatology, 2nd ed. Philadelphia, Mosby, 1998:9.1-9.8.
6. Bäckdahl M. The caput ulnae syndrome in rheumatoid arthritis. A study of morphology, abnormal anatomy and clinical picture. Acta Rheumatol Scand Suppl 1963;5:1-75.
7. Wilson RL, DeVito MC. Extensor tendon problems in rheumatoid arthritis. Hand Clin 1996;12:551-559.
8. Vaughan-Jackson OJ. Rupture of extensor tendons by attrition at the inferior radio-ulnar joint: report of two cases. J Bone Joint Surg Br 1948;30:528-530.
9. Mannerfelt L, Norman O. Attrition ruptures of flexor tendons in rheumatoid arthritis caused by bony spurs in the carpal tunnel: a clinical and radiological study. J Bone Joint Surg Br 1969;51:270-277.
10. Nørgaard F. Earliest roentgenological changes in polyarthritis of the rheumatoid type: rheumatoid arthritis. Radiology 1965;85:325-329.
11. Larsen A, Dale K, Eek M, et al. Radiographic evaluation of rheumatoid arthritis by standard reference films. J Hand Surg Am 1983;8:667-669.
12. Resnick D. Rheumatoid arthritis of the wrist: the compartmental approach. Med Radiogr Photogr 1976;52:50-88.
13. Michlovitz SL. The use of heat and cold in the management of rheumatic diseases. In Michlovitz S, ed. Thermal Agents in Rehabilitation, 2nd ed. Philadelphia, FA Davis, 1990:158-174.
14. Glowacki KA. Hemiresection arthroplasty of the distal radioulnar joint. Hand Clin 2005;21:591-601.
15. DiBenedetto MR, Lubbers LM, Coleman CR. Long term results of the minimal resection Darrach procedure. J Hand Surg Am 1991;16:445-450.
16. Leslie BM, Carlson G, Ruby LK. Results of extensor carpi ulnaris tenodesis in the rheumatoid wrist undergoing a distal ulna resection. J Hand Surg Am 1990;15:547-551.
17. Cobb TK, Beckenbaugh RD. Biaxial total-wrist arthroplasty. J Hand Surg Am 1996;21:1011-1021.
18. Bosco JA, Bynum DK, Bowers WH. Long-term outcome of Volz total wrist arthroplasties. J Arthroplasty 1994;9:25-31.
19. Anderson MC, Adams BD. Total wrist arthroplasty. Hand Clin 2005;21:621-630.
20. Barbier O, Saels P, Rombouts JJ, et al. Long-term functional results of wrist arthrodesis in rheumatoid arthritis. J Hand Surg Br 1999;24:27-31.
21. Jebson PJ, Adams BD. Wrist arthrodesis: review of current technique. J Am Acad Orthop Surg 2001;9:53-60.
22. Meads BM, Scougall PJ, Hargreaves IC. Wrist arthrodesis using a Synthes wrist fusion plate. J Hand Surg Br 2003;28:571-574.
23. Ishikawa H, Murasawa A, Nakazono K. Long-term follow-up study of radiocarpal arthrodesis for the rheumatoid wrist. J Hand Surg Am 2005;30:658-666.
24. Solem H, Berg NJ, Finsen V. Long term results of arthrodesis of the wrist: a 6-15 year follow up of 35 patients. Scand J Plast Reconstr Surg Hand Surg 2006;40:175-178.
25. Rauhaniemi J, Tiusanen H, Sipola E. Total wrist fusion: a study of 115 patients. J Hand Surg Br 2005;30:217-219.
26. Vincent KA, Szabo RM, Agee JM. The Sauvé-Kapandji procedure for reconstruction of the rheumatoid distal radioulnar joint. J Hand Surg Am 1993;18:978-983.
27. Fujita S, Masada K, Takeuchi E, et al. Modified Sauvé-Kapandji procedure for disorders of the distal radioulnar joint in patients with rheumatoid arthritis. J Bone Joint Surg Am 2005;87:134-139.

Thoracic Compression Fracture 38

Toni J. Hanson, MD

Synonyms

Thoracic compression fracture
Dorsal compression fracture
Wedge compression
Vertebral crush fracture[1,2]

ICD-9 Code

733.13   Fx vertebra compression thoracic closed

DEFINITION

A compression fracture is caused by forces transmitted along the vertebral body. The ligaments are intact, and compression fractures are usually stable.[3] Compression fractures in the thoracic vertebrae are commonly seen in osteoporosis with decreased bone mineral density. Such fractures may occur with trivial trauma and are usually stable.[4,5] Pathologic vertebral fractures may occur with metastatic cancer (commonly from lung, breast, or prostate) as well as with other processes affecting verte-brae. Trauma, such as a fall from a height or a motor vehicle accident, can also result in thoracic compression fracture. Considerable force is required to fracture healthy vertebrae, which are resistant to compression. In such cases, the force required to produce a fracture may cause extension of fracture components into the spinal canal with neurologic findings. There may be evidence of additional trauma, such as calcaneal frac-tures from a fall. Multiple thoracic compression frac-tures, as seen with osteoporosis, can produce a kyphotic deformity.[6-8]

SYMPTOMS

Pain in the thoracic spine over the affected vertebrae is the usual hallmark of the presentation. It may be se-vere, sharp, exacerbated with movement, and decreased with rest. Severe pain may last 2 to 3 weeks and then decrease during 6 to 9 weeks; however, pain may per-sist for months. Typically, in osteoporotic fractures, the mid and lower dorsal vertebrae are affected. Acute fractures in osteoporosis, however, may result in little

discomfort or poor localization.[9] Multiple fractures result in kyphosis (dowager's hump). A good history and physical examination are essential as there may be indicators of a more ominous underlying pathologic process.[10,11]

PHYSICAL EXAMINATION

Tenderness with palpation or percussion over the af-fected region of the thoracic vertebrae is the primary finding on examination. Spinal movements also pro-duce pain. Kyphotic deformity may be present in the patient who has had multiple prior compression frac-tures. Neurologic examination below the level of the fracture is recommended to assess for the presence of reflex changes, Babinski sign, and sensory alteration. Sacral segments can be assessed through evaluation of rectal tone, volitional sphincter control, anal wink, and pinprick if there is concern about bowel and bladder function.[12] The patient's height, weight, and chest ex-pansion are useful. It is also important to assess the patient's gait for stability. Comorbid neurologic and orthopedic conditions may contribute to gait dysfunc-tion and fall risk.[13,14]

FUNCTIONAL LIMITATIONS

Functional limitations in a patient with an acute painful thoracic compression fracture can be significant. The patient may experience loss of mobility and indepen-dence in activities of daily living, household activities, and social functioning. In patients with severe symp-toms, hospitalization may be necessary.[15]

DIAGNOSTIC TESTING

Anteroposterior and lateral radiographs of the thoracic spine can confirm the clinical impression of a thoracic compression fracture. On radiographic examination in a thoracic compression fracture, the height of the affected vertebrae is reduced, generally in a wedge-shaped fash-ion, with anterior height less than posterior vertebral height (Fig. 38-1). A bone scan may help localize (but not necessarily determine the etiology of) processes such

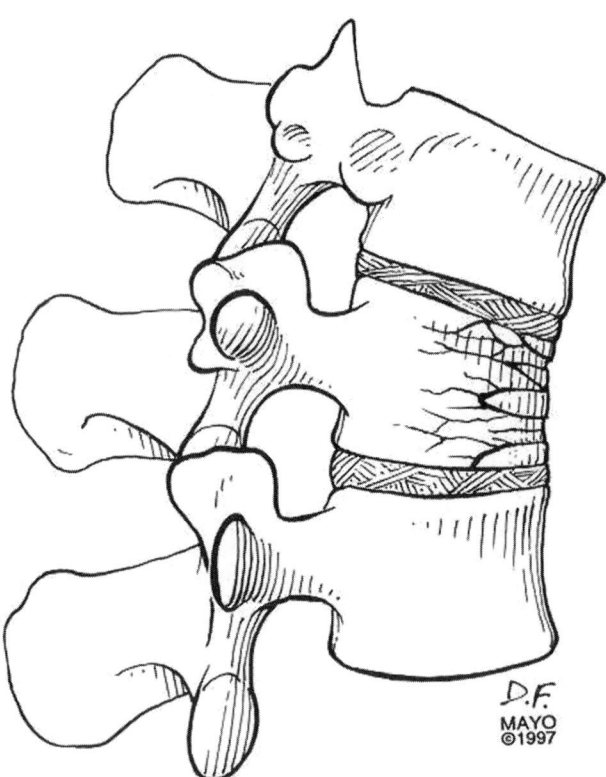

FIGURE 38-1. Thoracic compression fracture with reduction in anterior vertebral height and wedging of the vertebrae.

Differential Diagnosis

Thoracic sprain

Thoracic radiculopathy

Thoracic disc herniation

Metastatic malignant disease

Primary spine malignant neoplasm (uncommon, most frequently multiple myeloma)[18]

Benign spinal tumors

Infection, osteomyelitis (rare)[19]

Inflammatory arthritis

Musculoskeletal pain, other

Referred pain (pancreatic cancer, abdominal aortic aneurysm)

as metastatic cancer, occult fracture, and infection. Percutaneous needle biopsy of the affected vertebral body can be helpful diagnostically in selected cases. Spinal imaging, such as computed tomography or magnetic resonance imaging, may also elucidate further detail.[16] Laboratory tests, including serum calcium concentration, alkaline phosphatase activity, and 24-hour urine collection as well as bone mineral density testing,[17] may be helpful for metabolic processes. A complete blood count and sedimentation rate or C-reactive protein level (which are nonspecific but sensitive indicators of an occult infection or inflammatory disease) may also be helpful. Diagnostic testing is directed, as appropriate, on the basis of the entire clinical presentation.

TREATMENT

Initial

Initial treatment consists of activity modification, including limited bed rest. Cushioning with use of a mattress overlay (such as an egg crate) can also be helpful. Pharmacologic agents, including oral analgesics, muscle relaxants, and anti-inflammatory medications, as appropriate to the patient, are helpful. These include such agents as tramadol, 50 mg (one or two every 4 to 6 hours, not exceeding eight per day); propoxyphene napsylate, 100 mg; acetaminophen, 650 mg (one every 4 to 6 hours); and acetaminophen, 300 mg, and codeine 30 mg (one or two every 4 to 6 hours, not exceeding 4 grams per day). If pain is more severe or persistent, controlled-release oxycodone (10 mg or 20 mg every 12 hours) may be considered. Muscle relaxants such as cyclobenzaprine, 10 mg three times daily, may be helpful initially with muscle spasm. A variety of nonsteroidal anti-inflammatories, including celecoxib (Celebrex, a cyclooxygenase 2 inhibitor), can be considered, depending on the patient. Calcitonin (one spray daily in alternating nostrils, providing 200 IU/0.09 mL per spray) has also been used for painful osteoporotic fractures.[20] Stool softeners and laxatives may be necessary to reduce strain with bowel movements and constipation, particularly with narcotic analgesics. Avoidance of spinal motion, especially flexion, through appropriate body mechanics (such as log rolling in bed) and spinal bracing is helpful.

A variety of spinal orthoses reduce spinal flexion (Fig. 38-2). They must be properly fitted.[21,22] A lumbosacral orthosis may be sufficient for a low thoracic fracture. A thoracolumbosacral orthosis is used frequently (Fig. 38-2C and D). If a greater degree of fracture immobilization is required, an off-the-shelf orthosis (Fig. 38-2E) or a custom-molded body jacket may be fitted by an orthotist.

Proper diagnosis and treatment of underlying contributors to the thoracic compression fracture are necessary. Most thoracic compression fractures will heal.[23,24]

Rehabilitation

Physical therapy assists with gentle mobilization of the patient by employing proper body mechanics, optimizing transfer techniques, and training with gait aids (such as a wheeled walker) to reduce biomechanical stresses on the spine and to ensure gait safety.[25] Pain-relieving modalities, such as therapeutic heat or cold, and transcutaneous electrical stimulation may also be employed. Exercise should not increase spinal symptoms and should be implemented at the appropriate juncture. In addition to proper body mechanics and postural training emphasizing spinal extension and avoidance of flexion, spinal

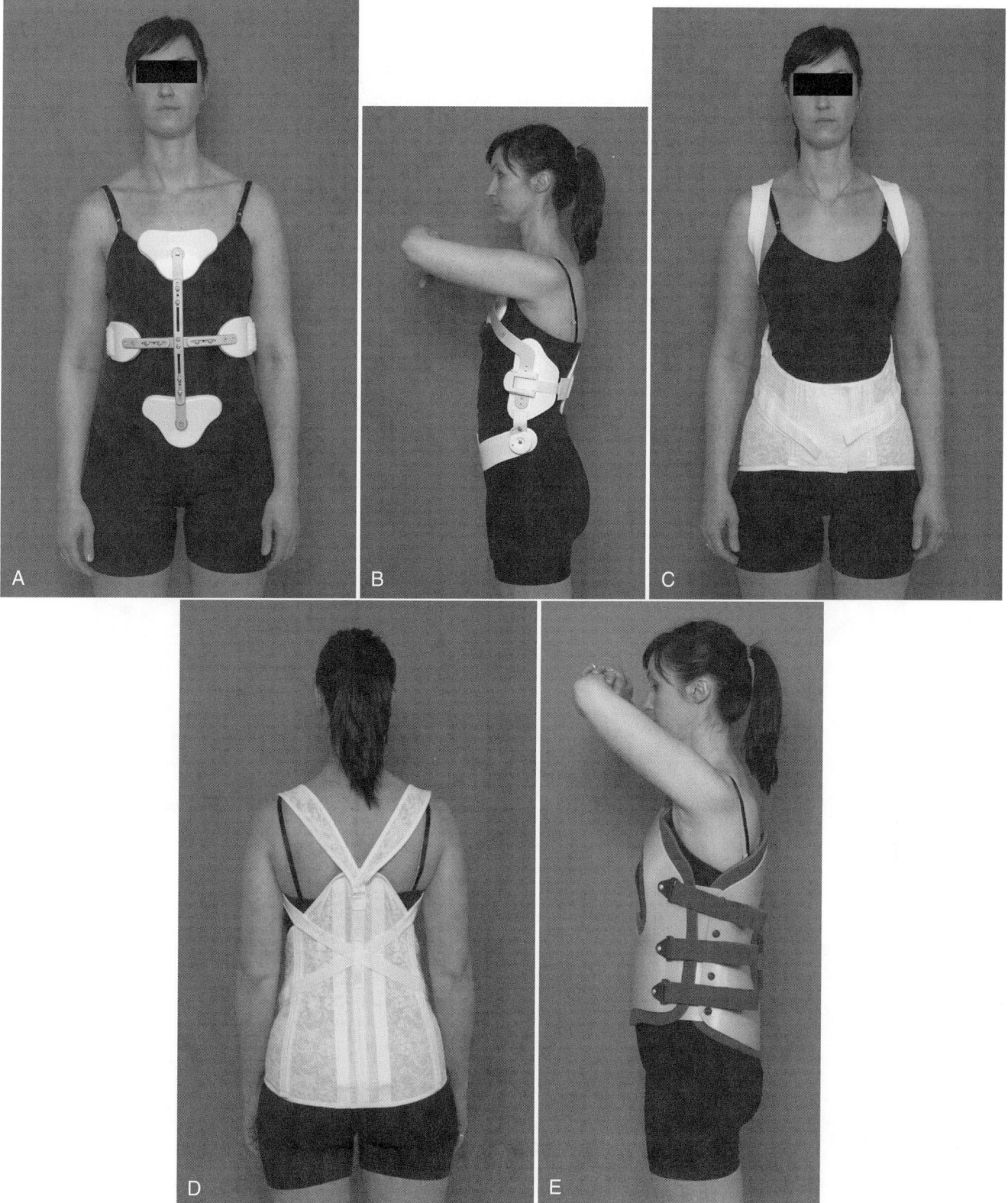

FIGURE 38-2. A, Cruciform anterior spinal hyperextension brace (to limit flexion). **B,** Three-point sagittal hyperextension brace (to limit flexion). **C,** Thoracolumbosacral orthosis, anterior view. **D,** Thoracolumbosacral orthosis, posterior view. **E,** Off-the-shelf molded spinal orthosis with Velcro closures.

extensor muscle strengthening, limb strengthening, stretching to muscle groups (such as the pectoral muscles, hips, and lower extremities), and deep breathing exercises may also be indicated. Weight-bearing exercises for bone health, balance, and fall prevention are also important.[26] Proper footwear, with cushioning inserts, can also be helpful. Occupational therapy can help the patient with activities of daily living, reinforce proper spinal ergonomics, address equipment needs, and prevent falls. Successful rehabilitation is targeted at increasing the patient's comfort, decreasing deformity, and decreasing resultant disability, and it is individualized to address specific needs of the patient.[27-29]

Procedures

Invasive procedures are generally not indicated. Percutaneous vertebroplasty or kyphoplasty with use of polymethyl methacrylate may help reduce fracture pain, reinforce thoracic vertebral strength, and improve function;

with kyphoplasty, some potential restoration of vertebral height has been reported.[25,30] Patients with imaging evidence of an acute or a subacute thoracic fracture who have correlating pain, who fail to improve with conservative management, and who are without contraindications may be candidates for such interventional procedures. Complications can include infection, bleeding, fracture, and systemic issues such as embolism. Cement leaks into surrounding tissues with spinal cord, spinal nerve, or vascular compression can occur. Figure 38-3 demonstrates a T11 vertebral fracture case study. The radiographs, T1 and T2 magnetic resonance images of the fracture, and post-vertebroplasty images are demonstrated.

Surgery

Surgery is rarely necessary. Surgical stabilization can be considered in patients with continued severe pain after compression fracture as a result of nonunion of the

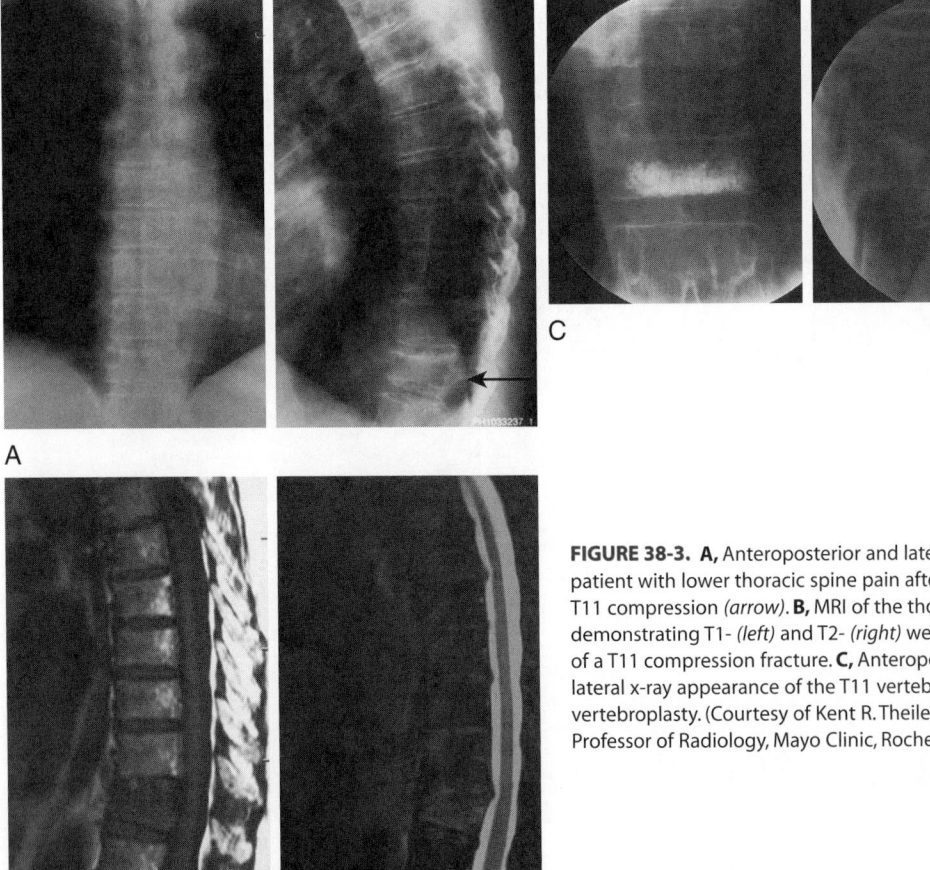

FIGURE 38-3. A, Anteroposterior and lateral x-rays of a patient with lower thoracic spine pain after a fall. Note T11 compression *(arrow)*. **B,** MRI of the thoracic spine demonstrating T1- *(left)* and T2- *(right)* weighted images of a T11 compression fracture. **C,** Anteroposterior and lateral x-ray appearance of the T11 vertebrae after vertebroplasty. (Courtesy of Kent R. Theilen, MD, Assistant Professor of Radiology, Mayo Clinic, Rochester, Minn.)

fracture, with spinal instability, or if neurologic complications occur. Referral to a spine surgeon is recommended in these cases for further assessment.[31]

POTENTIAL DISEASE COMPLICATIONS

Neurologic complications, including nerve or spinal cord compromise, as well as orthopedic complications with continued pain, nonunion, and instability can occur. Underlying primary disease, for example, metastatic thoracic compression, needs to be addressed. Patients with severe kyphosis may experience cardiopulmonary dysfunction. Severe kyphosis may also result in rib impingement on the iliac bones, producing more symptoms. Severe pain accompanying a fracture may further limit deep breathing and increase the risk of pulmonary complications, such as pneumonia. Progressive spinal deformity may produce secondary pain generators. The patient may have progressive levels of dependency as a result.

POTENTIAL TREATMENT COMPLICATIONS

Side effects with medications, particularly nonsteroidal anti-inflammatory medications as well as narcotic medications, can occur. It is important to select medications appropriately for individual patients. There may be difficulty with the use of spinal orthotics, such as intolerance in patients with gastroesophageal reflux disease. Kyphotic patients frequently do not tolerate orthoses, and fitting is problematic. Surgery can result in many complications, not only from general anesthesia risks but also from infection, bleeding, or thromboembolism. Poor mechanical strength of bone, as in osteoporosis with paucity of dense lamellar and cortical bone, may result in suboptimal surgical outcome.

References

1. Benson LS. Orthopaedic PEARLS. Philadelphia, FA Davis, 1999:369.
2. Goldie B. Fracture of a cervical vertebra; acute low back pain and sciatica; spinal stenosis; back pain associated with spinal instability; vertebral crush fracture; pelvic fracture (excluding pubic rami fracture of the elderly); fracture of the pubic rami. In Goldie B. Orthopaedic Diagnosis and Management: A Guide to the Care of Orthopaedic Patients, 2nd ed. London, Blackwell Scientific, 1998:183-209.
3. Bezel E, Stillerman C. The Thoracic Spine. St. Louis, Quality Medical, 1999:20.
4. Toh E, Yerby S, Bay B. The behavior of thoracic trabecular bone during flexion. J Exp Clin Med 2005;30:163-170.
5. Toyone T, Tanaka T, Wada Y, Kamikawa K. Changes in vertebral wedging rate between supine and standing position and its association with back pain: a prospective study in patients with osteoporotic vertebral compression fractures. Spine 2006;31:2963-2966.
6. Kesson M, Atkins E. The thoracic spine. In Kesson M, Atkins E, eds. Orthopaedic Medicine: A Practical Approach. Boston, Butterworth-Heinemann, 1998:262-281.
7. McRae R. The thoracic and lumbar spine. In Parkinson M, ed. Pocketbook of Orthopaedics and Fractures, vol 1. London, Churchill Livingstone/Elsevier, 1999:79-105.
8. Dandy D, Edwards D. Disorders of the spine. In Dandy D, Edwards D. Essential Orthopaedics and Trauma. New York, Churchill Livingstone, 1998:431-451.
9. Bonner F, Chesnut C, Fitzsimmons A, Lindsay R. Osteoporosis. In DeLisa J, Gans BM, eds. Rehabilitation Medicine: Principles and Practice, 3rd ed. Philadelphia, Lippincott-Raven, 1998:1453-1475.
10. Van de Velde T. Disorders of the thoracic spine: non-disc lesions. In Ombregt L, ed. A System of Orthopaedic Medicine. Philadelphia, WB Saunders, 1995:455-469.
11. Errico T, Stecker S, Kostuik J. Thoracic pain syndromes. In Frymoyer J, ed. The Adult Spine: Principles and Practice, 2nd ed. Philadelphia, Lippincott-Raven, 1997:1623-1637.
12. Huston C, Pitt D, Lane C. Strategies for treating osteoporosis and its neurologic complications. Appl Neurol 2005;1.
13. Hu S, Carlson G, Tribus C. Disorders, diseases, and injuries of the spine. In Skinner H, ed. Current Diagnosis and Treatment in Orthopedics, 2nd ed. New York, Lane Medical Books/McGraw-Hill, 2000:177-246.
14. Pattavina C. Diagnostic imaging. In Hart TJ. Uehara DT, eds. Handbook of Orthopaedic Emergencies. Philadelphia, Lippincott-Raven, 1999:32-47, 116-140.
15. Goldstein T. Treatment of common problems of the spine. In Goldstein T, ed. Geriatric Orthopaedics: Rehabilitative Management of Common Problems, 2nd ed.Gaithersburg, Md. Aspen, 1999:211-232.
16. Bisese J. Compression fracture secondary to underlying metastasis. In Bolger E, Ramos-Englis M, eds. Spinal MRI: A Teaching File Approach. New York, McGraw-Hill, 1992:73-129.
17. Genant H, Lang P, Steiger P, et al. Osteoporosis: assessment by bone densitometry. In Manelfe C, ed. Imaging of the Spine and Spinal Cord. New York, Raven Press, 1992:221-242.
18. Heller J, Pedlow F. Tumors of the spine. In Garfin S, Vaccaro AR, eds. Orthopaedic Knowledge Update. Spine. Rosemont, Ill, American Academy of Orthopaedic Surgeons, 1997:235-256.
19. Levine M, Heller J. Spinal infections. In Garfin S, Vaccaro A, eds. Orthopaedic Knowledge Update. Spine. Rosemont, Ill, American Academy of Orthopaedic Surgeons, 1997:257-271.
20. Kim D, Vaccaro A. Osteoporotic compression fractures of the spine: current options and considerations for treatment. Spine 2006;6:479-487.
21. Saunders H. Spinal orthotics. In Saunders R, ed. Evaluation, Treatment and Prevention of Musculoskeletal Disorders, vol 1. Bloomington, Minn, Educational Opportunities, 1993:285-296.
22. Bussel M, Merritt J, Fenwick L. Spinal orthoses. In Redford J, ed. Orthotics Clinical Practice and Rehabilitation Technology. New York, Churchill Livingstone, 1995:71-101.
23. Brunton S, Carmichael B, Gold D. Vertebral compression fractures in primary care. J Fam Pract 2005;Suppl:781-788.
24. Old J, Calvert M. Vertebral compression fractures in the elderly. Am Fam Physician 2004;69:111-116.
25. Rehabilitation of Patients with Osteoporosis-Related Fractures. Washington, DC, National Osteoporosis Foundation, 2003:4.
26. Sinaki M. Critical appraisal of physical rehabilitation measures after osteoporosis vertebral fracture. Osteoporosis Int 2003;14:773-779.
27. Browngoehl L. Osteoporosis. In Grabois M, Garrison SJ, Hart KA, Lehmkuhl LD, eds. Physical Medicine and Rehabilitation: The Complete Approach. Malden, Mass, Blackwell Science, 2000:1565-1577.
28. Eilbert W. Long-term care and rehabilitation of orthopaedic injuries. In Hart R, Rittenberry TJ, Uehara DT, eds. Handbook of Orthopaedic Emergencies. Philadelphia, Lippincott-Raven, 1999:127-138.
29. Barr J, Barr M, Lemley T, McCann R. Percutaneous vertebroplasty for pain relief and spinal stabilization. Spine 2000;25:923-928.
30. Kostuik J, Heggeness M. Surgery of the osteoporotic spine. In Frymoyer J, ed. The Adult Spine: Principles and Practice, 2nd ed. Philadelphia, Lippincott-Raven, 1997:1639-1664.
31. Snell E, Scarpone M. Orthopaedic issues in aging. In Baratz M, Watson AD, Imbriglia JE, eds. Orthopaedic Surgery: The Essentials. New York, Thieme, 1999:865-870.

Thoracic Radiculopathy **39**

Darren Rosenberg, DO

Synonyms

Thoracic radiculitis
Thoracic disc herniation

ICD-9 Code

724.4   Thoracic or lumbosacral neuritis or radiculitis, unspecified

DEFINITION

Thoracic radiculopathy is generally a painful syndrome caused by mechanical compression, chemical irritation, or metabolic abnormalities of the thoracic spinal nerve root. Thoracic disc herniation accounts for less than 5% of all disc protrusions.[1,2] The majority of herniated thoracic disc herniations (35%) occur between T8 and T12, with a peak (20%) at T11-12. Most patients (90%) present clinically between the fourth and seventh decades; 33% present between the ages of 40 and 49 years. Approximately 33% of thoracic disc protrusions are lateral, preferentially encroaching on the spinal nerve root; the remainder are central or central lateral, resulting primarily in various degrees of spinal cord compression. Synovial cysts, although rare (0.06% of patients requiring decompressive surgery) in the thoracic spine, may also be responsible for foraminal encroachment. These tend to be more common at the lower thoracic levels.[3] Natural degenerative forces and trauma are generally believed to be the most important factors in the etiology of mechanical thoracic radiculopathy. Foraminal stenosis from bone encroachment may also cause compression of the exiting nerve root and radicular symptoms. Perhaps one of the most common metabolic causes of thoracic radiculopathy is diabetes, often resulting in multilevel disease.[4] This may occur at any age but often appears with other neuropathic symptoms due to injury to the blood supply to the nerve root.

SYMPTOMS

The majority of patients (67%) present with complaints of "band-like" chest pain (Fig. 39-1). The second most common symptom (16%) is lower extremity pain.[5]

Injury to nerve roots T2-3 may present as axillary or midscapular pain. Injury to nerve roots T7-12 may manifest as abdominal pain.[6] Unlike thoracic radiculopathy, spinal cord compression produces upper motor neuron signs and symptoms consistent with myelopathy, whereas T11-12 lesions may damage the conus medullaris or cauda equina, causing bowel and bladder dysfunction and lower extremity symptoms.[7] Thus, in a true thoracic radiculopathy, pain is the primary complaint. It is important to include in the history any trauma or risk factors for non-neurologic causes of chest wall or abdominal pain. Because thoracic radiculopathy is not common, it is important in nontraumatic cases to be suspicious of more serious pathologic processes, such as malignant disease. Therefore, a history of weight loss, decreased appetite, and previous malignant disease should be elicited. Thoracic compression fractures that may mimic the symptoms of thoracic radiculopathy may be seen in young people with acute trauma, particularly falls—regardless of whether they land on their feet. In older people (particularly women with a history of osteopenia or osteoporosis) or in individuals who have prolonged history of steroid use, a compression fracture should be ruled out.

PHYSICAL EXAMINATION

The physical examination may show only limitations of range of motion—particularly trunk rotation, flexion, and extension—generally due to pain. In traumatic cases, location of ecchymosis or abrasions should be noted. *Range of motion testing should not be done if a spinal fracture is suspected.* Careful palpation for tenderness over the thoracic spinous and transverse processes as well as over the ribs and intercostal spaces is critical in localizing the involved level. Pain with percussion over the vertebral bodies should alert the clinician to the possibility of vertebral fracture.

Sensation may be abnormal in a dermatomal pattern. This will direct the examiner to more closely evaluate the involved level. Any abnormalities of the spine should be noted, including scoliosis, which is best detected when the patient flexes forward. Weakness or spasticity is seldom seen unless the spinal cord is compromised.

219

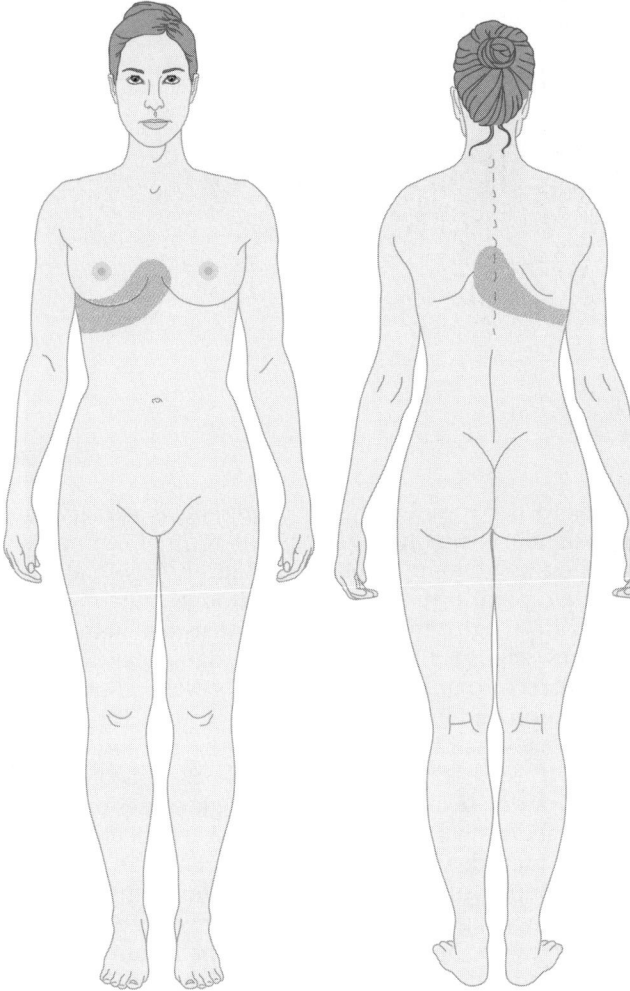

FIGURE 39-1. Typical pain pattern in a thoracic radiculopathy.

Deep tendon reflexes should be normal. A thorough examination of the cardiopulmonary system, abdominal organs, and skin should be performed, particularly in individuals who have sustained trauma.

FUNCTIONAL LIMITATIONS

The pain produced by thoracic radiculopathy often limits an individual's movement and activity. Patients may complain of pain with dressing and bathing, particularly during activities that include trunk movements, such as putting on shoes. Work activities may be restricted, such as lifting, climbing, and stooping. Even sedentary workers may be so uncomfortable that they are not able to perform their jobs. Anorexia may result from pain in the abdominal region.

DIAGNOSTIC STUDIES

Because of the low incidence of thoracic radiculopathy and the possibility of serious disease (e.g., tumor), the clinician should have a low threshold for ordering imaging studies in patients with persistent (more than 2 to

4 weeks) thoracic pain of unknown origin. Magnetic resonance imaging remains the imaging study of choice to evaluate the soft tissue structures of the thoracic spine. Computed tomography and computed tomographic myelography are alternatives if magnetic resonance imaging cannot be obtained.

The electromyographic evaluation of thoracic radiculopathy can be challenging because of the limited techniques available and lack of easily accessible muscles representing a myotomal nerve root distribution. The muscles most commonly tested are the paraspinals, intercostals, and abdominals. The clinician must investigate multiple levels of the thoracic spine to best localize the lesion. Techniques for intercostal somatosensory evoked potentials have also been shown to isolate individual nerve root levels.[8]

In patients who have sustained trauma, plain radiographs are advised to rule out fractures and spinal instability.

TREATMENT

Initial

Pain control is important early in the disease course. Patients should be advised to avoid activities that cause increased pain and to avoid heavy lifting. Nonsteroidal anti-inflammatory drugs are often the first line

Differential Diagnosis

Intercostal neuralgia

Cholecystitis

Compression fracture

Angina

Peptic ulcer disease

Rib fracture

Aortic aneurysm

Pyelonephritis

Pott disease

Esophageal disorders

Mastalgia

Malignant neoplasm (primary or metastatic)

Pleuritis

Postherpetic neuralgia

Adiposis dolorosa

Pulmonary embolism

Myofascial trigger point

Enthesopathy (ligament or tendon)

Costovertebral joint dysfunction

Costotransverse ligament sprain

of treatment and help control pain and inflammation. Oral steroids can be powerful anti-inflammatory medications and are typically used in the acute stages. This is generally done by starting at a moderate to high dose and tapering during several days. For example, a methylprednisolone (Medrol) dose pack is a prepackaged prescription that contains 21 pills. Each pill is 4 mg of Solu-Medrol. The pills are taken during the course of 6 days. On the first day, six tablets are taken, and then the dose is decreased by one pill each day. Care should be taken with use of steroids in diabetic patients because they may elevate blood glucose levels. In patients with uncontrolled diabetes who present with thoracic radiculopathy, glucose control should be attempted, although extremely elevated serum glucose levels have not been proved to cause the diabetic form of thoracic radiculopathy. Because of the risk of gastric ulceration, steroids are not typically used simultaneously with nonsteroidal anti-inflammatory drugs. Both non-narcotic and narcotic analgesics may be used to control pain. In subacute or chronic cases, other medications may be tried, such as tricyclic antidepressants and anticonvulsants (e.g., gabapentin and carbamazepine), which have been effective in treating symptoms of neuropathic origin.

Moist heat or ice can be used, as tolerated, for pain. Transcutaneous electrical nerve stimulation units may also help with pain.

Rehabilitation

Physical therapy can be used initially to assist with pain control. Modalities such as ultrasound and electrical stimulation may reduce pain and improve mobility. Physical therapy can then progress with spine stabilization exercises, back and abdominal strengthening, and a trial of mechanical spine traction. Some patients may benefit from a thoracolumbar brace to reduce segmental spine movement. Patients with significant spinal instability documented by imaging studies should be referred to a spine surgeon.

In addition, physical therapy should address postural retraining, particularly for individuals with habitually poor posture. Work sites can be evaluated, if indicated. All sedentary workers should be counseled on proper seating, including use of a well-fitting adjustable chair with a lumbar support. More active workers should be advised on appropriate lifting techniques and avoidance of unnecessary trunk rotation.

Finally, physical therapy can focus on improving biomechanical factors that may play a role in abnormal loads on the thoracic spine. These include flexibility exercises for tight hamstring muscles and orthotics for pes planus (flat feet).

Procedures

Paravertebral spinal nerve root blocks have been shown to significantly reduce radiating pain.[9] This is done under fluoroscopic guidance to minimize risk of injury to the lung and to ensure the accuracy of the level of injection.

Surgery

Thoracoscopic microsurgical excision of herniated thoracic discs has been shown to have excellent outcomes with less surgical time, less blood loss, fewer postoperative complications, and shorter hospitalizations than more traditional and invasive surgical approaches.[10] Traditionally, mechanical causes of thoracic radiculopathy have been treated with posterior laminectomy, lateral costotransversectomy, or anterior discectomy by a transthoracic approach. In three series of 91 surgically treated cases, pain resolved or improved in 67% to 94% of patients, and myelopathy improved in 71% to 97% of patients.[11]

POTENTIAL DISEASE COMPLICATIONS

If it is left untreated, thoracic radiculopathy can result in chronic pain and its associated comorbidities. Progressive thoracic spinal cord compression, if unrecognized, can lead to paraparesis, neurogenic bowel and bladder, and spasticity.

POTENTIAL TREATMENT COMPLICATIONS

Analgesics and nonsteroidal anti-inflammatory drugs have well-known side effects that most commonly affect the gastric, hepatic, and renal systems. Rarely, short-term oral steroid use may produce avascular necrosis of the hip and, more commonly, glucose intolerance. Tricyclic antidepressants may cause dry mouth and urinary retention. Along with anticonvulsants, they may also cause sedation. On occasion, physical therapy may exacerbate symptoms. The risks of invasive pain procedures and surgery, including bleeding, infection, and further neurologic compromise, are well documented.

References

1. Arce CA, Bohrmann GJ. Herniated thoracic discs. Neurol Clin 1985;3: 382-392.
2. Brown CW, Deffer PA, Akmakjian J, et al. The natural history of thoracic disc herniation. Spine 1992;17(Suppl):S97-S102.
3. Cohen-Gadol AA, White JB, Lynch JJ, et al. Synovial cysts of the thoracic spine. J Neurosurg Spine 2004;1:52-57.
4. Dumitru D. Electrodiagnostic Medicine. Philadelphia, Hanley & Belfus, 1995:558.
5. Bicknell JM, Johnson SF. Widespread electromyographic abnormalities in spinal muscles in cancer, disc disease, and diabetes. Univ Mich Med Center J 1976;42:124-127.
6. Devon R, Shuster E. Axillary pain as a heralding sign of neoplasm involving the upper thoracic root. Neurology 2006;66:1760-1762.
7. Tokuhashi Y, Matsuzaki H, Uematsu Y, Oda H. Symptoms of thoracolumbar disc herniation. Spine 2001;26:E512-E518.
8. Dreyfuss P, Dumitru D, Prewitt-Buchanan L. Intercostal somatosensory evoked potentials: a new technique. Am J Phys Med Rehabil 1993;72:144-150.
9. Richardson J, Jones J, Atkinson R. The effect of thoracic paravertebral blockade on intercostal somatosensory evoked potentials. Anesth Analg 1998;87:373-376.
10. Rosenthal D, Dickman CA. Thoracoscopic microsurgical excision of herniated thoracic discs. J Neurosurg 1998;89:224-235.
11. Dretze DD Jr, Fessler RG. Thoracic disc herniations. Neurosurg Clin North Am 1993;4:75-90.

Thoracic Sprain or Strain 40

Alexios Carayannopoulos, DO, MPH, and Darren Rosenberg, DO

Synonyms

Thoracic sprain
Pulled upper back
Benign thoracic pain

ICD-9 Codes

721.2   Thoracic spondylosis, aggravated
724.1   Thoracalgia (thoracic-mid back pain)
847.1   Sprains and strains of other unspecified parts of back (thoracic)
847.2   Thoracic strain

DEFINITION

Thoracic strain or sprain refers to the acute or subacute onset of pain in the region of the thoracic spine due to bone or soft tissue injury, including muscles, ligaments, tendons, and fascia, of an otherwise normal back. Because the thoracic cage is unified by the overlying fascia, injury or dysfunction of any one of these elements can translate into injury to the whole.

Epidemiology

Although literature on musculoskeletal pain in the cervical and thoracic spine is abundant, similar information about musculoskeletal pain in the thoracic region is sparse.[1-3] Patients with mechanical disorders of the thoracic spine amount to only 1.96% of all patients who experience common mechanical back pain.[4] Therefore, observation and characterization of such lesions are minimal, subsequently limiting the potential to improve treatment methods for thoracic sprain and strain disorders. Moreover, pain felt in the thoracic spine is often referred from the cervical spine, mistakenly giving the impression that the incidence is higher than it actually is.[5]

Thoracic strain or sprain may be the indirect result of disc lesions, the incidence of which has been reported to be evenly distributed between the sexes. These are most common in patients from the fourth to sixth decades. Protrusions have been found at every level of the thoracic spine.[6] Intervertebral disc prolapse necessitating surgery is not common according to DePalma and Rothman,[7] who reported in 1970 that of 1000 intervertebral disc operations, only one was for thoracic disc disease. Others have reported isolated cases of thoracic disc protrusion.[8,9]

As with most nonspecific mechanical disorders of the cervical and lumbar regions, the natural history of the majority of patients with nonspecific thoracic strain or sprain is resolution within several months.

Mechanisms

Thoracic sprain and strain injuries can occur in all age groups, but there is an increased prevalence among patients of working age.[10] Intrinsic mechanisms include bone disease as well as alteration of normal spine or upper extremity biomechanics. This includes cervical or thoracic deformity from neuromuscular or spinal disease as well as shoulder or scapular dysfunction. However, the most common intrinsic cause of thoracic strain is poor posture or excessive sitting. Poor posture may be related to development of Scheuermann disease in the young and osteoporosis in the elderly.

Poor posture is often manifested as excessive protraction or drooping of the neck and shoulders as well as decreased lumbar lordosis or "flat back." The thoracic spine is considered to be the least mobile area of the vertebral column secondary to the length of the transverse processes, the presence of costovertebral joints, the decrease in disc height compared with the lumbar spine, and the presence of the rib cage. Movements that occur in the thoracic spine include rotation with flexion or extension. With the classic "slouched position" encountered in children and adolescents and often carried on through adulthood, there is excessive flexion with a decrease in rotation and extension.

Postural alterations promote increased thoracic kyphosis, resulting in the "flexed posture." Excessive flexion results in excessive strain on the "core," including the small intrinsic muscles of the spine, the long paraspinal muscles, and the abdominal and rib cage muscles. Excessive flexion can increase the risk of rib stress fractures

223

as well as costovertebral joint irritation. This can cause referral of pain to the chest wall with subsequent development of trigger points in the erector spinae, levator scapulae, rhomboids, and trapezius. Poor motion in extension and rotation can place an increased load on nearby structures, such as the lumbar or cervical spine and shoulders.

Extrinsic or environmental mechanisms include repetitive strain, trauma, and obesity. Risk factors include repetitive motions such as lifting, twisting, and bending. Occupations requiring manual labor are predisposed to a higher incidence of such disorders. Traumatic causes include falls, violence, and accidents leading to vertebral fractures, chest wall contusions, or flail chest.

SYMPTOMS

Patients typically report pain in the mid back, which may be related to upper extremity or neck movements. Symptoms may be exacerbated by deep breathing, coughing, rotation of the thoracic spine, or prolonged standing. The pain can be generalized in the mid back area or focal. If it is focal, it is usually described as a "knot," which is deep and ache-like. It may radiate to the anterior chest wall, abdomen, shoulder-arm, cervical spine, or lumbosacral spine and may be accentuated with movement of the upper extremity or neck. As described by McKenzie,[5] the location of pain in mechanical disorders of the thoracic spine is either central (symmetric) or unilateral (asymmetric).

Like other regional musculoskeletal disorders, thoracic pain may derive from soft tissue, visceral, disc, or articular structures and is difficult to differentiate. Other symptoms include muscle spasm, tightness, and stiffness as well as pain or decreased range of motion in the mid back, low back, neck, or shoulder.

PHYSICAL EXAMINATION

As the thoracic cage and spine are the anchors for the limbs, the thoracic spine influences and is influenced by active and resisted movement of the extremities, cranium, and lumbar and cervical spine.[11] Therefore, a careful spinal and shoulder examination is essential to rule out restrictive movements, obvious deformity, soft tissue asymmetry, and skin changes (infection, tumor). Detailed examination of other systems is important because thoracic pain can be referred.

Examination includes static and dynamic assessment of posture. The examination of sitting and standing posture and the quality of mount must be established before dynamic evaluation. The patient should be observed in relaxed stance with the shirt removed. Viewing is from the posterior, lateral, and anterior perspectives, and deviations from an ideal posture, as described by Kendall and associates,[12] are noted. McKenzie[5] tests static positions to determine a direction of preference with the following positions: erect sitting flexion, erect sitting extension, erect sitting rotation, and extension

lying prone and supine. With dynamic assessment, it is important to affect the patient's symptoms by moving and stressing the structures from which pain is thought to originate.

Active range of motion of the cervical, thoracic, and trunk regions is assessed to determine pain-provoking movements.[13] Cervical and trunk active range of motion can be described on the basis of comparisons of pain-free motion in the opposite direction, if present, or an estimated range of normal.[14] It has been acknowledged that visual estimation of active range of motion for the cervical and trunk regions has no known reliability.[15] Shoulder range of motion can be estimated by visually comparing side to side, which has been shown to yield fair to good estimates of reliability for the shoulder joint.[16]

In addition, the presence of deformities and the site of pain and tenderness are noted. Pain is often felt between the scapulae, around the lower border of the scapula, and centrally in the area between T1 and T7. However, much of the pain felt in the thoracic area has been shown to originate in the cervical spine.[17] Pain in the region above an imaginary line drawn between the inferior borders of the scapulae is most likely secondary to the cervical region. Pain provocation with palpatory assessment or mobility testing has been found to yield reliable scores with assessment of the lumbar spine, and several authors have suggested that it may thereby be used as a basis of clinical decision-making in the assessment of the thoracic spine.[13,18,19]

Neurologic testing is important and should include motor, sensory, and reflex examination. Manual muscle testing as described by Hislop and Montgomery[20] can be used to test upper extremity strength and can be modified in the sitting position to avoid multiple position changes. Gross sensory examination by use of light touch over the upper extremity and thoracic dermatomes can be performed to determine whether nerve root or peripheral lesions are present; however, the reliability of data obtained during sensory testing by this method has not been determined.[21] In terms of reflexes, careful examination of the abdomen can be important. Because the abdominal muscles are innervated segmentally, the upper muscles from T7 to T10 and the lower muscles from T10 to L1, the presence or absence of this reflex may pinpoint the quadrant involved in a lower or upper motor neuron lesion at the respective spinal level.

Given the fact that the thoracic cage is unified by the overlying fascia and that injury or dysfunction of any one of these elements can translate into injury to the whole, assessment of accessory motion or joint play can be valuable. This can be performed in the prone position with pressure directed from posterior to anterior to assess joint play from C7 to T12.[21] In addition, accessory motion of the costovertebral, costotransverse, and costosternal joints can be evaluated. Costovertebral and costotransverse motion can be assessed with a posterior-directed force at each rib level.[22,23] Even though the costovertebral and costotransverse joints are two distinct articulations, they are often grouped together because it has been shown that movement at one joint cannot occur without movement at the other joint. Costosternal motion can be assessed with the patient in a supine position with pressure directed anterior to posterior at each rib level.[23] For each assessment, the presence of pain and relative mobility compared with the other side should be noted.[13] In addition, scapular mobility and motion should be examined with repeated bouts of shoulder flexion and abduction within the patient's available active range of motion to note the presence of pain and relative mobility.[20]

The essential finding in the physical examination of thoracic sprain or strain is thoracic muscle spasm with a normal neurologic examination. Pain may be exacerbated when the patient lifts the arms overhead, extends backward, or rotates. Rib motion may be restricted and may be assessed by examining excursion of the chest wall. This is accomplished by laying hands on the upper and lower chest wall and looking for symmetry and rhythm of movement. The upper ribs usually move in a bucket-handle motion, whereas the lower ribs move in a pump-handle motion. Restriction of specific ribs can be assessed by examining individual rib movements with respiration.

The position of comfort is usually flexion, but this is the position that should be avoided. Sensation and reflex examination findings should be normal. A finding of lower extremity weakness or neurologic deficit on physical examination suggests an alternative diagnosis and may warrant further investigation.[24]

FUNCTIONAL LIMITATIONS

Functional limitations include difficulty with bending, lifting, and overhead activities, such as throwing and reaching. These limitations affect both active and sedentary workers. Activities of daily living, such as upper extremity bathing and dressing, might be affected. General mobility may be impaired. As most sports-related or leisure activities involve use of the upper extremity, extension, or rotation of the thorax, athletic participation and functional capacity may be limited as well.

DIAGNOSTIC STUDIES

Thoracic sprain and strain injuries are typically diagnosed on the basis of the history and physical examination. No tests are usually necessary during the first 4 weeks of symptoms if the injury is nontraumatic. If there is suspicion of tumor (night pain, constitutional symptoms), infection (fever, chills, malaise), or fracture (focal tenderness with history of trauma or fall), earlier and more complete investigation is warranted.

Plain films are indicated if the injury is associated with recent trauma or to rule out osteoporosis or malignant disease. Magnetic resonance imaging is the study of choice in considering thoracic malignant neoplasia or when the patient has unilateral localized thoracic pain with sensory-motor deficits to rule out a thoracic disc herniation.[25] A computed tomographic scan or triple-phase bone scan can identify bone abnormalities if magnetic resonance imaging is contraindicated. However, magnetic resonance imaging can detect abnormalities unrelated to the patient's symptoms because many people who do not have pain have abnormal imaging findings.[26]

TREATMENT

Initial

The initial treatment of a thoracic sprain or strain injury generally involves the use of cold packs to decrease pain and edema during the first 48 hours after the injury. Thereafter, the application of moist heat to reduce pain

Differential Diagnosis

Thoracic back symptoms may also be due to pain referred from other organ systems or processes. Cancer, cardiac, pulmonary, gallbladder, hepatobiliary, renal, and gastroesophageal conditions are potential causes of referred thoracic or scapular pain.[27-30] Bone disease can also cause thoracic pain; this includes Paget disease, osteopenia or osteoporosis, and osteomalacia. Features requiring further consideration include nontraumatic pain or night pain (tumor); pulsatile abdominal mass (dissecting aortic aneurysm); constitutional symptoms of unexplained weight loss, night pain, fever, or chills (cancer); fever (possible soft tissue or bone infection); enlarging soft tissue mass (thoracolumbar hernia); previous use of systemic corticosteroids (osteoporotic collapse); immunosuppression (lymphoma, infection); and history of cancer (metastatic disease).[31,32]

Other spinal entities in the differential include the following:

> Thoracic radiculopathy
>
> Facet joint arthropathy
>
> Structural rib dysfunction
>
> Spinal stenosis
>
> Scheuermann disease
>
> Ankylosing spondylosis
>
> Discitis
>
> Vertebral fracture (trauma, insufficiency, pathologic)
>
> Scoliosis or kyphosis

Other extraspinal causes in the differential include the following:

> Peptic ulcer disease
>
> Pancreatitis
>
> Cholecystitis
>
> Nephrolithiasis
>
> Shingles[33,34]

and muscle spasm is indicated. Bed rest for up to 48 hours may be beneficial, but prolonged bed rest is discouraged. Relative rest by avoidance of activities that exacerbate pain is preferable to complete bed rest. Temporary use of a rib binder or elastic wrap may reduce pain as well as increase activity tolerance and mobility. A short course of nonsteroidal anti-inflammatory drugs, acetaminophen, muscle relaxants, or topical anesthetics such as Lidoderm patches may be beneficial. Capsaicin cream can be used topically for shingles or focal tenderness but may not be tolerated secondary to burning sensation of the skin. Narcotics are generally not necessary.

Rehabilitation

Most acute thoracic sprain or strain injuries will heal spontaneously with rest and physical modalities used at home, such as ice, heating pad, and massage. Body mechanics and postural training are important aspects of the rehabilitation program for thoracic sprain or strain.[35,36] A focus on correct posture at work and while driving is specifically important. In the car, patients can use a lumbar roll to promote proper posture; at work, patients are advised to sit upright at the computer in an adjustable, comfortable chair. Other workplace modifications include forearm rests (data arms) to support the arms and the use of a telephone earpiece or headset to prevent neck and upper thoracic strain.

For patients with abnormally flexed or slouched posture, household modifications can be made that might help encourage extension and subsequently decrease pain. These include pillows or lumbar rolls on chairs and replacement of sagging mattresses with firm bedding. Also, use of paper plates and lightweight cookware in the kitchen and reassignment of objects in overhead cabinets to areas that are more accessible can help if lifting or reaching is painful.

If pain persists beyond a couple of weeks, physical therapy may be indicated. In general, physical therapy will apply movements that centralize, reduce, or diminish the patient's symptoms while discouraging movements that peripheralize or increase the patient's symptoms.[5] In most cases, an active approach that encourages stretching, strengthening, and exercise is preferred to a more passive approach. To correct sitting posture, patients are advised to continue to use the lumbar roll in all sitting environments. To correct standing posture, patients are shown how to take the lumbar lordosis off end range and to move the lower part of the spine backward while at the same time moving the upper spine forward, raising the chest and retracting the head and neck. To correct lying posture, patients should use a firm mattress as previously indicated. In the case of patients who experience more pain in the thoracic spine when lying in bed, this advice often leads to worsening of the symptoms rather than a resolution. In these patients, advice should be given to deliberately sag the mattress by placing pillows under each end of the mattress so that it becomes dished. In this manner, the thoracic kyphosis is not forced into the extended range in lying supine, and the removal of this stress allows a comfortable night's sleep.

However, long-term goals still include improvement in extension range of motion.[5]

In persons with osteoporosis, research has shown that extension exercises performed regularly significantly reduce the number of compression fractures in the group exercising in this manner.[37] For this exercise, patients are instructed to lie down with a pillow under the abdomen and the hands clasped behind the back. The patient is instructed to lift the head, shoulders, and both legs simultaneously as high as possible; the position is held for a second, and then the patient relaxes. This is repeated as many times as possible in a progressive fashion, and patients are instructed to exercise in this manner for the rest of their lives.[5] Passive modalities, such as ultrasound, electrical stimulation, and light massage for pain control, should be used sparingly. Modalities that include superficial and deep heat or cold may help increase range of motion and decrease pain but should be used in moderation.

After a formal physical therapy program is completed, a home exercise or gym regimen is essential and should be prescribed and individualized for all patients to maintain gains made during physical therapy. Exercises at home are aimed at improvement in flexibility of the thoracic spine and may include extension in lying, standing, and sitting performed six to eight times throughout the day. In addition, alternating arm and leg lifts and active trunk extension in the prone position should be performed. Finally, regular stretching to improve extension and rotation with trigger pointing can decrease muscle tension over the affected muscles. A thoracic wedge, which is designed to increase extension range of motion, can be used. The wedge is a hard piece of molded plastic or rubber with a wedge cut out to accommodate the spine. The patient lies on the ground with the wedge placed in between the shoulder blades. The patient is instructed to arch over it. Alternatively, two tennis balls can be taped together for the same effect. These exercises can be done before regular stretching to increase excursion. Regular massage therapy can maintain flexibility and prevent tightening from more regular exercise.

At the gym, progressive isotonic movements such as rowing, lat pull-downs, and pull-ups and an abdominal crunch strengthening program should be emphasized. Instruction in proper positioning and technique should be provided to prevent further injury. Use of a "physioball" at home or at the gym can facilitate trunk extension as well as abdominal stretching and strengthening to increase overall conditioning of the thoracic cage and core musculature. This can be done in conjunction with use of Thera-Bands with progressive resistance to facilitate stretching of the arms and shoulders with mild strengthening of the shoulder, arm, and core muscles. Finally, a pool program can be prescribed. Swimming strokes such as the crawl, backstroke, and butterfly emphasize extension and can be very useful to prevent or to correct a flexion bias. With the crawl, patients are instructed to breathe on both sides to prevent unilateral strain in the neck and upper thoracic spine.

Manual medicine, which includes osteopathic manipulative medicine, chiropractic, and physical therapy mobilization, may also be used for acute and subacute thoracic pain. Specifically, techniques that actively engage restrictive movements, such as extension and rotation, can be used. These include muscle energy and high-velocity, low-amplitude techniques that engage the barrier or restriction to extend the patient's physiologic barrier. They can be performed at the micro segmental level of the spine or at the macro level of the thoracic cage, shoulder, and upper extremity. These techniques can temporarily reduce restriction of movement to improve overall range with subsequent restoration of proper posture and alignment. There can be a subsequent reduction in muscle spasm, increase in range of motion, and decrease of pain. In combination with an active physical therapy and exercise program, small gains with manual medicine can lead to sustained benefits in posture and overall conditioning.

Procedures

Trigger point injections may help reduce focal pain caused by taut bands of muscle, allowing the patient to exercise to restore range of motion, to correct postural imbalance, and to increase strength and balance of the dysfunctional segment.[38,39] Acupuncture can be used for local as well as for systemic treatment. Finally, botulinum toxin A (Botox) has been used for specific muscles, including rhomboids, trapezius, levator scapulae, and serratus, that often contribute to thoracic strain and sprain.

It is generally accepted that administration of botulinum toxin A may lead to diminished pain in patients with painful muscle spasm or cervical dystonia by decreasing muscle tone. Botulinum toxin A is a potent neurotoxin that blocks the release of acetylcholine at the neuromuscular junction and thereby inhibits muscle contraction.[40] It is also thought that botulinum toxin may itself possess analgesic properties, but these mechanisms are unknown. It is thought that botulinum toxin A–induced analgesia arises from reduction of muscle spasm by cholinergic chemodenervation at motor end plates through inhibition of gamma motor endings in muscle spindles.[41] In addition, it has been posited that subcutaneous injection of botulinum toxins may contribute to antinociception by inhibition of local neurotransmitter release from primary sensory neurons in the area of injection.[42] Although there are no studies specifically looking at use of botulinum toxin A for treatment of thoracic strain, there are studies that looked at treatment of regional myofascial pain disorders. One study showed effective pain relief for generalized myofascial pain syndrome.[43] In another study, there was no statistically significant improvement in pain with direct trigger point injections of patients with cervicothoracic myofascial pain syndrome.[44]

In general, doses of Botox should not exceed 400 units total, with 25 to 50 units for small muscles and 100 units for larger muscles. Typically, the muscle-paralyzing effectiveness of botulinum toxin A lasts 3 to 4 months.[45] Patients need to be warned of the possibility of excessive weakening, infection, bleeding, and development of antibodies.

Surgery

Surgery is not usually indicated unless focal disc herniation is involved or there is instability of particular spinal segments from fracture or dislocation.

POTENTIAL DISEASE COMPLICATIONS

Thoracic sprain and strain injuries can occasionally develop into myofascial pain syndromes.

POTENTIAL TREATMENT COMPLICATIONS

Possible complications include gastrointestinal side effects from nonsteroidal anti-inflammatory drugs. Other possible complications include somnolence or confusion from muscle relaxants; addiction from narcotics; bleeding, infection, postinjection soreness, and pneumothorax from trigger point injections; excessive weakness and development of antibodies from botulinum toxin; and temporary post-treatment exacerbation of pain from manual medicine.

References

1. Edmondston SJ, Singer KP. Thoracic spine: anatomical and biomechanical considerations for manual therapy. Man Ther 1997;2: 132-143.
2. McRae M, Cleland J. Differential diagnosis and treatment of upper thoracic pain: a case study. J Manual Manipulative Ther 2003; 11:43-48.
3. Schiller L. Effectiveness of spinal manipulative therapy in the treatment of mechanical thoracic spine pain: a pilot randomized clinical trial. J Manual Manipulative Ther 2001;24:394-401.
4. Kramer J. Intervertebral Disk Diseases. Causes, Diagnosis, Treatment and Prophylaxis. New York, Thieme, 1981.
5. McKenzie RA. The Cervical and Thoracic Spine: Mechanical Diagnosis and Therapy. Waikanae, NZ, Spinal Publications Ltd, 1990.
6. Love JG, Schorn VG. Thoracic-disk protrusions. JAMA 1965;191: 627-630.
7. DePalma A, Rothman RH. The Intervertebral Disc. Philadelphia, WB Saunders, 1970.
8. Chambers AA. Thoracic disk herniation. Semin Roentgenol 1988;23:111-117.
9. Chowdhary UM. Intradural thoracic disc protrusion. Spine 1987;12: 718-719.
10. Choi BC, Levitsky M, Lloyd RD, et al. Patterns and risk factors for sprains and strain in Ontario, Canada, 1990. J Occup Environ Med 1996;38:379-389.
11. Austin GP, Benesky WT. Thoracic pain in a collegiate runner. Man Ther 2000;7:168-172.
12. Kendall FP, McCreary EK, Provance PG. Muscles: Testing and Function, 4th ed. Philadelphia, Lippincott Williams & Wilkins, 1993:70-103.
13. Fruth SJ. Differential diagnosis and treatment in a patient with posterior upper thoracic pain. Phys Ther 2006;86:254-268.
14. Reese NB, Bandy WD. Joint Range of Motion and Muscle Length Testing. Philadelphia, WB Saunders, 2002.
15. Youdas JW. Reliability of measurements of cervical spine range of motion: comparison of three methods. Phys Ther 1991;71:98-104.
16. Hayes K, Walton JR, Szomor ZL, Murrell GA. Reliability of five methods of assessing shoulder range of motion. Aust J Physiother 2001;47:289-294.
17. Cloward RB. Cervical discography: a contribution to the etiology and mechanism of neck, shoulder, and arm pain. Ann Surg 1959;150:1052.

18. Boline PD, Haas M, Meyer JJ, et al. Interexaminer reliability of eight evaluative dimensions of lumbar segmental abnormality: part II. J Manipulative Physiol Ther 1995;75:212-222.
19. Maher C, Adams R. Reliability of pain and stiffness assessments in clinical examination measures for identification of lumbar segmental instability. Arch Phys Med Rehabil 2003;84:1858-1864.
20. Hislop HJ, Montgomery J. Daniels and Worthingham's Muscle Testing: Techniques of Manual Examination, 7th ed. Philadelphia, WB Saunders, 2002.
21. Magee DJ. Orthopedic Physical Assessment, 4th ed. Philadelphia, WB Saunders, 2002.
22. Bookhout MR. Evaluation of the thoracic spine and rib cage. In Flynn TW. The Thoracic Spine and Rib Cage: Musculoskeletal Evaluation and Treatment. Boston, Butterworth-Heinemann, 2000:244-256.
23. Maitland GD. Peripheral Manipulation, 3rd ed. Boston, Butterworth-Heinemann, 1991.
24. Acute low back problems in adults: assessment and treatment. Acute Low Back Problems Guideline Panel. Agency for Health Care Policy and Research. Am Fam Physician 1995;51:469-484.
25. Dietze DD Jr, Fessler RG. Thoracic disc herniations. Neurosurg Clin North Am 1993;4:75-90.
26. Wood KB, Garvey TA, Gundry C, et al. Magnetic resonance imaging of the thoracic spine. Evaluation of asymptomatic individuals. J Bone Joint Surg Am 1995;77:1631-1638.
27. Scaringe JG, Ketner C. Manual methods for the treatment of rib dysfunctions and associated functional lesions. Top Clin Chiropractic 1999;6:20-38.
28. Gerwin RD. Myofascial and visceral pain syndromes: visceral-somatic pain representations. J Musculoskeletal Pain 2002;10:165-175.
29. Lillegard WA. Medical causes of pain in the thoracic region. In Flynn TW. The Thoracic Spine and Rib Cage: Musculoskeletal Evaluation and Treatment. Boston, Butterworth-Heinemann, 1996:107-120.
30. Triano JJ, Erwin M, Hansen DT. Costovertebral and costotransverse joint pain: a commonly overlooked pain generator. Top Clin Chiropractic 1999;6:79-92.
31. Car J, Aziz S. Acute low back pain: 10 minute consultation. BMJ 2003;327:541-542.
32. Faraj AA, Medhian H. Thoracolumbar hernia: a rare cause of back pain. Eur Spine J 1997;6:203-204.
33. Snider RK. Essentials of Musculoskeletal Care. Rosemont, Ill, American Academy of Orthopaedic Surgeons, 1997.
34. Bruckner FE, Allard SA, Moussa NA. Benign thoracic pain. J R Soc Med 1987;80:286-289.
35. Guccione AA. Physical therapy for musculoskeletal syndromes. Rheum Dis Clin North Am 1996;22:551-562.
36. Turner JA. Educational and behavioral interventions for back pain in primary care. Spine 1996;21:2851-2859.
37. Sinaki M, Mikkelsen BA. Postmenopausal spinal osteoporosis: flexion versus extension exercises. Arch Phys Med Rehabil 1984;65:593-596.
38. Rosen NB. The myofascial pain syndromes. Phys Med Rehabil Clin North Am 1993;4:41-63.
39. Travell JG, Simons DJ. Myofascial Pain and Dysfunction: The Trigger Point Manual. Baltimore, Williams & Wilkins, 1991.
40. Smith J, Audette J, Royal M. Botulinum toxin in pain management of soft tissue syndromes. Clin J Pain 2002;18(Suppl):147-154.
41. Parpura V, Haydon PG. Physiological astrocytic calcium levels stimulate glutamate release to modulate adjacent neurons. Proc Natl Acad Sci USA 2000;97:8629-8634.
42. Cui M, Chaddock JA, Rubino J, et al. Retargeted clostridial endopeptidase: antinociceptive activity in preclinical models of pain. Arch Pharmacol 2002;365(Suppl 2):R16.
43. Graboski CL, Gray DS, Burnham RS. Botulinum toxin A versus bupivacaine trigger point injections for the treatment of myofascial pain syndrome: a randomized double blind crossover study. Pain 2005;118:170-175.
44. Ferrante FM, Bearn L, Rothrock R, et al. Evidence against trigger point injection technique for the treatment of cervicothoracic myofascial pain with botulinum toxin type A. Anesthesiology 2005;103:377-383.
45. Sellin LC. The action of botulinum toxin at the neuromuscular junction. Med Biol 1981;59:11-20.

Lumbar Degenerative Disease 41

Michael K. Schaufele, MD, and Aimee H. Walsh, MD

Synonyms

Osteoarthritis of the spine
Spondylosis
Lumbar arthritis
Degenerative joint disease of the spine
Degenerative disc disease

ICD-9 Codes

721.3   Lumbosacral spondylosis without myelopathy
721.90   Spondylosis of unspecified site (spinal arthritis)
722.52   Degeneration of lumbar or lumbosacral intervertebral disc
724.2   Low back pain

DEFINITION

Degeneration of the structures of the spine is a process associated with aging. It may be accelerated in patients with previous trauma or injury to the lumbar spine. L4-5 and L5-S1 are the most commonly involved lumbar levels, given that they undergo the greatest torsion and compressive loads. Degenerative processes may affect several anatomic structures, resulting in different clinical syndromes.

The facet (zygapophyseal) joints and sacroiliac joints, like other synovial joints in the body, may develop osteoarthritis.[1] The intervertebral disc experiences progressive disc dehydration as part of the normal aging process of the spinal structures. In certain patients, fissures in the annulus fibrosus may develop, causing an inflammatory response. Nociceptive pain fibers may grow into these fissures.[2] Further degeneration may result in progression of the disease or complete annular tears, which may be the source of discogenic low back pain, also referred to as internal disc disruption syndrome. Up to 39% of patients with chronic low back pain may suffer from internal disc disruption.[3] The loss of segmental integrity may lead to further degeneration of the disc, which results in narrowing of the intervertebral disc space. Because of increased loads on the posterior elements, facet degeneration may develop. Facet arthropathy may be an independent or concurrent source of low back pain. Further disc degeneration and subsequent loss of disc height may cause subluxation of the facet joints, resulting in degenerative spondylolisthesis, most commonly at the L4-5 level.[4]

Other conditions seen with lumbar degeneration include spondylosis deformans and diffuse idiopathic skeletal hyperostosis. Spondylosis deformans is a degenerative condition marked by formation of anterolateral osteophytes and is mainly a radiologic diagnosis. In spondylosis deformans, the intervertebral spaces are usually well preserved, unlike in degenerative disc disease. The initiating factor in the development of this condition may be degeneration of the annulus fibrosus, primarily in the anterolateral disc space.[5] Spondylosis may become clinically symptomatic if excessive osteophyte formation leads to neural compression, such as in spinal stenosis. Diffuse idiopathic skeletal hyperostosis involves ossification of the ligamentous attachments to the vertebral bones (entheses). Radiologic features consist of flowing, excessive anterior osteophyte formation. Diffuse idiopathic skeletal hyperostosis affects 5% to 10% of patients older than 65 years.[6] This diagnosis is typically an incidental finding on radiologic studies.[7]

Other factors associated with lumbar degeneration include environmental, occupational, and psychosocial influences. Environmental influences include cigarette smoking and occupational activities that involve repetitive bending and prolonged exposures to stooping, sitting, or vibrational stresses. These repetitive actions may result in degeneration of the lumbosacral motion segments.[6] Psychosocial factors are well known to contribute to significant disability in low back pain, often in patients with only minimal structural impairment.[8]

SYMPTOMS

Lumbar degenerative symptoms range from minor to debilitating. Common complaints include chronic back pain and stiffness. Patients may also report limited range of motion, especially with extension in the case of facet arthropathy or spinal stenosis. Symptoms of pain with lumbar flexion, coughing, sneezing, or Valsalva maneuver are often associated with disc disease. Should the degenerative changes result in compression of neural structures, patients may develop radicular symptoms into the leg. This can be seen in conditions such as lumbar disc herniations and spinal stenosis.

Lumbar degenerative disease is probably entirely asymptomatic in the majority of cases. Approximately one third of subjects have substantial abnormalities on magnetic resonance imaging despite being clinically asymptomatic.[9] Because of factors not well understood, such as leakage of inflammatory factors from the disc, a chronic pain syndrome may develop in some patients, possibly from repetitive sensitization of nociceptive fibers in the annulus fibrosus.[10]

Clinicians should inquire about atypical symptoms of back pain, including night pain, fever, and recent weight loss. These may lead to the diagnosis of malignant neoplasm or infection.

Symptoms of chronic pain, including sleep disturbances and depression, should be sought.

PHYSICAL EXAMINATION

The purpose of the physical examination is to direct further evaluation and therapy toward one of the five most common sources of low back pain: discogenic, facet arthropathy or instability, radiculopathy or neural compression, myofascial or soft tissue, and psychogenic. Combinations of these sources of back pain often exist. This distinction will allow the use of advanced diagnostic tests and therapeutic options in the most cost-effective approach.

A standardized low back examination should include assessment of flexibility (lumbosacral flexion, extension, trunk rotation, finger-floor distance, hamstring and iliopsoas range of motion, and hip range of motion). An inclinometer may assist in standardizing lumbar range of motion measurements.[11] A complete examination includes inspection of lower extremities for atrophy and vascular insufficiency, muscle strength testing, and assessment for sensory abnormalities and their distribution. It is important to note asymmetries in deep tendon reflexes (patellar tendon [L4], hamstring tendon [L5], and Achilles tendon [S1]), which may be the most objective finding. Upper motor neuron signs, such as Babinski and Hoffmann, should also be tested. Functional strength testing should include heel to toe walking, calf and toe raises, single-leg knee bends, and complete gait evaluation. Specific testing for lower back syndromes includes straight-leg raising, femoral stretch sign, dural tension signs, and sacroiliac joint provocative maneuvers (e.g., FABER, Gillet, Yeoman, and Gaenslen tests) as well as specific evaluation techniques, such as the McKenzie technique. Assessment of the patient for nonorganic signs of back pain (Waddell signs; Table 41-1) will help the clinician to recognize patients in whom psychological factors may contribute to the pain syndrome.[12]

FUNCTIONAL LIMITATIONS

Functional limitations in degenerative diseases of the lumbar spine depend on the anatomic structures involved. All aspects of daily living, including self-care, work, sports activities, and recreation, may be affected.

TABLE 41-1 Waddell Signs

Five nonorganic physical signs are described by Waddell.

Tenderness	Nonorganic tenderness may be either superficial or nonanatomic. Superficial tenderness can be elicited by lightly pinching over a wide area of lumbar skin. Nonanatomic pain is described as deep tenderness felt over a wide area rather than localized to one structure.
Simulation test	This is usually based on movement that produces pain. Two examples are axial loading, in which low back pain is reported on vertical loading over the standing patient's skull by the clinician's hands, and rotation, in which back pain is reported when the shoulder and pelvis are passively rotated in the same plane as the patient stands relaxed with feet together.
Distraction test	If a positive physical finding is demonstrated in a routine manner, this finding is checked while the patient's attention is distracted. Straight-leg raising is the most useful distraction test. There are several variations to this test; most commonly, however, straight-leg raise is done in the supine position and then, while the patient is distracted, in the sitting position. This is commonly referred to as the flip test. However, one should keep in mind that biomechanically, the two positions are very different.
Regional disturbances	Regional disturbances involve a widespread area, such as an entire quarter or half of the body. The essential feature of this nonorganic physical sign is divergence of the pain beyond the accepted neuroanatomy. Examples include give-away weakness in many muscle groups manually tested and sensory disturbances, such as diminished sensation to light touch, pinprick, or vibration, that do not follow a dermatomal pattern. Again, care must be taken not to mistake multiple root involvement for regional disturbance.
Overreaction	Waddell reported that overreaction during the examination may take the form of disproportionate verbalization, facial expression, muscle tension, tremor, collapsing, and even profuse sweating. Analysis of multiple nonorganic signs showed that overreaction was the single most important nonorganic physical sign. However, this sign is also the most influenced by the subjectivity of the observer.

Modified from Geraci MC Jr, Alleva JT. Physical examination of the spine and its functional kinetic chain. In Cole AJ, Herring SA, eds. The Low Back Pain Handbook. Philadelphia, Hanley & Belfus, 1997:58-59.

Symptoms are typically exacerbated during bending, twisting, stooping, and forward flexion in patients with primary discogenic pain. Patients with facet arthropathy or instability report increased pain with extension-based activity, including standing and walking. Pain is often relieved with sitting and other similar forward-flexed positions. Patients with myofascial or soft tissue syndromes report pain that is worsened with static and prolonged physical activity. Symptomatic improvement may be associated with rest and modalities including heat, cold, and pressure. Patients with contributing psychological factors, such as depression and somatization disorders, typically report pain out of proportion to the underlying pathologic process, poor sleep, and significant disability in their daily activities.

DIAGNOSTIC STUDIES

Diagnostic testing is directed by the history and physical examination and should be ordered only if the therapeutic plan will be significantly influenced by the results. Anteroposterior and lateral lumbar spine radiographs are helpful for identifying loss of disc height as a result of disc degeneration, spondylosis or osteophyte formation, and facet arthropathy (Fig. 41-1). Oblique views are helpful to identify spondylolysis. Flexion-extension films are necessary to identify dynamic instability and can assist in the selection of appropriate surgical candidates for fusion procedures. Significant degenerative instability usually does not occur before the age of 50 years, but it should

be included as a differential diagnosis in patients with clinical symptoms suggestive of advanced facet arthropathy and disc degeneration.[6] Magnetic resonance imaging of the lumbar spine is used because of its sensitivity for identification of abnormalities of the soft tissues and neural structures. It is particularly helpful in identifying various stages of degenerative disc disease as well as annular tears and disc herniation. Other significant sources of back pain, such as neoplasms, osteomyelitis, and fractures, can also be identified with magnetic resonance imaging. Computed tomography is a valuable diagnostic tool in assessing fractures and other osseous abnormalities of the lumbar spine. Computed tomographic imaging in combination with myelography (computed tomographic myelography) aids in presurgical planning by allowing identification of osseous structures causing neural compression, especially in spinal stenosis.

Discography is currently the only technique to correlate structural abnormalities of the intravertebral disc seen on advanced imaging studies with a patient's pain response. Reproduction of painful symptoms with intradiscal injection of radiopaque contrast material aids in the localization of specific disc levels as pain generators and can be useful in separating painful disc degeneration from painless degeneration. Electrodiagnostic studies may become necessary in cases of peripheral neurologic deficits not clarified by physical examination or imaging. They allow identification of compression neuropathy, radiculopathy, or systemic motor and sensory diseases.

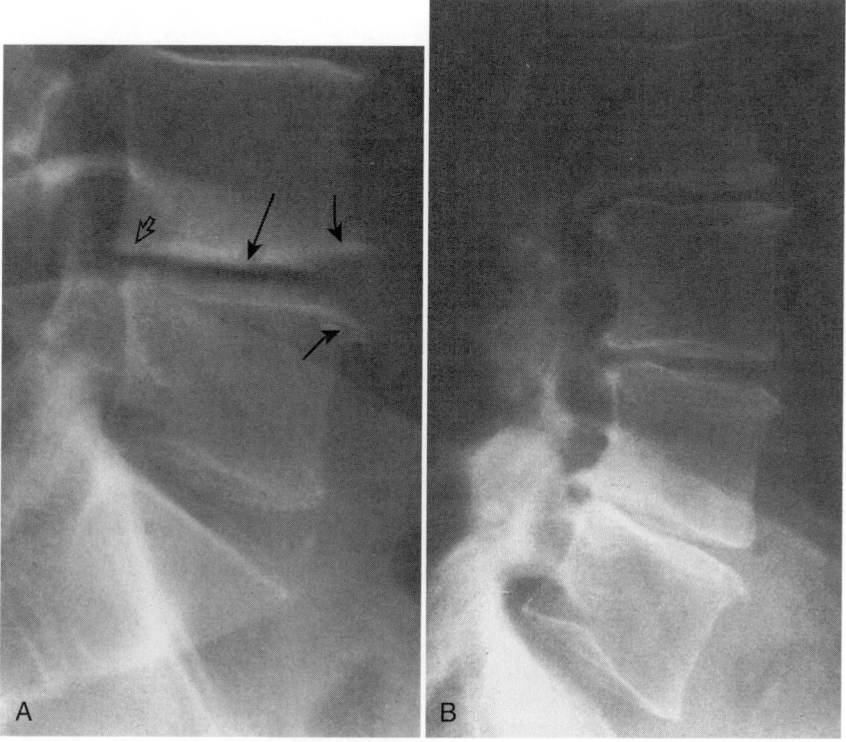

FIGURE 41-1. Chronic degenerative changes—plain film. **A,** On a coned down lateral film, the L4-5 motion segment shows a vacuum phenomenon in the disc *(large black arrow)*, end-plate remodeling with large anterior spurs *(curved arrows)*, and grade I retrolisthesis *(open arrow)*. **B,** A standing lateral film shows multilevel degenerative disc disease with large posterior spurs, small anterior osteophytes, end-plate remodeling, and moderately severe disc space narrowing at L2-3, L3-4, and L4-5. (Reprinted with permission from Cole AJ, Herzog RJ. The lumbar spine: imaging options. In Cole AJ, Herring SA, eds. The Low Back Pain Handbook. Philadelphia, Hanley & Belfus, 1997:176.)

Differential Diagnosis (see also Table 41-2)

Radiculopathy

Spondylolysis, spondylolisthesis

Spinal stenosis

Tumors

Fractures (e.g., osteoporotic compression fractures)

Osteomyelitis of the spine, discitis

TREATMENT

Initial

Probably the most important treatment of any low back pain condition is education and reassurance of the patient. Most of the acute low back symptoms are self-limited and typically resolve within 4 to 6 weeks. The mostly benign nature of degenerative conditions of the spine should be emphasized as well as the fact that acute exacerbations tend to improve over time regardless of therapy. Therapy is directed toward management of the symptoms rather than "cure" of the disease.

TABLE 41-2 Pseudospine Pain: Diagnostic Keys

	Condition	Diagnostic Keys
Vascular	Abdominal aortic aneurysm	Older than 50 years Abdominal and back pain Pulsatile abdominal mass
Gynecologic	Endometriosis	Woman of reproductive age Cyclic pelvic and back pain
	Pelvic inflammatory disease	Young, sexually active woman Systemically ill (fever chills) Discharge, dysuria
	Ectopic pregnancy	Missed period Abdominal or pelvic pain Positive pregnancy test result
Genitourinary	Prostatitis	Men older than 30 years Dysuria Low back and perineal pain
	Nephrolithiasis	Flank and groin pain Hematuria
Gastrointestinal	Pancreatitis	Abdominal pain radiating to back Systemic signs (fever, nausea, vomiting) Elevated serum amylase
	Penetrating or perforated duodenal ulcer	Abdominal pain radiating to back
Rheumatologic	Fibromyalgia	Young to middle-aged woman Widespread pain Multiple tender points Disrupted sleep, fatigue Normal radiographs and laboratory values
	Polymyalgia rheumatica	Older than 50-60 years Hip or shoulder girdle pain and stiffness Elevated erythrocyte sedimentation rate Dramatic response to low-dose prednisone
	Seronegative spondyloarthropathies (ankylosing spondylitis, Reiter syndrome, psoriatic, enteropathic)	Younger man (ankylosing spondylitis, Reiter syndrome) Lower lumbosacral pain Morning stiffness ("gel") Improvement with activity Radiographic sacroiliitis
	Diffuse idiopathic skeletal hyperostosis (DISH, Forestier disease)	Older than 50-60 years Thoracolumbar stiffness or pain Flowing anterior vertebral calcification
	Piriformis syndrome	Buttock and leg pain Pain on resisted hip external rotation and abduction Transgluteal or transrectal tenderness

TABLE 41-2 Pseudospine Pain: Diagnostic Keys—cont'd

	Condition	Diagnostic Keys
	Scheuermann kyphosis	Age 12-15 years Thoracic or thoracolumbar pain Increased fixed thoracic kyphosis 3 or more wedged vertebrae with end-plate irregularities
	Trochanteric bursitis, gluteal fasciitis	Pain or tenderness over greater trochanter
	Adult scoliosis	Back pain Uneven shoulders, scapular prominence Paravertebral hump with forward flexion
Metabolic	Osteoporosis	Woman older than 60 years Severe acute thoracic pain (fracture) Severe weight-bearing pelvic pain (fracture) Aching, dull thoracic pain; relieved in supine position (mechanical) Loss of height, increased thoracic kyphosis
	Osteomalacia	Diffuse skeletal pain or tenderness Increased alkaline phosphatase
	Paget disease	Bone pain: low back, pelvic, tibia Increased alkaline phosphatase Characteristic radiographic appearance
	Diabetic polyradiculopathy	Older than 50 years Diffuse leg pain, worse at night Proximal muscle weakness
Malignant neoplasia		Older than 50 years Back pain unrelieved by positional change—night pain Previous history of malignant disease Elevated erythrocyte sedimentation rate

Modified from Mazanec D. Pseudospine pain: conditions that mimic spine pain. In Cole AJ, Herring SA, eds. The Low Back Pain Handbook. Philadelphia, Hanley & Belfus, 1997:98.

Initial therapy for lumbar degenerative disease should consist of anti-inflammatory medications, muscle relaxants (Table 41-3), occasionally opioid medications for severe symptom exacerbation, and a functionally oriented physical therapy program. Most patients do well with these measures and do not require any invasive procedures. Other useful initial treatments may include trigger point injections as well as heat and cold modalities. Low-dose tricyclic antidepressants can help with improvement of sleep.

TABLE 41-3 Commonly Used Drugs for Muscle Relaxation

Generic Name	Brand Name	Common Doses
Cyclobenzaprine	Flexeril	5-20 mg po tid
Carisoprodol	Soma	350 mg po tid
Baclofen	Lioresal	10-20 mg po q6h
Methocarbamol	Robaxin	500-750 mg po tid
Chlorzoxazone	Parafon Forte	250-500 mg po tid
Orphenadrine	Norflex	100 mg po bid

Modified from Schofferman J. Medications for low back pain. In Cole AJ, Herring SA, eds. The Low Back Pain Handbook. Philadelphia, Hanley & Belfus, 1997:117.

Rehabilitation

Rehabilitation of lumbar degenerative disc disease includes a detailed assessment of functional limitations and functional goals for every patient. A full assessment of occupational and leisure activity demands and goals should also be implemented. For example, patients with advanced degenerative disc disease may benefit from early vocational rehabilitation and counseling with the goal of avoiding future occupational disability and surgical procedures.

On occasion, lumbar orthotics are prescribed, but these are generally not thought to be beneficial in the treatment of degenerative low back pain unless there is a significant spondylolisthesis or some other specific indication.

Therapy goals focus on normalization of impairments in flexibility, strength, and endurance and should emphasize healthy lifestyle modifications. A basic lumbar stabilization program with a focus on posture, footwear modifications (if necessary), workplace modifications (if appropriate), and general conditioning works for most patients. Modalities such as ultrasound and electrical stimulation can be used for acute low back pain; however, the focus of supervised therapy should be on an active program rather than the passive treatment that modalities provide.

In patients whose condition does not improve with the outlined initial therapeutic measures, a more intensive, functional restoration approach may be helpful. This commonly includes comprehensive physical rehabilitation with psychological support. These programs can be called many things (e.g., comprehensive spine program, chronic pain program, work conditioning program). Although most of these programs are traditionally considered later in the course of degenerative diseases, early referral may be helpful in decreasing related disability.[13] Another common functional rehabilitation technique is the dynamic lumbar stabilization approach.[14] This muscle stabilization program uses static and dynamic postural exercises to improve the patient's overall function. It includes education about proper body mechanics during activities of daily living, improved extremity strength and endurance, and muscle stabilization through gym training and healthy lifestyle activities. The hallmark of this program is that postural control is attained through pelvic tilting to control the degree of lumbar lordosis in a pain-free range. The program is designed to advance the patient toward increasingly demanding exercises and to incorporate these exercises into activities of daily living. The program progresses through the building of static strength into dynamic stabilization for patients with more physically demanding athletic activities and occupational demands. This program is supported by a home exercise program.

Core strengthening expands on the concept of lumbar stabilization and has become a key component of rehabilitation programs, not only for athletes. Core stability is the ability of the lumbopelvic-hip complex to prevent buckling and to return to equilibrium after perturbation. Although bone and soft tissues contribute, core stability is predominantly maintained by the dynamic function of the trunk musculature. Decreased core stability may predispose to injury, and appropriate training may reduce injury.[15,16]

Procedures

Spinal injection procedures have become an increasingly important part of the overall treatment program for lumbar degenerative disease. These procedures have diagnostic, therapeutic, and even prognostic benefits. It is now commonly agreed that injections should ideally be performed with x-ray guidance and contrast enhancement.[17] The most commonly used procedures are epidural steroid injections, which have shown benefit primarily for temporary relief of radicular symptoms.[18] Modern injection techniques, such as the transforaminal approach, ensure that the medication, usually a corticosteroid, is delivered into the anterior epidural space.[19] Facet joint injections are commonly performed intra-articularly or through medial branches. Intra-articular facet injections may allow temporary pain relief in cases of synovitis and facet joint cysts. Medial branch injections are used to establish the diagnosis of facet-mediated pain by temporary blockade of the supplying nerve branches of the affected joint.[20] Medial branch neurotomies ("facet rhizotomies") may provide longer symptomatic relief for patients with clearly identified facet pain.[21] On occasion, intradiscal steroid injections are applied, but their use is debated because intradiscal steroid may cause discitis, progression of disc degeneration, and calcification of the intervertebral disc.[22,23]

Minimally invasive intradiscal therapies (e.g., chemonucleolysis, laser, percutaneous disc decompression) have been used since the 1970s with various clinical successes. Newer treatment techniques have evolved in the last several years; intradiscal electrothermal therapy involves controlled thermal application to the posterior annulus through an intradiscal catheter. The currently available research data show conflicting results about the therapeutic efficacy of these treatment modalities.[24]

Surgery

The surgical indications for degenerative disc disease of the lumbar spine are highly debated and evolving. Surgery is considered when intensive nonsurgical therapy, including injection procedures and semi-invasive procedures, has failed and the patient continues to have functionally limiting pain. Confounding psychological factors and mental disorders should be excluded before any surgical procedure.[25] Current data are incomplete to judge the scientific validity of spinal fusion for low back pain syndromes.[26] However, if the intervertebral disc is clearly identified as the source of low back pain, interbody fusion with excision of the diseased disc appears to have favorable results. In general, surgical options include posterior fusion procedures with or without pedicle screw instrumentation, anterior interbody fusion with or without pedicle screws, and a combination of these procedures. In case of neural compression, additional decompression procedures may be required.

Disc arthroplasty ("artificial disc") has recently become available in the United States after more than a decade of positive experience in Europe.[27] The indication of this surgery is for patients with chronic low back pain due to symptomatic degenerative disc disease without significant radiographic instability, neural compression, and facet joint arthropathy. Current outcome studies do not show a clear benefit in pain and functional improvement over fusion surgeries, and questions about the longevity of the implants remain.

POTENTIAL DISEASE COMPLICATIONS

In general, degenerative lumbar disease is a benign condition. However, increasing functional limitations can occur, especially if advanced segmental degeneration leads to neural compression and symptoms of spinal stenosis, neural claudication, and segmental instability develop. Persistent neurologic deficits from these conditions are rare and can be avoided if the conditions are diagnosed early and appropriate treatment is begun. A small number of patients may develop chronic pain syndromes. Low back pain is the most common cause of the chronic pain syndrome. Not surprisingly, the incidence of mental disorders, such as depression and somatoform disorders, is high, and these disorders commonly respond better to a behavioral psychology approach than to disease-oriented medical treatment approaches. Early detection of patients with mental disorders will help avoid unnecessary medical treatment and allow appropriate psychological and psychiatric interventions.

POTENTIAL TREATMENT COMPLICATIONS

As with any medications, clinicians must be fully aware of their risks and unwanted side effects. Analgesics and nonsteroidal anti-inflammatory drugs have well-known side effects that most commonly affect the gastric, hepatic, and renal systems. Muscle relaxants can cause sedation. Low-dose tricyclic antidepressants can cause sedation and urinary retention in men with benign prostatic hypertrophy. Some patients require chronic opioid therapy, and issues of constipation and dependence arise. Risks associated with spinal injection include cortisone flare, hyperglycemia, dural puncture, and, rarely, hematoma, infection, and neurologic damage. All potential complications should be thoroughly discussed with the patient before treatment. Potential surgical complications will vary with the procedure but can be as high as 17% for lumbar fusion procedures for degenerative disc disease.[28]

References

1. Schwarzer AC, Aprill CN, Bogduk N. The sacroiliac joint in chronic low back pain. Spine 1995;20:31-37.
2. Freemont AJ, Peacock TE, Goupille P, et al. Nerve ingrowth into diseased intervertebral disc in chronic back pain. Lancet 1997;350:178-181.
3. Schwarzer AC, Aprill CN, Derby R, et al. The prevalence and clinical features of internal disc disruption in patients with chronic low back pain. Spine 1995;20:1878-1883.
4. Kirkaldy-Willis WH. Managing Low Back Pain. New York, Churchill Livingstone, 1999.
5. Schmorl G, Junghanns H. The Human Spine: Health and Disease, 2nd ed. New York, Grune & Stratton, 1971.
6. Fraser RD, Bleasel JF, Moskowitz RW. Spinal degeneration: pathogenesis and medical management. In Frymoyer JW, ed. The Adult Spine: Principles and Practice, 2nd ed. Philadelphia, Lippincott-Raven, 1997:735-759.
7. Helms CA. Fundamentals of Skeletal Radiology, 2nd ed. Philadelphia, WB Saunders, 1995.
8. Rainville J, Ahern DK, Phalen L, et al. The association of pain with physical activities in chronic low back pain. Spine 1992;17:1060-1064.
9. Boden SD, Davis DO, Dina TS, et al. Abnormal magnetic-resonance scans of the lumbar spine in asymptomatic subjects: a prospective investigation. J Bone Joint Surg Am 1990;72:403-408.
10. Saal JS. The role of inflammation in lumbar pain [see comments]. Spine 1995;20:1821-1827.
11. Rainville J, Sobel JB, Hartigan C. Comparison of total lumbosacral flexion and true lumbar flexion measured by a dual inclinometer technique. Spine 1994;19:2698-2701.
12. Waddell G, McCulloch JA, Kummel E, Venner RM. Nonorganic physical signs in low-back pain. Spine 1980;5:117-125.
13. Mayer TG, Gatchel RJ, Mayer H, et al. A prospective two-year study of functional restoration in industrial low back injury. An objective assessment procedure [published erratum appears in JAMA 1988;259:220]. JAMA 1987;258:1763-1767.
14. Saal JA. Dynamic muscular stabilization in the nonoperative treatment of lumbar pain syndromes. Orthop Rev 1990;19:691-700.
15. Bliss LS, Teeple P. Core stability: the centerpiece of any training program. Curr Sports Med Rep 2005;4:179-183.
16. Willson JD, Dougherty CP, Ireland ML, Davis IM. Core stability and its relationship to lower extremity function and injury. J Am Acad Orthop Surg 2005;13:316-325.
17. O'Neill C, Derby R, Kenderes L. Precision injection techniques for diagnosis and treatment of lumbar disc disease [review]. Semin Spine Surg 1999;11:104-118.
18. Carette S, Leclaire R, Marcoux S, et al. Epidural corticosteroid injections for sciatica due to herniated nucleus pulposus. N Engl J Med 1997;336:1634-1640.
19. Lutz GE, Vad VB, Wisneski RJ. Fluoroscopic transforaminal lumbar epidural steroids: an outcome study. Arch Phys Med Rehabil 1998;79:1362-1366.
20. Carette S, Marcoux S, Truchon R, et al. A controlled trial of corticosteroid injections into the facet joints for chronic low back pain. N Engl J Med 1998;325:1002-1007.
21. Buttermann GR. The effect of spinal steroid injections for degenerative disc disease. Spine J 2004;4:495-505.
22. Darmoul M, Bouhaouala MH, Rezgui M. Calcification following intradiscal injection, a continuing problem? [in French]. Presse Med 2005;34:859-860.
23. Dreyfuss P, Halbrook B, Pauza K, et al. Efficacy and validity of radiofrequency neurotomy for chronic lumbar zygapophysial joint pain. Spine 2000;25:1270-1277.
24. Saal JA, Saal JS. Intradiscal electrothermal treatment for chronic discogenic low back pain: a prospective outcome study with minimum 1-year follow-up [in process citation]. Spine 2000;25:2622-2627.
25. Carragee EJ, Tanner CM, Khurana S, et al. The rates of false-positive lumbar discography in select patients without low back symptoms. Spine 2000;25:1373-1380.
26. Bigos SJ. A literature-based review as a guide for generating recommendations to patients acutely limited by low back symptoms. In Garfin SR, Vaccaro AR, eds. Orthopaedic Knowledge Update. Spine. Rosemont, Ill, American Academy of Orthopaedic Surgeons, 1997:15-25.
27. Tropiano P, Huang RC, Girardi FP, et al. Lumbar total disc replacement. Seven- to eleven-year follow-up. J Bone Joint Surg Am 2005;87:490-496.
28. Fritzell P, Hagg O, Wessberg P, et al. 2001 Volvo Award Winner in Clinical Studies: Lumbar fusion versus nonsurgical treatment for chronic low back pain. Spine 2001;26:2521-2534

Lumbar Facet Arthropathy 42

Ted A. Lennard, MD

Synonyms

Z-joint pain
Zygapophyseal joint pain
Facet joint arthritis
Apophyseal joint pain
Posterior element disorder
Facet syndrome

ICD-9 Codes

721.3   Lumbosacral spondylosis without myelopathy
721.90   Spondylosis of unspecified site (spinal arthritis)
724.2   Low back pain

DEFINITION

Lumbar facet joints are formed by the articulation of the inferior and superior articular facets of adjacent vertebrae. These joints, located posteriorly in the spinal axis, are lined with synovium and have highly innervated joint capsules. Lumbar facet arthropathy refers to any acquired, degenerative, or traumatic process that changes the normal anatomy or function of a lumbar facet joint. These changes often disrupt the normal biomechanics of the joint, resulting in hyaline cartilage damage and periarticular hypertrophy. When they are painful, these joints may limit daily living activities, recreational sports, and work. Lumbar facet joints may be a primary source of pain, but they are often painful concomitantly with a degenerative or injured lumbar disc, fracture, or ligamentous injury.[1]

SYMPTOMS

Patients often complain of generalized or lateralized spinal pain, sometimes well localized. Pain may be provoked with spinal extension and rotation, from either a standing or a prone position. Relief with partial lumbar flexion is common. In the lumbar spine, these joints may refer pain into the buttock or posterior thigh but rarely below the knee.[2-4] Neurologic symptoms, such as lower extremity numbness, paresthesias, and weakness, would be unexpected from a primary facet joint disorder.

PHYSICAL EXAMINATION

A detailed examination of the lumbar spine and a lower extremity neurologic examination are considered standard procedure for those thought to have facet arthropathy. Although no portion of the examination has been shown to definitively correlate with the diagnosis of a facet joint disorder, the physical examination can be helpful in elevating the clinician's level of suspicion for this diagnosis.[5,6] The examination starts with simple observation of the patient's gait, movement patterns, posture, and range of motion. Generalized and segmental spinal palpation is followed by a detailed neurologic examination for sensation, reflexes, tone, and strength. In the absence of coexisting pathologic processes, such as lumbar radiculopathy, strength, sensation, and deep tendon reflexes should be normal.

Provocative maneuvers and nerve tension tests, including straight-leg raising, should accompany the evaluation to rule out any superimposed nerve root injury that might accompany a facet disorder. The clinician notes the patient's response when the lower extremity is raised with the hip flexed and the knee extended. This "tension" placed on inflamed or injured lower lumbosacral nerve roots will provoke pain, paresthesias, or numbness down the extremity. Typically, in isolated cases of lumbar facet disorders, this maneuver does not provoke radiating symptoms into the lower extremity, but it may cause lower back pain. Some physicians find that facet pain can be reproduced with prone extension with rotation and standing spinal extension.

Additional examination techniques may be necessary (e.g., vascular, peripheral joint), depending on the patient's presentation.

FUNCTIONAL LIMITATIONS

Patients with lumbar facet joint arthropathy may experience difficulty with prolonged walking, twisting, stair climbing, standing, and prone lying. Extreme flexion may also be problematic. Because facet problems are common with underlying disc disease, patients often have difficulty with lumbar flexion activities, such as lifting, bending, and stooping.

DIAGNOSTIC STUDIES

Fluoroscopy-guided, contrast-enhanced, anesthetic intra-articular or medial branch blocks are considered the "gold standard" for the diagnosis of a painful lumbar facet joint (Figs. 42-1 and 42-2).[7,8] Clinical history, examination findings, radiographic changes, computed tomography, magnetic resonance imaging, and bone scan have not been shown to correlate with facet joint pain.[5,6,9]

TREATMENT

Initial

Initial treatment emphasizes local pain control with ice, oral analgesics and nonsteroidal anti-inflammatory drugs, topical creams, local periarticular corticosteroid injections, and avoidance of exacerbating activities. Spinal manipulations and acupuncture may also reduce local pain. Temporary use of corsets and limited activity can be used.

Rehabilitation

Physical therapy may include modalities to control pain (e.g., ultrasound), traction, instruction in body mechanics, flexibility training (including hamstring stretching), spinal strengthening, articular mobilization techniques, generalized conditioning, and restoration of normal movement patterns. Critical assessment of the biomechanics of specific activities that may be job related (e.g., working on an assembly line, carpentry work) or sports related (e.g., running, cycling) is important. This assessment can result in prevention of recurrent episodes of pain because changes in a technique or activity may reduce the underlying forces at the joint level. Simple ergonomic measures that act to support the lumbar spine during sitting and standing may reduce the occurrence of low back pain from the facet joints. These measures include proper chair design and chair height, properly designed work table, and adjustable chair supports. While standing, the addition of a footrest and the ability to change body position routinely may reduce low back pain.

Differential Diagnosis

Radiculopathy

Spondylolysis or spondylolisthesis

Internal disc disruption

Lumbar stenosis

Myofascial pain syndrome

Spondylosis

Nerve root compression

Sacroiliac joint dysfunction

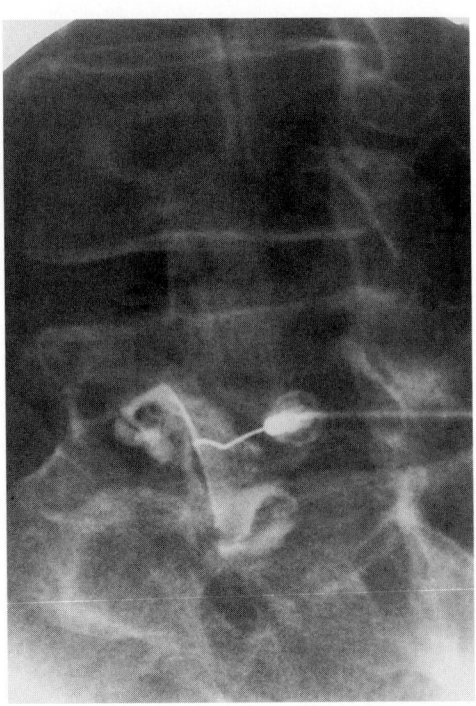

FIGURE 42-1. Oblique radiograph of an L5-S1 Z-joint arthrogram. Superior and inferior capsular recesses are demonstrated. (Reprinted with permission from Lennard TA. Pain Procedures in Clinical Practice. Philadelphia, Hanley & Belfus, 2000.)

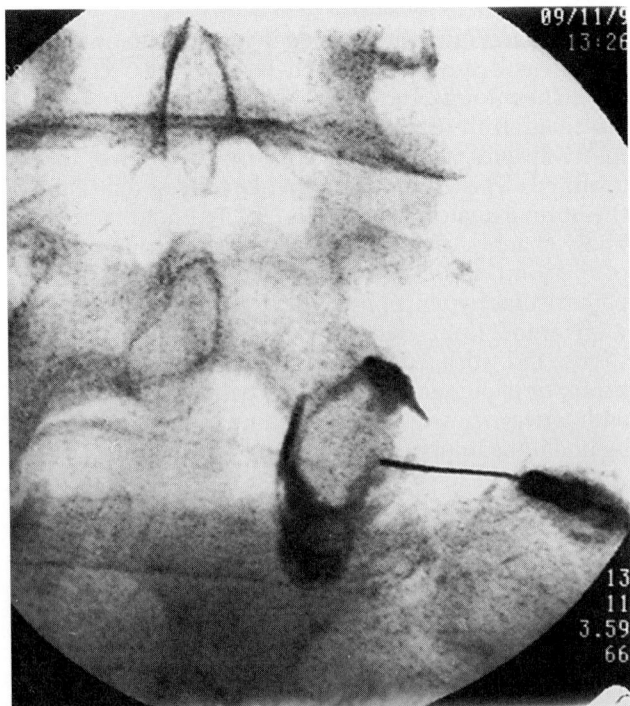

FIGURE 42-2. Anteroposterior radiograph of a needle placed into the L5-S1 facet joint with an arthrogram. (Reprinted with permission from Lennard TA. Pain Procedures in Clinical Practice. Philadelphia, Hanley & Belfus, 2000.)

Procedures

Intra-articular, fluoroscopy-guided, contrast-enhanced facet injections are considered essential in the proper diagnosis and treatment of a painful facet joint.[7,8,10-12] In some centers, ultrasound guidance is being used.[13,14] Patients can be evaluated before and after injection to determine what portion of their pain can be attributed to the joints injected. After confirmation with contrast material, 1 to 2 mL of an anesthetic-corticosteroid mix is injected directly into the joint. An alternative approach is to perform anesthetic medial branch blocks with small volumes (0.1 to 0.3 mL) of anesthetic. Recent data suggest that medial branch blocks may be the preferred method for diagnosis of facet joint pain.[12,15,16] If the facet joint is found to be the putative source of pain, a medial branch neurotomy may be desirable.[17-19]

Surgery

Surgery is rare in primary and isolated facet arthropathies. Surgical spinal fusion may be performed for discogenic pain, which may affect secondary cases of facet arthropathies.

POTENTIAL DISEASE COMPLICATIONS

Because a common cause of facet arthropathy is degenerative in nature, this disorder is often progressive, resulting in chronic, intractable spinal pain.[20,21] It often coexists with spinal disc abnormalities, further leading to chronic pain. This subsequently results in diminished spinal motion and weakness.

POTENTIAL TREATMENT COMPLICATIONS

Treatment-related complications may be caused from medications; nonsteroidal anti-inflammatory drugs may cause gastrointestinal and renal problems, and analgesics may result in liver dysfunction and constipation. Local periarticular injections and acupuncture may cause local transient needle pain. Local manual treatments or injections will often cause transient exacerbation of symptoms. Intra-articular facet injections will cause transient local spinal pain and swelling and possibly bruising. More serious injection-related complications include an allergic reaction to the medications, injury to a blood vessel or nerve, trauma to the spinal cord, and infection. When more serious injection complications occur, they can usually be attributed to poor procedure technique.[7]

References

1. Manchikanti L, Pampati V, Rivera J, et al. Role of facet joints in chronic low back pain in the elderly: a controlled comparative prevalence study. Pain Pract 2001;1:332-337.
2. Dreyer SJ, Dreyfuss P. Low back pain and the zygapophyseal joints. Arch Phys Med Rehabil 1996;77:290-300.
3. Dreyer S, Dreyfuss P, Cole A. Posterior elements and low back pain. Phys Med Rehabil State Art Rev 1999;13:443-471.
4. Fukui S, Ohseto K, Shiotani M, et al. Distribution of referred pain from the lumbar zygapophyseal joints and dorsal rami. Clin J Pain 1997;13:303-307.
5. Dolan AL, Ryan PJ, Arden NK, et al. The value of SPECT scans in identifying back pain likely to benefit from facet joint injection. Br J Rheumatol 1996;35:1269-1273.
6. Schwarzer AC, Scott AM, Wang S, et al. The role of bone scintigraphy in chronic low back pain: comparison of SPECT and planar images and zygapophyseal joint injection. Aust N Z J Med 1992;22:185.
7. Bogduk N. International Spinal Injection Society Guidelines for the performance of spinal injection procedures. Part I. Zygapophysial joint blocks. Clin J Pain 1997;13:285-302.
8. Dreyfuss P, Kaplan M, Dreyer SJ. Zygapophyseal joint injection techniques in the spinal axis. In Lennard TA, ed. Pain Procedures in Clinical Practice. Philadelphia, Hanley & Belfus, 2000:332-369.
9. Pneumaticos SG, Chatziioannou SN, Hipp JA, et al. Low back pain: prediction of short term outcomes of facet joint injection with bone scintigraphy. Radiology 2006;238:693-698.
10. Boswell MV, Colson JD, Spillane WF. Therapeutic facet joint interventions in chronic spinal pain: a systematic review of effectiveness and complications, Pain Physician 2005;8:101-114.
11. Sehgal N, Dunbar EE, Shah RV, Colson J. Systematic review of diagnostic utility of facet (zygapophysial) joint injections in chronic spinal pain: an update. Pain Physician 2007;10:213-228.
12. Lindner R, Sluijter ME, Schleinzer W. Pulsed radiofrequency treatment of the lumbar medial branch for facet pain: a retrospective analysis. Pain Med 2006;7:435-439.
13. Galiano K, Obwegeser AA, Bodner G, et al. Ultrasound guidance for facet joint injections in the lumbar spine: a computed tomography–controlled feasibility study. Anesth Analg 2005;101:579-583.
14. Shim JK, Moon JC, Yoon KB, et al. Ultrasound guided lumbar medial branch block: a clinical study with fluoroscopy control. Reg Anesth Pain Med 2006;32:451-454.
15. Bogduk N. Lumbar medial branch. In Bogduk N, ed. Practice Guidelines, Spinal Diagnostic and Treatment Procedures. San Francisco, International Spinal Intervention Society, 2004:47-65.
16. Birkenmaier C, Veihelmann A, Trouillier HH, et al. Medial branch blocks versus pericapsular blocks in selecting patients for percutaneous cryodenervation of lumbar facet joints. Reg Anesth Pain Med 2007;32:27-33.
17. Dreyfuss P, Halbrook B, Pauza K, et al. Lumbar radiofrequency neurotomy for chronic zygapophyseal joint pain: a pilot study using dual medial branch blocks. Int Spinal Injection Soc Sci Newslett 1999;3:13-31.
18. Dreyfuss P, Halbrook B, Pauza K, et al. Efficacy and validity of radiofrequency neurotomy for chronic lumbar zygapophyseal joint pain. Spine 2000;25:1270-1277.
19. Kleef M, Barendse G, Kessels A, et al. Randomized trial of radiofrequency lumbar facet denervation for chronic low back pain. Spine 1999;2-4:1937-1942.
20. Cavanaugh JM, Ozaktay AC, Yamashita T, et al. Mechanisms of low back pain: a neurophysiological and neuroanatomic study. Clin Orthop 1997;335:166-180.
21. Lewinnek GE, Warfield CA. Facet joint degeneration as a cause of low back pain. Clin Orthop Relat Res 1986;213:216-222.

Lumbar Radiculopathy 43

Maury Ellenberg, MD, and Joseph C. Honet, MD

Synonyms

Lumbar radiculitis
Sciatica
Pinched nerve
Herniated nucleus pulposus with nerve root irritation

ICD-9 Codes

722.52 Degeneration of lumbar or lumbosacral intervertebral disc
724.2   Low back pain

DEFINITION

Lumbar radiculopathy refers to a pathologic process involving the lumbar nerve roots. Lumbar radiculitis refers to an inflammation of the nerve root. These terms should not be confused with disc herniation, which is a displacement of the lumbar disc from its anatomic location between the vertebrae (often into the spinal canal) (Fig. 43-1). Although lumbar radiculopathy is often caused by a herniated lumbar disc, this is not invariably the case. Many pathologic processes, such as bone encroachment, tumors, and metabolic disorders (e.g., diabetes), can also result in lumbar radiculopathy. More important, disc herniation is often an incidental finding on imaging of the lumbar spine of asymptomatic individuals.[1,2]

When disc herniation results in radiculopathy, the precise cause of the pain is not fully understood. The two possibilities are mechanical compression and inflammation. It has been demonstrated that in a "nonirritated" nerve, mechanical stimulus rarely leads to pain; yet in an "irritated" nerve, it usually results in pain. Furthermore, inflammatory mediators have experimentally been shown to cause radicular pain in the absence of compression.[3] It is likely that both factors may be at work individually or together in any given patient. Because of this, it should be no surprise that disc herniations and nerve root compression can be present in asymptomatic patients[2] and that patients can have radiculopathy without visible disc herniations or nerve root compression.[4] The prevalence of lumbar radiculopathy varies from about 2.2% to 8%, depending on the study, and the incidence ranges from 0.7% to 9.6%.[5] One study found a higher incidence in men (67%) and an association with obesity and smoking. A correlation was also found with more strenuous occupations and radiculopathy,[5] with the highest prevalence in patients 45 to 65 years old.[6]

SYMPTOMS

The most common symptom in lumbar radiculopathy is pain. The pain may vary in severity and location. The pain may be severe and is often increased or precipitated by standing, sitting, coughing, and sneezing. The location of the pain depends on the nerve root involved, and there is a great deal of overlap among the dermatomes. Most commonly, S1 radiculopathy produces posterior thigh and calf pain; L5, buttocks and anterolateral leg pain; L4, anterior thigh, anterior or medial knee, and medial leg pain; and L3, groin pain. Usually, the patient cannot pinpoint the precise onset of pain. It may start in the back, but by the time the patient is evaluated, pain may be present only in the buttocks or limb.

Paresthesias are also common and occur in the dermatomal distribution of the involved nerve root (rarely is complete sensory loss present). The patient may occasionally present with weakness of a part of the limb. On rare occasion, there is bladder and bowel involvement, especially urinary retention.

PHYSICAL EXAMINATION

The most important elements in the evaluation of lumbar radiculopathy are the history and physical examination.[7]

A thorough musculoskeletal and peripheral neurologic examination should be performed. Examine the back for asymmetry or a shift over one side of the pelvis. Evaluate back motion and see whether radicular symptoms (pain radiating to an extremity) in the distribution of the patient's complaints are produced.

Manual muscle testing is a vital part of the examination for radiculopathy. The major muscle weakness in relation

241

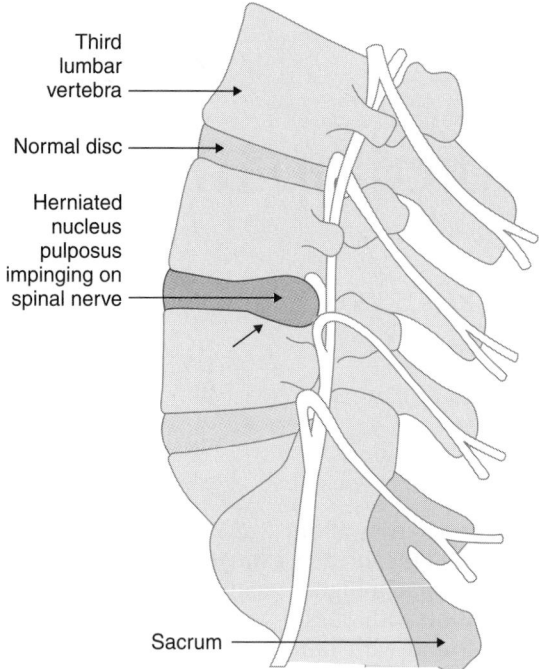

Third lumbar vertebra

Normal disc

Herniated nucleus pulposus impinging on spinal nerve

Sacrum

FIGURE 43-1. A herniated disc.

of radiculopathy; it is most often seen with nonspecific low back pain. On occasion, the process of lumbar radiculopathy may start with low back pain, and several days or weeks later, the symptom will occur in the leg. It is possible that the initial process of nucleus rupture through the annulus may result in the initial back pain, but the pathogenesis is not completely known at this time. Compare side to side to be sure not to confuse the pain produced with hamstring stretch. There are a number of variations on this test.

Rectal examination and perianal and inguinal sensory testing should be done if there is history of bowel or bladder incontinence or retention or recent onset of erectile dysfunction.

Waddell signs are a group of indicators that a nonorganic process is interfering with the accuracy of the physical examination. The signs are superficial, nonanatomic tenderness; simulation by axial loading or rotation of the head, causing complaints of back pain; distraction by sitting straight-leg raising versus supine; regional disturbance, that is, weakness or sensory loss in a region of the body that is in a nonanatomic distribution; and overreaction, what is described commonly as excessive pain behavior. These signs are often present in patients with compensation, litigation, or psychoemotional issues.[8] Evaluation for the presence of Waddell signs should be a routine part of the examination in patients with these issues.

FUNCTIONAL LIMITATIONS

The functional limitations depend on the severity of the problem. Limitations are usually due to pain but may occasionally occur because of weakness. Standing and walking may be limited, and sitting tolerance is often decreased. Patients with an L4 radiculopathy are at risk of falling down stairs if the involved leg is their "trailing" (power) leg on the stairs. Patients with a severe S1 radiculopathy will be unable to run because of calf weakness, even when the pain resolves. Patients with L5 radiculopathy may catch the foot on curbs or,

to the nerve root involved is as follows: L3, hip flexors; L4, knee extensors and hip adductors; L5, hip abductors, knee flexors, ankle dorsiflexors, foot everters, foot inverters, and great toe extensor; S1, ankle plantar flexors (Table 43-1). Try to detect weakness in the distribution of two peripheral nerves arising from the same nerve root. Proximal muscle weakness in the appropriate nerve root distribution is useful in distinguishing bilateral radiculopathy from peripheral neuropathy.

The straight-leg raising test can be performed with the patient sitting or supine. The leg is raised straight up by the examiner, and the test result is positive if the patient complains of pain in the extremity (not in the back), typically in a specific nerve root distribution. If the pain occurs only in the back, this is not an indicator

TABLE 43-1 Diagnosis of Lumbar Radiculopathy					
Nerve Root	**Pain Radiation**	**Gait Deviation**	**Motor Weakness**	**Sensory Loss**	**Reflex Loss**
L3	Groin and inner thigh	Sometimes antalgic	Hip flexion	Anteromedial thigh	Patellar (variable)
L4	Anterior thigh or knee, or upper medial leg	Sometimes antalgic; difficulty rising onto a stool or chair with one leg	Knee extension, hip flexion and adduction	Lateral or anterior thigh, medial leg and knee	Patellar
L5	Buttocks, anterior or lateral leg, dorsal foot	Difficulty heel walking; if more severe, then foot slap or steppage gait Trendelenburg gait	Ankle dorsiflexion, foot eversion and inversion, toe extension, hip abduction	Posterolateral thigh, anterolateral leg, and mid-dorsal foot	Medial hamstring (variable)
S1	Posterior thigh, calf, plantar foot	Difficulty toe walking or cannot rise on toes 20 times	Foot plantar flexion	Posterior thigh and calf, lateral and plantar foot	Achilles

if it is severe, on the ground. They may require a brace (ankle dorsiflexion assist). In patients with acute radiculopathy that is severe, the pain will usually preclude a whole range of activities—household, recreation, and work. The majority of patients, once the acute process is ameliorated, can return to most activities except for heavy household and work activity. After about 3 to 6 months, they can return to all activities unless there is residual weakness, in which case they are limited as noted before, depending on the radiculopathy level.

DIAGNOSTIC STUDIES

Diagnostic testing takes two forms: one to corroborate the diagnosis and the second to determine the etiology. For simple cases, diagnostic testing is usually not needed, and the clinical picture can guide the treatment. A history that includes trauma, cancer, infection, human immunodeficiency virus infection, diabetes, and the like is an indication for earlier diagnostic testing.

Electromyography

Electromyography and nerve conduction studies, when they are performed by an individual well versed in the diagnosis of neuromuscular disorders, can be valuable in the diagnosis of lumbar radiculopathy. They can also help with differential diagnoses and in patients whose physical examination is not reliable. Electromyography has the advantage over imaging techniques of high specificity, and recordings will rarely be abnormal in asymptomatic individuals.[9] These studies, however, do not give direct information about the *cause* of the radiculopathy.

Imaging

Imaging techniques in relation to lumbar radiculopathy usually refer to lumbosacral spine radiography, computed tomography (CT), and magnetic resonance imaging (MRI).

Plain radiography can be useful to exclude traumatic bone injury or metastatic disease. It allows visualization of the disc space but not of the contents of the spinal canal or the nerve roots. CT and MRI allow visualization of the disc, spinal canal, and nerve roots (Fig. 43-2). There is a high incidence of abnormal findings in asymptomatic people; rates of disc herniation range from 21% in the 20- to 39-year age group to 37.5% in the 60- to 80-year age group.[2] To be meaningful, CT and MRI must clearly correlate with the clinical picture. Perform these studies if tumor is suspected or surgery is contemplated. They also may be useful in precisely locating pathologic changes for selective epidural steroid injection. The most accurate study is MRI, and gadolinium enhancement is not needed unless tumor is suspected or the patient has undergone prior surgery. Gadolinium enhancement is useful postsurgically to distinguish disc herniation from scar tissue.

Differential Diagnosis

Trochanteric bursitis

Anserine bursitis

Hamstring strain

Lumbosacral plexopathy

Diabetic amyotrophy

Peripheral neuropathy: sciatic, tibial, peroneal, femoral

Avascular necrosis of the hip

Hip osteoarthritis

Shin splints

Lateral femoral cutaneous neuropathy (meralgia paresthetica)

Spinal stenosis

Cauda equina syndrome

Demyelinating disorder

Lumbar facet syndrome

Piriformis syndrome

TREATMENT

Initial

The treatment goal is to reduce inflammation and thereby relieve the pain and resolve the radiculopathy regardless of the underlying anatomic abnormalities. Bed rest, which had been the mainstay of nonoperative treatment, is now recommended only for symptom control. Studies have not shown bed rest to have an effect on the final outcome of the disorder.[10] As long as patients avoid activities such as bending and lifting, which tend to increase intradiscal pressures, they can carry on most everyday activities.

Use nonsteroidal anti-inflammatory drugs (NSAIDs) to help reduce inflammation and to provide pain relief. NSAIDs have been shown to be effective in acute low back pain.[11] However, a review that included pooling of three randomized controlled trials using NSAIDs showed no effectiveness over placebo.[12] It is still reasonable to give NSAIDs a short trial in acute lumbar radiculopathy. The use of oral steroids is more controversial and has not passed the scrutiny of well-controlled studies, even in acute low back pain.

Use opioids as needed for pain relief. There is little concern for addiction in the acute case, and sufficient medication should be provided. The needs range from none to high doses, such as the equivalent of 60 to 100 mg of morphine (e.g., MS Contin) a day. Start with hydrocodone or oxycodone and titrate up as needed. For more severe pain, use a long-acting opioid, such as oxycodone (OxyContin) or MS Contin;

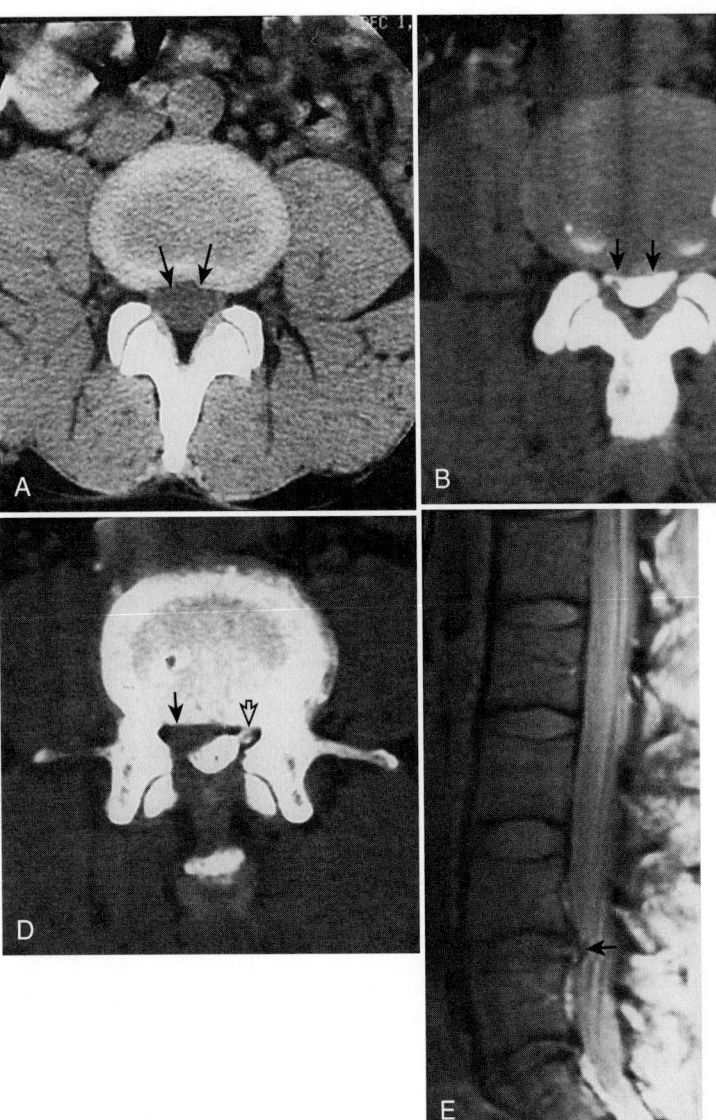

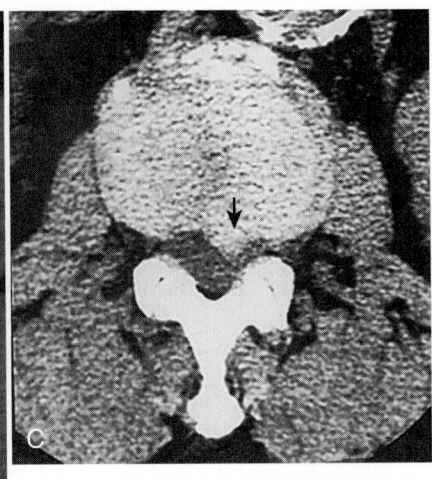

FIGURE 43-2. A, Normal disc. Note the concave posterior margin of the disc *(arrows)*. **B,** Bulging disc. Image from a CT myelogram shows the broad-based margin of the bulging disc *(arrows)* pushing on the anterior thecal sac. **C,** Left posterior disc herniation *(arrow)*. **D,** Right posterior disc herniation. The abnormal soft tissue from the herniated disc is seen in the right lateral recess on this CT myelogram *(arrow)*. Note the normally opacified nerve root sheath on the contralateral side *(open arrow)*. **E,** Herniated discs L4-5 and L5-S1; the L4-5 herniation is the larger of the two. There is posterior displacement of the low-signal posterior longitudinal ligament *(arrow)*. (Reprinted with permission from Barckhausen RR, Math KR. Lumbar spine diseases. In Katz DS, Math KR, Groskin SA, eds. Radiology Secrets. Philadelphia, Hanley & Belfus, 1998:322-335.)

for breakthrough pain, use a shorter acting opioid, such as hydrocodone, oxycodone, or short-acting morphine. There are scanty data on the use of other medication in acute lumbar radiculopathy. Medications such as cyclobenzaprine, metaxalone, methocarbamol, and chlorzoxazone, some of which may have effectiveness in acute low back pain,[13] have not been shown to be effective in acute radiculopathy. Anticonvulsants and tricyclic antidepressants, which demonstrate pain-relieving activity in peripheral neuropathy and postherpetic neuralgia, have not been well studied in lumbar or cervical radiculopathy. In an uncontrolled study, lamotrigine has shown effectiveness in radiculopathies of 12- to 36-month duration.[14] Clinically, it is reasonable to try both an anticonvulsant, such as gabapentin or lamotrigine, and a tricyclic, such as doxepin or nortriptyline, in a longer standing radiculopathy. Start with a low dose and titrate up gradually to determine the minimally effective dose.

Rehabilitation

With an acute painful radiculopathy, it is generally best to wait for some of the acute stage to subside before physical therapy is ordered. In a longer standing problem, therapy may be the best first approach.

Physical methods are a useful adjunct to the medication treatment. Various methods, including flexion and extension exercises (often called a lumbosacral stabilization program), have been tried. Whatever method is used, if radicular pain is produced, the exercises should be stopped. After the radiculopathy resolves, the patient is prescribed a proper exercise regimen to improve flexibility and strength. Lumbar stabilization exercises and remaining active may be the most effective of the various methods studied carefully in lumbar radiculopathy. One study showed no effectiveness of lumbar traction.[15] Other modalities, such as transcutaneous electrical nerve stimulation, acupuncture, massage, and manipulation, are not well studied with randomized controlled trials in lumbar radiculopathy.[4] Because they are not likely to cause injury, they can be given a short trial. The manipulation should be done cautiously.

Procedures

Epidural steroid injection can be very effective in lumbar radiculopathy with or without disc herniation, especially in patients with acute radiculopathy.[15,16] A much lower response rate has been found in patients with long-standing problems and in those with secondary reinforcers, such as litigation or workers' compensation claims. Although it is unclear whether long-term outcomes are altered, epidural steroids are beneficial during the first 3 months and can allow more rapid pain relief and return to function.[15] These procedures should be performed under fluoroscopic guidance.[17] It is reasonable practice to perform a translaminar epidural even before imaging techniques. If there is no effect with the first injection, selective nerve root injection (transforaminal injection) can be attempted.[17] The transforaminal injection will be most effective if it is based on MRI results, particularly if a far lateral disc herniation corresponding to the level of the radiculopathy is present. It is advisable to perform one injection and to reevaluate the patient to determine whether more injections are required. A maximum of three injections should be performed for one episode of radiculopathy, but it is reasonable to repeat this procedure for recurrent episodes of radiculopathy after 3 to 6 months.

Nonoperative treatment allows resolution of the radiculopathy in up to 90% of cases.[18] More interestingly, studies have demonstrated that when radiculopathy is the result of disc herniation, the actual herniation will resolve in the majority of cases, and even when the herniation remains, the symptoms often will still abate.[19-21]

Surgery

Surgery is appropriate under two conditions. First, surgery is performed on an emergency basis when a patient presents with a central disc herniation with bowel and bladder incontinence or retention and bilateral lower extremity weakness. In this very rare condition, a neurosurgeon or orthopedic spine surgeon must be consulted immediately and the patient operated on, preferably within 6 hours. Second, surgery is an option if a patient continues to have pain that limits function after an adequate trial of nonoperative treatment.

Selection of patients is extremely important for a good surgical outcome to be achieved. The best outcomes occur in patients with single-level root involvement; when pain is experienced more in the limb than in the back; and with an anatomic abnormality on imaging that corresponds to the patient's symptoms, physical examination findings, and electromyographic findings in patients without psychological or secondary gain issues.[22]

The type of surgery depends on the cause of the radiculopathy. For cases of disc herniation, simple laminectomy and discectomy suffice. Fusion should be avoided in these instances. With spinal stenosis, a more extensive laminectomy with foraminotomy may be needed. Fusion should be reserved for the relatively infrequent case of well-demonstrated spinal instability together with radiculopathy or if the surgical procedure will result in spinal instability.

POTENTIAL DISEASE COMPLICATIONS

Complications relate to involvement of the nerve roots in the cauda equina. The most serious is the "paraplegic disc." In this case, the herniated disc can cause paralysis, but this is very rare. More common, but still unusual, is a disc that causes weakness and involvement of bowel and bladder function. Residual weakness may occur either spontaneously or after surgery. Patients may progress to a chronic low back pain syndrome; this is particularly likely to occur in patients with secondary gain issues.

POTENTIAL TREATMENT COMPLICATIONS

NSAIDs can cause gastrointestinal bleeding, mouth ulcers, and renal and hepatic complications. Newer cyclooxygenase 2 (COX-2) inhibitors avoid the gastrointestinal bleeding. Some questions have been raised about the contribution of COX-2 inhibitors and other NSAIDs to cardiovascular disease. These medications should always be used cautiously, in proper doses, and for limited periods.

Epidural steroid injections can (rarely) result in epidural abscess and epidural hematoma. Patients should not take aspirin for 5 days before the injection. Some centers recommend that NSAIDs not be taken for 3 to 5 days before the procedure, although there is no literature documenting an increased incidence of bleeding complications from epidural or spinal injections when patients are taking NSAIDs. Warfarin should be discontinued; if in doubt, the international normalized ratio should be checked. Clopidogrel bisulfate (Plavix) and similar antiplatelet agents should be discontinued for a week before injection. The injection can produce local pain, and if it is performed without fluoroscopy, it can often result in spinal headache from piercing of the dura and resultant spinal fluid leak. This occurs considerably less often when fluoroscopic guidance is used.

Surgical complications include infection, nerve root injury, paralysis, local back pain, and the usual postoperative complications (e.g., thrombophlebitis, bladder infection). More serious surgical complications include nerve root or cauda equina injury, arachnoiditis, and post-laminectomy pain syndromes.

References

1. Jensen MC, Brant-Zawadzki MN, Obuchowski N, et al. Magnetic resonance imaging of the lumbar spine in people without back pain. N Engl J Med 1994;331:69-73.
2. Boden SD, Davis DO, Dina TS, et al. Abnormal magnetic-resonance scans of the lumbar spine in asymptomatic subjects. J Bone Joint Surg Am 1990;72:403-408.
3. Murata Y, Olmarker K, Takahashi I, et al. Effects of selective tumor necrosis factor-alpha inhibition to pain—behavioral changes caused by nucleus pulposus–induced damage to the spinal nerve in rats. Neurosci Lett 2005;382:148-152.
4. Rhee JM, Schaufele M, Abdu W. Radiculopathy and the herniated lumbar disc. Controversies regarding pathophysiology and management. J Bone Joint Surg Am 2006;88:2070-2080.
5. Younes M, Bejia I, Aguir Z, et al. Prevalence and risk factors of disk-related sciatica in an urban population in Tunisia. Joint Bone Spine 2006;72:538-542.
6. Praemer A, Furner S, Rice DP. Musculoskeletal Conditions in the United States, 2nd ed. Rosemont, Ill, American Academy of Orthopaedic Surgeons, 1999.
7. Deyo RA, Rainville J, Kent DL. What can the history and physical examination tell us about low back pain? JAMA 1992;268:760-765.
8. Waddell G, McCulloch JA, Kummel E, Venner RM. Nonorganic physical signs in low-back pain. Spine 1980;5:117-125.
9. Robinson LR. Electromyography, magnetic resonance imaging, and radiculopathy: it's time to focus on specificity. Muscle Nerve 1999;22:149-150.
10. Vroomen P, de Krom M, Wilmink JT, et al. Lack of effectiveness of bed rest for sciatica. N Engl J Med 1999;340:418-423.
11. van Tulder MW, Scholten RJ, Koes BW, Deyo RA. Nonsteroidal anti-inflammatory drugs for low back pain. A systematic review within the framework of the Cochrane Collaboration Back Review Group. Spine 2000;25:2501-2513.
12. Vroomen PCAJ, de Krom MC, Slofstra PD, Knottnerus JA. Treatment of sciatica: a systematic review. J Spinal Disord 2000;13:463-469.
13. van Tulder MW, Touray T, Furlan AD, et al. Cochrane Back Review Group. Muscle relaxants for nonspecific low back pain: a systematic review within the framework of the Cochrane Collaboration. Spine 2003;28:1978-1992.
14. Eisenberg E, Damunni G, Hoffer E, et al. Lamotrigine for intractable sciatica: correlation between dose, plasma concentration and analgesia. Eur J Pain 2003;7:485-491.
15. Carette S, Leclaire R, Marcoux S, et al. Epidural corticosteroid injections for sciatica due to herniated nucleus pulposus. N Engl J Med 1997;336:1634-1637.
16. Thomas E, Cyteval C, Abiad L, et al. Efficacy of transforaminal versus interspinous corticosteroid injection in discal radiculalgia—a prospective randomised, double-blind study. Clin Rheumatol 2003;22:299-304.
17. Lutz GE, Vad VB, Wisneski RJ. Fluoroscopic transforaminal lumbar epidural steroids: an outcome study. Arch Phys Med Rehabil 1998;79:1362-1366.
18. Saal JA, Saal JS. Nonoperative treatment of herniated lumbar intervertebral disc with radiculopathy: an outcome study. Spine 1997;14:431-437.
19. Ellenberg M, Reina N, Ross M, et al. Regression of herniated nucleus pulposus: two patients with lumbar radiculopathy. Arch Phys Med Rehabil 1989;70:842-844.
20. Ellenberg M, Ross M, Honet JC, et al. Prospective evaluation of the course of disc herniations in patients with proven radiculopathy. Arch Phys Med Rehabil 1993;74:3-8.
21. Saal JA, Saal JS, Herzog J. The natural history of intervertebral disc extrusions treated nonoperatively. Spine 1990;7:683-686.
22. Finneson BE, Cooper VR. A lumbar disc surgery predictive score-card. A retrospective evaluation. Spine 1979;4:141-144.

Low Back Strain or Sprain 44

Omar El Abd, MD

DEFINITION

Lumbar strain or sprain is a term used by clinicians to describe an episode of reported acute low back pain. The patients report pain in the low back at the lumbosacral region accompanied by contraction of the paraspinal muscles (hence, the expression "muscle sprain" or "strain"). The definite cause is unknown in most cases. It most likely is secondary to a chemical or mechanical irritation of the sensory nociceptive fibers in the intervertebral discs, facet joints, sacroiliac joints, or muscles and ligaments at the lumbosacral junction area.

Painful spine conditions are common among the general population. Episodes of back pain constitute the second leading symptom prompting patients to seek evaluation by a physician.[1] Waddell[2] reported that 60% to 70% of people have had an episode of back pain at a certain point in their life. Deyo and Tsui-Wu[3] reported that the cumulative lifetime prevalence of low back pain lasting at least 2 weeks is 13.8%. The incidence of radiculopathy is reported to be much lower than the incidence of axial back pain at 2% to 6%.[3] Several studies suggest that 90% of patients with an acute episode of back pain recover within 6 weeks.[4,5] On the other hand, a study by Waxman and associates[6] demonstrated that there might be a higher incidence of recurrence and persistence of pain after the initial acute episode. As studies vary, clinicians encounter a number of patients who convert from acute pain to chronic pain.

Consequently, the goals of the clinician evaluating patients with an episode of acute low back pain are to have a working differential diagnosis of the condition and its etiology, to rule out radiculopathy or other medical causes, to have a rehabilitation plan that aims to prevent recurrence of this episode, and to formulate a management plan if the condition does not improve promptly.

SYMPTOMS

The pain develops spontaneously or after events such as sports participation, repetitive bending, lifting, motor vehicle accidents, and falls. Pain is predominantly located in the lumbosacral area (axial) overlying the lumbar spinous processes and along the paraspinal muscles. There may be an association with pain in the lower extremities; however, the lower extremity pain is less intense than the low back pain. Pain is described as sharp and shooting in character.

Trunk rotation, sitting, and bending forward usually exacerbate pain. Lying down with application of modalities (heat or ice) usually mitigates it.

Red flags that require prompt medical response are outlined in Table 44-1.

ETIOLOGY

Axial Pain (Pain Overlying the Lumbosacral Area)

Degenerative disc disease is the most common known cause of axial pain. The pain from the intervertebral discs is located in proximity to the degenerated disc. Multiple inflammatory products are found in the painful disc tissue that may increase the excitability of the sensory neurons. These products are phospholipase A_2 (present in high levels),[7] prostaglandin E, histamine-like substances, potassium ions, lactic acid, substance P, calcitonin gene–related peptide, vasoactive intestinal peptide, and other polypeptide amines.[8,9] The pain is referred from the disc to the surrounding back muscles.

Facet (zygapophyseal) joint arthropathy is another source of axial pain, present in about 30% to 50% of patients describing axial pain in the lumbar as well as in the cervical spine.[10-12] The facets are paired synovial joints adjacent to the neural arches. The facet joints are

TABLE 44-1 Red Flags

Symptom	Concern
Pain in the lower extremities (including the buttocks) more than pain in the lower back	Radiculopathy
Weakness in one or both lower extremities	Radiculopathy and the possibility of cauda equina syndrome (especially if there is bilateral involvement of the lower extremities)
Bowel or bladder changes; saddle anesthesia	Cauda equina
Severe pain in the low back, including pain while lying down	Malignant neoplasm
Fever, chills, night sweats, recent loss of weight	Infection and malignant neoplasm

innervated through the medial branch of the dorsal rami of the spinal nerve exiting at the level of the facet and the medial branch of the dorsal ramus of the spinal nerve cephalad to the joint; innervation possibly extends two or three levels or more cephalad and caudal to the joint. Pain is predominantly in the paraspinal area and is accompanied by contractions of the muscles that guard around the facet joints. The pain from the facet joints can be unilateral or bilateral.

Sacroiliac joint arthropathy is a cause of axial back pain as well. The pain is located in the lumbosacral-buttock junction with referral to the lower extremity and to the groin area. Painful conditions of the sacroiliac joint are known to result from spondyloarthropathies, infection, malignant neoplasms, pregnancies, and trauma and even to occur spontaneously.

Radicular Pain

Involvement of nerve roots causes radicular pain. Nerve roots are affected secondary to mechanical pressure and inflammation. Mechanical pressure is usually secondary to disc protrusion (herniation) or due to spinal stenosis. In disc herniation, the nucleus pulposus protrudes through the annulus fibrosus and causes mechanical compression of the nerve root either in the central canal or in the foramen. Multiple inflammatory products (listed before) that play an important role in producing pain accompany acute disc herniations. Disc herniations involve all age groups, with predominance in the young and middle aged. Spinal stenosis, on the other hand, predominantly affects the elderly; it is a combination of disc degeneration, ligamentum hypertrophy, and facet arthropathy or spondylolisthesis. In radiculopathy, symptoms are present along a nerve root distribution. This causes pain in the lower extremities. Predominant buttocks area pain is a common presentation of lumbar radicular pain. Sensory symptoms include pain, numbness, and tingling that follow the distribution of a particular nerve root. The symptoms may be accompanied by motor weakness in a myotomal distribution.

Myofascial Pain

There are different theories explaining muscular reasons for acute low back pain, but they remain unproved.[13,14] These theories are as follows: inflammation—failure at the myotendinous junction and the production of an inflammatory repair response; ischemia—postural abnormalities causing chronic muscle activation and ischemia; trigger points secondary to repetitive strain of muscles (this theory remains the most attractive[14]); and muscle imbalance.

Referred Pain

Musculoskeletal structures in proximity to the spine and organs in the abdomen and pelvis are potential sources of pain with referral to the spine and the paraspinal area.

Occult Lesions

These lesions may present with axial or radicular symptoms or with both. Spine metastasis[15] and spine and paraspinal infections are considered a rare possibility. Skilled history taking and physical examination are necessary in diagnosis of these dangerous conditions.

PHYSICAL EXAMINATION

The physical examination starts with a thorough history to ascertain the pain's onset, character, location, and aggravating and mitigating factors. Inquiry about associated symptoms, such as weakness, bowel or bladder symptoms, fever, and abnormal loss of weight, and past medical history are important. Examination includes inspection of the lower back and the lower extremities. Palpation of the paraspinal muscles, lumbar facet joints, inguinal lymph nodes, and lower extremity pulses is performed. Hip examination, root tension signs, discogenic provocative maneuvers, and sacroiliac joint maneuvers are performed (Table 44-2). Gait examination, with heel and toe walking, is assessed. Sensory examination and thorough manual muscle testing are performed. Deep tendon reflexes are examined.

DIAGNOSTIC STUDIES

Radiologic studies are not necessary unless certain red flags are present[16]: history of trauma, constitutional symptoms, suspicion of radiculopathy, history of cancer, or persistent symptoms lasting longer than 1 month

TABLE 44-2 Spine Physical Examination Maneuvers

Maneuver	Description	Significance
Pelvic rock	In a supine position, flex the patient's hips until the flexed knees approximate to the chest; then, rotate the lower extremities from one side to the other.	Lumbar discogenic pain provocation
Sustained hip flexion	In a supine position, raise the patient's extended lower extremities to approximately 60 degrees. Ask the patient to hold the lower extremities in that position and release. The test result is positive on reproduction of low lumbar or buttock pain. Then lower the extremities successively approximately 15 degrees and, at each point, note the reproduction and intensity of pain.	Lumbar discogenic pain provocation
Root tension signs—upper extremity	Contralateral neck lateral bending and abduction of the ipsilateral upper extremity	Reproduces cervical radicular pain in the periscapular area or in the upper extremity
Spurling maneuver	Passively perform cervical extension, lateral bending toward the side of symptoms, and axial compression.	Reproduces cervical radicular pain in the periscapular area or in the upper extremity
Straight-leg raise	While the patient is lying supine, the involved lower extremity is passively flexed to 30 degrees with the knee in full extension.	Reproduces pain in the buttock, posterior thigh, and posterior calf in conditions with S1 radicular pain
Reverse straight-leg raise	While the patient is lying prone, the involved lower extremity is passively extended, the knee flexed.	Reproduces pain in the buttock and anterior thigh in conditions with high lumbar (such as L3 and L4) radicular pain
Crossed straight-leg raise	While the patient is lying supine, the contralateral lower extremity is passively flexed to 30 degrees with the knee in full extension.	Reproduces pain in the ipsilateral buttock, posterior thigh, and posterior calf in conditions with S1 radicular pain
Sitting root test	While the patient is sitting, the involved lower extremity is passively flexed with the knee extended.	Reproduces pain in the buttock, posterior thigh, and posterior calf in conditions with S1 radicular pain
Lasègue sign	While the patient is lying supine, the involved lower extremity is passively flexed to 90 degrees.	Reproduces pain in the buttock, posterior thigh, and posterior calf in conditions with S1 radicular pain
Bragard sign	While the patient is lying supine, the involved lower extremity is passively flexed to 30 degrees, with dorsiflexion of the foot.	Reproduces pain in the buttock, posterior thigh, and posterior calf in conditions with S1 radicular pain
Gaenslen maneuver	The patient is placed in a supine position with the affected side flush with the edge of the examination table. The hip and knee on the unaffected side are flexed, and the patient clasps the flexed knee to the chest. The examiner then applies pressure against the clasped knee, extends the lower extremity on the ipsilateral side, and brings it under the surface of the examination table.	Reproduces pain in patients with sacroiliac joint syndrome
Sacroiliac joint compression	Apply compression to the joint with the patient lying on the side.	Reproduces pain in patients with sacroiliac joint syndrome
Pressure at sacral sulcus	Apply pressure on the posterior superior iliac spine (dimple).	Reproduces pain in patients with sacroiliac joint syndrome
Patrick test (FABER test)	While the patient is supine, the knee and hip are flexed. The hip is abducted and externally rotated.	Reproduces pain in patients with sacroiliac joint syndrome, facet joint arthropathy (pain is reproduced in the low back), degenerative joint disease of the hip (pain is reproduced in the groin)
Yeoman test	While the patient is in the prone position, the hip is extended and the ilium is externally rotated.	Reproduces pain in patients with sacroiliac joint syndrome
Iliac gapping test	Distraction can be performed to the anterior sacroiliac ligaments by applying pressure to the anterior superior iliac spines.	Reproduces pain in patients with sacroiliac joint syndrome

Differential Diagnosis

Degenerative disc disease

Facet joint arthropathy

Lumbar radiculopathy

Sacroiliac joint syndrome

Acute vertebral compression fracture

Sacral stress fracture

Referred pain from abdomen or pelvis

Occult lesions in the spine, such as metastasis or infection

without improvement. Other reasons include rheumatologic conditions, use of steroids, and litigations.

The "gold standard" for evaluation of painful spine conditions is magnetic resonance imaging (MRI), which allows good visualization of discs and nerves as well as provides valuable information necessary for further management if the condition does not improve. MRI evaluation is required only if symptoms persist for longer than 1 month or if radicular pain or weakness is noted. It is also used in the workup for back pain accompanied by constitutional symptoms.

TREATMENT

Initial

Inflammation is a major culprit of pain. Nonsteroidal anti-inflammatory drugs (NSAIDs) are a cornerstone of pain management and should be provided in adequate doses. Muscle relaxants are commonly used for pain management along with NSAIDs. These medications do not target a particular pathologic process and should be used in conjunction with NSAIDs. They are particularly helpful in improving sleep and relieving muscles "spasms" in patients with low back pain.

Tramadol and opioid medications can be used in cases of severe pain. If there is a need for extended use of these medicines, imaging studies should be performed promptly and other management modalities should be considered. If medical management of pain is ineffective, spine manipulation,[17] acupuncture, and massage can be helpful in providing pain management.[18] Modalities such as heat and ice can also be used. Bed rest is not recommended in management of acute low back pain. It is advisable to remain active as much as possible.[19]

Rehabilitation

The cornerstone for a complete recovery and the prevention of a recurrence of acute low back pain or the transformation to chronic low back pain is participation in a regular spine stabilization program. The program should begin immediately after the pain starts to improve. Initiation of an exercise program while the patient is experiencing severe symptoms is not helpful because the patient's ability to participate is limited by pain. A lumbar stabilization exercise program consists of stretching the lower extremities and pelvis and lumbosacral muscles as well as performing exercises to strengthen the lumbosacral muscles. Postural training and learning proper body mechanics are essential. Patients are taught to perform these exercises and are advised to incorporate them into their daily routine.

Procedures

Spinal injections are not considered a first-line management of acute low back pain. If progressive radiculopathy is suspected and confirmed by MRI, therapeutic spinal nerve root blocks should be promptly considered. In axial acute low back pain, if conservative management fails in 4 weeks, MRI is performed. If the MRI findings and the clinical findings suggest intervertebral disc disease, transforaminal epidural steroid injections or interlaminar epidural steroid injections are used. In this context, if MRI findings are normal and clinical findings suggest abnormality, therapeutic facet joint injections or sacroiliac joint injections are used.

Surgery

Surgical intervention is not indicated in the management of acute low back pain.

POTENTIAL DISEASE COMPLICATIONS

Most patients will recover within 2 weeks. However, if symptoms change from axial low back pain to radicular pain, weakness develops in one or both lower extremities, or pain persists, the clinician should promptly order imaging studies. Further management is required as soon as possible to prevent deterioration of the patient's condition.

POTENTIAL TREATMENT COMPLICATIONS

NSAIDs used in management have known gastrointestinal complications, such as peptic ulcer disease. Patients must take the medications with food, antacids, or ulcer-preventing medications.

Muscle relaxants, tramadol (Ultram), and opioids have sedative side effects. Patients are advised to refrain from driving and operating machinery while taking these medications.

References

1. Cypress BK. Characteristics of physician visits for back symptoms: a national perspective. Am J Public Health 1983;73:389-395.
2. Waddell G. The epidemiology of low back pain. In Waddell G. The Back Pain Revolution. New York, Churchill Livingstone, 1998: 69-84.

3. Deyo RA, Tsui-Wu YJ. Descriptive epidemiology of low back pain and its related medical care in the United States. Spine 1987;12:264-268.

4. Shekelle PG, Markovich M, Louie R. An epidemiologic study of episodes of back pain care. Spine 1995;20:1668-1673.

5. Manchikanti L. Epidemiology of low back pain. Pain Physician 2000;3:167-192.

6. Waxman R, Tennant A, Helliwell P. A prospective follow up study of low back pain in the community. Spine 2000;25:2085-2090.

7. Saal JS, Franson RC, Dobrow R, et al. High levels of inflammatory phospholipase A_2 activity in lumbar disc herniations. Spine 1990;15:674-678.

8. Coppes MA, Marani E, Thomeer R, Groen G. Innervation of "painful" lumbar discs. Spine 1997;22:2342-2350.

9. Freemont AJ, Peacock TE, Goupille P, et al. Nerve ingrowth into diseased intervertebral disc in chronic back pain. Lancet 1997;350:178-181.

10. Aprill C, Bogduk N. The prevalence of cervical zygapophyseal joint pain. A first approximation. Spine 1992;17:744-747.

11. Bogduk N, Marsland A. The cervical zygapophyseal joint as a source of neck pain. Spine 1988;13:610-617.

12. Schwarzer AC, Wang S, Bogduk N, et al. Prevalence and clinical features of lumbar zygapophysial joint pain: a study in an Australian population with chronic low back pain. Ann Rheum Dis 1995;54:100-106.

13. Bogduk N. Low back pain. In Bogduk N. Clinical Anatomy of the Lumbar Spine and Sacrum, 3rd ed. New York, Churchill Livingstone, 1997;187-214.

14. Manchikanti L, Singh V, Fellows B. Structural basis of chronic low back pain. In Manchikanti L, Slipman CW, Fellows B, eds. Low Back Pain: Diagnosis and Treatment. Paducah, Ky, American Society of Interventional Pain Physicians, 2002:77-95.

15. Slipman CW, Patel RK, Botwin K, et al. Epidemiology of spine tumors presenting to musculoskeletal physiatrists. Arch Phys Med Rehabil 2003;84:492-495.

16. Deyo RA, Diehl AK. Lumbar spine films in primary care: current use and effects of selective ordering criteria. J Gen Intern Med 1986;1:20-25.

17. El Abd OH, Slipman CW. Chiropractic care. Physicians' Information and Education Resource. American College of Physicians. Available at: http://pier.acponline.org/.

18. Cherkin DC, Sherman KJ, Deyo RA, Shekelle PG. A review of the evidence for the effectiveness, safety, and cost of acupuncture, massage therapy, and spinal manipulation for back pain. Ann Intern Med 2003;138:898-906.

19. Hagen KB, Jamtvedt G, Hilde G, Winnem MF. The updated Cochrane review of bed rest for low back pain and sciatica. Spine 2005;30:542-546.

Lumbar Spondylolysis and Spondylolisthesis 45

James Spinelli, DO, and James Rainville, MD

James Spinelli, DO, and James Rainville, MD

Synonym

Slipped vertebra

ICD-9 Codes

738.4   Lumbar spondylolisthesis
756.11 Lumbar spondylolysis

DEFINITION

Spondylolysis refers to a bone defect in the pars interarticularis. The term *pars interarticularis* translates to "bridge between the joints"; as such, it is the isthmus or bone bridge between the inferior and superior articular surfaces of the neural arch of a single vertebra. When bilateral spondylolysis is present, the posterior aspects of the neural arch including the inferior articular surfaces are no longer connected by bone to the rest of the vertebra (Fig. 45-1).

Spondylolysis is an acquired condition; it has never been found at birth.[1] Spondylolysis is most commonly acquired early in life[2,3] and is identified by lumbar radiographs in 4.4% of children 5 to 7 years of age.[2,4] By 18 years of age, 6% of the population has spondylolysis[2]; few additional cases are thought to occur thereafter. Accordingly, the prevalence remains steady at 6% in radiographic screening of adult spines.[5]

Spondylolysis most commonly occurs at the L5 vertebra, where about 90% of the cases are found. It is found with decreasing frequency at progressively higher lumbar levels.[2,6,7] It is more common in males than in females (7.7% vs. 4.6%),[6] can be unilateral or bilateral, and has a suspected genetic predisposition.[2,8-10]

The most likely cause of spondylolysis is a stress fracture of the pars that remains un-united.[11] This is consistent with the higher incidence of spondylolysis suspected in adolescents and young adults who aggressively participate in sports requiring repetitive flexion-extension movements, such as gymnastics,[12-14] throwing sports,[14] football,[15] wrestling,[16] dance,[12] and swimming breast and butterfly strokes.[17] Further supporting an acquired stress fracture as the cause is the lack of spondylolysis in the lumbar spines of individuals who have never walked.[18]

Spondylolisthesis refers to displacement of a vertebral body in relation to the one below it. The most common type of spondylolisthesis, and the alignment abnormality implied when the term is used in this chapter, is an anterior displacement, also called anterolisthesis. Spondylolisthesis can also occur in a posterior direction, called retrolisthesis, or laterally, called laterolisthesis. Spondylolisthesis is an abnormal finding. Whenever spondylolisthesis is present, it is pathognomonic of structural and functional failure of the neural arch and facet joints, which are responsible for maintaining normal vertebral alignment.

Spondylolisthesis is classified by etiology and grade. The five etiologic types are dysplastic, isthmic or spondylolytic, degenerative, traumatic, and pathologic. Dysplastic spondylolisthesis results from congenital dysplasia of one or more facet joints. Isthmic or spondylolytic spondylolisthesis (see Fig. 45-1) results from bilateral pars defects (bilateral spondylolysis). Degenerative spondylolisthesis results from degeneration of the facet joints and intervertebral discs (most common at L4-5 and with advancing age). Traumatic spondylolisthesis results from fractures of posterior elements other than the pars, such as facet joints, laminae, or pedicles. Pathologic spondylolisthesis results from pathologic changes in posterior elements due to malignant disease, infection, or primary bone disease.

The grade of spondylolisthesis is rated by the percentage of slippage of the posterior corner of the vertebral body above over the superior surface of the vertebral body below. At least 5% slippage must be present for a diagnosis of spondylolisthesis to be conferred. Slippage can be further categorized into five grades. Grade I indicates slippage from 5% to 25%; grade II is 26% to 50%; grade III is 51% to 75%; grade IV is more than 75% (Fig. 45-2)[19]; and grade V is complete dislocation of adjacent vertebrae, also called spondyloptosis. The majority of cases (60% to 75%) are classified as grade I; 20% to 38% are classified as grade II; and less than 2% of all cases are graded III, IV, and V.[5,6,20,21]

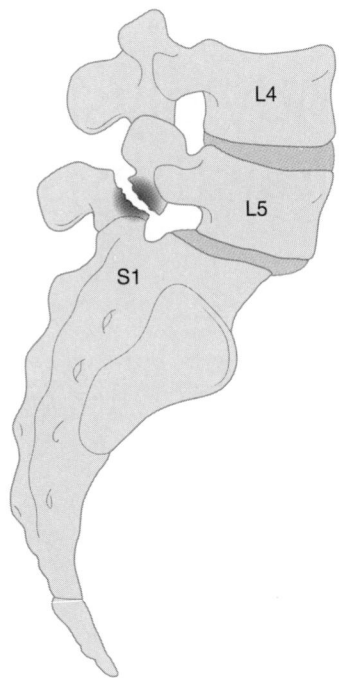

FIGURE 45-1. Spondylolysis of L5 with L5-S1 spondylolisthesis. (Reprinted with permission from Herkowitz HN. The Lumbar Spine, 3rd ed. Philadelphia, Lippincott Williams & Wilkins, 2004:558.)

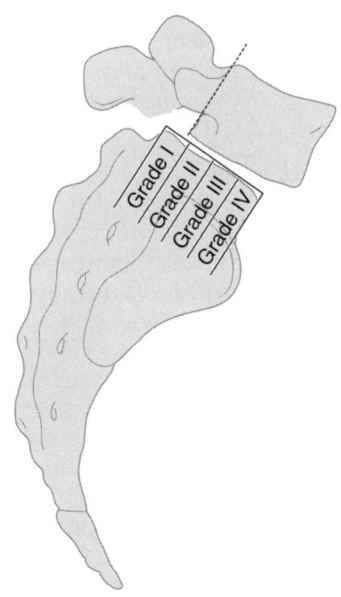

FIGURE 45-2. Meyerding classification of spondylolisthesis into grades based on the amount of slippage of the superior vertebral body on the vertebral body below. (Reprinted with permission from Herkowitz HN. The Lumbar Spine, 3rd ed. Philadelphia, Lippincott Williams & Wilkins, 2004:560.)

Spondylolisthesis is present in 50% to 75 % of children and adolescents at the time that spondylolysis is diagnosed[9,22,23] and increases with age.[20] After diagnosis, concern about the progression of spondylolisthesis is common, but prognostic factors are lacking.[23] In general, progression occurs before and during the early teenage years,[2,24] and only minor progression occurs after skeletal maturity. Advancing age may lead to slight

additional progression of spondylolytic spondylolisthesis, which is usually attributed to progressive degeneration of the disc and facet joints.[20,25,26] Participation in competitive sports has not been found to influence the progression of spondylolisthesis.[27]

SYMPTOMS

Most people with spondylolysis or spondylolisthesis are asymptomatic. For the symptomatic minority, the most common complaint is low back pain, which can range from mild to severe.[22] Back pain is frequently described as a dull, aching pain in the back, buttocks, and posterior thigh, the characteristics of which are not distinct compared with other degenerative back disorders.[2]

For children, adolescents, and adults with established spondylolysis and spondylolisthesis, it is difficult to attribute pain symptoms to these abnormalities. Most people with these findings are asymptomatic, and the incidence of back pain in this population is generally similar to that in the population without spondylolysis and spondylolisthesis.[2,6,8,10,28,29] In addition, the degree of spondylolisthesis is not associated with the prevalence of back pain,[29] and no study has linked progression with pain symptoms. Disability because of back pain is no more prevalent in the population with spondylolysis and spondylolisthesis than in the general public.[22,29] Therefore, patients with spondylolysis and spondylolisthesis should be evaluated and treated like others with back pain, and health care providers should be cautious in attributing symptoms to these findings.

Spondylolisthesis combined with disc degeneration may result in significant narrowing of the neuroforamina at the affected level. This can cause compression or irritation of the exiting nerve roots and results in radiation of pain into the lower extremity and neurologic symptoms within the affected dermatome and myotome. Because spondylolytic spondylolisthesis most commonly involves the L5-S1 level, the L5 nerve root is most often affected by this problem.

PHYSICAL EXAMINATION

The physical examination in spondylolysis and spondylolisthesis has few specific or sensitive findings. Painful trunk range of motion is often noted in children and adolescents with symptoms from acute spondylolysis. This is especially noted for trunk extension, as this motion shifts load to the posterior vertebral elements and thus through the region of the pars.[30] Limited range of motion for trunk extension has been observed,[21,31] and palpation of the back may reveal local tenderness at the lumbosacral junction, the level at which spondylolysis is most common.[21] Unfortunately, these findings are common to other spinal disorders and are not specific for spondylolysis.

Detection of spondylolisthesis on physical examination is difficult except in the rare cases of grade III or greater slips. Here, a "step-off" of the spinous processes can be seen or palpated at the level of the spondylolisthesis. In grade I and grade II spondylolisthesis, the step-off is much more difficult to detect and has never been shown to be a reliable finding. Neurologic deficits and positive results of straight-leg raising tests are rarely found in cases of spondylolisthesis, including cases with sciatica.[21] When neurologic deficits are noted, they usually involve the L5 roots, which can become irritated within their neuroforamina.[21,32,33] Lumbar tenderness and restricted range of motion were noted in some cases of spondylolisthesis[21] but are general signs present in most back disorders.

DIAGNOSTIC STUDIES

The lateral oblique radiograph may reveal the classic "collar on the Scottie dog" finding of spondylolysis (Fig. 45-3). This represents the bone defect between the inferior and superior articulating processes. The sensitivity of this approaches only 33% because the plane of the pars defect must be close to the plane of the radiographic image to be clearly visualized.[34] The lateral radiograph reveals the presence and grade of spondylolisthesis.

Computed tomography is considered superior to magnetic resonance imaging for direct visualization of the pars interarticularis. Therefore, some advocate axial computed tomography as the test of choice for identifying spondylolysis.[35] If spondylolysis is suspected when computed tomography is ordered, scanning can be done by use of thin sections or reverse gantry angle to ensure optimal visualization of the pars.[35] On axial views, pars defects can be difficult to identify because

they can simulate the adjacent facet joints. However, they usually lack the regular cortical surfaces of the facets.[36] It is also useful to try to identify an intact cortical ring for each vertebra, including the vertebral body, the pedicles, the pars, and the posterior neural arch. If the intact ring is not found in any of the cuts through the levels of the pedicles, a defect in the ring at the appropriate position suggests the diagnosis of spondylolysis[37] (Fig. 45-4). Sagittal reconstruction images are often helpful for confirming the presence of spondylolysis (Fig. 45-5).

Magnetic resonance imaging with fat saturation technique can identify subtle bone marrow edema of early stress injury to the pars.[38] This provides greater detection sensitivity for early stress reactions or fractures in the pars that are not yet detectable by radiography or computed tomography.[39] Magnetic resonance imaging is also useful for grading spondylolisthesis and for visualizing the neuroforamina. As spondylolisthesis progresses, the neuroforamen becomes horizontally oriented, and the exiting nerve root becomes situated between the pedicle above and the uncovered disc below. With further narrowing because of disc degeneration, the nerve root becomes increasingly entrapped within the foramen. This is well visualized on T2 sagittal and axial images as the high fat signal that normally surrounds the nerve root becomes obliterated.[32]

Bone scintigraphy uses radioisotopes that accumulate in metabolically hyperactive bone to identify abnormal bone activity. In acute spondylolysis, the stress fracture usually results in increased metabolic bone activity as the fracture attempts to heal (Fig. 45-6). This is detected

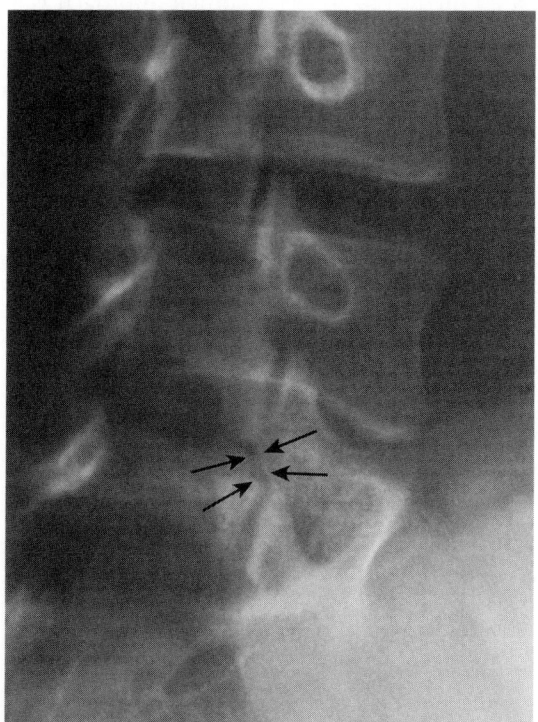

FIGURE 45-3. Spondylolysis defect of pars interarticularis of L5 noted on oblique radiograph.

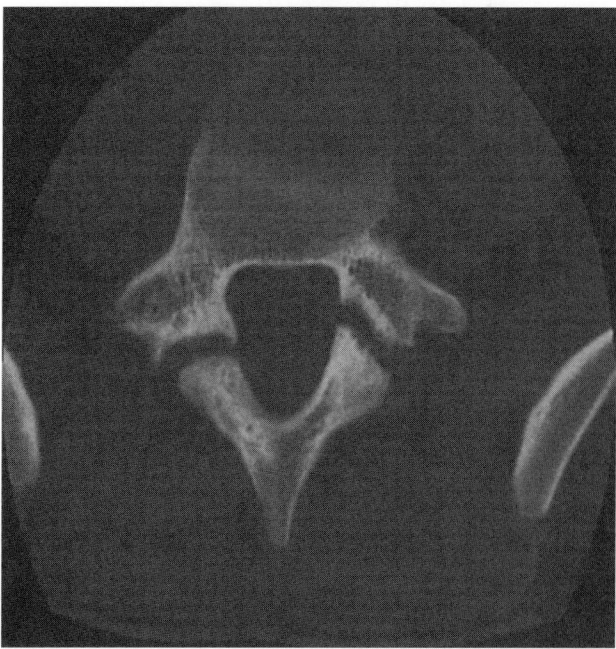

FIGURE 45-4. Spondylolysis defect of L5 as seen on axial computed tomographic scan. Note the lack of a complete ring of vertebrae because of bilateral spondylolysis.

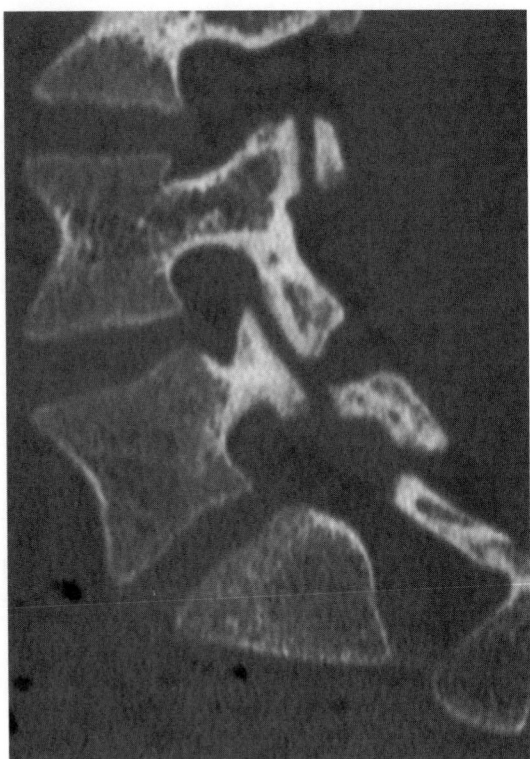

FIGURE 45-5. Spondylolysis of L5 as seen on sagittal reconstruction of computed tomographic image. Observe the continuity of bone from the pedicle of the L4 vertebra into the superior articular process (facet), then along the pars interarticularis to the inferior articular process. Now repeat this for L5 and note the defect in the pars interarticularis that separates the inferior articular process from the rest of the vertebra.

early in the course of spondylolysis by the accumulation of radioisotope at the fracture site. Long-standing spondylolysis with an established nonunion usually reveals no such increased radioisotope uptake.[40] Single-photon emission computed tomography (SPECT) improves the localizing ability of bone scintigraphy. SPECT creates a series of slices through the target structure, permitting spatial separation of overlapping bone. Because of these abilities, SPECT imaging has established a place in the evaluation of adolescent athletes with back pain.[41,42]

TREATMENT

Acute Spondylolysis

A child or adolescent with acute symptomatic spondylolysis, with or without spondylolisthesis, will complain of pain. The first step is always to determine the cause of pain symptoms through history taking, physical examination, and the judicious use of diagnostic studies as reviewed before.

In children or adolescents with acute symptomatic spondylolysis as suggested by bone scintigraphy, SPECT, or magnetic resonance imaging, attempts to induce or to aid healing are warranted. Rigid antilordotic thoracolumbosacral orthosis bracing for 23 hours a day for a period of 6 months is advocated to reduce stress on the pars interarticularis, although this treatment has not been assessed in randomized controlled trials.[43-45] Activity modification that allows modest physical activities while wearing the brace is usually recommended until symptoms subside, and physical therapy for trunk strengthening has been used. With this approach, symptoms improve in 75% of children, and many lytic defects are noted to heal.[43-45] A similar approach is advocated in children and adolescents with concurrent spondylolisthesis. However, once spondylolisthesis is present, healing of the pars defect becomes improbable. In this situation, the goal is symptom reduction, and good results are observed in many patients.[44,45] To date, there is no evidence to support bracing for the prevention of slip progression. In cases of incidental findings of spondylolisthesis, there is no need for treatment or restriction of activities, including aggressive sports participation.[11,27,46]

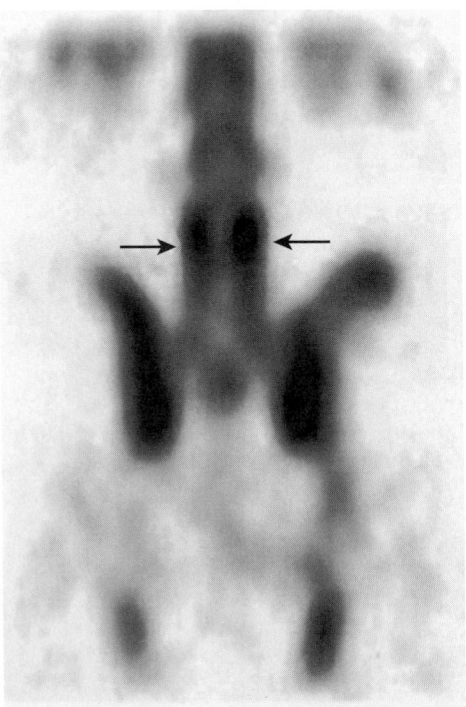

FIGURE 45-6. Bone scan of axial skeleton revealing increased radioactive isotope uptake in pars interarticularis on both sides of neural arch of L4 vertebra.

Differential Diagnosis

Degenerative low back pain

Lumbar disc herniation

Discitis

Lumbar radiculopathy

Spinal stenosis (central versus neuroforaminal)

Vertebral fracture (by compression, tumor, infection)

Lumbar sprain or strain

In adults with spondylolysis, with or without spondylolisthesis, back pain complaints are treated like other nonspecific back pain disorders. This includes education, analgesics, nonsteroidal anti-inflammatory drugs,[47-49] exercise, avoidance of bed rest, and rapid return to activities.[50-52]

Rehabilitation

Exercise has received some study as a treatment of spondylolysis and spondylolisthesis. One study has advocated flexion over extension exercises,[53] although methodologic shortcomings limit the strength of these recommendations. A spinal stabilization exercise program was found to be superior to uncontrolled treatment at short- and long-term follow-up.[54] Aggressive physical therapy programs for those with back pain, spondylolysis, or spondylolisthesis have been shown to provide significant short-term benefit in terms of flexibility, strength, endurance, pain tolerance, and level of disability. This type of program consists of stretching and high-intensity, progressively resistive training performed in a non-pain-contingent manner.[55,56] Stretching targets the hip flexors, hamstrings, quadriceps, and gastrocnemius-soleus muscles. Strengthening targets the abdominals and the various back muscles. Modalities, including ultrasound and electrical stimulation, have not been shown to improve symptoms and are generally of limited value.

Procedures

Various types of spinal injections are performed with use of fluoroscopy to ensure proper needle placement. Anesthetic agents may be used for short-term pain relief, usually for diagnostic purposes. Injection of steroids may be tried for longer term therapeutic purposes in adults with symptomatic spondylolysis or spondylolisthesis. For radicular pain, epidural injections may be used if the site of nerve root compression lies within the spinal canal, whereas selective nerve root blocks may be used if compression lies within the transforaminal space. For axial pain, facet injections may be used if the facet joints themselves are thought to be the source of pain.

Surgery

Surgery is indicated in cases of spondylolisthesis causing progressive neurologic deficit; cauda equina compression with leg weakness, sensory loss, or bladder or bowel incontinence; and persistent and severe back and leg pain despite aggressive conservative treatment. Surgery usually includes lumbar spinal decompression of the affected nerve roots and fusion of the spondylolisthesis. Results are generally favorable.[57]

POTENTIAL DISEASE COMPLICATIONS

Most cases of spondylolysis and spondylolisthesis are asymptomatic and remain that way.[58] The intervertebral disc and facet degeneration that occurs naturally with age is accelerated in the presence of spondylolysis. Because of this, spondylolytic spondylolisthesis can progress and result in nerve root compression or spinal stenosis.[59]

POTENTIAL TREATMENT COMPLICATIONS

Nonsteroidal anti-inflammatory drugs can cause gastric bleeding and renal and hepatic toxicity. Acetaminophen, in large amounts, can cause hepatic toxicity. Narcotic analgesics are potentially addictive, and because studies of the low back pain population have not found significant differences between narcotics and nonsteroidal anti-inflammatory drugs in terms of pain relief, extreme caution should be used beyond the short term.[60-62] Exercise can irritate spinal tissue already inflamed. Spinal injections may result in a temporary increase in pain, spinal headache, infection, nerve root damage, or spinal cord damage. Surgical decompression or fusion can lead to infection, failed fusion, persistent back pain, nerve root damage, or spinal cord damage.

References

1. Lonstein JE. Spondylolisthesis in children. Cause, natural history, and management. Spine 1999;24:2640-2648.
2. Fredrickson BE, Baker D, McHolick WJ, et al. The natural history of spondylolysis and spondylolisthesis. J Bone Joint Surg Am 1984;66:699-707.
3. Wertzberger KL, Peterson HA. Acquired spondylolysis and spondylolisthesis in the young child. Spine 1980;5:437-442.
4. Baker DR, McHolick WJ. Spondylolysis and spondylolisthesis in children. J Bone Joint Surg Am 1956;38:933-934.
5. Virta L, Rönnemaa T, Österman K, et al. Prevalence of isthmic lumbar spondylolisthesis in middle-aged subjects from eastern and western Finland. J Clin Epidemiol 1992;45:917-922.
6. Österman K, Schlenzka D, Poussa M, et al. Isthmic spondylolisthesis in symptomatic and asymptomatic subjects, epidemiology, and natural history with special reference to disk abnormalities and mode of treatment. Clin Orthop Relat Res 1993;297:65-70.
7. Rothman SL, Glenn WV. CT multiplanar reconstruction in 253 cases of lumbar spondylolysis. Am J Neuroradiol 1984;5:81-90.
8. Albanese M, Pizzutillo PD. Family study of spondylolysis and spondylolisthesis. J Pediatr Orthop 1982;4:495-499.
9. Shahriaree H, Sajadi KM, Rooholamini SA. A family with spondylolisthesis. J Bone Joint Surg Am 1979;61:1256-1258.
10. Wynne-Davies R, Scott JHS. Inheritance and spondylolysis. J Bone Joint Surg Br 1979;61:301-305.
11. Wiltse LL, Widell EH, Jackson DW. Fatigue fracture: the basic lesion in isthmic spondylolisthesis. J Bone Joint Surg Am 1975;57:17-22.
12. Hutchinson MR. Low back pain in elite rhythmic gymnasts. Med Sci Sports Exerc 1999;31:1686-1688.
13. Jackson DW, Wiltse LL, Cirincoine RJ. Spondylolysis in the female gymnast. Clin Orthop 1976;117:68-73.
14. Soler T, Calderon C. The prevalence of spondylolysis in the Spanish elite athletes. Am J Sports Med 2000;28:57-61.
15. McCarroll JR, Miller JM, Ritter MA. Lumbar spondylolysis and spondylolisthesis in college football players. A prospective study. Am J Sports Med 1986;14:404-406.
16. Granhed H, Morelli B. Low back pain among retired wrestlers and heavyweight lifters. Am J Sports Med 1988;16:530-533.
17. Nyska M, Constantini N, Cale-Benzoor M. Spondylolysis as a cause of low back pain in swimmers. Int J Sports Med 2000;21:3775-3779.
18. Rosenberg NJ, Bargar WL, Friedman B. The incidence of spondylolysis and spondylolisthesis in nonambulatory patients. Spine 1981;6:35-38.

19. Meyerding HW. Spondylolisthesis. Surg Gynecol Obstet 1932;54: 371-377.
20. Ishida Y, Ohmori K, Inoue H, et al. Delayed vertebral slip and adjacent disc degeneration in isthmic defect of the fifth lumbar vertebra. J Bone Joint Surg Br 1999;81:240-244.
21. Möller H, Hedlund R. Surgery versus conservative management in adult isthmic spondylolisthesis—a prospective randomized study: part I. Spine 2000;25:1711-1715.
22. Frennered AK, Danielson BI, Nachemson AL. Natural history of symptomatic isthmic low-grade spondylolisthesis in children and adolescents: a seven-year follow-up study. J Pediatr Orthop 1991;11:209-213.
23. Danielson BI, Frennered AK, Irstam LKH. Radiologic progression of isthmus lumbar spondylolisthesis in young patients. Spine 1991;16:422-425.
24. Seitsalo S, Österman K, Hyvarinen H, et al. Progression of spondylolisthesis in children and adolescents: a long-term follow-up of 272 patients. Spine 1991;16:417-421.
25. Ikata T, Miyake R, Katoh S, et al. Pathogenesis of sports-related spondylolisthesis in adolescents: radiographic and magnetic resonance imaging study. Am J Sports Med 1996;24:94-98.
26. Fredrickson BE, Baker D, Murtland AM, et al. The natural history of spondylolysis and spondylolisthesis: 45-year follow-up. Presented at the 15th annual meeting of the North American Spine Society; New Orleans, La; October 26, 2000.
27. Muschik M, Hahnel H, Robinson PN. Competitive sports and the progression of spondylolysis. J Pediatr Orthop 1996;16:364-369.
28. Congeni J, McCulloch J, Swanson K. Lumbar spondylolysis: a study of natural progression in athletes. Am J Sports Med 1997;25: 248-253.
29. Virta L, Rönnemaa T. The association of mild-moderate isthmic lumbar spondylolisthesis and low back pain in middle-age patients is weak and it only occurs in women. Spine 1993;18:1496-1503.
30. Yamane T, Yosida T, Mimatsu K. Early diagnosis of lumbar spondylolysis by MRI. J Bone Joint Surg Br 1993;75:764-768.
31. McGregor AH, Cattermole HR, Hughes SPF. Global spinal motion in subjects with lumbar spondylolysis and spondylolisthesis: does the grade or type of slip affect global spinal motion? Spine 2001;26:282-286.
32. Jinkins JR, Rauch A. Magnetic resonance imaging of entrapment of lumbar nerve roots in spondylolytic spondylolisthesis. J Bone Joint Surg Am 1994;76:1643-1648.
33. Jinkins JR, Matthews JC, Sener RN, et al. Spondylolysis, spondylolisthesis, and associated nerve entrapment in the lumbosacral spine: MR evaluation. Am J Roentgenol 1992;159:799-803.
34. Saifuddin A, White J, Tucker S. Orientation of lumbar pars defects: implications for radiological detection and surgical management. J Bone Joint Surg Br 1998;80:208-211.
35. Harvey CJ, Richenberg JL, Saifuddin A. The radiological investigation of lumbar spondylolysis. Clin Radiol 1998;53:723-728.
36. Grogan JP, Hemminghytt S, Williams AL, et al. Spondylolysis studied with computer tomography. Radiology 1982;145:737-742.
37. Langston JW, Gavant ML. Incomplete ring sign: a simple method for CT detection of spondylolysis. J Comput Assist Tomogr 1985;9:728-729.
38. Sauryo K, Katoh S, Takata Y, et al. MRI signal changes of the pedicle as an indicator for early diagnosis of spondylolysis in children and adolescents; a clinical and biomechanical study. Spine 2006;31:206-211.
39. Hollenberg GM, Beatie PF, Meyers SP, et al. Stress reaction of the lumbar pars interarticularis: the development of a new MRI classification system. Spine 2002;27:181-186.
40. Lowe J, Schachner E, Hirschberg E, et al. Significance of bone scintigraphy in symptomatic spondylolysis. Spine 1984;9:653-655.
41. Bellar RD, Summerville DA, Treves ST, et al. Low-back pain in adolescent athletes: detection of stress injuries to the pars interarticularis with SPECT. Radiology 1991;180:509-512.
42. Itol K, Hashimoto T, Shigenobu K. Bone SPECT of symptomatic lumbar spondylolysis. Nucl Med Commun 1996;17:389-396.
43. Morita T, Ikata T, Katoh S, et al. Lumbar spondylolysis in children and adolescents. J Bone Joint Surg Br 1995;81:620-625.
44. Blanda J, Bethem D, Moats W, et al. Defect of pars interarticularis in athletes: a protocol for nonoperative treatment. J Spinal Disord 1993;6:406-411.
45. Steiner ME, Micheli LJ. Treatment of symptomatic spondylolysis and spondylolisthesis with the modified Boston brace. Spine 1985;10:937-942.
46. Semon RL, Spengler D. Significance of lumbar spondylolysis in college football players. Spine 1981;6:172-174.
47. Postacchini F, Facchini M, Palieri P. Efficacy of various forms of conservative treatment in low back pain: a comparative study. Neuroorthopedics 1988;6:28-35.
48. Amlie E, Weber H, Holme I. Treatment of acute low-back pain with piroxicam: results of a double-blind placebo-controlled trial. Spine 1987;12:473-476.
49. Berry H, Bloom B, Hamilton EBD, et al. Naproxen sodium, diflunisal, and placebo in the treatment of chronic back pain. Ann Rheum Dis 1983;41:129-132.
50. Deyo RA, Diehl AK, Rosenthal M. How many days of bed rest for acute low back pain? A randomized clinical trial. N Engl J Med 1986;315:1064-1070.
51. Gilbert JR, Taylor DW, Hildebrand A, Evans C. Clinical trial of common treatments for low back pain in family practice. Br Med J (Clin Res Ed) 1985;291:791-794.
52. Malmivaara A, Hakkinen U, Aro T, et al. The treatment of acute low back pain—bed rest, exercises or ordinary activity? N Engl J Med 1995;332:351-355.
53. Sinaki M, Lutness MP, Ilstrup DM, et al. Lumbar spondylolisthesis: retrospective comparison and three-year follow-up of two conservative treatment programs. Arch Phys Med Rehabil 1989;70:594-598.
54. O'Sullivan PB, Twomey LT, Allison GT. Evaluation of specific stabilizing exercise in the treatment of chronic low back pain with radiologic diagnosis of spondylolysis and spondylolisthesis. Spine 1997;22:2959-2967.
55. Rainville J, Mazzaferro R. Evaluation of outcomes of aggressive spine rehabilitation in patients with back pain and sciatica from previously diagnosed spondylolysis and spondylolisthesis. Arch Phys Med Rehabil 2001;82:1309.
56. Rainville J, Sobel J, Hartigan C, et al. The effect of compensation involvement on the reporting of pain and disability by subjects referred for rehabilitation of chronic low back pain. Spine 1997;22:2016-2024.
57. Jacobs WC, Vreeling A, De Kleuver M. Fusion for low-grade adult isthmic spondylolisthesis: a systematic review of the literature. Eur Spine J 2006;15:391-402.
58. Torgerson WR, Dotter WE. Comparative roentgenographic study of the asymptomatic and symptomatic lumbar spine. J Bone Joint Surg Am 1976;58:850-853.
59. Floman Y. Progression of lumbosacral spondylolisthesis in adults. Spine 2000;25:342-347.
60. Brown FL, Bodison S, Dixon J, et al. Comparison of diflunisal and acetaminophen with codeine in the treatment of initial or recurrent acute low back strain. Clin Ther 1986;9(Suppl C):52-58.
61. Muncie HL, King DE, DeForge B. Treatment of mild to moderate pain of acute soft tissue injury: diflunisal vs acetaminophen with codeine. J Fam Pract 1986;23:125-127.
62. Wiesel SW, Cuckler JM, Deluca F, et al. Acute low-back pain: an objective analysis of conservative therapy. Spine 1980;5:324-330.

Lumbar Spinal Stenosis 46

Zacharia Isaac, MD, and David Wang, DO

Synonyms

Pseudoclaudication
Neurogenic claudication
Spinal claudication
Low back pain

ICD-9 Code

724.02 Spinal stenosis, lumbar region

DEFINITION

Lumbar spinal stenosis is classically defined as narrowing of the spinal canal, nerve root canals, or tunnels of the intervertebral foramina at the lumbar level.[1] However, a significant portion of the general population may have anatomic spinal stenosis without symptoms. Numerous imaging studies have indicated that 20% to 25% of asymptomatic people older than 40 years have significant narrowing of the lumbar spinal canal.[2-4] This stenosis causes symptoms only when there is sufficient impingement on neural structures, including the cauda equina or exiting nerve roots. Therefore, spinal stenosis as a clinical entity is considered significant only if it results in symptomatic pain and compromised function.

The significant anatomic elements of the lumbosacral spine include the five lumbar vertebrae L1 to L5, the sacrum, the intervertebral discs, the ligamentum flavum, the zygapophyseal joints, the lumbar spinal nerve rootlets, the spinal nerve roots, and the cauda equina (Fig. 46-1).

Various schemes for classification of spinal stenosis have been devised and are listed in Table 46-1.

Congenital lumbar spinal stenosis is uncommon, representing 9% of cases[5]; symptoms first appear in patients during their 30s. Achondroplastic dwarves often develop stenosis secondary to hypoplasia of the pedicles.[6,7] Acromegaly may cause spinal stenosis by enlargement of the synovium and cartilage, which results in decreased cross-sectional area of the canal. Symptomatic spinal stenosis secondary to purely isolated congenital causes is rare. More commonly, patients will have a combination of congenital and acquired stenosis; a developmentally smaller canal predisposes them to symptoms once acquired changes occur to the surrounding anatomy. Developmental factors that lead to a small canal include statistically significantly shorter pedicles[8] and a trefoil-shaped canal.[9,10]

The acquired types of spinal stenosis are numerous, but degenerative is the most common. The first stage in the degenerative process is generally degradation of the hydrophilic proteoglycans within the intervertebral disc, attendant disc desiccation, and loss of disc height. This causes a shift of load onto the posterior structures of the canal, in particular the facet joints, which normally provide 3% to 25% of the support during axial loading but may bear up to 47% with degeneration of the disc.[11] As the facets bear more of the burden, they undergo degeneration, one aspect of which is osteophyte formation.[10] This further diminishes the cross-sectional area of the canal and can also result in stenosis of the neural foramina (termed foraminal stenosis). The ligamentum flavum also undergoes degenerative hypertrophic change as well as buckling with decreased intervertebral disc height, leading to further encroachment of the canal. Epidural fat may also contribute to reduced canal space in some patients.[12] Patients with acquired lumbar spinal stenosis usually develop symptoms during their 50s and 60s.

Spinal stenosis can be differentiated by anatomic location, including central canal, lateral recess, foraminal, and extraforaminal (Table 46-2). Additional subcategorization includes division of the lateral canal into three regions: entrance zone, mid-zone, and exit zone.[13]

Canal Measurements

The normal adult central canal has a midsagittal diameter of at least 13 mm.[14] Relative stenosis is defined as a canal diameter between 10 and 13 mm; patients may or may not be symptomatic. Absolute stenosis occurs at a diameter of less than 10 mm, and patients are usually symptomatic.[15] Extraforaminal nerve root compression can occur with disc herniation, degenerative scoliosis, or isthmic spondylolisthesis. Far-out syndrome, described by Wiltse and colleagues,[16] involves L5 root

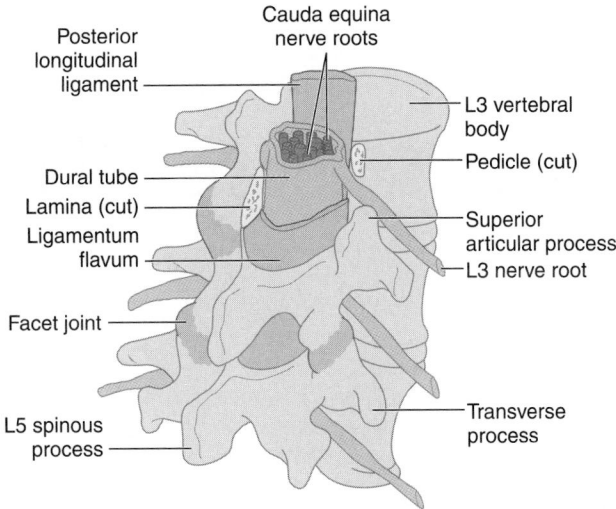

FIGURE 46-1. Normal anatomic structures of the lumbar spine at the third through the fifth lumbar levels. Note the close association between the nerve roots and the dural tube, the ligamentum flavum, the facet joints, the pedicles, and the lamina. The ligamentum flavum (interlaminar ligament) attaches laterally to the facet capsules.

TABLE 46-2 Anatomic Classification of Spinal Stenosis
Central canal
Lateral canal
Entrance zone (lateral recess)
Mid-zone (underneath pars interarticularis and pedicle)
Exit zone (intervertebral foramen)
Foraminal
Extraforaminal

impingement between the L5 transverse process and sacral ala in patients with spondylolisthesis. Extension of the spine can reduce foraminal cross-sectional area by 20%[17] and central canal volume by up to 67%.[18]

Finally, spinal stenosis has been categorized according to the patient's presenting pain syndrome of mechanical back pain, radicular pain, or neurogenic claudication.[19] The symptomatic pain pattern can be an indication of the anatomic and pathophysiologic mechanism of the patient's particular case of spinal stenosis.

SYMPTOMS

Symptomatic lumbar spinal stenosis may result in both back pain (from axial components, such as facet degeneration) and leg pain (from radicular components of nerve root compression both central and lateral). Leg

TABLE 46-1 Etiologic Classification of Spinal Stenosis
Congenital
Achondroplastic
Acromegaly
Acquired
Degenerative
Post-traumatic
Spondylolytic (isthmic spondylolisthesis)
Iatrogenic
Metabolic (Paget disease, chlorosis, fluorosis, diffuse interstitial skeletal hypertrophy, pseudogout, oxalosis)
Combined congenital and acquired

pain is often greater than back pain, and depending on which nerve roots are impinged, leg pain can be unilateral or bilateral and monoradicular or polyradicular. Patients with acquired, degenerative lumbar spinal stenosis tend to have a history of chronic low back pain and develop leg pain later in their course. In a study of 100 patients with lumbar spinal stenosis, back pain had been present for an average of 14 years and leg pain for an average of 2 years.[20] The classic symptom of lumbar spinal stenosis is neurogenic claudication, also known as pseudoclaudication, which typically presents as buttock, thigh, and calf pain exacerbated with walking, standing, or lumbar extension and alleviated with sitting, lying, or lumbar flexion. Symptoms also commonly involve cramping, numbness, tingling, heaviness, and spasms. Because the spinal canal and neuroforamina widen with flexion and become narrower with extension, pain often improves with squatting and walking tolerance increases with a flexed posture, such as while walking uphill or on an inclined treadmill or while pushing a shopping cart. Neurogenic claudication was found in one study to have a sensitivity of 63% and a specificity of 71% compared with a combination of clinical, radiologic, and imaging test findings.[21]

Symptoms that have been reported to have high sensitivity for lumbar spinal stenosis are as follows: best posture with regard to symptoms is sitting (89%),[22] worst posture with regard to symptoms is standing or walking (89%),[22] pain below buttocks (88%),[23] pain in legs worsened by walking and relieved by sitting (81%),[22] radiating leg pain (81%),[21] and age older than 65 years (77%).[23] Symptoms with high specificity for lumbar spinal stenosis include no pain when seated (93%) and symptoms improved when seated (83%).[23]

PHYSICAL EXAMINATION

Unlike the history, no physical examination findings are considered classic for lumbar spinal stenosis. Abnormal findings in lumbar spinal stenosis are similar to those in other disorders that cause peripheral neurologic deficits, but they are often not present. In the study by Amundsen and colleagues,[20] abnormal findings within the 100-subject cohort included sensory dysfunction (51%), diminished deep tendon reflexes (47%), positive Lasègue test result (24%), and leg weakness (23%), among others. As such, the physical examination tends to have higher specificity for lumbar spinal stenosis than the history does, whereas the patient's history has higher sensitivity. Physical and functional findings with high sensitivity include longer recovery time after level versus inclined treadmill walking (82%)[22] and no pain with lumbar flexion (79%).[23] Highly specific aspects of examination and testing include improved walking tolerance on inclined versus level treadmill (92%), earlier onset of symptoms on level versus inclined treadmill (83%),[22] absent Achilles reflex (78%), lower extremity weakness (78%), pinprick or vibration deficit (>75%), wide-based gait (>75%), and presence of Romberg sign (>75%).[23]

FUNCTIONAL LIMITATIONS

Worsening leg and back pain from walking, back extension, and prolonged standing is the primary contributor to activity limitation. As such, patients with lumbar spinal stenosis tend to have difficulties with walking long distances, going down stairs, and household or yard work (e.g., dishwashing, lawn mowing, and vacuuming)[24] as well as with tasks that require overhead work (which may induce spinal extension). Balance deficits from sensory deficits may increase fall risk.

DIAGNOSTIC STUDIES

Diagnostic studies can provide useful information on structural and neurologic changes associated with spinal stenosis, but they must be interpreted in the context of the patient's clinical presentation. Several studies have demonstrated that there is no correlation between radiologic findings and clinical or functional outcomes.[25-27] However, another study found that severity of lumbar spinal stenosis as measured on functional myelography predicted long-term disability independent of therapeutic intervention.[28] The various qualities of the diagnostic tests are summarized in Table 46-3.

TREATMENT

Initial

There is an overall lack of high-quality prospective controlled studies examining the efficacy of various noninvasive treatments of lumbar spinal stenosis. Moreover, many of the existing recommendations are in regard to back pain in general, without differentiation of pain associated specifically with lumbar spinal stenosis. Therefore, much of clinical practice is based on extrapolation of recommendations, anecdotal experience, and expert opinion.

The oral analgesics used in lumbar spinal stenosis are acetaminophen, nonsteroidal anti-inflammatory drugs, muscle relaxants, anti-neuropathic pain medications in-

Differential Diagnosis

Lumbar spondylosis without spinal stenosis

Cervical and thoracic spinal stenosis

Herniated nucleus pulposus

Lumbar facet syndrome

Vertebral fracture with significant deformity or retropulsed fragments

Peripheral vascular disease

Venous claudication after thrombosis

Myxedema claudication

Inferior vena caval obstruction

Sacroiliac dysfunction

Osteoarthritis of the hips and knees

Trochanteric bursitis

Anterior tibial compartment syndrome

Spinal tumors

Conus medullaris and cauda equina neoplasms

Neurofibromas, ependymomas, hemangioblastomas, dermoids, epidermoids, lipomas

Metastatic spread of tumor

Peripheral neuropathy

Peripheral nerve entrapment

Restless legs syndrome

Stroke

Myofascial pain syndrome

Epidural abscess

Inflammatory arachnoiditis

cluding anticonvulsants and antidepressants, tramadol, and opioids. However, a number of systematic reviews have evaluated the use of pain medications in nonspecific low back pain. The review by Mens[36] stated that acetaminophen, nonsteroidal anti-inflammatory drugs, and mild opioids are potential first-line drugs, but there is no evidence that one is more effective than another. Non-benzodiazepine muscle relaxants were listed as second-line drugs for acute low back pain. The efficacy of these medications for the treatment of symptomatic lumbar spinal stenosis is still unclear, and the sedating quality of these medications poses an increased risk of adverse events in elderly patients. Antidepressants with mixed-receptor or predominantly noradrenergic activity, including tricyclics, bupropion, venlafaxine, and duloxetine, are somewhat effective.[37] First-generation (e.g., carbamazepine and phenytoin) and second-generation (e.g., gabapentin and pregabalin) antiepileptic drugs are also somewhat effective.

TABLE 46-3 Comparison of Various Diagnostic Tests for Lumbar Spinal Stenosis

Imaging Method	Pertinent Findings	Advantages	Disadvantages	Accuracy
Plain radiography	Anteroposterior view: narrow interpedic-ular distance (normally 23-30 mm)[20] Lateral view: decreased canal width Ferguson view: far-out syndrome[19] Facet degeneration, cyst formation Ligamentum flavum ossification Intervertebral disc space narrowing Vertebral body end plate osteophyte	Inexpensive Easy to obtain Can rule out gross bone disease	Poor soft tissue visualization	Sensitivity 66% and specificity 93% compared with plain CT as reference[19]
Plain myelography	Ventral extradural defects: caused by disc protrusions and vertebral end plate osteophytes Lateral or posterior extradural defects: caused by facet osteophytes Hourglass constriction: indicates central stenosis	Shows sagittal plane	Invasive May need several dye in-jections for high-grade stenosis Limited view of foramen Contraindicated in patients with contrast allergy, al-coholism, seizures, phe-nothiazine intake[19]	71.8% correlation with surgical findings[29] Sensitivity 54%-100%, equivocal compared with CT or MRI Specificity slightly higher than that of CT or MRI
Plain computed to-mography (CT)	Fat plane obliteration at exiting root Canal shape (trefoil vs. round or ovoid) Pedicle length-direct measurement	Relatively inex-pensive Axial view Superior bone detail	Poor soft tissue visualization Higher radiation exposure vs. other imaging techniques	83% correlation with surgical findings[29] Sensitivity 74%-100%
Computed tomographic myelography	As above Useful in degenerative scoliosis or history of prior instrumentation	Visualization of central and lateral canals	Invasive Higher radiation exposure vs. other imaging techniques	Sensitivity 87%[30] Comparable with MRI
Magnetic reso-nance imaging (MRI)	Disc degeneration: dark on T2 Annular tears: bright on T2 Stenosis and herniations in central and foraminal zones well visualized Evaluation of spine and spinal cord tumors	Noninvasive Shows sagittal plane Good soft tissue visualization	Interference from ferro-magnetic implants Limitations on patient's body size, need to lie still, claustrophobia Expensive and time-consuming	83% correlation with surgical findings[29] Sensitivity 77%-87% Three-dimensional magnetic reso-nance myelography sensitivity 100% As accurate as CT myelography[32]
Electrodiagnostics	Bilateral multilevel lumbosacral radicu-lopathy is most common diagnosis Paraspinal mapping EMG score>4[33] Tibial F wave and soleus H reflex latencies after exercise[34,35]	Can evaluate for peripheral neuropathy and entrapments as well as progres-sion of neuro-logicimpairment Can rule out other neuromuscular disease	Significant interpretation bias May be difficult to differ-entiate lumbar spinal stenosis from other multiroot diseases (e.g., arachnoiditis) Patient discomfort or pain Expensive and time-consuming	Abnormal study in 78%-97% of pa-tients with stenosis Paraspinal mapping EMG score>4: specificity 100% and sensitivity 30%

Rehabilitation

To our knowledge, there are no randomized controlled trials evaluating the effectiveness of physical or manual therapies in treating patients specifically with lumbar spinal stenosis. General recommendations include rela-tive rest (avoidance of pain-exacerbating activities while staying active to minimize deconditioning) and a flex-ion-biased exercise program, including inclined tread-mill and exercise bicycle. Flexion biasing increases the cross-sectional area of the spinal canal compared with exercises performed in neutral or extension, thereby maximizing activity tolerance.[38] Whitman and associ-

ates[24] reported a case series of three patients who dem-onstrated significant improvements in pain and func-tion at 18 months after undergoing specialized physical therapy programs that included spinal manipulation, flexion and rotation spine mobilization exercises, hip joint mobilization, hip flexor stretching, muscle retrain-ing (lower abdominal, gluteal, and calf muscles), body weight-supported ambulation, and daily walking with properly prescribed orthotics. Body weight-supported ambulation acts to decrease the axial loading of the spine to increase the cross-sectional area of the neural foramina, and studies have provided some support of this strategy.[24,39] Physical modalities such as cold or hot packs, ultrasound, iontophoresis, and transcutaneous electrical nerve stimulation may be helpful, but data of clinical efficacy are lacking.[40] Physicians and therapists must be aware of any medical comorbidities, such as cardiovascular and pulmonary disease, osteoporosis, cognitive deficits, and other musculoskeletal or neuromuscular conditions, that may have an impact on therapy tolerance.

Procedures

Recommendations for the use of nonsurgical interventional procedures in the symptomatic control of lumbar spinal stenosis, particularly fluoroscopically guided epidural steroid injections, are somewhat controversial. A systematic review by Abdi and colleagues[41] concluded that for interlaminar, transforaminal, and caudal epidural steroid injections, there is strong evidence for short-term relief and limited to moderate evidence for long-term relief of lumbar radicular pain. A number of studies have cited short-term success rates of 71% to 80%[42,43] and long-term success rates of 32% to 75%.[42,44] Furthermore, symptomatic management with epidural steroid injections may delay surgery an average of 13 to 28 months.[45,46] In general, epidural steroid injections can be considered a safe and reasonable therapeutic option for symptomatic management before surgical intervention is pursued.

Surgery

Patients with persistent symptoms despite conservative measures may benefit from surgical treatment. There are no universally accepted indications for and contraindications to surgery. A key feature in the selection of patients is ensuring that the symptoms indeed arise from nerve root compression. Surgery generally consists of decompressive laminectomy with medial facetectomy. The decompression relieves central canal stenosis; the medial facetectomy and attendant dissection along the lateral recesses decompress areas of foraminal stenosis.

The Maine Lumbar Spine Study[47] prospectively examined the outcome of initial surgical versus nonsurgical treatment in 148 patients at 1, 4, and 8 to 10 years. Rates of improvement in predominant symptom, low back pain, and leg pain at 1 year ranged from 77% to 79% in the surgery group and 42% to 45% in the nonsurgical group. At 8- to 10-year follow-up, the rates dropped to 53% to 67% in the surgery group and remained essentially stable at 41% to 50% in the nonsurgical group. As such, the benefits from surgery diminished over time, although improvements in leg pain and back-related functional status were maintained. A time-dependent decrease in benefit among older patients was evident in another study by Yamashita and colleagues.[48] In patients requiring surgery, earlier intervention is associated with improved long-term outcomes.[47,49]

Two key controversies in the surgical management of lumbar spinal stenosis are the appropriate role for a concomitant arthrodesis (lumbar fusion) and the utility of instrumentation. A comprehensive multipart systematic review by Resnick and colleagues[50,51] concluded that the literature consistently supports the addition of arthrodesis, particularly posterior lumbar fusion, to decompression surgery only in patients with lumbar spinal stenosis secondary to spondylolisthesis.

POTENTIAL DISEASE COMPLICATIONS

The natural history of lumbar spinal stenosis is not well understood, but existing literature seems to indicate that the majority of cases do not lead to significant deterioration. Johnsson and coworkers[52] examined the symptomatic and functional outcomes of 19 patients with moderate stenosis who did not undergo surgery. Average follow-up was 31 months, at which time 26% were worse, 32% unchanged, and 42% improved. Another study by Johnsson and colleagues[53] observed 32 patients with spinal stenosis who did not receive treatment, 75% of whom had neurogenic claudication. At a mean follow-up period of 49 months, 70% were unchanged, 15% were worse, and 15% were better. In patients with worsening symptomatic stenosis, there may be a progressive increase in back or leg pain and a decrease in walking tolerance. Severe stenosis may lead to a neurogenic bladder, especially in patients with narrowed dural sac anteroposterior diameter.[54] Cauda equina syndrome is a rare but serious complication,[55,56] in which case emergent surgical decompression is generally required.

POTENTIAL TREATMENT COMPLICATIONS

Exacerbation of symptoms is possible, particularly with functional restoration programs that may attempt to condition patients to painful activities through safe repetition of pain-inducing motions. In addition, patients with significant comorbidities, such as cardiopulmonary disease, are at risk for activity-induced adverse events. Complications from medication use include liver toxicity with acetaminophen; gastritis, gastrointestinal bleeds, renal toxicity, and platelet inhibition with nonsteroidal anti-inflammatory drugs; increased risk of cardiovascular events with some cyclooxygenase 2 (COX-2) inhibitors; nausea and lowering of seizure threshold with tramadol; anticholinergic effects including dry mouth and urinary retention with tricyclic antidepressants; sedation, ataxia, and other cognitive side effects with anticonvulsants (although gabapentin and pregabalin are relatively safe); and sedation, constipation, urinary retention, tolerance, and central pain sensitization with opioids. Adverse gastrointestinal events related to nonsteroidal anti-inflammatory drugs can be minimized with the use of a COX-2 inhibitor or concomitant use of a gastroprotective agent such as a proton pump inhibitor or H_2 blocker.[57]

Quantified data on complications associated with nonsurgical interventional procedures, including epidural steroid injections, are limited. A retrospective study of

207 patients receiving transforaminal epidural steroid injections[58] reported the following adverse events: transient nonpositional headaches that resolved within 24 hours (3.1%), increased back pain (2.4%), facial flushing (1.2%), increased leg pain (0.6%), vasovagal reaction (0.3%), increased blood glucose concentration in an insulin-dependent diabetic (0.3%), and intraoperative hypertension (0.3%). Other potential complications are infection at the injection site, dural puncture potentially with associated spinal headache, chemical or infectious meningitis, epidural hematoma, intravascular penetration, anaphylaxis, and nerve root or spinal cord injury leading to paresis or paralysis.[59,60]

Complications of decompressive surgery include infection (0.5% to 3%), epidural hematoma, vascular injury (0.02%), thromboembolism including pulmonary embolism (0.5%), dural tears <1% to 15%), nerve root injury, postsurgical spinal instability, nonunion or hardware failure, adjacent segment degeneration, recurrence of symptoms (10% to 15%), and death (0.35% to 2%).[40,61]

References

1. Arnoldi CC, Brodsky AE, Cauchoix J, et al. Lumbar spinal stenosis and nerve root entrapment syndromes: definition and classification. Clin Orthop Relat Res 1976;115:4-5.
2. Wiesel SW, Tsourmas N, Feffer HL, et al. A study of computer-assisted tomography. I. The incidence of positive CAT scans in an asymptomatic group of patients. Spine 1984;9:549-551.
3. Boden SD, Davis DO, Dina TS, et al. Abnormal magnetic-resonance scans of the lumbar spine in asymptomatic subjects: a prospective investigation. J Bone Joint Surg Am 1990;72:403-408.
4. Hitselberger WE, Witten RM. Abnormal myelograms in asymptomatic patients. J Neurosurg 1968;28:204-206.
5. Getty CJ. Lumbar spinal stenosis: the clinical spectrum and the results of operation. J Bone Joint Surg Br 1980;62:481-485.
6. Bergstrom K, Laurent U, Lundberg PO. Neurological symptoms in achondroplasia. Acta Neurol Scand 1971;47:59-70.
7. Bethem D, Winter RB, Lutter L, et al. Spinal disorders of dwarfism: review of the literature and report of eighty cases. J Bone Joint Surg Am 1981;63:1412-1425.
8. Singh K, Samartzis D, Vaccaro AR, et al. Congenital lumbar spinal stenosis: a prospective, control-matched, cohort radiographic analysis. Spine J 2005;5:615-622.
9. Eisenstein S. The trefoil configuration of the lumbar vertebral canal: a study of South African skeletal material. J Bone Joint Surg Br 1980;62:73-77.
10. Rothman R. The Spine. Philadelphia, WB Saunders, 1991.
11. Yang KH, King AI. Mechanism of facet load transmission as a hypothesis for low-back pain. Spine 1984;9:557-565.
12. Herzog RJ, Kaiser JA, Saal JA, Saal JS. The importance of posterior epidural fat pad in lumbar central canal stenosis. Spine 1991;16(Suppl):S227-S233.
13. Lee CK, Rauschning W, Glenn W. Lateral lumbar spinal canal stenosis: classification, pathologic anatomy and surgical decompression. Spine 1988;13:313-320.
14. Ullrich CG, Binet EF, Sanecki MG, Kieffer SA. Quantitative assessment of the lumbar spinal canal by computed tomography. Radiology 1980;134:137-143.
15. Verbiest H. Pathomorphologic aspects of developmental lumbar stenosis. Orthop Clin North Am 1975;6:177-196.
16. Wiltse LL, Guyer RD, Spencer CW, et al. Alar transverse process impingement of the L5 spinal nerve: the far-out syndrome. Spine 1984;9:31-41.
17. Panjabi MM, Takata K, Goel VK. Kinematics of lumbar intervertebral foramen. Spine 1983;8:348-357.
18. Sortland O, Magnaes B, Hauge T. Functional myelography with metrizamide in the diagnosis of lumbar spinal stenosis. Acta Radiol Suppl 1977;355:42-54.
19. Truumees E. Spinal stenosis: pathophysiology, clinical and radiologic classification. Instr Course Lect 2005;54:287-302.
20. Amundsen T, Weber H, Lilleas F, et al. Lumbar spinal stenosis: clinical and radiologic features. Spine 1995;20:1178-1186.
21. Roach KE, Brown MD, Albin RD, et al. The sensitivity and specificity of pain response to activity and position in categorizing patients with low back pain. Phys Ther 1997;77:730-738.
22. Fritz JM, Erhard RE, Delitto A, et al. Preliminary results of the use of a two-stage treadmill test as a clinical diagnostic tool in the differential diagnosis of lumbar spinal stenosis. J Spinal Disord 1997;10:410-416.
23. Katz JN, Dalgas M, Stucki G, et al. Degenerative lumbar spinal stenosis: diagnostic value of the history and physical examination. Arthritis Rheum 1995;38:1236-1241.
24. Whitman JM, Flynn TW, Fritz JM. Nonsurgical management of patients with lumbar spinal stenosis: a literature review and a case series of three patients managed with physical therapy. Phys Med Rehabil Clin North Am 2003;14:77-101, vi-vii.
25. Haig AJ, Tong HC, Yamakawa KS, et al. Spinal stenosis, back pain, or no symptoms at all? A masked study comparing radiologic and electrodiagnostic diagnoses to the clinical impression. Arch Phys Med Rehabil 2006;87:897-903.
26. Moon ES, Kim HS, Park JO, et al. Comparison of the predictive value of myelography, computed tomography and MRI on the treadmill test in lumbar spinal stenosis. Yonsei Med J 2005;46: 806-811.
27. Borenstein DG, O'Mara JW Jr, Boden SD, et al. The value of magnetic resonance imaging of the lumbar spine to predict low-back pain in asymptomatic subjects: a seven-year follow-up study. J Bone Joint Surg Am 2001;83:1306-1311.
28. Hurri H, Slatis P, Soini J, et al. Lumbar spinal stenosis: assessment of long-term outcome 12 years after operative and conservative treatment. J Spinal Disord 1998;11:110-115.
29. Modic MT, Masaryk T, Boumphrey F, et al. Lumbar herniated disk disease and canal stenosis: prospective evaluation by surface coil MR, CT, and myelography. AJR Am J Roentgenol 1986;147:757-765.
30. Bischoff RJ, Rodriguez RP, Gupta K, et al. A comparison of computed tomography-myelography, magnetic resonance imaging, and myelography in the diagnosis of herniated nucleus pulposus and spinal stenosis. J Spinal Disord 1993;6:289-295.
31. Jia LS, Shi ZR. MRI and myelography in the diagnosis of lumbar canal stenosis and disc herniation: a comparative study. Chin Med J (Engl) 1991;104:303-306.
32. Schnebel B, Kingston S, Watkins R, Dillin W. Comparison of MRI to contrast CT in the diagnosis of spinal stenosis. Spine 1989;14:332-337.
33. Haig AJ, Tong HC, Yamakawa KS, et al. The sensitivity and specificity of electrodiagnostic testing for the clinical syndrome of lumbar spinal stenosis. Spine 2005;30:2667-2676.
34. Adamova B, Vohanka S, Dusek L. Dynamic electrophysiological examination in patients with lumbar spinal stenosis: is it useful in clinical practice? Eur Spine J 2005;14:269-276.
35. Bal S, Celiker R, Palaoglu S, Cila A. F wave studies of neurogenic intermittent claudication in lumbar spinal stenosis. Am J Phys Med Rehabil 2006;85:135-140.
36. Mens JM. The use of medication in low back pain. Best Pract Res Clin Rheumatol 2005;19:609-621.
37. Maizels M, McCarberg B. Antidepressants and antiepileptic drugs for chronic non-cancer pain. Am Fam Physician 2005;71:483-490.
38. Sikorski JM. A rationalized approach to physiotherapy for low-back pain. Spine 1985;10:571-579.
39. Fritz JM, Erhard RE, Vignovic M. A nonsurgical treatment approach for patients with lumbar spinal stenosis. Phys Ther 1997;77:962-973.
40. Yuan PS, Booth RE Jr, Albert TJ. Nonsurgical and surgical management of lumbar spinal stenosis. Instr Course Lect 2005;54:303-312.
41. Abdi S, Datta S, Lucas LF. Role of epidural steroids in the management of chronic spinal pain: a systematic review of effectiveness and complications. Pain Physician 2005;8:127-143.
42. Delport EG, Cucuzzella AR, Marley JK, et al. Treatment of lumbar spinal stenosis with epidural steroid injections: a retrospective outcome study. Arch Phys Med Rehabil 2004;85:479-484.

43. Papagelopoulos PJ, Petrou HG, Triantafyllidis PG, et al. Treatment of lumbosacral radicular pain with epidural steroid injections. Orthopedics 2001;24:145-149.

44. Botwin KP, Gruber RD, Bouchlas CG, et al. Fluoroscopically guided lumbar transformational epidural steroid injections in degenerative lumbar stenosis: an outcome study. Am J Phys Med Rehabil 2002;81:898-905.

45. Riew KD, Yin Y, Gilula L, et al. The effect of nerve-root injections on the need for operative treatment of lumbar radicular pain: a prospective, randomized, controlled, double-blind study. J Bone Joint Surg Am 2000;82:1589-1593.

46. Narozny M, Zanetti M, Boos N. Therapeutic efficacy of selective nerve root blocks in the treatment of lumbar radicular leg pain. Swiss Med Wkly 2001;131:75-80.

47. Atlas SJ, Keller RB, Wu YA, et al. Long-term outcomes of surgical and nonsurgical management of lumbar spinal stenosis: 8 to 10 year results from the Maine Lumbar Spine Study. Spine 2005;30:936-943.

48. Yamashita K, Ohzono K, Hiroshima K. Five-year outcomes of surgical treatment for degenerative lumbar spinal stenosis: a prospective observational study of symptom severity at standard intervals after surgery. Spine 2006;31:1484-1490.

49. Niggemeyer O, Strauss JM, Schulitz KP. Comparison of surgical procedures for degenerative lumbar spinal stenosis: a meta-analysis of the literature from 1975 to 1995. Eur Spine J 1997;6:423-429.

50. Resnick DK, Choudhri TF, Dailey AT, et al. Guidelines for the performance of fusion procedures for degenerative disease of the lumbar spine. Part 10: fusion following decompression in patients with stenosis without spondylolisthesis. J Neurosurg Spine 2005;2:686-691.

51. Resnick DK, Choudhri TF, Dailey AT, et al. Guidelines for the performance of fusion procedures for degenerative disease of the lumbar spine. Part 9: fusion in patients with stenosis and spondylolisthesis. J Neurosurg Spine 2005;2:679-685.

52. Johnsson KE, Uden A, Rosen I. The effect of decompression on the natural course of spinal stenosis: a comparison of surgically treated and untreated patients. Spine 1991;16:615-619.

53. Johnsson KE, Rosen I, Uden A. The natural course of lumbar spinal stenosis. Clin Orthop Relat Res 1992;279:82-86.

54. Inui Y, Doita M, Ouchi K, et al. Clinical and radiologic features of lumbar spinal stenosis and disc herniation with neuropathic bladder. Spine 2004;29:869-873.

55. Rauschning W. Pathoanatomy of lumbar disc degeneration and stenosis. Acta Orthop Scand Suppl 1993;251:3-12.

56. Johnsson KE, Sass M. Cauda equina syndrome in lumbar spinal stenosis: case report and incidence in Jutland, Denmark. J Spinal Disord Tech 2004;17:334-335.

57. Physicians' Desk Reference, 59th ed. Montvale, NJ, Thomson Healthcare, 2005.

58. Botwin KP, Gruber RD, Bouchlas CG, et al. Complications of fluoroscopically guided transforaminal lumbar epidural injections. Arch Phys Med Rehabil 2000;81:1045-1050.

59. Rydevik BL, Cohen DB, Kostuik JP. Spine epidural steroids for patients with lumbar spinal stenosis. Spine 1997;22:2313-2317.

60. Huntoon MA, Martin DP. Paralysis after transforaminal epidural injection and previous spinal surgery. Reg Anesth Pain Med 2004;29:494-495.

61. Jansson KA, Blomqvist P, Granath F, Nemeth G. Spinal stenosis surgery in Sweden 1987-1999. Eur Spine J 2003;12:535-541.

Sacroiliac Joint Dysfunction 47

Zacharia Isaac, MD, and Jennifer Devine, MD

Synonyms

Sacroiliac joint syndrome
Sacroiliac joint pain
Sacroiliac joint injury
Sacroiliac subluxation
Sacroiliac joint instability
Sacroiliac joint ankylosis
Sacroiliac joint sprain and strain

ICD-9 Codes

724.6   Disorders of sacrum
846.1   Sprain and strain of sacroiliac ligament
846.8   Sprain and strain of sacroiliac region

DEFINITION

The sacroiliac joint is a small but significant cause of low back, buttock, groin, and lower extremity pain. Sacroiliac joint dysfunction is a diagnosis that should be arrived at only after careful consideration of other diagnoses that can often cause similar symptoms and examination findings. Sacroiliac joint dysfunction occurs with structural change to the joint or changes to the relative positions of the sacrum and pelvis.[1] Pain can be mediated by intra-articular, capsular, and ligamentous structures. The prevalence of sacroiliac joint dysfunction in the general population is reported between 15% and 38%.[2-4] Differentiation of sacroiliac joint pain from other causes is complicated by the joint's anatomy. Because of its redundant and variable innervation, the dysfunctional sacroiliac joint can present as a variety of referred pain syndromes.[5] Moreover, sacroiliac joint pain can arise from both hypermobility and hypomobility, making definitive diagnosis even more elusive. Sacroiliac joint syndrome may be more common in women than in men; various studies demonstrate a ratio of approximately 3 or 4:1.[5-8]

The sacroiliac joints are the bilateral weight-bearing joints that connect the articular surface of the sacrum with the ilium, joining the axial and appendicular skeletons. The anterior and inferior third of the joint is synovial; the remainder of the joint space is syndesmotic.

The sacroiliac joint is bordered on its ventral and superior edges by the ventral sacroiliac ligament and on its dorsal and inferior surfaces by the interosseous and dorsal sacroiliac ligaments. The articular capsule of the sacroiliac joint is thin and stabilized anteriorly by the ventral sacroiliac ligament. The strong extracapsular fibers of the dorsal sacroiliac and interosseous ligaments contribute principally to the stability of the joint. Further anchoring of the sacroiliac joint is conferred by the sacrotuberous and sacrospinous ligaments, which provide additional connections between the pelvis and sacrum. Innervation of the sacroiliac joint remains incompletely studied, and several anatomic studies have reported different innervation. The dorsal branch of S1 and fibers from L4, L5, and even L3 can provide sensory input to the joint.[9] Other studies have described innervation predominantly through dorsal rami of spinal nerve roots L5-S4.[10,11]

The sacroiliac joint undergoes changes throughout life that affect the biomechanics of the joint. During childhood and adolescence, the joint is more mobile, absorbing forces throughout the gait cycle. With normal aging, the joints develop uneven opposing surfaces, and the joints are thought to gradually fuse in later years.[12-14] Movements around the sacroiliac joints are small in magnitude yet complex in nature. As body weight is transmitted downward through the first sacral vertebra, the sacrum is pushed downward and forward, causing its lower end to rotate upward and backward.[12] Although there are no muscles that directly control movements around the joint, imbalance of the musculature surrounding the sacroiliac joint can affect stresses through the joint. Muscles anterior to the sacroiliac joint, including the psoas and iliacus, can influence movement of the sacrum.[2] Weakness in posterior muscles, such as the gluteus maximus and medius, can affect pelvic posture during weight bearing, thereby altering stresses through the joint.

SYMPTOMS

By far the most common presenting symptom of sacroiliac joint dysfunction is low back pain and gluteal pain, which can be indolent and refractory to traditional interventions

267

and therapies. Pain referral from sacroiliac joint dysfunction is not limited to the lumbosacral region or buttocks. Presenting complaints often include pain that is aggravated by prolonged standing, asymmetric weight bearing, or stair climbing. Pain can also stem from running, large strides, or extreme postures.[15] Because sacroiliac joint pain is thought to arise from a variety of causes (hypermobility, hypomobility, osteologic deformity, joint inflammation, and erosion), joint dysfunction can present with a wide variety of specific complaints. In a retrospective study of 50 patients with positive diagnostic response to fluoroscopically guided sacroiliac joint injection, investigators sought to characterize the most common presenting symptoms experienced by the cohort. In their study, the most common symptoms were buttock pain (94%), lower lumbar pain (72%), and lower extremity pain (50%). Pain in the distal leg and pain in the foot were also reported, as was groin pain.[5]

Sacroiliac joint dysfunction is not a cause of neuropathic pain. However, because of the anatomic proximity of spinal nerve roots as well as the lumbar and sacral plexuses, pain referral patterns can mimic a variety of neurologic pathologic processes.

PHYSICAL EXAMINATION

A thorough assessment of the low back, hips, and pelvis, including musculoskeletal and neurologic testing, is essential in isolating back pain caused by sacroiliac joint dysfunction and to exclude other common diagnoses. Examination should include measurement of leg length and assessment of pelvic symmetry by inspection of the posterior superior iliac spine, anterior superior iliac spine, gluteal folds, pubic tubercles, ischial tuberosities, and medial malleoli. The sacral sulcus is palpated and inspected with the patient prone, and any muscle atrophy in the gluteal muscles or distal extremity is noted. Atrophy in the limb implicates a lumbar radiculopathy more than sacroiliac joint syndrome. Palpation of the bony sacrum, subcutaneous tissues, muscles, and ligaments is performed.

Provocative tests have long been used by clinicians to differentiate sacroiliac joint–derived back pain from other regional pain generators. However, repeated clinical studies have suggested that when they are considered separately, the most commonly used provocative tests have low specificity for sacroiliac dysfunction[4,9,16,17] One possible explanation for this is interrater unreliability. Others suggest that both the minimal range of motion around the joints and the difficulty in simulating physiologic stresses through the joints make it more likely that provocative tests will elicit pain from surrounding structures.[15] Such structures include the lumbar intervertebral disc, zygapophyseal joint, and hip joint. Several investigators have shown that in the diagnosis of sacroiliac joint disease, a multitest regimen is more clinically useful than any individual test finding. Recent research suggests that three or more positive findings on provocative tests are 85% sensitive and 79% specific for sacroiliac joint disease.[4]

Provocative Tests

Gaenslen Test

With the patient supine, lying close to the edge of the examination table with the buttock of the tested side over the edge of the table, the patient's leg is dropped off the table such that the thigh and hip are in hyperextension. The contralateral knee is then maximally flexed. Pain or discomfort with this maneuver suggests sacroiliac joint disease, although a false-positive result can be seen in patients with an L2-4 nerve root lesion,[18,19] spondylolisthesis, sacral fractures, lumbar compression fractures, or spinal stenosis.

Patrick Test (Also Called FABER Test)

With the patient supine on a level surface, the thigh is flexed and the ankle placed above the patella of the opposite extended leg. Downward pressure is applied simultaneously to the flexed knee and the opposite anterior superior iliac spine, as the ankle maintains its position above the knee. Pain or discomfort in the gluteal region reflects sacroiliac disease; pain in the groin or thigh may be suggestive of hip disease.

Distraction Test (Also Called the Gapping Test)

With the patient supine, pressure is applied downward and laterally to the bilateral anterior superior iliac spines. This maneuver stretches the ventral sacroiliac ligaments and joint capsule while placing pressure on the dorsal sacroiliac ligaments.

Compression Test

With the patient lying in the lateral recumbent position, the examiner stands behind the patient and applies pressure downward on the uppermost iliac crest, compressing the pelvis. This stretches the dorsal sacroiliac ligaments and compresses the ventral sacroiliac ligaments.

Pressure over the Sacral Sulcus

Application of pressure to the gluteal region causing familiar gluteal pain can be suggestive of sacroiliac joint dysfunction. This is commonly seen and is a nonspecific finding; it is often seen in discogenic axial pain, radicular pain, sacral fractures, facet syndrome, and piriformis syndrome.

FUNCTIONAL LIMITATIONS

Patients with sacroiliac joint dysfunction syndrome can have a range of functional limitations. There can often be difficulty with sitting, standing, walking, lying, bending, lifting, or sustained position. These functional limitations can be mild or incapacitating. Sequelae of chronic pain conditions, including sacroiliac joint dysfunction, are insomnia, depression, globalization of pain syndrome, psychological pain behavior, and symptom magnification. These sequelae can have additional or disproportionate associated functional limitations.

DIAGNOSTIC STUDIES

Plain radiography can reveal osteologic causes of sacroiliac joint–mediated pain, such as infection and inflammatory or degenerative arthritis. Plain radiographic views, including Ferguson views and anteroposterior views, can help identify sacroiliac joint erosions. Bone scan and computed tomography can detect bone changes caused by entities such as fracture, infection, tumor, sacroiliac joint erosions, and arthritis. Magnetic resonance imaging can reveal these entities as well as show soft tissue disease and marrow changes in sacroiliitis with its associated erosions. True sacroiliac joint dysfunction can often be seen in the presence of normal imaging and is a clinical syndrome separate from these diagnoses.

Fluoroscopically guided diagnostic anesthetic injection remains the "gold standard" for diagnosis of sacroiliac joint–derived low back pain.[7,8,17,20] However, numerous investigators have shown anesthetic leakage from the joint space after injection, and there is speculation that overlap to adjacent neural structures may yield erroneous diagnoses of sacroiliac dysfunction.[11] A placebo effect and other nonspecific factors also can lead to erroneous diagnosis. For these reasons, confirmatory studies can be performed after informed consent has been obtained and the patient is educated about the reasons for confirmatory studies. These confirmatory studies include a patient-blinded, placebo versus anesthetic injection and a variable-duration anesthetic time-dependent block.

Differential Diagnosis

Discogenic low back pain

Lumbar radicular pain

Lumbar facet syndrome

Seronegative spondyloarthropathy

Piriformis syndrome

Sacral fractures

Spondylolisthesis

Spinal stenosis

Hip osteoarthritis

TREATMENT

Initial

Sacroiliac joint dysfunction is treated initially with relative rest and avoidance of provocative activities. Local modalities such as ice and heat or topical analgesics such as Lidoderm patch can be applied for symptomatic relief. Manipulative therapy can alleviate pain and help with muscle spasms but does not change joint alignment significantly. No significant muscle groups cross the sacroiliac joint. Approximately 2 degrees of rotation and 0.77 mm of translation occur with stress or manipulation.[21,22] Commonly used pharmacologic measures include acetaminophen, nonsteroidal anti-inflammatory medications, and muscle relaxants. Chronic use of nonsteroidal anti-inflammatory drugs should be avoided because of gastric, renal, and possibly cardiac side effects. Opiates in rare instances can be considered for short-term use but carry potential risks of sedation, constipation, physical dependence, and addiction. Patients with true sacroiliitis related to a seronegative spondyloarthropathy may be candidates for the use of disease-modifying antirheumatic drugs.

Rehabilitation

Physical therapy is directed toward lumbar core muscle strength and lower extremity flexibility; modalities such as ice massage, heat, electrical stimulation for the alleviation of pain or muscle spasm, sacroiliac joint mobilization techniques, and postural education exercises are employed. Sacroiliac joint belts can be helpful and are worth an initial trial to address symptoms. Addressing hip girdle muscle strength, hip range of motion, tight iliotibial band, hip or knee osteoarthritis, trochanteric bursitis, leg length discrepancy, or pelvic obliquity can have adjunctive benefit.

Procedures

Fluoroscopically guided intra-articular steroid injection can have therapeutic benefit.[6] Injection therapy should be complemented with a therapeutic exercise regimen. Radiofrequency denervation has been described as effective for the treatment of sacroiliac joint dysfunction.[23] Neuromodulatory therapies with an electrical stimulator implanted at the third sacral nerve root in a limited number of subjects with sacroiliac joint pain have also been effective in the management of refractory cases.[24] Prolotherapy has also been described for the treatment of sacroiliac joint dysfunction.[16,25-27] Well-designed randomized controlled trials are lacking for nearly all sacroiliac joint dysfunction treatments.

Surgery

Surgery is very rarely performed for sacroiliac joint dysfunction and requires thorough workup with minimally invasive diagnostic anesthetization of the sacroiliac joint with comparative blocks of variable anesthetic duration or placebo-controlled blocks and exclusion of discogenic, facet, radicular, and hip-mediated pain. Surgical intervention involves fusion of the sacroiliac joint with hardware.

POTENTIAL DISEASE COMPLICATIONS

Sacroiliac joint dysfunction, like other causes of chronic pain, can produce pain-related insomnia, depression, anxiety, globalization of pain, and disability. Older patients with gluteal pain should be evaluated for fracture or tumor, and younger patients should be evaluated for seronegative spondyloarthropathy.

POTENTIAL TREATMENT COMPLICATIONS

Pharmacologic measures can have numerous side effects. Acetaminophen can be hepatotoxic in large doses. Nonsteroidal anti-inflammatory drug therapy is well known to be associated with gastrointestinal and renal side effects. Manipulation therapy or therapeutic exercise can increase pain in some patients. Intra-articular steroid injection can be associated with temporary increase in pain. Potential systemic steroid effects include increase in serum blood glucose concentration, hypertension, and fluid retention. Local steroid injection can cause fatty atrophy, potential infection, and skin depigmentation.

References

1. Dreyfuss P, Dryer S, Griffin J, et al. Positive sacroiliac screening tests in asymptomatic adults. Spine 1994;19:1138-1143.
2. Greenman PE. Principles of Manual Medicine, 2nd ed. Baltimore, Williams & Wilkins, 1996:305-367, 530-532.
3. Ebraheim NA, Xu R, Nadaud M, et al. Sacroiliac joint injection: a cadaveric study. Am J Orthop 1997;26:338-341.
4. van der Wurff P, Meyne W, Hagmeijer RH. Clinical tests of the sacroiliac joint. Man Ther 2000;5:89-96.
5. Slipman CW, Jackson HB, Lipetz JS, et al. Sacroiliac joint pain referral zones. Arch Phys Med Rehabil 2000;81:334-338.
6. Slipman CW, Lipetz JS, Plastaras CT, et al. Fluoroscopically guided therapeutic sacroiliac joint injections for sacroiliac joint syndrome. Am J Phys Med Rehabil 2001;80:425-432.
7. Broadhurst N, Bond MJ. Pain provocation tests for the assessment of sacroiliac joint dysfunction. J Spinal Disord 1998;11:341-345.
8. van der Wurff P, Buijs EJ, Groen GJ. A multitest regimen of pain provocation tests as an aid to reduce unnecessary minimally invasive sacroiliac joint procedures. Arch Phys Med Rehabil 2006;87:10-14.
9. Berthelot JM, Labat JJ, Le Goff B, et al. Provocative sacroiliac joint maneuvers and sacroiliac joint block are unreliable for diagnosing sacroiliac joint pain. Joint Bone Spine 2006;73:17-23.
10. Grob KR, Neuhuber WL, Kissling RO. Innervation of the sacroiliac joint of the human [in German]. Z Rheumatol 1995;54:117-122.
11. Fortin JD, Kissling RO, O'Connor BL, Vilensky JA. Sacroiliac joint innervation and pain. Am J Orthop 1999;28:687-690.
12. Rosse C, Gaddum-Rosse P. Hollinshead's Textbook of Anatomy, 5th ed. Philadelphia, Lippincott-Raven, 1997:312-313.
13. Beal MC. The sacroiliac problem: review of anatomy, mechanics, and diagnosis. J Am Osteopath Assoc 1982;81:667-679.
14. Mierau DR, Cassidy JD, Hamin T, Milne RA. Sacroiliac joint dysfunction and low back pain in school aged children. J Manipulative Physiol Ther 1984;7:81-84.
15. Dreyfuss P, Dreyer SJ, Cole A, Mayo K. Sacroiliac joint pain. J Am Acad Orthop Surg 2004;12:255-265.
16. Linetsky FS, Manchikanti L. Regenerative injection therapy for axial pain. Tech Reg Anesth Pain Manage 2005;9:40-49.
17. Dreyfuss P, Michaelsen M, Pauza K, et al. The value of medical history and physical examination in diagnosing sacroiliac joint pain. Spine 1996;21:2594-2602.
18. Daum WJ. The sacroiliac joint: an underappreciated pain generator. Am J Orthop 1995;24:475-478.
19. Magee DJ. Orthopedic Physical Assessment, 3rd ed. Philadelphia, WB Saunders, 1997:434-459.
20. Slipman CW, Sterenfeld EB, Chou LH, et al. The predictive value of provocative sacroiliac joint stress maneuvers in the diagnosis of sacroiliac joint syndrome. Arch Phys Med Rehabil 1998;79:288-292.
21. Egund N, Olsson TH, Schmid H, Selvik G. Movements in the sacroiliac joints demonstrated with roentgen stereophotogrammetry. Acta Radiol Diagn (Stockh) 1978;19:833-846.
22. Sturesson B, Selvik G, Uden A. Movements of the sacroiliac joints. A roentgen stereophotogrammetric analysis. Spine 1989;14:162-165.
23. Yin W, Willard F, Carreiro J, Dreyfuss P. Sensory stimulation–guided sacroiliac joint radiofrequency neurotomy: technique based on neuroanatomy of the dorsal sacral plexus. Spine 2003;28:2419-2425.
24. Calvillo O, Esses SI, Ponder C, et al. Neuroaugmentation in the management of sacroiliac joint pain: report of two cases. Spine 1998;23:1069-1072.
25. Dorman T. Pelvic mechanics and prolotherapy. In Vleeming A, Mooney V, Dorman T, et al, eds. Movement, Stability, and Low Back Pain: The Essential Role of the Pelvis. New York, Churchill Livingstone, 1997:501-522.
26. Gedney EH. Hypermobile joint. Osteopath Prof 1937;4:30-31.
27. Hackett GS. Ligament and Tendon Relaxation Treated by Prolotherapy, 3rd ed. Springfield, Ill, Charles C Thomas, 1958.

Hip Osteoarthritis 48

Patrick M. Foye, MD, and Todd P. Stitik, MD

Synonyms

Hip osteoarthritis
Hip degenerative joint disease
Degenerative hip joint
Coxarthrosis

ICD-9 Codes

715.15   Primary (idiopathic) osteoarthritis of the hip
715.25   Secondary osteoarthritis of the hip
716.15   Traumatic osteoarthritis of the hip

DEFINITION

Hip osteoarthritis (OA, also called degenerative joint disease) is the most prevalent pathologic condition at the hip joint. The hip joint (femoroacetabular joint) is a ball-and-socket joint, with the femoral head situated within the concavity formed by the acetabulum and labrum. This anatomic arrangement allows movements in multiple planes, including flexion, extension, adduction, abduction, internal rotation, and external rotation. Significant mechanical forces (three to eight times body weight)[1,2] are exerted on the hip joint during weight-bearing activities such as walking, running, jumping, and lifting. Additional stresses are created by recreational activities (e.g., impacts and falls during sports) and severe trauma (e.g., motor vehicle collisions). Hip trauma is significantly associated with unilateral but not bilateral hip OA, whereas obesity is associated with bilateral but not unilateral hip OA.[3] Occupational heavy lifting and frequent stair climbing seem to increase the risk of hip OA.[4]

In a study of 2490 subjects aged 55 to 74 years, the prevalence of hip OA was 3.1%; 58% of hip OA cases were unilateral, and 42% were bilateral.[3] The prevalence of hip OA is about 3% to 6% in the white population, but by contrast, it is far lower in Asian, black, and East Indian populations.[5] Total hip replacement in patients with hip OA is twice as common in women.[6]

A central feature of hip OA is cartilage breakdown, thus compromising the femoroacetabular articulation. In addition to cartilage, other tissues affected by the disease process include subchondral bone, synovial fluid, ligaments, synovial membrane, joint capsule, and adjacent muscles. Eventually, the joint develops osteophytes (exostosis), joint space narrowing, bone sclerosis adjacent to the joint, and potentially even joint fusion (arthrosis).

OA can be classified as either primary (idiopathic) or secondary.[7] The most common form of hip OA is primary,[8] which represents the "wear and tear" degenerative changes that occur over time. Hip OA is considered secondary if a specific underlying cause can be identified, such as significant prior hip trauma, joint infection, or preexisting congenital or other deformities.[7] Among patients undergoing total hip replacement, the likelihood that the hip OA was primary (rather than secondary) is highest among white individuals (66%), followed by black subjects (54%), Hispanics (53%), and Asians (28%).[9] Unlike rheumatoid arthritis, OA is relatively noninflammatory during most stages of the disease process. Symptomatic acetabular structural abnormalities can occur in patients with hip instability from classic developmental dysplasia or post-traumatic acetabular dysplasia as well as with retroversion of the acetabulum.[10]

SYMPTOMS

Groin pain is the classic manifesting symptom for hip OA. Other presenting symptoms of hip OA include hip pain, stiffness, and associated functional limitations. Many patients report "hip" pain when really they are referring to the superior lateral thigh region (e.g., greater trochanteric bursitis rather than hip joint disease). Hip joint pain typically presents as groin pain, perhaps with some referred pain down toward (and even beyond) the medial knee. Questioning the patient about lumbosacral, sacroiliac, or coccyx pain may reveal that the "hip" symptoms are actually referred from the spine.

Hip OA pain usually has an insidious onset, is worse with activity (particularly weight bearing and rotational loading of the joint), and is somewhat relieved with rest.[7] Advanced OA may be painful even at rest.[7] The physician should specifically ask about any constitutional symptoms that might suggest infection or malignant disease and also about any history of hip trauma[11] (recent or remote).

PHYSICAL EXAMINATION

Antalgic gait is characterized by a limp with decreased single-limb stance time on the painful limb, a shortened stride length for the contralateral limb, and an increased double support time.

Range of motion should be evaluated not only at both hip joints (in multiple planes) but also at the lumbosacral spine, knees, and ankles to more thoroughly evaluate the kinetic chain. The earliest sign of hip OA is loss of hip internal rotation.[12,13] Limping, groin pain, or limited hip internal rotation supports a diagnosis of a hip (rather than spine) disorder,[14] but it still remains prudent also to perform a lumbosacral physical examination when lumbosacral pain generators are being considered.

The Patrick test is performed by having the patient supine with the ipsilateral heel on the contralateral knee, thus forming the "figure-four" position, also referred to by the acronym FABER maneuver (hip flexed, abducted, and externally rotated; Fig. 48-1). The physician pushes the raised leg toward the table, producing groin pain that suggests intra-articular hip disease or back or buttock pain that suggests sacroiliac joint disease.

Palpation of the greater trochanteric bursae, iliotibial bands, sacroiliac joints, and ischial bursae may reveal pain generators other than the hip joint itself.

Weak hip muscles may be due to pain or disuse, but radiculopathy and neuropathy can also be considered. Hip abductor weakness may be manifested with a Trendelenburg gait.[13] With hip OA, the remainder of the neurologic examination in the lower limbs is normal (e.g., muscle stretch reflexes and sensory testing).

On inspection of the fingers, hypertrophic degenerative changes (exostoses), such as Heberden nodes at the distal interphalangeal joints,[12] are independent risk factors for hip OA.[11] Their presence thus increases the likelihood of similar findings at the hip joint.

FUNCTIONAL LIMITATIONS

Patients with hip OA often report functional limitations in weight-bearing activities such as walking, running, and climbing stairs. The hip range of motion restrictions may cause difficulties with activities such as donning or doffing of socks and shoes, picking up clothing from the floor,[15] and getting in and out of cars. Hip pain and weakness may necessitate use of the upper limbs to arise from a chair.[15] A careful history can elicit details of occupational, recreational, and other functional activities that the patient has decreased or ceased because of the hip OA.

DIAGNOSTIC STUDIES

Plain radiography is the primary diagnostic study for hip OA[16] (Fig. 48-2). The severity of radiographic hip OA findings can be categorized on the basis of the minimal joint space (MJS), defined as the shortest distance on the radiograph between the femoral head margin and the acetabular edge.[15] MJS is determined by four joint space measurements (medial, lateral, superior, and axial). Croft's MJS grades are 0 (MJS > 2.5 mm), 1 (MJS > 1.5 mm and ≤ 2.5 mm), and 2 (MJS ≤ 1.5 mm).[15] MJS

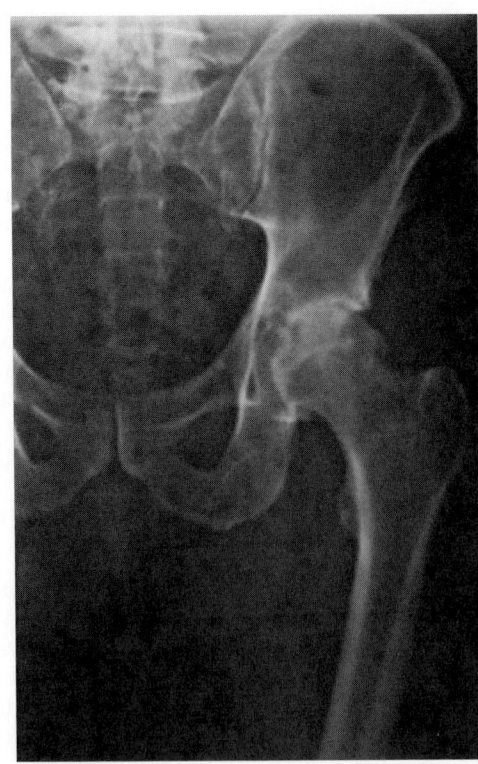

FIGURE 48-2. Radiograph demonstrating hip OA, including joint space narrowing, superior migration of the femur within the acetabulum, and subchondral sclerosis.

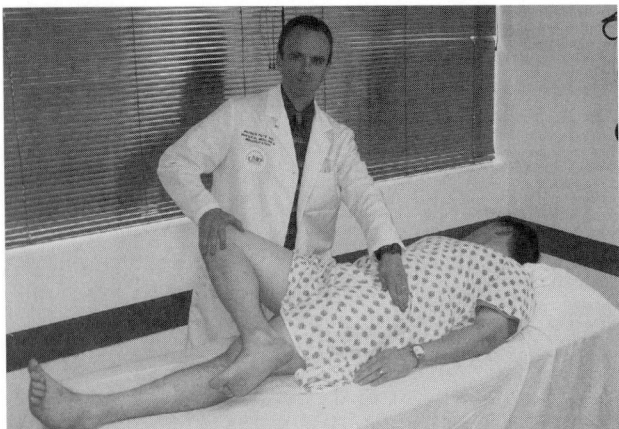

FIGURE 48-1. FABER maneuver (Patrick test). Pain produced in the groin suggests intra-articular disease, such as hip OA; pain produced in the back or buttock suggests sacroiliac disease.

is predictive of hip pain, is strongly associated with other radiographic features of hip OA, and has interrater reliability.[17] Alternatively, the Kellgren-Lawrence grading system of hip OA is a scale of 0 to 5 that considers not only joint space narrowing but also three additional factors: osteophytes, subchondral sclerosis, and subchondral cysts.[15] Both MJS and Kellgren-Lawrence grade are associated with clinical symptoms of hip OA.[15]

Magnetic resonance imaging is generally not needed to diagnose hip OA, but it is superior to radiography or bone scan when the differential diagnosis includes avascular necrosis or hip labral tear.[18] Hip joint arthrography is also generally unnecessary for the diagnosis of hip OA but may help define labral tears. Symptom relief through intra-articular injection of local anesthetic (e.g., with fluoroscopic or ultrasound guidance) can help confirm that the patient's symptoms are arising from the hip joint.

Electrodiagnostic studies should be considered when the differential diagnosis includes lumbosacral radiculopathy or peripheral nerve disease.

Differential Diagnosis

Intra-articular
Avascular necrosis

Protrusio acetabuli

Hip labral (cartilage) tear

Hip joint infection

Acetabular fracture

Rheumatoid arthritis

Extra-articular
Femur fracture

Trochanteric bursitis

Iliotibial band tendinitis

Snapping hip syndrome

Muscle or tendon groin strain

Lumbosacral radiculopathy

Sacroiliac pain

Coccydynia

TREATMENT

Initial

Patients with OA should be educated about their diagnosis, prognosis, and available treatments. Patients are encouraged to take an active role in managing their OA and maximizing their outcomes.[19]

Weight loss is very important because body weight is an independent risk factor for the development and progression of hip OA,[20,21] although it is less clearly established at the hip than at the knee.[12] Forces on the hip joint are roughly three to five times the patient's body weight during ambulation[2] and up to eight times body weight during jogging.[1] Loss of even modest amounts of excess body weight can significantly decrease lower extremity joint forces, OA progression, and related symptoms.[20,21]

The initial medication of choice for OA is acetaminophen,[22,23] at a maximum dose of 1000 mg four times a day. Although OA is primarily considered a noninflammatory arthritis (at least in early stages), prescription of nonsteroidal anti-inflammatory drugs in addition to the acetaminophen can provide further analgesic benefit.[12] In appropriately selected patients, tramadol or more traditional opioid analgesics may also be used for pain relief and associated functional benefits.[12]

Rehabilitation

The American College of Rheumatology (ACR) guidelines for the medical management of hip and knee OA recommend exercise as an important component of treatment.[21,22] The ACR guidelines recommend an exercise program consisting of range of motion, strengthening, and aerobic conditioning by walking or aquatic therapy.[21,22] Water-based exercise for lower limb OA decreases pain and increases function in the short term and also at 1 year.[24]

Stretching programs can address the range of motion restrictions in patients with hip OA, which are, in order of severity, extension, internal rotation, abduction, external rotation, adduction, and flexion.[19] Flexibility programs often begin with patients gently moving their joints through the available range of motion (to maintain range of motion) and then progress to regaining of lost range of motion.[12] Proper stretching should be sustained for at least 30 seconds while avoiding the sudden, jerky, or ballistic stretching that would be likely to exacerbate OA.[12]

Strengthening programs should address all planes of hip movement.[19] OA patients may begin with static strengthening exercises[12] to minimize joint movements that could exacerbate the OA symptoms.[12] Eventually, incorporation of dynamic exercises can maximize strength and function.[12]

Patients with hip OA are often deconditioned, thus suggesting a role for aerobic exercises.[19] Because OA particularly affects the elderly, it is especially important to screen for cardiovascular or other precautions before an exercise program is begun. Many patients with hip OA may have difficulty tolerating high-impact aerobics, such as jogging and stair climbing,[19] so activities such as cycling and aquatic exercises may be substituted. It is important to encourage ongoing exercise compliance.[8,12]

There is little clinical scientific evidence supporting passive modalities (e.g., cryotherapy, thermotherapy, transcutaneous electrical nerve stimulation) for hip

OA,[19] although theoretically they may facilitate better tolerance of the active therapy program.[12]

Hip OA pain may be decreased by use of a cane in the contralateral hand,[8,13] presumably by shifting the center of gravity medially, away from the involved hip. In cases of bilateral hip OA, the cane can be used contralateral to the more severely involved hip. A shoe lift can correct a leg length discrepancy[8] caused by hip joint space narrowing or superior migration of the femoral head within the acetabulum.

An occupational therapy evaluation of activities of daily living may identify difficulties with hand activities (e.g., due to hand OA) and difficulties with donning and doffing of footwear (due to restricted hip range of motion). Adaptive equipment (e.g., reachers, sock donners, long-handled shoe horns, elastic shoelaces) may help maximize independence despite persistent physical impairments.[12]

Procedures

Nonsurgical procedures for hip OA primarily include intra-articular injections with corticosteroids or viscosupplements.

Corticosteroid Injections

Although early OA is considered noninflammatory, end-stage OA may have an inflammatory component,[7] which may provide a basis for anti-inflammatory intra-articular injections with corticosteroids. It is difficult to obtain true intra-articular hip joint injection without fluoroscopy[8,12] or other image guidance, particularly because OA can decrease the targeted joint space and osteophytes can obstruct needle entry.[25] A randomized controlled trial of fluoroscopically guided intra-articular hip joint injections has shown that compared with local anesthetic, corticosteroids decrease hip OA pain (at 3- and 12-week follow-ups), improve hip range of motion in all directions, and significantly improve functional abilities.[26] Ultrasonography-guided hip joint corticosteroid injection for hip OA has shown significant relief of pain during walking compared with saline injection.[27] Despite the benefits shown in prospective, randomized controlled trials,[26,27] it is notable that one retrospective study seems to show that combined injections of corticosteroid, contrast agent, and anesthetic before total hip arthroplasty may increase the risk of postoperative infection and surgical revision.[28] Despite the limitations of that study (inherent flaws of a retrospective review and data lacking statistical power to determine the role of the time interval between steroid injection and subsequent total hip arthroplasty),[28] the possibility of infection should be discussed with patients before corticosteroid injection. Hip joint injection under fluoroscopic guidance is shown in Figure 48-3.

Viscosupplementation Injections

True intra-articular placement is even more important with viscosupplementation than with corticosteroids because viscosupplements have high molecular weights

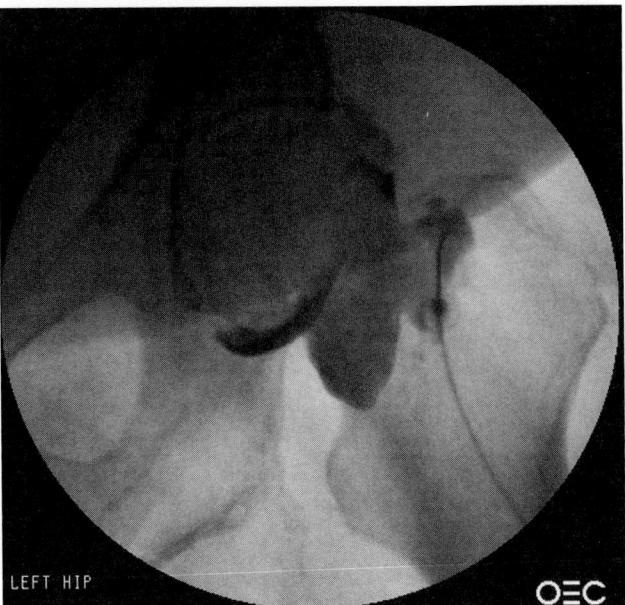

FIGURE 48-3. Fluoroscopic image showing intra-articular injection of contrast material (before corticosteroid), which can be seen spreading within the joint capsule along the proximal aspect of the femoral neck and also up into the space between the femoral head and the acetabulum. The image guidance helps ensure appropriate intra-articular placement of the injectate.

and are unlikely to permeate to the joint capsule.[25] Thus, when it is available, image guidance with fluoroscopy[25] or ultrasonography seems prudent for viscosupplementation injections.[28]

At the time of this writing, viscosupplements are approved by the Food and Drug Administration only for use at the knee. Some pilot studies indicate that image-guided hip joint viscosupplementation injections are well tolerated, safe, and beneficial for hip OA.[29]

Surgery

Surgical treatment of hip OA includes joint realignment (realignment osteotomy, such as for hip dysplasia[13]), joint fusion (arthrodesis), and, most commonly, joint replacement (arthroplasty).[23] Hip joint arthroplasty can be categorized as either hemiarthroplasty (prosthetic replacement of the proximal femur while the acetabulum is left intact) or total hip arthroplasty (also called total hip replacement, with surgical replacement of both the acetabulum and the proximal femur).[23] Hip hemiarthroplasty is often performed after proximal femur fractures, when the acetabulum is relatively intact. Conversely, in OA, there is usually degeneration of both the acetabulum and the femur; thus, the definitive surgery is to replace both of these through total hip arthroplasty. An arthroplasty can also be categorized on the basis of the specific prosthetic hardware used (e.g., unipolar or bipolar) and whether cement is used to hold the hardware in place.[23] Comparisons of the posterior and direct lateral surgical approaches for total hip arthroplasty show similar rates of postoperative dislocation (1% to 4%), postoperative Trendelenburg gait, and sciatic nerve injury.[30]

Customized preoperative exercises are well tolerated even in patients with end-stage hip OA and improve early recovery of physical function after eventual total hip arthroplasty is performed.[31]

Postoperative rehabilitation with physical therapy (and perhaps occupational therapy) generally includes therapeutic exercise, transfer training, gait training, and instruction in activities of daily living.[32] After total hip arthroplasty, early ambulation (even within the first 1 to 2 days postoperatively)[8] may maximize recovery and minimize complications such as deep venous thrombosis and symptomatic thromboembolism.[32]

The patient is taught how to follow the weight-bearing status specified by the orthopedic surgeon,[8] which depends on factors such as whether the prosthesis was cemented in place or not.[32] Many patients may safely bear weight as tolerated.[32] A cane or walker should be used until hip abductors are strong enough that the patient no longer limps during unassisted gait.[8]

After a posterior approach total hip arthroplasty, prevention of hip dislocation often involves "hip precautions" (e.g., teaching the patient to carefully avoid positions of hip adduction, flexion, and internal rotation).[8] Patients are taught to use elevated chair seats and elevated toilet seats and to avoid crossing the legs.[8] The recommended duration for hip precautions varies widely from 6 weeks to 6 months. Postoperative patients with a significant fall or sudden onset of pain should undergo radiography for evaluation of dislocation.

Prophylaxis against deep venous thrombosis and related venous thromboembolism may include early ambulation, intermittent pneumatic compression stockings, inferior vena cava filters, and pharmacologic methods (such as unfractionated heparin, low-molecular-weight heparin, warfarin, or synthetic pentasaccharides).[32] The optimal duration of thromboprophylaxis is not known, but a 4- to 6-week course has been suggested after total hip arthroplasty.[32]

After the acute care hospital, total hip arthroplasty patients are discharged to either inpatient rehabilitation (acute or subacute) or directly home, depending on postoperative pain, functional status, and home environment.[8,32]

POTENTIAL DISEASE COMPLICATIONS

Hip OA is a degenerative process characterized by gradual progressive worsening of femoroacetabular joint destruction and resultant symptoms. Hip OA can produce severe pain, stiffness, functional limitations, and associated compromise of quality of life. The decrease in mobility can subsequently result in weakness, osteoporosis, obesity, and cardiovascular deconditioning.

POTENTIAL TREATMENT COMPLICATIONS

Acetaminophen can cause hepatic side effects; nonsteroidal anti-inflammatory drugs are associated with gastrointestinal, renal, and cardiovascular risks. Tramadol can cause sedation and dizziness. Hip injections carry risks of infection and postprocedure exacerbation of symptoms. Hip replacement surgeries can be complicated by infection, nerve injury, dislocation, hardware loosening, deep venous thrombosis, and anesthesia-related side effects.[32]

References

1. Anderson K, Strickland SM, Warren R. Hip and groin injuries in athletes. Am J Sports Med 2001;29:521-533.
2. Hashimoto N, Ando M, Yayama T, et al. Dynamic analysis of the resultant force acting on the hip joint during level walking. Artif Organs 2005;29:387-392.
3. Tepper S, Hochberg MC. Factors associated with hip osteoarthritis: data from the First National Health and Nutrition Examination Survey (NHANES-I). Am J Epidemiol 1993;137:1081-1088.
4. Coggon D, Kellingray S, Inskip H, et al. Osteoarthritis of the hip and occupational lifting. Am J Epidemiol 1998;147:523-528.
5. Hoaglund FT, Steinbach LS. Primary osteoarthritis of the hip: etiology and epidemiology. J Am Acad Orthop Surg 2001;9: 320-327.
6. Croft P, Lewis M, Wynn Jones C, et al. Health status in patients awaiting hip replacement for osteoarthritis. Rheumatology (Oxford) 2002;41:1001-1007.
7. Stitik TP, Kaplan RJ, Kamen LB, et al. Rehabilitation of orthopedic and rheumatologic disorders. 2. Osteoarthritis assessment, treatment, and rehabilitation. Arch Phys Med Rehabil 2005;86(Suppl 1): S48-S55.
8. Nicholas JJ. Rehabilitation of patients with rheumatic disorders. In Braddom RL, ed. Physical Medicine and Rehabilitation. Philadelphia, WB Saunders, 1996:711-727.
9. Hoaglund FT, Oishi CS, Gialamas GG. Extreme variations in racial rates of total hip arthroplasty for primary coxarthrosis: a population-based study in San Francisco. Ann Rheum Dis 1995;54:107-110.
10. Trousdale RT. Acetabular osteotomy: indications and results. Clin Orthop Relat Res 2004;429:182-187.
11. Cooper C, Inskip H, Croft P, et al. Individual risk factors for hip osteoarthritis: obesity, hip injury, and physical activity. Am J Epidemiol 1998;147:516-522.
12. Stitik TP, Foye PM, Stiskal D, Nadler RR. Osteoarthritis. In DeLisa JA, ed. Physical Medicine and Rehabilitation Principles and Practice, vol 1. 4th ed. Philadelphia, Lippincott Williams & Wilkins, 2005:765-786.
13. Lieberman JR, Berry DJ, Bono JV, Mason JB. Hip and thigh. In Snider RJ, ed. Essentials of Musculoskeletal Care. Rosemont, Ill, American Academy of Orthopaedic Surgeons, 1998:264-303.
14. Brown MD, Gomez-Marin O, Brookfield KF, Li PS. Differential diagnosis of hip disease versus spine disease. Clin Orthop Relat Res 2004;419:280-284.
15. Reijman M, Hazes JM, Pols HA, et al. Validity and reliability of three definitions of hip osteoarthritis: cross sectional and longitudinal approach. Ann Rheum Dis 2004;63:1427-1433.
16. Boegard T, Jonsson K. Hip and knee osteoarthritis. Conventional X-ray best and cheapest diagnostic method [in Swedish]. Lakartidningen 2002;99:4358-4360.
17. Croft P, Cooper C, Wickham C, Coggon D. Defining osteoarthritis of the hip for epidemiologic studies. Am J Epidemiol 1990;132: 514-522.
18. Bluemke DA, Zerhouni EA. MRI of avascular necrosis of bone. Top Magn Reson Imaging 1996;8:231-246.

19. Arokoski JP. Physical therapy and rehabilitation programs in the management of hip osteoarthritis. Eura Medicophys 2005;41: 155-161.
20. Foye PM. Weight loss in the treatment of osteoarthritis. Phys Med Rehabil State Art Rev 2001;15:33-41.
21. Foye PM, Stitik TP, Chen B, Nadler SF. Osteoarthritis and body weight. Nutrition Res 2000;20:899-903.
22. Recommendations for the medical management of osteoarthritis of the hip and knee: 2000 update. American College of Rheumatology Subcommittee on Osteoarthritis Guidelines. Arthritis Rheum 2000;43:1905-1915.
23. Stitik TP, Foye PM. eMedicine: Osteoarthritis. Physical Medicine and Rehabilitation: Arthritis and Connective Tissue Disorders. April 8, 2005. Available at: http://www.emedicine.com/PMR/topic93.htm. Accessed June 26, 2005.
24. Cochrane T, Davey RC, Matthes Edwards SM. Randomised controlled trial of the cost-effectiveness of water-based therapy for lower limb osteoarthritis. Health Technol Assess 2005;9:iii-iv, ix-xi, 1-114.
25. Foye PM, Stitik TP. Fluoroscopic guidance during injections for osteoarthritis. Arch Phys Med Rehabil 2006;87:446-447.
26. Kullenberg B, Runesson R, Tuvhag R, et al. Intraarticular corticosteroid injection: pain relief in osteoarthritis of the hip? J Rheumatol 2004;31:2265-2268.
27. Qvistgaard E, Christensen R, Torp-Pedersen S, Bliddal H. Intra-articular treatment of hip osteoarthritis: a randomized trial of hyaluronic acid, corticosteroid, and isotonic saline. Osteoarthritis Cartilage 2006;14:163-170.
28. Kaspar S, de V de Beer J. Infection in hip arthroplasty after previous injection of steroid. J Bone Joint Surg Br 2005;87:454-457.
29. Pourbagher MA, Ozalay M, Pourbagher A. Accuracy and outcome of sonographically guided intra-articular sodium hyaluronate injections in patients with osteoarthritis of the hip. J Ultrasound Med 2005;24:1391-1395.
30. Jolles BM, Bogoch ER. Posterior versus lateral surgical approach for total hip arthroplasty in adults with osteoarthritis. Cochrane Database Syst Rev 2004;1:CD003828.
31. Gilbey HJ, Ackland TR, Wang AW, et al. Exercise improves early functional recovery after total hip arthroplasty. Clin Orthop Relat Res 2003;408:193-200.
32. Bitar AA, Kaplan RJ, Stitik TP, et al. Rehabilitation of orthopedic and rheumatologic disorders. 3. Total hip arthroplasty rehabilitation. Arch Phys Med Rehabil 2005;86(Suppl 1):S56-S60.

Femoral Neuropathy 49

Earl J. Craig, MD, and Daniel M. Clinchot, MD

Synonym

Diabetic amyotrophy

ICD-9 Codes

355.2   Other lesion of femoral nerve
355.8   Mononeuritis of lower limb, unspecified
355.9   Mononeuritis of unspecified site
782.0   Disturbance of skin sensation

DEFINITION

Femoral neuropathy is the focal injury of the femoral nerve causing various combinations of pain, weakness, and sensory loss in the anterior thigh. Diabetic amyotrophy is the most common cause of focal femoral neuropathy; hemorrhage, most often due to anticoagulation therapy, also is common. Table 49-1 lists other possible causes of femoral neuropathy.

The femoral nerve arises from the anterior rami of the lumbar nerve roots 2, 3, and 4. After forming, the nerve passes on the anterolateral border of the psoas muscle, between the psoas and iliacus muscles, down the posterior abdominal wall, and through the posterior pelvis until it emerges under the inguinal ligament lateral to the femoral artery (Fig. 49-1).[1,2,10] The course continues down the anterior thigh, innervating the anterior thigh muscles. The sensory-only saphenous nerve branches off the femoral nerve distal to the inguinal ligament and courses through the thigh until the Hunter subsartorial canal, where the nerve dives deep. The femoral nerve innervates the psoas and iliacus muscles in the pelvis and the sartorius, pectineus, rectus femoris, vastus medialis, vastus lateralis, and vastus intermedius muscles in the anterior thigh. The femoral nerve provides sensory innervation to the anterior thigh. The saphenous nerve provides sensory innervation to the anterior patella, anteromedial leg, and medial foot (Fig. 49-2).

SYMPTOMS

The symptoms depend on how acute the injury is and what caused the injury. A patient will often first complain of a dull, aching pain in the inguinal region, which may intensify within hours. Shortly thereafter, the patient may note difficulty with ambulation secondary to leg weakness. The patient may or may not complain of weakness in the hip or thigh but will often notice difficulty with functional activities, such as getting out of a chair and traversing stairs or inclines.

Numbness over the anterior thigh and medial leg is common. The numbness may extend into the anteromedial leg and the medial aspect of the foot.

PHYSICAL EXAMINATION

The examination includes a complete neuromuscular evaluation of the low back, hips, and both lower limbs. This should include inspection for asymmetry or atrophy, manual muscle testing, muscle stretch reflexes, and sensory testing for light touch and pinprick.

In the case of femoral neuropathy, the clinician may see atrophy or asymmetry of the quadriceps muscles and weakness of hip flexion and/or knee extension. Strength testing may be limited because of pain. Quadriceps strength should be compared with adductor strength, which typically is normal. Palpation over the inguinal ligament may reveal a fullness and/or exacerbate the patient's pain symptoms. There is often a decreased or loss of quadriceps reflex and decreased sensation to the anterior thigh and anterior and medial leg. Palpation may be tender in the thigh and groin. Pain may be exacerbated with hip extension (Fig. 49-3).[1,2]

FUNCTIONAL LIMITATIONS

Functional limitations due to femoral neuropathy are generally a result of weakness and vary according to the severity of the injury and the functional reserve of the patient. Individuals may have difficulty getting up from a seated position and walking without falling. Inclines and stairs often magnify the limitations. Recreational

TABLE 49-1 Possible Causes of Focal Femoral Neuropathy[1,2]

Open injuries

Retraction during abdominal-pelvic surgery[3,4]

Hip surgery—heat used by methyl methacrylate, especially in association with leg lengthening[5,6]

Penetration trauma (e.g., gunshot and knife wounds, glass shards)

Closed injuries

Retroperitoneal bleeding after femoral vein or artery puncture[7]

Cardiac angiography

Central line placement

Retroperitoneal fibrosis

Injury during femoral nerve block

Diabetic amyotrophy

Infection

Cancer[8]

Pregnancy

Radiation

Acute stretch injury due to a fall or other trauma

Hemorrhage after a fall or other trauma

Spontaneous hemorrhage—generally due to anticoagulant therapy

Idiopathic

Hypertrophic mononeuropathy[9]

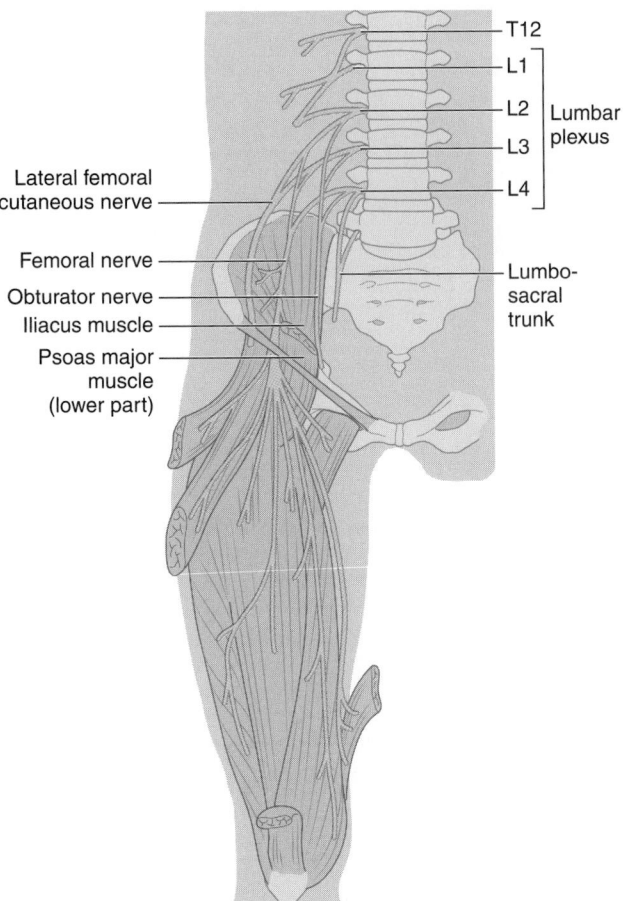

FIGURE 49-1. Anatomy of the femoral nerve.

and work-related activities are often affected, such as running, climbing, and jumping.

DIAGNOSTIC STUDIES

Electrodiagnostic studies (nerve conduction studies and electromyography) are the "gold standard" to confirm the presence of a femoral nerve injury. These should be performed no earlier than 3 to 4 weeks after the injury. Obviously, in cases of suspected hemorrhage, imaging studies should be done immediately. Imaging studies may include magnetic resonance imaging or computed tomography of the pelvis to look for a hemorrhage or a mass causing impingement.[10-13]

In terms of electrodiagnostic studies, nerve conduction studies of the femoral motor component are routinely used. Routine nerve conduction studies are not available for the sensory component of the femoral nerve. Saphenous nerve sensory evaluation is available in routine study but is technically difficult and unreliable.[2] The needle electromyography should evaluate muscles innervated by the femoral, obturator, tibial, and peroneal nerves. The needle evaluation therefore should include evaluation of the iliopsoas, at least two of the four quadriceps femoris muscles, one or two adductor muscles, gluteus minimus, three muscles between the knee and the ankle, and paraspinal muscles. Electromyography should be performed to rule out other causes of

neuropathic thigh pain, including upper and mid lumbar radiculopathy, polyradiculopathy, and plexopathy. Serial electromyographic studies may help with evaluation of the recovery process.

Somatosensory evoked potentials may also be useful.

Differential Diagnosis

Lumbar radiculopathy

Lumbar polyradiculopathy

Lumbar plexopathy

Avascular necrosis of the femoral head

Polymyalgia rheumatica

TREATMENT

Initial

Treatment of femoral neuropathy is focused on three separate areas: relief of symptoms, facilitation of nerve healing, and restoration of function. In acute cases in which hemorrhage or trauma is the cause, surgical

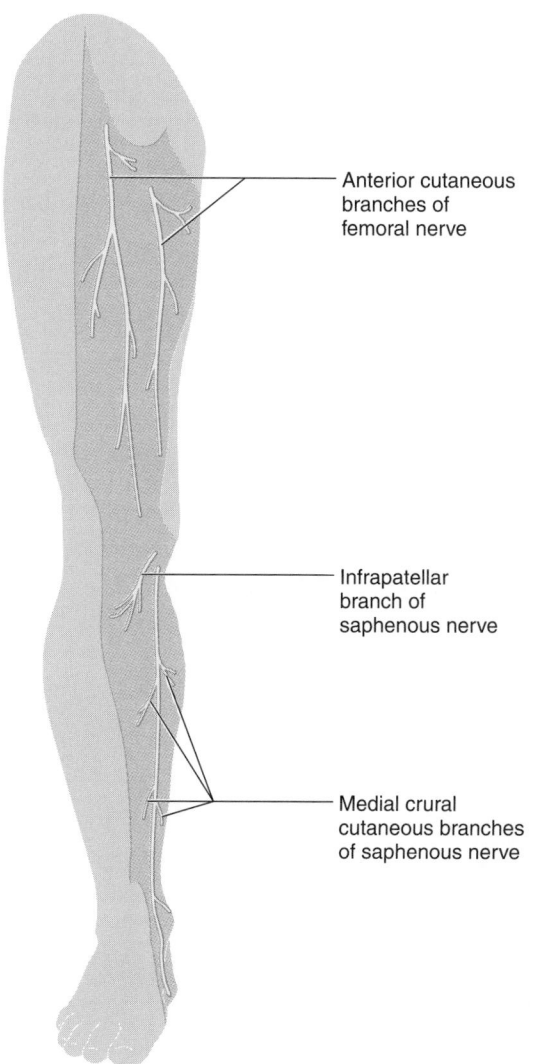

Anterior cutaneous branches of femoral nerve

Infrapatellar branch of saphenous nerve

Medial crural cutaneous branches of saphenous nerve

FIGURE 49-2. Sensory innervation of the femoral nerve.

Nerves that have sustained a less severe injury (neurapraxia injury) often heal during hours to weeks once the irritant is removed. Nerves that have sustained a more serious injury (neurotmesis or axonotmesis) typically have a much longer healing course because of the time required for wallerian degeneration and regeneration. It is important to educate the patient about the potential for a prolonged (sometimes more than 1 year) course of healing. Also, it is important to counsel patients that healing may not be complete and that there may be permanent loss of strength and sensation as well as continued pain symptoms.

Rehabilitation

Once the damage has been stopped or reversed, the focus turns to improvement of hip flexion and knee extension strength by maximizing the function of the available neuromuscular components. This is accomplished with physical therapy instruction and a home exercise program. Improvement of strength in all lower extremity muscle groups is important. Aggressive strengthening should be limited in a nerve that is acutely injured because it may promote further injury and delay healing.

It is also essential to work on proper gait mechanics. The physical therapist can help the patient with gait training and gait aids to prevent falls and to improve energy use. Range of motion in all lower extremity joints should be addressed. Neuromuscular electrical stimulation may be of benefit in improving strength in some individuals.

Procedures

Procedures are not indicated for this disease process.

Surgery

In the case of femoral nerve injury due to impingement, mass lesion, or hemorrhage, surgery may be required to remove the pressure. Early surgical evacuation in patients with femoral nerve compression secondary to retroperitoneal hemorrhage can reduce the likelihood of prolonged neurologic impairment.[14] In the case of a penetrating injury to the femoral nerve, surgery to align the two ends of the nerve and to remove scar tissue may be required.

POTENTIAL DISEASE COMPLICATIONS

Potential complications include continued pain, numbness, and weakness despite treatment. In addition, the weakness in the hip and knee increases the risk for falls.

POTENTIAL TREATMENT COMPLICATIONS

Analgesics and nonsteroidal anti-inflammatory drugs have well-known side effects that most commonly affect the gastric, hepatic, and renal systems. Narcotics have the potential for addiction and sedation. Carbamazepine

intervention may be the initial treatment. Likewise, this is the case when the injury is due to a mass lesion, such as a tumor.

Acute, subacute, and chronic relief of the pain and numbness is attempted with modalities and medications. Ice may be helpful acutely, and heat may be helpful in the subacute stage. If an inflammatory component is suspected, nonsteroidal anti-inflammatory drugs may help both pain and inflammation. Alternatively, oral corticosteroids may be used. Narcotics are used when acetaminophen and nonsteroidal anti-inflammatory drugs do not control the pain. Antiseizure medications, such as carbamazepine and gabapentin, are also of benefit for the neuropathic pain in some individuals. Transcutaneous electrical stimulation may also help with pain control.

Facilitation of healing depends on the cause of the injury to the nerve. In the case of diabetes, improved blood glucose control may help recovery. Injury due to impingement may be improved by removal of the mass. Often, little can be done to facilitate healing.

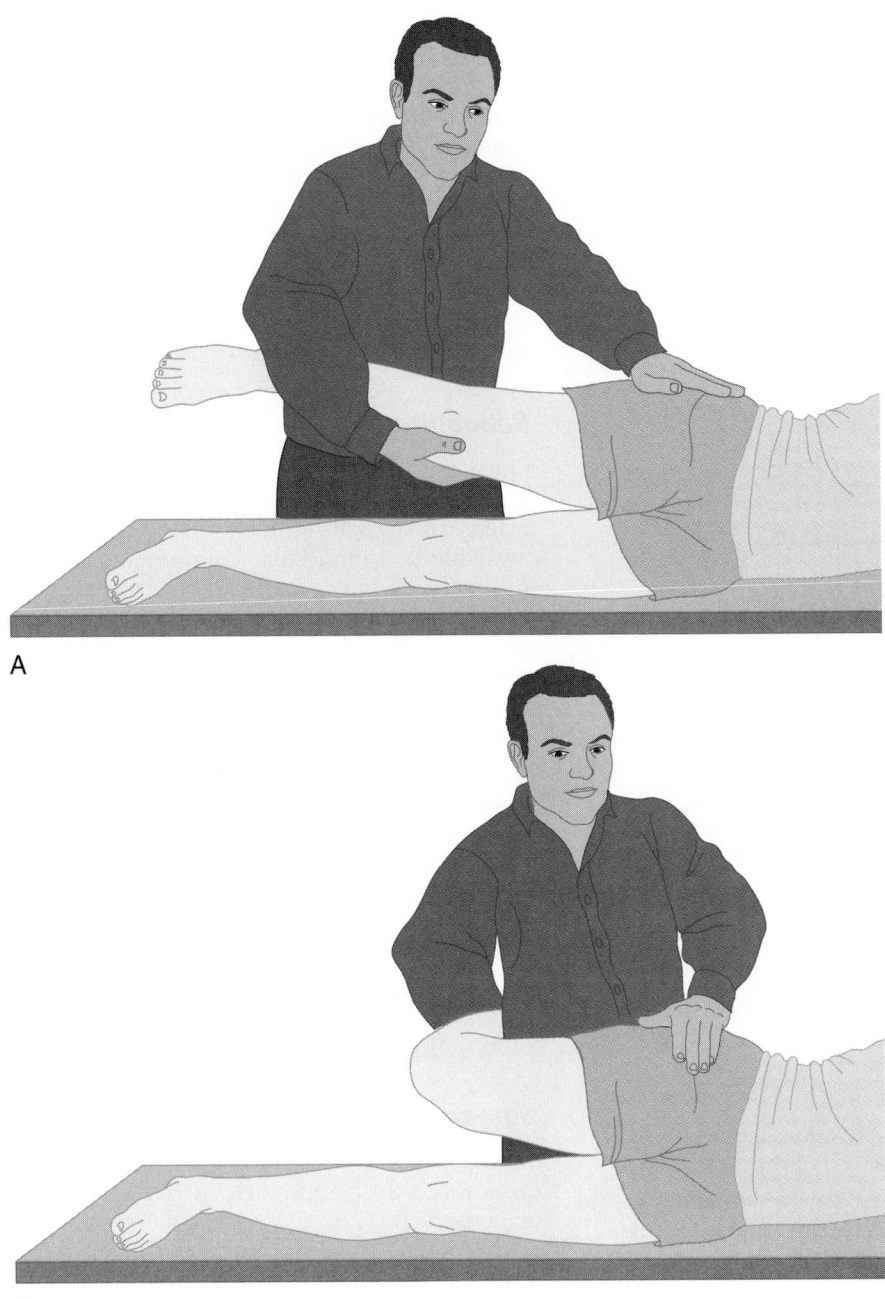

A

B

FIGURE 49-3. Traction on the femoral nerve may be accomplished with hip and knee extension initially **(A)** and then gentle knee flexion **(B)**.

can cause sedation and aplastic anemia. The patient taking carbamazepine should be evaluated with serial complete blood counts and checking of carbamazepine level. Gabapentin can cause sedation. The potential risks of surgical intervention include bleeding, infection, and adverse reaction to the anesthetic agent.

References

1. Kimura J. Electrodiagnosis in Diseases of Nerve and Muscle: Principles and Practice, 2nd ed. Philadelphia, FA Davis, 1989.
2. Dumitru D. Electrodiagnostic Medicine. Philadelphia, Hanley & Belfus, 1995.
3. Donovan PJ, Zerhouni EA, Siegelman SS. CT of psoas compartment of the retroperitoneum. Semin Roentgenol 1981;16:241-250.
4. Simeone JF, Robinson F, Rothman SLG, et al. Computerized tomographic demonstration of retroperitoneal hematoma causing femoral neuropathy. J Neurosurg 1977;47:946-948.
5. Dillavou ED, Anderson LR, Bernert RA, et al. Lower extremity iatrogenic nerve injury due to compression during intraabdominal surgery. Am J Surg 1997;173:504-508.
6. Kvist-Poulson H, Borel J. Iatrogenic femoral neuropathy subsequent to abdominal hysterectomy: incidence and prevention. Obstet Gynecol 1982;60:516-520.
7. Tysvaer AT. Computerized tomography and surgical treatment of femoral compression neuropathy. J Neurosurg 1982;57:137-139.
8. Ho KM, Lim HH. Femoral nerve palsy: an unusual complication after femoral vein puncture in a patient with severe coagulopathy. Anesth Analg 1999;89:672.

9. Eggli S, Hankemayer S, Muller ME. Nerve palsy after leg lengthening in total replacement arthroplasty for developmental dysplasia of the hip. J Bone Joint Surg Br 1999;81:843-845.

10. Moore KL. Clinically Oriented Anatomy, 2nd ed. Baltimore, Williams & Wilkins, 1985.

11. Oldenburg M, Muller RT. The frequency, prognosis and significance of nerve injuries in total hip arthroplasty. Int Orthop 1997;21:1-3.

12. Gieger D, Mpinga E, Steves MA, et al. Femoral neuropathy: unusual presentation for recurrent large-bowel cancer. Dis Colon Rectum 1998;41:910-913.

13. Takao M, Fukuuchi Y, Koto A, et al. Localized hypertrophic mononeuropathy involving the femoral nerve. Neurology 1999;52:389-392.

14. Parmer SS, Carpenter JP, Fairman RM, et al. Femoral neuropathy following retroperitoneal hemorrhage: case series and review of the literature. Ann Vasc Surg 2006;20:536-540.

Lateral Femoral Cutaneous Neuropathy 50

Earl J. Craig, MD, and Daniel M. Clinchot, MD

DEFINITION

Lateral femoral cutaneous neuropathy, commonly called meralgia paresthetica, is the focal injury of the lateral femoral cutaneous nerve causing pain and sensory loss in the lateral thigh of the affected individual.

The lateral femoral cutaneous nerve is a pure sensory nerve that receives fibers from L2-3 (Fig. 50-1; see also Fig. 49-1). After forming, the nerve passes through the psoas major muscle and around the pelvic brim to the lateral edge of the inguinal ligament, where it passes out of the pelvis in a tunnel created by the inguinal ligament and the anterior superior iliac spine.[1-3] A number of anatomic variations have described the exit of the lateral femoral cutaneous nerve from the pelvis.[4] Approximately 25% of the population has an anomalous course of the lateral femoral cutaneous nerve out of the pelvis.[5] Approximately 12 cm below the anterior superior iliac spine, the nerve splits into anterior and posterior branches. The nerve provides cutaneous sensory innervation to the lateral thigh. The size of the area innervated varies among individuals.

The nerve may be injured as a result of a number of causes, as outlined in Table 50-1. Lateral femoral cutaneous neuropathy is more commonly seen in overweight individuals because of compression of the nerve (due to abdominal girth) when the thigh is flexed in a seated position.

SYMPTOMS

Patients typically complain of lateral thigh pain and numbness. The numbness may be described as tingling or a decrease in sensation. The pain is often burning in quality but may be sharp, dull, or aching. The patient may also complain of an itching sensation. In some instances, there will be a precipitating event, such as a long car ride in which the patient was seated for a prolonged period, putting stress on the nerve. This is especially true in individuals who wear the seat belt snugly. The patient should not complain of weakness in the lower extremities. The diagnosis requires a high index of suspicion by the evaluating clinician.

PHYSICAL EXAMINATION

Because the lateral femoral cutaneous nerve is purely sensory, the only finding typical of this condition is decreased sensation, which should be limited to an area of variable diameter in the lateral thigh. In adult men, the clinician may also see an area on the lateral thigh in which the hair has rubbed off. Palpation over the anterior superior iliac spine may exacerbate symptoms.

The physical examination is also used to exclude other possible causes of pain and weakness of the hip, thigh, and knee. The examination should include a complete neuromuscular evaluation of the low back, the hips, and the entire lower extremities. This should include inspection for asymmetry or atrophy, manual muscle testing, muscle stretch reflexes, and sensory testing for light touch and pinprick. In the case of lateral femoral cutaneous neuropathy, the clinician should not see muscle atrophy or asymmetry or weakness of lower extremities. Reflexes should remain intact.

FUNCTIONAL LIMITATIONS

Typically, there are no functional limitations because this injury is more an annoyance than truly disabling. No true weakness is seen, although prolonged standing and extension at the hip may exacerbate the pain and thus limit

283

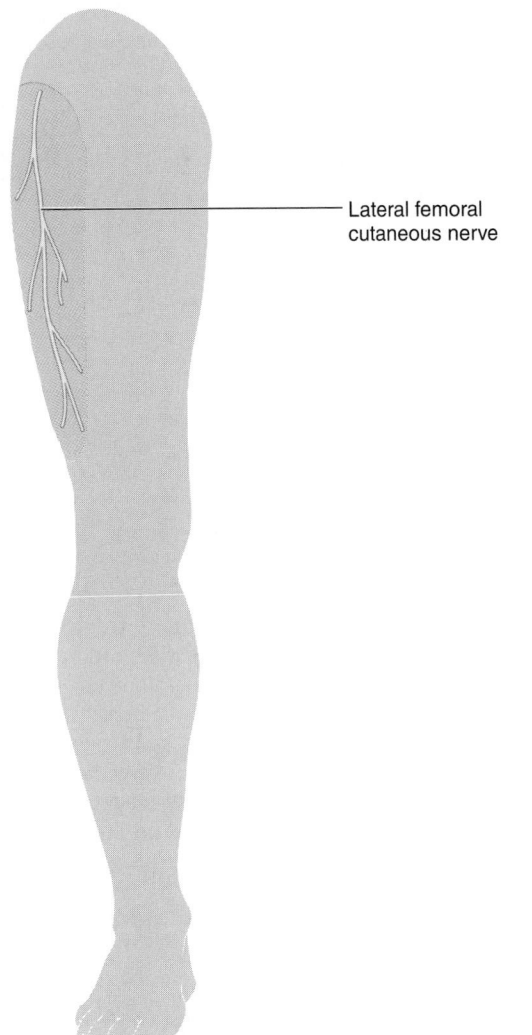

Lateral femoral cutaneous nerve

FIGURE 50-1. The lateral femoral cutaneous nerve is purely sensory and innervates the anterolateral thigh.

TABLE 50-1 Causes of Lateral Femoral Cutaneous Neuropathy

Operative and postoperative complications and scarring
Retroperitoneal tumor
Retroperitoneal fibrosis
Spinal tumor
Infection
Pregnancy
Penetrating injury
Iliac bone graft
Pressure injury
Tight clothing
Seat belt
Obesity
Idiopathic

firm the diagnosis.[9] Shin and colleagues[10] documented the utility of recording from two sites within the lateral femoral cutaneous dermatome. This technique facilitates use of a more realistic amplitude in the side-to-side comparison. Controversy exists in regard to the best site of stimulation of the lateral femoral cutaneous nerve. Classically, the stimulation electrode is placed 1 cm medial to the anterior superior iliac spine. More recently, a stimulation site of 4 cm distal to the anterior superior iliac spine has been suggested as a means to obtain a more reliable response.[11] The needle electromyography is done to rule out other pathologic processes, and the recording should be normal. Serial electromyographic studies may help with evaluation of the recovery process.

Somatosensory evoked potentials may also be used, but a study reported that sensory conduction studies are a more reliable method of evaluation of the lateral femoral cutaneous nerve.[12] Once the diagnosis is made, magnetic resonance imaging or computed tomography of the pelvis may be required to look for a mass causing impingement.

TREATMENT

Initial

Treatment of lateral femoral cutaneous neuropathy is focused on symptom relief and facilitation of nerve healing.

the patient in performing tasks such as standing and walking. The nerve may be further compressed and the symptoms exacerbated when the patient is seated, so long car or plane rides may be difficult. Similarly, individuals who are sedentary at work may experience painful symptoms that limit their ability to function.

DIAGNOSTIC STUDIES

History and physical examination are the most important diagnostic tools, and all other testing should be used as an extension of these. Electromyography is the primary diagnostic tool and should include lateral femoral cutaneous sensory nerve conduction studies and needle electromyography of the lower extremity.[2,3] Although routine lateral femoral cutaneous nerve conduction studies have standard normal values with which an individual's study result can be compared, it is generally recommended to do comparison studies on the unaffected side, as the studies are technically difficult.[3,6-8] The side-to-side amplitude ratio has been shown to be a better way to con-

Differential Diagnosis

Lumbar radiculopathy

Lumbar polyradiculopathy

Lumbar plexopathy

Lumbar facet syndrome

Retroperitoneal mass

Femoral neuropathy

Both early and late symptomatic relief of the pain and numbness is attempted with modalities and medications. Both heat and ice can be used. If an inflammatory component is suspected, nonsteroidal anti-inflammatory drugs or corticosteroids may be used. Narcotics are used when acetaminophen and anti-inflammatory medications do not control the pain. Antiseizure medications, such as carbamazepine and gabapentin, are also of benefit in some individuals.

Facilitation of healing varies according to the cause of the injury to the nerve. For most individuals, this entails removal of the cause of the pressure over the anterior iliac region. The pressure may be caused by tight clothing, belts, seat belts, or excess weight. Elimination of the pressure may include weight loss or clothing adjustment. Nerves that have sustained a less serious (neurapraxic) injury often heal during hours to weeks once the irritant is removed. Nerves that have sustained a more severe injury (neurotmesis or axonotmesis) typically have a much longer healing course because of the time required for wallerian degeneration and regeneration. The use of anti-inflammatory medications may also be of benefit in the healing process.

Rehabilitation

Physical therapy may facilitate healing of the injured nerve. Gentle stretching of the anterior thigh and groin is indicated. The application of hot packs or ultrasound often facilitates the stretching process. Ice may be helpful when the patient continues to have swelling and inflammation around the pelvic brim. In some individuals, a general conditioning program to help with weight loss may also be useful. A dietitian can assist the patient with weight loss. A skilled therapist may be able to use soft tissue mobilization to help free an impinged and inflamed nerve. Augmented soft tissue mobilization is one of several techniques that may be useful. Electrical stimulation and transcutaneous nerve stimulation may be helpful in reducing the perception of pain by the patient during therapy treatments. Transcutaneous electrical nerve stimulation can be used on a daily basis for pain control.

Procedures

When conservative treatment fails, injection of the nerve at or near the anterior superior iliac spine with steroids and local anesthetic may be helpful (Fig. 50-2). If the steroid injection is helpful but short lasting, the nerve can be injected with phenol or other neurotoxic agents as a last resort.

Under sterile conditions, the pelvis is palpated and the anterior superior iliac spine and inguinal ligament are identified. A 25-gauge, 2-inch needle is placed perpendicular to the skin approximately 1 inch medial to the anterior superior iliac spine and inferior to the inguinal ligament. The needle is advanced into the soft tissue approximately 1 inch (this depends on the patient's size and amount of excess subcutaneous tissue). At times, paresthesias may be elicited, thereby

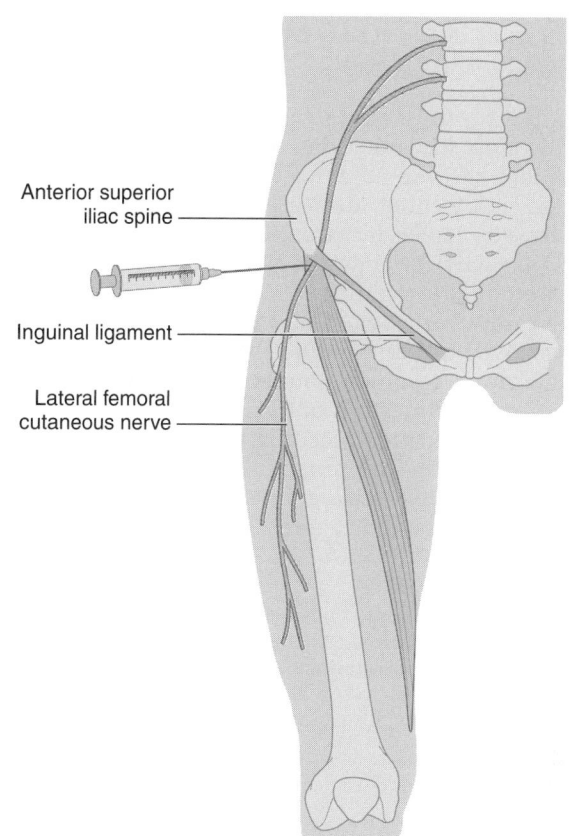

FIGURE 50-2. The nerve injection site for steroids and local anesthetic is at or near the anterior superior iliac spine.

verifying needle placement; however, it is important not to inject directly into the nerve. Once the area to be injected is located, inject a 5- to 10-mL solution of local anesthetic and steroid (e.g., 2.5 mL of triamcinolone, 40 mg/mL, mixed with 2.5 mL of 0.5% bupivacaine).

Postinjection care may include icing of the injected area for 10 to 15 minutes and counseling of the patient to avoid pressure on the nerve.

Surgery

In the case of lateral femoral cutaneous nerve injury due to impingement, surgery may be required to remove the pressure. Surgical removal of neuroma or neurectomy proximal to the neuroma may also be helpful if a neuroma is found. In individuals with severe symptoms, neurolysis has been shown to result in a good outcome. This holds true even for individuals with prolonged symptoms. However, obesity has been associated with a poorer outcome when neurolysis is performed.[13]

POTENTIAL DISEASE COMPLICATIONS

Potential complications include continued pain and numbness despite treatment.

POTENTIAL TREATMENT COMPLICATIONS

Complications of treatment are well recognized. Each medication has potential adverse side effects. Nonsteroidal anti-inflammatory drugs have the potential of gastric bleeding, decreased renal blood flow, and decreased platelet function. Cyclooxygenase 2 inhibitors may have fewer gastric side effects. Narcotics have the potential for addiction and sedation. Carbamazepine can cause sedation and aplastic anemia. The patient taking carbamazepine should be evaluated with serial complete blood counts. Gabapentin can cause sedation. The injection of the nerve also has potential risks, which include bleeding, infection, and worsening of the pain. The potential risks of surgical intervention include bleeding, infection, and adverse reaction to the anesthetic agent.

References

1. Moore KL. Clinically Oriented Anatomy, 2nd ed. Baltimore, Williams & Wilkins, 1985.
2. Kimura J. Electrodiagnosis in Diseases of Nerve and Muscle: Principles and Practice, 2nd ed. Philadelphia, FA Davis, 1989.
3. Dumitru D. Electrodiagnostic Medicine. Philadelphia, Hanley & Belfus, 1995.
4. Williams PH, Trzil KP. Management of meralgia paresthetica. J Neurosurg 1991;74:76-80.
5. de Ridder VA, de Lange S, Popta JV. Anatomic variations of the lateral femoral cutaneous nerve and the consequences for surgery. J Orthop Trauma 1999;13:207-211.
6. Butler ET, Johnson EW, Kaye ZA. Normal conduction velocity in the lateral femoral cutaneous nerve. Arch Phys Med Rehabil 1974;55:31-32.
7. Lagueny A, Deliac MM, Deliac P, et al. Diagnostic and prognostic value of electrophysiologic tests in meralgia paresthetica. Muscle Nerve 1991;14:51-56.
8. Sarala PK, Nishihara T, Oh SJ. Meralgia paresthetica: electrophysiologic study. Arch Phys Med Rehabil 1979;60:30-31.
9. Seror P, Seror R. Meralgia paresthetica: clinical and electrophysiological diagnosis in 120 cases. Muscle Nerve 2006;33:650-654.
10. Shin YB, Park JH, Kwon DR, Park BY. Variability in conduction of the lateral femoral cutaneous nerve. Muscle Nerve 2006;33:645-649.
11. Russo MJ, Firestone LB, Mandler RN, Kelly JJ. Nerve conduction studies of the lateral femoral cutaneous nerve. Implications in the diagnosis of meralgia paresthetica. Am J Electroneurodiagnostic Technol 2005;45:180-185.
12. Seror P. Lateral femoral cutaneous nerve conduction v somatosensory evoked potentials for electrodiagnosis of meralgia paresthetica. Am J Phys Med Rehabil 1999;78:313-316.
13. Siu TLT, Chandran KN. Neurolysis for meralgia paresthetica: an operative series of 45 cases. Surg Neurol 2005;63:19-23.

Piriformis Syndrome 51

Thomas H. Hudgins, MD, and Joseph T. Alleva, MD

Synonyms

Hip pocket neuropathy
Wallet neuritis

ICD-9 Code

719.45   Pain in joint, pelvic region, and thigh

DEFINITION

The piriformis muscle and sciatic nerve both exit the pelvis through the greater sciatic notch. Numerous anatomic variations of this relationship have been well documented (Fig. 51-1). Cadaver studies have described the sciatic nerve passing below the piriformis muscle, through the muscle belly, as a divided nerve above and through the muscle, and as a divided nerve through and below the muscle.[1,2] More recently, a case report of piriformis syndrome described a fifth variation of an undivided nerve passing above an undivided piriformis muscle.[3] Yeoman[4] was the first to describe the relationship of these two structures in 1928, and Robinson[5] first coined the term *piriformis syndrome* in 1947.

Piriformis syndrome describes a clinical situation whereby the piriformis muscle is compressing the sciatic nerve, resulting in a sciatic neuropathy. This may be an intrinsic injury to the piriformis muscle (primary syndrome) or a compression at the pelvic outlet (secondary syndrome).[6]

Although the anatomic relation of these two structures is well documented, this remains a controversial diagnosis. There is no consensus among clinicians on the validity of this entity and therefore no documentation of the incidence.[7] Nevertheless, Goldner[8] predicted an incidence of less than 1% in an orthopedic practice. The incidence is the same for men and women.

SYMPTOMS

The patient with piriformis syndrome will complain of buttock pain with or without radiation into the leg. This may be seen in chronic as well as in acute situations. Often, a history of minor trauma may be described, such as falling onto the buttock. Sitting on hard surfaces will exacerbate the symptoms of pain and occasional numbness and paresthesias without weakness. Activities that produce a motion of hip adduction and internal rotation, such as cross-country skiing and the overhead serve in tennis, may also exacerbate the symptoms.[9,10] Because of the relationship of the piriformis muscle with the lateral pelvis wall, patients may also experience pain with bowel movements, and women may complain of dyspareunia.[11]

PHYSICAL EXAMINATION

The physical examination will reveal normal neurologic findings with symmetric strength and reflexes. Tenderness to palpation is experienced from the sacrum to the greater trochanter, representing the area of the piriformis muscle.[12] A palpable taut band is tender with both rectal and pelvic examination because the piriformis muscle sits in the deep pelvic floor.[10] Passive hip abduction and internal rotation may compress the sciatic nerve, reproducing pain (a Freiberg sign). Contraction of the piriformis with resistance to active hip external rotation and abduction may also reproduce pain or asymmetric weakness (a Pace sign).[13] A positive result of the straight-leg test may also be appreciated.[14] Rectal examination may be performed to palpate a taut band but is not recommended.

FUNCTIONAL LIMITATIONS

The patient with piriformis syndrome will experience pain with prolonged sitting and with activities that produce hip internal rotation and adduction. This may include cross-country skiing and one-legged motions, such as the overhead serve in tennis and the kicking motion in soccer. Sitting on hard surfaces such as benches, church pews, or wallets kept in a back pocket ("wallet neuritis") may exacerbate symptoms.

DIAGNOSTIC TESTING

Piriformis syndrome is a clinical diagnosis. Magnetic resonance imaging and computed tomography are primarily reserved to rule out other disorders associated

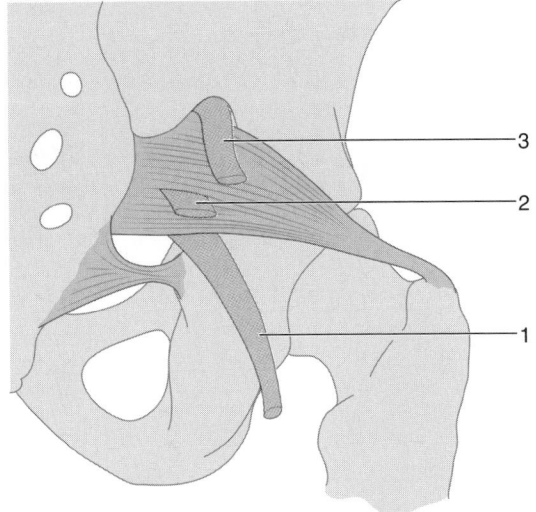

FIGURE 51-1. Three variations in the course of the sciatic nerve as related to the piriformis muscle. The sciatic nerve is shown above *(3)*, through *(2)*, and below *(1)* the piriformis muscle.

with sciatic neuropathy. A few case reports have demonstrated hypertrophy of the piriformis muscle on both computed tomography and magnetic resonance imaging.[15] Electrodiagnostic testing may reveal a prolonged H reflex in symptomatic cases.[16] This was validated by demonstration of a prolongation of the H wave with hip flexion, adduction, and internal rotation (the FAIR test) in symptomatic cases. Patients diagnosed with piriformis syndrome by this FAIR test demonstrated successful treatment outcomes with physical therapy and injections in 70% of the cases. Surgery was successful in recalcitrant cases directed at the piriformis.[17] Electrodiagnosis is also helpful in differentiating piriformis syndrome from a lumbosacral radiculopathy.

TREATMENT

Initial

Nonsteroidal anti-inflammatory drugs and analgesic medications are prescribed to reduce local prostaglandin-mediated inflammation, pain, and spasm.[10] Judicious

Differential Diagnosis

Secondary causes of piriformis syndrome:

Superior and inferior gluteal artery aneurysm

Benign pelvic tumor

Endometriosis

Myositis ossificans

Diagnoses that mimic piriformis syndrome:

Lumbar facet syndrome

L5-S1 radiculopathy[13]

use of modalities such as heat therapy may be beneficial to increase collagen distensibility and compliance with a physical therapy program. Avoidance of exacerbating activities and use of soft cushions for prolonged sitting are also advocated initially.

Rehabilitation

The use of heat therapy such as ultrasound is followed by a gentle stretch of the piriformis muscle. The piriformis is stretched with hip internal rotation above 90 degrees of hip flexion and with external rotation below 90 degrees of hip flexion.[17] Strengthening of the hip abductors, in particular the gluteus medius, should be emphasized. This is performed with Thera-Band around the ankles and walking sideways. The gluteus medius may also be isolated with lunges in a transverse and coronal plane. Correction of biomechanical imbalances that may predispose the individual to piriformis syndrome should also be initiated; these include increased pronation, hip abductor weakness, lower lumbar spine dysfunction, sacroiliac joint hypomobility, and hamstring tightness.[9,10] These imbalances may lead to a gait with hip in external rotation, shortened stride length, and functional leg length discrepancy.

Procedures

Recalcitrant cases may require a perisciatic injection of corticosteroid.[14] An approach of 1 cm caudal and 2 cm lateral to the lower border of the sacroiliac joint correlated to successful distribution in the sciatic nerve area confirmed by fluoroscopic guidance.[18] Caudal epidural steroid injections to bathe the lower sacral nerve roots in corticosteroid has been described with mixed results. Injection of botulinum toxin type B (12,500 U) has also been reported. No single technique is universally accepted.

Surgery

Rarely, surgical release of the piriformis muscle is performed to relieve the compression.[12] Piriformis syndrome carries a favorable prognosis; most patients will respond to a nonoperative approach.[9]

POTENTIAL DISEASE COMPLICATIONS

This is a clinical diagnosis that is often overlooked. The primary complication is chronic sciatica.

POTENTIAL TREATMENT COMPLICATIONS

Bleeding and gastrointestinal and renal side effects of nonsteroidal anti-inflammatory drugs are well documented. Complications of local corticosteroid injections include infection, hematoma or bleeding, and soft tissue atrophy at the site. Surgical techniques must be careful to avoid inadvertent injury to the nerves in the buttock. The functional loss of sectioning of the piriformis muscle is inconsequential as the other hip abductors may compensate for this movement.[12,18]

References

1. Pecina M. Contribution to the etiological explanation of the piriformis syndrome. Acta Anat (Basel) 1979;105:181-187.
2. Beaton LE, Anson BJ. Sciatic nerve and the piriformis muscle: their interrelation as a possible cause of coccydynia. J Bone Joint Surg 1938;20:686-688.
3. Ozaki S, Hamabe T, Muro T. Piriformis syndrome resulting from an anomalous relationship between the sciatic nerve and piriformis muscle. Orthopedics 1999;22:771-772.
4. Yeoman W. The relation of arthritis of the sacroiliac joint to sciatica. Lancet 1928;2:1119-1122.
5. Robinson D. Piriformis syndrome in relation to sciatic pain. Am J Surg 1947;73:355-358.
6. Papadopoulos EC, Khan SN. Piriformis syndrome and low back pain: a new classification and review of the literature. Orthop Clin North Am 2004;35:65-71.
7. Silver JK, Leadbetter WB. Piriformis syndrome: assessment of current practice and literature review. Orthopedics 1998;21:1133-1135.
8. Goldner JL. Piriformis compression causing low back and lower extremity pain. Am J Orthop 1997;26:316-318.
9. Douglas S. Sciatic pain and piriformis syndrome. Nurse Pract 1997;22:166-180.
10. Parziale JR, Hudgins TH, Fishman LM. The piriformis syndrome. Am J Orthop 1996;25;819-823.
11. Barton PM. Piriformis syndrome: a rational approach to management. Pain 1991;47:345-352.
12. McCrory P, Bell S. Nerve entrapment syndromes as a cause of pain in the hip, groin and buttock. Sports Med 1999;27:261-274.
13. Yuen EC, So YT. Sciatic neuropathy. Neurol Clin 1999;17:617-631.
14. Hanania M, Kitain E. Perisciatic injection of steroid for the treatment of sciatica due to piriformis syndrome. Reg Anesth Pain Med 1998;23:223-228.
15. Jankiewicz JJ, Hennrikus WL, Hookum JA. The appearance of the piriformis muscle syndrome in computed tomography and magnetic resonance imaging. A case report and review of the literature. Clin Orthop 1991;262:205-209.
16. Fishman LM, Zybert PA. Electrophysiologic evidence of piriformis syndrome. Arch Phys Med Rehabil 1992;73:359-364.
17. Fishman LM, Dombi GW, Michaelsen C, et al. Piriformis syndrome: diagnosis, treatment, and outcome—a 10-year study. Arch Phys Med Rehabil 2002;83:295-301.
18. Benzon HT, Katz JA, Benzon HA, Iqbal MS. Piriformis syndrome: anatomic considerations, a new injection technique, and a review of the literature. Anesthesiology 2003;98:1442-1448.

Quadriceps Contusion 52

Seneca A. Storm, MD, and J. Michael Wieting, DO

Synonym

Traumatic quadriceps strain

ICD-9 Codes

924.00 Contusion of lower limb (thigh)
924.9   Contusion of lower limb (unspecified site)

DEFINITION

Muscle contusions and strains account for 90% of contact sport–related injuries.[1,2] Quadriceps muscle contusions result from blunt trauma to the anterior thigh and are encountered most commonly in contact sports such as football, soccer, basketball, and wrestling; injury is caused by a direct hit from a helmet, shoulder pad, elbow, or knee. The acute trauma damages muscle tissue, causing hemorrhage and subsequent inflammation. Quadriceps contusions are graded mild, moderate, or severe between 12 and 24 hours. A mild contusion has more than 90 degrees of knee flexion; moderate, between 45 and 90 degrees of knee flexion; and severe, less than 45 degrees of knee flexion.[3]

SYMPTOMS

Quadriceps contusions may not be immediately evident after the contact injury. Pain, swelling, and decreased range of motion of the knee, particularly flexion, are seen within 24 hours. Symptoms may worsen with active muscle contraction and with passive stretch. Loss of knee range of motion can be the result of muscle and articular edema as well as of physiologic inhibition of the quadriceps muscle group and "splinting." After injury, the quadriceps muscle group often becomes stiff, and the athlete may have difficulty bearing weight on the affected extremity, resulting in an antalgic gait. Hemorrhage and resultant hematoma are described as either intermuscular or intramuscular.

PHYSICAL EXAMINATION

Visual inspection of quadriceps contusion shows a variable amount of swelling and discoloration over the anterior thigh due to hematoma formation and intramuscular bleeding. Pain of varying intensity is present on palpation of the quadriceps muscle group. A firm palpable mass may be noted in the anterior thigh and is usually due to hematoma formation; if the hematoma formation is large, a knee effusion may also be present. Bone incongruity and tenderness may indicate fracture of the femur, patella, or tibial plateau. Check for the presence of distal pulses and capillary refill and assess range of motion of adjacent joints to be sure that the injury is localized to the anterior thigh.

Evaluation of range of motion reveals decreased knee flexion, especially past 90 degrees; knee extension will be less painful than flexion.[4] Extension lag or complete lack of extension is noted in partial or complete quadriceps rupture. With quadriceps tendon rupture, a palpable defect may be present. Quadriceps rupture is a relatively rare injury more common in patients older than 50 years, and it is typically associated with underlying metabolic or inflammatory disease.[5] Muscle stretch reflexes of the patellar tendon may be inhibited, and serial measurements of thigh circumferences should be made during the initial 24- to 72-hour postinjury period to assess for possible compartment syndrome. Paresthesias, loss of pulses, distal pallor, intense pain, and decreased temperature should alert the clinician to consider this diagnosis. See Chapter 58 for more information. Sensory testing should include the femoral and saphenous nerve distribution of the distal leg.

An intermuscular hematoma with septal or fascial sheath hemorrhage may be more likely to disperse and to result in distal ecchymosis. If the contusion is in the distal third of the quadriceps, discoloration and swelling will often track into the knee region because of gravity. An intramuscular hematoma may resolve more slowly and be associated with myositis ossificans and scar contracture.

FUNCTIONAL LIMITATIONS

Initially, gait will be antalgic and weight bearing difficult on the involved extremity. Rehabilitation typically occurs in three phases. In the first phase (first 24 hours), pain usually limits activity, and the patient may require crutches.[6] During a period of days to weeks, running and "kicking" activities will be limited secondary to knee stiffness and pain associated with terminal knee flexion and extension. Most patients recover uneventfully.

DIAGNOSTIC STUDIES

Plain radiographs are initially obtained in moderate to severe quadriceps contusions to rule out a coexisting fracture. Magnetic resonance imaging is the diagnostic imaging study of choice and allows visualization of the involved quadriceps muscles. Resolution of the injury, as detected by magnetic resonance imaging, lags behind functional recovery.[7] Ultrasonography may be helpful if tendon injury is suspected.[8] Nuclear bone scan may be ordered in the days to weeks after injury to assess for the development of myositis ossificans traumatica, heterotopic bone formation that may develop in up to 20% of injuries. Bone scans are more sensitive than plain films for detection of heterotopic bone formation and can be useful in monitoring its resolution. Suspicion of compartment syndrome warrants consideration of intracompartmental pressure monitoring, although conservative management in cases without concomitant fracture has been reported.[7,9] Compartment syndrome may be more likely in a patient with associated fracture or suspected large-vessel injury. For severe contusions or in a patient who appears ill, laboratory work is indicated, including creatine kinase activity, hematocrit determination, and possibly coagulation studies.[10]

TREATMENT

Initial

Immediately, the patient should cease activity. The knee is gently elevated and flexed to 120 degrees, and ice is applied to the anterior thigh (for 20 minutes at a time every 2 or 3 hours). An elastic bandage should be placed around the injured leg and thigh and gentle compression applied to reduce hematoma formation. If the injury is mild, icing is repeated for 2 or 3 days; the patient should ambulate with crutches, either non–weight bearing or partial weight bearing. In between icing, a thigh pad is applied. Temporary bed rest may be appropriate if the injury is severe. However, rehabilitation should be aggressive to the limit of pain tolerance. Avoid massage for the first 1 to 2 weeks after injury to lessen the chance of additional hemorrhage. Whirlpool, heat, and ultrasound modalities are avoided for the same reason until the edema stabilizes. If edema persists or becomes severe or warning signs of compartment syndrome develop, surgical referral is made to evaluate the possibility of compartment syndrome or ongoing hemorrhage. Needle aspiration of a formed hematoma may be indicated to relieve pressure and pain.[11]

Determination of the appropriate time to progress the amount of activity performed and readiness for return to activity is important for recovery from injury. Animal models of muscle contusion suggest that continued use of the extremity promotes circulation and venous drainage, minimizing postinjury swelling. Because of the risk of hematoma formation, nonsteroidal anti-inflammatory drugs (NSAIDs) are avoided in the first 24 hours after injury. The role of NSAIDs in the treatment of muscle injuries is unclear because inflammatory cells are an important part of clearing away necrotic muscle followed by the regeneration and scar formation phase, leading to the question of whether NSAIDs help or delay the healing process.[12] The inflammatory response may be a necessary phase in soft tissue healing. Clinically, NSAIDs are used, but alternative analgesics like acetaminophen may be considered. However, in the animal model of quadriceps contusion, continued use of the contused muscle was more predictive of recovery than whether the animal received acetaminophen or NSAIDs.[12] Steroids should be avoided.[1] Medication use should facilitate continued rehabilitation and tolerance of activity progression.

Rehabilitation

Rehabilitation consists of three phases. The goals of the first phase are to limit bleeding, to immobilize the knee in full flexion, to elevate the leg for 24 hours, and to prescribe relative rest; excessive activity or alcohol ingestion, which could aggravate the injury, is avoided. Phase two involves restoration of motion, modalities, and return to weight bearing. Crutches and partial weight bearing are used during immobilization and until the patient has at least 90 degrees of knee flexion, good quadriceps control, and limited limp. After 48 hours from the injury and for the next 2 to 5 days, test range of motion with the patient in the prone position. Perform knee flexion exercises in the "pain-free range" with associated hip flexion. This can be followed with active-assisted range of motion exercises. It is important to avoid forced stretching because this may aggravate the injury and slow healing. Static quadriceps exercises can be instituted. Animal models of muscle contusion

---

Differential Diagnosis

Quadriceps tear or strain

Quadriceps tendon rupture

Soft tissue tumors

Compartment syndrome

Fracture of femur, patella, or tibial plateau

Referred pain from hip or knee

Metabolic abnormalities leading to tendon injuries (hypocalcemia, steroid use)

demonstrate that early mobilization increases tensile strength of muscle compared with immobilization.[13]

Proprioceptive neuromuscular facilitation exercises using reciprocal inhibition of the quadriceps and hamstrings can be done as well.[14] Modalities may include pulsed ultrasound or high-velocity galvanic stimulation, with continuous pulses of 80 to 120 per second, at the patient's level of sensory perception for 20- to 25-minute periods. Interferential electrical stimulation may assist in further edema resolution, but both ultrasound and electrical stimulation should be used once edema has stabilized. Cautious use of ultrasound can help increase blood resorption.[14] Cold compression may be useful.

Phase three starts when the patient has 120 degrees of pain-free range of motion and excellent quadriceps control. Noncontact sports may be resumed at this point, along with active knee range of motion, progressive resistive exercises, and cycling. Pain-free knee range of motion within 10 degrees of the unaffected extremity should be the goal before return to activity is considered. Jumping, springing, and cutting activities should be incorporated into the rehabilitation program, at which point functional testing to assess safe return to activity can be done. A protective pad larger than the original contusion should be worn during play for 3 to 6 months after injury. Most quadriceps contusions resolve within a few weeks, and complications are rare.

If the patient does not have painless, full range of motion 3 to 4 weeks after injury, radiographic imaging should be performed to detect whether myositis ossificans is present. Time to return to activity is variable and depends on severity of injury; full recovery is expected in severe contusions by 5 to 8 weeks.

Procedures

On occasion, needle aspiration of a formed hematoma is performed to alleviate pressure and pain.

Surgery

Surgery is rarely indicated with these injuries, except in association with a concomitant compartment syndrome or fracture. Untreated compartment syndrome may lead to muscle necrosis, fibrosis, scarring, and contractures. However, even in severe quadriceps muscle contusion, there is some indication that treatment should be conservative with pain management and maintenance of knee range of motion.[7]

POTENTIAL DISEASE COMPLICATIONS

If the quadriceps region becomes extremely warm with marked increased edema and the patient complains of paresthesias with abnormal findings on neurovascular examination and significant quadriceps weakness, consideration must be given to the development of a potential compartment syndrome. A case of osteomyelitis has been reported in an otherwise healthy athlete who sustained a quadriceps contusion.[15]

Myositis ossificans traumatica usually stabilizes and is resorbed spontaneously by 6 months after injury with conservative care.[16] Plain films may show ectopic bone formation 2 to 4 weeks after injury; the most common location is in the midshaft of the femur. Serial bone scans can be performed to monitor resolution of ectopic bone in a symptomatic athlete. Surgical removal of ectopic bone is rarely indicated and should not be performed for at least 12 months after injury to allow adequate maturation; this is to prevent enlargement of ectopic bone and recurrence.

POTENTIAL TREATMENT COMPLICATIONS

Analgesics and NSAIDs have well-known side effects that most commonly affect the gastric, hepatic, and renal systems. Avoid vigorous soft tissue massage and passive stretch in the acute postinjury period to prevent further bleeding and hematoma formation (this occurs frequently in a field setting after hamstring injury).

References

1. Beiner JM, Jokl P, Cholewicki J, Panjabi MM. The effect of anabolic steroids and corticosteroids on healing of muscle contusion injury. Am J Sports Med 1999;27:2-9.
2. Canale ST, Cantler ED Jr, Sisk TD, Freeman BL 3rd. A chronicle of injuries of an American intercollegiate football team. Am J Sports Med 1981;9:384-389.
3. Reid D. Sports Injury Assessment and Rehabilitation. New York, Churchill Livingstone, 1992.
4. Ryan JB, Wheeler JH, Hopkinson WJ, et al. Quadriceps contusions. West Point update. Am J Sports Med 1991;19:299-304.
5. Katz T, Alkalay D, Rath E, et al. Bilateral simultaneous rupture of the quadriceps tendon in an adult amateur tennis player. J Clin Rheumatol 2006;12:32-33.
6. Schenck RC Jr. Athletic Training and Sports Medicine, 3rd ed. Rosemont, Ill, American Academy of Orthopaedic Surgeons, 1999.
7. Diaz JA, Fischer DA, Rettig AC, et al. Severe quadriceps muscle contusions in athletes. A report of three cases. Am J Sports Med 2003;31:289-293.
8. Heyde CE, Mahlfeld K, Stahel PF, Kayser R. Ultrasonography as a reliable diagnostic tool in old quadriceps tendon ruptures: a prospective multicentre study. Knee Surg Sports Traumatol Arthrosc 2005;13:564-568.
9. Robinson D, On E, Halperin N. Anterior compartment syndrome of the thigh in athletes—indications for conservative treatment. J Trauma 1992;32:183-186.
10. DeBerardino T, Milne L, DeMaio M. Quadriceps injury. Available at: http://www.emedicine.com. Accessed June 21, 2006.
11. DeLee JC, Drez D. Orthopaedic Sports Medicine: Principles and Practice. Philadelphia, WB Saunders, 1994.
12. Rahusen FT, Weinhold PS, Almekinders LC. Nonsteroidal anti-inflammatory drugs and acetaminophen in the treatment of an acute muscle injury. Am J Sports Med 2004;32:1856-1859.
13. Jarvinen MJ, Lehto MU. The effects of early mobilisation and immobilisation on the healing process following muscle injuries. Sports Med 1993;15:78-89.
14. Geraci M. Rehabilitation of the hip, pelvis, and thigh. In Kibler WB, Herring SA, Press JM, eds. Functional Rehabilitation of Sports and Musculoskeletal Injuries. Gaithersburg, Md, Aspen, 1998.
15. Bonsell S, Freudigman PT, Moore HA. Quadriceps muscle contusion resulting in osteomyelitis of the femur in a high school football player. A case report. Am J Sports Med 2001;29:818-820.
16. Young JL, Laskowski ER, Rock MG. Thigh injuries in athletes. Mayo Clin Proc 1993;68:1099-1106.

Total Hip Replacement 53

Robert S. Skerker, MD, and Gregory J. Mulford, MD

Synonyms

Total hip replacement
Bipolar hemiarthroplasty
Unipolar hemiarthroplasty
Revision arthroplasty
Austin Moore endoprosthesis
Birmingham hip resurfacing

ICD-9 Codes

715.95   Osteoarthritis, hip
733.42   Aseptic necrosis of bone, head and neck of femur
820.09   Fracture of neck of femur, other (head of femur, subcapital)
820.8   Fracture of neck of femur, unspecified part of neck femur, closed
835.00   Dislocation of hip
996.59   Loosening of total hip replacement
V43.64   Total hip replacement

DEFINITION

Arthroplasty, commonly called joint replacement, involves the reconstruction of a diseased, damaged, or ankylosed joint by natural modification or artificial materials. The most common causes of adult hip disease are osteoarthritis, rheumatoid arthritis, avascular necrosis, post-traumatic degenerative joint disease, congenital hip disease, and infectious diseases within the joint or adjacent bone. The modern era of hip joint replacement began in the late 1960s when Sir John Charnley combined a stainless steel femoral component with a polyethylene socket fixed to the adjacent bone with polymethyl methacrylate. Since that time, arthroplasty of the hip joint has become an accepted and standard treatment of common adult hip joint disease. Modern hip arthroplasty surgery has resulted in the restoration of pain-free motion and improved quality of life for millions.[1] Joint arthroplasty has become the most common elective surgical procedure performed in the United States; annually, there are more than 200,000 hip replacements. If one includes partial hip replacements and revision arthroplasty along with unclassified hip arthroplasties, the figure increases to more than 350,000

hip surgeries per year. Statistics from 1990 through 2003 show a dramatic increase in yearly hip arthroplasty in the new millennium.[2]

The primary indications for total hip arthroplasty (THA) include progressive pain and dysfunction or a decline in mobility, self-care, and daily living activities despite conservative treatment. Relative contraindications include active or recent joint infection, neurotrophic joints, inability of the patient to cooperate in the immediate postoperative period or with the rehabilitation program after joint implantation, serious comorbid medical conditions that result in a higher surgical risk or compromised postoperative medical status, rapidly progressive or terminal cancer with shortened survival or severe debility, and severe nutritional depletion that jeopardizes postoperative wound healing.

A survey of the opinions of orthopedic surgeons about indications for THA found no clear consensus. Most surgeons required severe pain on a daily basis, rest pain several days per week, and destruction of most of the joint space on a radiograph. Younger age, comorbidity, technical difficulties, and lack of motivation also factored in the decision against surgery, whereas the desire to return to work and an independent lifestyle swayed the decision for surgery.[3]

SYMPTOMS

The primary symptom of hip disease is groin pain and occasionally pain that radiates to the knee. Lateral proximal thigh pain in the region of the greater trochanter is usually not an indicator of hip joint disease. Pain in this location typically reflects local muscle or bursal inflammation or is referred from the pelvis or lumbosacral spine. The primary sign of hip disease is a gait disturbance, such as limp. Patients may complain of difficulty in walking because of pain, limp, or both. Numbness and paresthesias should be absent; but if they are present, they suggest an alternative diagnosis (e.g., lumbar radiculopathy). Patients with hip osteoarthritis often complain of morning stiffness or stiffness after sitting and have difficulty with stair climbing.

Negative   Positive

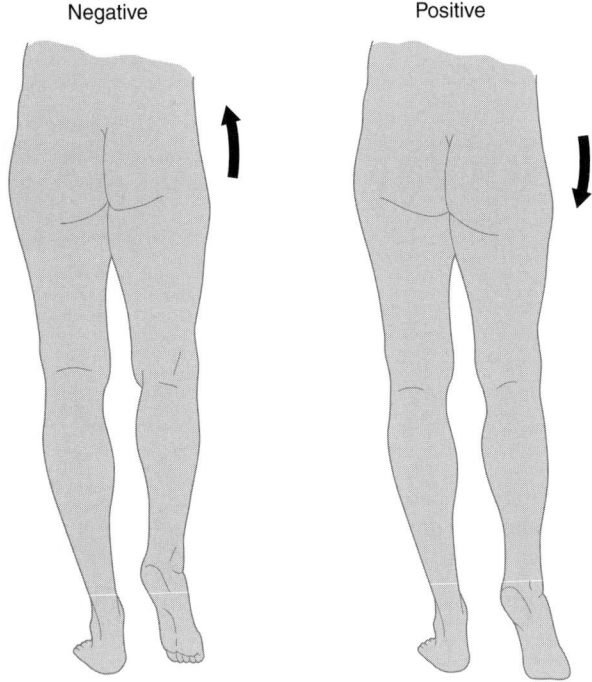

FIGURE 53-1. Trendelenburg sign. (Reprinted with permission from Goldstein B, Chavez F. Applied anatomy of the lower extremities. Phys Med Rehabil State Art Rev 1996;10:601-630.)

PHYSICAL EXAMINATION

Candidates for THA are likely to have antalgic (painful) gait patterns representing a combination of pain that inhibits motion, structural loss of joint motion, and weakness. Hip pain or weakness of the hip abductors results in contralateral pelvic tilt or drop (Trendelenburg sign) with ipsilateral weight bearing (Fig. 53-1).

Passive hip range of motion usually demonstrates significant loss of rotation and moderate loss of abduction and flexion of the involved hip. End ranges of motion are often painful. The manual muscle examination demonstrates mild to moderate weakness of hip flexion, abduction, and extension. Hip weakness is not true weakness but represents a disuse weakness usually associated with pain and decreased mobility. Functionally, it may be difficult for the affected individual to rise from a low seat, to cross the affected leg, and to reach the affected foot. A hip flexion contracture may be observed with the Thomas test (Fig. 53-2), and accentuated lumbar lordosis may be seen in those with a hip flexion contracture, which may result in secondary mechanical low back pain due to alteration of normal spine mechanics. Neurologic examination findings are typically normal, except for hip girdle weakness due to guarding or disuse.

FUNCTIONAL LIMITATIONS

Functional limitations from severe hip disease include difficulty in walking and with all mobility, even rising from a seated position, because of pain and weakness. This may affect a patient's ability to dress, to bathe, to perform household chores, to participate in recreational activities, and to work outside the home.

DIAGNOSTIC STUDIES

Plain radiography remains the primary imaging tool for evaluation of the person with hip disease. On radiographic examination, significant loss of joint cartilage as demonstrated by joint space narrowing, joint incongruity, osteophyte formation, subchondral cysts, and sclerosis

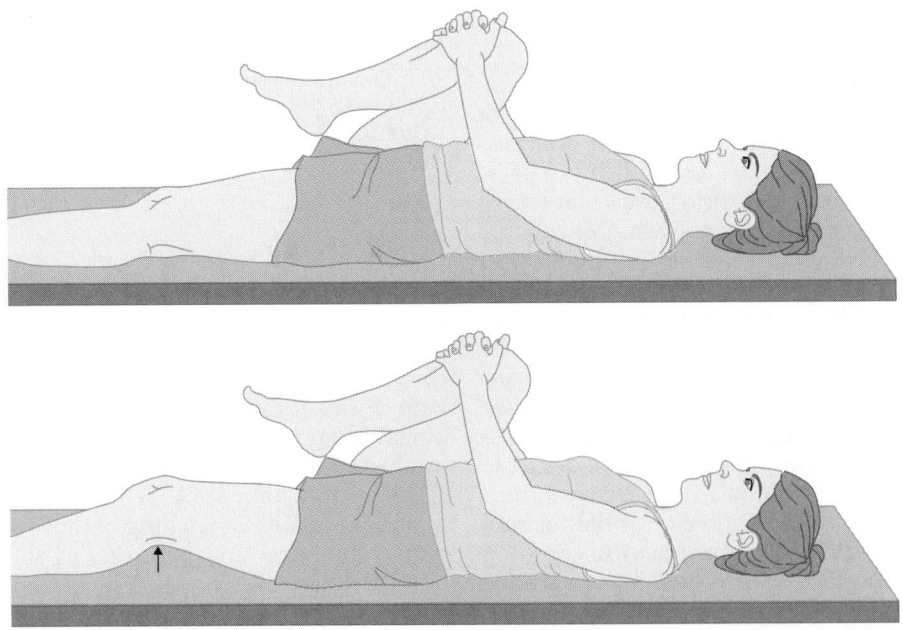

FIGURE 53-2. Thomas test to assess a hip flexion contracture. The patient lies supine while the clinician flexes one of the patient's hips, bringing the knee to the chest to flatten the lumbar spine. The patient holds the flexed knee and hip against the chest. If there is a flexion contracture of the hip, the patient's other leg will rise off the table.

are seen in individuals who are candidates for THA (Fig. 53-3). In patients thought to have a dislocation after THA, radiographs should be obtained urgently because a true dislocation must be relocated expediently (Fig. 53-4). Plain radiographs are also obtained in patients thought to have prosthetic loosening (Fig. 53-5).

On occasion, a bone scan may be needed to rule out an occult femoral neck fracture, infection, or other bone disorder. Magnetic resonance imaging is often useful in assessment for avascular necrosis as the cause of hip pain.[4,5] Postoperative limb swelling should trigger deep venous thrombosis surveillance screening with venous ultrasonography and Doppler wave signal analysis (commonly referred to as duplex scanning). Minor calf clots are observed by repeated study within 7 days to evaluate for propagation.

Laboratory parameters should be monitored for anemia and metabolic abnormalities. Wound cultures are performed only in patients with atypical drainage or erythema at the operative site.

TREATMENT

Initial

On the day of surgery, the patient often receives perioperative prophylactic antibiotics, autologous blood transfusions for blood loss–induced anemia, and pain

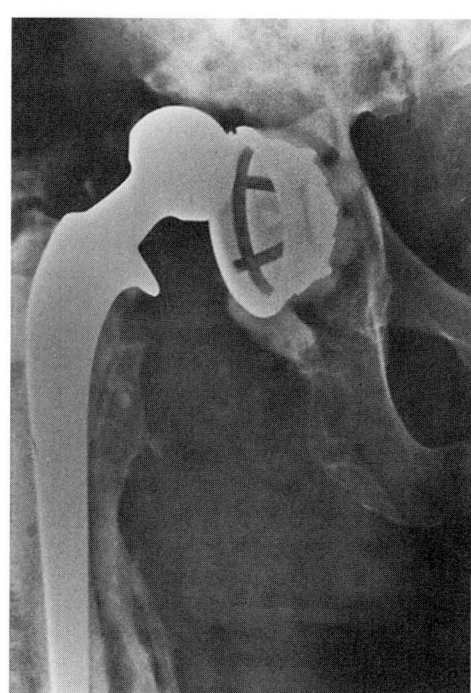

FIGURE 53-4. Total hip replacement—dislocation. The femur has dislocated superiorly and laterally relative to the acetabulum. This dislocation is due to abnormal (vertical) position of the acetabular cup that occurred from loosening (see widened cement-bone interface). (Reprinted with permission from Katz DS, Math KR, Groskin SA. Radiology Secrets. Philadelphia, Hanley & Belfus, 1998:317.)

Differential Diagnosis

Prosthetic loosening

Periprosthetic fracture

Infection

Component failure

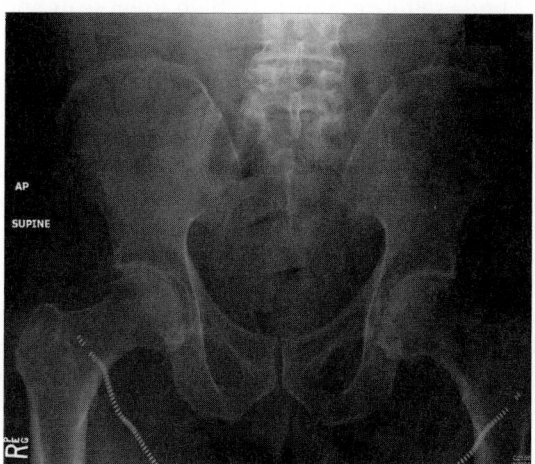

FIGURE 53-3. AP pelvis radiograph showing moderate to severe degenerative changes of the hips. Notice the sclerotic changes at the acetabular and femoral heads. Note the loss of joint space, especially inferiorly, and osteophytes.

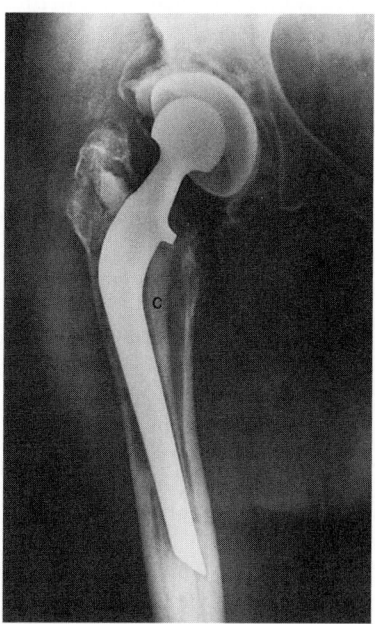

FIGURE 53-5. Total hip replacement—loose femoral component. There is a wide area of lucency between the opaque cement (C) and the adjacent bone at the medial aspect of the proximal femur in addition to the area of lucency at the metal-bone interface surrounding the acetabular prosthesis. These were new findings indicative of loosening of both components. (Reprinted with permission from Katz DS, Math KR, Groskin SA. Radiology Secrets. Philadelphia, Hanley & Belfus, 1998:317.)

control with narcotics (delivered orally, intravenously, or by a patient-controlled analgesia pump). Within 24 hours postoperatively, to prevent deep venous thrombosis, a regimen of pharmacologic treatment (usually a vitamin K antagonist, a low-molecular-weight heparin, or fondaparinux) and mechanical compression with antithrombotic calf pumps begins. If the patient's condition is stable, the patient is ready for discharge from the acute care hospital by the third or fourth postoperative day.[6] By that time, surgical drains have been removed, all perioperative antibiotics have ceased, transfusion therapy has concluded, and the patient-controlled analgesia pump has been discontinued in favor of oral analgesic medications. Outpatient, inpatient, or home rehabilitation typically ensues. Adequate pain management must be continually reevaluated as the patient progresses through postoperative rehabilitation and recovery. Long-acting oral narcotics combined with rescue doses of immediate-release narcotics 30 to 60 minutes before a therapy session work well. Thereafter, non-narcotic analgesics and nonsteroidal anti-inflammatory drugs can be used for pain control if necessary.

Careful attention is given to treatment of anemia because patients with adequate hemoglobin levels generally tolerate activity well and progress in rehabilitation more readily than do those with low hemoglobin levels. Adequate nutrition, iron supplements, vitamins, and, if needed, erythropoietin can be used. Blood transfusions may be necessary if the hemoglobin level continues to drift downward and there is concern of hemodynamic instability or if the patient becomes symptomatic with lightheadedness or delirium. Patients with coronary artery disease should be transfused to a hemoglobin level above 10 g/dL.

It is also essential to monitor for deep venous thrombosis, which can occur at the time of surgery or any time within the first 6 weeks after surgery. The incidence of deep venous thrombosis after total hip implantation without prophylactic anticoagulation is 40% to 70%; the incidence of proximal clot (defined as any thrombosis in the popliteal vein or more proximal) is between 10% and 20%; and the incidence of fatal pulmonary embolism is between 0.5% and 5%.[7-10] Prophylaxis with warfarin (keeping the international normalized ratio between 2 and 3) is ideal. However, many orthopedic surgeons are concerned about bleeding complications and prefer an international normalized ratio of 1.8 to 2.0. Another accepted prophylactic agent is enoxaparin at a dose of 30 mg subcutaneously every 12 hours.[11-13] Propagating calf clots may be treated with full anticoagulation for 6 weeks to 3 months. Major proximal deep venous thrombosis is definitively treated with full anticoagulation for 3 to 6 months.

In the absence of deep venous thrombosis, edema is common after hip arthroplasty from a combination of disruption of local lymphatic drainage around the hip, dissection of blood and fluids through tissue planes, and loss of the local muscle pump due to pain inhibition.

Elevation and compression are the mainstays of treatment. More severe swelling may require transient diuretic therapy and more aggressive compression wraps.

Wound care of the incision line is accomplished with dry sterile dressing changes once or twice a day. Once wound drainage ceases, a dressing is no longer essential. Painting the incision with povidone-iodine (Betadine) provides a drying effect and reduces cutaneous bacterial flora; then a nonstick gauze is applied. Tape burns around the surgical incision are a common problem and are treated with a hydrogel pad such as DuoDerm for approximately 1 week. Serous drainage without signs of erythema or induration is usually commonplace for 3 to 4 days postoperatively, but persistent drainage deserves oral prophylactic antibiotics to prevent secondary infection. Surgical clips are routinely left in place for 12 to 14 days and then removed, at which point the wound is reinforced with Steri-Strips. If the incision develops erythema around the staples, they are removed sooner. More serious wound problems should be communicated to the operative surgeon for collaboration on additional management including cultures, antibiotics, and more invasive intervention if necessary.

Rehabilitation

Hip precautions should be followed and are taught to patients to minimize the possibility of hip dislocation. Patients with weak periarticular tissues, revision surgeries, or previous dislocations are at the highest risk for a dislocation, which is greatest during the first postoperative week. Most surgeons use a posterolateral approach to the hip joint and dislocate the joint by hyperflexion, adduction, and internal rotation. After hip replacement, that combination of movements may increase the risk of dislocation. Therefore, an abduction pillow or wedge is placed between the legs to maintain safe alignment. Patients are taught not to reach forward by flexing at the hip. Alternatively, adaptive equipment such as sock aids, reachers, and dressing sticks are used to perform lower body self-care. Similarly, high toilet seats and tub benches for bathing serve to prevent hip flexion beyond 90 degrees.

A hip dislocation is not subtle and should be suspected if the patient cannot endure weight bearing, the limb is acutely shortened or externally rotated, or the patient is intolerant of gentle hip motion because of excessive pain. A dislocation often results in a significant functional setback as the patient is often more cautious and fearful of performing activities of daily living and mobility training. If an abduction hip brace is ordered to prevent recurrent dislocation, this must be worn at all times and severely restricts motion, mobility, and toileting ability. There is little information in the literature to guide the duration of hip precautions. It is probably wise to enforce strict precautions for 6 weeks.

Rarely, a significant leg length discrepancy ($^3/_4$ inch or more) may require a lift. Most cases result from pelvic obliquity from muscle imbalances or hip contractures (such as adductor tightness) and can be ameliorated with ongoing therapy.[14]

A typical total hip replacement clinical pathway or protocol for inpatient rehabilitation is now a 7- to 10-day program.[15] Most patients successfully complete this pathway, provided there are no major medical complications (Table 53-1). Many published sources outline the benefits as well as the elements of the total hip replacement clinical pathway.[16-18] There is also a shift toward rapid discharge to home from acute care with an outpatient rehabilitation program, especially in the era of minimally invasive surgery.[19] Individuals who undergo THA revision surgery have a more difficult postoperative rehabilitation experience; they often show less progress in functional independence measures, longer rehabilitation length of stay, and greater hospital charges compared with primary hip replacement surgery. These differences in outcomes are even more pronounced if an infected prosthesis is the cause of the revision arthroplasty.[20]

Therapeutic exercises to improve hip and knee mobility and strength begin on the first day of the rehabilitation program and continue daily thereafter. Ankle pumps, heel slides, gluteal squeezes, and quadriceps setting exercises are taught.[21] The therapy staff undertakes daily review of hip precautions, proper bed mobility, and bed transfers. By the third postoperative day, the patient should be able to tolerate 2 to 3 hours of therapy a day unless severe anemia or other medical problems result in further functional limitations. Active-assisted range of motion and strengthening exercises are progressed as tolerated. Strengthening of hip abductors is important, but caution must be taken to avoid overly aggressive abductor strengthening if a trochanteric osteotomy has been performed.

TABLE 53-1 Goals of Rehabilitation after Total Hip Arthroplasty

Successful postoperative pain management

Maintain medical stability

Achieve successful surgical incision healing

Guard against dislocation of the implant

Prevent bed rest hazards (e.g., thrombophlebitis, pulmonary embolism, decubiti, pneumonia)

Obtain pain-free range of motion within precaution limits

Strengthen hip and knee musculature

Gain functional strength

Teach transfers and ambulation with assistive devices

Successful progression to prior living situation

Modified from Cameron H, Brotzman SB, Boolos M. Rehabilitation after total joint arthroplasty. In Brotzman SB, ed. Clinical Orthopaedic Rehabilitation. St. Louis, Mosby, 1996:284-311.

Activities of daily living are assessed, and each individual's unique needs and goals drive the specific, individualized plan of care and treatments given. For instance, a patient may have assistance from a spouse or other family member at home to help don and doff shoes and socks. Therefore, it may not be reasonable or necessary to teach the use of a sock aid or long-handled shoehorn for lower body dressing. Upper and lower body bathing and dressing within hip and weight-bearing precautions are essential components of the rehabilitation program. Appropriate adaptive equipment is provided. Bathroom transfers and kitchen activities are also incorporated into the rehabilitation program. Often, raised toilet seats or commodes and tub transfer benches are helpful and necessary to prevent excessive hip flexion in the sitting position.

Early protected ambulation progresses toward independent mobility as tolerated on the basis of the individual's response and weight-bearing restrictions. Weight-bearing aids (walkers, crutches, armrests) are used during all phases of mobility training. Progressive stair climbing is pursued until the patient is safe with or without standby assistance.

Discharge planning to the next level of care, including durable medical equipment, medical follow-up, and follow-up rehabilitation services (either in the home or in the community), must be communicated to the patient and family.

Most patients should be able to ambulate community distances, initially with a walker or a cane, and then advance to ambulation without an assistive device or return to their presurgical baseline within 4 to 12 weeks after hip arthroplasty. The rate of advancement in gait training is usually limited by the weight-bearing status established at the time of surgery. Most people are able to return to activities such as dancing, low-impact sports, and presurgical exercise regimens within 12 weeks.[22] Elderly, less active patients should also be able to return to their baseline level of function and in many instances progress to higher levels of activity that had been limited by pain before surgery.[23,24] Activities such as cycling, golfing, and bowling after THA should be encouraged, whereas running, jogging, water-skiing, cross-country skiing, football, baseball, handball, hockey, karate, soccer, and racket sports (activities that result in high stress or torque through the femur) should be minimized or avoided.[25,26]

Procedures

Wound care, staple removal, and Steri-Strip application are typically performed after THA.

Surgery

There are three common types of hip arthroplasty components: unipolar endoprosthesis, bipolar endoprosthesis, and true total hip (separate femoral and acetabular) components. The unipolar implant (Moore endoprosthesis or Austin Moore endoprosthesis) is a single, machined metal alloy component comprising a femoral stem, neck, and head. The implant head articulates with native acetabular cartilage. This type of prosthesis often finds use in the minimally mobile elderly patient who sustains an intracapsular (subcapital) displaced femoral neck fracture. The bipolar endoprosthesis includes a polished metal alloy acetabular component that is anatomically matched to the patient's acetabulum to provide surface bearing (Fig. 53-6). Within this large spherical head sits a polyethylene liner into which the femoral component is snap fit. This creates an outer bearing interface between the implant and the native acetabulum and an inner bearing interface between the polyethylene liner and the femoral component. This design principle theoretically reduces motion at the native acetabulum (cartilage-metal interface) by increasing motion within the movable prosthetic parts, thereby reducing stress, wear, or erosion of the acetabular cartilage. It can be used instead of the simpler unipolar (Moore) prosthesis for the same indications. It may also be used for revision arthroplasty. The THA components include a femoral stem (in various sizes and shapes), a femoral neck (in various angles and lengths), a femoral head, and an acetabular shell or cup with a polyethylene liner of various sizes and inclinations (Fig. 53-7). This allows resurfacing of both sides of the hip joint and allows the highest degree of "customization" for each individual. It is the most complex device of the three to insert properly but is used most commonly.

Surgical technique is beyond the scope of this text. However, the rehabilitation will be affected by the two common fixation techniques: cemented and cementless or press fit. In general, the cemented technique is used only on the femoral component. After a cement restrictor plug is placed in the distal femoral canal, polymethyl methacrylate cement is freshly made and inserted into the femoral canal by pressurized cementing technique. Insertion of the femoral stem creates an

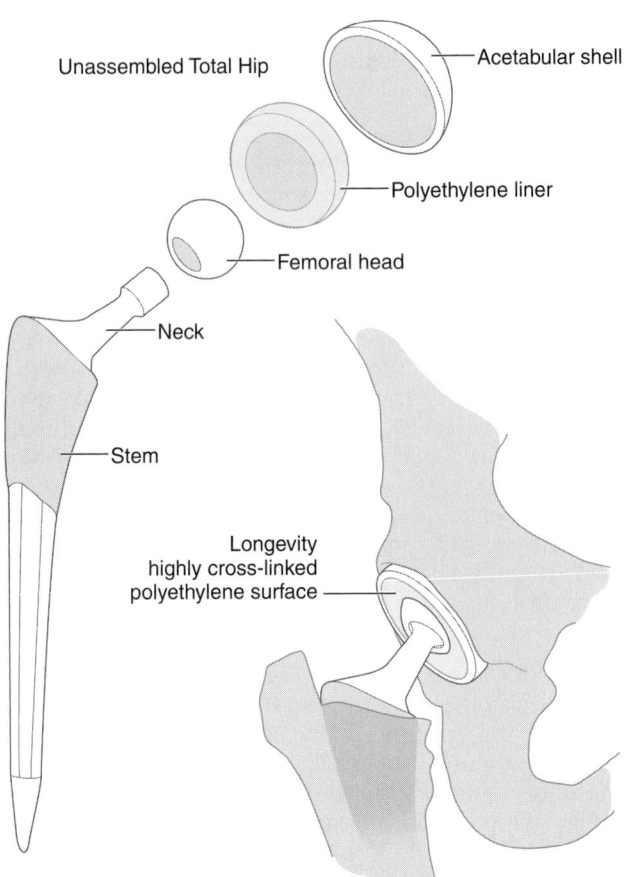

FIGURE 53-7. The components of a total hip replacement.

intimate fit of the prosthesis to the intramedullary canal with a small circumferential cement mantle. Cement polymerization rigidly fixates the femoral component. A press-fit femoral component usually employs porous surface coating to allow bone ingrowth and stability. The press-fit technique is most commonly used in the younger, more active patient. Frequently, the patient with a cemented prosthesis is allowed to bear weight as tolerated immediately, whereas the individual with a noncemented press-fit prosthesis often must wait for 6 to 8 weeks before fully bearing weight to allow stability by bone ingrowth.

In most instances, the acetabular cup is press fit. Porous coating components have given excellent clinical results, whereas nonporous coated acetabular implants have proved unsatisfactory. One or two screws may be placed for added stability. If a trochanteric osteotomy is performed during the surgery, hip abduction resistance exercises are usually restricted.

Two newer THA surgical techniques are now or soon will be available to the younger, more active population.[27,28] The first, often referred to as the mini–hip replacement, is a standard THA done with minimally invasive surgical technique. Requiring two small hip incisions, the surgery causes much less soft tissue and muscle trauma and results in early hospital discharge to home, less blood loss, and quicker return to full

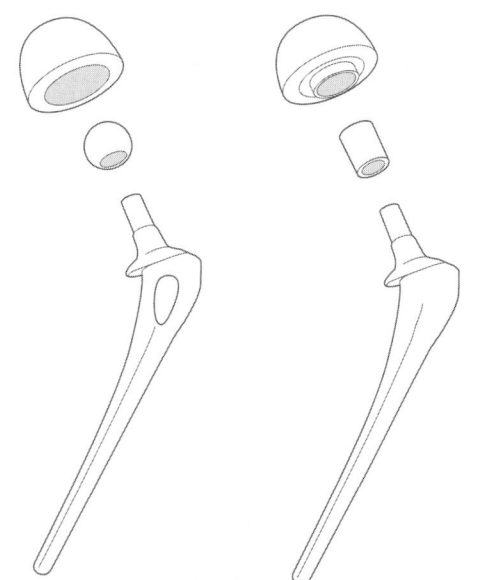

FIGURE 53-6. The components of a bipolar endoprosthesis.

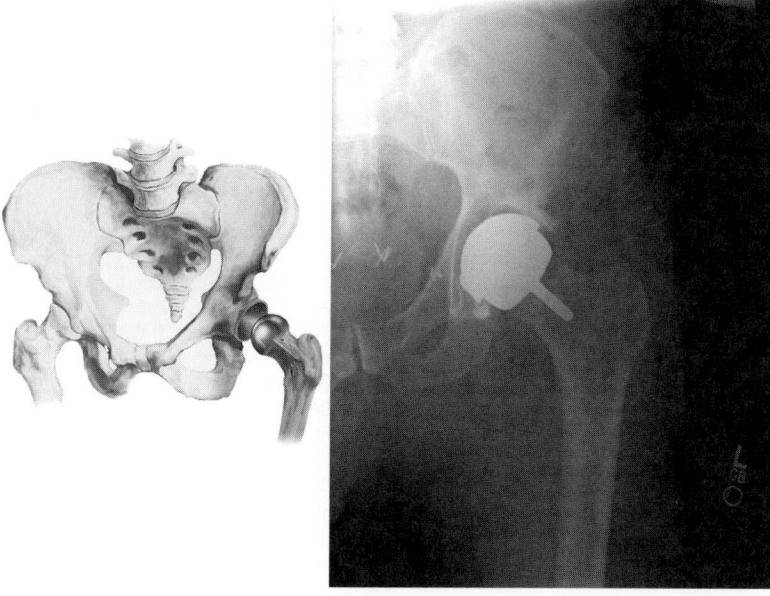

FIGURE 53-8. Birmingham Hip Resurfacing System available from Smith & Nephew.

activities. The second, called the Birmingham Hip Resurfacing System, is designed to resurface the socket and the femoral head with minimal bone removal (Fig. 53-8). It uses a metal on metal construct for end bearing. In addition to activity advantages, it may also increase prosthetic longevity and decrease the risk of perioperative thromboembolic disease.

POTENTIAL DISEASE COMPLICATIONS

Pain and functional limitations, including gait deviations and demonstrable hip girdle weakness, may persist past the immediate postoperative period (12 weeks). A body of literature suggests that many individuals can benefit from longer rehabilitation programs that address those impairments.[29,30] The short-term prognosis for modern cemented or uncemented THA is excellent.[31,32] The long-term prognosis remains good to excellent in most cases.[33,34] A general rule of thumb suggests that a total hip implant should last 10 to 15 years. Lower levels of daily activity often result in an extended life expectancy of the prosthetic components, whereas increased activity may lead to earlier wear and loosening.

Common physical impairments after THA include decreased muscle strength, limited hip range of motion, limited flexibility, and abnormalities of gait. Hip joint weakness has been shown to persist at 2 years after surgery, indicating a need for prolonged exercise. Current data suggest that THA patients continue to experience physical and functional limitations lasting at least 1 year postoperatively. Therefore, it is reasonable to have patients continue with therapeutic exercises to address these limitations well beyond the early recovery period (first 12 weeks).[35,36]

POTENTIAL TREATMENT COMPLICATIONS

Late prosthetic hip infection by a hematogenous source can be a serious complication, often requiring extensive hospitalization, intravenous administration of antibiotics, and explantation of the hardware. Eventual reimplantation is done after the infection is eradicated. Therefore, prophylactic antibiotics (with use of the guidelines for endocarditis prophylaxis) are essential when a THA patient has dental work or any other invasive procedure (e.g., colonoscopy). Overly aggressive anticoagulation can lead to hemorrhage. Analgesics can lead to constipation and dependency. Nonsteroidal anti-inflammatory drugs have well-known side effects inclusive of increased cardiovascular morbidity and thus must be used cautiously and only for a short duration. The surgical treatment itself can lead to iatrogenic problems, such as postoperative wound infections, deep venous thrombosis, or nerve injury. Significant limb length discrepancy may lead to awkward gait or tripping.

References

1. Ethgen O, Bruyere O, Richy F, et al. Health-related quality of life in total hip and total knee arthroplasty. J Bone Joint Surg Am 2004;86:963-974.
2. Data obtained from U.S. Department of Health and Human Services Centers for Disease Control and Prevention; National Center for Health Statistics.
3. Mancuso CA, Ranawat CS, Esdaile JM, et al. Indications for total hip and total knee arthroplasties: results of orthopaedic surveys. J Arthroplasty 1996;11:34-46.
4. Khanna AJ, Yoon TR, Mont MA, et al. Femoral head osteonecrosis: detection and grading by using a rapid MR imaging protocol. Radiology 2000;217:188-192.
5. Koo KH, Ahn IO, Kim R, et al. Bone marrow edema and associated pain in early stage osteonecrosis of the femoral head: prospective study with serial MR images. Radiology 1999;213:715-722.

6. Munnin MC, Ruby TE, Glynn NW, et al. Early inpatient rehabilitation after elective hip and knee arthroplasty. JAMA 1998;279;847-852.

7. Turpie AG, Levine MN, Hirsh J, et al. A randomized controlled trial of a low-molecular-weight heparin (enoxaparin) to prevent deep-venous thrombosis in patients undergoing elective hip surgery. N Engl J Med 1986;315:925-929.

8. Lieberman JR, Geerts WH. Prevention of venous thromboembolism after total hip and knee arthroplasty. J Bone Joint Surg Am 1994;76:1239-1250.

9. Merli GJ. Deep vein thrombosis and pulmonary embolism prophylaxis in orthopedic surgery. Med Clin North Am 1993;77:397-411.

10. Geerts WH, Pineo GF, Heit JA, et al. Prevention of venous thromboembolism: the Seventh ACCP Conference on Antithrombotic and Thrombolytic Therapy. Chest 2004;126(suppl):338-400.

11. Levine MN, Hirsh J, Gent M, et al. Prevention of deep vein thrombosis after elective hip surgery. Ann Intern Med 1991;114:545-551.

12. Spiro TE, Johnson GJ, Christie MJ, et al. Efficacy and safety of enoxaparin to prevent deep venous thrombosis after hip replacement surgery. Ann Intern Med 1994;121:81-87.

13. Lieberman JR, Hsu WK. Prevention of venous thromboembolic disease after total hip and knee arthroplasty [Current Concepts Review]. J Bone Joint Surg Am 2005;87:2097-2112.

14. Edeen J, Sharkey PF, Alexander AH. Clinical significance of leg-length inequality after total hip arthroplasty. Am J Orthop 1995;24:347-351.

15. Wang A, Hall S, Gilbey H, Ackland T. Patient variability and the design of clinical pathways after primary total hip replacement surgery. J Qual Clin Pract 1997;17:123-129.

16. Clinical Pathways for Medical Rehabilitation. Aspen Reference Group. Gaithersburg, Md, Aspen, 1998.

17. Cameron H, Brotzman SB, Boolos M. Rehabilitation after total joint arthroplasty. In Brotzman SB, ed. Clinical Orthopaedic Rehabilitation. St. Louis, Mosby, 1996:284-311.

18. Dowsey MM, Kilgour ML, Santamaria NM, Choong PF. Clinical pathways in hip and knee arthroplasty: a prospective randomized controlled study. Med J Aust 1999;170:59-62.

19. Oldmeadow LB, McBurney H, Robertson VJ, et al. Targeted postoperative care improves discharge outcome after hip or knee arthroplasty. Arch Phys Med Rehabil 2004;85:1424-1427.

20. Vincent KR, Vincent HK, Lee LW, et al. Outcomes after inpatient rehabilitation of primary and revision total hip arthroplasty. Arch Phys Med Rehabil 2006;87:1026-1032.

21. Bitar AA, Kaplan RJ, Stitik TP, et al. Rehabilitation of orthopedic and rheumatologic disorders. 3. Total hip arthroplasty rehabilitation. Arch Phys Med Rehabil 2005;86(Suppl 1):S56-S60.

22. Mont MA, LaPorte DM, Mullick T, et al. Tennis after total hip arthroplasty. Am J Sports Med 1999;27:60-64.

23. Brander VA, Malhotra S, Jet J, et al. Outcome of hip and knee arthroplasty in persons aged 80 years and older. Clin Orthop Relat Res 1997;345:67-78.

24. Gogia PP, Christensen CM, Schmidt C. Total hip replacement in patients with osteoarthritis of the hip: improvement in pain and functional status. Orthopedics 1994;17:145-150.

25. McGrory BJ, Stuart MJ, Sim FH. Participation in sports after hip and knee arthroplasty: review of literature and survey of surgeon preferences. Mayo Clin Proc 1995;70:342-348.

26. Yun AG. Sports after total hip replacement. Clin Sports Med 2006;25:359-364.

27. Berger RA, Jacobs JJ, Meneghini RM, et al. Rapid rehabilitation and recovery with minimally invasive total hip arthroplasty. Clin Orthop Relat Res 2004;429:239-247.

28. Berger RA, Dorr LD. Minimally invasive total hip arthroplasty. In Barrack RL, ed. American Academy of Orthopaedic Surgeons Orthopaedic Knowledge Update. Hip and Knee Reconstruction, 3rd ed. Rosemont, Ill, American Academy of Orthopaedic Surgeons, 2006:427-438.

29. Braeker AM, Lochhaas-Gerlach JA, Gollish JD, et al. Determinants of 6-12 month postoperative functional status and pain after elective total hip replacement. Int J Qual Health Care 1997;9:413-418.

30. Shih C, Du Y, Lin Y, Wu C. Muscular recovery around the hip joint after total hip arthroplasty. Clin Orthop Relat Res 1994;302:115-120.

31. Towheed TE, Hochberg MC. Health related quality of life after total hip replacement. Semin Arthritis Rheum 1996;26:483-491.

32. Aarons H, Hall G, Hughes S, Salmon P. Short-term recovery from hip and knee arthroplasty. J Bone Joint Surg Br 1996;78:555-558.

33. Rissanen P, Aro S, Sintonen H, et al. Quality of life and functional ability in hip and knee replacements: a prospective study. Qual Life Res 1996;5:56-64.

34. Lieberman JR, Dorey F, Shekelle P, et al. Differences between patients' and physicians' evaluations of outcome after total hip arthroplasty. J Bone Joint Surg Am 1996;78:835-838.

35. Long WT, Dorr LD, Healy B, Perry J. Functional recovery of noncemented total hip arthroplasty. Clin Orthop Relat Res 1993;228:73-77.

36. Brander VA, Stulberg SD, Chang RW. Rehabilitation following hip and knee arthroplasty. Phys Med Rehabil Clin North Am 1994;5:815-836.

Trochanteric Bursitis 54

Michael Fredericson, MD, and Kelvin Chew, MD

DEFINITION

Trochanteric bursitis is a common cause of pain over the lateral aspect of the hip. Its peak incidence is between the fourth and sixth decades of life; it occurs four times more frequently in women than in men, which may be due to gender differences in lower limb biomechanics.[1,2] It may be associated with trauma after contusions from falls, but it is often due to repetitive microtrauma to the soft tissue structures around the greater trochanter of the femur.[3] It has been suggested that gluteal tendon degeneration and tears at the greater trochanter attachment induce inflammation in the bursae.[4] Trochanteric bursitis is also seen after hip surgery, especially in osteotomies, as a result of either the subcutaneous position of the implant on the greater trochanter or postoperative hip abductor weakness.[5] Less common causes are infection[6,7] and rheumatoid arthritis.[8] Other contributing factors include hip abductor–external rotator weakness from other causes, hip osteoarthritis, lumbar spondylosis, obesity, leg length discrepancies, and iliotibial band tightness.[9] Alteration of gait pattern due to back pain may also be a cause.

Three main bursae surround the greater trochanter of the femur: the subgluteal maximus, medius, and minimus bursae.[10] Figure 54-1 illustrates the bursae around the greater trochanter of the femur. The subgluteus maximus bursa is the largest bursa that lies lateral to the greater trochanter and beneath the gluteus maximus and iliotibial tract. The subgluteal medius bursa lies deep beneath the gluteus medius tendon and posterosuperior to the lateral facet of the greater trochanter. The subgluteus minimus bursa lies beneath the gluteus minimus tendon at the anterosuperior edge of the greater trochanter. The subgluteus maximus bursa is most often involved in trochanteric bursitis, but the other deeper bursae can also give rise to symptoms.[4]

SYMPTOMS

The main presentation of trochanteric bursitis is pain at the greater trochanteric region, usually overlying the subgluteus maximus bursa over the lateral aspect of the hip. The pain can radiate down the lateral aspect of the thigh but seldom extends beyond the knee. There may be associated paresthesia that does not follow any specific dermatomal segment. The symptoms are exacerbated by hip movements, in particular external rotation and abduction. Pain also may be brought on by walking, running, and other weight-bearing activities as well as by prolonged standing. Sleep may be affected because pain is aggravated by lying in the lateral decubitus position on the affected bursa; pain on the contralateral side in the decubitus position could be due to hip adduction.

PHYSICAL EXAMINATION

A localized area of tenderness is found on palpation at the region of the greater trochanter, with maximal tenderness typically at the site of insertion of the gluteal medius at the greater trochanter. Bursal swelling may be difficult to palpate, but bruising may be seen with recent trauma. The Trendelenburg sign has been found to be a sensitive test for trochanteric bursitis.[11] The sign is present when excessive pelvic tilt occurs with the patient in single-leg stance or when walking as illustrated in Figure 54-2. The gluteus medius and minimus form the abductor apparatus that plays an important role in hip abduction and stabilization of the pelvis during gait.[12] In weight bearing on the affected hip, the abductor apparatus is unable to stabilize the pelvis; thus, the contralateral hip drops.[13] Balance is often maintained by shifting the trunk to the affected side.

Symptoms also may be reproduced with resisted hip abduction, with the patient in a side-lying position and the hip at 45 degrees of abduction. Pain can also be elicited with resisted hip internal rotation, with the patient

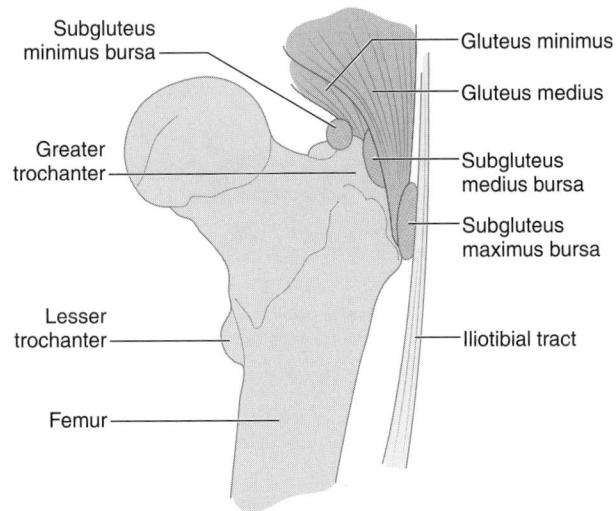

FIGURE 54-1. Diagram of bursae around the greater trochanter of the femur.

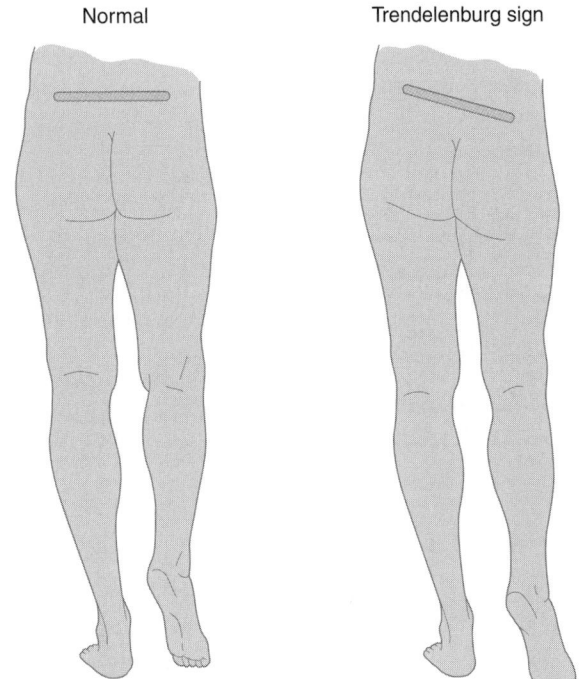

FIGURE 54-2. Trendelenburg sign. The pelvis tilts and collapses toward the normal side of the hip, with single-leg stance on the affected side.

in a supine position and the hip starting at 45 degrees of flexion and maximal external rotation.

Activity-related pain, particularly in the anterior hip or groin, along with limited range of motion of the hip is indicative more often of an intra-articular hip pathologic process, such as osteoarthritis. Lumbosacral radiculopathy should be ruled out with a detailed neurologic examination, which is typically normal with trochanteric bursitis. Examination for and potential discovery of associated conditions (e.g., leg length discrepancies,

hip muscle weakness, arthritis, and lumbar spondylosis) may affect treatment decisions.

FUNCTIONAL LIMITATIONS

Chronic pain can limit activity and cause muscle deconditioning and associated weakness. This can affect the basic activities of daily life, including walking and stair climbing. Pain may occur on lying in the lateral decubitus position on the affected side and may interrupt sleep.

DIAGNOSTIC STUDIES

Laboratory studies, although seldom required, may detect suspected infection or connective tissue disease. Imaging studies are used mainly to exclude associated musculoskeletal conditions as well as other underlying diseases; there are no specific radiologic findings for trochanteric bursitis.

Calcifications around the greater trochanter may be seen in radiographs of the hip; however, it is unclear whether these calcifications occur in the bursa or at the tendon insertion of the gluteus muscles.[14] In patients with leg length discrepancy, pelvic tilting may be seen with a standing anteroposterior pelvis film. Ultrasonography over the lateral aspect of the affected hip may demonstrate well-defined fluid collection consistent with bursal enlargement.[15] Multiple fibrin-coated lesions within the enlarged bursa have also been demonstrated.[16] Bone scan may demonstrate increased linear uptake at the greater trochanter in the early blood pool phase and delayed images.[14,17]

Magnetic resonance imaging may show high signal intensity within a distended bursa on fluid-sensitive sequences and may demonstrate thickening and irregularity of the synovial lining.[18] Subgluteal bursal distention with associated gluteus medius and minimus tendinopathy is well demonstrated with magnetic resonance imaging.[19,20]

Differential Diagnosis

Osteoarthritis of the hip

Lumbosacral radiculopathy

Leg length discrepancy

Gluteal tendinopathy and tear

Avascular necrosis of the femoral head

Iliotibial band syndrome

Hip stress fractures

Tumors

TREATMENT

Initial

Initial treatment entails ice, anti-inflammatory medications, and activity modification, such as avoidance of stair climbing. Direct pressure on the affected site must be avoided; as such, advice on bed positioning should be given. Weight loss is advised in obese individuals. Gentle stretching is encouraged but with avoidance of excessive hip range of motion in the initial phase.

Rehabilitation

Physical therapy entails a combination of strengthening and stretching modalities and correction of abnormal biomechanics. Strengthening exercises should focus particularly on the hip abductors, extensors, and external rotators. Myofascial soft tissue therapy and contraction-relaxation exercises to lengthen shortened muscle groups are also advocated, especially for the tensor fascia lata–iliotibial band complex.

Ice massage and iontophoresis may be useful at the outset of the injury. Thereafter, heat, phonophoresis, and therapeutic ultrasound may be used during the subacute to chronic phases (but avoided during the acute phase of the disease).

Biomechanical evaluation of any leg length discrepancies or underlying gait abnormalities should be performed. Correction of these may be facilitated through orthotics or lifts. Other assistive devices, such as canes and walkers, may be prescribed, depending on the severity of injury.

Procedures

Corticosteroid injections of the bursa, usually combined with local anesthetic, are effective in the comprehensive treatment of this condition.[21,22] In preparation for this procedure, the patient lies in the supine or lateral decubitus position on the unaffected side. The tender area over the greater trochanter is identified and marked. Then, under sterile conditions, a syringe with a 22- or 25-gauge needle, containing triamcinolone (20 to 40 mg) with 1% lidocaine (3 to 4 mL), is advanced until contact is made with the bone of the greater trochanter. The solution is introduced after a lack of resistance is detected. This procedure also may be carried out in two stages with introduction of lidocaine before the steroid. It has been shown that fluoroscopic guidance may enhance precision of the placement of the cortisone injections.[23] In general, a series of no more than three injections spaced 6 weeks apart can be given. However, caution must be exercised with repeated injection because it may be associated with muscle and tendon weakening.[24] Patients are reevaluated within a month to assess therapeutic response.

Surgery

In refractory cases, surgery (including arthroscopic bursectomy[25] and tendon release[26,27]) may be considered. In patients with associated gluteal tendon tears, surgical débridement and repair may be necessary.[28]

POTENTIAL DISEASE COMPLICATIONS

The disease may progress to persistent pain and a myofascial pain syndrome, which can affect mobility and result in subsequent muscle deconditioning and associated hip weakness. Particularly in elderly persons, catastrophic injury may result from falls.

POTENTIAL TREATMENT COMPLICATIONS

Complications due to anti-inflammatory medications include drug hypersensitivity, gastric ulceration, and hepatotoxicity. Heat modalities may cause burns and may aggravate the condition during the acute phase.

General complications from injections include bleeding, bruising, infection, and drug hypersensitivity reactions. With cortisone injections to the greater trochanter, necrotizing fasciitis has been reported.[29] Other complications with steroid injections are tendon ruptures, nerve injury, lipoatrophy, and skin depigmentation.[30]

References

1. Butcher JD, Salzman KL, Lillegard WA. Lower extremity bursitis. Am Fam Physician 1996;53:2317-2324.
2. Ferber R, Davis IM, Williams DS. Gender differences in lower extremity mechanics during running. Clin Biomech (Bristol, Avon) 2003;18:350-379.
3. Haller CC, Coleman PA, Estes NC, Grisolia A. Traumatic trochanteric bursitis. Kans Med 1989;90:17-18, 22.
4. Dunn T, Heller CA, McCarthy SW, Dos Remedios C. Anatomical study of the "trochanteric bursa." Clin Anat 2003;16:233-240.
5. Glassman AH. Complications of trochanteric osteotomy. Orthop Clin North Am 1992;23:321-333.
6. Jaovisidha S, Chen C, Ryu KN, et al. Tuberculous tenosynovitis and bursitis: imaging findings in 21 cases. Radiology 1996;201:507-513.
7. Yamamoto T, Iwasaki Y, Kurosaka M. Tuberculosis of the greater trochanteric bursa occurring 51 years after tuberculous nephritis. Clin Rheumatol 2002;21:397-400.
8. Tanaka H, Kido K, Wakisaka A, et al. Trochanteric bursitis in rheumatoid arthritis. J Rheumatol 2002;29:1340-1341.
9. Shbeeb ML, Matteson EL. Trochanteric bursitis (greater trochanteric pain syndrome). Mayo Clin Proc 1996;71:565-569.
10. Bencardino JT, Palmer WE. Imaging of hip disorders in athletes. Radiol Clin North Am 2002;40:267-287.
11. Bird PA, Oakley SP, Shnier R. Prospective evaluation of magnetic resonance imaging and physical examination findings in patients with greater trochanteric pain syndrome. Arthritis Rheum 2001;44:2138-2145.
12. Kumagai M, Shiba N, Nishimara H, Inoue A. Functional evaluation of hip abductor muscles with use of magnetic resonance imaging. J Orthop Res 1997;15:888-893.
13. Hardcastle P, Nade S. The significance of the Trendelenburg test. J Bone Joint Surg Br 1985;67:741-746.
14. Caruso FA, Toney MA. Trochanteric bursitis: a case report of plain film, scintigraphic and MRI correlation. Clin Nucl Med 1994;19:393-395.

15. Chhem R, Cardinal E, Aubin B. Adult hip. In Chhem R, Cardinal E, eds. Guidelines and Gamuts in Musculoskeletal Ultrasound. New York, Wiley, 1999:125-160.

16. Huang CC, Ko SF, Weng LH, et al. Sonographic demonstration of hyperechoic fibrin coating of rice bodies in trochanteric bursitis: the "fried rice" pattern. J Ultrasound Med 2006;25:667-670.

17. Allwright SJ, Cooper RA, Nash P. Trochanteric bursitis: bone scan appearance. Clin Nucl Med 1988;13:561-564.

18. Dwek J, Pfirrmann C, Stanley A, et al. MR imaging of the hip abductors: normal anatomy and commonly encountered pathology at the greater trochanter. Magn Reson Imaging Clin North Am 2005;13:691-704.

19. Kingzett-Taylor A, Tirman PF, Feller J, et al. Tendinosis and tears of the gluteus medius and minimus muscles as a cause of hip pain. Am J Roentgenol 1999;173:1123-1126.

20. Walsh G, Archibald CG. MRI in greater trochanter pain syndrome. Australas Radiol 2003;47:85-87.

21. Shbeeb MI, O'Duffy JD, Michet CJ Jr, et al. Evaluation of glucocorticosteroid injection for the treatment of trochanteric bursitis. J Rheumatol 1996;23:2104-2106.

22. Lievense A, Bierma-Zeinstra S, Schouten B, et al. Prognosis of trochanteric pain in primary care. Br J Gen Pract 2005;55:199-204.

23. Cohen SP, Narvaez JC, Lebovits AH, Stojanovic MP. Corticosteroid injections for trochanteric bursitis: is fluoroscopy necessary? A pilot study. Br J Anaesth 2005;94:100-106.

24. Speed CA. Fortnightly review; corticosteroid injections in tendon lesions. BMJ 2001;323:382-386.

25. Fox JL. The role of arthroscopic bursectomy in the treatment of trochanteric bursitis. Arthroscopy 2002;18:E34.

26. Slawski DP, Howard RF. Surgical management of refractory trochanteric bursitis. Am J Sports Med 1997;25:86-89.

27. Bradley DM, Dillingham MF. Bursoscopy of the trochanteric bursa. Arthroscopy 1998;14:884-887.

28. Kagan A 2nd. Rotator cuff tears of the hip. Clin Orthop Relat Res 1999;368:135-140.

29. Hofmeister E, Engelhardt S. Necrotizing fasciitis as complication of injection into greater trochanteric bursa. Am J Orthop 2001;30:426-427.

30. Basford JR. Physical agents. In Delisa JA, Gans BM, eds. Rehabilitation Medicine: Principles and Practice. Philadelphia, Lippincott-Raven, 1993:973-995.

Anterior Cruciate Ligament Tear 55

Eduardo Amy, MD, and William Micheo, MD

Synonyms

Anterior cruciate ligament (ACL) tear
ACL sprain
ACL-deficient knee

ICD-9 Codes

717.83 Old disruption of anterior cruciate ligament
844.2 Cruciate injury, acute

DEFINITION

The anterior cruciate ligament (ACL) is an intra-articular structure essential for the normal function of the knee. It is commonly injured during activities that involve complex movements, such as cutting and pivoting. It is estimated than one in 3000 individuals sustains an ACL injury each year in the United States, corresponding to an overall injury rate of approximately 100,000 injuries annually.[1] The injury usually results from a sudden deceleration during high-velocity movements in which a forceful contraction of the quadriceps muscle is required. Other mechanisms of injury are valgus stress, hyperextension, and external rotation, as in landing from a jump, and severe internal rotation of the knee with varus or hyperextension.[1] It has been reported that 70% of the acute ACL injuries are sports related and affect women more than men, particularly in basketball and soccer.[2] In the last two decades, there has also been an increase in the incidence and appropriate diagnosis of ACL injuries in children associated with more participation in high-demand contact and noncontact sports, increased awareness of the injury, and better imaging techniques.[3] Risk factors associated with ACL injuries include generalized joint laxity, anatomic differences between men and women, hormonal changes, training techniques, and biomechanical variations in landing from a jump or cutting.[4]

The ACL may be partially or completely torn. It also may be injured in combination with other structures, most commonly tears of the medial collateral ligament and medial meniscus.

The ACL is a collagenous structure approximately 38 mm in length and 10 mm in width. The ligament arises from a wide base in the tibia anterolateral to the anterior tibial spine. It then traverses the knee in a posterolateral direction, attaching in a broad fan-like fashion at the posterolateral corner of the intercondylar notch of the femur. According to Fu and collaborators, it is organized in two major bundles named after their insertion sites on the tibia.[5] The anteromedial bundle, which tightens in flexion and is the longer of the two, controls anterior translation of the tibia on the femur. The posterolateral bundle, which tightens in extension and internal rotation, controls rotation.[6-8]

Biomechanical studies with use of cadaver specimens have evaluated the forces that affect the ACL.[9] These forces are highest in the last 30 degrees of extension, in hyperextension, and under other load conditions, including anterior tibial translation, internal rotation, and varus. The ACL is a static stabilizer of the knee with a primary function of resisting hyperextension and anterior tibial translation in flexion and providing rotatory control. It is also a secondary restraint to valgus and varus forces in all degrees of flexion.

SYMPTOMS

Individuals usually present with pain, immediate swelling, and limited range of motion. They may give a history of hearing a "pop." In an acute injury, the individual will have severe pain and difficulty with walking. In a chronic injury, a patient may have a history of recurrent episodes of knee instability associated with swelling and limited motion. Patients may describe locking or a "giving way" phenomenon. They may also give a history of a remote injury to the knee that was not rehabilitated.

PHYSICAL EXAMINATION

The physical examination has been found to be sensitive and specific in the diagnosis of ACL tears and correlates with arthroscopically documented knee injuries.[10] The clinician should observe the knee for asymmetry, palpate for areas of tenderness, measure active and passive range of motion, and document muscle atrophy. The apprehension test to rule out

307

patellar instability, valgus and varus testing with the knee in full extension and 30 degrees of flexion to evaluate the collateral ligaments, and joint line palpation as well as the McMurray test to evaluate the meniscus should be performed before the ACL is assessed.

The key test in evaluating the integrity of the ACL in the patient with an acute injury is the Lachman test, in which an anterior force is applied to the tibia with the knee in 30 degrees of flexion while the clinician tries to reproduce anterior migration of the tibia on the femur. Another important test in the acute setting is the lateral pivot shift maneuver, in which the examiner attempts to reproduce anterolateral instability by internally rotating the leg, applying a valgus stress to the knee as it is flexed, and feeling for anterior migration of the tibia on the femur (Fig. 55-1). In the patient who is able to flex the knee to 90 degrees, particularly in chronic or recurrent injury, the anterior drawer test, in which an anterior force is applied

to the tibia, should be performed (Fig. 55-2). It is important to complete the examination by performing the posterior drawer test, which evaluates the posterior cruciate ligament; a torn posterior cruciate ligament with posterior tibial subluxation may give a false-positive result of the anterior drawer maneuver as the tibia is reduced. In general, findings should be normal on the neurologic examination, including muscle strength, sensation, and reflexes; however, there may be some associated weakness (particularly of the knee extensors) due to pain or disuse.

FUNCTIONAL LIMITATIONS

Limitations include reduced knee motion, muscle weakness, and pain that interferes with activities involving pivoting and jumping. Recurrent episodes of instability may limit participation in strenuous sports, such as basketball, soccer, tennis, and volleyball.[11,12] These episodes

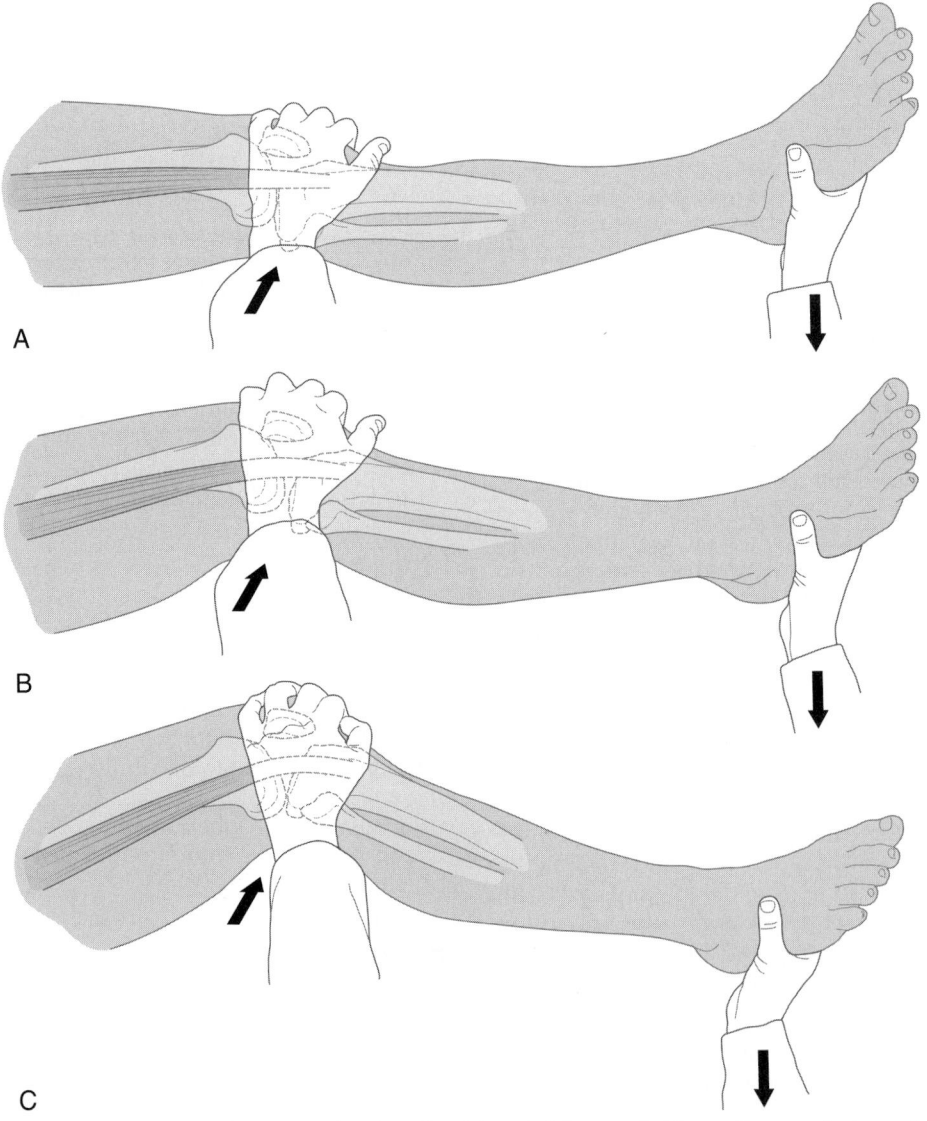

FIGURE 55-1. Position for the lateral pivot shift test. Note that the patient's knee is fully extended. Internally rotate the leg and apply a valgus stress. As you begin to flex the knee, the lateral tibial plateau is subluxed. As tension in the iliotibial band is lessened at 45 degrees of flexion, a pivot shift is felt as the tibia is reduced. This test identifies a rupture of the anterior cruciate ligament.

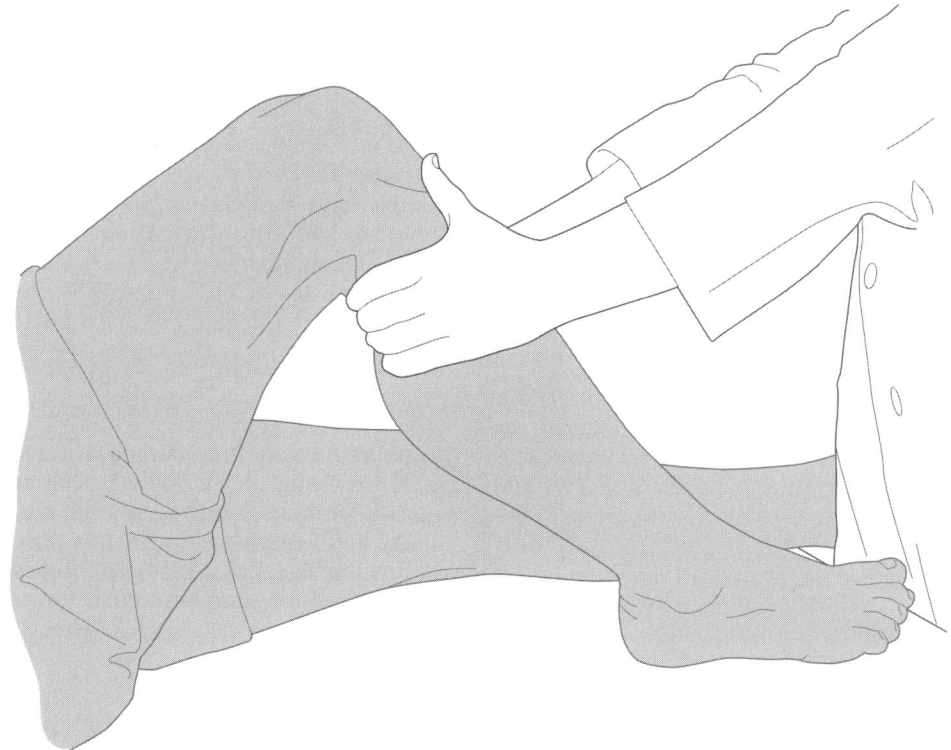

FIGURE 55-2. Position for the anterior drawer test. The hip is flexed 45 degrees, the knee is flexed 90 degrees, and the tibia is in neutral rotation. Anterior pull can be applied to the proximal tibia with both hands.

of the knee's giving way may result in increased ligamentous laxity, leading to limitations with activities of daily living, such as going down stairs and changing directions while walking.

DIAGNOSTIC STUDIES

Diagnostic studies include plain radiographs to rule out intra-articular fractures, loose bodies, and arthritic changes. These include the standing anteroposterior view, lateral view, tunnel view, standing posteroanterior 45-degree flexion view, and Merchant view of the patella. Magnetic resonance imaging may be indicated in the acute setting to evaluate associated pathologic changes, such as bone bruises, meniscal tears, and other ligamentous injuries, and to aid in treatment planning of combined injuries. In the pediatric and adolescent athlete, magnetic resonance imaging may also give information about physical injuries that may otherwise go unnoticed.

TREATMENT

Initial

Immediately after injury, the management of an ACL tear includes relative rest, ice, compression, elevation, and analgesic or anti-inflammatory medication. Many patients will initially benefit from use of a knee immobilizer and crutches. If the knee is very swollen and painful with limited motion that restricts participation in treatment, arthrocentesis may be performed. It is

Differential Diagnosis

Isolated ACL tear

Combined lesions

       Posterolateral ligamentous complex tear

       Medial collateral ligament and medial meniscus

Intra-articular fracture

Patellar dislocation

Meniscal tear

important to establish an accurate diagnosis and the presence of associated injuries as these may necessitate prompt surgery. These include chondral or osteochondral fractures, meniscal tears, and other injured capsular structures. In general, in the absence of associated injuries, the acute management can be conservative with early protected rehabilitation.

Treatment of ACL injuries depends on a number of factors, including the patient's age, level of activity, presence of associated injuries, and importance of returning to athletic activities that involve acceleration and deceleration and cutting moves. Surgery is the only definitive treatment of complete ACL injuries, but it is generally not necessary for older individuals who do not complain of knee instability with recreational activities or work.

In general, younger patients and those with a high activity level should be considered for ACL reconstruction. Surgical referral is not necessary in the immediate postinjury period but should be facilitated as soon as it is clear that an individual desires surgery as a definite treatment measure. When associated injuries are present, especially if these cause mechanical symptoms, or in the case of the elite competitive athlete, surgical treatment should be considered as soon as the initial inflammatory phase has passed.[13]

Rehabilitation

The rehabilitation of an ACL tear begins as soon as the injury occurs. Rehabilitation management focuses on reducing pain, restoring full motion, correcting muscle strength deficits, achieving muscle balance, and returning the patient to full activity free of symptoms.[14] The rehabilitation program consists of acute, recovery, and functional phases.

Anterior Cruciate Ligament Injury

The patient with an ACL-deficient knee that has not been reconstructed may present with an acute or a recurrent injury. In the acutely injured knee, protection of secondary structures is of paramount importance, and progression of rehabilitation will depend on the extent of damage to other knee structures. Early use of closed kinetic chain exercises, in which the distal segment of the extremity is flexed and the proximal segments are free to move, has allowed functional progression of strengthening. These exercises allow quadriceps strengthening with hamstring muscle co-contraction, which reduces the strain in the ACL and minimizes patellofemoral joint reaction forces (Table 55-1).[14,15]

The individual with a recurrently unstable knee will benefit from a trial of rehabilitation. Correction of muscle weakness and proprioceptive deficits and functional retraining in combination with activity modification could reduce episodes of instability and should be considered before surgery in the individual with low activity levels.

Acute Phase

This phase focuses on treatment of tissue injury, clinical signs, and symptoms. The goal in this stage is to allow tissue healing while reducing pain and inflammation. Reestablishment of nonpainful range of motion, prevention of muscle atrophy, and maintenance of general fitness should be addressed. This phase may last 1 to 2 weeks.

Recovery Phase

This phase focuses on obtaining normal passive and active knee motion, improving knee muscle function, achieving normal hamstrings and quadriceps muscle balance, and working on proprioception. Biomechanical and functional deficits, including inflexibilities and inability to run or jump, should begin to be addressed. This phase may last 2 to 8 weeks after the injury occurs.

Functional Phase

This phase focuses on increasing power and endurance of the lower extremities while improving neuromuscular control. Rehabilitation at this stage works on the entire kinetic chain, addressing specific functional deficits. This program should be continuous with the ultimate goal of prevention of recurrent injury and safe return to competition. The functional phase may last 8 weeks to 6 months after the injury occurs.

If the patient completes a rehabilitation program and is willing to modify the activity level, including the limitation of sports activity that involves cutting and pivoting maneuvers, the functional prognosis for daily living activities is good.[9,16] In this group of patients, functional braces may be used for sports participation that involves

TABLE 55-1 Anterior Cruciate Ligament Tear Rehabilitation

	Acute Phase	Recovery Phase	Functional Phase
Therapeutic intervention	Modalities: cryotherapy, electrical stimulation	Modalities: superficial heat, pulsed ultrasound, electrical stimulation	General flexibility, strengthening training
	Active-assisted flexion and extension	Range of motion, flexibility exercises	Power and endurance of lower extremities: diagonal and multiplanar motions, plyometrics
	Static quadriceps and hamstring exercise	Dynamic lower extremity strengthening	Neuromuscular control, proprioceptive training
	General conditioning: bicycle and pool exercises	Closed kinetic chain exercises, multiplanar lower extremity joint exercises	Return to sports-specific participation with functional bracing
	Ambulation with crutches	General conditioning	
		Gradual return to sports-specific training with functional bracing	
Criteria for advancement	Pain reduction	Full nonpainful motion	No clinical symptoms
	Recovery of pain-free motion	Symmetric quadriceps and hamstring strength	Normal running and jumping mechanics
	Adequate knee muscle control	Correction of inflexibility	Normal kinetic chain integration
	Tolerance for strengthening exercises	Symptom-free progression in a sports-specific program	Completed sports-specific program

changes of direction. These braces may reduce symptoms of instability in individuals who use them and appear to reduce some strain in the ACL in low-demand activities.

Postsurgical Rehabilitation

In the patient who is a candidate for ACL reconstruction, rehabilitation should start before surgery. Reduction of pain and swelling as well as achievement of full range of motion should be attempted before reconstruction. After surgery, rehabilitation should begin on the first postoperative day. Early use of cryotherapy, compression, and elevation has been shown to reduce swelling postoperatively. It is important to achieve full extension and to initiate early active flexion in the first few days after surgery. Weight bearing with crutches is usually started immediately after the operation.[17]

Rapid progression of the rehabilitation program has reduced complications usually associated with ACL knee surgery, which included stiffness, muscle atrophy, muscle weakness, and patellofemoral pain. In the early rehabilitation period, special precautions need to be taken to avoid excessive strain of the reconstructed ligament with terminal (0 to 30 degrees) extension-resisted quadriceps exercises. Early use of closed kinetic chain exercises, such as mini-squats, steps, and leg press, has allowed quadriceps strengthening with tolerable shear forces to the graft[14,15,17] (Table 55-2). Aquatic exercises that allow progressive weight bearing with benefit from the effects of buoyancy can be started as soon as the sutures are removed.

Individuals will vary in the rate in which they achieve full motion, normal strength, normal proprioception, and adequate sports-specific skills. Achievement of these goals should be accomplished before the individual is allowed to return to sports activity. With accelerated rehabilitation programs, patients usually return to activity in 6 months after surgery. These accelerated rehabilitation programs do not lead to an increase in anterior knee laxity compared with nonaccelerated rehabilitation, and both accelerated and nonaccelerated rehabilitation appear to have the same effect in terms of clinical assessment, satisfaction of patients, and functional performance.[18]

Procedures

Knee joint aspiration may be attempted in the first 24 to 48 hours after the injury to document hemarthrosis and to assist in the diagnosis. If the injured individual is not progressing in treatment because of swelling and significant limitation of motion, aspiration may be performed at later stages of treatment for symptom relief. Under sterile conditions, with a 25-gauge, 1-inch sterile disposable needle, infiltrate the skin with a local anesthetic approximately 2 cm proximal and lateral (or medial) to the patella. Follow this injection with a second injection by use of an 18-gauge, 1½-inch needle into the joint capsule. Aspirate any fluid and note the color and consistency. Without withdrawal of the needle, take off the syringe and empty it. Repeat this until all of the fluid is aspirated. Use one hand to compress the suprapatellar area to be sure all of the fluid is out before the procedure is completed.

Postinjection care includes icing of the knee for 15 minutes after the injection and then for 20 minutes two or three times daily for several days.

TABLE 55-2 Postsurgical Anterior Cruciate Ligament Tear Rehabilitation

	Acute Phase	Recovery Phase	Functional Phase
Therapeutic intervention	Modalities: cryotherapy, electrical stimulation Active-assisted flexion, passive extension Static quadriceps (90 to 45 degrees), dynamic hamstrings exercises, straight-leg raise exercises General conditioning: upper extremity ergometer Ambulation with crutches	Modalities: superficial heat, pulsed ultrasound, electrical stimulation Active flexion and extension exercises Dynamic quadriceps (90 to 30 degrees), hamstring strengthening Closed kinetic chain exercises, multiplanar lower extremity joint exercises General conditioning: bicycle, swimming, aquatic exercises Gradual return to sports-specific training with optional functional brace use	General flexibility training, strengthening exercise program Power and endurance of lower extremities: diagonal and multiplanar motions with tubings, light weights, medicine balls, plyometrics Neuromuscular control, proprioceptive training Return to sports-specific participation Optional functional brace use
Criteria for advancement	Pain reduction Recovery of 90 degrees of flexion, full extension Adequate knee muscle control Tolerance for strengthening exercises	Full flexion, knee hyperextension Symmetric quadriceps and hamstring strength Symptom-free progression in a sports-specific program	No clinical symptoms Normal running and jumping mechanics Normal kinetic chain integration Completed sports-specific program

Surgery

Surgery is indicated in patients with recurrent episodes of instability in activities of daily living and in active recreational athletes who are symptomatic and do not wish to modify their activities. Surgery is definitely indicated in the high-demand competitive athlete.

The surgical procedure of choice is the arthroscopically assisted autograft by full endoscopic or two-incision techniques, with use of either patellar bone–tendon–bone graft or four strands of hamstring tendon graft. A debate exists between the proponents of each graft source and fixation, and although both seem to be fairly equal in long-term studies, they each have pros and cons.[19,20] The hamstring tendon group tends to recover faster initially and to have less pain and swelling. However, although the graft strength is good, the fixation of the graft as well as the incorporation of the graft to bone seems to be weaker than with the patellar tendon.[12,21,22]

The patellar tendon group, on the other hand, has better fixation and incorporation because it heals bone to bone faster and behaves biomechanically like a single unit; the sum of these gives it a more reproducible result, making it the preferred graft for the high-demand athlete.[3,23] The downside of its use is that it tends initially to produce more morbidity, such as swelling, pain, and difficulty in gaining motion. It also has a higher incidence of postoperative patellofemoral pain. Other grafts used are the quadriceps tendon and contralateral patellar tendon. Allograft tendon material, such as patellar tendon and tibialis anterior tendon, has also gained popularity. The advantages of these are clear and include less donor site morbidity. The disadvantages are the possibility of disease transmission, slower graft incorporation, potential for stretching of the graft, and higher cost. A new modality of reconstruction, the anatomic ACL reconstruction, has been popularized by Fu and coworkers.[12] In fact, this tries to address the reconstruction of both the anteromedial and the posterolateral bundles of the ACL. Fu and others have shown in vitro that this double-bundle anatomic ACL reconstruction better controls the important aspect of rotational instability of ACL deficiency; however, in vivo, it has not been shown to be better than the standard single-bundle ACL reconstruction.[12,24]

POTENTIAL DISEASE COMPLICATIONS

An untreated ACL injury can lead to changes in the knee joint that may be associated with significant alterations in the patient's lifestyle. The patients who continue participation in strenuous sports have recurrent episodes secondary to anterior laxity and rotatory instability. These may lead to damage of associated structures, such as the meniscus and other secondary restraints. A significant number of patients develop joint space narrowing with evidence of osteoarthritis.[9,16]

Attention has recently been given to prevention of initial or recurrent ACL injury by modifying neuromuscular risk factors such as muscle weakness and imbalance, correcting proprioceptive deficits, and working on sports-specific techniques such as cutting and jumping. These programs combine strengthening, balance, and plyometric exercises with apparent improved dynamic stability and a reduction in the incidence of injury.[25]

POTENTIAL TREATMENT COMPLICATIONS

Medication complications include gastric, cardiovascular, and renal toxicity with nonsteroidal anti-inflammatory drugs. Injections carry the risk of infection (in approximately 1% to 2% of cases). Surgery has the risks of venous thrombosis and complications from the anesthesia. Fibrous ankylosis and significant loss of motion can be seen in the early rehabilitation stages secondary to poor progression of therapy or compliance of the patient.[25]

Poor graft placement and fixation can lead to loss of motion and subsequent graft failure with recurrent instability. In patients in whom chondral lesions or meniscal tears are identified at the time of surgery, long-term sequelae include the development of arthritis even after the reconstruction.[4,6,24,26]

References

1. Hernandez L, Micheo W, Amy E. Rehabilitation update for the anterior cruciate ligament injured patient: current concepts. Bol Asoc Med P R 2006;1:62-72.
2. Arendt E, Dick R. Knee injury patterns among men and women in collegiate basketball and soccer: NCAA data and review of literature. Am J Sports Med 1995;23:694-701.
3. Utukuri MM, Somayaji HS, Khanduja V, et al. Update on paediatric ACL injuries. Knee 2006;13:345-352.
4. Huston LJ, Greenfield ML, Wotjys EM. Anterior cruciate ligament injuries in the female athlete: potential risk factors. Clin Orthop 2002;372:50-63.
5. Thore Z, Petersen W, Fu F. Anatomy of the anterior cruciate ligament: a review. Oper Tech Orthop 2005;15:20-28.
6. Amis A, Bull A, Denny T, et al. Biomechanics of rotational instability and anterior cruciate reconstruction. Oper Tech Orthop 2005;15:29-35.
7. Yasuda K, Kondo E, Ichiyama H, et al. Surgical and biomechanical concepts of anatomic ACL reconstruction. Oper Tech Orthop 2005;15:96-102.
8. Yagi M, Kuroda R, Yoshiya S, et al. Anterior cruciate ligament reconstruction: the Japanese experience. Oper Tech Orthop 2005;15:116-122.
9. Fithian DC, Paxton LW, Goltz DH. Fate of the anterior cruciate ligament-injured knee. Orthop Clin North Am 2002;33:621-636.
10. O'Shea KJ, Murphy KP, Heekin D, Hernzwurm PJ. The diagnostic accuracy of history, physical examination, and radiographs in the evaluation of traumatic knee disorders. Am J Sports Med 1996;24:164-167.
11. Boden BP, Griffin LY, Garrett WE. Etiology and prevention of noncontact ACL injury. Phys Sports Med 2000;28:53-62.
12. Fu F, Bennett CH, Ma B, et al. Current trends in anterior cruciate ligament reconstruction. Part 2. Operative procedures and clinical correlations. Am J Sports Med 2000;28:124-130.
13. Shelbourne KD, Foulk DA. Timing of surgery in acute anterior cruciate ligament tears on the return of quadriceps muscle strength after reconstruction using an autogenous patellar tendon graft. Am J Sports Med 1995;23:686-689.
14. Gotlin RS, Huie R. Anterior cruciate ligament injuries: operative and rehabilitative options. Phys Med Rehabil Clin North Am 2000;11:895-924.

15. Escamilla RF, Fleisig GS, Zheng N, et al. Biomechanics of the knee during closed kinetic chain and open kinetic chain exercises. Med Sci Sports Exerc 1998;30:556-569.

16. Daniel DM, Stone ML, Dobson BE, et al. Fate of the ACL-injured patient: a prospective outcome study. Am J Sports Med 1994;22:632-644.

17. Arnold T, Shelbourne KD. A perioperative rehabilitation program for anterior cruciate ligament surgery. Phys Sports Med 2000;28:31-49.

18. Beynnon BD, Uh BS, Johnson RJ, et al. Rehabilitation after anterior cruciate ligament reconstruction: a prospective, randomized, double-blind comparison of programs administered over 2 different time intervals. Am J Sports Med 2005;33:347-359.

19. Cha P, Chhabra A, Harner C. Single bundle anterior cruciate ligament reconstruction using the medial portal technique. Oper Tech Orthop 2005;15:89-95.

20. Herrington L, Wrapson C, Matthews M, et al. Anterior cruciate ligament reconstruction, hamstrings versus BTB patella grafts: a systematic literature review of outcome from surgery. Knee 2005;12:41-50.

21. Roe J, Pinczewski LA, Russell VJ, et al. A 7-year follow-up of patella tendon and hamstring tendon grafts for arthroscopic anterior cruciate ligament reconstruction: differences and similarities. Am J Sports Med 2005;33:1337-1345.

22. Freedman KB, D'Amato MJ, Nedeff DD, et al. Arthroscopic anterior cruciate ligament reconstruction: a metaanalysis comparing patellar tendon and hamstring tendon autografts. Am J Sports Med 2003;31:2-11.

23. Foster MC, Foster IW. Patella tendon or four strand hamstring? A systematic review of autografts for ACL reconstruction. Knee 2005;12:225-230.

24. Aglietti P, Cuomo P, Giron F, Boerger T. Double bundle ACL reconstruction. Oper Tech Orthop 2005;15:111-115.

25. Wilk KE, Reinhold MM, Hooks TR. Recent advances in the rehabilitation of isolated and combined anterior cruciate ligament injuries. Orthop Clin North Am 2003;34:107-137.

26. Brown CH, Carson EW. Revision anterior cruciate ligament surgery. Clin Sports Med 1999;18:109-171.

Baker's Cyst 56

Ed Hanada, MD, Meryl Stein, MD, and Darren Rosenberg, DO

Synonym

Popliteal cyst

ICD-9 Code

727.51   Synovial cyst of popliteal space (Baker's cyst)

DEFINITION

Baker's cyst, the most common cyst in the posterior knee, affects approximately 19% of asymptomatic adults (especially adults older than 50 years)[1] and 6% of children.[2] Two age incidence peaks exist: 4 to 7 years and 35 to 70 years.[3,4] Three factors are key to the formation of Baker's cyst: (1) communication between the knee joint and popliteal bursae, (2) one-way valve effect, and (3) unequal pressure between the joint and bursae during varying degrees of knee movement.[4] Chronic irritation in the knee joint may increase production of synovial fluid, which may flow from the knee joint into the bursae under higher intra-articular pressure until the one-way valve formed by the gastrocnemius-soleus complex "closes," trapping the fluid in one of the popliteal bursae. This bursa then distends and forms a palpable mass, more commonly in the posteromedial aspect of the popliteal fossa.[5] Cysts detected by ultrasonography extend between the deep fascia and the medial head of the gastrocnemius muscle.[5] Anatomically, the lack of supporting structures in this area may predispose this region of the popliteal space to cyst formation.[5] Most commonly, the source of this chronic irritation is an inflammatory or degenerative joint disease, such as rheumatoid arthritis or osteoarthritis, respectively. In fact, in a study of 40 patients with radiographic evidence of primary osteoarthritis of the knee, 22% had Baker's cyst diagnosed by ultrasonography.[6] Chondromalacia patellae, chronic ligamentous or meniscal tear, chronic low-grade infection, pigmented villonodular synovitis, and persistent capsulitis are also commonly associated with Baker's cysts.[7] Noncommunicating cysts often have no associated knee disease and may be primary bursal enlargements from repeated trauma to the bursa itself related to muscle activation. Direct trauma is the most common cause of these cysts in children.[2]

SYMPTOMS

Baker's cysts are often nontender and may present as a fluctuant mass in the popliteal fossa (Fig. 56-1). Typical symptoms, if present, include swelling, pain, and stiffness exacerbated by activity such as walking. Symptoms are most readily elicited when knee flexion compresses the fluid-filled cyst, although knee extension may also cause tension on the cyst by the extended gastrocnemius-soleus muscles. The mass is often accompanied by leg swelling or diffuse calf tenderness. Numbness and tingling may be present if there is neural or vascular involvement.

PHYSICAL EXAMINATION

Baker's cysts are often visible or at least palpable along the medial aspect of the popliteal fossa. The cyst may be identified with the patient prone with the knee first extended and then flexed while the popliteal fossa is inspected and palpated. The round, smooth, fluctuant, and often tender cyst will be firm on palpation with knee extension and may soften or disappear with 45 degrees of knee flexion, a phenomenon known as Foucher sign.[8] The cyst can extend into the thigh or leg, or it can have multiple satellites along the calf and even into the foot. These satellite cysts may or may not be connected to the primary cyst through channels. When a joint effusion accompanies the cyst, it is worthwhile to search for the source of chronic irritation. Examine the knee's range of motion, test patellar and tibiofemoral and cruciate ligamentous laxity, and evaluate for potential patellofemoral pain and meniscal tears.[7] Furthermore, because of the proximity of the sciatic nerve or its branches to the popliteal region where cysts may be present, nerve compression may be manifested as decreased sensation and muscle atrophy.[9,10]

FUNCTIONAL LIMITATIONS

The degree of impairment produced by the cyst depends on its size and amount of tenderness. Baker's cysts are usually painless and limit movement minimally, if at all, unless there is an underlying meniscal injury. However,

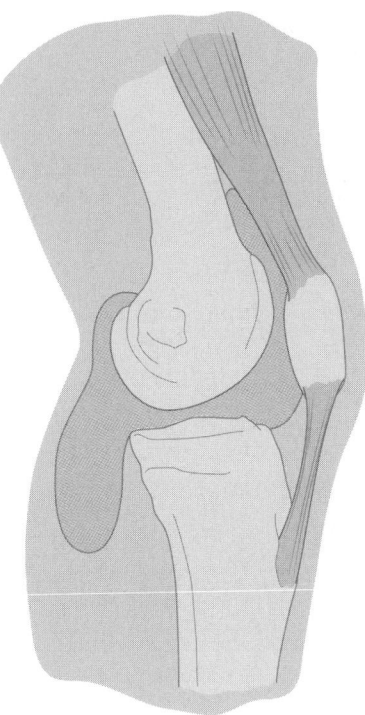

FIGURE 56-1. Schematic diagram of Baker's cyst.

Differential Diagnosis

Venous complexes

Inflammatory arthritis (rheumatoid)

Fat pads

Liposarcoma

Hematoma

Ganglionic cysts

Synovial hemangioma

Abscess

Malignant fibrous histiocytoma

Neoplasms (sarcoma)

Thrombophlebitis

Arterial aneurysms

Pseudothrombophlebitis

Compartment syndrome

larger cysts may be associated with moderate limitations in physical activity, particularly walking.

DIAGNOSTIC STUDIES

Imaging can help by defining underlying pathologic processes associated with ongoing pain despite medical treatment. Plain films of the knee can be used to diagnose underlying degenerative joint disease but are rarely necessary to diagnose Baker's cyst. Ultrasonography distinguishes solid from cystic masses and is therefore especially helpful in detecting Baker's cysts when extensive joint deformities, such as those present with rheumatoid arthritis, obscure the cyst.[11] Furthermore, ultrasonography is an economical and helpful method of differentiating thrombophlebitis from Baker's cysts if there is diagnostic uncertainty. Arthrography, through the injection of contrast dye into the knee joint or bursa, may clearly demonstrate the enlarged bursal structure. In addition, computed tomography may differentiate cysts from lipomas and malignant neoplasms and may show noncommunicating cysts or cysts that are not in the typical locations. Magnetic resonance imaging outlines the anatomy of the entire joint and is a sensitive test to identify Baker's cyst as well as its likely cause. Magnetic resonance imaging also helps in ruling out suspected solid tumors and defining pathologic changes for possible surgical excision. On these scans, Baker's cysts appear as well-circumscribed masses with low signal intensity on T1-weighted images and high signal intensity on T2-weighted images. In general, ultrasonography and magnetic resonance imaging are the two most common radiologic methods for evaluation of suspected Baker's cysts, each with its strengths and drawbacks.[12] Testing of the erythrocyte sedimentation rate may also be helpful if an inflammatory process is suspected.

TREATMENT

Initial

Intervention is needed only when Baker's cyst is symptomatic. The simplest treatment is to aspirate the fluid because aspiration collapses the cyst, and the symptoms consequently disappear. However, treatment of the cyst alone may not be adequate, and treatment of the underlying joint disease may be necessary. Ice and anti-inflammatory agents (nonsteroidal anti-inflammatory drugs), for example, can reduce the inflammatory effusions produced by degenerative joint disease. Quadriceps strengthening exercises can be used for patellofemoral syndrome. In some cases, venous sclerosants are used to prevent recurrence.[8] The cysts tend to involute spontaneously in children.

Rehabilitation

Treatment is directed toward the cause of Baker's cyst. Rehabilitation may include compression and range of motion exercises as a means of decreasing swelling in addition to physical modalities (such as ice) and pharmacotherapy (such as nonsteroidal anti-inflammatory drugs). Furthermore, in cases of degenerative or inflammatory arthropathy and cruciate ligament or meniscal injuries, resistance exercises to maintain and to improve lower extremity muscle strength may be helpful, especially in cases of compromised gait from painful loading. A comprehensive rehabilitation program may lead to progress in gait and in function to perform daily activities.

Procedures

Needle aspiration of the cyst is the most effective therapy, and provided the predisposing cause of the cyst resolves, it generally results in improvement of symptoms and function. Furthermore, if knee joint effusion is present, joint aspiration, accompanied by intra-articular corticosteroid injection, may be beneficial. In cases of noncommunicating cysts, corticosteroid injection directly into the cyst may help decrease swelling. The effect of this intervention may be followed serially through ultrasonography.[13] The possibility of a vascular malformation must be eliminated either by auscultation of the mass with a stethoscope to listen for bruits or by palpation of it to feel for a pulse before cyst aspiration.[14] In addition, imaging techniques such as ultrasonography may assist in detecting cysts.

Surgery

Surgical excision is attempted only after all other methods have failed and the cyst is sufficiently large and symptomatic.[15] Furthermore, arthroscopic disruption of the posterior wall of the capsule has been described.[16] On occasion, surgery is necessary to correct the underlying pathologic process (e.g., arthroscopic surgery for meniscal tears or total knee replacement for intractable degenerative joint disease).

POTENTIAL DISEASE COMPLICATIONS

The most common complications of Baker's cysts are dissection into the calf and rupture, leading to calf, ankle, and foot ecchymoses.[8] When the cyst ruptures, it produces a "pseudothrombophlebitis syndrome," meaning that it results in intense calf pain and swelling without associated deep venous thrombosis. Less commonly, Baker's cyst produces compartment syndrome,[16] peripheral neuropathy,[9,10] or lower extremity claudication.[17] More rarely, if the cyst is infected, it can result in septic arthritis of the knee if an intra-articular–bursal communication exists.[18] Moreover, a possible sequela of Baker's cysts may be intramuscular dissection, both distally[19] and less commonly proximally.[20]

POTENTIAL TREATMENT COMPLICATIONS

Analgesics and nonsteroidal anti-inflammatory drugs have well-known side effects that most commonly affect the gastric, hepatic, and renal systems. Aspiration can result in recurrence, infection, bleeding, and neurovascular compromise.

References

1. Tshirch F, Schmid M, Pfirrmann C, et al. Prevalence of size of meniscal cysts, ganglionic cysts, synovial cysts of the popliteal space, fluid-filled bursae, and other fluid collections in asymptomatic knees on MR imaging. AJR Am J Roentgenol 2003;180:1431-1436.
2. De Maeseneer M, Debaere C, Desprechins B, Osteaux M. Popliteal cysts in children: prevalence, appearance and associated findings at MR imaging. Pediatr Radiol 1999;29:605-609.
3. Gristina A, Wilson P. Popliteal cysts in adults and children. Arch Surg 1964;88:357-363.
4. Handy J. Popliteal cysts in adults: a review. Semin Arthritis Rheum 2001;31:108-118.
5. Labropoulos N, Shifrin DA, Paxinos O. New insights into the development of popliteal cysts. Br J Surg 2004;91:1313-1318.
6. Naredo E, Cabero F, Palop M, et al. Ultrasonographic findings in knee osteoarthritis: a comparative study with clinical and radiographic assessment. Osteoarthritis Cartilage 2005;13:568-574.
7. Tinker R. Orthopaedics in Primary Care. Baltimore, Williams & Wilkins, 1979.
8. Langsfeld M, Matteson B, Johnson W, et al. Baker's cysts mimicking the symptoms of deep vein thrombosis: diagnosis with venous duplex scanning. J Vasc Surg 1997;25:658-662.
9. Ginanneschi F, Rossi A. Lateral cutaneous nerve of calf neuropathy due to peri-popliteal cystic bursitis. Muscle Nerve 2006;34: 503-504.
10. Willis JD, Carter PM. Tibial nerve entrapment and heel pain caused by a Baker's cyst. J Am Podiatr Med Assoc 1998;88:310-311.
11. Katz WA. Diagnosis and Management of Rheumatic Diseases, 2nd ed. Philadelphia, JB Lippincott, 1988.
12. Jacobson J. Musculoskeletal ultrasound and MRI: which do I choose? Semin Musculoskeletal Radiol 2005;9:135-149.
13. Acebes JC, Sanchez-Pernaute O, Diaz-Oca A, Herrero-Beaumont G. Ultrasonographic assessment of Baker's cysts after intra-articular corticosteroid injection in knee osteoarthritis. Clin Ultrasound 2006;34:113-117.
14. Birnbaum J. The Musculoskeletal Manual. New York, Academic Press, 1982.
15. Takahashi M, Nagano A. Arthroscopic treatment of popliteal cyst and visualization of its cavity through the posterior portal of the knee. Arthroscopy 2005;21:638.e1-638.e4.
16. Schimizzi A, Jamali A, Herbst K, Pedowitz R. Acute compartment syndrome due to ruptured Baker cyst after nonsurgical management of an anterior cruciate ligament tear: a case report. Am J Sports Med 2006;34:657-660.
17. Zhang W, Lukan J, Dryjski M. Nonoperative management of lower extremity claudication caused by a Baker's cyst: case report and review of the literature. Vascular 2005;13:244-247.
18. Drees C, Lewis T, Mossad S. Baker's cyst infection: case report and review. Clin Infect Dis 1999;29:276-278.
19. Fang CS, McCarthy CL, McNally EG. Intramuscular dissection of Baker's cysts: report on three cases. Skeletal Radiol 2004;33: 367-371.
20. Rubman MH, Schultz E, Sallis JG. Proximal dissection of a popliteal giant synovial cyst: a case report. Am J Orthop 1997;26:33-36.

Collateral Ligament Sprain 57

Paul Lento, MD, and Venu Akuthota, MD

DEFINITION

The medial and lateral collateral ligaments are important structures that predominantly prevent valgus and varus forces, respectively, through the knee (Fig. 57-1).

Like other ligamentous injuries, knee collateral ligament sprains can be defined by three grades of injury. With a first-degree sprain, there is localized tenderness without frank laxity. Anatomically, only a minimal number of fibers are torn. On physical examination, the joint space opens less than 5 mm (i.e., 1+ laxity). With a moderate or second-degree sprain, there is more generalized tenderness without frank laxity. Grade 2 sprains can cover the gamut from a few fibers torn to nearly all fibers torn. The joint may gap 5 to 10 mm (i.e., 2+ laxity) when force is applied. A severe or grade 3 sprain, by definition, is a complete disruption of all ligamentous fibers with a joint space gap of more than 10 mm (i.e., 3+ laxity) on stressing of the ligament.[1]

Medial Complex Injury and Resultant Instability

The medial collateral ligament (MCL) is the most commonly injured ligament of the knee.[2] This ligament is usually injured when valgus forces are applied to the knee. Contact injuries produce grade 3 MCL deficits; noncontact MCL injuries typically result in lower grade injuries. Although MCL injury can occur in isolation, valgus forces typically instigate injury to other medial structures.[3] Findings of a rotational component to medial joint instability should prompt a search for cruciate ligament, meniscal, or posterior oblique ligament involvement.[4,5]

Lateral Complex Injury and Resultant Instability

The lateral collateral ligament (LCL) is much less frequently injured than the MCL. True isolated injury to the LCL is rare. True straight lateral instability requires a large vector force. Thus, a complete knee dislocation with possible damage to neurovascular structures should be suspected if straight lateral instability is present.[6] Posterolateral rotatory instability appears to be a more frequent cause of lateral instability than of straight lateral instability. Most authors believe that posterolateral rotatory instability requires disruption of the arcuate complex, the posterior cruciate ligament, and the LCL. The usual mechanism of posterolateral rotatory instability is forcing of the knee into hyperextension and external rotation.[6,7]

SYMPTOMS

Medial or lateral knee pain is the most common symptom related to knee collateral ligament injury. Interestingly, grade 1 and grade 2 injuries cause more pain than grade 3 injuries do.[2,3] Pain is often accompanied by a sensation of knee locking.[5] This may be due to hamstring spasm or concomitant meniscal injury. Patients may also report an audible pop, although it is more common with anterior cruciate ligament injuries.[2] A giving way sensation or a feeling of instability is often reported with high-grade injuries. Moreover, patients with high-grade injuries may also have neurovascular damage.[8] Therefore, these individuals may complain of a loss of sensation or muscle strength below the level of the knee.[6]

PHYSICAL EXAMINATION

Physical examination begins with the uninjured knee to obtain a baseline. Palpatory examination can be as important as laxity testing. Palpation can reveal tenderness

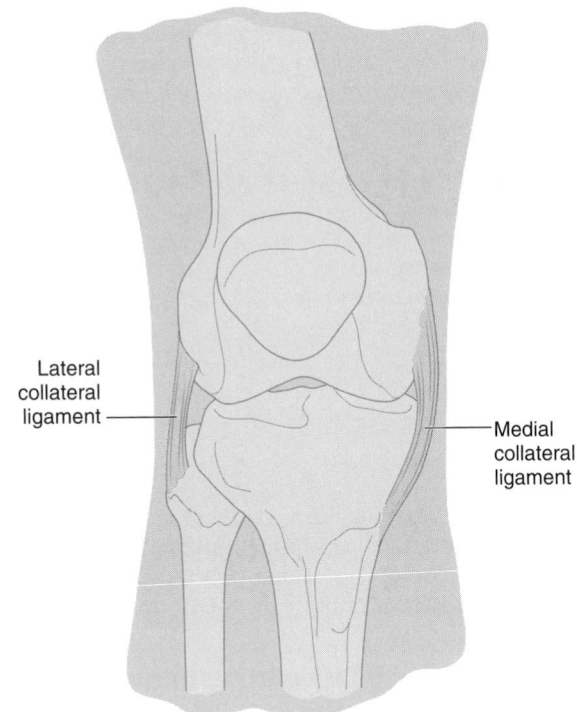

Lateral collateral ligament

Medial collateral ligament

FIGURE 57-1. Medial and lateral collateral ligaments.

knee with a valgus force not only implies damage to the superficial and deep fibers of the MCL but also indicates rupture of the posterior cruciate ligament or posterior oblique ligament.[11,12] If laxity occurs at 30 degrees but not at 0 degrees, one may confidently conclude that MCL injury is present with sparing of the posterior capsule and posterior cruciate ligament.[3,10] Although the anterior drawer test is classically used for chronic anterior cruciate ligament tears, it can be a useful adjunctive test for detection of MCL or posterior oblique ligament injury.[3]

Laxity of the lateral knee joint ligaments is determined by the adduction stress test, which is also performed at 0 degrees and 30 degrees of knee flexion and compared with the opposite "normal" knee (Fig. 57-2B). Gapping of the lateral joint line at 30 degrees of knee flexion indicates damage to the LCL and arcuate ligament complex.[9,12] However, joint opening with the knee in full extension indicates damage not only to the LCL but also to the middle third of the capsular ligament, cruciate ligaments, iliotibial band, or arcuate ligament complex.[7,13] When LCL injury is associated with rotational instability, the reverse pivot shift may be helpful.[14] This maneuver is performed by application of a varus force to an initially flexed knee. A positive test result reveals a clunk as the knee is passively extended from a flexed position. The clunk is a result of the relocation with extension of a knee subluxed in flexion,.[8,12] Rotational instability may also be detected by the external rotation recurvatum test (Fig. 57-3).

along the length of the collateral ligament, localized swelling, or a tissue defect.[5] With pure joint line tenderness, an underlying meniscal injury should be suspected. A true knee joint effusion may also be present with collateral ligament injuries; however, it is more prevalent with meniscal or cruciate injury.[9]

Instability of the medial joint ligaments is determined by the abduction stress test (Fig. 57-2A), performed by examination of the knee at 0 degrees and 30 degrees of joint flexion. If the test result is negative, a firm endpoint will be reached. If the test result is grossly positive, the femur and tibia will gap with valgus stress and "clunk" back when the stress is removed.[10] Although it is controversial, increased medial joint laxity of the fully extended

FUNCTIONAL LIMITATIONS

The functional limitations for patients with medial and lateral collateral ligament injuries result from instability. In general, sagittal plane movements are better tolerated than frontal or transverse plane motions. Most patients with grade 3 tears of the MCL are able to walk comfortably without an assistive device. Few, however, are able to traverse steps or to do a full knee squat.[3] Patients may also report difficulty with transfers and "cutting" sports activities. Some individuals with

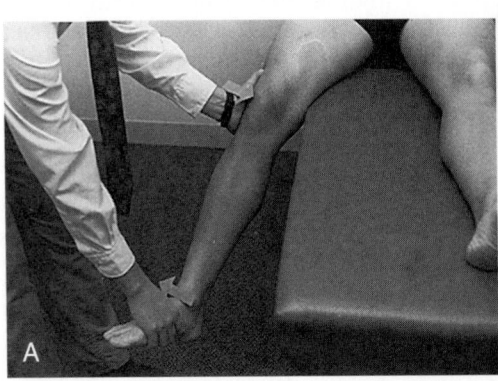
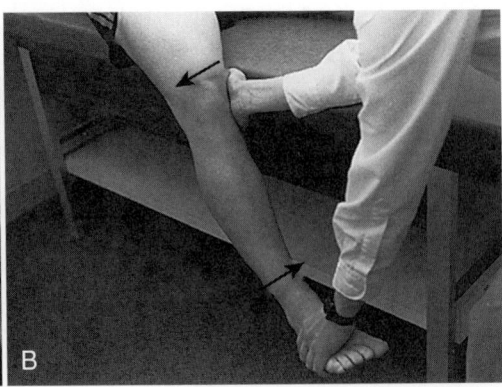

FIGURE 57-2. A, Abduction stress of the knee at 30 degrees tests for medial collateral ligament injury. **B,** Adduction stress of the knee at 30 degrees tests for lateral collateral ligament injury. (Reprinted with permission from Mellion MB, Walsh WM, Shelton GL. The Team Physician's Handbook, 2nd ed. Philadelphia, Hanley & Belfus, 1997:558-559.)

well as the severity of collateral ligament damage.[15] Bone bruises not evident on plain films may be detected by magnetic resonance imaging. This can be an important finding, particularly in patients who are experiencing persistent pain.

TREATMENT

Initial

After it has been determined whether concomitant injury is present, all grades of collateral ligament injuries are treated initially in the same manner. The basic principles of PRICE (*protect, rest, ice, compression, elevation*) apply. Patients with grade 2 and grade 3 injuries may need crutches or a hinged knee brace locked between 20 and 60 degrees to provide additional support for an unstable knee. Allowable brace range of motion is increased as tolerated to prevent arthrofibrosis.[4,9,16] Nonsteroidal anti-inflammatory medications may be prescribed to provide pain relief as well as to reduce local inflammation associated with acute injury.

Rehabilitation

The goals of rehabilitation for the knee with a collateral ligament injury are to restore range of motion, to increase stability, and to return pain-free activity. Within the first

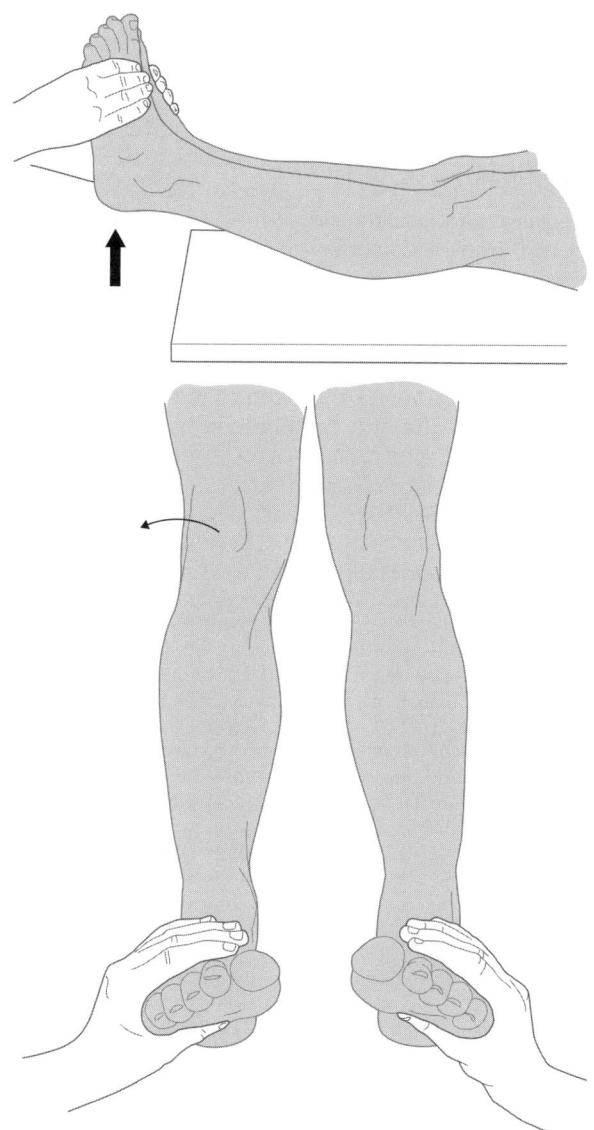

FIGURE 57-3. External rotation recurvatum test. Both knees are passively held in extension by holding the forefoot. If the tibia on the affected side externally rotates more than the normal side, the test result is considered positive and indicates damage to the posterolateral knee structures.

posterolateral ligament injuries may have pain with prolonged standing or knee hyperextension. This posterolateral laxity may eventually result in significant genu recurvatum as well as tibia vara, producing pain with even basic activities such as walking and standing.[7]

DIAGNOSTIC TESTING

Plain radiographs are usually normal in acute sprains of the collateral ligaments. Radiographs may be particularly useful to detect avulsion and tibial plateau fractures.[4] For example, an avulsion fracture of the proximal fibula can be detected after a varus-type injury, the so-called Segond fracture.[10] The current "gold standard" diagnostic test is magnetic resonance imaging. Magnetic resonance imaging can detect concomitant injury as

Differential Diagnosis

Medial Knee Differential

Medial meniscus injury

Anterior cruciate ligament injury

Medial compartment osteoarthritis

Pes anserine bursitis

Medial tibial plateau fracture

Vastus medialis obliquus injury

Medial plica band syndrome

Medial or Lateral Pain

Patella subluxation or dislocation

Bone bruise

Osteochondral injury

Referred or radicular pain

Lateral Knee Differential

Lateral meniscus tear

Iliotibial band syndrome

Lateral compartment osteoarthritis

Popliteus or biceps tendinitis

Lateral gastrocnemius strain

24 to 48 hours after injury, isometric quadriceps contractions and electrical stimulation can be instituted to reduce local tissue swelling and to retard muscle atrophy.[10,16] Range of motion and gentle stretching activities are introduced after the first day.[4] Early weight bearing is also encouraged. Aerobic conditioning can be maintained by use of upper body ergometry, stationary bicycle, or swimming with gentle flutter kicks. Maintenance-phase rehabilitation should emphasize exercise in multiple planes. Rehabilitation should eventually progress to functional or sport-specific activity. A combination of closed and open kinetic chain exercises is used.[17] Typically, individuals with mild collateral ligament injuries return to activity after 3 to 4 weeks; patients with severe injuries typically return to activity after 8 to 12 weeks.[18] Prophylactic hinged knee brace use has been advocated, although effectiveness remains controversial.[19-21] Postsurgical rehabilitation for grade 3 LCL and MCL injuries with concomitant anterior cruciate ligament, posterior cruciate ligament, or meniscal repair should be at the discretion of the individual surgeon. Variability occurs with each surgeon in respect to immediate weight bearing, protected range of motion, and return to full activity.

Procedures

Procedures such as corticosteroid injections have not been studied in collateral ligament injuries.[22]

Surgery

The treatment of grade 1 and grade 2 injuries of the medial and collateral ligaments is nonsurgical. Grade 3 injuries, especially when they are associated with concomitant injuries, may be treated surgically. However, most practitioners treat isolated grade 3 MCL injuries nonsurgically secondary to the high healing rates.[10,16,23,24] Repair of an MCL tear without repair of an associated anterior cruciate ligament injury may lead to a high failure rate.[5] In contrast, grade 3 LCL injuries or posterolateral complex tears with or without associated cruciate ligament injuries have been shown to heal poorly with nonsurgical measures.[4,25,26] In this case, surgical intervention within 2 weeks, addressing deficits of the arcuate ligament complex, lateral meniscus, and cruciates, provides optimal outcomes.[4]

POTENTIAL DISEASE COMPLICATIONS

The most significant disease complication is chronic knee instability. This most commonly occurs with undetected injury to the posterolateral joint complex. Another cited complication is an increased risk of osteoarthritis. Osteoarthritis occurs more frequently with combined MCL and anterior cruciate ligament ruptures than with pure MCL injury.[27] Pellegrini-Stieda disease may also be a rare complication. This condition consists of focal calcium deposition in the area of the injured ligament, typically on the femoral insertion of the MCL. Massage or manipulation may worsen this condition.

Instead, calcium reabsorption may be stimulated by dry needling.[4,9]

POTENTIAL TREATMENT COMPLICATIONS

Analgesics and nonsteroidal anti-inflammatory drugs have well-known side effects that most commonly affect the gastric, hepatic, and renal systems. If the injured knee is immobilized for too long or if range of motion does not proceed in an appropriate fashion, stiffness may result with possible loss of full extension. Similarly, if a surgeon reattaches the deep or superficial components of the MCL to the femoral condyle as opposed to the epicondyle, ankylosis of the joint may result, restricting flexion as well as extension.[5]

References

1. Committee on the Medical Aspects of Sports, American Medical Association. Standard Nomenclature of Athletic Injuries. Chicago, American Medical Association, 1966:99-101.
2. Linton RC, Indelicato PA. Medial ligament injuries. In DeLee JC, Drez D, eds. Orthopaedic Sports Medicine: Principles and Practice, vol 2. Philadelphia, WB Saunders, 1994:1261-1274.
3. Hughston JC, Andrews JR, Cross MJ, et al. Classification of knee ligament instabilities. Part I. The medial compartment and cruciate ligaments. J Bone Joint Surg Am 1976;58:159-172.
4. LaPrade RF. Medial ligament complex and the posterolateral aspect of the knee. In Arendt EA, ed. Orthopaedic Knowledge Update. Rosemont, Ill, American Academy of Orthopedic Surgeons, 1999:327-347.
5. Bocell JR. Medial collateral ligament injuries. In Baker CL, ed. The Hughston Clinic Sports Medicine Book. Baltimore, Williams & Wilkins, 1995:516-525.
6. Jakob RP, Warner JP. Lateral and posterolateral rotatory instability of the knee. In DeLee JC, Drez D, eds. Orthopaedic Sports Medicine: Principles and Practice, vol 2. Philadelphia, WB Saunders, 1994:1275-1312.
7. Hughston JC, Andrews JR, Cross MJ, et al. Classification of knee ligament instabilities. Part II. The lateral compartment. J Bone Joint Surg Am 1976;58:173-183.
8. DeLee JC, Riley MB, Rockwood CA. Acute posterolateral rotatory instability of the knee. Am J Sports Med 1983;11:199-207.
9. Simon RR, Koenigsknecht SJ. The knee. In Simon RR, Koenigsknecht SJ, eds. Emergency Orthopedics, The Extremities. East Norwalk, Conn, Appleton & Lange, 1995:437-462.
10. Reider B. Medial collateral ligament injuries in athletes. Sports Med 1996;21:147-156.
11. Swenson TM, Harner CD. Knee ligament and meniscal injuries: current concepts. Orthop Clin North Am 1995;26:529-546.
12. Magee DJ. Knee. In Magee DJ. Orthopedic Physical Examination, 2nd ed. Philadelphia, WB Saunders, 1992:372-447.
13. Grood ES, Noyes FR, Butler DL, et al. Ligamentous and capsular restraints preventing straight medial and lateral laxity in intact human cadaver knees. J Bone Joint Surg Am 1981;63:1257-1269.
14. LaPrade RF, Glenn TC. Injuries to the posterolateral aspect of the knee. Am J Sports Med 1997;25:433-438.
15. Stoller DW, Cannon WD, Anderson LJ. The knee. In Stoller DW, ed. Magnetic Resonance Imaging in Orthopaedics and Sports Medicine, 2nd ed. Philadelphia, JB Lippincott, 1997:203-442.
16. Richards DB, Kibler BW. Rehabilitation of knee injuries. In Kibler BW, Herring SA, Press JM, eds. Functional rehabilitation of sports and musculoskeletal injuries. Gaithersburg, Md, Aspen, 1998:244-253.
17. Shelbourne KD, Klootwyk TE, DeCarlo MS. Ligamentous injuries. In Griffin LY, ed. Rehabilitation of the Injured Knee, 2nd ed. St. Louis, Mosby, 1995:149-164.
18. Brukner P, Kahn K. Acute knee injuries. In Brukner P, Kahn K, eds. Clinical Sports Medicine. New York, McGraw-Hill, 1997:337-371.

19. Rovere GD, Haupt HA, Yates CS. Prophylactic knee bracing in college football. Am J Sports Med 1986;14:262-266.
20. Teitz CC, Hermanson BK, Kronmal RA, et al. Evaluation of the use of braces to prevent injury to the knee in collegiate football players, J Bone Joint Surg Am 1988;70:422-427.
21. Hewson GF, Mendini RA, Wang JB. Prophylactic knee bracing in college football. Am J Sports Med 1986;14:262-266.
22. Cole B, Schumacher HR. Injectable corticosteroids in modern practice. J Am Acad Orthop Surg 2005;13:37-46.
23. Indelicato PA. Nonoperative treatment of complete tears of the medial collateral ligament of the knee. J Bone Joint Surg Am 1983;65:323-329.
24. Reider B, Sathy MR, Talkington J, et al. Treatment of isolated medial collateral ligament injuries with early functional reha-bilitation. A five-year follow-up study. Am J Sports Med 1994;22:470-477.
25. Kannus P. Nonoperative treatment of grade II and III sprains of the lateral ligament compartment of the knee. Am J Sports Med 1989;17:83-88.
26. LaPrade RF, Hamilton CD, Engebretson L. Treatment of acute and chronic combined anterior cruciate ligament and posterolat-eral knee ligament injuries. Sports Med Arthroscopy Rev 1997;5:91-99.
27. Lundberg M, Messner K. Ten-year prognosis of isolated and combined medial collateral ligament ruptures. Am J Sports Med 1997;25:2-6.

Compartment Syndrome 58

Karen P. Barr, MD

DEFINITION

Compartment syndrome can be either an acute or chronic condition caused by increased tissue pressure within an enclosed fascial space. The focus of this chapter is compartment syndrome of the leg, although it can also affect the thighs or upper extremities.

Acute Compartment Syndrome

Acute compartment syndrome is a serious condition caused by a rapid rise in pressure in an enclosed space. If the pressure is high enough and maintained long enough, decreased blood flow causes necrosis of the muscles and nerves in the involved compartment. If fasciotomy is not performed, patients may suffer contractures, paralysis, infection, and gangrene in the limb as well as systemic problems, such as myoglobinuria and kidney failure.[1] Acute compartment syndrome is most commonly caused by a tibial fracture[2,3] and can occur in as many as 17% of these fractures.[3] The anterior compartment is most commonly affected, although multiple compartments are often involved. Other forms of trauma, such as crush injuries, muscle rupture, direct blow to a muscle, and circumferential burns, can also lead to compartment syndrome. Direct pressure, such as from a cast or anti-shock garment, can increase the risk for compartment syndrome.[4]

Nontraumatic causes of acute compartment syndrome are more rare. These include hemorrhage into a compartment, as can occur in anticoagulated patients,[4] and compartment syndrome after diabetic muscle infarction.[5]

Another cause of compartment syndrome is ischemia and then hyperperfusion caused by prolonged surgery in the lithotomy position. This is also known as well-leg compartment syndrome and is most often seen after pelvic and perineal surgery. Risk factors include the length of the procedure, the amount of leg elevation, the amount of perioperative blood loss, and the presence of peripheral vascular disease and obesity. The overall incidence in complex pelvic surgeries may be as high as 1 in 500.[6]

Chronic Compartment Syndrome

This is also known as chronic exertional compartment syndrome (CECS) and is an overuse injury most commonly seen in runners,[7] cyclists, and other athletes in sports that demand running, such as basketball and soccer. In CECS, the fascia in the lower leg does not accommodate to the increase in blood flow and fluid shifts that may occur with heavy exercise.[2] An increase in compartmental pressure then interferes with blood flow, leading to ischemia and pain.[8]

SYMPTOMS

The area in which symptoms occur and the type of complaints depend on which compartment is involved.

Acute Compartment Syndrome

Patients may present with pain out of proportion to the injury and swelling or tenseness in the area. Other symptoms include severe pain with passive movement of the muscles within the compartment, loss of voluntary movement of the muscles involved, and sensory changes and paresthesias in the area supplied by the nerve involved.[2,3]

Chronic Compartment Syndrome

In chronic compartment syndrome, symptoms start gradually, usually with an increase in training load or training on hard surfaces. The pain is described as aching, burning, or cramping and occurs with repetitive movements, most commonly running but also with dancing, cycling, and hiking. The pain usually occurs around the same time each time the patient participates in the activity (e.g., after 15 minutes of running) and increases or stays constant if the activity continues. The pain disappears or dramatically lessens after a few minutes of rest.

As symptoms progress, a dull aching pain may persist. Pain may be localized to a particular compartment, although multiple compartments can often be involved. Numbness and tingling may occur in the nerves that travel within the involved compartment. Chronic compartment syndrome can be seen with other overuse syndromes (e.g., concurrent with tibial stress fractures).

PHYSICAL EXAMINATION

The examination is focused on the following four compartments of the leg (Fig. 58-1).

Anterior compartment contains the tibialis anterior, which dorsiflexes the ankle; the long toe extensors, which dorsiflex the toes; the anterior tibial artery; and the deep peroneal nerve, which supplies sensation to the first web space.

Lateral compartment contains the peroneus longus and brevis, which evert the foot, and the superficial peroneal nerve, which supplies sensation to the dorsum of the foot.

Superficial posterior compartment contains the gastrocnemius and soleus muscles, which plantar flex the foot, and part of the sural nerve, which supplies sensation to the lateral foot and distal calf.[1,9,10]

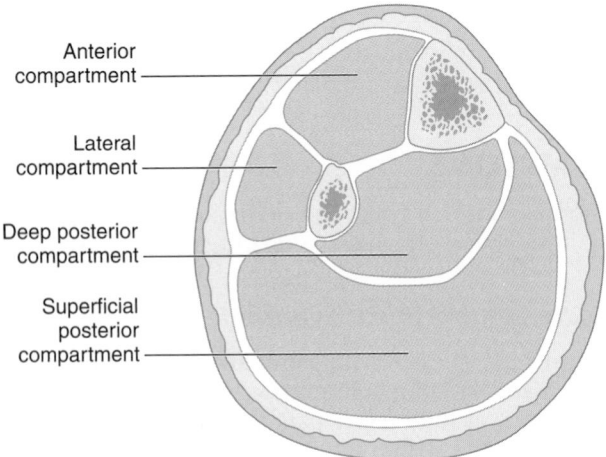

FIGURE 58-1. The focus of the physical examination in compartment syndrome is the anterior, lateral, superficial posterior, and deep posterior compartments.

Anterior compartment

Lateral compartment

Deep posterior compartment

Superficial posterior compartment

Deep posterior compartment contains the tibialis posterior, which plantar flexes and inverts the foot; the long toe flexors, which plantar flex the toes; the peroneal artery; and the tibial nerve, which supplies sensation to the plantar surface of the foot. This compartment may contain several subcompartments.[11]

Acute Compartment Syndrome

In acute compartment syndrome, patients present with a swollen, tense leg. They have weakness or paralysis of the muscles involved in the affected compartment and numbness in the area supplied by the nerve involved in the affected compartment. Pulses and capillary refills are generally normal, as these are involved only with extremely high pressures.[2,3,12,13]

Chronic Compartment Syndrome

In chronic compartment syndrome, patients may have pain with palpation of the muscles involved or may be asymptomatic at rest. The compartment may feel firm. In approximately 40% of cases, muscle herniation in the compartment can be palpated, especially in the anterior and lateral compartments where the superficial peroneal nerve pierces the fascia.[14] In severe cases, numbness may occur in the area supplied by the nerve involved, but this is usually normal at rest.[2] Weakness may be present, depending on the compartment involved: dorsiflexion weakness if the anterior compartment is involved, foot eversion weakness if the lateral compartment is involved, and plantar flexion weakness if one of the posterior compartments is involved.

Pain is reproduced by repetitive activity, such as toe raises, or running in place. Compartment syndrome occurs more commonly in patients who pronate during running; thus, pronation is a common finding on physical examination.[1,2,15]

FUNCTIONAL LIMITATIONS

Acute Compartment Syndrome

The sequelae of new compartment syndrome may be nerve and muscle injury with resulting footdrop, severe muscle weakness, and contractures. This can lead to an abnormal gait and all the limitations that this can cause, including difficulties with stairs, sports participation, and activities of daily living.

Chronic Compartment Syndrome

With chronic compartment syndrome, functional limitations usually occur around the same point each time during exercise, at that individual's ischemic threshold. For example, symptoms may start to develop each time a runner reaches the half-mile mark or each time a cyclist climbs a large hill. This may significantly limit sports participation and occasionally even interferes with activities of daily living, such as prolonged walking.

DIAGNOSTIC STUDIES

The "gold standard" for diagnosis is compartmental tissue pressure measurement. The devices most commonly used to measure intracompartmental pressures were traditionally the slit and wick catheters (Fig. 58-2).[2] Newer devices, such as the transducer-tipped probe (Fig. 58-3), are now gaining popularity.[16]

Acute Compartment Syndrome

Traditionally, tissue pressure above 30 mm Hg was considered the cutoff value for fasciotomy to be performed.[2,16] Normal pressure is less than 10 mm Hg. However, it is likely that many unnecessary fasciotomies were performed by use of this measure alone. Currently, continuous monitoring of compartment pressures is used in high-risk cases, such as leg trauma with tibial fractures. The differential pressure, calculated as the intramuscular pressure subtracted from the diastolic blood pressure, determines whether fasciotomy is indicated. Studies have shown that if this number remains consistently above 30, even with markedly elevated tissue pressures, patients have excellent clinical outcomes and fasciotomy is not necessary.[17,18]

Because of the invasive nature of compartmental pressure measurements, other diagnostic tools have been sought. Magnetic resonance imaging may be helpful in making the diagnosis. Changes seen with acute compartment syndrome include loss of normal muscle architecture on T1-weighted images, edema within the compartment, and strong enhancement of the affected compartment with the contrast agent gadolinium-DTPA.[19]

Chronic Compartment Syndrome

For CECS, absolute pressure measurements obtained at rest and during and after exercise are used to make the diagnosis. Interestingly, there does not seem to be a particular threshold compartmental pressure at which

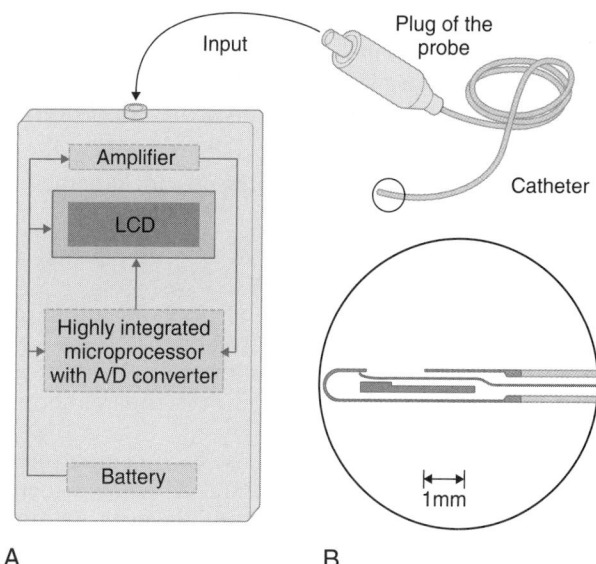

FIGURE 58-3. Transducer-tipped probe. **A,** Handheld device. **B,** Catheter tip with pressure-sensing mechanics. (From Willy C, Gerngross H, Sterk J. Measurement of intracompartmental pressure with use of a new electronic transducer-tipped catheter system. J Bone Joint Surg Am 1999;81:158-168.)

symptoms occur, and patients with higher pressures do not necessarily have worse symptoms than those of patients with less abnormal pressures.[8]

The following is one set of values[2,13] commonly used to diagnose *anterior compartment* syndrome:

- Pre-exercise pressure >15 mm Hg
- 1 minute after exercise >30 mm Hg
- 5 minutes after exercise >20 mm Hg

Values for *posterior compartments* are more controversial. Normal resting pressures are less than 10 mm Hg, and values should return to resting levels after 1 to 2 minutes of exercise.[13]

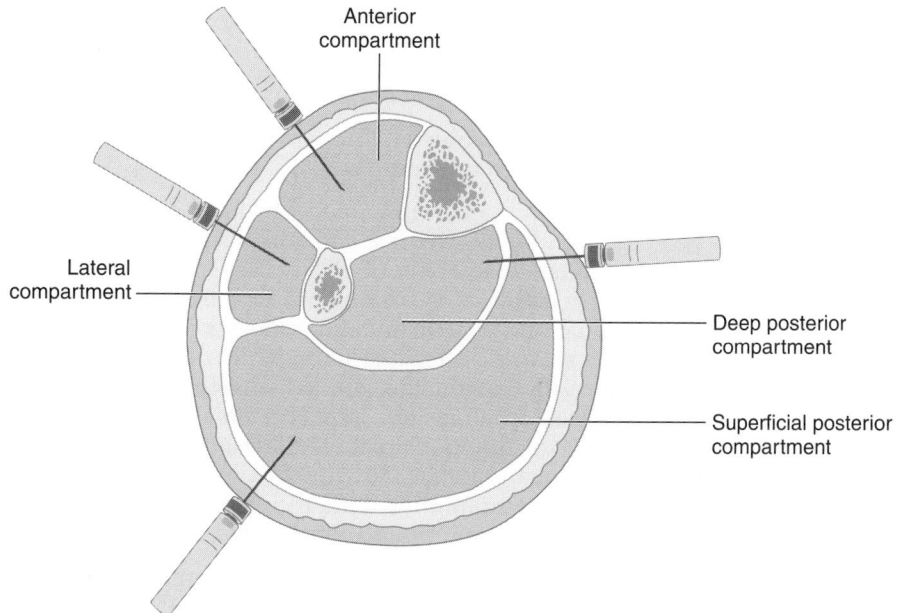

FIGURE 58-2. Compartmental tissue pressure measurements for the diagnosis of compartment syndrome with the use of slit and wick catheters.

It is important that the patient's symptoms correlate with the compartment in which there is elevated pressure. Pressure should increase in the symptomatic compartment with exercise and remain elevated for an abnormal time.[8,10]

Drawbacks to measurement of pressures include the following:

- They are invasive and can be complicated by bleeding or infection.
- Because of the anatomy, it is more difficult to test the deep posterior compartment.
- Pressures are dependent on the position of the leg and the technique used, so strict standards should be followed.
- It is time-consuming because each compartment must be tested separately, and all compartments should be tested because multiple areas are often involved.
- It is often difficult for patients to exercise with the catheter in place.[15,20]

Because of these drawbacks, alternative tests to confirm the diagnosis are sometimes used. Magnetic resonance imaging done before and after exercise can show increased signal intensity throughout the affected compartment in the T2-weighted images after exercise in patients with compartment syndrome.[21,22] Near-infrared spectroscopy measures hemoglobin saturation and has shown evidence of ischemia in patients with CECS. These diagnostics appear similar to compartmental pressure measurements in sensitivity and specificity.[22]

Differential Diagnosis

Acute Compartment Syndrome

Arterial occlusion

Severe muscle trauma

Neurapraxia of the common, deep, or superficial peroneal or tibial nerve

Deep venous thrombosis

Cellulitis

Chronic Compartment Syndrome

Tibial or fibular stress fractures

Shin splints

Atherosclerosis with vascular claudication

Popliteal artery compression from aberrant insertion of the medial gastrocnemius

Muscle hyperdevelopment causing compression of the popliteal artery

Cystic adventitial disease[23]

TREATMENT

Initial

Acute Compartment Syndrome

Initial treatment of acute compartment syndrome is surgery.

Chronic Compartment Syndrome

For chronic compartment syndrome, the initial treatment consists of rest, ice, and nonsteroidal anti-inflammatory drugs. Control of pronation with orthotics is important. The patient should be counseled to avoid running on hard surfaces and to wear running shoes with the appropriate amount of cushion and a flared heel.[2] Massage has been shown in small studies to be promising, but more research needs to be done in this area to see whether long-term significant changes can be made with either manual therapy or massage.[24]

Rehabilitation

Acute Compartment Syndrome

The rehabilitation of acute compartment syndrome is limited to the post-fasciotomy stage. Rehabilitation depends on the extent of the injury. Proper skin care for either the open area left to close by secondary intent or the skin grafts that have been applied is imperative. An ankle-foot orthotic to correct footdrop is often needed. Physical therapy is needed for gentle range of motion exercises to prevent contractures and should begin as soon after surgery as possible and as allowed by wound healing issues. Other measures include strengthening in muscles that may be only partially affected and gait training, possibly with an assistive device. There is no literature to support any specific rehabilitation protocols, and so programs should be individualized on the basis of the particular patient's needs. If the patient has deficits in activities of daily living, such as dressing or transfers, occupational therapy may be helpful in addressing these areas.

Chronic Compartment Syndrome

The rehabilitation of chronic compartment syndrome has not been fully explored.

Because it is an overuse injury, the first line of treatment is generally relative rest and analysis to correct the underlying cause. For example, it is generally thought that CECS occurs more commonly in those with excessive pronation, so rehabilitation focuses on establishing normal muscle lengths throughout the kinetic chain, especially lengthening through stretching exercises for the gastrocnemius and posterior tibialis, and strengthening the anterior tibialis.[24] Shoe orthoses to address overpronation may also be helpful. Training errors, such as too rapid increases in intensity or duration of running, are addressed and corrected.

If fasciotomy is done for chronic compartment syndrome, postsurgical rehabilitation should follow. Weight bearing is permitted as tolerated, and gentle range of motion exercises are begun 1 to 2 days postoperatively. Strengthening and gradual return to activity begin at 1 to 2 weeks. Full return to activity such as running usually takes 8 to 12 weeks.[25]

Procedures

Procedures are not typically done in compartment syndrome except as stated earlier to measure compartmental pressures as a diagnostic procedure.

Surgery

Acute Compartment Syndrome

Fasciotomy should be performed for acute compartment syndrome as soon as possible. Large longitudinal incisions are made in the affected compartment. These incisions are left open to be closed gradually, or split-thickness skin grafts are applied. Results of the surgery are variable and depend on the length of time of ischemia and other injuries involved.[26]

If treatment is delayed for more than 12 hours, it is assumed that permanent damage has occurred to the muscles and nerves in the involved compartment. Sometimes, patients are managed with supportive care: pain management, observation of renal status, and monitoring of fluids. This is because increased morbidity, especially infection and loss of limb, and increased mortality have been shown with delayed fasciotomy. Late reconstruction procedures can be done, if necessary, to correct muscle contractures or to perform tendon transfers for footdrop.[26]

Chronic Compartment Syndrome

Fasciotomy is also the mainstay for surgical treatment of chronic compartment syndrome, and some authors state that there is a 100% failure rate with conservative treatment. This may be because the population of patients that specialists see for this problem has already had failed conservative management by the time the diagnosis is made. The average time from the onset of symptoms to the time that the diagnosis is made is 22 months.[2]

For chronic compartment syndrome, different techniques for fasciotomy have been described. Most consist of making a small incision in the skin and then releasing the fascia as far proximally and distally as possible while avoiding nerves and vessels.

Results of surgery are usually good, with average success rates of 80% to 90% as defined by a decrease in symptoms and a return to sports.[25]

POTENTIAL DISEASE COMPLICATIONS

Acute Compartment Syndrome

In acute compartment syndrome, ischemia of less than 4 hours usually does not cause permanent damage. If ischemia lasts more than 12 hours, severe damage is expected. Ischemia of 4 to 12 hours can also cause significant damage, including muscle necrosis, muscle contractures, loss of nerve function, infection, gangrene, myoglobinuria, and renal failure. Amputation of the affected limb is sometimes necessary, and even death may occur from the systemic effects of necrosis or infection.[1-3] Recurrence has also been known to develop. Calcific myonecrosis can also be a late side effect.[27]

Chronic Compartment Syndrome

Chronic compartment syndrome may cause some damage to the muscle and nerves, but this has not been definitively proved.

POTENTIAL TREATMENT COMPLICATIONS

Fasciotomy for acute compartment syndrome has serious complications. Mortality rates are 11% to 15%, and serious morbidity is common, including amputation rates of 10% to 20% and diminished limb function in 27%.[28]

Fasciotomy for chronic compartment syndrome is generally a much less extensive surgery on a much healthier population, and complications are uncommon. They may include bleeding, infection, and nerve injury, particularly to the superficial peroneal nerve, and nonrelief or recurrence of symptoms. Case series report a recurrence rate of 3% to 20%. The most common reasons for recurrence are excessive scar tissue formation, causing the compartment to become tight again, and inadequate fascial release. A case series exploring the outcome of repeated fasciotomy for recurrence of symptoms reported that 70% of patients had good or excellent outcomes.[29]

One potential long-term complication of fasciotomy is an increased risk for development of chronic venous insufficiency caused by the loss of the calf musculovenous pump.[30]

References

1. Swain R, Ross D. Lower extremity compartment syndrome. When to suspect acute or chronic pressure buildup. Postgrad Med 1999;105: 159-162, 165, 168.
2. DeLee JC, Drez D. Orthopaedic Sports Medicine: Principles and Practice. Philadelphia, WB Saunders, 2002:1612-1619.
3. Gulli B, Templeman D. Compartment syndrome of the lower extremity. Orthop Clin North Am 1994;25:677-684.
4. Horgan AF, Geddes S, Finlay IG. Lloyd-Davies position with Trendelenburg—a disaster waiting to happen? Dis Colon Rectum 1999;42:916-919; discussion 919-920.
5. Woolley SL, Smith DR. Acute compartment syndrome secondary to diabetic muscle infarction: case report and literature review. Eur J Emerg Med 2006;13:113-116.
6. Simms MS, Terry TR. Well leg compartment syndrome after pelvic and perineal surgery in the lithotomy position. Postgrad Med J 2005;81:534-536.
7. Edwards PH Jr, Wright ML, Hartman JF. A practical approach for the differential diagnosis of chronic leg pain in the athlete. Am J Sports Med 2005;33:1241-1249.
8. Mannarino F, Sexson S. The significance of intracompartmental pressures in the diagnosis of chronic exertional compartment syndrome. Orthopedics 1989;12:1415-1418.

9. Blackman PG. A review of chronic exertional compartment syndrome in the lower leg. Med Sci Sports Exerc 2000;32(Suppl): S4-S10.

10. Styf JR, Korner LM. Diagnosis of chronic anterior compartment syndrome in the lower leg. Acta Orthop Scand 1987;58:139-144.

11. Cheney RA, Melaragno PG, Prayson MJ, et al. Anatomic investigation of the deep posterior compartment of the leg. Foot Ankle Int 1998;19:98-101.

12. Mars M, Hadley GP. Failure of pulse oximetry in the assessment of raised limb intracompartmental pressure. Injury 1994;25:379-381.

13. Mubarak SJ, Hargens AR, Owen CA, et al. The wick catheter technique for measurement of intramuscular pressure. A new research and clinical tool. J Bone Joint Surg Am 1976;58:1016-1020.

14. Detmer DE, Sharpe K, Sufit RL, Girdley FM. Chronic compartment syndrome: diagnosis, management, and outcomes. Am J Sports Med 1985;13:162-170.

15. Hayes AA, Bower GD, Pitstock KL. Chronic (exertional) compartment syndrome of the legs diagnosed with thallous chloride scintigraphy. J Nucl Med 1995;36:1618-1624.

16. Elliott KG, Johnstone AJ. Diagnosing acute compartment syndrome. J Bone Joint Surg Br 2003;85:625-632.

17. White TO, Howell GE, Will EM, et al. Elevated intramuscular compartment pressures do not influence outcome after tibial fracture. J Trauma 2003;55:1133-1138.

18. McQueen MM, Court-Brown CM. Compartment monitoring in tibial fractures. The pressure threshold for decompression. J Bone Joint Surg Br 1996;78:99-104.

19. Rominger MB, Lukosch CJ, Bachmann GF. MR imaging of compartment syndrome of the lower leg: a case control study. Eur Radiol 2004;14:1432-1439.

20. Takebayashi S, Takazawa H, Sasaki R, et al. Chronic exertional compartment syndrome in lower legs: localization and follow-up with thallium-201 SPECT imaging. J Nucl Med 1997;38:972-976.

21. Lauder TD, Stuart MJ, Amrami KK, Felmlee JP. Exertional compartment syndrome and the role of magnetic resonance imaging. Am J Phys Med Rehabil 2002;81:315-319.

22. van den Brand JG, Nelson T, Verleisdonk EJ, van der Werken C. The diagnostic value of intracompartmental pressure measurement, magnetic resonance imaging, and near-infrared spectroscopy in chronic exertional compartment syndrome: a prospective study in 50 patients. Am J Sports Med 2005;33:699-704.

23. Ni Mhuircheartaigh N, Kavanagh E, O'Donohoe M, Eustace S. Pseudo compartment syndrome of the calf in an athlete secondary to cystic adventitial disease of the popliteal artery. Br J Sports Med 2005;39:e36.

24. Blackman PG, Simmons LR, Crossley KM. Treatment of chronic exertional anterior compartment syndrome with massage: a pilot study. Clin J Sport Med 1998;8:14-17.

25. Schepsis AA, Gill SS, Foster TA. Fasciotomy for exertional anterior compartment syndrome: is lateral compartment release necessary? Am J Sports Med 1999;27:430-435.

26. Finkelstein JA, Hunter GA, Hu RW. Lower limb compartment syndrome: course after delayed fasciotomy. J Trauma 1996;40: 342-344.

27. Snyder BJ, Oliva A, Buncke HJ. Calcific myonecrosis following compartment syndrome: report of two cases, review of the literature, and recommendations for treatment. J Trauma 1995;39:792-795.

28. Heemskerk J, Kitslaar P. Acute compartment syndrome of the lower leg: retrospective study on prevalence, technique, and outcome of fasciotomies. World J Surg 2003;27:744-747.

29. Schepsis AA, Fitzgerald M, Nicoletta R. Revision surgery for exertional anterior compartment syndrome of the lower leg: technique, findings, and results. Am J Sports Med 2005;33:1040-1047.

30. Singh N, Sidawy AN, Bottoni CR, et al: Physiological changes in venous hemodynamics associated with elective fasciotomy. Ann Vasc Surg 2006;20:301-305.

Hamstring Strain 59

Carole S. Vetter, MD, and Anne Z. Hoch, DO, PT

DEFINITION

Hamstring strains are among the most common muscle injuries, particularly in athletes. The hamstrings consist of three muscles: the semimembranosus and semitendinosus muscles medially, and the long and short heads of the biceps femoris muscle laterally. The term *hamstring* comes from slaughterhouses, where hogs are hung up by these strong tendinous muscles when slaughtered.[1]

Hamstring strains constitute a range of injuries from delayed-onset muscle soreness to partial tears to complete rupture of the muscle-tendon unit.[2] Injuries can occur from direct or indirect forces. Direct forces refer to lacerations and contusions. Complete avulsion of the proximal hamstring origin from the ischial tuberosity has been described, most commonly in water-skiers.[3,4] These injuries occur when a forced hip flexion is sustained while the knee remains in complete extension.

The majority of hamstring injuries, however, occur from indirect forces with exertional use of the muscles, such as running, sprinting, and hurdling. Most hamstring injuries occur at the myotendinous junction during eccentric actions when the muscle lengthens while developing force, most commonly in the lateral hamstrings.[1] The biceps femoris has two heads with different origins and dual innervation and is therefore considered a "hybrid" muscle.[5] Dyssynergic contraction of the muscles is one of many proposed etiologic factors predisposing the hamstrings to strain. Other proposed etiologic factors include the hamstring's being a two-joint muscle,

insufficient hamstring flexibility (Fig. 59-1), insufficient warm-up and stretching before activity, strength imbalance between the hamstrings and quadriceps, strength imbalances between the right and left hamstrings, previous injury to the hamstring, higher running speeds, and poor strength or endurance of the hamstrings. Hamstring strains can occur in a variety of patients from young to old and in any level of athletics from the "weekend warrior" to the elite athlete.

The hamstrings function over two joints. Like other biarticular muscle groups, such as the quadriceps femoris, the gastrocnemius, and the biceps brachii, the hamstrings are more susceptible to injury. The hamstrings cross the hip and knee joint (with the exception of the short head of the biceps femoris). During the later part of the swing phase of gait, the hamstrings act eccentrically to decelerate knee extension; and at heel strike, the hamstrings act concentrically to extend the hip. During running, this rapid change in function puts the muscle at risk for injury; the higher the running speed and angular velocity, the greater the forces at heel strike.[6,7] Any large strength imbalance between the larger and stronger quadriceps and the hamstrings will put the hamstrings at a disadvantage. If the synergy of antagonists is altered, a vigorous contraction of the weaker muscle may result in injury. Any factor that adversely affects the neuromuscular coordination during running, such as lack of proper warm-up, poor training, or muscle fatigue, may result in a strain injury.

Hamstring strains can be divided into three grades according to their severity:

1. Grade I or first-degree strain: mild strain with minimal muscle damage (less than 5% of muscle fiber disruption). There is associated pain but little or no loss of muscle strength.
2. Grade II or second-degree strain: moderate strain with more severe partial tearing of the muscle but no complete disruption of the myotendinous unit. Pain is present with loss of knee flexion strength.
3. Grade III or third-degree strain: severe strain involving complete tearing of the myotendinous unit. This injury presents with severe pain and marked loss of knee flexion strength.[2,8]

331

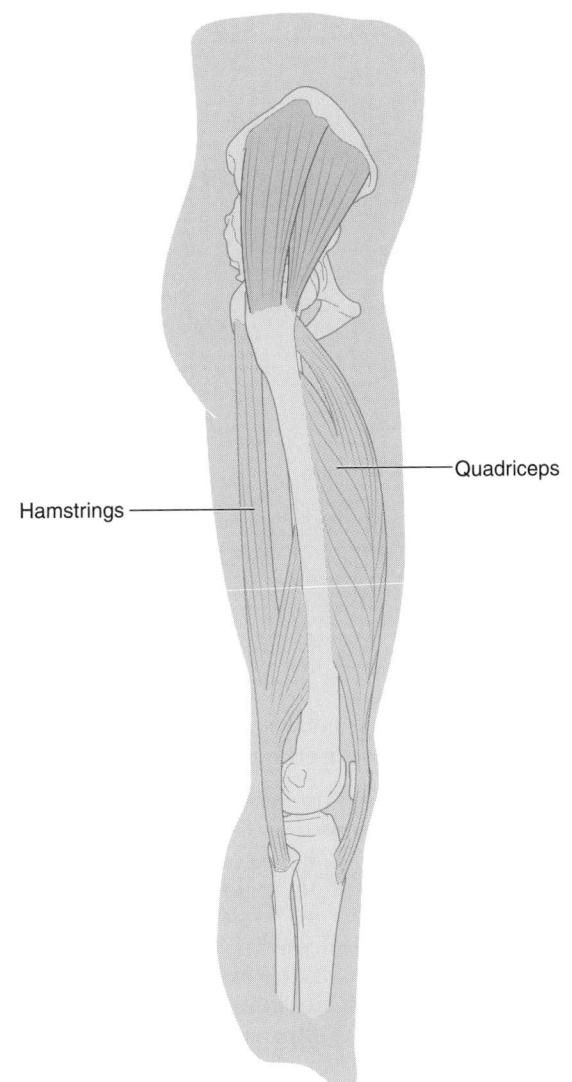

FIGURE 59-1. Tight hamstring muscles may lead to an imbalance between the quadriceps and hamstring muscles, placing an athlete at increased risk for injury.

Avulsion of the hamstrings tendon from its origin on the ischium or distally from the tibia or fibula is not graded like the classic myotendinous strains. These injuries are usually complete or partial avulsion injuries and described as such.

SYMPTOMS

At the time of injury, patients typically report a sudden, sharp pain in the back of the thigh. Some describe a "popping" or tearing sensation. There is generalized pain and point tenderness at the site of injury. The patient may complain of tightness, weakness, and impaired range of motion. Depending on the severity of the injury, the individual may or may not be able to continue the activity and occasionally is unable to bear weight on the affected limb. Swelling and ecchymosis are variable and may be delayed for several days. The ecchymosis may descend to the thigh and present at the distal thigh

or back of the knee, calf, or ankle. The injury may occur in the early or late stages of activity, and patients may give a history of inadequate warm-up or fatigue.

Rarely the patient may complain of symptoms of numbness, tingling, and distal extremity weakness. If these are present, further investigation into a sciatic nerve irritation is warranted. Complete tears and proximal hamstring avulsion injuries can cause a large hematoma or scar tissue to form around the sciatic nerve.[9,10]

Alternatively, any change in training patterns and increased eccentric exercise in a previously untrained subject can lead to hamstring injury with delayed-onset muscle soreness. This is believed to be the result of microscopic damage followed by a local inflammatory response.[11]

PHYSICAL EXAMINATION

The physical examination begins with assessment of gait abnormalities. Patients with hamstring injuries often have a shortened walking gait or running stride associated with a limp. Swelling and ecchymosis may not be detectable for several days after the initial injury, and the amount of bleeding depends on the severity of the strain. Unlike direct muscle contusions, in which the ecchymosis remains confined to the muscle proper, the bleeding in a hamstring strain can escape through the ruptured fascia with resultant ecchymosis into interfascial spaces, explaining the common finding of ecchymosis distal to the site of injury.[12]

The posterior thigh is inspected for visible defects and deformity, asymmetry, swelling, and ecchymosis (Fig. 59-2). The entire length of the hamstrings should

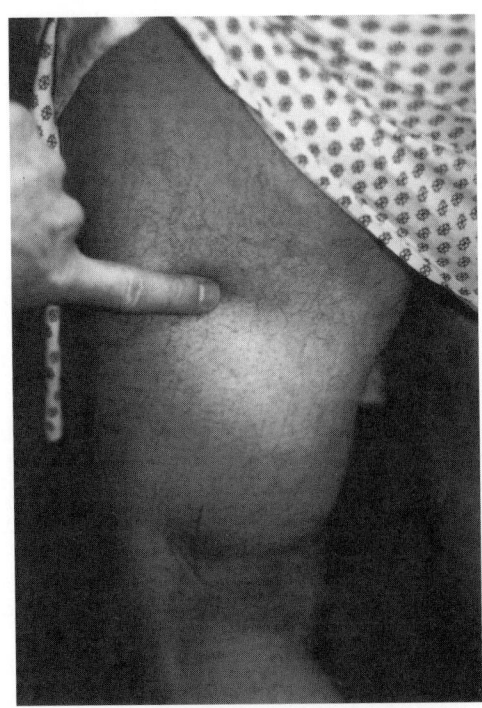

FIGURE 59-2. Clinical photograph of posterior thigh deformity after complete tear of the hamstrings.

be palpated, including the proximal origin near the ischial tuberosity and distal insertions at the posterior knee. A palpable defect in the posterior thigh indicates a more severe injury with possible complete rupture of the muscle.

Active and passive range of motion of the hamstrings should be tested and compared with the contralateral side. Range of motion of the knee can be measured with the hip at 90 degrees in the supine position or sitting position. Deficits in knee and hip range of motion are common, and the point at which pain limits range of motion should be noted (Fig. 59-3). Concentric and eccentric muscle strength testing of the hamstrings should also be performed with the patient both sitting and prone. Weakness of knee flexion and hip extension is common. Asymmetry of the hamstrings can sometimes be accentuated with active-resisted static muscle contraction. A soft tissue defect with distal bulging of the retracted muscle belly indicates a partial or complete rupture.

Neurologic examination findings should be normal except for strength testing of the hamstring group and in rare cases when there is an associated sciatic nerve irritation. In these cases, there may be weakness, particularly notable in plantar flexion, and loss of the affected Achilles reflex.

FUNCTIONAL LIMITATIONS

Most patients sustaining a hamstring strain have no residual deficits and return to their previous level of function. However, others may experience difficulty with walking or running, time lost from occupation, and delayed return to sports. Hamstring strains heal slowly and are at high risk for reinjury if return to activities is too early. With severe injuries, it may take up to 1 year for patients to resume preinjury activities; in some cases

of complete ruptures, patients never return to the previous level of function.[13]

DIAGNOSTIC STUDIES

The common hamstring strain usually requires no additional testing because the diagnosis is made by history and clinical examination. However, more severe cases may warrant diagnostic imaging. If the injury localizes near the origin of the hamstrings, plain radiographs may help identify irregularities of the ischial tuberosity, such as a bone avulsion of the ischial tuberosity (especially in the adolescent). Other radiographic findings may include ectopic calcification consistent with chronic myositis ossificans.[1,8] Magnetic resonance imaging is being used more commonly to determine the degree of injury and to identify complete proximal avulsion injuries (Fig. 59-4).

TREATMENT

Initial

Initial management of a hamstring strain consists of the PRICE principle (*p*rotection, *r*est, *i*ce, *c*ompression, and *e*levation). Relative rest and protection may involve weight bearing as tolerated or, with higher grade injuries (grade II or grade III injuries), cane or crutch walking. Ambulatory aids help prevent tissue irritation and the resulting inflammation, both of which prolong recovery. Assistive devices should be used until the patient can walk without a limp in a normal heel-toe gait. The application of ice as often as every 2 or 3 hours for 20 minutes the first few days is indicated to limit the amount of pain and swelling. Ice provides an anti-inflammatory effect and helps reduce swelling. Icing is continued through the recovery to inhibit inflammation and to allow muscle healing. Compression by taping or elastic wrapping of the thigh combined with elevation reduces hemorrhage, thereby helping control edema and pain. Nonsteroidal anti-inflammatory drugs and other analgesics are commonly used to limit the inflammatory reaction and for pain control in the first few days. Soft tissue mobilization to the site of pain should

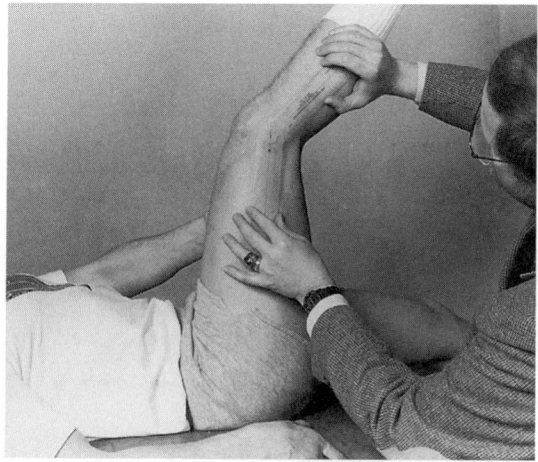

FIGURE 59-3. Measurement of hamstring tightness. With the patient supine and the hip flexed 90 degrees, the knee should extend fully if the hamstrings are flexible. If the knee will not extend completely, the residual knee flexion angle is measured and recorded as hamstring tightness. (Reprinted with permission from Mellion MB. Office Sports Medicine, 2nd ed. Philadelphia, Hanley & Belfus, 1996:275.)

Differential Diagnosis

S1 radiculopathy

Piriformis syndrome

Referred pain from sacroiliac joint or lumbar spine

Bone avulsion or apophysitis of the ischial tuberosity

Ischial bursitis (weaver's bottom)

Stress fracture in the pelvis, femoral neck, or femoral shaft

Adductor magnus strain

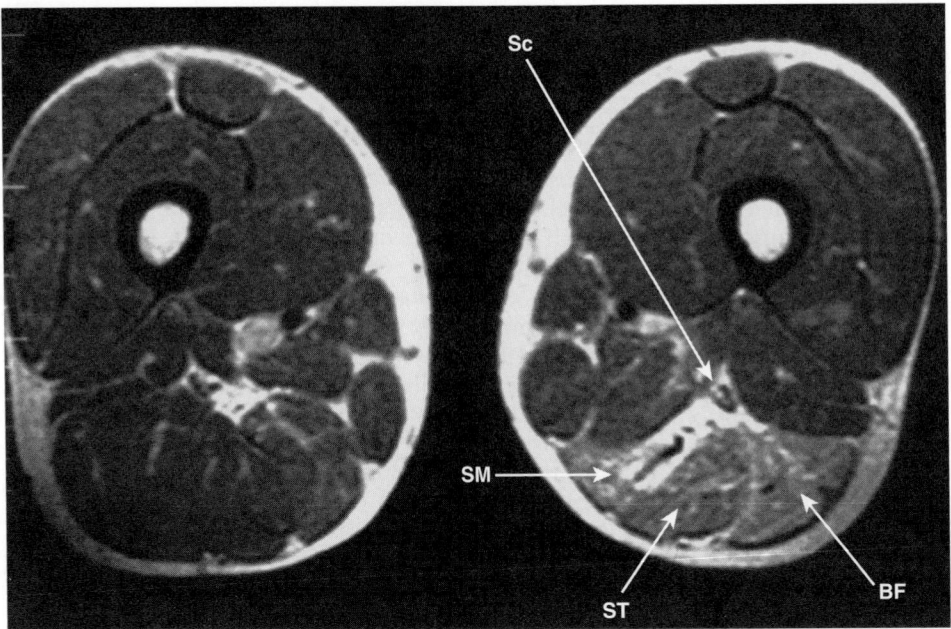

FIGURE 59-4. Axial magnetic resonance image demonstrating injury to the semitendinosus (ST), semimembranosus (SM), and biceps femoris (BF) muscles. The sciatic nerve (Sc) is shown anterior to the muscles and within the hematoma of injury.

be avoided for at least 5 days because this may exacerbate the inflammatory response.

Rehabilitation

The elements of a hamstring rehabilitation program involve a pain-free progression of stretching, strengthening, and sports-specific activities. In the acute phase, pain-free range of motion should be achieved as soon as possible to prevent adhesions and scarring in the muscle tissue. Patients should start with pain-free active range of motion and progress to pain-free passive range of motion and gentle stretching. For a full stretch of the hamstring muscle to be achieved, the hip must be flexed to 90 degrees and the knee fully extended. This stretch is best achieved in the supine position; a towel can facilitate hamstring lengthening (Fig. 59-5). It is also critical to improve flexibility throughout the spine and lower extremities. Strengthening can begin when the patient achieves full active extension without pain. It is best to start with static contractions, such as multiple-angle submaximal isometric exercises.[14] Once these are performed at 100% effort without pain, the patient may progress to isotonic exercise, such as prone hamstring strengthening and isokinetic exercise. These concentric strength exercises are followed by eccentric strength exercises and sports-specific activities as tolerated. Return to sport is allowed when full motion is restored, strength is at least 90% that of the uninjured side, and hamstring-quadriceps strength ratio is symmetric.[6] Hamstring flexibility must be maintained throughout the rehabilitation process to prevent reinjury. Aerobic conditioning should continue throughout the rehabilitation process. Bicycling *without* toe clips (toe clips increase use of hamstrings), swimming or jogging in a pool, and upper body ergometry are recommended.

Rehabilitation programs incorporating progressive agility and trunk stabilization exercising have been shown to decrease reinjury rates.[15]

It is critical to educate patients about how to prevent recurrent hamstring injuries. This includes a good warm-up period before engaging in sports. Full return to play must be gradual because the risk of recurrent injury is high. In addition, training errors, such as an abrupt switch to a hard surface or an increase in training intensity, should be avoided.

Procedures

Procedures are not typically performed in hamstring strain injuries.

Surgery

Routine hamstring strains do not require surgical intervention and respond well to a conservative rehabilitation program. However, in the case of complete hamstring avulsion from the ischial tuberosity, surgical repair is recommended because of the residual loss of power and function in nonoperatively treated patients.[3,4,16] Surgical neurolysis is also recommended for the rare complication of symptomatic scarring around the sciatic nerve.[9,10]

POTENTIAL DISEASE COMPLICATIONS

The most common complication of hamstring strain is recurrent injury. Loss of hamstring flexibility and strength as well as neuromuscular coordination puts the patient at risk for reinjury, especially if the return to activity is before full recovery.

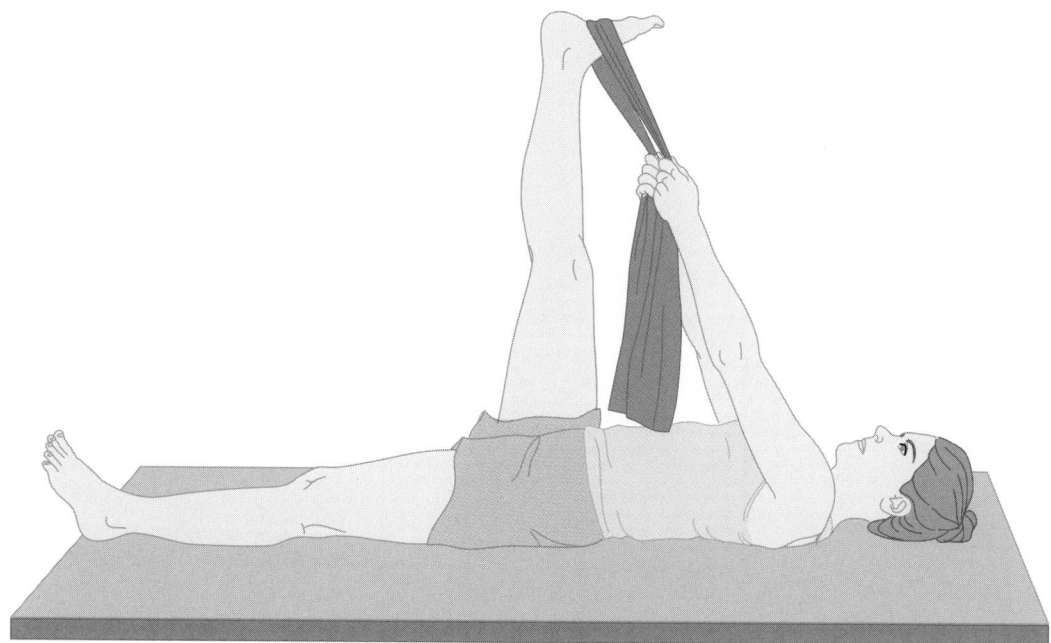

FIGURE 59-5. Stretching the hamstring fully requires the hip to be at 90 degrees with the ankle dorsiflexed. However, forceful stretching should be avoided.

Two cases of posterior thigh compartment syndrome have been reported with complete hamstring tears, one resulting from injury alone and one complicated by anticoagulation therapy.[17,18] Complete hamstring tears can also result in substantial scar formation around the sciatic nerve within the posterior thigh. Patients may present with radicular-type symptoms ranging from sensory paresthesias to footdrop.

Patients with chronic complete hamstring avulsion off the ischial tuberosity may complain of pain, weakness, and cramping as well as difficulty in running and walking and poor leg control, especially walking downhill.[3]

POTENTIAL TREATMENT COMPLICATIONS

Nonsteroidal anti-inflammatory drugs are known to have gastrointestinal, renal, and liver side effects. Ultrasound therapy should be avoided in the acute treatment of high-degree strains, especially if hematoma formation is suspected, because it may extend the hematoma.[18]

References

1. Morris AF. Sports Medicine: Prevention of Athletic Injuries. Dubuque, William C. Brown Publishers, 1984:162-163.
2. Kujala UM, Orava S, Järvinen M. Hamstring injuries: current trends in treatment and prevention. Sports Med 1997;23:397-404.
3. Brewer BJ. Athletic injuries; musculotendinous unit. Clin Orthop 1962;23:30-38.
4. Blasier RB, Morawa LG. Complete rupture of the hamstring origin from a water skiing injury. Am J Sports Med 1990;18:435-437.
5. Burkett LN. Investigation into hamstring strains: the case of the hybrid muscle. J Sports Med 1976;3:228-231.
6. Young JL, Laskowski ER, Rock M. Thigh injuries in athletes. Mayo Clin Proc 1993;68:1099-1106.
7. Agre JC. Hamstring injuries: proposed aetiological factors, prevention, and treatment. Sports Med 1985;2:21-33.
8. Zarins B, Ciullo JV. Acute muscle and tendon injuries in athletes. Clin Sports Med 1983;2:167-182.
9. Street CC, Burks RT. Chronic complete hamstring avulsion causing foot drop. Am J Sports Med 2000;28:1-3.
10. Hernesman SC, Hoch AZ, Vetter CS, Young CC. Foot drop in a marathon runner from chronic complete hamstring tear. Clin J Sport Med 2003;13:365-368.
11. Brockett CL, Morgan DL, Proske U. Predicting hamstring strain injury in elite athletes. Med Sci Sports Exerc 2004;36:379-387.
12. Best TM. Soft-tissue injuries and muscle tears. Clin Sports Med 1997;16:419-434.
13. Salley PI, Friedman RL, Coogan PG, et al. Hamstring muscle injuries among water skiers: functional outcome and prevention. Am J Sports Med 1996;24:130-136.
14. Worrel TW. Factors associated with hamstring injuries: an approach to treatment and preventative measures. Sports Med 1994;17:338-345.
15. Sherry MA, Best TM. A comparison of 2 rehabilitation programs in the treatment of acute hamstring strains. J Orthop Sports Phys Ther 2004;34:116-125.
16. Cross MG, Vandersluis R, Wood D, Banff M. Surgical repair of chronic complete hamstring tendon rupture in the adult patient. Am J Sports Med 1998;26:785-788.
17. Oseto MC, Edwards JC, Acus RW. Posterior thigh compartment syndrome associated with hamstring avulsion and chronic anticoagulation therapy. Orthopedics 2004;27:229-230.
18. Kwong Y, Patel J. Spontaneous complete hamstring avulsion causing posterior thigh compartment syndrome. Br J Sports Med 2006;40:723-724.

Iliotibial Band Syndrome 60

Venu Akuthota, MD, Sonja K. Stilp, MD,
Paul Lento, MD, and Peter Gonzalez, MD

Synonyms

Iliotibial band friction syndrome
Iliotibial tract friction syndrome
Snapping hip

ICD-9 Codes

719.65   Snapping hip
728.89   Iliotibial band syndrome

DEFINITION

The iliotibial band (ITB) is a dense fascia on the lateral aspect of the knee and hip.[1] Traditionally, the gluteus maximus and tensor fascia lata were thought to be the proximal origin of the ITB. Further anatomic dissections have demonstrated that the gluteus medius also has direct and indirect contributions to the ITB (Fig. 60-1).[2] In the distal thigh, the ITB passes over the lateral femoral epicondyle and separates into two components. The iliotibial tract of the distal ITB attaches to Gerdy tubercle of the anterolateral proximal tibia. The iliopatellar band of the ITB has aponeurotic connections to the patella and the vastus lateralis.[3] An anatomic pouch can be found underlying the posterior ITB at the level of the lateral femoral epicondyle. Controversy exists as to whether this pouch is a bursa, a synovial extension of the knee joint, or degenerative tissue.[4] Others have reported that a highly innervated fat pad overlies the lateral femoral epicondyle.[5]

Iliotibial band syndrome (ITBS) or iliotibial band friction syndrome is an overuse injury typically referring to lateral knee pain as a result of impingement of the distal ITB over the lateral femoral epicondyle. Less commonly, ITBS may refer to hip pain associated with movement of the ITB across the greater trochanter. This chapter deals primarily with distal ITBS. The suspected pain generator in ITBS is as controversial as the anatomy around the lateral epicondyle. It has been postulated to be bursitis, synovitis, or irritation of the fat pad.[6] Although the anatomic pain generator may not be fully known, pain at the distal aspect of the ITB is thought to be caused by the fibers of the ITB passing over the lateral femoral epicondyle with knee flexion and extension.[6]

Friction has been implicated as the most important factor in ITBS.[7,8] Maximum friction occurs when the posterior fibers of the ITB pass over the lateral femoral epicondyle at 20 to 30 degrees of knee flexion, the putative "impingement zone." Repeated knee flexion and extension, particularly with increased running mileage per week, creates friction and has been shown to predispose an individual to lateral knee pain.[9] Friction has been shown to play a role in cycling activities as well. Cycling-induced ITBS is thought to result from the repetitive activity of cycling, as less time is spent in the impingement zone than during running activities.[10] Other authors have theorized that pain is due not only to friction but also to compression of the fat pad between the ITB and the lateral femoral epicondyle. The compression of the fat pad was found to be greatest at 30 degrees of flexion, similar to previous reports, and increased with internal rotation of the tibia during knee flexion.[5]

Although it has not been extensively studied, poor neuromuscular control appears to be an important *modifiable* risk factor for ITBS. Weakness of hip abductors has been implicated in ITBS.[6] Specifically, neuromuscular control is needed to attenuate the valgus–internal rotation vectors at the knee after heel strike. If appropriate control is not available, the ITB may have an abrupt increase in tension at its insertion site. Strengthening of the gluteus medius and tensor fascia lata, decelerators of the valgus–internal rotation vectors at the knee, has been shown to reduce symptoms of ITBS.[11] Lack of dynamic flexibility, particularly of the ITB, has been implicated with ITB injury susceptibility. Yet, no research study to date has revealed a correlation between ITB tightness and ITB injury. Theoretically, however, tightness of the ITB or its constituent muscles increases impingement of the ITB on the lateral femoral epicondyle.[7] Other risk factors that may be attenuated with proper shoe wear or foot orthoses include excessive foot-ankle pronation and supination.[9,12,13] Increased ground reaction force, as with running in old shoes, may also increase frictional forces at the knee and exacerbate symptoms.[7] Intrinsic or nonmodifiable factors, such as bone malalignment or a wide distal ITB, may contribute to

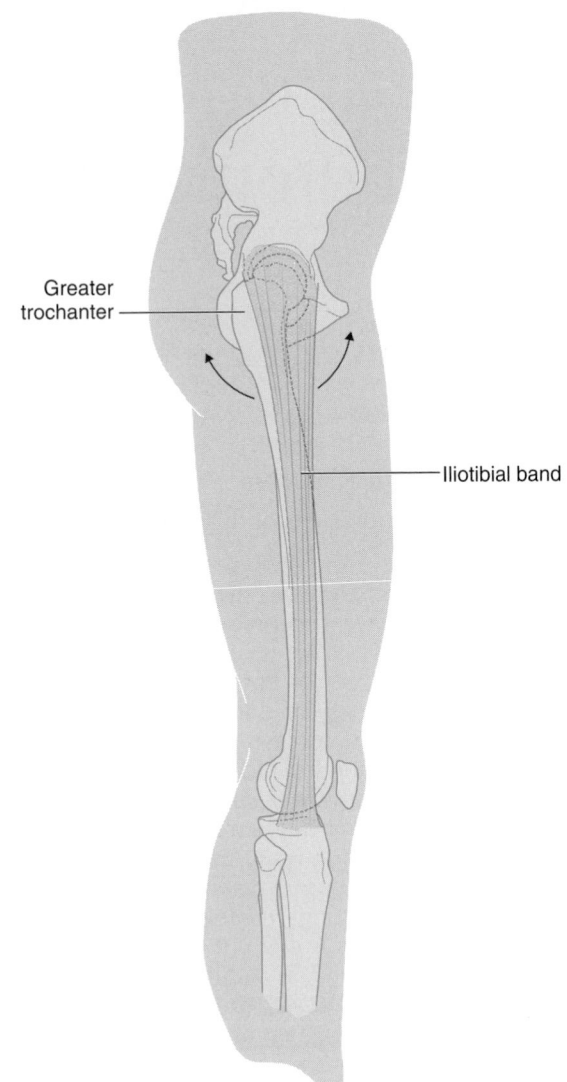

Greater trochanter

Iliotibial band

FIGURE 60-1. Anatomy of the iliotibial band, which can cause "snapping" as it slips anteriorly and posteriorly over the prominent greater trochanter.

the development of ITBS. Finally, repeated direct trauma to the lateral knee, particularly with soccer goalies, appears to be injurious to the ITB impingement area.[14]

SYMPTOMS

Symptoms of ITBS occur typically at the lateral femoral epicondyle but may emanate from the distal attachment of the ITB at Gerdy tubercle on the tibia. ITBS is the most common cause of lateral knee pain in runners.[15] Individuals present with sharp or burning lateral knee pain that is aggravated during repetitive activity. This pain may radiate up into the lateral thigh or down to Gerdy tubercle.[16] Runners often describe a specific, reproducible time when the symptoms commence.[17] Pain usually subsides after a run; however, in severe cases, persistent pain may cause restriction in distance.[18,19] Runners also note more pain with downhill running because of the increased time spent in the

impingement zone.[7] Paradoxically, runners state that faster running and sprinting often does not produce pain. Fast running allows the athlete to spend more time in knee angles greater than 30 degrees.[7] Cyclists present with rhythmic, stabbing pain with pedaling. Specifically, they complain of pain at the end of the downstroke or the beginning of the upstroke. Bikers with improper saddle height and cleat position may experience greater symptoms.[20]

ITBS symptoms may also occur as a lateral snapping hip. An external or lateral snapping hip occurs as the ITB rapidly passes anteriorly over the greater trochanter as the femur passes from extension to flexion.[21] Athletes, particularly dancers, sometimes experience an audible painful snap on landing in poor turnout (decreased external rotation at the hip) and with excessive anterior pelvic tilt.[22,23]

PHYSICAL EXAMINATION

Physical examination begins with a screening examination of the joints above and below the site of injury. Hip girdle examination includes an assessment for joint range of motion, asymmetries,[24] muscle strength (particularly hip abductors),[11] and lumbopelvic somatic dysfunctions.[25] The modified Thomas and Ober tests are used to assess flexibility of the ITB and related musculature at the hip and knee (Figs. 60-2 and 60-3).[26,27]

The knee examination includes palpation, patellar accessory motion,[28] and the Noble compression test (Fig. 60-4).[8] Knee tenderness is noted either at the lateral femoral epicondyle (above the lateral joint line) or at Gerdy tubercle. Palpatory examination should also include a thorough assessment for myofascial restrictions and trigger points along the lateral thigh musculature.[17,18] On rare occasion, ITB swelling and crepitus accompany tenderness. Pain can also be frequently elicited by the Noble compression test.[8] Other conditions are effectively ruled out by performing a relevant physical examination.

The foot and ankle examination is particularly useful in the determination of gastrocnemius-soleus inflexibility, subtalar motion restrictions, and specific foot type (e.g., hindfoot varus). Finally, a biomechanical assessment of sports-specific activity can be done. Walkers and runners are observed for abnormalities such as excessive foot-ankle pronation, inability to attenuate shock at the knee, Trendelenburg frontal plane gait at the pelvis, and forward trunk lean. Bicyclers are observed for proper foot placement on the pedal, saddle height, and knee angles with pedaling revolution.[20] Dancers can be observed performing *rond de jambe* or *grand plié* for proper turnout and pelvic stabilization.[22]

The findings of the neurologic examination, including strength, sensation, and reflexes, are typically normal. Strength may be affected by disuse or guarding due to pain, particularly in the hip abductors and external rotators.

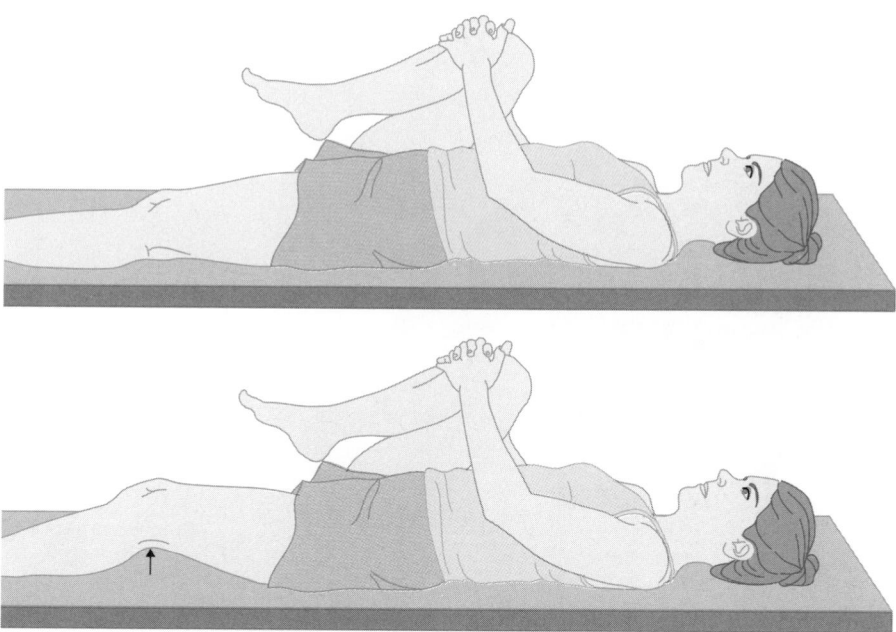

FIGURE 60-2. Thomas test to assess hip flexion contracture. The patient lies supine while the clinician flexes one of the patient's hips, bringing the knee to the chest to flatten the lumbar spine. The patient holds the flexed knee and hip against the chest. If there is a flexion contracture of the hip, the patient's other leg will rise off the table.

FUNCTIONAL LIMITATIONS

ITBS pain usually restricts athletes from their sports activity but does not typically cause limitations of daily activities. Yet, a vicious circle is set forth in which biomechanical deficits (e.g., gluteal weakness and ITB tightness) cause ITB tissue injury with resultant functional adaptations to avoid the pain of the tissue injury (e.g., external rotation of the hip).[24]

DIAGNOSTIC STUDIES

Imaging has a limited role in ITBS because it is usually a clinical diagnosis. Radiographs are rarely helpful. Diagnostic ultrasonography has been used in some centers to confirm injuries.[29] Dynamic sonography may also be helpful in identifying abnormal motion of the proximal ITB in diagnosis of external snapping hip syndrome.[30] When definitive diagnosis is needed or other diagnoses need to be excluded, magnetic resonance imaging has emerged as a potentially useful test.[31] Magnetic resonance imaging may show a thickened ITB or high intensity on axial T2-weighted images.[31,32]

TREATMENT

Initial

Acute-phase treatment is akin to that of other musculoskeletal injuries. Relative rest consists of activity modification, particularly with restriction of those activities that exacerbate the pain symptoms. In most instances, this does not mean a complete cessation of activity. The clinician needs to emphasize the positive aspects of relative rest and provide alternative training regimens. The ITB can be relatively off-loaded if an individual can

keep his or her activity below the threshold of pain. Frequently, this can be achieved by simply decreasing intensity or training duration. Medications such as nonsteroidal anti-inflammatory drugs may help reduce

Differential Diagnosis

ITB: Hip

Hip joint disease

Meralgia paresthetica

Trochanteric bursitis

Internal snapping hip

Referred or radicular pain from lumbar spine

Primary myofascial pain

ITB: Knee

Popliteus tendinitis

Lateral collateral ligament injury

Lateral hamstring strain

Lateral meniscus tear

Patellofemoral pain

Common peroneal nerve injury

Fabella syndrome

Lateral plica

Stress fracture

Primary myofascial pain

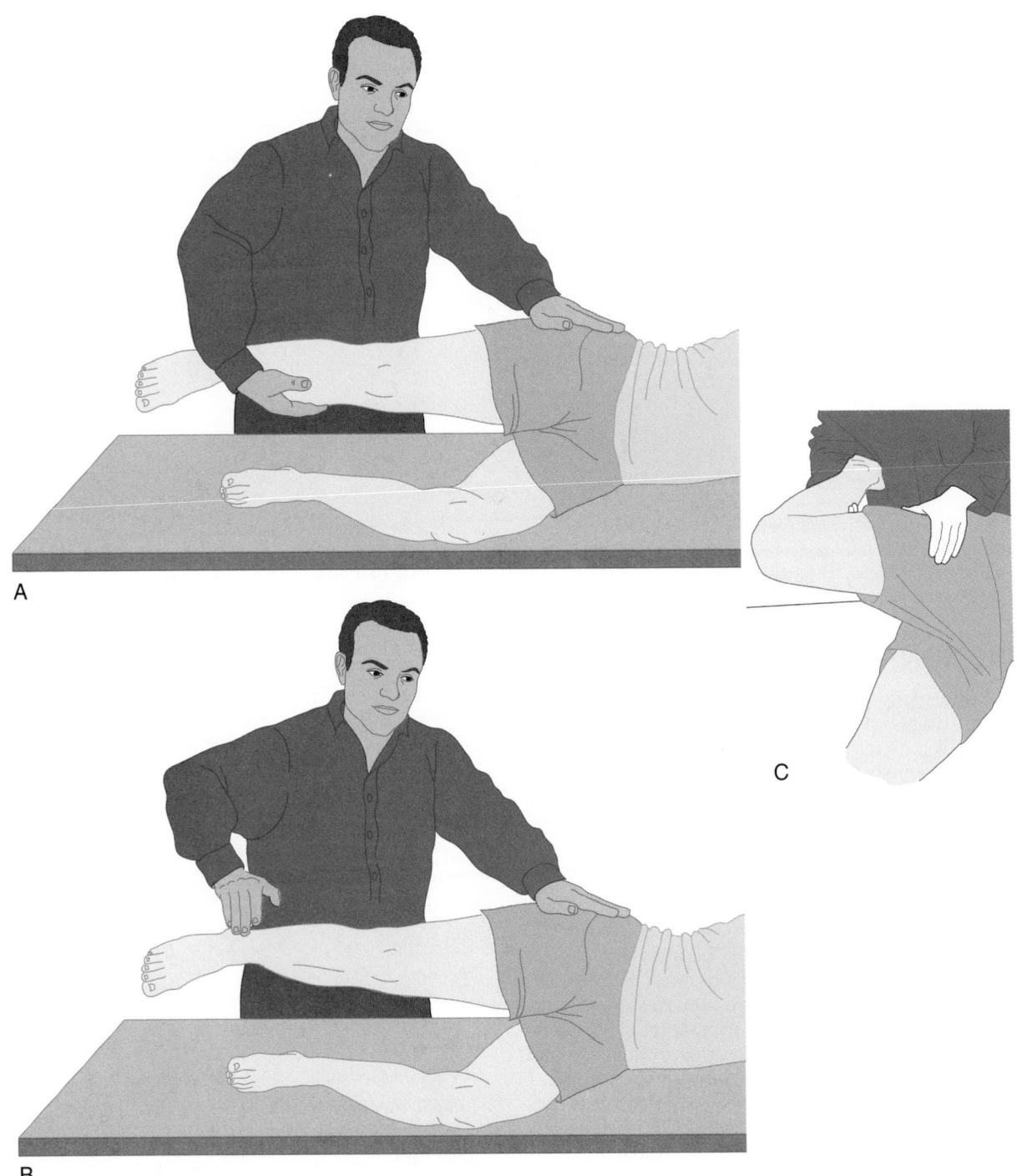

FIGURE 60-3. Ober test to assess contracture of the ITB. The patient is side-lying with the lower leg flexed at the hip and knee. The clinician passively abducts and extends the patient's upper leg with the knee straight **(A)** or flexed to 90 degrees **(C)**. The test result is positive if the leg remains abducted and does not fall to the table **(B)**.

pain and inflammation in the first few weeks of injury. If swelling is present, some authors advocate a local corticosteroid injection in the initial stages.[17,18] As well, modalities such as ice massage can be helpful in the early period.

It is critical early on to address the biomechanical cause of ITB injury.

Rehabilitation

Ultrasound, phonophoresis, iontophoresis, and electrical stimulation may also be used to reduce early inflammation and pain.

The subacute phase of rehabilitation addresses the biomechanical deficits found on physical examination.

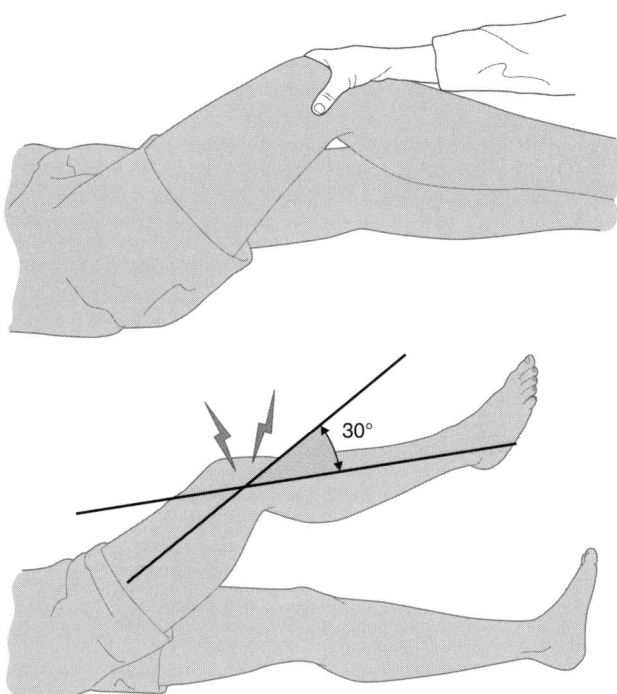

FIGURE 60-4. Noble compression test to determine whether there is ITB friction at the knee. The patient lies supine, and the knee is flexed to 90 degrees (the hip flexes as well). The clinician applies pressure with the thumb at the lateral femoral epicondyle while the patient slowly extends the knee. The test result is positive if the patient complains of severe pain over the lateral femoral epicondyle at 30 degrees.

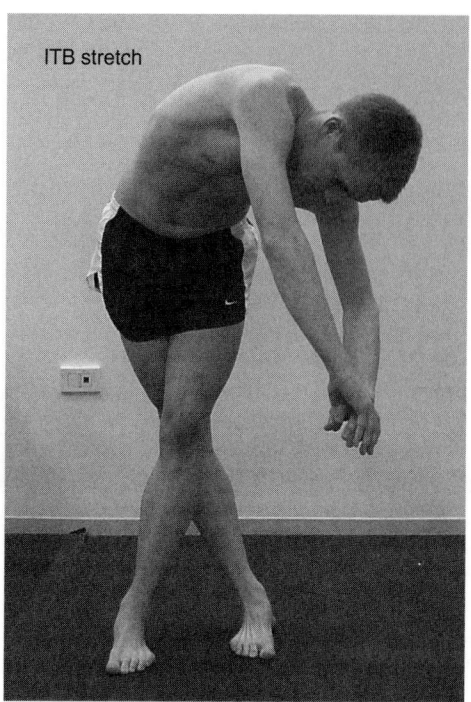

FIGURE 60-5. ITB stretch.

Typically, flexibility deficits are seen in the ITB, iliopsoas, quadriceps, and gastrocnemius-soleus.[17,18] Proper stretching addresses all three planes and incorporates proximal and distal musculotendinous fibers. Fredericson and colleagues[33] studied the relative effectiveness of three commonly prescribed standing ITB stretches. The authors concluded that when overhead arm extension is added to the standing ITB stretch, the ITB length and average external adduction moments could be increased.[33] This stretch is performed standing with the symptomatic leg extended and adducted across the uninvolved leg. The subject laterally flexes the trunk toward the contralateral side and extends both arms overhead (Fig. 60-5). A study evaluated the effectiveness of the Ober test (see Fig. 60-3) and the modified Ober test in stretching the ITB and the most distal component, the iliotibial tract. The modified test is performed the same as the Ober test except the knee remains extended at 0 degrees. The investigators used ultrasonography to assess the soft tissue changes of the iliotibial tract and concluded that both tests are effective in the initial stages of stretching. However, the modified Ober test may afford a greater stretch of the iliotibial tract of the ITB when additional adduction of the hip is allowed.[34] Some muscle groups do not respond to stretch unless myofascial and joint restrictions are concomitantly addressed by experienced therapists or by self-administered techniques.[17,18] Proper facilitation of hip girdle musculature can be achieved by addressing antagonistic tight structures, such as tight hip flexors or anterior hip capsule.[35] Subtalar mobilizations are often needed to prevent excessive valgus–internal rotation forces from transferring to the knee and ITB.[36] In conjunction with a flexibility and joint mobilization program, strengthening of weak or inhibited muscles can be started. Strengthening regimens ultimately need to move away from the plinth to more functional activities, such as single squats and lunges, with an emphasis on proper pelvic and core stabilization.

Finally, the maintenance phase focuses on returning patients to their respective activities with confidence in their functional abilities. In this phase, athletes are ideally observed or videotaped in their sporting environment. Frequently, runners have form deviations that lead to uncontrolled valgus–internal rotation of the knee. These abnormalities include excessive pronation, inability to shock attenuate at the knee, and Trendelenburg frontal plane gait at the pelvis. A change to shock-absorbing or motion-control shoes can accommodate supination and overpronation, respectively.[37] Foot orthoses have also been advocated for runners with lower limb injuries. Their benefit is as yet empirical. Cyclists can often correct their ITB problems with equipment and bicycle adjustments.[16] Dancers performing *rond de jambe* or *grand plié* can be cued on maintaining turnout and neutral pelvic position.[35] After sports-specific adjustments have been made, athletes need to be reintroduced to activity gradually and individually.

Procedures

Corticosteroid injections may be performed at different locations along the ITB. Injection into the anatomic pouch at the lateral femoral epicondyle is a relatively simple procedure and is advocated for patients with persistent pain and swelling[17] (Fig. 60-6). A mixture of

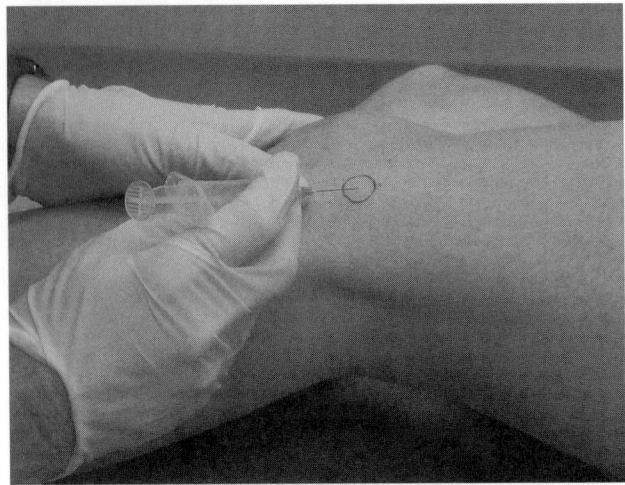

FIGURE 60-6. Distal ITB injection technique at the lateral epicondyle of the femur.

anesthetic (e.g., 1 mL of 1% lidocaine) and long-acting steroid (e.g., 1 mL of betamethasone) is instilled to the affected site. A randomized controlled study evaluating the efficacy of corticosteroid injections in runners with acute symptoms of ITB-mediated pain showed that runners in the injection group experienced less pain during running activities.[38] Steroid injections should be repeated only if adequate relief is obtained after the initial injection. Patients can return to play as their pain allows.

Surgery

Surgical treatment of ITBS is rarely needed. Surgery involves either excision of the posterior half of the ITB where it passes over the lateral femoral epicondyle or removal of the underlying putative bursa.[39] These procedures appear to have mixed results and should be contemplated only for patients who have exhausted all other options, including a comprehensive rehabilitation program as previously outlined.

POTENTIAL DISEASE COMPLICATIONS

If ITBS is not properly addressed, biomechanical adaptations can occur.[24] Chronic pain, leading to progressive disability, is a potential complication.

POTENTIAL TREATMENT COMPLICATIONS

Rehabilitation complications are rare. Nonsteroidal anti-inflammatory drugs and analgesics have well-known side effects that may affect gastrointestinal, hepatic, or renal function. Corticosteroid injections have the potential complications of infection, depigmentation of skin, and flare of symptoms at the site of injection. Surgical procedures for ITBS carry inherent risks. Postoperative infection and other standard risks should be explained to patients before surgical interventions.

Overall, interventional procedures for the ITB carry few risks or complications.

References

1. Porterfield J, DeRosa C. Mechanical Low Back Pain: Perspectives in Functional Anatomy, 2nd ed. Philadelphia, WB Saunders, 1998.
2. Gottschalk F, Kourosh S, Leveau B. The functional anatomy of tensor fasciae latae and gluteus medius and minimus. J Anat 1989;166:179-189.
3. Terry GC, Hughston JC, Norwood LA. The anatomy of the iliopatellar band and iliotibial tract. Am J Sports Med 1986;14:39-45.
4. Nemeth WC, Sanders BL. The lateral synovial recess of the knee: anatomy and role in chronic iliotibial band friction syndrome. Arthroscopy 1996;12:574-580.
5. Fairclough J, Hayashi K, Toumi H, et al. The functional anatomy of the iliotibial band during flexion and extension of the knee: implications for understanding iliotibial band syndrome. J Anat 2006;208:309-316.
6. Fredericson M, Weir A. Practical management of iliotibial band friction syndrome in runners. Clin J Sport Med 2006;16:261-268.
7. Orchard JW, Fricker PA, Abud AT, Mason BR. Biomechanics of iliotibial band friction syndrome in runners. Am J Sports Med 1996;24:375-379.
8. Noble CA. The treatment of iliotibial band friction syndrome. Br J Sports Med 1979;13:51-54.
9. Messier SP, Edwards DG, Martin DF, et al. Etiology of iliotibial band friction syndrome in distance runners. Med Sci Sports Exerc 1995;27:951-960.
10. Farrell KC, Reisinger KD, Tillman MD. Force and repetition in cycling: possible implications for iliotibial band friction syndrome. Knee 2003;10:103-109.
11. Fredericson M, Cookingham CL, Chaudhari AM, et al. Hip abductor weakness in distance runners with iliotibial band syndrome. Clin J Sport Med 2000;10:169-175.
12. James SL. Running injuries to the knee. J Am Acad Orthop Surg 1995;3:309-318.
13. Schwellnus MP. Lower limb biomechanics in runners with iliotibial band friction syndrome [abstract]. Med Sci Sports Exerc 1993;25:S68.
14. Xethalis J, Lorei M. Soccer injuries. In Nicholas J, Hershman E, eds. The Lower Extremity and Spine in Sports Medicine. St. Louis, Mosby, 1995:1509-1557.
15. Paluska S. An overview of hip injuries in running. Sport Med 2005;35:991-1014.
16. Holmes J, Pruitt A, Whalen N. Cycling injuries. In Nicholas J, Hershman E, eds. The Lower Extremity and Spine in Sports Medicine. St. Louis, Mosby, 1995:1559-1579.
17. Fredericson M, Guillet M, DeBenedictis L. Quick solutions for iliotibial band syndrome. Physician Sportsmed 2000;28:53-68.
18. Fredericson M, Wolf C. Iliotibial band syndrome in runners: innovations in treatment. Sport Med 2005;35:451-459.
19. Lindenberg G, Pinshaw R, Noakes T. Iliotibial band friction syndrome in runners. Physician Sportsmed 1984;12:118-130.
20. Holmes JC, Pruitt AL, Whalen NJ. Lower extremity overuse in bicycling. Clin Sports Med 1994;13:187-205.
21. Allen WC, Cope R. Coxa saltans: the snapping hip revisited. J Am Acad Orthop Surg 1995;3:303-308.
22. Khan K, Brown J, Way S, et al. Overuse injuries in classical ballet. Sports Med 1995;19:341-357.
23. Sammarco GJ. Dance injuries. In Nicholas J, Hershman E, eds. The Lower Extremity and Spine in Sports Medicine. St. Louis, Mosby, 1995:1385-1410.
24. Press J, Herring S, Kibler W. Rehabilitation of the combatant with musculoskeletal disorders. In Dillingham T, Belandres P, eds. Rehabilitation of the Injured Combatant. Washington, DC, Office of the Surgeon General, 1999:353-415.
25. Greenman P. Principles of Manual Medicine, 2nd ed. Baltimore, Williams & Wilkins, 1996.
26. Geraci M, Alleva J. Physical examination of the spine and its functional kinetic chain. In Cole A, Harring S, eds. The Low Back Pain Handbook. Philadelphia, Hanley & Belfus, 1996.

27. Kendall F, McCreary E, Provance P. Muscles: Testing and Function, 4 ed. Baltimore, Williams & Wilkins, 1993.

28. Puniello MS. Iliotibial band tightness and medial patellar glide in patients with patellofemoral dysfunction. J Orthop Sports Phys Ther 1993;17:144-148.

29. Martens M, Libbrecht P, Burssens A. Surgical treatment of the iliotibial band friction syndrome. Am J Sports Med 1989;17:651-654.

30. Choi YS, Lee SM, Song BY, et al. Dynamic sonography of external snapping hip syndrome. J Ultrasound Med 2002;21:753-758.

31. Bergman AG, Fredericson M. MR imaging of stress reactions, muscle injuries, and other overuse injuries in runners. Magn Reson Imaging Clin North Am 1999;7:151-174, ix.

32. Ekman EF, Pope T, Martin DF, Curl WW. Magnetic resonance imaging of iliotibial band syndrome. Am J Sports Med 1994;22:851-854.

33. Fredericson M, White JJ, Macmahon JM, Andriacchi TP. Quantitative analysis of the relative effectiveness of 3 iliotibial band stretches. Arch Phys Med Rehabil 2002;83:589-592.

34. Wang TG, Jan MH, Lin KH, Wang HK. Assessment of stretching of the iliotibial tract with Ober and modified Ober tests: an ultrasonographic study. Arch Phys Med Rehabil 2006;87:1407-1411.

35. Geraci M. Rehabilitation of the hip, pelvis, and thigh. In Kibler W, Herring S, Press J, eds. Functional Rehabilitation of Sports and Musculoskeletal Injuries. Gaithersburg, Md, Aspen, 1998:216-243.

36. Gray G. Chain Reaction Festival. Adrian, Mich, Wynn Marketing, 1999.

37. Barber FA, Sutker AN. Iliotibial band syndrome. Sports Med 1992;14:144-148.

38. Gunter P, Schwellnus MP. Local corticosteroid injection in iliotibial band friction syndrome in runners: a randomized controlled trial. Br J Sports Med 2004;38:269-272.

39. Drogset JO, Rossvoll I, Grontvedt T. Surgical treatment of iliotibial band friction syndrome. A retrospective study of 45 patients. Scand J Med Sci Sports 1999;9:296-298.

Knee Osteoarthritis 61

Allen N. Wilkins, MD, and Edward M. Phillips, MD

Synonyms

Degenerative joint disease of the knee joint
Degenerative arthritis
Joint destruction of the knee
Osteoarthrosis

ICD-9 Codes

715.16   Osteoarthrosis, localized, primary, lower leg
715.26   Osteoarthrosis, localized, secondary, lower leg
716.16   Traumatic arthropathy, lower leg

DEFINITION

Osteoarthritis is steadily becoming the most common cause of disability for the middle-aged and has become the most common cause of disability for those older than 65 years.[1] Before the age of 50 years, men have a higher prevalence and incidence than women do. However, after the age of 50 years, women have a higher overall prevalence and incidence.[2] For these individuals, the knee is the body part most commonly involved by osteoarthritis. Symptomatic knee osteoarthritis is found in approximately 10% of the population older than 65 years.[3] In addition to the growing population of elderly patients with knee osteoarthritis, an increasing number of former athletes with previous knee injuries may experience post-traumatic knee osteoarthritis. Osteoarthritis of the knee results from mechanical and idiopathic factors. Osteoarthritis alters the balance between degradation and synthesis of articular cartilage and subchondral bone.

Osteoarthritis can involve any or all of the three major knee compartments: medial, patellofemoral, or lateral. The medial compartment is most often involved and often leads to medial joint space collapse and thus to a genu varum (bowleg) deformity. Lateral compartment involvement may lead to a genu valgum (knock-knee) deformity. Isolated disease of the patellofemoral joint occurs in up to a tenth of patients with osteoarthritis of the knee. Arthritis in one compartment might, through altered biomechanical stress patterns, eventually lead to involvement of another compartment.

Osteoarthritis affects all structures within and around a joint. Hyaline articular cartilage is lost. Bone remodeling occurs, with capsular stretching and weakness of periarticular muscles. Synovitis is present in some cases. Ligamentous laxity also occurs. Lesions in the bone marrow may also develop, which may suggest trauma to bone.[4] Osteoarthritis involves the joint in a nonuniform and focal manner. Localized areas of loss of cartilage can increase focal stress across the joint, leading to further cartilage loss. With a large enough area of cartilage loss or with bone remodeling, the joint becomes tilted, and malalignment develops.

With regard to obesity, being overweight at an average age of 36 years is a risk factor for development of knee osteoarthritis in later life (>70 years). Loss of 5 kg of weight reduced the risk of symptomatic knee osteoarthritis in women (of average height) by 50%.[5]

Sports injuries and vigorous physical activity are considered to be important risk factors in knee osteoarthritis. Elite athletes who take part in high-impact sports do have an increased risk of knee osteoarthritis.[6] It is unclear whether the increased risk in this particular study was directly related to traumatic injury. However, it has been suggested in another study that subjects with a history of knee injury are at a fivefold to sixfold increased risk for development of knee osteoarthritis.[7] Knee osteoarthritis is common in those performing heavy physical work, especially if this involves knee bending, squatting, kneeling, or repetitive use of joints.[8,9] It is unclear if the association of knee osteoarthritis with these work-related activities is secondary to the nature of the work or the increased likelihood of injury.

Malalignment is the most potent risk factor for structural deterioration of the knee joint.[10] By further increasing the degree of focal loading, it creates a vicious circle of joint damage that ultimately can lead to joint failure.

SYMPTOMS

Knee osteoarthritis is characterized by joint pain, tenderness, decreased range of motion, crepitus, occasional effusion, and often inflammation of varying degrees.

345

Initial osteoarthritis symptoms are generally minimal, given the gradual and insidious onset of the condition. Pain typically occurs around the knee, particularly during weight bearing, and decreases with rest. With progression of the disease, pain can persist even at rest. Activities associated with osteoarthritic pain are climbing stairs, getting out of a chair, getting in and out of a car, and walking long distances.

Joint stiffness may occur after periods of inactivity, such as after awakening in the morning or prolonged sitting. Patients often report higher pain levels in the morning, but usually for less than 30 minutes. Patients often experience limitation of movement because of joint stiffness or swelling. Many patients report a "locking" or a "catching" sensation, which is probably due to a variety of causes, including debris from degenerated cartilage or meniscus in the joint, increased adhesiveness of the relatively rough articular surfaces, muscle weakness, and even tissue inflammation. Stiffness can discourage mobility. This initiates a cycle that results in deconditioning, decreased function, and increased pain.

Barometric changes, such as those associated with damp, rainy weather, will often increase pain intensity. Patients often note that their knees "give way" or feel unstable at times.

Pain may also radiate to adjacent sites as osteoarthritis indirectly alters the biomechanics of other anatomic structures, such as ligaments, muscles, nerves, and veins.

PHYSICAL EXAMINATION

Examination of the patient includes testing for various possible causes of knee pain (see the section on differential diagnosis). Therefore, the entire limb from the hip to the ankle is examined. It is important to identify findings such as quadriceps weakness or atrophy and knee and hip flexion contractures. Gait should be observed for presence of a limp, functional limb length discrepancy, or buckling. Genu varum or valgum is often better appreciated when the patient is standing.

The affected knee should be compared with the contralateral uninvolved knee. Knee examination may reveal decreased knee extension or flexion secondary to effusion or osteophytes (both of which may be palpable). Osteophytes along the femoral condyles may be palpated, especially along the medial distal femur. Palpation may reveal patellar or parapatellar tenderness. Crepitation, resulting from juxtaposition of roughened cartilage surfaces, may be appreciated along the joint line when the knee is flexed or extended. A mild effusion and tenderness may be appreciated along the medial joint line or at the pes anserine bursa. Ligament testing may reveal laxity of one or both of the collateral ligaments. Lateral subluxation of the patella may be found in patients with genu valgum (Table 61-1).

The findings of the neurologic examination are typically normal, with the exception of decreased muscle strength, particularly in the quadriceps, due to disuse or guarding secondary to pain.

TABLE 61-1 Typical Physical Examination Findings in Knee Osteoarthritis	
Inspection	Bone hypertrophy
	Varus deformity from preferential medial compartment involvement
Palpation	Increased warmth
	Joint effusion
	Joint line tenderness
Range of motion	Painful knee flexion
	Decreased joint flexion secondary to pain
	Crepitus (coarse)
Joint stability	Mediolateral instability

Another clue on examination that the patient probably has knee osteoarthritis is the finding of visible bone enlargements (exostoses) of the fingers. At the distal interphalangeal joints, these are referred to as Heberden nodes; at the proximal interphalangeal joints, they are known as Bouchard nodes, usually a slightly later finding.

FUNCTIONAL LIMITATIONS

Joint stiffness and pain during weight bearing lead directly to difficulties with prolonged standing, transfers, walking, and participation in physical activity or exercise programs. Involvement of the patellofemoral compartment may lead to difficulty with climbing stairs as well as to a buckling sensation. Disability is further compounded by secondary factors such as depression, poor aerobic capacity, and coexisting chronic conditions.[11] Radiographic evidence of knee osteoarthritis, even without symptoms, is associated with an increased risk for dependence with activities of daily living.[12] The risk for dependence with stair climbing and walking attributed to knee osteoarthritis is comparable to that with cardiovascular disease and greater than with any other medical condition in elders.[13]

DIAGNOSTIC STUDIES

Radiographic abnormalities can be found both in joint areas subjected to excessive pressure and in joint areas subjected to diminished pressure. These changes include joint space narrowing, subchondral sclerosis, and bone cysts in weight-bearing regions of the joint and osteophytes in low-pressure areas, especially along the marginal regions of the joint. Joint space narrowing is the initial finding, followed by subchondral sclerosis, then by osteophytes, and finally by cysts with sclerotic margins (known as synovial cysts, subchondral cysts, subarticular pseudocysts, or necrotic pseudocysts).

Radiographic evidence of osteoarthritis is not well correlated with symptoms.[14] Results have been conflicting, probably because of the differences in populations studied and radiographic and clinical criteria used. The presence of osteophytes had a strong association with knee pain, whereas the absence or presence of joint space narrowing was not associated with pain.[15] Knee pain severity was a more important determinant of functional impairment than radiographic severity of osteoarthritis.[16,17] There was no correlation between joint space narrowing and a disability score (Western Ontario and McMaster Universities Osteoarthritis index, WOMAC) at a single time point.[17]

Osteophytes *alone* are associated with aging rather than with osteoarthritis. Indications for plain x-ray films include trauma, effusion, symptoms not readily explainable by physical examination findings, severe pain, presurgical planning, and failure of conservative management.

Recommended films are weight-bearing (standing) anteroposterior, lateral, and patellar views. Radiographs taken during weight bearing with the knee in full extension and partial flexion may reveal a constellation of findings associated with osteoarthritis, including asymmetric narrowing of the joint space (typically medial compartment), osteophytes, sclerosis, and subchondral cysts (Fig. 61-1). A Merchant view specifically evaluates the patellofemoral space. Non–weight-bearing lateral views may help in the evaluation of the patellofemoral and tibiofemoral joint spaces. Tunnel views can help visualize loose osteochondral bodies.

Magnetic resonance imaging usually adds little but cost to the entire evaluation of osteoarthritis of the knee. It may reveal changes that suggest the presence of osteoarthritis. However, it is not indicated in the initial evaluation of older persons with chronic knee pain. Magnetic resonance imaging findings of osteoarthritis, such as meniscal tears, are common in middle-aged and older adults with and without knee pain.

Musculoskeletal ultrasonography has potential for detecting bone erosions, synovitis, tendon disease, and enthesopathy. It has a number of distinct advantages over magnetic resonance imaging, including good patient tolerability and ability to scan multiple joints in a short time. However, there are scarce data about its validity, reproducibility, and responsiveness to change, making interpretation and comparison of studies difficult. In particular, there are limited data describing standardized scanning methodology and standardized definitions of ultrasound pathologic changes.[18]

Laboratory test results are typically normal, but analysis may be undertaken especially for elder patients to establish a baseline (e.g., blood urea nitrogen concentration, creatinine concentration, or liver function tests before use of nonsteroidal anti-inflammatory drugs or acetaminophen) or to exclude other conditions such as rheumatoid arthritis. Synovial fluid analysis should not be undertaken unless destructive, crystalline, or septic arthritis is suspected.

TREATMENT

Initial

The PRICE regimen may help provide initial relief for patients in pain: *p*rotection with limited weight bearing by use of a cane or modification of exercise to reduce stress; relative *r*est (or taking adequate rests throughout the day, avoiding prolonged standing, climbing of stairs, kneeling, deep knee bending); *i*ce (applied while the skin is protected with a towel for up to 15 minutes at a time several times a day; note, however, that some patients with chronic pain may find better relief with moist heat); *c*ompression (if swelling exists, wrapping with an elastic bandage or a sleeve may help); and *e*levation (may help diminish swelling, if it is present).

There are a wide variety of treatment options for knee arthritis. Such options include oral and topical nonsteroidal anti-inflammatory drugs; topical capsaicin cream; acetaminophen; and nutritional intervention, such as glucosamine sulfate, chondroitin sulfate, and vitamin C (Table 61-2). Orthotics and footwear are also included in the list of treatment options and are discussed further in the next section.

Rehabilitation

Exercise

Exercises are likely to be most effective if they train muscles for the activities a person performs daily.[29] Randomized studies support the benefits of exercise, even if it is home based, on pain and function in patients with osteoarthritis.[30-32] Because there is currently no cure for osteoarthritis, most research continues to evaluate the use of exercise as a treatment to alleviate symptoms of the disease and to enhance functional capacity. Two meta-analyses published in 2004 focus specifically on the efficacy of strengthening[33] and aerobic exercise[34] for osteoarthritis.

With regard to muscle strengthening, improvements in strength, pain, function, and quality of life were noted. However, there was no evidence that the type of strengthening exercise influences outcome. Static or dynamic

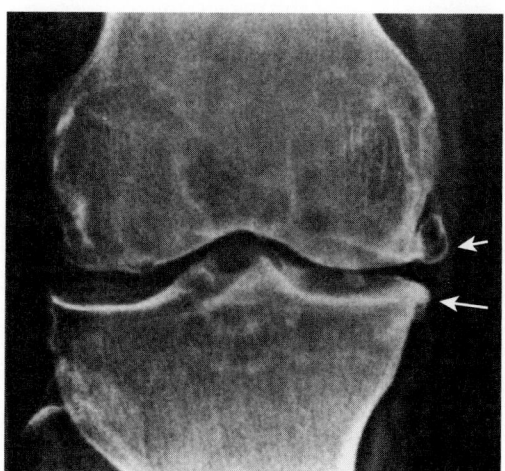

FIGURE 61-1. Knee radiograph demonstrating osteophytes *(arrows)* and medial joint space narrowing consistent with degenerative arthritis. (Reprinted with permission from West SG. Rheumatology Secrets. Philadelphia, Hanley & Belfus, 1997:58.)

TABLE 61-2 Pharmacologic and Supplemental Nutrition Treatment Options

Medication	Related Details
Acetaminophen	Acetaminophen appears to be less effective among patients who have already received treatment with NSAIDs.[19] The maximum dosage is 4 g/day in patients with normal hepatic function.
Oral NSAIDs	Studies show almost equal efficacy among traditional NSAIDs.[20,21] A randomized prospective study demonstrated equal efficacy between selective cyclooxygenase 2 inhibitors and traditional NSAIDs.[22]
Tramadol-acetaminophen	American Pain Society guidelines recommend tramadol-acetaminophen for treatment of osteoarthritis pain when NSAIDs alone cannot provide adequate relief. It is considered safe and effective in a subset of elderly patients.[23]
Oxycodone	Patients with moderate to severe pain from osteoarthritis can achieve effective pain relief without deterioration in function when opioids are included as part of a comprehensive pain management program.[24]
Topical NSAIDs	A quantitative systematic review of 86 trials evaluating the efficacy of topical NSAIDs in osteoarthritis and tendinitis found them significantly more effective than placebo.[25]
Topical capsaicin	Limited data from controlled trials have shown improvements with capsaicin.[26]
Glucosamine sulfate (1500 mg orally qd) and chondroitin sulfate (1200 mg orally qd)	One large randomized clinical trial found that glucosamine and chondroitin sulfate alone or in combination did not reduce pain effectively in the overall group of patients with osteoarthritis of the knee. However, the combination of glucosamine and chondroitin sulfate was effective in the subgroup of patients with moderate to severe knee pain.[27]
Vitamin C	Vitamin C was associated with reduced progression of radiographic osteoarthritis and pain in one study.[28]

NSAIDs, nonsteroidal anti-inflammatory drugs.

Differential Diagnosis

Common Causes of Knee Pain by Age Group

Children and adolescents	Patellar subluxation Osgood-Schlatter disease Patellar tendinitis Referred pain (e.g., slipped capital femoral epiphysis) Osteochondritis dissecans Subchondral fracture Genetic or congenital defect Septic arthritis Tumor
Adults	Patellofemoral pain syndrome (chondromalacia patellae) Medial plica syndrome Pes anserine bursitis Trauma: ligamentous sprains Meniscal tear Inflammatory arthropathy: rheumatoid arthritis, Reiter syndrome Septic arthritis Midlumbar radiculopathy Tumor
Older adults	Osteoarthritis Crystal-induced inflammatory arthropathy: gout, pseudogout Rheumatoid arthritis Popliteal cyst Tumor

Differential Diagnosis of Knee Pain by Anatomic Site

Anterior knee pain	Patellar subluxation or dislocation Tibial apophysitis (Osgood-Schlatter lesion) Jumper's knee (patellar tendinitis) Patellofemoral pain syndrome (chondromalacia patellae)
Medial knee pain	Medial collateral ligament sprain Medial meniscal tear Pes anserine bursitis Medial plica syndrome
Lateral knee pain	Lateral collateral ligament sprain Lateral meniscal tear Iliotibial band tendinitis
Posterior knee pain	Popliteal cyst (Baker's cyst) Posterior cruciate ligament injury

strengthening exercises can maintain or improve periarticular muscle strength, thereby reversing or preventing biomechanical abnormalities and their contribution to joint dysfunction and degeneration.

With regard to aerobic exercise, results indicated that aerobic exercise alleviates pain and joint tenderness and promotes functional status and respiratory capacity. Aerobic exercise improves activity tolerance, increases pain threshold, and can have positive effects on mood and motivation for participation in other activities.

Whereas strengthening appears superior to aerobic exercise in the short term for specific impairment-related outcomes (e.g., pain), aerobic exercise appears more effective for functional outcomes in the longer term. There is also evidence that exercise can improve proprioception,[29] thus improving biomechanics and protective responses.

Attempts to maintain function can be helped through non–weight-bearing strengthening, especially of the quadriceps. For patients with greater pain, this can be done with static exercise or through water aerobics, which allows motion at the knee with reduced joint loads. Exercise bicycles and walking should be recommended to enhance aerobic capacity. Deep knee bends in the presence of effusion should be avoided. Particular attention must be paid to strengthening of the medial quadriceps in patients with genu valgum who have lateral subluxation of the patella. Maintaining activity is critical to maintaining function. Even those patients scheduled for total knee arthroplasty should pursue static and dynamic strengthening as well as cardiovascular conditioning preoperatively to ease the postoperative rehabilitation.

Modalities

The use of transcutaneous electrical nerve stimulation (TENS) is supported by a few small, short-term trials. In a small-scale, randomized, double-blind crossover trial comparing active and placebo TENS for symptomatic knee osteoarthritis in subjects who were considered to be candidates for total knee replacement, patients reported significantly more pain relief and less medication use with active TENS therapy than with the placebo.[35] For most patients, pain relief was experienced only during periods of active use of the device, although the beneficial effect was sustained for several hours in a few.

Additional therapeutic modalities, such as electrical stimulation or massage, may also be used. Therapists may also review postural alignment and joint positioning techniques, especially for when the patient is sleeping. In particular, the use of a pillow under bent knees, much favored by many patients when they are supine, should be avoided because resulting knee flexion contractures, even if small, can significantly increase stresses on the knee during gait. Stretching of the hamstrings and quadriceps may also prove beneficial. Patients should be counseled against prolonged wearing of high heels, which is associated with medial knee osteoarthritis.[36]

Adaptive Equipment

Adaptive equipment, such as a cane or walker, can reduce hip or knee loading, thereby reducing pain. It may also prevent falls in patients with impaired balance. Proper training in the use of a cane is important because it reduces joint loading in the contralateral hip but amplifies forces in the ipsilateral hip.

Bracing and Footwear

The basic rationale for a knee brace for unicompartmental knee osteoarthritis is to improve function by reducing the patient's symptoms. This can be accomplished, in theory, by reducing the biomechanical load on the affected compartment of the knee. Clinical trials are generally small and difficult to control adequately because of the nature of knee braces and the difficulty in designing a trial with a true placebo. Also, each brace has a unique design and may have features that make it more or less acceptable to the patient. Therefore, clinical trials done with one brace design may not be applicable to all osteoarthritis knee braces.

A review of the published literature on knee bracing for osteoarthritis points out some of the limitations of the clinical trials to date but acknowledges the limited evidence for improvement in pain and function in patients using osteoarthritis braces compared with medical treatment or neoprene sleeves.[37]

In patients with osteoarthritis and varus malalignment of the knees, a shoe wedge (thicker laterally) moves the center of loading laterally during walking, a change that extends from foot to knee, lessening medial load across the knee. Although such modifications to footwear decrease varus malalignment,[38] one randomized trial[39] showed no reduction in pain compared with a neutral insert. However, a review of the published literature on the efficacy of laterally wedged foot orthotics for improving these symptoms does indicate a strong scientific basis for applying wedged insoles in an attempt to reduce pain in patients with medial compartment knee osteoarthritis.[40]

Tilting or malalignment of the patella may cause patellofemoral pain. Patellar realignment with the use of braces or tape to pull the patella back into the trochlear sulcus of the femur or to reduce its tilt may lessen pain. In clinical trials using tape to reposition the patella into the sulcus without tilt, knee pain was reduced compared with placebo.[41,42] However, patients may find it difficult to apply tape, and skin irritation is common. Commercial patellar braces are also available, but their efficacy has not been studied formally.

Heel lifts or built-up shoes may be required in the presence of leg length discrepancy to prevent compensatory knee flexion gait on the longer side. In the presence of knee deformity, therapists can also evaluate for altered biomechanics (e.g., genu varum may lead to femoral internal torsion, resulting in compensatory external rotation of the tibia, which predisposes the patient to increased arthritic changes). Therapists can also visit the homes and workplaces of patients to

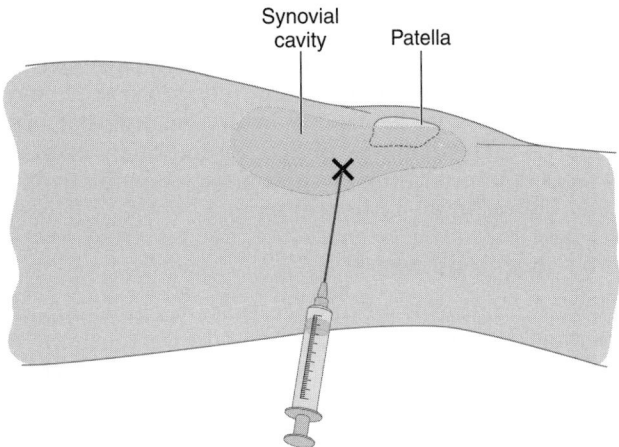

FIGURE 61-2. Location for needle insertion.

suggest adjustments, such as raised toilet seats, grab bars, reachers, and the like.

Acupuncture

Acupuncture, a technique in existence for thousands of years, has gained renewed interest as a treatment of osteoarthritis. A multicenter, 26-week National Institutes of Health–funded randomized controlled trial found acupuncture to be effective as adjunctive therapy for reducing pain and improving function in patients with knee osteoarthritis.[43]

Procedures

Intra-articular corticosteroid injections may help in reduction of local inflammation and improvement of symptoms. Injection is most often used as an adjunctive therapy for acute or severe symptom flares (Fig. 61-2). Because the corticosteroid is delivered directly, systemic toxicity is minimized. Intra-articular corticosteroid injections should be given no more than two or three times a year to reduce potential damage to cartilage from the steroids. Table 61-3 lists potential systemic side effects of corticosteroid injections. Administration of steroids through iontophoresis

may be an alternative for patients hesitant to undergo injections.

The authors' preferred technique for intra-articular injection of the knee is as follows. With the patient supine, under sterile conditions with use of a 25-gauge needle, 2 or 3 mL of local anesthetic (e.g., 1% lidocaine) is injected just posterior to the upper lateral pole of the patella. Alternatively, ethyl chloride spray can be used. Then, by use of a 1½-inch, 22- to 25-gauge needle, either local steroid (e.g., methylprednisolone, 20 to 40 mg/mL) or hyaluronic acid is injected in the same region (these products are available in 2-mL vials or prefilled syringes, one injection per vial).

If a knee effusion exists, it may be necessary to drain the effusion to avoid dilution of the medications. This is ideally done with an 18- to 20-gauge needle. Switching of the syringes while the needle remains in place prevents additional trauma.

Postinjection care includes local icing for 5 to 10 minutes. Patients are advised to avoid excessive weight bearing for 24 to 48 hours after an injection.

Viscosupplementation with hyaluronic acid, available as naturally occurring hyaluronan or synthetic hylan G-F 20, may be helpful. Hyaluronan is administered in a series of five weekly injections; hylan G-F 20 is given in three weekly injections. Treatments are typically repeated two to four times per year.

Clinical trials of hyaluronan injections have focused on patients with knee osteoarthritis. However, data on efficacy are inconsistent. Two meta-analyses[23,44] reported statistically significant but limited clinical efficacy. One meta-analysis showed publication bias in the form of preferential publication of positive studies. Two large, unpublished trials showed no efficacy with hyaluronan injections.[44]

Side effects included local inflammation and increased pain at the injection site. There is no evidence that hyaluronan injection in humans alters biologic processes or progression of cartilage damage. The hyaluronic acid is injected into the knee in the same manner as the intra-articular steroid is administered.

TABLE 61-3 Minimizing Potential Side Effects of Intra-articular Corticosteroid

Side Effect	Ways to Minimize Risk
Systemic effects	Avoid high doses and multiple simultaneous injections; use accurate injection techniques
Tendon rupture, fat atrophy, muscle wasting, skin pigment changes	Avoid misdirected injections
Septic arthritis	Use sterile technique; withhold therapy in at-risk patients
Nerve and blood vessel damage	Use accurate injection techniques
Postinjection symptom flare or synovitis	Avoid the same preparation for future injections
Flushing	Avoid high doses
Anaphylaxis	Take careful drug allergy history
Steroid arthropathy	Avoid high doses and overly frequent injections

Surgery (Table 61-4)

Most would agree that the term *arthroscopic débridement* includes lavage and the removal of loose bodies, debris, mobile fragments of articular cartilage, unstable torn menisci, and impinging osteophytes. However, it is clear from the literature that drilling, abrasion chondroplasty, microfracture, saucerization, notchplasty, osteophyte removal, synovectomy, and arthrolysis are also performed simultaneously in many clinical series.

Patients who have a short history and a sudden onset of mechanical symptoms and also have knee effusions are likely to do best.[45] Meniscal symptoms and signs, synovitis or synovial impingement, osteophytic impingement, and catching or locking caused by loose bodies favor a good outcome. Significant instability and malalignment are poor prognostic factors. Patients who have radiographic signs of advanced degeneration are unlikely to benefit.[45]

Most of the orthopedic published literature on knee osteoarthritis has reported retrospective studies. Most authors report improvement in 50% to 80% of patients; however, as one would expect with a degenerative condition, results deteriorate with time. There is evidence supporting the therapeutic value of arthroscopic débridement of the knee.[46-48] However, there is a need for better-designed clinical trials comparing arthroscopic débridement with established alternative treatments.

Up to a quarter of patients with osteoarthritis of the knee have predominantly arthritis of the medial compartment. The surgical options for such patients are medial unicompartmental knee replacement, proximal tibial or distal femoral osteotomy, and total knee replacement.

Osteotomy is a less drastic measure than knee replacement and is often favored by younger, active patients with unicompartmental symptoms. In osteotomy, a wedge-shaped piece of bone is removed from either the femur or tibia to bring the knee joint back into a more physiologic alignment. This procedure moves the weight-bearing axis to the less damaged compartment. Recovery is prolonged and relief of symptoms often incomplete, but osteotomy may delay the need for total knee replacement for 5 to 10 years.[49,50] Successful treatment could allow a return to sport. The risks specific to this surgery depend on the technique and include nonunion at the osteotomy site, common peroneal nerve injury, pain from the proximal tibiofibular joint, and overcorrection or undercorrection of the deformity. Part of an ongoing debate within the orthopedic community concerns the relative merits of high tibial osteotomy compared with unicompartmental knee replacement in younger patients.

Unicompartmental knee replacement requires a smaller surgical approach than for total knee replacement, leading to less blood loss and quicker rehabilitation. The range of knee motion after unicompartmental knee replacement is generally superior to that after total knee replacement. Finally, revision of a unicompartmental knee replacement to a total knee replacement is potentially more straightforward than revision of a total knee replacement.[51]

The prerequisites for a unicompartmental knee replacement include stability of the joint, correctable varus deformity, fixed flexion deformity of less than 10 degrees, and minimal lateral compartment disease. Radiographic evidence of patellofemoral osteoarthritis is not necessarily a problem, provided patients do not have major anterior knee pain. Two studies have reported survivorship rates for implants of 95% and 98% at 10 years.[52,53] These rates are comparable to the best reported for total knee replacement and are an improvement on rates previously reported for unicompartmental knee replacement.

The relative merits of unicompartmental knee replacement over total knee replacement or proximal tibial osteotomy in young (<60 years) active patients continue to be debated. Unicompartmental knee replacement has

TABLE 61-4 Surgical Options for Osteoarthritis of the Knee

Established Techniques	Indications	Outcome
Arthroscopic débridement	Knee effusions Meniscal signs and symptoms Synovitis Osteophytic impingement Catching or locking caused by loose bodies	Most reports show improvement in 50% to 80% of patients; however, results deteriorate with time
Osteotomy of the proximal tibia or distal femur	Predominantly medial compartment involvement	Recovery is prolonged Relief of symptoms often incomplete
Unicompartmental knee replacement	Predominantly medial compartment involvement Minimal lateral compartment disease No major anterior knee pain Stable knee joint Correctable varus deformity Fixed flexion deformity of less than 10 degrees	Survivorship rates for implants of 95% and 98% at 10 years
Patellofemoral replacement	Isolated patellofemoral joint involvement	Results have been variable
Total knee replacement	Tricompartmental disease	Survival rates of between 84% and 98% at 15 years

now become an accepted treatment for older patients with medial compartment arthritis. The results of unicompartmental knee replacement in lateral compartment disease have yet to be fully determined.

Patients considered for patellofemoral replacement must be assessed for degenerative changes in the rest of the knee joint. Several types of patellofemoral arthroplasties are available, but the results have been variable, highlighting the need for careful selection of patients.[51,54,55] The most common problems are maltracking of the patella, excessive wear of the polyethylene implant, and disease progression in the rest of the knee joint.

Total knee replacements, with a quarter-century track record, have generally provided most patients with good pain relief (see Chapter 71). Whereas joint replacement surgery has been found in numerous studies to provide pain relief, it paradoxically may lead to increase of services as patients become more mobile.[56]

Severe chondromalacia may necessitate patellectomy (patella excision). Knee arthrodesis today is generally reserved for patients in whom knee replacement surgery fails. Other less commonly used surgical options, such as synovectomy and small prostheses (to correct deformity), are also possible.

POTENTIAL DISEASE COMPLICATIONS

Progressive knee osteoarthritis may result in reduced mobility and the general systemic complications of immobility and deconditioning. Antalgic gait can result in contralateral hip disease (e.g., greater trochanteric bursitis). The risk of falls will be increased by decreased mobility at the knee. Complaints of chronic pain may result from the initial knee osteoarthritis if it is inadequately treated.

POTENTIAL TREATMENT COMPLICATIONS

Complications of anti-inflammatory medication and steroid injections are well known. Repeated steroid injections can lead to further cartilage destruction as well as to sepsis. Infection is a rare but possible result of joint injection or surgery. Cryotherapy or heat therapy can, of course, lead to frostbite or burns. Hyaluronic acid injections may result in localized transient pain or effusion.

Arthroscopy may damage the articular surface membrane, thus initiating damage to uninvolved cartilage. Excessive arthroscopic scraping has sometimes been associated with persistent pain. The possibility of infection and deep venous thrombosis and the small but real possibility of intraoperative mortality limit the use of surgery to a last-line option. One series of patients *not* taking anticoagulants experienced a 50% rate of deep venous thrombosis, 14.5% of which was proximal deep venous thrombosis,[57] thus indicating the importance of anticoagulation, which reduces the risk to less than 5%. In any case, mechanical wear and prosthesis loosening, especially for cement prostheses, often lead to the need for revision after a decade or so.

References

1. Bashaw RT, Tingstad EM. Rehabilitation of the osteoarthritic patient: focus on the knee. Clin Sports Med 2005;24:101-131.
2. Felson DT, Zhang Y. An update on the epidemiology of knee and hip osteoarthritis with a view to prevention. Arthritis Rheum 1998;41:1343-1355.
3. Krohn K. Footwear alterations and bracing for knee osteoarthritis. Curr Opin Rheumatol 2005;17:653-656.
4. Felson DT, McLaughlin S, Goggins J, et al. Bone marrow edema and its relation to progression of knee osteoarthritis. Ann Intern Med 2003;139:330-336.
5. Pai Y-C, Rymer WZ, Chang RW, et al. Effect of age and osteoarthritis on knee proprioception. Arthritis Rheum 1997;40:2260-2265.
6. Oiveria SA, Felson DT, Reed JI, et al. Incidence of symptomatic hand, hip and knee osteoarthritis among patients in a health maintenance organisation. Arthritis Rheum 1995;38:1134-1141.
7. Felson DT, Zhang Y, Hannan MT, et al. The incidence and natural history of knee osteoarthritis in the elderly: the Framingham Osteoarthritis Study. Arthritis Rheum 1995;38:1500-1505.
8. Hunter DJ, March L, Sambrook PN. Knee osteoarthritis: the influence of environmental factors. Clin Exp Rheumatol 2002;20: 93-100.
9. Maetzel A, Makela M, Hawker G, et al. Osteoarthritis of the hip and knee and mechanical occupational exposure: a systematic overview of the evidence. J Rheumatol 1997;24:599-607.
10. Sharma L, Song J, Felson DT, et al. The role of knee alignment in disease progression and functional decline in knee osteoarthritis. JAMA 2001;286:188-195.
11. Felson DT, Lawrence RC, Dieppe PA, et al. Osteoarthritis: new insights. Part 1: the disease and its risk factors. Ann Intern Med 2000;133:635-646.
12. Guccione A, Felson D, Anderson J. Defining arthritis and measuring functional status in elders: methodological issues in the study of disease and physical disability. Am J Public Health 1990;80:945-949.
13. Guccione A, Felson D, Anderson J, et al. The effects of specific medical conditions on the functional limitation of elders in the Framingham Study. Am J Public Health 1994;84:351-358.
14. Lawrence J, Bremner J, Bier F. Osteo-arthrosis. Prevalence in the population and relationships between symptoms and x-ray changes. Ann Rheum Dis 1966;25:1-24.
15. Cicuttini F, Baker J, Hart D, et al. Association of pain with radiological changes in different compartments and views of the knee joint. Osteoarthritis Cartilage 1996;4:143-147.
16. Bruyere O, Honore A, Giacovelli G, et al. Radiologic features poorly predict clinical outcomes in knee osteoarthritis. Scand J Rheumatol 2002;31:13-16.
17. McAlindon T, Cooper C, Kirwan J, et al. Determinants of disability in osteoarthritis of the knee. Ann Rheum Dis 1993;52:258-262.
18. Wakefield RJ, Balint PV, Szkudlarek M, et al. Musculoskeletal ultrasound including definitions for ultrasonographic pathology. J Rheumatol 2005;32:2485-2487.
19. Pincus T, Koch GG, Sokka T, et al. A randomized, double-blind, crossover clinical trial of diclofenac plus misoprostol versus acetaminophen in patients with osteoarthritis of the hip or knee. Arthritis Rheum 2001;44:1587-1598.
20. Towheed TE, Hochberg MC. A systematic review of randomized controlled trials of pharmacological therapy in osteoarthritis of the hip. J Rheumatol 1997;24:349-357.
21. Goldberg SH, Von Feldt JM, Lonner JH. Pharmacologic therapy for osteoarthritis. Am J Orthop 2002;31:673-680.
22. Cannon GW, Caldwell JR, Holt P, et al. Rofecoxib, a specific inhibitor of cyclooxygenase 2, with clinical efficacy comparable with that of diclofenac sodium: results of a one-year, randomized, clinical trial in patients with osteoarthritis of the knee and hip. Rofecoxib Phase III Protocol 035 Study Group. Arthritis Rheum 2000;43:978-987.
23. Rosenthal NR, et al, for the CAPSS-105 Study Group. Tramadol/acetaminophen combination tablets for the treatment of pain associated with osteoarthritis flare in an elderly patient population. J Am Geriatr Soc 2004;52:374-380.

24. Apgar B. Controlled-release oxycodone for osteoarthritis-related pain. Am Fam Physician 2000;62:1405-1406.

25. Moore RA, Tramer MR, Carroll D, et al. Quantitative systematic review of topically applied non-steroidal anti-inflammatory drugs. BMJ 1998;316:333-338.

26. Zhang WY, Po ALW. The effectiveness of topically applied capsaicin: a meta-analysis. Eur J Clin Pharmacol 1994;46:517-522.

27. Clegg DO, Reda DJ, Harris CL, et al. Glucosamine, chondroitin sulfate, and the two in combination for painful knee osteoarthritis. N Engl J Med 2006;354:795-808.

28. McAlindon TE, Jacques P, Zhang Y, et al. Do antioxidant micronutrients protect against the development and progression of knee osteoarthritis? Arthritis Rheum 1996;39:648-656.

29. Felson D. Osteoarthritis of the knee. N Engl J Med 2006;354:841-848.

30. O'Reilly SC, Muir KR, Doherty M. Effectiveness of a home exercise on pain and disability from osteoarthritis of the knee: a randomised controlled trial. Ann Rheum Dis 1999;58:15-19.

31. Ettinger WH Jr, Burns R, Messier SP, et al. A randomized trial comparing aerobic exercise and resistance exercise with a health education program in older adults with knee osteoarthritis: the Fitness Arthritis and Seniors Trial (FAST). JAMA 1997;277:25-31.

32. Baker KR, Nelson ME, Felson DT, et al. The efficacy of home based progressive strength training in older adults with knee osteoarthritis: a randomized controlled trial. J Rheumatol 2001;28:1655-1665.

33. Pelland L, Brosseau L, Wells G, et al. Efficacy of strengthening exercises for osteoarthritis. Part I: a meta-analysis. Phys Ther Rev 2004;9:77-108.

34. Brosseau L, Pelland L, Wells G, et al. Efficacy of aerobic exercises for osteoarthritis. Part II: a meta-analysis. Phys Ther Rev 2004;9:125-145.

35. Puett DW, Griffin MR. Published trials of nonmedicinal and noninvasive therapies for hip and knee osteoarthritis. Ann Intern Med 1994;121:133-140.

36. Kerrigan D, Todd M, O'Reilly P. Knee osteoarthritis and high heeled shoes. Lancet 1998;351:1399-1401.

37. Brouwer R, Jakma T, Verhagen A, et al. Braces and orthoses for treating osteoarthritis of the knee. Cochrane Database Syst Rev 2005;1:CD004020.

38. Kerrigan DC, Lelas JL, Goggins J, et al. Effectiveness of a lateral-wedge insole on knee varus torque in patients with knee osteoarthritis. Arch Phys Med Rehabil 2002;83:889-893.

39. Maillefert JF, Hudry C, Baron G, et al. Laterally elevated wedged insoles in the treatment of medial knee osteoarthritis: a prospective randomized controlled study. Osteoarthritis Cartilage 2001;9:738-745.

40. Marks R, Penton L. Are foot orthotics efficacious for treating painful medial compartment knee osteoarthritis? A review of the literature. Int J Clin Pract 2004;58:49-57.

41. Hinman RS, Crossley KM, McConnell J, Bennell KL. Efficacy of knee tape in the management of osteoarthritis of the knee: blinded randomised controlled trial. BMJ 2003;327:135.

42. Cushnaghan J, McCarthy C, Dieppe P. Taping the patella medially: a new treatment for osteoarthritis of the knee joint? BMJ 1994;308:753-755.

43. Hochberg M, Lixing L, Bausell B, et al. Traditional Chinese acupuncture is effective as adjunctive therapy in patients with osteoarthritis of the knee [abstract]. Arthritis Rheum 2004;50:S644.

44. Lo GH, LaValley M, McAlindon T, et al. Intra-articular hyaluronic acid in treatment of knee osteoarthritis: a metaanalysis. JAMA 2003;290:3115-3121.

45. Day B. The indications for arthroscopic débridement for osteoarthritis of the knee. Orthop Clin North Am 2005;36:413-417.

46. Jackson RW, Dieterichs C. The results of arthroscopic lavage and débridement of osteoarthritic knees based on the severity of degeneration: a 4- to 6-year symptomatic follow-up. Arthroscopy 2003;19:13-20.

47. Fond J, Rudin D, Ahmad S, et al. Arthroscopic débridement of osteoarthritis of the knee: 2- and 5-year results. Arthroscopy 2002;18:829-834.

48. Pearse EO, Craig DM. Partial meniscectomy in the presence of severe osteoarthritis does not hasten the symptomatic progression of osteoarthritis. Arthroscopy 2003;19:963-968.

49. Naudie D, Bourne RB, Rorabeck CH, Bourne TJ. The Install Award. Survivorship of the high tibial valgus osteotomy. A 10- to 22-year followup study. Clin Orthop Relat Res 1999;367:18-27.

50. Billings A, Scott DF, Camargo MP, et al. High tibial osteotomy with a calibrated osteotomy guide, rigid internal fixation, and early motion. Long-term follow-up. J Bone Joint Surg Am 2000;82:70-79.

51. Deshmukh RV, Scott RD. Unicompartmental knee arthroplasty: long-term results. Clin Orthop Relat Res 2001;392:272-278.

52. Murray DW, Goodfellow JW, O'Connor JJ. The Oxford medial unicompartmental arthroplasty: a ten-year survival study. J Bone Joint Surg Br 1998;80:983-989.

53. Svard UC, Price AJ. Oxford medial unicompartmental knee arthroplasty. A survival analysis of an independent series. J Bone Joint Surg Br 2001;83:191-194.

54. Smith AM, Peckett WR, Butler-Manuel PA, et al. Treatment of patellofemoral arthritis using the Lubinus patellofemoral arthroplasty: a retrospective review. Knee 2002;9:27-30.

55. Tauro B, Ackroyd CE, Newman JH, Shah NA. The Lubinus patellofemoral arthroplasty. A five- to ten-year prospective study. J Bone Joint Surg Br 2002;84:696-701.

56. Orbell S, Espley A, Johnston M, Rowley D. Health benefits of joint replacement surgery for patients with osteoarthritis. J Epidemiol Community Health 1998;52:564-570.

57. Fujita S, Hirota S, Oda T, et al. Deep venous thrombosis after total hip or total knee arthroplasty in patients in Japan. Clin Orthop Relat Res 2000;375:168-174.

Knee Bursitis 62

Ed Hanada, MD, Florian S. Keplinger, MD, and Navneet Gupta, MD

Synonyms

Prepatellar bursitis (housemaid's knee)
Infrapatellar bursitis (vicar's knee)
Anserine bursitis
Medial (tibial) collateral ligament bursitis
Semimembranosus bursitis

ICD-9 Codes

726.60   Enthesopathy of knee, unspecified bursitis of knee
726.61   Pes anserinus tendinitis or bursitis
726.62   Tibial collateral ligament bursitis
726.63   Fibular collateral ligament bursitis
726.65   Prepatellar bursitis
726.69   Other bursitis: infrapatellar; subpatellar

DEFINITION

Knee bursitis can arise from inflammation of any bursa in the region of the knee joint and is a common clinical disorder that may lead to functional difficulties. Eleven bursae are found within this region (Fig. 62-1).[1] Three bursae communicate with the knee joint: quadriceps or suprapatellar, popliteus, and medial gastrocnemius. Four bursae are associated with the patella: superficial and deep prepatellar, and superficial and deep infrapatellar. Two are related to the semimembranosus tendons, and two are related to the collateral ligaments of the knee (one of which is under the pes anserinus, or the conjoined tendons of the sartorius, gracilis, and semitendinosus muscles).[1]

In the popliteal fossa, a bursa is located between the medial head of the gastrocnemius and semimembranosus tendon. Swelling in this area is also called Baker's cyst and may actually be due to other inflammatory or degenerative conditions (see Chapter 56). For this chapter's purpose, discussion is limited to knee bursitis arising from inflammation of the previously mentioned bursae.

The most common knee bursitis conditions are the following.

Prepatellar bursitis (housemaid's knee) is caused by direct trauma, such as falling on a bent knee or frequent kneeling on a hard surface.[1] A case of a massive prepatellar bursitis from chronic crawling as a means of household ambulation in an adult man with cerebral palsy has been reported.[2] In 376 subjects with knee pain and radiographic evidence of knee osteoarthritis, 3.1% had evidence of prepatellar bursitis on magnetic resonance imaging.[3]

Infrapatellar bursitis (vicar's knee) is usually due to repetitive knee flexion in weight bearing, such as deep knee bends, squatting, or jumping; it can be associated with patellar-quadriceps tendinitis.[4,5] In 376 subjects undergoing routine magnetic resonance imaging who had knee pain and radiographic evidence of knee osteoarthritis, 10.6% had evidence of superficial infrapatellar bursitis.[3]

Anserine bursitis is commonly seen in overweight older women who also have osteoarthritis of the knees and in individuals who participate in sports that require running, side-to-side movement, and cutting.[5,6] In a study involving persons with a symptomatic knee presenting to an orthopedic clinic with suspected internal knee derangement who had magnetic resonance imaging, only 2.5% of these patients had radiologic evidence of pes anserine bursitis, with no gender preference.[7]

Medial collateral ligament bursitis refers to inflammation of a bursa located between the deep and superficial parts of the medial collateral ligament.[5] It has been associated with degenerative disease of the medial joint compartment, with marginal osteophytic spur formation.[8] Furthermore, this bursitis may be seen in equestrian and motorcycle athletes because of the friction applied to the medial side of the knee.[8]

Semimembranosus bursitis is usually seen in runners and may be associated with hamstring tendinitis.[4] This was seen in 4.4% of symptomatic subjects undergoing routine magnetic resonance imaging.[3]

SYMPTOMS

The patient will usually complain of local pain, tenderness, or swelling in the affected site. The pain is worse with flexion and usually occurs at night or after activity.

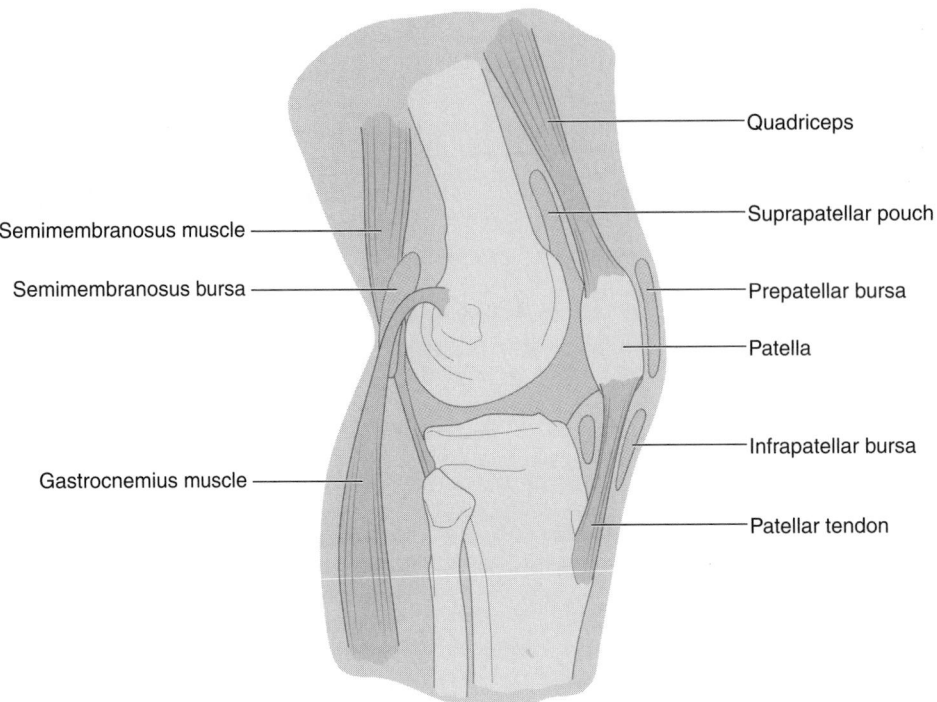

FIGURE 62-1. Bursae around knee joint.

Labels: Quadriceps, Suprapatellar pouch, Prepatellar bursa, Patella, Infrapatellar bursa, Patellar tendon, Semimembranosus muscle, Semimembranosus bursa, Gastrocnemius muscle

The pain also may be more prominent and accompanied by stiffness on waking in the morning. Limping may or may not be present.

PHYSICAL EXAMINATION

The patient may have an antalgic gait, with a shortened stance phase on the affected side. There is discrete tenderness to palpation associated with fullness at the site of the bursa involved, and there may be associated redness and increased temperature. If the bursa connects with the knee joint, there may be an associated effusion. There is often limited range of motion in the knee. Neurologic examination findings should be normal.

FUNCTIONAL LIMITATIONS

The patient may have difficulty with prolonged walking. Decreased balance is often seen in older patients, sometimes necessitating assistive devices (e.g., walker, crutches, cane, or wheelchair). If there is limitation in knee range of motion, patients may have difficulty bending the knees to drive or sitting at a desk at work. They will also have problems stooping, kneeling, crawling, or climbing, which may interfere with vocational and recreational activities. Athletes such as runners may have diminished performance or may be sidelined altogether.

DIAGNOSTIC STUDIES

The diagnosis is based mainly on history and clinical examination. Aspiration is rarely needed but may be necessary if an infection is suspected. Radiologic studies are usually performed to rule out other diagnoses but may show exostosis in areas related to the bursa. Ultrasound imaging may be helpful to visualize the swelling in the bursal sac and may be augmented by use of an air-steroid-saline mixture as a contrast medium.[9] Plain radiographs should be obtained if a bone tumor is suspected, particularly in patients with night pain. Arthrography, which is rarely done, may show the connection to the knee joint, if it is involved. Magnetic resonance imaging may be needed to rule out a tumor or malignant neoplasm and may show a fluid collection in the involved bursa.[1,4]

TREATMENT

Initial

Restriction of activity that provokes or aggravates symptoms is important.[1,4-6,10] In athletes, this may mean a substitution of the usual athletic activities while the

Differential Diagnosis

Infection (e.g., septic knee)

Arthritis (osteoarthritis, rheumatoid arthritis, psoriatic arthritis)

Tumor

Patellar fracture

Meniscal tear

Collateral ligament sprain or tear

Saphenous nerve entrapment

healing process proceeds. Local application of ice helps decrease pain and inflammation. The patient can be taught to use superficial heat for chronic bursitis. This can be done with moistened warm compresses or with a microwaveable or electric heating pad. Precautions should be observed and given to the patient to prevent burns and other complications (see section on potential treatment complications).

Nonsteroidal anti-inflammatory drugs can be prescribed to decrease pain and inflammation. Oral steroids are generally not indicated as initial treatment.

Rehabilitation

Use of an orthosis in the affected knee may assist in preventing painful movement and further inflammation as well as provide comfort. Shoe inserts unilaterally or bilaterally, depending on the pathologic process, may also lead to positively altered biomechanics of the lower extremities to improve symptoms. For example, for those individuals with associated medial compartment knee osteoarthritis, a lateral wedge insole may improve symptoms and function.[11] However, long-term use of splints is not advised because it may be associated with muscle weakness.

Formal physical therapy may address stretching of the quadriceps, hamstrings, iliotibial band, and hip adductor muscles if these muscles are tight. Strengthening exercises are often needed in chronic knee bursitis

because of disuse weakness Correction of gait abnormalities (e.g., leg length discrepancy with a heel lift or pes planus with orthotics) is also important. Patients should also be counseled to protect their knees from further trauma (e.g., by avoidance of bending or kneeling or by use of knee pads).

Modalities such as ultrasound have not been proved to be more effective than a combination of the aforementioned measures. Ultrasound should be avoided when an effusion is present because it can worsen an effusion. Phonophoresis and iontophoresis may have merit, but they are still controversial.[12]

Procedures

Intrabursal corticosteroid injection is appropriate if there is no response to conservative management or if the patient demonstrates significant functional limitations (Fig. 62-2). Typically, no more than three injections are done in a 6- to 12-month period. Alternative diagnoses should be considered for patients with refractory symptoms.

The patient is generally advised to avoid activity involving the area injected for approximately 2 weeks to promote retention of the corticosteroid in the bursa and to avoid systemic absorption.[13] There is some evidence to suggest that persons who have pes anserine bursitis that is demonstrated with ultrasonography may have the best outcome after corticosteroid injection.[14,15]

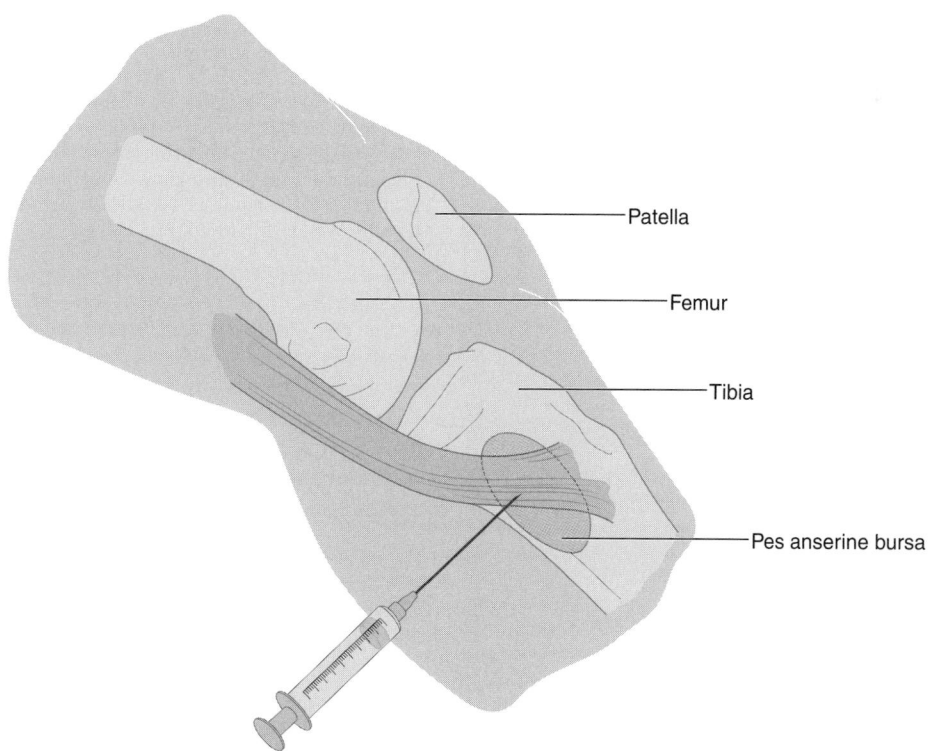

Patella

Femur

Tibia

Pes anserine bursa

FIGURE 62-2. Under sterile conditions, with use of a 1$^1/_2$-inch, 22-gauge needle, inject the bursa at the point of maximal tenderness. A 1- to 3-mL combination of local anesthetic and corticosteroid is used (e.g., 1 mL of 1% lidocaine mixed with 1 mL of 40 mg/mL triamcinolone acetonide). Local anesthetics may be injected just before the steroid to diminish pain and to prevent postinjection steroid flare.[1,4-6,13] Application of ice is helpful in decreasing pain at the site after injection.

Surgery

Surgery is generally not indicated and should be undertaken only in refractory cases. Excision of a bursa can be considered if the disease does not respond to conservative measures, despite treatment, and it greatly limits the patient's activities. Successful surgical resection of bursae has been reported in the literature.[16-19]

POTENTIAL DISEASE COMPLICATIONS

Possible complications include chronic pain, deconditioning, disuse muscle atrophy, and knee flexion contracture. Furthermore, this may lead to decreased walking ability and postural instability over time, especially in older adults.

POTENTIAL TREATMENT COMPLICATIONS

Potential complications from medications include drug hypersensitivity and prolonged bleeding; nonsteroidal anti-inflammatory drugs have gastric, renal, and hepatic side effects. Hyperglycemia, electrolyte imbalance, and gastric irritation or ulceration from intrabursal steroid injection are not as common as with orally administered corticosteroids but can still occur from systemic absorption of the injectant. Local ice application may produce hypersensitivity and vasoconstriction in patients with Raynaud disease and peripheral vascular disease, and local heat application may produce burns, sedation, skin discoloration, and vascular compromise. Moreover, injections may result in drug hypersensitivity, sterile abscess, infection, nerve injury, tendon rupture, and lipoatrophy from intralesional steroids.[13,14]

References

1. Cailliet R. Knee Pain and Disability, 3rd ed. Philadelphia, FA Davis, 1992.
2. Thompson T, Simpson B, Burgess D, Wilson R. Massive prepatellar bursa. J Natl Med Assoc 2006;98:90-92.
3. Hill CL, Gale DR, Chaisson CE, et al. Periarticular lesions detected on magnetic resonance imaging: prevalence in knees with and without symptoms. Arthritis Rheum 2003;48:2836-2844.
4. Larson R, Grana W. The Knee: Form, Function, Pathology, and Treatment. Philadelphia, WB Saunders, 1993.
5. Biundo J. Regional Rheumatic Pain Syndromes, 10th ed. Atlanta, Arthritis Foundation, 1993.
6. Alvarez-Nemegyei J, Canosa JJ. Evidence-based soft tissue rheumatology IV: Anserine bursitis. J Clin Rheumatol 2004;10:205-206.
7. Rennie WJ, Saifuddin A. Pes anserine bursitis: incidence in symptomatic knees and clinical presentation. Skeletal Radiol 2005;34:395-398.
8. McCarthy CL, McNally EG. The MRI appearance of cystic lesions around the knee. Skeletal Radiol 2004;33:187-209.
9. Koski J, Saarakkala S, Heikkinen J, Hermunen H. Use of air-steroid-saline mixture as contrast medium in greyscale ultrasound imaging: experimental study and practical applications in rheumatology. Clin Exp Rheumatol 2005;23:373-378.
10. Kang I, Han S. Anserine bursitis in patients with osteoarthritis of the knee. South Med J 2000;93:207-209.
11. Toda Y, Tsukimura N. A six-month followup of a randomized trial comparing the efficacy of a lateral-wedge insole with subtalar strapping and an in-shoe lateral wedge insole in patients with varus deformity osteoarthritis of the knee. Arthritis Rheum 2004;50:3129-3136.
12. Basford J. Physical agents. In Delisa J, Gans B, eds. Rehabilitation Medicine: Principles and Practice. Philadelphia, JB Lippincott, 1993:404-424.
13. Neustadt D. Intra-articular corticosteroids and other agents: aspiration techniques. In Katz W, ed. The Diagnosis and Management of Rheumatic Disease. Philadelphia, JB Lippincott, 1988:812-825.
14. Yoon H, Kim S, Suh Y, et al. Correlation between ultrasonographic findings and the response to corticosteroid injection in pes anserinus tendinobursitis syndrome in knee osteoarthritis patients. J Korean Med Sci 2005;20:109-112.
15. Handy J. Anserine bursitis: a brief review. South Med J 1997;90:376-377.
16. Yamamoto T, Akisue T, Marui T, et al. Isolated suprapatellar bursitis: computed tomographic and arthroscopic findings. Arthroscopy 2003;19:E10.
17. Klein W. Endoscopy of the deep infrapatellar bursa. Arthroscopy 1996;12:127-131.
18. Kerr DR, Carpenter CW. Arthroscopic resection of olecranon and prepatellar bursae. Arthroscopy 1990;6:86-88.
19. Hennrikus WL, Champa JR, Mack GR. Treating septic prepatellar bursitis. West J Med 1989;151:331-332.

Meniscal Injuries 63

Paul Lento, MD, and Venu Akuthota, MD

Synonyms

Cartilage tears
Locked knee

ICD-9 Codes

717.3	Other and unspecified derangement of medial meniscus
717.4	Derangement of lateral meniscus
717.40	Derangement of lateral meniscus, unspecified
717.41	Bucket-handle tear of lateral meniscus
717.42	Derangement of anterior horn of lateral meniscus
717.43	Derangement of posterior horn of lateral meniscus
717.49	Derangement of lateral meniscus, other
717.5	Derangement of lateral meniscus, not elsewhere classified
717.9	Unspecified internal derangement of the knee
836.0	Acute tear of medial meniscus of knee
836.1	Acute tear of lateral meniscus of knee

DEFINITION

The menisci serve important roles in maintaining proper joint health, stability, and function.[1] The anatomy of the medial and lateral menisci helps explain functional biomechanics. Viewed from above, the medial meniscus appears C shaped and the lateral meniscus appears O shaped[1] (Fig. 63-1). Each meniscus is thick and convex at its periphery (the horns) but becomes thin and concave at its center. This contouring serves to provide a larger area for the rounded femoral condyles and the relatively flat tibia. As well, menisci do not move in isolation. They are connected to each other anteriorly and to the anterior cruciate ligament, the patella, the femur, and the tibia by ligaments.[2,3]

The medial meniscus is less mobile than the lateral meniscus. This is due to its firm connections to the knee joint capsule and the medial collateral ligament. This decreased mobility, in conjunction with the fact that the medial meniscus is wider posteriorly, is cited as the usual reason for the higher incidence of tears within the medial meniscus than within the lateral meniscus.[1] The semimembranosus muscle (through attachments from the joint capsule) helps retract the medial meniscus posteriorly, serving to avoid entrapment and injury to the medial meniscus as the knee is flexed.[3]

The lateral meniscus is not as adherent to the joint capsule. Unlike the medial meniscus, the lateral meniscus does not attach to its respective collateral ligament. The posterolateral aspect of the lateral meniscus is separated from the capsule by the popliteus tendon. Therefore, the lateral meniscus is more mobile than the medial meniscus.[1,3] The attachment of the popliteus tendon to the posterolateral meniscus ensures dynamic retraction of the lateral meniscus when the knee internally rotates to return out of the screw-home mechanism.[2] Therefore, both the medial and the lateral menisci, by having attachments to muscle structures, share a common mechanism that helps avoid injury.

The architecture of the vascular supply to the meniscus has important implications for healing.[1,4] Capillaries penetrate the menisci from the periphery to provide nourishment. After 18 months of age, as weight bearing increases, the blood supply to the central part of the menisci recedes. In fact, research has shown that eventually only the peripheral 10% to 30% of the menisci, or the red zone, receives this capillary network (Fig. 63-2).[5] Therefore, the central and internal portion or white zone of these fibrocartilaginous structures becomes avascular with age, relying on nutrition received through diffusion from the synovial fluid. Because of this vascular arrangement, the peripheral meniscus is more likely to heal than are the central and posterolateral aspects.[4]

The primary but not sole function of the menisci is to distribute forces across the knee joint and to enhance stability.[1,6-8] Multiple studies have shown that the ability of the joint to transmit loads is significantly reduced if the meniscus is partially or wholly removed.[1,6,7,9] Fairbank[10] published a seminal article in 1948 suggesting that the menisci are vital in protecting the articular surfaces. He reported that individuals who had undergone total meniscectomies demonstrated premature osteoarthritis.

Meniscal tears are classified by their complexity, plane of rupture, direction, location, and overall shape. Tears are commonly defined as vertical, horizontal, longitudinal, or oblique in relation to the tibial surface[11] (Fig. 63-3). Most meniscal tears in young patients will be vertical-longitudinal, whereas horizontal cleavage tears are more commonly found in older patients.[12] The bucket-handle

359

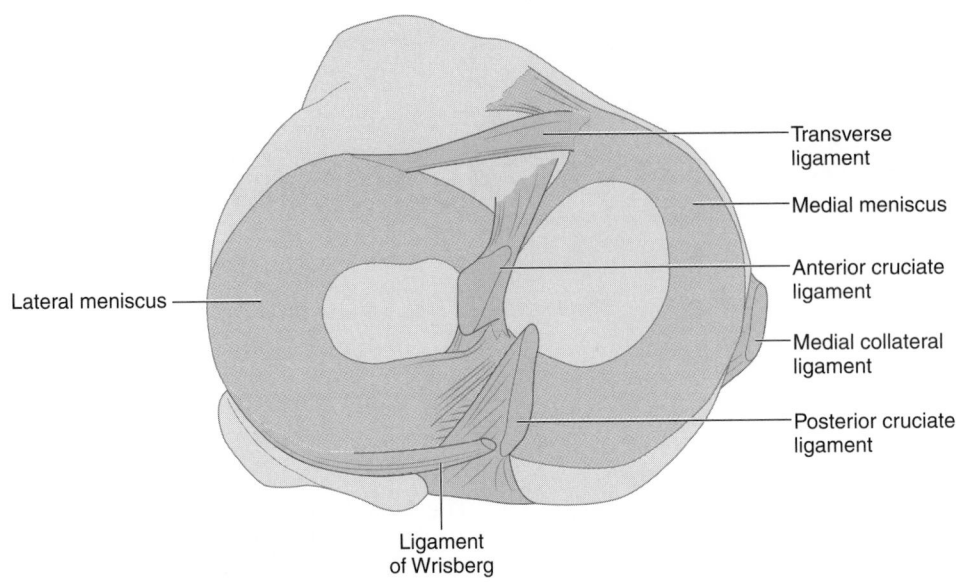

FIGURE 63-1. Superior view of medial and lateral menisci.

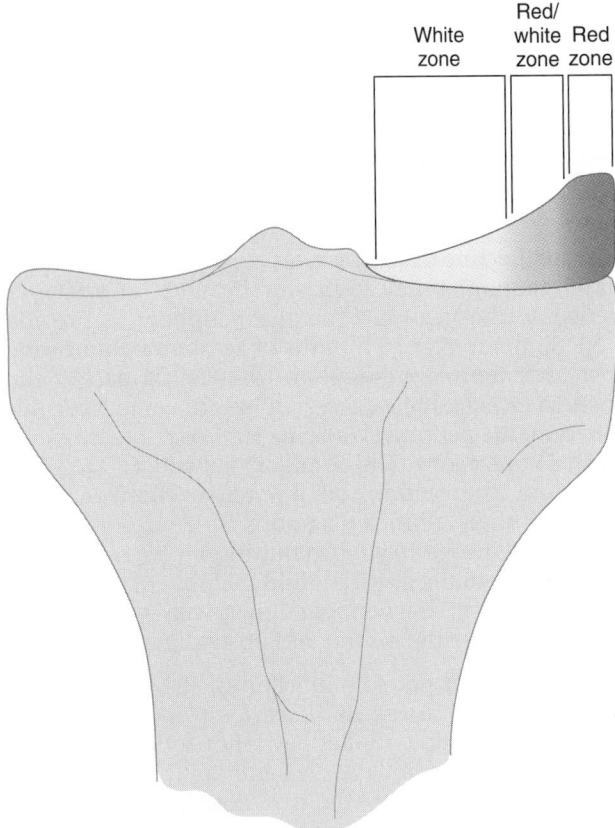

FIGURE 63-2. Vascular zones of the meniscus. Tears within the red zone have a higher healing potential.

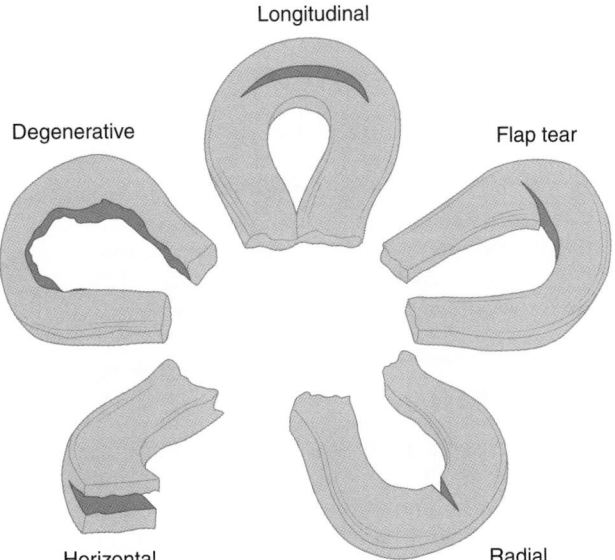

FIGURE 63-3. Types of meniscal tears.

tear is the most common type of vertical (or longitudinal) tear[13] (Fig. 63-4). Tears are also described as complete, full-thickness or partial tears. Complete, full-thickness tears are so named as they extend from the tibial to femoral surfaces. In addition, medial meniscus tears outnumber lateral meniscus tears from 2:1 to 5:1.[14,15]

Meniscal injuries may result from an acute injury or from gradual degeneration with aging.[16] Vertical tears (e.g., bucket-handle tears) tend to occur acutely in individuals 20 to 30 years of age and are usually located in the posterior two thirds of the meniscus.[13,17] Sports commonly associated with meniscal injuries are soccer, football, basketball, baseball, wrestling, skiing, rugby, and lacrosse. Injury commonly occurs when an axial load is transmitted through a flexed or extended knee that is simultaneously rotating.[16] Degenerative tears, in contrast, are usually horizontal and are seen in older individuals with concomitant degenerative joint changes.[13,18]

On the basis of arthroscopic examination, the majority of acute peripheral meniscal injuries are associated with some degree of occult anterior cruciate ligament laxity.[19]

Longitudinal

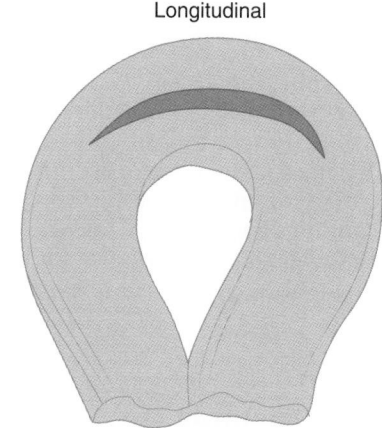

FIGURE 63-4. Bucket-handle type of meniscal tear.

In addition, true anterior cruciate ligament tears are associated with lesions of the posterior horns of the menisci.[19] Lateral meniscal tears appear to occur with more frequency with acute anterior cruciate ligament injuries, whereas medial meniscal tears have a higher incidence with chronic anterior cruciate ligament injuries. With chronic anterior cruciate ligament injuries, the medial meniscus may be more frequently damaged because its posterior horn serves as an important secondary stabilizer of anterior-posterior instability.[20]

SYMPTOMS

The history will help diagnose a meniscal injury 75% of the time.[12,21] Young patients who experience meniscal tears will recall the mechanism of injury 80% to 90% of the time and may report a "pop" or a "snap" at the time of injury. Deep knee bending activities are often painful, and mechanical locking may be present in 30% of patients.[22] Bucket-handle tears should be suspected in cases of mechanical locking with loss of full extension.[16] If locking is reported approximately 1 day after the injury, this may be due to "pseudolocking," which results from hamstring contracture.[14] Knee hemarthrosis may

also occur acutely, especially if the vascularized, peripheral portion of the meniscus is involved. In fact, 20% of all acute traumatic knee hemarthroses are caused by isolated meniscal injury.[23] More typically, however, knee swelling occurs approximately 1 day later as the meniscal tear causes mechanical irritation within the intra-articular space, creating a reactive effusion. Typically, this effusion is secondary to a lesion more in the central portion of the meniscus.[16]

In contrast, degenerative meniscal tears are not classically associated with a history of trauma. In fact, the mechanism of injury, which may not be reported by the patient, can be simple daily activities, such as rising from a chair and pivoting on a planted foot.[16] Patients with degenerative tears often also report recurrent knee swelling, particularly after activity.

PHYSICAL EXAMINATION

Physical examination aids in diagnosis of a meniscal injury accurately in 70% of patients.[24] Gait evaluation may reveal an antalgic gait with decreased stance phase and knee extension on the symptomatic side.[23] A knee effusion is observed in about half of individuals with a known meniscal tear.[25] Quadriceps atrophy may be noted a few weeks after injury. Palpation of the joint line frequently results in tenderness. Posteromedial or lateral tenderness is most suggestive of a meniscal tear.[12] The result of a "bounce home" test may be positive. This test result is positive when pain or mechanical blocking is appreciated as the patient's knee is passively forced into full extension.[14] Classically, the result of the McMurray test is positive 58% of the time in the presence of a tear but is also reported to be positive in 5% of normal individuals (Fig. 63-5).[13] The Apley compression test is an insensitive indicator of meniscal injury. With this test, the prone knee is flexed to 90 degrees and an axial load is applied (Fig. 63-6). A painful response is considered a confirmatory test result with a reported sensitivity of 45%.[23] No singular meniscal provocation test has been shown to be predictive of meniscal injury compared with findings on arthroscopy. Physical examination

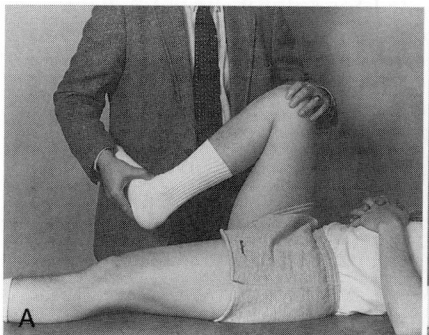 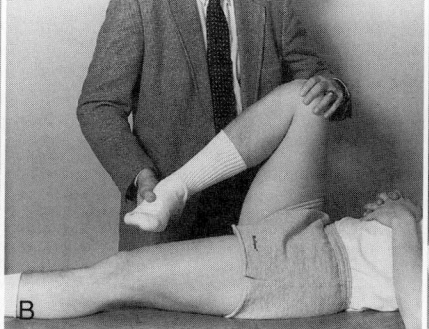 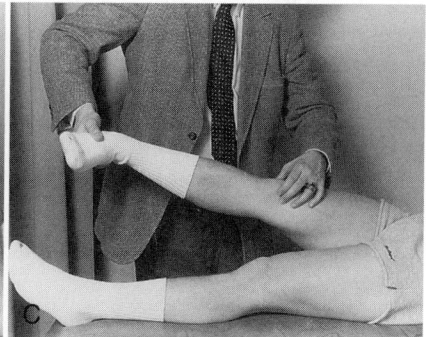

FIGURE 63-5. McMurray test. **A,** Starting position for testing of the medial meniscus. The knee is acutely flexed, with the foot and tibia in external rotation. **B,** Starting position for testing of the lateral meniscus. The knee is acutely flexed, and the foot and tibia are internally rotated. **C,** Ending position for the lateral meniscus. The knee is brought into extension while rotation is maintained. Ending position for the medial meniscus is the same but with the external rotation. If pain or a "clunk" is elicited, the test result is considered positive. (Reprinted with permission from Mellion MB. Office Sports Medicine, 2nd ed. Philadelphia, Hanley & Belfus, 1996:28.)

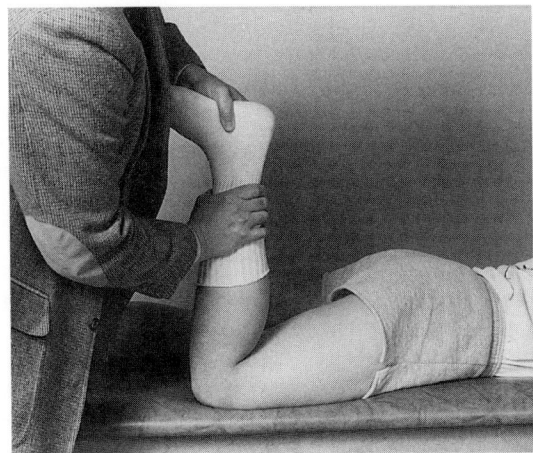

FIGURE 63-6. Apley compression test. The patient is prone. The examiner applies pressure on the sole of the foot toward the examination table. The tibia is internally and externally rotated. (Reprinted with permission from Mellion MB. Office Sports Medicine, 2nd ed. Philadelphia, Hanley & Belfus, 1996:259.)

findings become even less reliable in patients with concomitant anterior cruciate ligament deficiencies.[14]

Neurologic examination findings, including sensation and deep tendon reflexes, should be normal unless there is associated guarding due to pain or diffuse weakness, particularly with knee extension (quadriceps muscle).

FUNCTIONAL LIMITATIONS

Patients with meniscal injuries may have difficulty with deep knee bending activities, such as traversing stairs, squatting, or toileting. In addition, jogging, running, and even walking may become problematic, particularly if any rotational component is involved. Laborers who repetitively squat may report mechanical locking with loss of full knee extension on rising.

DIAGNOSTIC STUDIES

Standing plain radiographs are usually normal in isolated meniscal injuries. Presence of osteoarthritis, as with degenerative meniscal tears, can be detected with weight-bearing anteroposterior and lateral knee films. With nondegenerative tears, magnetic resonance imaging (MRI) has largely replaced plain radiographic examination in detecting injury.[12] Sagittal views demonstrate the anterior and posterior horns of the menisci; coronal images can be vital in diagnosis of bucket-handle and parrot-beak tears.[1,14] There are three grades of meniscal injury as determined by the location of T2 signal intensity within the black cartilage. By definition, only grade 3 tears qualify as true meniscal tears; however, a few grade 2 lesions seen on MRI will be found to be true tears on arthroscopy[26] (Fig. 63-7). With use of arthroscopy as the "gold standard," the sensitivity of MRI varies from 64% to 95%, with an accuracy of 83% to 93%.[16] MRI appears to have a false-positive rate of 10%.[1,24] A 5% false-negative rate is also

reported and may be due to the incidence of missed tears at the meniscosynovial junction.[27]

Interestingly, despite the recent accessibility and advancement in MRI, clinical examination by experienced physicians is cheaper and appears to be as accurate as MRI for the diagnosis of meniscal tears.[26] However, MRI may be particularly helpful when history and physical examination findings are equivocal and the physician is required to establish an expedient diagnosis.[13,23]

Differential Diagnosis

Anterior or posterior cruciate ligament tear

Medial collateral ligament tear

Osteoarthritis

Plica syndromes

Popliteal tendinitis

Osteochondritic lesions

Loose bodies

Patellofemoral pain

Fat pad impingement syndrome

Inflammatory arthritis

Physeal fracture

Tumors

TREATMENT

Initial

The truly locked knee resulting from a meniscal tear should be reduced within 24 hours of injury. Otherwise, acute tears of the meniscus may initially be treated with rest, ice, and compression, with weight bearing as tolerated. Patients may need to use crutches acutely. A knee splint may be applied for comfort of the patient, particularly in unstable knees with underlying ligamentous injury.[22]

Analgesics such as acetaminophen or opioids can be used for pain. Nonsteroidal anti-inflammatory drugs can be used for pain and inflammation.

Arthrocentesis can be performed (ideally in the first 24 to 48 hours) for both diagnostic and treatment purposes when there is a significant effusion.

Rehabilitation

Not all meniscal injuries necessitate surgical intervention or resection. In fact, some meniscal lesions have gradual resolution of symptoms during a 6-week period and may have normal function by 3 months.[11]

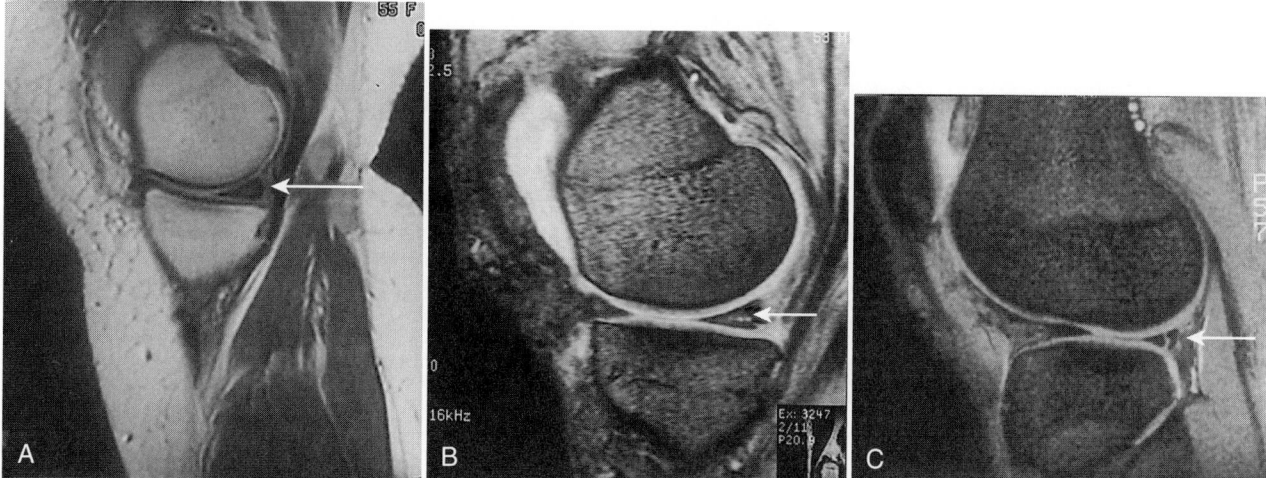

FIGURE 63-7. MRI grading of meniscal tears. **A,** Poorly defined "globular" zone of increased signal intensity *(arrow),* corresponding to grade 1 change. **B,** Linear zone of hyperintensity *(arrow)* not communicating with the articular surfaces, corresponding to grade 2 change. **C,** Linear band of hyperintensity *(arrow)* communicating with both articular surfaces, corresponding to grade 3 change, that is, a complete tear. (Reprinted with permission from Mellion MB. Office Sports Medicine, 2nd ed. Philadelphia, Hanley & Belfus, 1996:263.)

Types of tears that may be treated with nonsurgical measures include partial-thickness longitudinal tears, small (<5 mm) full-thickness peripheral tears, and minor inner rim or degenerative tears.[28] Healing potential is greatest for tears within the red zone.[29] In general, only meniscal injuries that are persistently symptomatic should be referred for surgical intervention.

Both nonsurgical and partial meniscectomy patients undergo similar rehabilitation protocols. Crutches may be used to off-load the affected limb. These can usually be discontinued when patients are ambulating without a limp.[30] The goal during the first week is to decrease pain and swelling while increasing range of motion and muscle strength and endurance. Institution of static strengthening in conjunction with electrical stimulation can retard quadriceps atrophy.[27] Aerobic conditioning can begin as long as the patient can tolerate bicycle training or aqua jogging. As time progresses, a combination of open and closed kinetic chain exercises in all three planes (sagittal, coronal, and transverse) can be performed in conjunction with stretching of the lower limb. Gradually, during the ensuing weeks, more functional activities are introduced. More challenging proprioceptive and balancing activities also can be started as deemed appropriate. Finally, plyometric training is begun, and the individual is gradually introduced back into sport-specific activities.

Multiple rehabilitation protocols for the surgically repaired meniscus have been described. Rehabilitation programs ideally need to be individualized to the specific type of repair performed. In addition, there has been considerable controversy among physicians about the patient's weight-bearing and immobilization status soon after surgical repair.[27,31-33] In general, however, initial exercises are nonaggressive, avoiding dynamic shear forces that may occur from joint active range of motion. Therefore, exercises are initially static, targeting hip abductors, adductors, and extensors. Static quadriceps exercises are performed with care to avoid terminal knee extension. While superior and medial patella mobilization is begun, stretching of the lower limb musculature in multiple planes is emphasized. After 2 to 3 weeks, goals are to increase range of motion and to advance weight-bearing status while a resistance exercise program is introduced. With the absence of effusion and significant pain, improved knee range of motion from 5 to 110 degrees should be achieved. More aggressive active range of motion may be started, particularly if the repair was to the outer peripheral or vascular zone of the meniscus, because the success rate for healing here is higher.[27] Gradually, more functional activities with use of resistive bands may be introduced. With time and success of the patient, resistance can be increased and proprioceptive neuromuscular facilitation activities can be implemented, ensuring that the individual is rehabilitated in the coronal, transverse, and sagittal planes.[34]

By 6 to 8 weeks, low-impact functional activities that entail components of the patient's sport or activity are introduced. Brace protection, if it was initially employed, may be discontinued, particularly when the patient demonstrates success with proprioceptive testing. Running, cutting, and rotational activities are avoided. Athletes may be able to return to their individual activities at about 16 weeks for those with repairs in the vascular zone and 24 weeks for those with repairs in the nonvascular zone.

Procedures

Patients presenting after an acute injury with an effusion may benefit from a joint aspiration not only to help relieve discomfort and stiffness but also to aid in discerning whether a hemarthrosis or marrow fat (to rule out an occult fracture) is present.

Surgery

Specific types of tears may not require surgical repair; these include longitudinal partial-thickness tears, stable full-thickness peripheral tears (<5 mm long), and short (<5 mm) radial tears.[30] These are usually stable and may not require either suture fixation or immobilization. However, arthroscopy may still be necessary to determine stability and to stimulate healing through perimeniscal abrasion.[11] Some larger longitudinal, radial, and degenerative meniscal tears are less likely to heal without surgical intervention. Although first-line treatment for these lesions is aggressive rehabilitation, recalcitrant cases may require a partial meniscectomy that preserves as much of the meniscus as possible.[32] In addition, the inner aspect of the cartilage, which may be ragged, may be rasped or shaved, providing a smooth surface that eliminates mechanical symptoms.

On occasion, other tears of the menisci, because of their size and location, are best treated by primary approximation with sutures and primary repair.[35] Typically, longitudinal tears longer than 5 mm in the periphery of the meniscus are best suited for this because they have a high rate of successful healing.[30] In older individuals, the mere presence of a horizontal or degenerative cleavage tear is insufficient to justify removal because these meniscal portions may still participate in significant load transmission but not necessarily cause symptoms.[11] Treatment of these degenerative tears is usually nonsurgical; however, unstable portions may be removed during arthroscopy.

POTENTIAL DISEASE COMPLICATIONS

Once a meniscal tear occurs, the joint inherently becomes less stable. This instability may promote further extension of the initial tear, turning a nonsurgical lesion into one in which arthroscopic repair may be necessary. Chronically, the resultant increased abnormal motion that occurs secondary to the meniscal injury may also lead to damage of the articular surface and predispose to premature osteoarthritis.[12]

POTENTIAL TREATMENT COMPLICATIONS

Analgesics such as acetaminophen and nonsteroidal anti-inflammatory drugs have well-known side effects that may affect the gastric, hepatic, and renal systems. If the clinician is unfamiliar with appropriate rehabilitation strategies, an overly aggressive regimen may lead to extension of the tear or failure of the meniscus to heal. A rehabilitative program that is too conservative, in contrast, may also lead to a significant loss of strength with muscle atrophy and decreased range of motion. If the surgical approach resulted in a significant amount of cartilage removed, the knee may be predisposed to

development of osteoarthritis as originally described by Fairbank.[10] Saphenous nerve injuries as well as infections are also common complications after meniscal repair surgery and arthroscopy.[12]

References

1. Renstrom P. Anatomy and biomechanics of the menisci. Clin Sports Med 1990;9:523-538.
2. Norkin C, Levangie P. The knee complex. In Norkin C, Levangie P, eds. Joint Structure and Function, 2nd ed. Philadelphia, FA Davis, 1992:337-378.
3. Maitra RS, Miller MD, Johnson DL. Meniscal reconstruction. Part I: indications, techniques, and graft considerations. Am J Orthop 1999;28:213-218.
4. Gray JC. Neural and vascular anatomy of the menisci of the human knee. J Orthop Sports Phys Ther 1999;29:23-30.
5. Arnoczky SP, Warren RF. The microvasculature of the meniscus and its response to injury. Am J Sports Med 1983;11:131-141.
6. Walker PS, Erkman MJ. The role of the menisci in force transmission across the knee. Clin Orthop Relat Res 1975;109:184-192.
7. Seedholm BB. Transmission on the load in the knee joint with special reference to the role of the menisci: I. Anatomy, analysis and apparatus. Eng Med 1979;8:207-219.
8. Ahmed AM, Burke DL. In vitro measurement of static pressure distribution in synovial joints: I. Tibial surface of the knee. J Biomech Eng 1983;105:216-225.
9. Krause WE, Pope MD, Johnson RJ, et al. Mechanical changes in the knee after meniscectomy. J Bone Joint Surg Am 1976;58:599-604.
10. Fairbank TJ. Knee joint changes after meniscectomy. J Bone Joint Surg Br 1948;30:664-670.
11. Newman AP, Daniels AU, Burke RT. Principles and decision making in meniscal surgery. Arthroscopy 1993;9:33-51.
12. Fu FH, Baratz M. Meniscal injuries. In DeLee JC, Drez D, eds. Orthopaedic Sports Medicine: Principles and Practice, vol 2. Philadelphia, WB Saunders, 1994:1146-1162.
13. Oberlander MA, Pryde JA. Meniscal injuries. In Baker CL, ed. The Hughston Clinic Sports Medicine Book. Baltimore, Williams & Wilkins, 1995:465-472.
14. Hardin GT, Farr J, Bach BR Jr. Meniscal tears: diagnosis, evaluation, and treatment. Orthop Rev 1992;21:1311-1317.
15. Metcalf RW. The torn medial meniscus. In Parisien JS, ed. Arthroscopic Surgery. New York, McGraw-Hill, 1988:93-110.
16. Tuerlings L. Meniscal injuries. In Arendt EA, ed. Orthopaedic Knowledge Update. Sports Medicine 2. Rosemont, Ill, American Academy of Orthopaedic Surgeons, 1999:349-354.
17. Baker BE, Peckham AC, Pupparo F. Review of meniscal injury and associated sports. Am J Sports Med 1983;11:8-13.
18. Rodkey WG. Basic biology of the meniscus and response to injury. Instr Course Lect 2000;49:189-193.
19. Poehling GG, Ruch DS, Chabon SJ. The landscape of meniscal injuries. Clin Sports Med 1990;9:539-549.
20. Bellabarba C, Bush-Joseph CA, Bach BR Jr. Patterns of meniscal injury in the anterior cruciate-deficient knee: a review of the literature. Am J Orthop 1997;26:18-23.
21. Casscells SW. The place of arthroscopy in the diagnosis and treatment of internal derangement of the knee: an analysis of 1000 cases. Clin Orthop Relat Res 1980;151:135-142.
22. Simon RR, Koenigsknecht SJ. The knee. In Simon RR, Koenigsknecht SJ, eds. Emergency Orthopedics: The Extremities. Norwalk, Conn, Appleton & Lange, 3rd ed., 1995:437-462.
23. Muellner T, Nikolic A, Vecsei V. Recommendations for the diagnosis of traumatic meniscal injuries in athletes. Sports Med 1999;27:337-345.
24. Rose NE, Gold SM. A comparison of accuracy between clinical examination and magnetic resonance imaging in the diagnosis of meniscal and anterior cruciate ligament tears. Arthroscopy 1996;12:398-405.
25. Anderson AF, Lipscomb AB. Clinical diagnosis of meniscal tears. Description of a new manipulative test. Am J Sports Med 1986;14:291-293.

26. Baratz ME, Rehak DC, Fu FH, et al. Peripheral tears of the meniscus. The effect of open versus arthroscopic repair on intra-articular contact stresses in the human knee. Am J Sports Med 1988;16:1-6.

27. Auberger SS, Mangine RE. Innovative approaches to surgery and rehabilitation. In Mangine RE, ed. Physical Therapy of the Knee, 2nd ed. New York, Churchill Livingstone, 1995:233-249.

28. DeHaven KE. Injuries to the menisci of the knee. In Nicholas JA, Hershman EB, eds. The Lower Extremity and Spine in Sports Medicine. St. Louis, Mosby, 1986:905-928.

29. Urquhart MW, O'Leary JA, Griffin JR, Fu FH. Meniscal injuries in the adult. In DeLee JC, Drez D, eds. Orthopaedic Sports Medicine: Principles and Practice, vol 2, 2nd ed. Philadelphia, WB Saunders, 2003:1668-1686.

30. DeHaven KE, Bronstein RD. Injuries to the menisci of the knee. In Nicholas JA, Hershman EB, eds. The Lower Extremity and Spine in Sports Medicine, 2nd ed. St. Louis, Mosby, 1995:813-823.

31. Brukner P, Khan K. Acute knee injuries. In Brukner P, Khan K, eds. Clinical Sports Medicine. New York, McGraw-Hill, 2nd ed., 2001:426-463.

32. Rispoli DM, Miller MD. Options in meniscal repair. Clin Sports Med 1999;18:77-90.

33. Shelbourne KD, Patel DV, Adsit WS, et al. Rehabilitation after meniscal repair. Clin Sports Med 1996;15:595-612.

34. Gray GW. Lunge tests. In Gray GW, ed. Lower Extremity Functional Profile. Adrian, Mich, Wynn Marketing, 1995:100-108.

35. Swenson TM, Harner CD. Knee ligament and meniscal injuries. Orthop Clin North Am 1995;26:535-546.

Jumper's Knee 64

Thomas H. Hudgins, MD

DEFINITION

Jumper's knee, first described by Blazina and colleagues[1] in 1973, is primarily a chronic overuse injury of the patellar tendon resulting from excessive stress on the knee extensor mechanism. Athletes involved in sports requiring repetitive jumping, running, and kicking (e.g., volleyball, basketball, tennis, track) are at greatest risk. For example, the incidence ranges from 22% to 39% in volleyball players.[2] Acceleration, deceleration, takeoff, and landing generate eccentric forces that can be three times greater than conventional concentric and static forces. These eccentric forces may exceed the inherent strength of the patellar tendon, resulting in microtears anywhere along the bone-tendon interface.[2-4] With continued stress, a cycle of microtearing, degeneration, and regeneration weakens the tendon and may lead to tendon rupture.

As in other overuse injuries, the predisposing factors in jumper's knee include extrinsic causes, such as errors in training, and intrinsic causes, such as biomechanical flaws. Training errors include improper warm-up or cool-down, rapid increase in frequency or intensity of activity, and training on hard surfaces.[3,4] Biomechanical flaws, such as muscle strength or flexibility imbalances (in jumper's knee, tight hamstrings and increased femoral anteversion[3]), and jumping mechanics[2,5] have also been implicated by many authors. Finally, an increased incidence of Osgood-Schlatter disease and idiopathic anterior knee pain during adolescence has been identified in patients with jumper's knee.[3]

Because histologic studies of the patellar tendon reveal collagen degeneration with little or no evidence of acute inflammation, many authors argue that "patellar tendinosis" is a more accurate description than "patellar tendinitis."[6-8] This distinction has important implications for rehabilitation. In treatment of patellar tendinosis and other chronic overuse tendinopathies, the treatment team should emphasize restoration of function rather than control of inflammation. This is an overuse syndrome that has no age or gender predilection.

SYMPTOMS

Patients typically report a dull, aching anterior knee pain, initially noted after a strenuous workout or competition, that is insidious in onset and well localized.[7] The bone-tendon junction at the inferior pole of the patella is most frequently affected (65% of cases), followed by the superior pole of the patella (25%) and the tibial tubercle (10%).[6] Other symptoms may include stiffness or pain after prolonged sitting or climbing stairs,[3] a feeling of swelling or fullness over the patella, and knee extensor weakness.[1] Mechanical symptoms of instability, such as locking, catching, and give-away weakness, are uncommon.

Four phases have been described in the progression of jumper's knee: phase 1, pain is present after activity only and is not associated with functional impairment; phase 2, pain is present during and after activity but does not limit performance and resolves with rest; phase 3, pain is present continually and is associated with progressively impaired performance; and phase 4, complete tendon rupture.[1]

As the disease progresses, the pain becomes sharper, more severe, and constant (present not only with athletic endeavor but also with walking and other everyday activities). If it is not treated, the disorder may result in tendon rupture, a sudden painful event associated with immediate inability to extend the knee.[7]

PHYSICAL EXAMINATION

The hallmark of jumper's knee is tenderness at the site of involvement, usually the inferior pole of the patella.[7] This sign is best elicited on palpation of the knee in full extension,[7] and the pain typically increases when the knee is extended against resistance.[3] On occasion, there may be swelling of the tendon or the fat pad, although a frank knee joint effusion is not typically present.[3] Mild patellofemoral crepitus and pain with compression of the patellofemoral joint have been noted.[3] In advanced disease, patients may have quadriceps atrophy without detectable weakness on manual muscle testing and hamstring tightness.[3,7] Test results for knee ligamentous laxity are negative. The examiner should also expect a normal, nonfocal neurologic examination.

FUNCTIONAL LIMITATIONS

Most patients experience little functional limitation in the early stages of jumper's knee. As the disease progresses, however, increasing disability from persistent pain and inhibition of knee extension impairs athletic performance. Eventually, walking and the ability to perform basic activities of living, such as ascending or descending stairs, may be compromised. In the event of patellar tendon rupture, complete functional impairment with inability to extend the affected knee, limiting weight bearing and ambulation, necessitates surgical repair.

DIAGNOSTIC TESTING

Radiographic changes are rarely present during the first 6 months of patellar tendinosis, limiting the usefulness of radiographs during initial evaluation.[4] When radiography is performed, the examination generally includes anteroposterior, lateral, intercondylar, and skyline tracking patellar views.[3] Documented findings include radiolucency at the site of involvement, elongation of the involved pole, and occasionally a fracture at the junction of the elongation with the main portion of the patella. On occasion, calcification of the involved tendon and irregularity or even avulsion of the involved pole may be seen.[1]

Ultrasonography has the advantage of allowing early diagnosis and dynamic imaging of the tendon while remaining inexpensive, noninvasive, reproducible, and sensitive to changes as small as 0.1 mm.[4] Some authors believe ultrasonography to be the preferred method for evaluation of jumper's knee. It has been used to confirm the diagnosis, to guide steroid injections, and to observe tendons after surgery.[4] It should be considered in cases that do not respond to a trial of conservative treatment after 4 to 6 weeks and when the diagnosis is questioned. Findings on ultrasound examination include thickening of the tendon.[4,9] A hypoechoic focal lesion at the area of greatest thickening correlates well with the lesion on magnetic resonance imaging (MRI), computed tomography, and histologic examination.[3,10] However, critics of ultrasonography have noted abnormalities in asymptomatic athletes. This phenomenon may be explained by a preclinical or postclinical stage of the disease.[4] Plain MRI, MRI with intravenous administration of gadolinium, and MRI arthrography with gadolinium

have been used to corroborate the clinical diagnosis of jumper's knee. Increased thickening of the patellar tendon on MRI is present in all patients resistant to conservative therapy.[11,12] MRI is also advantageous in excluding other intrinsic joint disease. MRI arthrography is particularly useful in examining the chondral surfaces of the patella and femur when osteochondritis dissecans or other pathologic processes in these areas are suspected. My recommendation is to begin with three views of the knee on radiographic scintigraphy to rule out bone pathologic changes and to evaluate joint space. If patients do not respond to physical therapy in 4 to 6 weeks, ultrasound examination is the preferred study at that time to confirm the diagnosis.

Differential Diagnosis

Patellofemoral maltracking

Retinacular pain

Fat pad lesion

Lipoma arborescens

Infrapatellar bursitis

Partial anterior cruciate ligament tear

Meniscal injuries

Chondromalacia patellae

Plica syndrome

Entrapment of the saphenous nerve

Osgood-Schlatter lesion

Sinding-Larsen syndrome[3,4,7]

TREATMENT

Initial

Because the syndrome is progressive and associated with difficult and slow rehabilitation, the importance of early diagnosis and treatment cannot be overemphasized.[13] Initial interventions include control of pain with nonsteroidal anti-inflammatory drugs, ice, and relative rest. Passive modalities such as ultrasound and iontophoresis are also used judiciously to control pain.

Rehabilitation

A comprehensive rehabilitation program should address the biomechanical flaws found on the musculoskeletal examination. These include the functional deficits (inflexibilities that lead to altered biomechanics) and subclinical adaptations (substitution patterns that compensate for the functional deficits).[14] This approach may be used in addressing all overuse syndromes. In patellar tendinosis, hamstring and quadriceps tightness and weakness need to be addressed.[14] As the rehabilitation program advances and pain abates, eccentric strengthening exercises should be emphasized. This type of strengthening exercise is optimal for rehabilitation of tendinopathies because it places maximal tensile load on the muscle and tendon unit (Fig. 64-1).[15] There is a paucity of randomized controlled studies supporting this type of exercise, but I think that this is the most optimal method.[16] This type of exercise may provoke pain initially, given the increased load placed on the muscle-tendon unit. This final phase of rehabilitation should also encompass sports-specific drills and training. Knee supports and straps such as the Cho-Pat strap have been used to alleviate pain and to change the force dynamics through the patellar tendon with good results.[4,17]

Procedures

Some authors recommend a peritendinous injection of steroid if noninvasive conservative therapy fails.[3,4] This is performed with ultrasound guidance to delineate accurate placement of the needle. Decreased pain with injection of the fat pad rather than of the tendon itself has been documented.[3] Because histologic studies have shown a minimal inflammatory component in surgical specimens, the mechanism of action of these approaches is unknown.[4] In addition, studies have associated tendon ruptures with steroid injection.[4,18]

Surgery

In the advanced stage of jumper's knee, if a well-documented conservative therapy trial has failed or if the tendon ruptures, surgery has been indicated. Several approaches have had mixed success; resection of the tendon disease with resuturing of the tendon is most often cited, and authors report 77% to 93% good or excellent results.[19,20]

However, when more invasive treatments, such as injections or surgery, are contemplated, it is incumbent on the practitioner to ensure that a comprehensive rehabilitation program has been followed thoroughly, as outlined earlier, before one declares a "conservative management failure." Criteria for conservative management failure are often ill-defined in the literature. In my experience, invasive procedures are rarely necessary for the management of jumper's knee. Postoperative rehabilitation begins with isometric strengthening of the quadriceps, restoring range of motion and advancing to eccentric strengthening in 6 to 12 weeks.

POTENTIAL DISEASE COMPLICATIONS

Stress reaction of the patella, stress fracture, and patellar tendon rupture are some of the advanced complications. Others include formation of accessory ossicles, avulsion apophysis, and bone growth acceleration or arrest in adolescents.[21]

POTENTIAL TREATMENT COMPLICATIONS

Gastrointestinal bleeding and renal side effects of nonsteroidal anti-inflammatory drugs are well documented. Complications of corticosteroid injections include bleeding, infection, and soft tissue atrophy at the site of injection. Tendon weakening with possible increased incidence of tendon rupture has also been cited. Surgery can lead to inadvertent tibial or peroneal nerve injury.

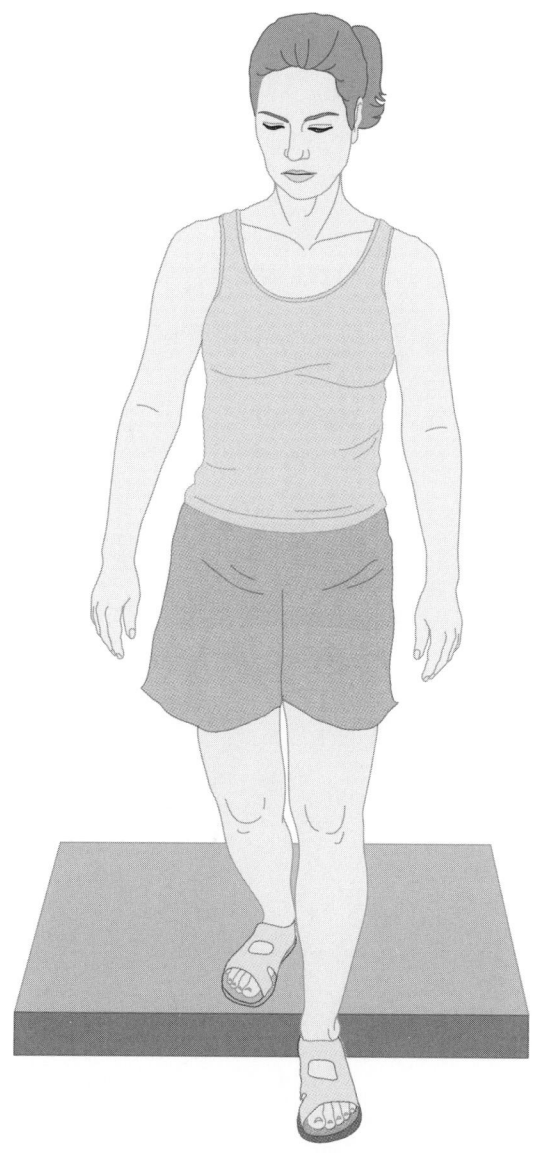

FIGURE 64-1. Eccentric strengthening, left quadriceps.

References

1. Blazina ME, Kerlan RK, Jobe FW, et al. Jumper's knee. Orthop Clin North Am 1973;4:665-678.
2. Ferretti A, Puddu G, Mariani PP, Neri M. The natural history of jumper's knee. Int Orthop 1985;8:239-242.
3. Duri ZA, Aichroth PM, Wilkins R, Jones J. Patellar tendonitis and anterior knee pain. Am J Knee Surg 1999;12:99-108.
4. Fredberg U, Bolvig L. Jumper's knee. Scand J Med Sci Sports 1999;9:66-73.
5. Colosimo AJ, Bassett FH. Jumper's knee diagnosis and treatment. Orthop Rev 1990;19:139-149.

6. Popp JE, Yu JS, Kaeding CC. Recalcitrant patellar tendinitis. Am J Sports Med 1997;25:218-222.

7. Lian O, Engebretsen L, Ovrebo RV, Bahr R. Characteristics of the leg extensors in male volleyball players with jumper's knee. Am J Sports Med 1996;24:380-385.

8. Richards DP, Ajemian SV, Wiley JP, Zernicke RF. Knee joint dynamics predict patellar tendinitis in elite volleyball players. Am J Sports Med 1996;24:676-683.

9. Visentini PJ, Khan KM, Cook JL, et al. The VISA score: an index of severity of symptoms in patients with jumper's knee (patellar tendinosis). J Sci Med Sport 1998;1:22-28.

10. Khan KM, Cook JL, Kiss ZS, et al. Patellar tendon ultrasonography and jumper's knee in female basketball players: a longitudinal study. Clin J Sport Med 1997;7:199-206.

11. Davies SG, Baudouin CJ, King JB, Perry JD. Ultrasound, computed tomography, and magnetic resonance imaging in patellar tendinitis. Clin Radiol 1991;43:52-56.

12. Khan KM, Bonar F, Desmond PM, et al. Patellar tendinosis (jumper's knee): findings at histopathologic examination, US, and MRI Imaging. Radiology 1996;200:821-827.

13. Jensen K, Di Fabio R. Evaluation of eccentric exercise in treatment of patellar tendinitis. Phys Ther 1989;69:211-216.

14. Gotlin RS. Effective rehabilitation for anterior knee pain. J Musculoskeletal Med 2000;17:421-432.

15. Stanish WD, Rubinovich RM, Curwin S. Eccentric exercise in chronic tendinitis. Clin Orthop Relat Res 1985;285:65-68.

16. Rabin A. Is there evidence to support the use of eccentric strengthening exercises to decrease pain and increase function in patients with patellar tendinopathy? Phys Ther 2006;86:450-456.

17. Palumbo PM. Dynamic patellar brace: a new orthosis in the management of patellofemoral disorders. Am J Sports Med 1981;9:45-49.

18. Ismail AM, Balakrishnan R, Rajakumar MK, Lumpur K. Rupture of patellar ligament after steroid infiltration. J Bone Joint Surg Br 1969;51:503-505.

19. Verheyden F, Geens G, Nelen G. Jumper's knee: results of surgical treatment. Acta Orthop Belg 1997;63:102-105.

20. Pierets K, Verdonk R, De Muynck M, Lagast J. Jumper's knee: postoperative assessment. Knee Surg Sports Traumatol Arthrosc 1999;7:239-242.

21. Cook JL, Khan KM, Harcourt PR, et al. A cross sectional study of 100 athletes with jumper's knee managed conservatively and surgically. Br J Sports Med 1997;31:332-336.

Patellofemoral Syndrome 65

Thomas H. Hudgins, MD

DEFINITION

Patellofemoral syndrome is the most common ailment involving the knee in both the athletic and the nonathletic population.[3-5] In sports medicine clinics, 25% of patients complaining of knee pain are diagnosed with this syndrome, and it affects women twice as often as men.[3] Yet despite the common occurrence of this disorder, there is no clear consensus on the definition, etiology, and pathophysiology.[6] The most common theory is that the syndrome is an overuse injury from repetitive overload at the patellofemoral joint. This increased stress results in physical and biomechanical changes of the patellofemoral joint.[6] The literature has focused on identification of risk factors leading to altered biomechanics to produce maltracking of the patella in the femoral trochlear groove and thus stress at the patellofemoral joint. Possible pain generators include the subchondral bone, retinacula, capsule, and synovial membrane.[7] Historically, the histologic diagnosis of chondromalacia had been associated with patellofemoral syndrome. However, chondromalacia is poorly associated with the incidence of patellofemoral syndrome.[5]

SYMPTOMS

The patient with patellofemoral syndrome will complain of diffuse, vague ache of insidious onset.[3] The anterior knee is the most common location for pain, but some patients describe posterior knee discomfort in the popliteal fossa.[4] The discomfort is aggravated by prolonged sitting with knees flexed ("theater" sign) as well as on ascending or descending of stairs and squatting because these positions place the greatest force on the patellofemoral joint.[8] The patient may also experience pseudolocking when the knee momentarily locks in an extended position.[9,10]

PHYSICAL EXAMINATION

The examination focuses on identification of risk factors that contribute to malalignment and rules out other pathologic processes associated with anterior knee pain. Tenderness to palpation at the medial and lateral borders of the patella may be appreciated.[3] A minimal effusion may also be present. The results of manual testing for intra-articular disease, such as the Lachman (anterior cruciate ligament) and McMurray (menisci) maneuvers, will be negative.

The presence of femoral anteversion, tibia internal rotation, excessive pronation at the foot, increased Q angle, and inflexibility of the hip flexors, quadriceps, iliotibial band, and gastrocnemius-soleus should be determined.[11] The patella position (baja or alta, squinting or grasshopper) should also be assessed with the patient sitting and standing. Each of these factors has either a direct or an indirect influence on the tracking of the patella with the femur (Fig. 65-1).

The Q angle is the intersection of a line from the anterior superior iliac spine to the patella with a line from the tibial tubercle to the patella (Fig. 65-2). This angle is typically less than 15 degrees in men and less than 20 degrees in women. An increased angle is associated with increased femoral anteversion and thus patellofemoral joint torsion.[9] However, a consensus on the importance of an increased Q angle is lacking.[6] Tight hip flexors, quadriceps, hamstrings, and gastrocnemius-soleus will increase knee flexion and thus patellofemoral joint reaction force. A tight iliotibial band will increase the lateral pull of the patella through the lateral retinacular fibers.[12,13] It is imperative to assess each of these components in the lower extremity kinetic chain to prescribe a tailored physical therapy program for each individual.

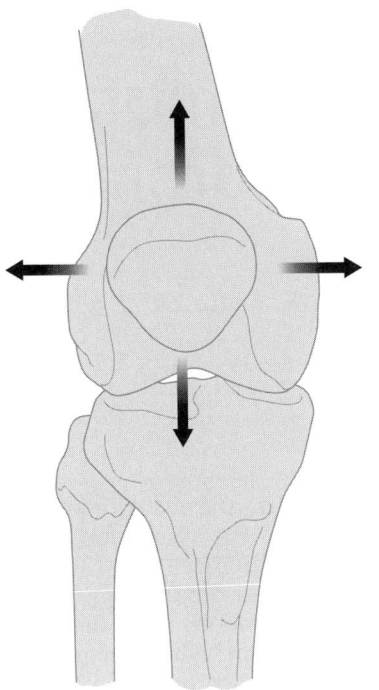

FIGURE 65-1. Forces on the patella in patellofemoral syndrome.

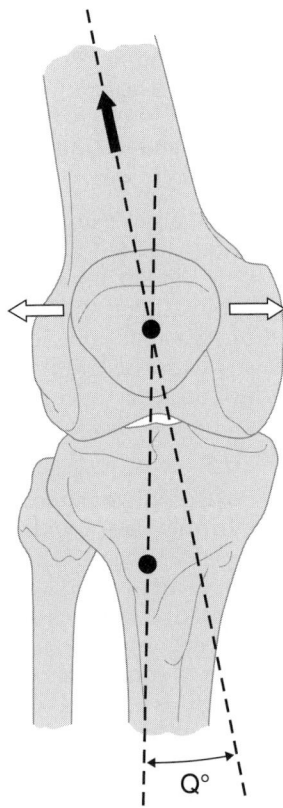

FIGURE 65-2. Measurement of Q angle. A line is drawn from the anterior iliac spine to the center of the patella. A second line is drawn from the center of the patella to the tibial tubercle. An angle between these two lines is called the Q angle.

FUNCTIONAL LIMITATIONS

The patient with the patellofemoral syndrome will avoid activities that provoke the discomfort initially, such as stair climbing. Prolonged sitting in a car may be difficult. In chronic, progressive cases, ambulation may be enough to incite the pain, making all activities of daily living difficult.

DIAGNOSTIC TESTING

Patellofemoral syndrome is a clinical diagnosis. Plain films may be used to evaluate Q angle and patella alta or baja. Advanced imaging, such as magnetic resonance imaging, is reserved for recalcitrant cases that do not respond to conservative care to rule out intra-articular disease. Bone scintigrams revealed diffuse uptake in the patellofemoral joint in 50% of patients diagnosed with patellofemoral syndrome.[14]

TREATMENT

Initial

As in other overuse injuries, the initial treatment focuses on decreasing pain. Icing is beneficial, particularly after activities. Nonsteroidal anti-inflammatory drugs may be used in a judicious manner. Relative rest with non–weight-bearing aerobic activity may also be necessary. A neoprene knee sleeve with patella cutout is helpful to increase proprioceptive feedback. McConnell's taping method can be used during the acute phase to reduce pain and to increase tolerance of a therapeutic exercise program.[13,15-17] Patella bracing was shown to reduce pain and to improve function in patients with patellofemoral syndrome but no more successfully than therapeutic exercise.[18]

Rehabilitation

With no consensus on the etiology and pathophysiology of patellofemoral syndrome, numerous treatment protocols and therapies have been used in the literature.[19]

Differential Diagnosis

Patella fracture

Patella dislocation

Quadriceps rupture

Patella tendinitis

Peripatellar bursitis

Osgood-Schlatter disease

Meniscal lesions

Ligamentous lesions

Plica syndromes

Osteochondritis dissecans

Nevertheless, most patients respond to a directed rehabilitation approach with therapeutic exercise.[12,13] The rehabilitation program should address deficiencies in strength, flexibility, and proprioception. Strength training can be achieved with both open kinetic chain and closed kinetic chain exercises. Open kinetic chain exercises occur when the distal link, the foot, is allowed to move freely in space. During closed kinetic chain exercises, the foot maintains contact with the ground, resulting in a multiarticular closed kinetic exercise.[13] An example of an open kinetic chain exercise is a leg extension. A closed kinetic chain exercise is a leg press or a wall sit. Closed kinetic chain exercises are also less stressful than open chain exercises at the patellofemoral joint in the functional range of 0 to 45 degrees of knee flexion.[20]

These exercises can be performed in multiple planes in a "functional" rehabilitation program (Figs. 65-3 and 65-4). This may entail having the patient perform a lunge (a closed kinetic chain exercise) in the coronal, sagittal, and transverse planes, simulating positions applied during activities. These exercises can also stress the patient's balance by performance of the lunges with eyes closed. Through this functional or skill training, the patient is being prepared for all functional tasks by achieving efficient nerve-muscle interactions.[8]

Many studies have focused on selective strengthening of the vastus medialis obliquus (VMO) as a dynamic medial stabilizer on the patella. Selective VMO strengthening may be achieved with combined hip adduction because the fibers of the VMO originate on the adductor magnus tendon and, to a lesser extent, the adductor longus. However, attempts at proving isolated recruitment of the VMO in relation to the vastus lateralis have failed.[3] Nevertheless, quadriceps strengthening in general should be incorporated in the rehabilitation program through closed kinetic chain and functional exercises as mentioned previously.

Procedures

Injections are not indicated because this is primarily a maltracking phenomenon without a clear consensus on the pain generator.

Surgery

Surgery is rarely indicated, and a directed rehabilitation program is often successful.[4] However, several techniques have been illustrated in the literature. These include lateral retinacular release to decrease the lateral force, proximal and distal realignment procedures, and elevation of the tibial tubercle.[1]

POTENTIAL DISEASE COMPLICATIONS

Recalcitrant chronic cases of anterior knee pain may show progressive degenerative changes at the patellofemoral joint, such as severe (grade IV) chondromalacia patellae.

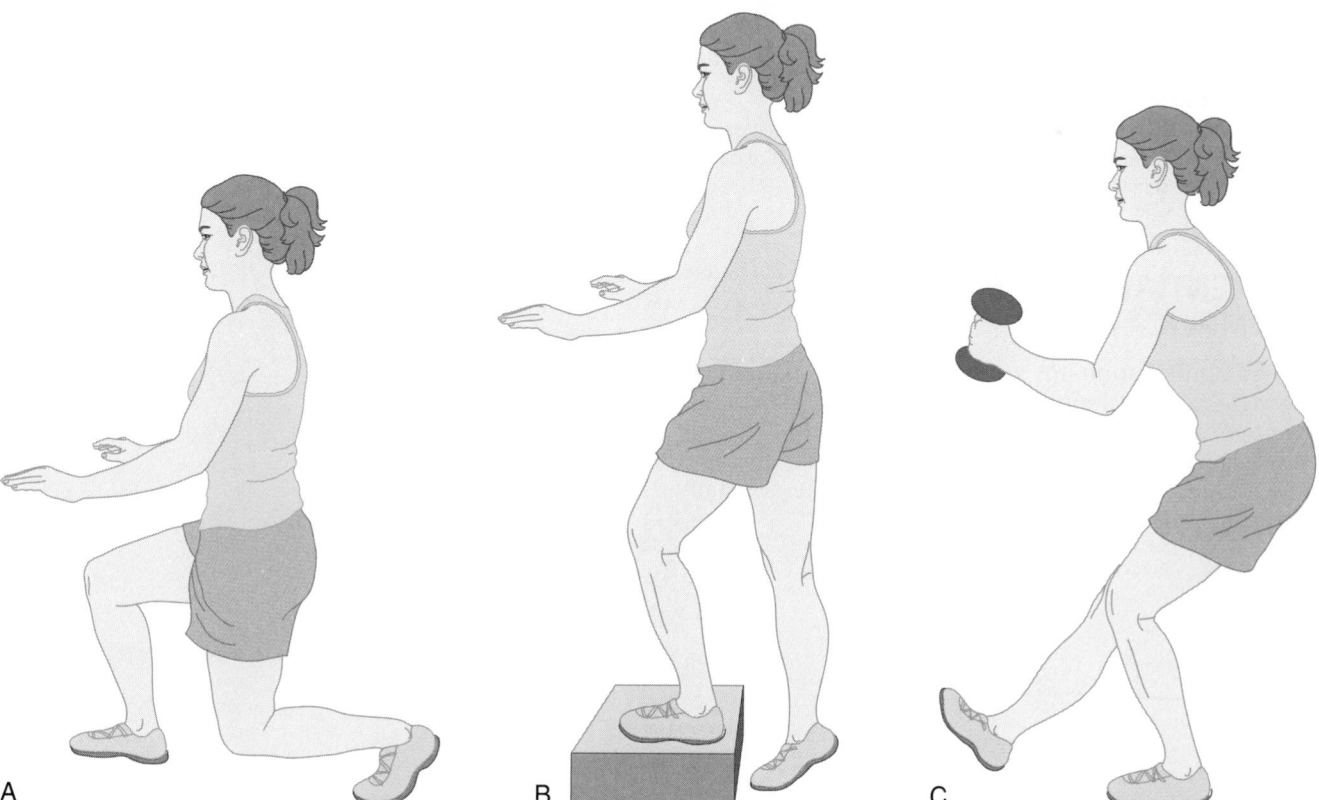

FIGURE 65-3. Skill training can help resolve anterior knee pain by improving strength and neuromuscular coordination. The lunge (**A**), step-down (**B**), and knee bend (**C**) are examples of force-absorbing skill-training exercises that are particularly valuable for improving strength, which in turn promotes stability. For the most benefit during the knee bend, the patient's knee should be aligned with the shoelaces.

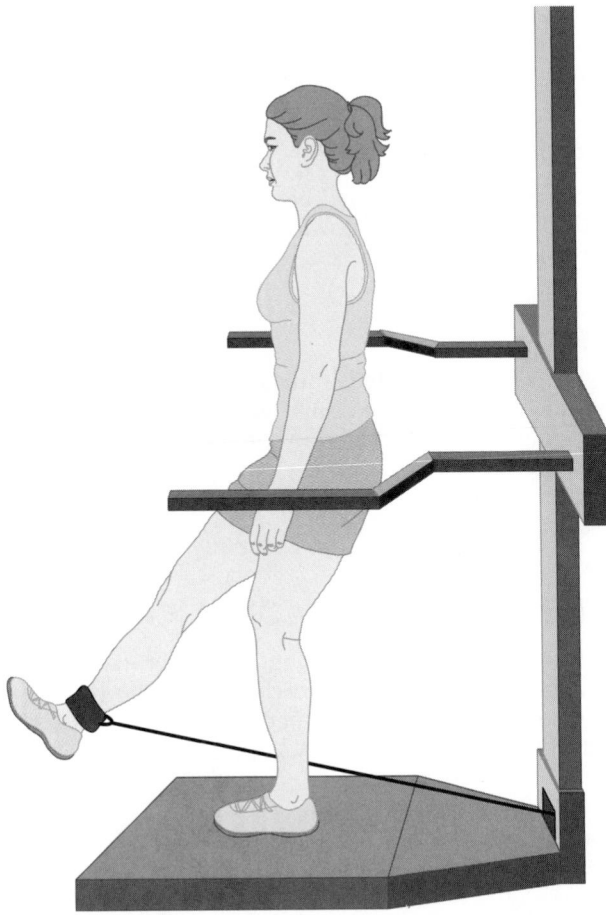

FIGURE 65-4. The standing cable column is an example of a skill-training exercise. The patient uses strength to exercise against resistance offered by a cable and simultaneously refines balancing skills.

References

1. Thomee R, Augustsson J, Karlsson J. Patellofemoral pain syndrome: a review of current issues. Sports Med 1999;28:245-262.
2. Beckman M, Craig R, Lehman RC. Rehabilitation of patellofemoral dysfunction in the athlete. Clin Sports Med 1989;8:841-860.
3. Powers CM. Rehabilitation of patellofemoral disorders: a critical review. J Orthop Sports Phys Ther 1998;5:345-354.
4. Goldberg B. Patellofemoral malalignment. Pediatr Ann 1997;26: 32-35.
5. Sanchis-Alfonso V. Pathogenesis of anterior knee pain syndrome and functional patellofemoral instability in the active young. Am J Knee Surg 1999;12:29-40.
6. Baker MM, Juhn MS. Patellofemoral pain syndrome in the female athlete. Clin Sports Med 2000;19:314-329.
7. Papagelopoulos PJ, Sim FH. Patellofemoral pain syndrome: diagnosis and management. Orthopedics 1997;20:148-157.
8. Gotlin RS. Effective knee rehabilitation for anterior knee pain. J Musculoskeletal Med 2000;17:421-432.
9. Hilyard A. Recent developments in the management of patellofemoral pain. Physiotherapy 1990;76:559-565.
10. Kannus P, Niittymaki S. Which factors predict outcome in the nonoperative treatment of patellofemoral pain syndrome? A prospective follow-up study. Med Sci Sports Exerc 1993;26:289-296.
11. Insall J, Falvo KA, Wise DW. Chondromalacia patellae. J Bone Joint Surg Am 1976;58:1-8.
12. Juhn MS. Patellofemoral pain syndrome: a review and guidelines for treatment. Am Fam Physician 1999;60:2012-2018.
13. Press JM, Young JA. Rehabilitation of patellofemoral pain syndrome. In Kibler WB, Herring SA, Press JM. Functional Rehabilitation of Sports and Musculoskeletal Injuries. Gaithersburg, Md, Aspen, 1998:254-264.
14. Naslund JE. Diffusely increased bone scintigraphic uptake in patellofemoral syndrome. Br J Sports Med 2005;39:162-165.
15. McConnell J. The management of chondromalacia patellae: a long term solution. Aust J Physiother 1986;32:215-233.
16. Kowall MG, Kolk G, Nuber GW. Patellar taping in the treatment of patellofemoral pain. Am J Sports Med 1996;24:61-65.
17. Larsen B. Patellar taping: a radiographic examination of the medial glide technique. Am J Sports Med 1995;23:465-471.
18. Lun VM, Wiley JP, Meeuwisse WH, Yanagawa TL. Effectiveness of patellar bracing for treatment of patellofemoral pain syndrome. Clin J Sport Med 2005;15:235-240.
19. Arroll B. Patellofemoral pain syndrome. Am J Sports Med 1997;25: 207-212.
20. Steinkamp LA. Biomechanical considerations in patellofemoral joint rehabilitation. Am J Sports Med 1993;21:438-442.

POTENTIAL TREATMENT COMPLICATIONS

Overcompensation for the malalignment may occur with surgical techniques such as the lateral retinacular release. The surgeon may lyse too many fibers, leading to increased medial tracking. Many of the realignment procedures should also be reserved for the skeletally mature patient.[1]

Peroneal Neuropathy 66

John C. King, MD

DEFINITION

Peroneal neuropathy is compromise of the peroneal nerve. This can be from its origins within the sciatic nerve, in which it remains distinct from the tibial portion of the sciatic nerve, throughout the course of the sciatic nerve, to its terminations in the leg and foot. The common peroneal nerve completely separates from the tibial nerve in the upper popliteal fossa and then traverses laterally to curve superficially around the fibular head. Before the fibular head, the lateral cutaneous nerve of the calf branches off to supply cutaneous sensation to the upper lateral leg. Near the fibular head, the common peroneal nerve bifurcates into the superficial peroneal nerve and deep peroneal nerve, which describes their relative locations as they wrap around the fibular head. Because the deep portion is immediately adjacent to the hard bony surface, it is more susceptible to compression injuries at the fibular head. This is the most common site of peroneal nerve compromise.[1]

The common peroneal nerve provides the lateral cutaneous nerve of the calf and the motor branch to the short head of the biceps femoris above the fibular head. The superficial peroneal nerve is predominantly sensory, providing cutaneous sensation to the lateral lower leg and most of the foot dorsum. The superficial peroneal nerve also innervates the foot everters, peroneus longus and brevis. The deep peroneal nerve is predominantly motor, innervating the foot and toe dorsiflexors, but it has a small cutaneous representation at the dorsal first web space of the foot.

Predisposing factors for peroneal mononeuropathy at the fibular head, the most common site of compromise, include weight loss,[1,2] diabetes,[1,3] peripheral polyneuropathy,[1] and positioning and localized prolonged pressure. Positioning and prolonged pressure issues can arise through recent anesthesia and surgery; recent prolonged hospitalization, especially bed rest or coma[1,4]; orthopedic casts, braces, and orthotics[5]; habitual leg crossing[1]; or prolonged squatting.[1,6]

A history of sustained pressure or trauma should be solicited as these are the most common causes of acute lesions. Figure 66-1 shows the most common causes of lesions of acute and nonacute onset. Iatrogenic causes should be considered; these include anesthesia for surgery leading to immobility and possible positioning issues, prolonged imposed bed rest with decreased sensorium due to sepsis or coma,[1] intermittent sequential pneumatic compression,[7] acupuncture,[8] plaster casts,[1] and, ironically, ankle-foot orthoses.[5] A history of severe inversion ankle sprain or blunt trauma to the ankle, leg, or fibular head can be helpful in identifying likely pathophysiologic mechanisms.

Stretch injury commonly occurs at the hip region and may be associated with hip surgery (e.g., total hip arthroplasty) or traumatic hip dislocation. The peroneal portion of the sciatic nerve is more susceptible than the tibial portion to stretch injuries because of its more lateral positioning and shorter distance between the piriformis and the fibular head than between the piriformis and the tarsal tunnel, the sites of relative fixation of these two nerves. Distal peroneal nerve stretch injury can also occur at the point where it passes through the peroneus longus muscle.

SYMPTOMS

Peroneal neuropathy typically presents with acute footdrop, but this can sometimes occur insidiously during several days to weeks. The footdrop can be complete or partial, often with increased tripping or falls as the primary complaint. Numbness or dysesthesias frequently occur in the lower lateral leg and dorsum of the foot, although pain is rare. When pain is present, it is usually

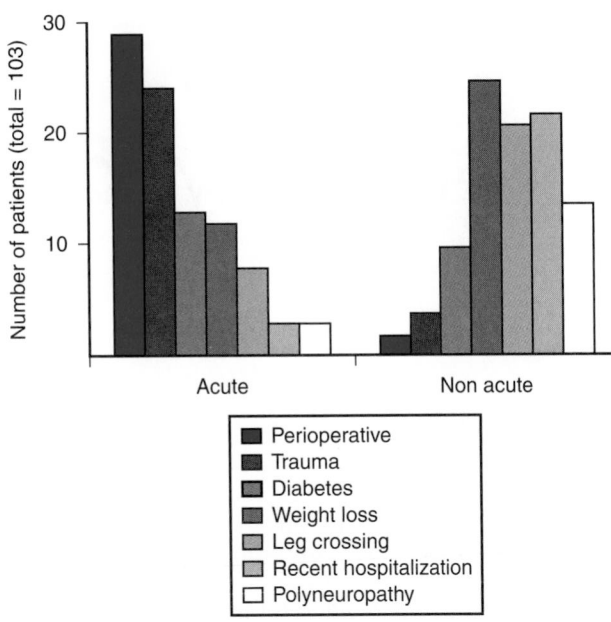

FIGURE 66-1. Predisposing factors in 103 patients with peroneal mononeuropathy divided between acute onset and nonacute onset. (Reprinted with permission from Katirji MB, Wilbourn AJ. Common peroneal mononeuropathy: a clinical and electrophysiologic study of 116 lesions. Neurology 1988;38:1723-1728.)

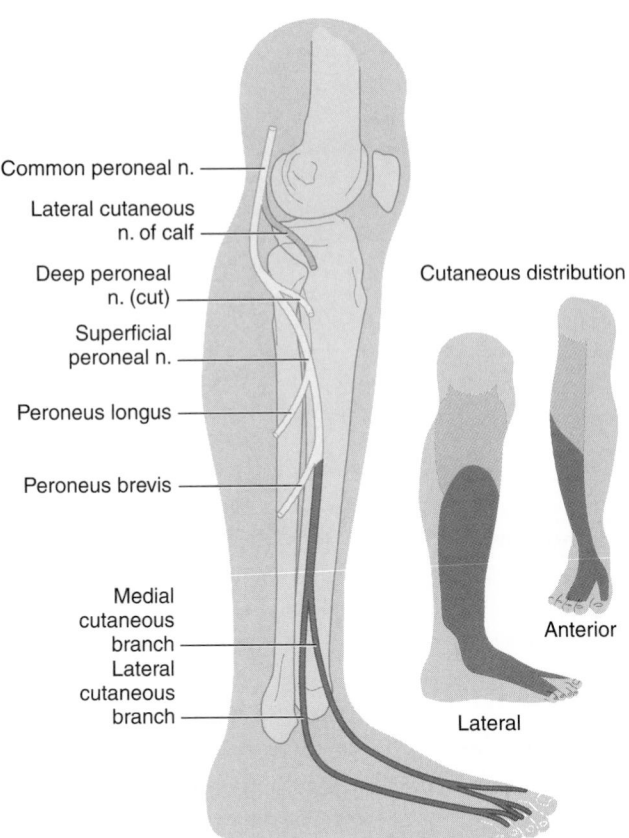

FIGURE 66-2. Common (light blue) and superficial (dark blue) peroneal nerve branch cutaneous distributions and motor branches. (Reprinted with permission from Haymaker W, Woodhall B. Peripheral Nerve Injuries: Principles of Diagnosis. Philadelphia, WB Saunders, 1953:292.)

located around the knee and felt as deep and ill-defined.[1] When pain is prominent and neuropathic in character, stretch injury of the peroneal portion of the sciatic nerve should be considered.

PHYSICAL EXAMINATION

The examination should be guided by a close understanding of the relevant anatomy, with focused study of the elements of each component of the peroneal nerve.

Sensory deficits in the upper lateral leg (Fig. 66-2) suggest a lesion proximal to the fibular head. Testing of foot inversion, to rule out concomitant tibial nerve compromise and therefore sciatic nerve as the likely site of injury, must be performed with the foot passively slightly dorsiflexed for optimal strength testing (often the foot will initially, at rest, be in a plantar flexed position during examination as a result of the existing footdrop) because inversion is weak normally when the foot is relatively plantar flexed.[1] With the long head of the biceps femoris intact, knee flexion strength will test normal despite a compromise to the short head of the biceps femoris strength. Palpation may reveal a lack of tissue tensing where the short head of the biceps femoris should be located. This is, however, challenging to discern and helpful only in the case of acute complete proximal peroneal nerve compromise with relative sparing of the tibial-innervated hamstring muscles. The function and innervation of the long and short heads of the biceps femoris can be more accurately determined electrodiagnostically. If both are compromised, knee flexion will test weak, as will plantar flexion and toe flexion, suggesting a sciatic nerve lesion. Muscle stretch reflexes will

usually be normal unless the sciatic nerve is severely compromised, when the medial hamstring and Achilles reflexes could be reduced or absent.

Sensory deficit or dysesthesia in the lower lateral leg and over most of the dorsum of the foot suggests involvement of the superficial peroneal or this portion of the sciatic nerve (see Fig. 66-2). Eversion weakness is consistent with superficial peroneal nerve compromise. If the superficial peroneal nerve lesion is isolated, then Achilles, quadriceps, and medial hamstring muscle stretch reflexes will be normal.

If eversion is strong but dorsiflexion is very weak, a more focal deep peroneal nerve compromise is suggested. There may be sensory deficits or dysesthesias along the isolated area of the dorsum of the first web space of the foot on the affected side (Fig. 66-3). A combination of deep and superficial peroneal nerve branch compromise often occurs, usually affecting the deep branch more severely than the superficial branch, especially with lesions at the fibular head.

FUNCTIONAL LIMITATIONS

The most common limitation is due to footdrop. This can lead to frequent tripping or falls and altered gait with foot slapping, circumduction, or hip hiking. These

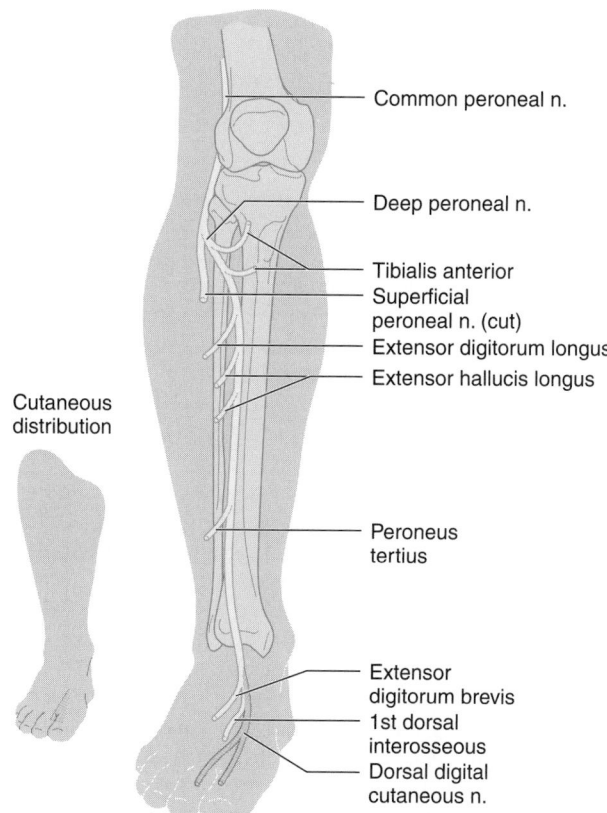

Cutaneous distribution

Common peroneal n.

Deep peroneal n.

Tibialis anterior

Superficial peroneal n. (cut)

Extensor digitorum longus

Extensor hallucis longus

Peroneus tertius

Extensor digitorum brevis

1st dorsal interosseous

Dorsal digital cutaneous n.

FIGURE 66-3. Deep *(blue area)* peroneal nerve cutaneous distribution and motor branches. (Reprinted with permission from Haymaker W, Woodhall B. Peripheral Nerve Injuries: Principles of Diagnosis. Philadelphia, WB Saunders, 1953:293.)

gait compensations require more energy per distance for walking and place one at a greater fall risk than if they are corrected by an ankle-foot orthosis. Any task requiring dynamic foot eversion or dorsiflexion muscle activity, such as walking and running or balance activities such as occur during lower extremity dressing, bathing, sports activities, or driving (especially when the right side is affected[9]), can be impaired.

DIAGNOSTIC STUDIES

Electrophysiologic studies are the "gold standard" for diagnosis of suspected peroneal neuropathy.[10,11] These studies can help distinguish site and severity of compromise from other possible causes of footdrop (see the section on differential diagnosis).[1,10] This includes both sensory nerve conduction studies of the superficial peroneal nerve and motor nerve conduction studies of the common, deep, and superficial peroneal nerve to the functionally deficient muscles, such as the tibialis anterior or peroneus longus. Although the peroneal motor nerve is commonly studied to the extensor digitorum brevis for polyneuropathy screening, this is not the targeted muscle to evaluate footdrop, or dorsiflexion weakness, as the tibialis anterior is the more relevant and germane motor conduction study.[1,10] Needle electromyography, especially of the short head of the biceps femoris, can help determine if the lesion is proximal to the

fibular head. Additional prognostic and severity data can be obtained by needle study as well as by comparison nerve conduction studies between the involved and uninvolved sides.

If the etiology cannot be determined with reasonable certainty, imaging studies can help identify less common, nontraumatic causes of peroneal neuropathy. These include ganglia, nerve tumors (primary nerve sheath, benign or malignant, or metastatic tumors), hematomas (especially with anticoagulation or bleeding dyscrasias),[1] aneurysms, venous thromboses,[12,13] and knee osteoarthritis.[14,15] The most common imaging study is magnetic resonance imaging along the course of the nerve, but imaging studies could include plain radiography or ultrasonography.

Differential Diagnosis

Cerebral lesions, especially midline cortical

Spinal cord lesions, Brown-Séquard syndrome

Lumbosacral radiculopathy, especially L5

Lumbosacral plexopathy

Compartment syndromes in the leg (especially anterior compartment)

Acute or subacute polyneuropathy

Motor neuron disease

TREATMENT

Initial

Treatment depends on lesion site and prognostic factors found on electrophysiologic studies. If a good prognosis is predicted, watchful waiting is indicated with temporary adaptations and preventive measures to minimize functional impact until complete recovery occurs. Removal of pressure to the involved area is important, and this may require bed rail modifications or protective padding around the knees, especially for sleep. Work or sports activities and clothing that could result in pressure to the involved areas should be assessed and modified to eliminate any unnecessary pressure or padding added to minimize blunt trauma effects. Habitual leg crossers must modify this behavior. With pressure relief, neurapraxic injuries often significantly improve by 6 weeks. If the lesion is more axon stretch, recovery can take as long as 1 mm/day. Completely denervated muscles need reinnervation by 18 months for recovery; the higher the lesion, the more likely a poor outcome will result for distal muscles. If prognosis is poor, such as with a severe high sciatic nerve injury, longer term adaptations and home preventive programs should be planned as well as possible surgical considerations, especially in children.[16]

If pain is neuropathic in nature (burning, tingling, or associated with hyperpathia), neuropathic pain medications such as the anticonvulsants or tricyclic antidepressants should be considered. These must be started in low dosage, taken routinely, and slowly titrated up; a steady-state level is needed to help block the new aberrant sodium channels of injured nerves, which is one mechanism by which these medications decrease neuropathic pain. These medications are not used on an as-needed basis like other more typical analgesics. When they are effective, the neuropathic pain medications tend to continue to be effective chronically and are often needed 6 months to 2 years, if not indefinitely.

Rehabilitation

Adaptive devices include an ankle-foot orthosis, which can be a simple fixed ankle off-the-shelf model if no other comorbidities exist. This brace helps with footdrop and improves foot clearance during the leg swing-through phase of gait. If the peroneal neuropathy occurs in isolation, then no plantar sensory loss is present, and concerns for contact pressure of skin to orthosis are lessened. If the patient presents with comorbid tibial nerve deficits, custom molding of the ankle-foot orthosis to minimize contact pressures to the skin should be considered. If the prognosis is poor or recovery not forthcoming, the addition of dorsiflexion assist to the ankle-foot orthosis may be helpful toward restoring an even more normal gait than is achievable with a fixed ankle. With significant obesity or edema or in the face of severe polyneuropathy requiring special accommodative shoe wear, a dual upright ankle-foot orthosis may be indicated. The addition of dorsiflexion assist can easily be accomplished by adding springs to the posterior channels of a dual upright ankle-foot orthosis. The addition of dorsiflexion assist may be mandatory if the patient is having difficulty driving and right foot involvement is the cause. Most patients will have a stable and safe gait with an ankle-foot orthosis without additional gait aids, such as walkers, crutches, or canes; but when needed, gait training with any necessary gait aids should be ordered through physical therapy.

Because of the unbalanced weakness of the dorsiflexors, the lesser or unopposed plantar flexors must be actively stretched on a daily basis to prevent contracture development, which can occur in a matter of weeks. Similarly, the inverters may also need to be stretched in a home exercise program if the eversion function has been compromised. Splinting can also assist with contracture prevention and treatment.

As the muscle recovers function, which may occur during a few months if it is due to axonotmetic compression at the fibular head, strengthening can be initiated once manual muscle strength greater than 3/5 returns. It is probably not prudent to exercise the newly reinnervated muscle to exhaustion, but moderate strengthening can be well tolerated. Patients may begin household ambulation without their ankle-foot orthoses before going long community distances. Patients should be advised to use their ankle-foot orthoses whenever prolonged walking is anticipated, even when manual muscle testing initially reveals 5/5 strength, because of early fatigue on initial strengthening.

Procedures

Although common peroneal neuropathy at the fibular head is rarely complicated by severe pain, sciatic or more distal superficial peroneal nerve stretch with axonotmesis can result in neuropathic pain. Medications focused on neuropathic pain are the mainstays of treatment, but additional nerve block is occasionally needed to resolve the associated pain adequately.

Surgery

Most compromise at the fibular head is due to transient pressure or trauma issues, and watchful waiting is often all that is needed with a good prognosis anticipated. Even incomplete proximal stretch injuries may recover over time, given enough remaining innervation to allow collateral sprouting to maintain the existing denervated muscle to avoid its atrophy and transformation to fatty connective tissue. When expected improvement does not occur or imaging studies reveal structures creating possible compromise of the nerve's function, surgical exploration, compression relief, or neurotomy or resection of compromising tumors, synovial cysts or ganglia, or other structures may be needed.[17-19] For poor-prognosis, high sciatic near-complete or complete peroneal lesions, a new technique of transplanting some tibial nerve elements into the denervated tibialis anterior muscle has been successful, especially in children, in restoring function where previous footdrop existed.[16] Tendon transfers have also been used with variable success.[17]

POTENTIAL DISEASE COMPLICATIONS

A common complication of peroneal neuropathy is footdrop and its deleterious effects on gait and balance, leading to falls and additional trauma. The sensory impairments place portions of the lateral leg and foot dorsum at risk for pressure ulcers or acute injuries that are not adequately treated due to lack of pain and sensation in those areas. If range of motion of the ankle is not adequately addressed, ankle contractures can result, further impairing gait and ankle-foot orthosis use.

POTENTIAL TREATMENT COMPLICATIONS

Any surgical treatment has the potential for infection, excessive bleeding, anesthetic death, and making the condition worse. Procedures likewise could worsen the condition and are used only when pain is intolerable and recalcitrant to medication interventions. Pain medications are most typically neuropathic pain–focused medications, such as tricyclic antidepressants (e.g., amitriptyline) and anticonvulsants (e.g., gabapentin). These have unique contraindications and side effect profiles. These medications must be initiated at a low dose and built up over time to minimize the occurrence of side effects. They are not used in an as-needed fashion like the more typical analgesics (such as nonsteroidal anti-inflammatory drugs) or opioids. Opioids tend to be less often used because of the chronic and neuropathic nature of most associated pain. Nonsteroidal anti-inflammatory and opioid drugs also have unique side effect profiles. Physical dependence and development of tolerance with opioids must be considered because the neuropathic pain from peroneal nerve lesions is most often chronic.

References

1. Katirji B. Peroneal neuropathy. Neurol Clin 1999;17:567-591.
2. Cruz-Martinez A, Arpa J, Palau F. Peroneal neuropathy after weight loss. J Peripher Nerv Syst 2000;5:101-105.
3. Stamboulis E, Vassilopoulos D, Kalfakis N. Symptomatic focal mononeuropathies in diabetic patients: increased or not? J Neurol 2005;252:448-452.
4. Aprile I, Padua L, Padua R, et al. Peroneal mononeuropathy: predisposing factors, and clinical and neurophysiological relationships. Neurol Sci 2000;21:367-371.
5. Ryan MM, Darras BT, Soul JS. Peroneal neuropathy from ankle-foot orthoses. Pediatr Neurol 2003;29:72-74.
6. Toğrol E, Colak A, Kutlay M, et al. Bilateral peroneal nerve palsy induced by prolonged squatting. Milit Med 2000;3:240-242.
7. McGrory BJ, Burke DW. Peroneal nerve palsy following intermittent sequential pneumatic compression. Orthopedics 2000;23:1103-1105.
8. Sato M, Katsumoto H, Kawamura K, et al. Peroneal nerve palsy following acupuncture treatment. J Bone Joint Surg Am 2003;85:916-918.
9. Fann AV. Peroneal neuropathy. In Frontera WR, Silver JK, eds. Essentials of Physical Medicine and Rehabilitation. Philadelphia, Hanley & Belfus, 2002:363-366.
10. Wilbourn AJ. AAEM case report #12: common peroneal mononeuropathy at the fibular head. Muscle Nerve 1986;9:825-836.
11. Marciniak C, Armon C, Wilson J, Miller R. Practice parameter: utility of electrodiagnostic techniques in evaluating patients with suspected peroneal neuropathy: an evidence-based review. Muscle Nerve 2005;31:520-527.
12. Yamamoto N, Koyano K. Neurovascular compression of the common peroneal nerve by varicose veins. Eur J Vasc Endovasc Surg 2004;28:335-338.
13. Bendszus M, Reiners K, Perez J, et al. Peroneal nerve palsy caused by thrombosis of crural veins. Neurology 2002;58:1675-1677.
14. Flores LP, Koerbel A, Tatagiba M. Peroneal nerve compression resulting from fibular head osteophyte-like lesions. Surg Neurol 2005;64:249-252.
15. Fetzer GB, Prather H, Gelberman RH, Clohisy JC. Progressive peroneal nerve palsy in a varus arthritic knee. J Bone Joint Surg Am 2004;86:1538-1540.
16. Gousheh J, Babaei A. A new surgical technique for the treatment of high common peroneal nerve palsy. Plast Reconstr Surg 2002;109:994-998.
17. Kim DH, Murovic JA, Tiel RL, Kline DG. Management and outcomes in 318 operative common peroneal nerve lesions. Neurosurgery 2004;54:1421-1428.
18. Thoma A, Fawcett S, Ginty M, Veltri K. Decompression of the common peroneal nerve. Plast Reconstr Surg 2001;107:1183-1188.
19. Hersekli MA, Akpinar S, Demirors H, et al. Synovial cysts of proximal tibiofibular joint causing peroneal nerve palsy: report of three cases and review of the literature. Arch Orthop Trauma Surg 2004;124:711-714.

Posterior Cruciate Ligament Sprain 67

Christine Curtis, BS, Peter Bienkowski, MD, and Lyle J. Micheli, MD

Synonym

Posterior cruciate ligament tear

ICD-9 Codes

717.84 Old disruption of posterior cruciate ligament
844.2   Acute posterior cruciate ligament tear

DEFINITION

Posterior cruciate ligament (PCL) tears represent 5% to 20% of all knee ligament injuries.[1] The PCL arises from the posterior aspect of the tibial plateau, crosses ("cruciate") behind the anterior cruciate ligament (ACL), and inserts into the lateral portion of the medial femoral condyle (Fig. 67-1). The main function of the PCL is to resist posterior displacement of the tibia on the femur. It also acts as a secondary restraint to external tibial rotation. Together with the ACL, it functions in the "screw-home" mechanism of the knee by which the tibia glides to its exact position at terminal knee extension. In general, PCL tears occur in a flexed knee when the tibia is displaced posteriorly. This can occur in a motor vehicle accident–dashboard injury or during a fall on a flexed knee with the foot in plantar flexion. The PCL may also rupture from hyperextension and rotation on a planted foot or on forced hyperflexion. PCL injuries may occur in isolation, but they generally occur with other injuries (e.g., ACL tear, collateral ligament tear, and meniscal injuries).

The long-term sequelae of posterior instability of the knee may include the development of degenerative arthritis.[2] In contrast to ACL injuries, most series of PCL injuries have reported a higher incidence of injury to men.[3]

SYMPTOMS

It is important to obtain information about the nature of the injury. Typically, patients report that they have fallen on a flexed knee or have sustained a blow to the anterior knee when it was flexed (e.g., on the dashboard of a car). Some patients may recall feeling or hearing a "pop" at the time of injury.

Patients may report pain along the medial and patellofemoral regions of the knee, instability, and an inability to bear weight and to walk. Swelling can range from insignificant to very swollen.

PHYSICAL EXAMINATION

In an acute injury, there may be contusions of the anterior tibia, and popliteal ecchymosis may be present. Swelling and effusions will vary and may not be present at all. See Table 67-1 for the general classifications of PCL injuries.

It is essential during the examination of the knee to evaluate all knee ligaments thoroughly to identify combined ligamentous injury. The goal of PCL evaluation is to exploit posterior subluxation of the tibia, which occurs with PCL insufficiency.

The "gold standard" of PCL examination is the posterior drawer test (Fig. 67-2). During this test, the knee is flexed at 90 degrees with the hip held at 45 degrees of flexion. It is essential to appreciate a normal 1-cm step-off of the medial tibial plateau anterior to the medial femoral condyle. The absence of the step-off should alert the clinician to a possibility of PCL injury. Posterior pressure is applied to the tibia while the amount of displacement of the medial tibial step-off and the quality of the endpoint in comparison with the contralateral knee are noted. Posterolateral instability may be evaluated by the posterior drawer test with the foot externally rotated 15 degrees. Similarly, posteromedial instability is assessed by the posterior drawer test with the foot internally rotated 15 degrees.

The posterior Lachman test involves positioning of the knee at 30 degrees of flexion with posterior pressure applied to the proximal tibia (Fig. 67-3). The extent of displacement and the quality of the endpoint are evaluated and compared with the contralateral knee.

The posterior sag test is performed with the patient supine with the hips and knees at 90 degrees of flexion (Fig. 67-4). The clinician grasps both heels and inspects

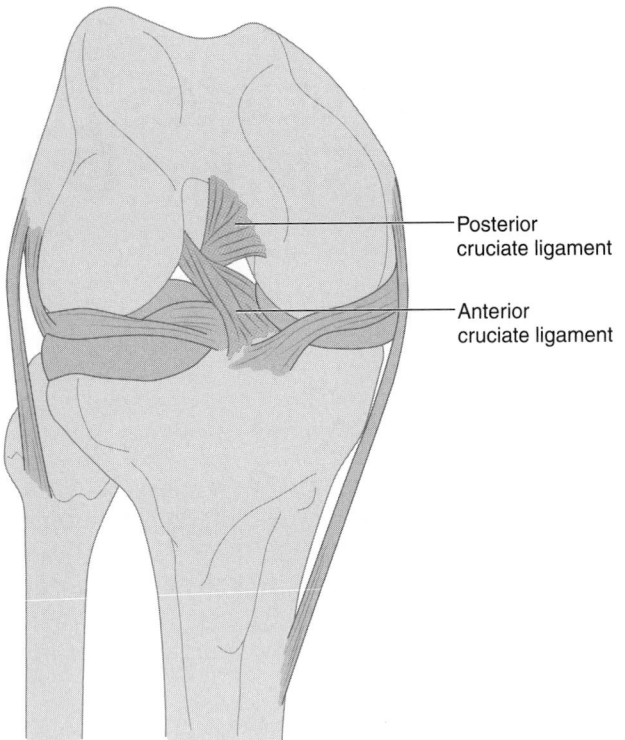

Posterior
cruciate ligament

Anterior
cruciate ligament

FIGURE 67-1. Anterior and posterior cruciate ligament structures.

TABLE 67-1 Classification of Posterior Cruciate Ligament Injuries

Grade	Definition	Laxity (mm)
I	PCL partially torn	<5
II	PCL partially torn	5-9
III	PCL completely torn	>10
IVa	PCL and LCL, posterolateral injury	>12
IVb	PCL and MCL, posteromedial injury	>12
IVc	PCL and ACL injury	>15

Note: grades I to III are isolated injuries; grade IV is a combined injury.
ACL, anterior cruciate ligament; LCL, lateral collateral ligament; MCL, medial collateral ligament; PCL, posterior cruciate ligament.
Modified from Janousek AT, Jones DG, Clatworthy M, et al. Posterior cruciate ligament injuries of the knee joint. Sports Med 1999;28:429-441.

for posterior tibial translation consistent with an insufficient PCL.

The reverse pivot shift includes a valgus-loaded, externally rotated knee moved from 90 degrees of flexion to full extension (Fig. 67-5). A positive test result is indicated by a pivot shift felt at 20 to 30 degrees when the posteriorly subluxated tibia is reduced.

The dynamic posterior shift test is implemented by extending the knee from 90 degrees of flexion to full extension with 90 degrees of hip flexion. A positive result is indicated if the tibia is reduced with a "clunk" near full extension.

The quadriceps active test is achieved with the knee flexed at 60 degrees while the foot is secured by the clinician. The patient attempts to extend the knee isometrically. PCL insufficiency is demonstrated by anterior tibial translation from a subluxated position.

The neurologic examination findings should be normal, with the possible exception of apparent weakness with strength testing as a result of pain.

FUNCTIONAL LIMITATIONS

Functional limitations of PCL tears may include difficulty with walking and a decrease in the level of functioning because of pain as well as apprehension of instability. Athletes may be unable to complete cutting movements. However, PCL injury is often less debilitating than ACL injury; many athletes are still able to participate effectively in running sports.

DIAGNOSTIC STUDIES

Diagnostic testing is useful as an adjunct to the clinical examination. The KT-1000 arthrometer is highly specific in the detection of high-grade (grade II, grade III) PCL tears.[4] Stress radiographs may be obtained to document the extent of posterior instability but are rarely done in settings where magnetic resonance imaging is readily available. After an acute injury, plain radiographs must be performed to rule out fractures, including PCL avulsions (the tunnel view is best to visualize this). Magnetic resonance imaging assessment is highly specific and sensitive in assessment of PCL injuries, particularly when newer fat suppression and "fast spin" techniques are used.[5-7] Finally, diagnostic arthroscopy allows direct visualization of the PCL.

Differential Diagnosis

Anterior cruciate ligament tear

Collateral ligament tear

Meniscal tear

Osteochondral fracture

Patellar tendon rupture

Patellofemoral dislocation

Tibial plateau fracture

TREATMENT

Initial

Initial treatment consists of protection, rest, ice, compression, and elevation (PRICE), crutches, and short-term nonsteroidal anti-inflammatory drugs. Analgesics may be used to control pain if this is an issue. Currently,

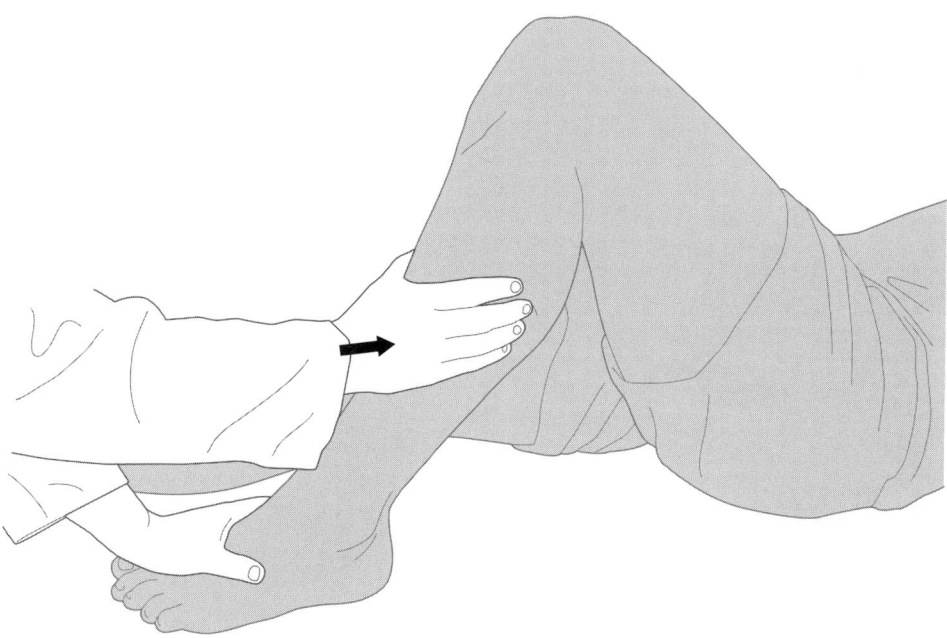

FIGURE 67-2. Posterior drawer test.

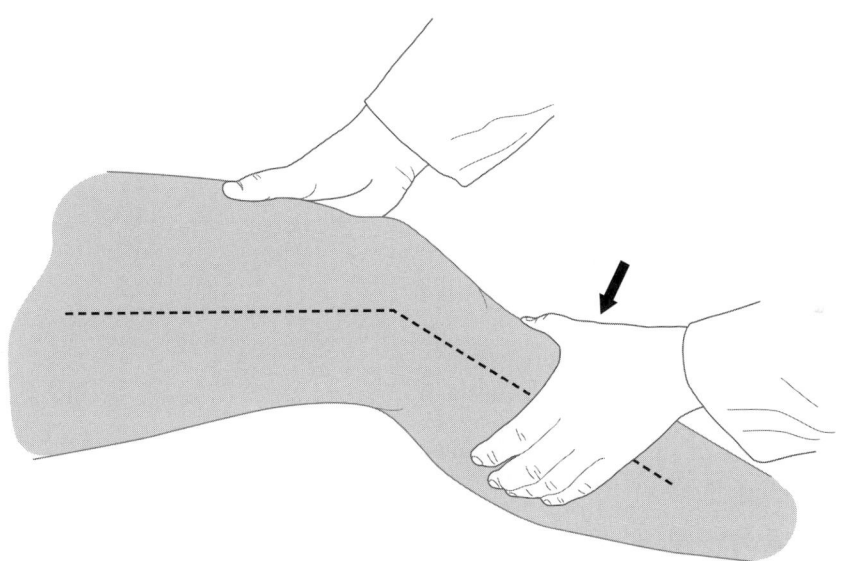

FIGURE 67-3. Correct position for posterior Lachman test.

nonoperative treatment is advocated for those with isolated PCL injuries with mild (grade I or grade II) laxity.[4] Some recommend conservative treatment for all acute isolated PCL injury as well as for chronic, isolated, asymptomatic PCL injury when it is newly diagnosed with no history of prior rehabilitation.[8]

Surgical intervention is advocated for patients with bone avulsion fractures, combined ligament injuries, and chronic symptomatic PCL laxity, particularly if this interferes with athletic participation in elite athletes.[9] In a high percentage of cases, athletic participation is still possible with PCL insufficiency.[3] Management includes immobilization in extension with a Velcro knee immobilizer and avoidance of hamstring exercise.

Rehabilitation

Nonoperative rehabilitation begins after the signs and symptoms of acute injury have subsided (7 to 10 days). Range of motion and progressive resistance quadriceps training is initiated while posterior tibial sag is prevented. The use of a PCL functional brace has not been proved to be effective, although some may find it useful.[9] After acute symptoms have subsided, or

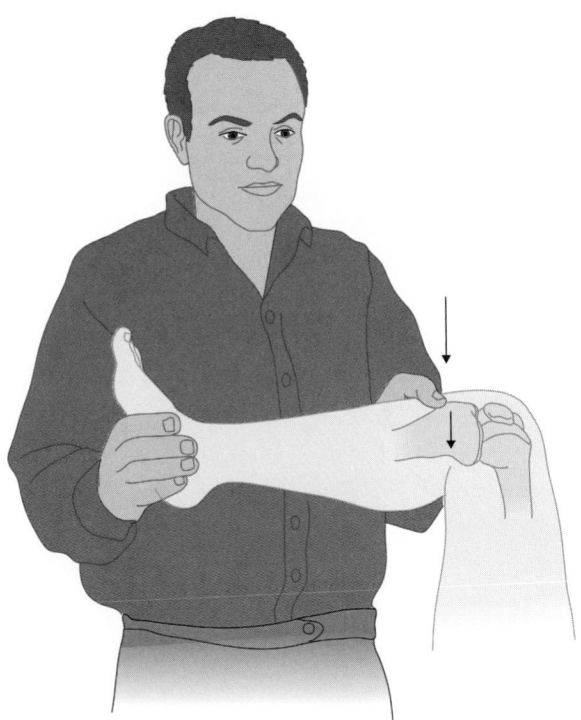

FIGURE 67-4. Posterior tibial sag test.

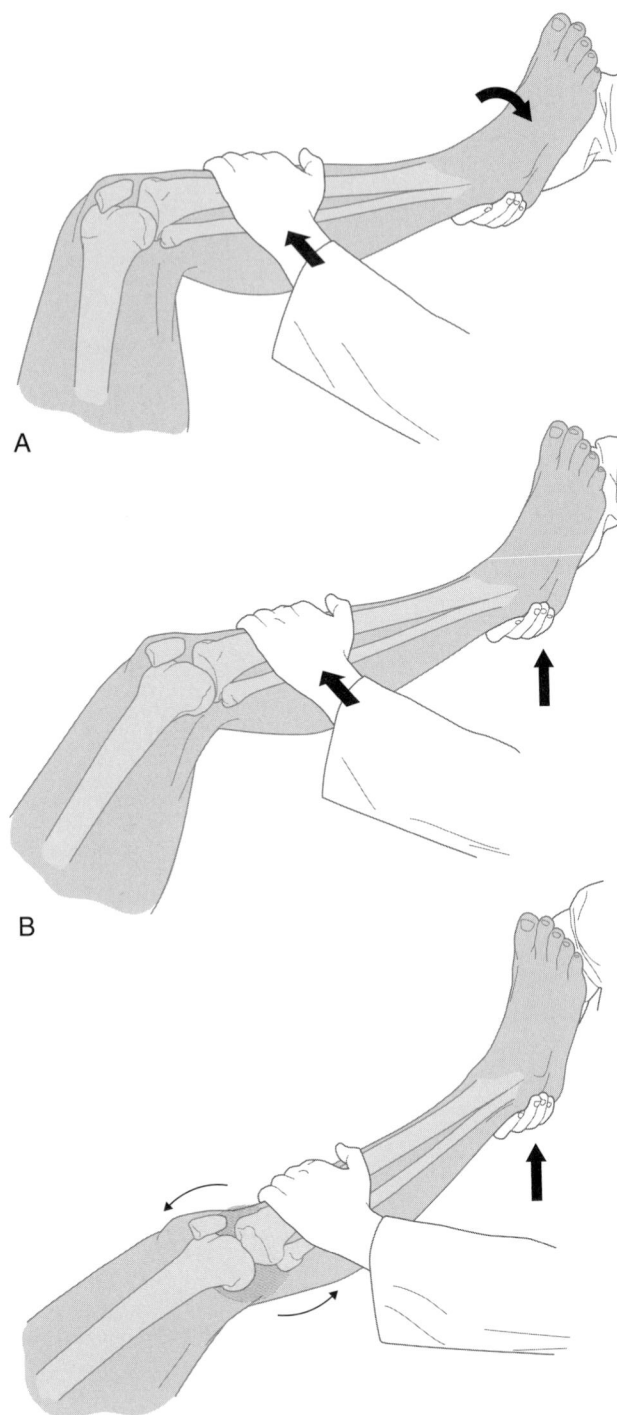

FIGURE 67-5. Reverse pivot shift test. **A,** The knee is flexed to 90 degrees. A valgus, external rotation force is applied to the knee. **B,** The knee is extended while the valgus, external rotation is maintained. **C,** Near full extension, the lateral tibia shifts forward, reducing the knee and confirming PCL deficiency.

immediately in dealing with a chronic tear, daily stationary bicycle exercises can be initiated. After 3 months, closed chain exercises are started, with the exception of isolated hamstring strengthening, which is done later in the course.[10]

Postoperative PCL rehabilitation includes initial bracing in full extension to prevent posterior tibial translation. Continuous passive motion, straight-leg raising, and quadriceps static exercises are initiated immediately after surgery. The day after surgery, partial weight bearing with crutches is initiated as tolerated. In the early phase of rehabilitation, gravity-assisted flexion exercises to 90 degrees and closed chain exercises emphasizing quadriceps strengthening are pursued. The progression to more than 90 degrees of flexion is delayed until 6 weeks after surgery.

Two studies by Italian investigators have documented the frequent clinical observation that the PCL, in contrast to the ACL, can undergo in situ healing of partial lesions, with improved stability and function.[11-13] This has been attributed to the capsular contiguity of the ligament, with better opportunity for revascularization than in the ACL.[1] It is thus imperative that the ligament be protected from undue stress during the rehabilitative phase of treatment.

At 9 to 12 months after surgical intervention, the patient with full range of motion, equal strength compared with the contralateral leg, and a stable knee is allowed to return to full activity.

Procedures

Arthrocentesis is performed for painful effusions (hemarthrosis). As mentioned earlier, KT-1000 arthrometer testing is done for diagnostic purposes and to document the degree of instability.[4]

Surgery

Various surgical techniques have been developed for the repair of the PCL. Controversy exists as to the most effective procedure.[10] The aim of surgery is to replace the PCL with a graft inserted into a tunnel drilled through the tibia and femur. Allograft or autograft tissue is most commonly used. Donor sites include the patellar tendon, hamstring tendons, and rarely the quadriceps tendon. Achilles tendon allograft is also useful. PCL reconstruction is performed arthroscopically, arthroscopically assisted, or open.[8]

POTENTIAL DISEASE COMPLICATIONS

Potential disease complications include pain, limitation of function and activity, and onset of degenerative arthritis. Patients with isolated PCL tears tend to fare better than do patients with combined ligamentous injuries.[14] Studies suggest that nonoperatively treated PCL injuries allow many athletes to return to their sport independent of level of laxity.[14] However, late degenerative arthritis has been reported as a consequence of PCL instability.[15]

POTENTIAL TREATMENT COMPLICATIONS

Treatment complications include the well-known side effects of nonsteroidal anti-inflammatory drugs. Prolonged bracing or immobilization can lead to significant muscle weakness and atrophy. The risks of surgery, although uncommon, are also well known. These include the risks of anesthesia. In addition, bleeding is controlled with a tourniquet and surgical hemostasis. Infection is limited with diligent sterile technique as well as with antibiotics. Damage to nerve and vascular structures, the popliteal vessels in particular, is a slight risk. Postoperative laxity of the PCL graft may occur. The theoretical risk of disease transmission with the use of allograft tissues is extremely low.

References

1. Kannus P, Bergfeld J, Jarvinen M, et al. Injuries to the posterior cruciate ligament of the knee. Sports Med 1991;12:110-131.
2. Janousek AT, Jones DG, Clatworthy M, et al. Posterior cruciate ligament injuries of the knee joint. Sports Med 1999;28:429-441.
3. Parolie JM, Bergfeld JA. Long-term results of nonoperative treatment of isolated posterior cruciate ligament injuries in the athlete. Am J Sports Med 1986;14:35-38.
4. Rubinstein RA Jr, Shelbourne KD, McCarroll JR, et al. The accuracy of the clinical examination in the setting of posterior cruciate ligament injuries. Am J Sports Med 1994;22:550-557.
5. Gross ML, Grover JS, Bassett LW, et al. Magnetic resonance imaging of the posterior cruciate ligament: clinical use to improve diagnostic accuracy. Am J Sports Med 1992;20:732-737.
6. Schaefer F, Schaefer P, Brossmann J, et al. Value of fat-suppressed PD-weighted TSE-sequences for detection of anterior and posterior cruciate ligament lesions—comparison to arthroscopy. Eur J Radiol 2006;58:411-415.
7. Ilaslan H, Sundaram M, Miniaci A. Imaging evaluation of the postoperative knee ligaments. Eur J Radiol 2005;54:178-188.
8. Margheritini F, Mariani PF, Mariani PP. Current concepts in diagnosis and treatment of posterior cruciate ligament injury. Acta Orthop Belg 2000;66:217-228.
9. St. Pierre P, Miller MD. Posterior cruciate ligament injuries. Clin Sports Med 1999;18:199-221.
10. Barber FA, Fanelli GC, Matthews LS, et al. The treatment of complete posterior cruciate ligament tears. Arthroscopy 2000;16:725-731.
11. Bellelli A, Mancini P, Polito M, et al. Magnetic resonance imaging of posterior cruciate ligament injuries: a new classification of traumatic tears. Radiol Med (Torino) 2006;111:828-835.
12. Mariani P, Margheritini F, Christel P, et al. Evaluation of posterior cruciate ligament healing: a study using magnetic resonance imaging and stress radiography. Arthroscopy 2005;21:1354-1361.
13. Margheritini F, Mancini L, Mauro CS, et al. Stress radiography for quantifying posterior cruciate ligament deficiency. Arthroscopy 2003;19:706-711.
14. Shelbourne KD, Davis TJ, Patel DV. The natural history of acute, isolated, nonoperatively treated posterior cruciate ligament injuries. Am J Sports Med 1999;27:276-283.
15. Boynton MD, Tietjens BR. Long-term follow-up of untreated isolated posterior cruciate deficient knees. Am J Sports Med 1996;24:306-310.

Quadriceps Tendinitis 68

Christine Curtis, BS, Peter Bienkowski, MD, and Lyle J. Micheli, MD

Synonym

Quadriceps tendinosis

ICD-9 Codes

726.60   Enthesopathy of knee, unspecified

844.8   Sprains and strains of knee and leg, other specified sites

959.7   Injury, other and unspecified, knee, leg, ankle, and foot

DEFINITION

The quadriceps tendon is located at the insertion of the quadriceps muscle into the patella and functions as part of the knee extensor mechanism. Quadriceps tendinitis (or, as named in the more recent literature, tendinosis) is an overuse syndrome characterized by repetitive overloading of the quadriceps tendon. The common mechanism of injury is microtrauma, in which the basal ability of the tissue to repair itself is outpaced by the repetition of insult.[1] Quadriceps tendinitis often occurs in athletes participating in running and jumping sports as well as in persons who perform frequent kneeling, squatting, and stair climbing.[2] The superior strength, mechanical advantage, and better vascularity of the quadriceps tendon make quadriceps tendinopathy much less frequent than patellar tendinopathy.[3]

SYMPTOMS

Patients usually report an insidious onset of knee pain and may note painful clicking. Patients are not physicians; their chief complaint is "knee pain." A burning sensation at the bone-tendon junction may be experienced.[4] The pain is aggravated by activity that challenges the extensor mechanism, including bending, stair climbing, running, and jumping. Severe weakness, an inability to extend the knee, or the report of acute trauma with a "pop" should alert the clinician to the possibility of a quadriceps tendon partial or complete rupture. On occasion, a single episode of overload may elicit symptoms.

PHYSICAL EXAMINATION

On examination of the knee, point tenderness is localized along the superior pole of the patella and along the quadriceps tendon. Quadriceps tendon pain may be elicited with extreme knee flexion and by resisted knee extension. The clinician should also be on the lookout for a palpable defect, suggesting partial rupture of the quadriceps tendon. Neurologic examination findings should be normal, with the possible exception of strength testing, which may be limited by pain or partial tendon rupture. Ligamentous examination of the knee is normal unless there is associated trauma.

FUNCTIONAL LIMITATIONS

Quadriceps tendinitis may interfere with activities of daily living. Pain is usually felt with stair climbing, kneeling, and rising from a chair. Athletes may be unable to participate in running and jumping activities.

DIAGNOSTIC STUDIES

Quadriceps tendinitis is a clinical diagnosis, and diagnostic investigations are not generally necessary. If a partial tear of the quadriceps tendon is suspected but not apparent clinically, magnetic resonance imaging may be of assistance in confirming the diagnosis. Ultrasonography and Doppler study have also been found to be helpful.[5]

TREATMENT

Initial

Initial treatment includes rest from aggravating activities. Activity modification should include protection from eccentric or high-load knee extension (e.g., going up and down stairs, bending, jumping). Proper warm-up and stretching should be conducted before activity. Also, the application of ice to the injured area for 20 minutes, two or three times daily and before and after athletics, can be useful. Nonsteroidal anti-inflammatory drugs may be used for pain and inflammation. In some instances,

387

Differential Diagnosis

Patellar tendinitis

Patellar fracture

Patellofemoral syndrome

Prepatellar bursitis

Apophysitis

Anterior fat pad syndrome

Chondromalacia patellae

Osteochondritis dissecans

Plica

Quadriceps tendon rupture

Quadriceps strain

Quadriceps contusion

Quadriceps tear

knee immobilizers are used but may promote weakness and disuse atrophy.

Rehabilitation

The main treatment modality includes muscle strengthening and stretching. All muscle strengthening exercises are conducted in the pain-free range. Static exercises may be used to minimize compressive forces across the patellofemoral joint.[2] Eccentric strengthening exercises may be useful.[6] Therapeutic modalities including ultrasonography, phonophoresis, and iontophoresis may be employed.[2] The use of icing immediately after activity or work has been advocated.[7] A general conditioning program is recommended.

Procedures

Local corticosteroid injections are not typically done because of the risk of tendon rupture, but they may be necessary in some cases unresponsive to treatment. Care should be taken to inject circumferential to the tendon and not in the tendon itself.

Surgery

Quadriceps tendinitis is mostly managed nonoperatively. Surgical intervention may be necessary in rare cases of partial rupture. Tendocalcinosis may reflect a chronic partial tear.[8] If partial tendon rupture is suspected, surgical consultation is advised.

POTENTIAL DISEASE COMPLICATIONS

Functional deterioration with the development of chronic symptoms may occur. A high level of functioning in patients with quadriceps tendinitis is usually regained and maintained.[2] In rare cases of progressive microtrauma to the injured area, rupture of tendon may result.

POTENTIAL TREATMENT COMPLICATIONS

The complications related to the use of nonsteroidal anti-inflammatory drugs include the development of gastritis as well as renal and hepatic involvement. Corticosteroid injection may predispose the tendon to rupture. Repeated injections of corticosteroids may increase the risk for mucoid degeneration, fibrinoid necrosis, mineralization, fibroblastic degeneration, and capillary proliferation within the tendon.[9]

References

1. Micheli LJ, Fehlandt AF Jr. Overuse injuries to tendons and apophyses in children and adolescents. Clin Sports Med 1992;11: 713-726.
2. Westrich GH, Haas SB, Bono JV. Occupational knee injuries. Orthop Clin North Am 1996;27:805-814.
3. Won J, Maffulli N. Tendinopathy of the extensor apparatus of the knee. In Micheli LJ, Kocher MS, eds. The Pediatric and Adolescent Knee. Philadelphia, WB Saunders, 2006:181-197.
4. Yost JG Jr, Ellfeldt HJ. Basketball injuries. In Nicholas JA, Hershman EB, eds. The Lower Extremity and Spine in Sports Medicine. St. Louis, Mosby, 1986:1440-1466.
5. Silvestri E, Biggi E, Molfetta L, et al. Power Doppler analysis of tendon vascularization. Int J Tissue React 2003;25:149-158.
6. Stanish WD, Curwin S, Mandel S. Exercise and the muscle tendon unit. In Stanish WD, Curwin S, eds. Tendinitis: Etiology and Treatment. New York, Oxford University Press, 2000:43-47.
7. Antich TJ, Randall CC, Westbrook RA, et al. Treatment of knee extensor mechanism disorders: comparison of four treatment modalities. J Orthop Sports Phys Ther 1986;8:225-259.
8. Varghese B, Radcliffe GS, Groves C. Calcific tendonitis of the quadriceps. Br J Sports Med 2006;40:652-654.
9. Key J, Johnson D, Jarvis G, Ponsonby D. Knee and thigh injuries. In Subotnick SI. Sports Medicine of the Lower Extremity. New York, Churchill Livingstone, 1989:297-310.

Shin Splints 69

Michael F. Stretanski, DO

DEFINITION

"Shin splints" is best thought of as a clinical syndrome defined in terms of pain and discomfort in the anterior portion of the leg from repetitive activity on hard surfaces or forcible, excessive use of the foot flexors. The diagnosis should be limited to musculoskeletal inflammations, excluding stress fractures and ischemic disorders.[1]

Shin splints most commonly occur in athletes who have sudden increases or changes in their training activity. This disorder occurs in runners and in athletes who participate in high-impact court or field sports as well as in gymnasts and particularly ballet dancers, alone or in conjunction with other overuse syndromes,[2] but it has also been well documented and studied in military personnel.[3-5] The etiology of shin splints is not clearly defined, but it is likely to be multifactorial with biomechanical abnormalities of the foot and ankle, poor footwear and shock absorption, hard playing surfaces, and training errors. Other contributing factors may include weakness of anterior and posterior compartment musculature, inadequate warm-up, leg length discrepancy, tibial torsion, excessive femoral anteversion, and increased Q angle.[6,7]

One prospective study[5] in military cadets looked at seven anatomic variables and identified greater internal and external hip range of motion and lower mean calf girth to be associated with a higher incidence of exertional medial tibial pain in men. It also showed a high rate of injury among women, but no intrinsic factor was specifically identified. Nutritional and endocrine factors are more likely to play an etiologic role in stress reactions. In school-age athletes and adults who participate

in seasonal sports, shin splints can occur when they resume their sport or start a new land-based sport (e.g., high-school or college athletes who go from playing basketball to cross-country or track).

It is important for the clinician to differentiate shin splints, which is a fairly benign condition, from acute compartment syndrome, which is a true emergency, and from the different types of stress fractures described in this region, which are more serious conditions. Further discussion of these diagnoses may be found in their respective chapters. Tibial periostitis has been described as an initial manifestation of polyarteritis nodosa.[8]

Primary adamantinoma,[9] a rare low-grade primary bone tumor, and hydatid bone disease[10] have also been reported in this region.

SYMPTOMS

Patients presenting with shin splints usually complain of a dull and aching pain near the junction of the mid and distal thirds of the posteromedial or anterior tibia (Fig. 69-1). Symptoms are commonly bilateral, occur with exercise, and are relieved with rest.[11] Initially, the pain may ease with continued running and recur after prolonged activity. Those with more severe shin splints may have persistent pain with normal walking, with activities of daily living, or at rest.

PHYSICAL EXAMINATION

Physical examination typically reveals generalized tenderness along the medial tibia. Mild swelling may be present. Resisted plantar flexion, toe flexion, or toe raises may aggravate symptoms, and pain-inhibitory weakness may be evident. Striking a 128-Hz tuning fork and placing it on the tibia may reproduce the pain associated with stress fractures. Patients with stress fractures will usually have point tenderness over the bone at the site of stress fracture. Lower extremity idiopathic osteonecrosis is most common in the fifth decade of life at the medial tibial plateau,[12] whereas those with shin splints will have more widespread tenderness to palpation that is more distal than these other pathologic

389

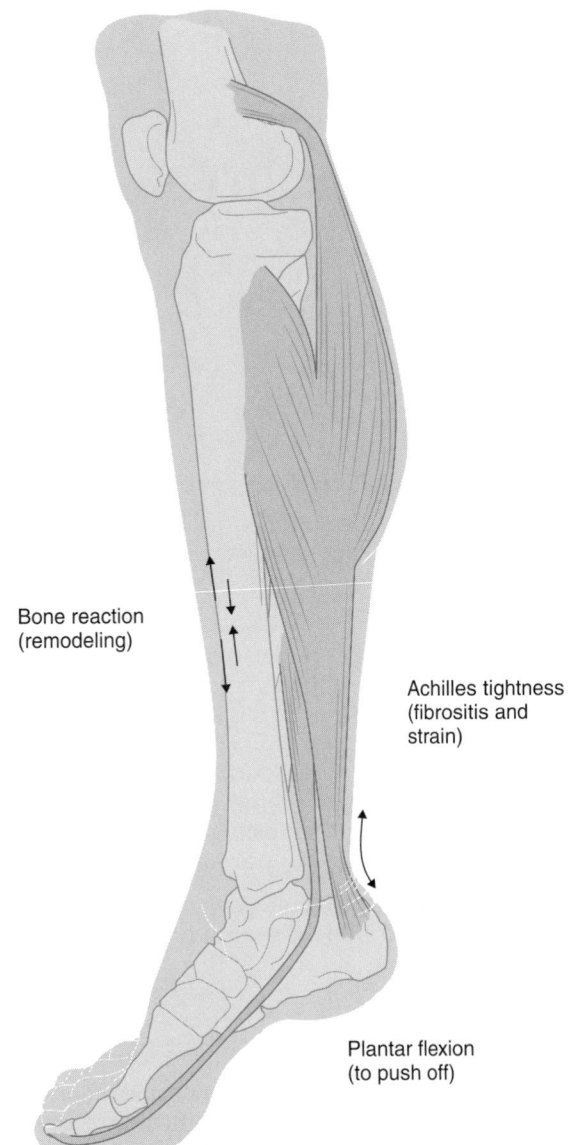

Bone reaction
(remodeling)

Achilles tightness
(fibrositis and
strain)

Plantar flexion
(to push off)

FIGURE 69-1. Repetitive microtrauma and overuse in running lead to soft tissue and even bone breakdown, a process commonly called shin splints. Muscle overpull can lead to periostitis, strain, or trabecular breakdown. The area approximately 13 cm proximal to the tip of the medial malleolus along the posterior tibial cortex appears to be maximally at risk.

processes. However, longitudinal tibial stress reactions may share a common anatomic pain distribution, and one study[13] showed tibial stress reactions in this same distal-third region.

The lower extremity examination focuses on static and dynamic components of the kinetic chain to uncover signs of coexisting lower extremity issues that may be contributing factors. These include forefoot pronation, pes cavus, pes planus, and excessive heel valgus or varus. Comparatively tight or weak lower extremity muscle groups should be noted for later rehabilitation goals. In particular, relative ankle plantar flexion, dorsiflexion, inversion, and eversion strength should be examined. Careful review of systems should be negative for fever, chills, night sweats, unintentional weight loss, and loss

of bowel or bladder control. The neurologic portion of the examination, including sensation and muscle stretch reflexes, is normal.

FUNCTIONAL LIMITATIONS

In early stages of shin splints, activity limitations occur most often during running or participation in ballistic activities. When symptoms are more severe, they may occur with walking or at rest, thus causing further functional limitations. Athletes may be unable to participate in their sport, and attempts to cross-train into other sports may result in worsening of symptoms.

DIAGNOSTIC STUDIES

Plain radiographs are typically normal early in the disease process but may be of use in ruling out more ominous disease, especially if symptoms present unilaterally. Later, there may be evidence of periosteal thickening. Radionuclide bone scanning helps differentiate shin splints from stress fracture. Diffuse radioisotopic uptake along the medial or posteromedial tibia on the delayed phase is the pattern usually seen with shin splints. A focal defined area of uptake in all phases is more consistent with a stress fracture.[14] Fat-suppressed magnetic resonance imaging may also be useful for discrimination between stress fracture and shin splints before plain radiography shows detectable periosteal reaction.[15] Exertional compartment syndrome is uncommon, but if clinical suspicion is high, compartment pressure measurements must be done to rule it out. Magnetic resonance imaging of the lumbar spine may be indicated if lumbar radiculopathy is in the differential diagnosis or lumbar spinal stenosis is suspected in older athletes or younger athletes with a congenitally narrow spinal canal.

TREATMENT

Initial

As with many overuse syndromes, relative rest—that is, participation only in those activities that can be done without pain—is the key to initial management. If reducing mileage, court, or studio time or just reducing intensity allows the athlete to remain pain free, continuation of the activity may be acceptable. In general, however, even in mild cases, the athlete should avoid repetitive lower extremity stress for at least 1 to 2 weeks. In more serious cases, athletes may need to stop running entirely for a longer time. If walking is painful, crutches are indicated. An air stirrup brace may also decrease pain associated with weight bearing.[7]

Stretching and ice or ice massage to the involved areas can be helpful. Nonsteroidal anti-inflammatory drugs can reduce inflammation and help manage pain. Analgesics can be taken for pain as well. Whirlpool, phonophoresis, iontophoresis, and ultrasound are

Differential Diagnosis

Stress fracture

Chronic exertional compartment syndrome

Tendinitis

Muscle strain

Muscle herniation

Vascular and muscular abnormalities

Lumbar radiculopathy

Pregnancy

Longitudinal tibial fatigue fracture

Hematoma

Primary muscle disease

Peroneal nerve entrapment

Fascial defect

Deep venous thrombosis

Sarcoma or osteosarcoma

Hydatid bone disease

traditionally attempted and may have a role in early symptomatic management. Electrical stimulation should probably be considered contraindicated in this diagnosis, in which the pathoetiology points toward excessive muscle contraction and a reactive periostitis in the first place.

In addressing malalignments of the lower extremities, orthoses, such as longitudinal arch supports with or without a medial heel wedge, may be indicated in select patients. Although review of the literature fails to yield any objective evidence for the widespread use of any of these interventions, the most encouraging evidence seems to be the use of shock-absorbing insoles.[3,16] Custom orthotic inserts, in one study of healthy female runners, have been shown to decrease rearfoot eversion angle and velocity and internal inversion moment as well as to decrease ankle dynamics in the frontal and sagittal planes. Whereas the particular relevance to shin splints is unclear, the ability to affect these measurements seems promising.[17]

Rehabilitation

In individuals who continue to have pain despite initial conservative treatment, physical therapy may be indicated to decrease pain and further educate the patient about the disorder. Advising the patient to ice after and to take nonsteroidal anti-inflammatory drugs before exercise may help in enabling the rehabilitation program.

Once the symptoms have diminished, the rehabilitation program focuses on improving muscle strength, flexibility, and endurance and preventing recurrence of injury.[18]

The primary muscles believed to be involved in shin splints are the flexor digitorum longus and the soleus. Others have implicated the tibialis posterior, but its attachment is more posterior than the area of typical shin splint symptoms, and it actually attaches to the interosseous membrane more than to the medial tibia.[19] The deep crural fascia also attaches to the posteromedial tibia. Long-term rehabilitation for shin splints involves improvement of the flexibility, strength, and endurance of the involved muscles and avoidance of contributing factors.

Anterior compartment stretching exercises, Achilles tendon stretching, and overall lower extremity flexibility exercises are important. Eccentric strengthening of antagonistic muscle groups is also useful. Pain can be a guide in the advancement of the rehabilitation program.

Athletes should have full range of motion that is symmetric to the uninvolved side and have nearly full strength before returning to their prior activity or to competition. Plyometrics should be avoided until a high level of strength, endurance, and flexibility has been attained.

Cardiovascular fitness should be maintained if possible through lower impact activities, such as biking, swimming, or water running.

Return to previous activity level should be a gradual process, individualized, and based on the athlete's response to increasing intensity of training. Proper footwear for the sport is believed to be essential. Running shoes lose more than 60% of their shock absorption after 250 miles of use.[6] Orthotic devices are often necessary in those individuals with foot abnormalities, such as pes planus. A plyometric program of strengthening and conditioning has been suggested as early as the third phase of rehabilitation,[20] but return to sport outcomes have not been reported.

Procedures

There is no proven benefit noted in the literature to support any injection-based procedure, such as local exogenous glucocorticoid injection. Limited empirical opinions exist on a role for sclerotherapeutic solutions. Great care must be taken in ensuring the correct diagnosis, as potentially disastrous results may occur in dealing with a coexistent compartment syndrome. Theoretically, a palliative role may exist for either in chronic recalcitrant cases with functional decline.

Surgery

Surgery is rarely indicated but involves a posteromedial fasciotomy with release of the fascial bridge of the medial soleus and the fascia of the deep posterior compartment, with periosteal cauterization.[14] Surgery is effective in relieving pain, but it frequently leaves the patient with persistent strength deficits, and full return to sports is not always achieved.[21]

POTENTIAL DISEASE COMPLICATIONS

If shin splints are not treated and biomechanical malalignments are not addressed, stress fractures and potentially true fractures may occur. This would result in further morbidity and more time lost from the desired physical activity as well as potential function decline.

POTENTIAL TREATMENT COMPLICATIONS

Complications involving the gastrointestinal and renal systems may result from treatment with nonsteroidal anti-inflammatory drugs. Fasciotomy may result in residual weakness. Overly aggressive rehabilitation or rehabilitation of the incorrect diagnosis may progress the injury or cause secondary injury. This author has experience with a case of severe reflex sympathetic dystrophy and peripheral nerve injury after sclerotherapy.

References

1. Subcommittee on Classification of Injuries in Sports and Committee on the Medical Aspects of Sports. Standard Nomenclature of Athletic Injuries. Chicago, American Medical Association, 1966.
2. Stretanski MF, Weber GJ. Medical and rehabilitation issues in classical ballet. Am J Phys Med 2002;81:383-391.
3. Johnston E, Flynn T, Bean M, et al. A randomized controlled trial of a leg orthosis versus traditional treatment for soldiers with shin splints: a pilot study. Milit Med 2006;171:40-44.
4. Larsen K, Weidich F, Leboeuf-Yde C. Can custom-made biomechanic shoe orthoses prevent problems in the back and lower extremities? A randomized, controlled intervention trial of 146 military conscripts. J Manipulative Physiol Ther 2002;25:326-331.
5. Burne SG, Khan KM, Boudville PB, et al. Risk factors associated with exertional medial tibial pain—a 12 month prospective clinical study. Br J Sports Med 2004;38:441-445.
6. Touliopolous S, Hershman EB. Lower leg pain: diagnosis and treatment of compartment syndromes and other pain syndromes of the leg. Sports Med 1999;27:193-204.
7. Reid DC. Sports Injury Assessment and Rehabilitation. New York, Churchill Livingstone, 1992:269-300.
8. Vedrine L, Rault A, Debourdeau P, et al. Polyarteritis nodosa manifesting as tibial periostitis [in French]. Ann Med Interne (Paris) 2001;152:213-214.
9. Ulmar B, Delling G, Werner M, et al. Classical and atypical location of adamantinomas—presentation of two cases. Onkologie 2006;29:276-278.
10. Kalinova K, Proichev V, Stefanova P, et al. Hydatid bone disease: a case report and review of the literature. J Orthop Surg 2005;13:323-325.
11. Andrish JA. The leg. In DeLee JC, Drez D, eds. Orthopaedic Sports Medicine: Principles and Practice. Philadelphia, WB Saunders, 1994:1603-1607.
12. Valenti JR, Illescas JA, Bariga A, Dlöz R. Idiopathic osteonecrosis of the medial tibial plateau. Knee Surg Sports Traumatol Arthrosc 2005;13:293-298.
13. Ruohola JS, Kiuru MJ, Pihlajamaki HK. Fatigue and bone injuries causing anterior lower leg pain. Clin Orthop Relat Res 2006;444:216-223.
14. Barry NN, McGuire JL. Acute injuries and specific problems in adult athletes. Rheum Dis Clin North Am 1996;22:531-549.
15. Aoki Y, Yasuda K, Tohyama H, et al. Magnetic resonance imaging in stress fractures and shin splints. Clin Orthop Relat Res 2004;421:260-267.
16. Thacker SB, Gilchrist J, Stroup DF, Kimsey CD. The prevention of shin splints in sports: a systematic review of the literature. Med Sci Sports Exerc 2002;34:32-40.
17. MacLean C, Davis IM, Hamill J. Influence of a custom foot orthotics intervention on lower extremity dynamics in healthy runners. Clin Biomech 2006;21:623-630.
18. Windsor RE, Chambers K. Overuse injuries of the leg. In Kibler WB, Herring SA, Press JM, eds. Functional Rehabilitation of Sports and Musculoskeletal Injuries. Gaithersburg, Md, Aspen, 1998:265-267.
19. Beck BR, Osternig LR. Medial tibial stress syndrome: the location of muscles in the leg in relation to symptoms. J Bone Joint Surg Am 1994;76:1057-1061.
20. Herring KM. A plyometric training model used to augment rehabilitation from tibial fasciitis. Curr Sports Med Rep 2006;5:147-154.
21. Yates B, Allen MJ, Barnes MR. Outcome of surgical treatment of medial tibial stress syndrome J Bone Joint Surg Am 2003;85:1974-1980.

Stress Fractures 70

Sheila Dugan, MD

Synonyms
Insufficiency fractures
Fatigue fractures
March fractures

ICD-9 Codes
821.0 Fracture of other and unspecified parts of femur, shaft or unspecified part, closed
823.8 Fracture of tibia and fibula, unspecified part, closed
824.8 Fracture of ankle, unspecified, closed
825.2 Fracture of tarsal and metatarsal bones, closed

DEFINITION

Stress fractures are complete or partial bone fractures caused by the accumulation of microtrauma.[1] Normal bone accommodates to stress through ongoing remodeling. If this remodeling system does not keep pace with the force applied, stress reaction (microfractures) and, finally, stress fracture can result. Stress fracture is the end result of a continuum of biologic responses to stress placed on bone. Adolescent, young adult, and premenopausal women athletes have a higher incidence of stress injuries to bone than men do.[2,3] Stress fractures in juveniles are rare.[4] Both extrinsic and intrinsic factors have been implicated in this imbalance between bone resorption and bone deposition.[5] Malalignment and poor flexibility of the lower extremities (intrinsic factors) and inadequate footwear, changes in training surface, and increases in training intensity and duration without an adequate ramp-up period (extrinsic factors) can lead to stress fractures.[6]

Stress fractures in athletes vary by sports and are most common in the lower extremities.[2,7] The most common sites are the tibia, metatarsals, and fibula, and they affect most commonly runners and dancers. The fracture site is the area of greatest stress, such as the origin of lower leg muscles along the medial tibia.[8] A narrower mediolateral tibial width was a risk factor for femoral, tibial, and foot stress fractures in a study of military recruits.[9] Studies of female runners demonstrated greater loading rates in those with history of tibial stress fractures compared with those without injury.[10,11] In contrast, in comparison of runners with and without history of tibial stress fracture, no difference in ground reaction forces, bone density, or tibial bone geometric parameters was found between groups.[12]

Military recruits have been extensively studied in regard to lower extremity stress fractures. In a study of 179 Finnish military recruits aged 18 to 20 years, tall height, poor physical conditioning, low hip bone mineral content and density, and high serum parathyroid hormone level were risk factors for stress fractures.[13] The authors postulated that given the poor vitamin D status, intervention studies of vitamin D supplementation to lower serum parathyroid hormone levels and possibly to reduce the incidence of stress fractures are warranted. A database of systematic reviews, including 13 randomized prevention trials, concluded that shock-absorbing insert use in footwear probably reduces the incidence of stress fractures in military personnel.[14] There was insufficient evidence to determine the best design of such inserts.

Stress fractures may be related to abnormalities of the bone, such as in female athletes with low bone density due to exercise-induced menstrual abnormalities.[15-18] Premature osteoporosis leads to an increased risk for stress fractures. One study looked at premenopausal women runners and collegiate athletes and concluded that those with absent or irregular menses were at increased risk for musculoskeletal injuries while engaged in active training.[16] Muscle deficits in the gastrocnemius-soleus complex in jumping athletes have also been implicated in causing tibial stress fractures. Bone injury may be a secondary event after a primary failure of muscle function.[19]

Individuals who are nonambulatory or have limited ambulation due to disability represent another population with abnormal bone and premature osteoporosis. In stroke patients, there is significant bone loss on the paretic side, which is greatest in those patients with the most severe functional deficits.[20] Spinal cord injury may not only cause bone loss but also alter bone structure and microstructure.[21] Practitioners caring for individuals with limited mobility should consider stress fracture in the differential diagnosis of overuse injuries.

393

SYMPTOMS

Patients may report an increase in training or activity level or a change in training conditions preceding the onset of symptoms. Because of pain in the affected region of the bone, patients may seek medical attention during the microfracture or stress reaction phase of injury. Should they forego relative rest (avoidance of the pain-provoking activity), they can progress to stress fracture or even complete fracture. The pain will gradually increase with activity and may occur with less intense exercise, such as walking, or even at rest. In general, however, the pain will improve with rest. The pain can lead to a decline in performance. The individual may also note swelling in the affected region of the bone. Symptoms of paresthesias and numbness should alert the clinician that an alternative diagnosis should be considered.

PHYSICAL EXAMINATION

On physical examination, the clinician will find an area of exquisite, well-localized tenderness, warmth, and edema over the affected region of the bone. Ecchymosis along the plantar aspect may be present with foot involvement. Percussion of the nearby region can cause pain. Placement of a vibrating tuning fork over the fracture site intensifies the pain.[22] In the tibia, stress fractures primarily occur along the medial border; the frequency, in order, is upper, lower, and midshaft. In the fibula, they usually occur one handbreadth proximal to the lateral malleolus.[5] Tarsal or metatarsal stress fractures present with localized foot tenderness. Weight-bearing activity, such as a one-legged hop test, can provoke the pain by increasing the ground reaction forces. For a presumed femoral stress fracture, the clinician can provoke pain by applying a downward force on the distal femur while the affected individual is seated with the distal femur extending beyond the edge of the seat (Fig. 70-1).

The physical examination must include an examination of the lumbar spine and lower limbs to evaluate for any anatomic malalignment or biomechanical abnormalities. For instance, an individual with rigid supinated feet or weak foot intrinsic muscles may transmit more ground reaction forces to the tibia. On physical examination, one can identify problems that must be addressed in treatment planning.

Strength should be normal but occasionally limited by pain. Sensation and muscle stretch reflexes should also be normal.

FUNCTIONAL LIMITATIONS

Recreational and athletic activities requiring weight bearing through the affected lower limb may be limited by pain. For instance, running results in the transmission of increased ground reaction forces through the leg. These forces can increase if one runs on a concrete surface versus an all-weather track. In acute cases, ambulation can be painful.

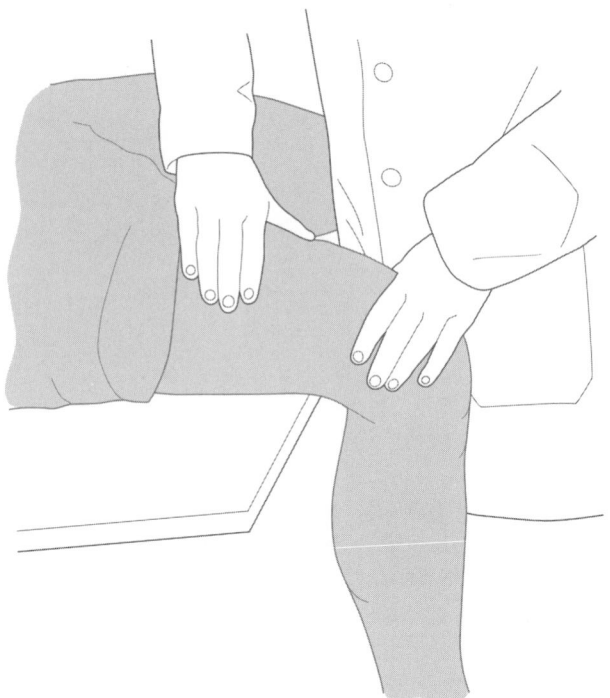

FIGURE 70-1. Physical examination technique to evaluate for femoral stress fracture. The examiner applies a downward pressure on the distal femur, using the examination table as a fulcrum, to increase the force across the fracture site. A positive test result reproduces the individual's pain.

DIAGNOSTIC STUDIES

Plain films may take as long as 6 weeks to demonstrate fracture, and films are initially normal in up to two thirds of patients.[23] Technetium Tc 99m diphosphonate bone scanning will yield the earliest confirmatory data for stress fractures, demonstrating a "hot spot" 1 to 4 days after fracture.[17] The fracture site may not return to normal on a bone scan for 5 months or longer, so it is not clinically useful to assess recovery. Computed tomography is necessary to differentiate stress fractures of the sacrum and the tarsal navicular bone.[24] Magnetic resonance imaging (MRI) delineates the fracture location and status of healing (Fig. 70-2). MRI provides soft tissue definition, which can be helpful in the setting of stress reaction or tendinitis. Although it can confirm the diagnosis in the acute phase, it is generally not indicated initially. MRI findings can help with clinical decision-making about return to activity or play. A retrospective review of military recruits presenting with anterior lower leg pain showed that only 56% had positive findings on MRI testing, implicating tissues other than bone as the pain generator.[25] In a study, 12% of asymptomatic feet in male college basketball players demonstrated bone marrow edema on MRI; the authors noted that this early detection might lead to preventive strategies to avoid injury.[26]

MRI grading systems have been developed with short T1 inversion recovery (STIR) sequences. Four grades of abnormality have been described from grade 1 (demonstration of periosteal edema on STIR or T2-weighted images) through grade 4 (visible injury line on T1- or

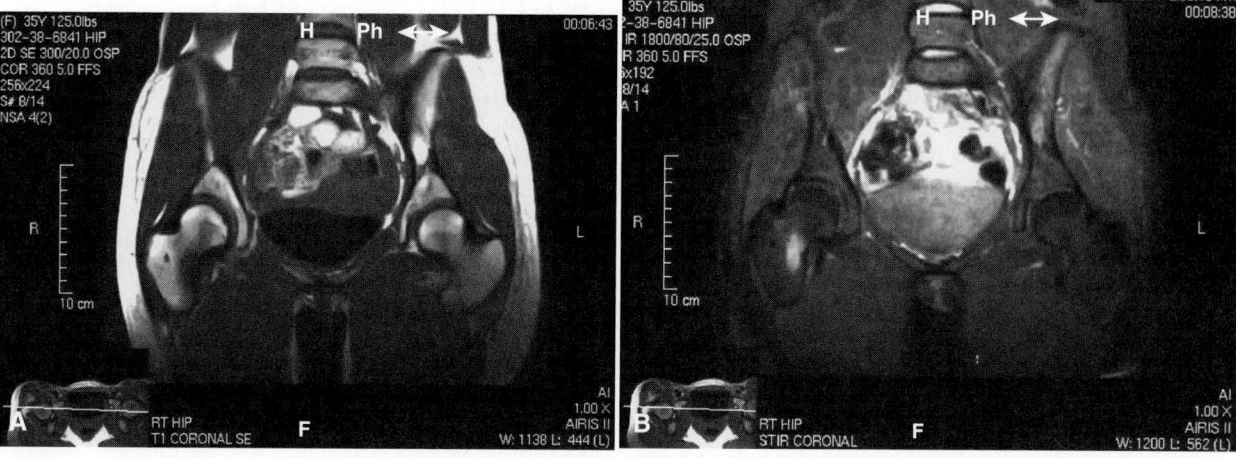

FIGURE 70-2. Femoral stress fracture on the compression side of the right femoral neck in a 35-year-old female marathon runner demonstrated on T1 **(A)** and STIR **(B)** coronal magnetic resonance images. (Images courtesy of David A. Turner, MD, Chairman, Department of Radiology, Rush University Medical Center, Chicago.)

T2-weighted images).[27,28] Radiographic grading scales of stress injuries to bone can be useful in clinical trials to more specifically delineate response to management. One should consider bone density testing in a female patient with a history of amenorrhea.[3]

Differential Diagnosis

Medial tibial stress syndrome

Osteoid osteoma

Compartment syndromes

Deep venous thrombosis

Knee disease (e.g., pes anserine bursitis)

Bone neoplasm

Osteomyelitis

TREATMENT

Initial

Pain and edema should be managed initially with PRICE (*p*rotection, *r*est, *i*ce, *c*ompression, and *e*levation). Use of nonsteroidal anti-inflammatory drugs (NSAIDs) is discouraged by several authors because of the negative impact of NSAIDs on tissue healing; in addition, masking of pain can compromise healing by reducing symptomatic feedback.[29-32] Acetaminophen may be helpful in patients who are resting but still have pain. Activities that provoke pain are eliminated. If ambulation is painful, athletes are placed on non–weight-bearing status or full crutch walking to eliminate painful weight bearing.[33] In non–weight-bearing subjects, a trial of walking is performed every 2 days, and once walking is pain free, full ambulation with crutches is begun. Fractures with

the propensity to progress to nonunion, such as midshaft tibial stress fractures and tarsal navicular fractures, may require immediate immobilization with a bivalved orthotic boot. Femoral neck fractures on the tension (superior) aspect can become displaced and require strict non–weight-bearing status with axillary crutches initially.[34] Metatarsal stress fractures can be treated with a stiff shoe and a straight cane or a rigid orthosis. Navicular fractures may require immobilization in a short leg cast.[29]

In the setting of female athletes with exercise-induced amenorrhea, nutritional counseling and correction of any energy debt must be included in the stress fracture treatment program. If the menstrual cycle does not return with these interventions, there is controversy about the use of an oral contraceptive pill to restore menses. Fewer athletes with fractures were using oral contraceptive pills than were athletes without fractures in one study.[35] In addition, women without stress fractures had a higher intake of calcium than did those with stress fractures. Nine elite runners with stress fractures were compared with matched control subjects without stress fractures, and significant differences in the number of menses per year (less in the fracture group) and the age at onset of menses (delayed in the fracture group) were identified.[36]

Rehabilitation

Physical therapy modalities such as heat and interferential electrical stimulation are used to increase local blood flow and to promote healing; however, there is a lack of controlled studies to prove their efficacy. Deep soft tissue massage, including transverse friction massage, may be indicated and complement stretching for the muscles that originate along the medial tibia. Ongoing cardiovascular and strengthening activities should continue if they produce no pain; aqua jogging, stationary bicycling, or use of the elliptical machine can be substituted for running.

Athletes can return to running once they are pain free with ambulation and cross-training activities; however, training schedules should be modified, and pain should be used as the guide to progression of the program.[37] In the setting of low-risk stress fractures, athletes may continue to participate if activity can be modified to minimize stress at the fracture site.[38] Sports-specific training must be addressed before return to play.

Careful attention to the training surface and equipment is mandatory. In the setting of significant forefoot or rearfoot biomechanical abnormalities, custom foot orthotics may be indicated. Taping may be used temporarily to provide stability of the ankle and foot. Local lower extremity strengthening is progressed from static exercises to concentric to eccentric training on the basis of symptoms. Plyometric (weight-bearing eccentric) training should precede return to play. Shock-absorbing insoles and running on shock-absorbing surfaces are recommended and thought to decrease the ground reaction forces transmitted to the bones of the lower extremity.[14,39] In a prospective study of athletes without control subjects, immobilization with a pneumatic leg brace was used to allow participation in a modified training schedule earlier. The authors concluded that the brace promoted healing and limited the forces across the fracture site.[40]

Rocker-bottom shoes and steel shanks can be used to prevent and to treat lower extremity stress fractures in susceptible disabled individuals.

Procedures

There is no specific nonsurgical procedure for this injury.

Surgery

Conservative management successfully treats lower extremity stress fractures with a few exceptions. Femoral neck stress fractures on the tensile (superior) aspect may require pinning if they do not heal after a course of non–weight bearing. Midshaft tibial fractures are at risk for nonunion and must be immobilized and observed closely; an open bone grafting procedure may be indicated in the setting of nonunion. Tarsal navicular stress fractures that do not respond to conservative treatment and demonstrate displacement, comminution, or nonunion may require open reduction with internal fixation.[41] In 26 subjects with 32 fractures treated for 2 years or more, surgical fixation of navicular stress fractures appears to be as effective as conservative management in the longer term.[42]

POTENTIAL DISEASE COMPLICATIONS

If biomechanical and training principles are not addressed during treatment, stress fractures can recur. In female athletes with menstrual abnormalities and premature osteoporosis, failure to treat these conditions might also lead to recurrent stress fractures.

POTENTIAL TREATMENT COMPLICATIONS

Immobilization can lead to loss of joint range of motion and reduced muscle strength. Treatment risks with NSAIDs include gastrointestinal, hepatic, and renal side effects; in addition, detrimental effects on bone healing must be considered. A large retrospective study found that use of NSAIDs was associated with a 1.47 relative risk of fractures (nonvertebral) compared with control subjects who did not receive NSAIDs.[43] Treatment of amenorrhea with oral contraceptive pills involves increased risk for blood clots and their sequelae. Treatment of premature osteoporosis with bisphosphonates includes risk for esophageal erosion or ulceration. Complications of surgery include nonunion and other typical infrequent complications (e.g., infection, bleeding). Subjects who underwent surgical treatment for tarsal navicular stress fracture were more likely to continue to be tender over the navicular than were nonoperative subjects.[42]

References

1. McBryde AM. Stress fractures in runners. Clin Sports Med 1985;4: 737-752.
2. Bennell KL, Brukner PD. Epidemiology and site specificity of stress fractures. Clin Sports Med 1997;16:179-196.
3. Nattiv A, Armsey TD. Stress injury to bone in the female athlete. Clin Sports Med 1997;16:197-219.
4. Niemeyer P, Weinberg A, Schmitt H, et al. Stress fractures in the juvenile skeletal system. Int J Sports Med 2006;27:242-249.
5. Reid DC. Exercise induced leg pain. In Reid DC, ed. Sports Injury Assessment and Rehabilitation. New York, Churchill Livingstone, 1992:269.
6. Sullivan D. Stress fractures in 51 runners. Clin Orthop 1984; 187:188.
7. Sanderlin BW, Raspa RF. Common stress fractures. Am Fam Physician 2003;68:1527-1532.
8. Markey KL. Stress fractures. Clin Sports Med 1987;6:405-425.
9. Giladi M, Milgrom C, Simkin A, et al. Stress fractures: identifiable risk factors. Am J Sports Med 1991;19:647-652.
10. Grimston SK, Engsberg JR, Kloiber R, Hanley DA. Bone mass, external loads and stress fractures in female runners. Int J Sports Biomech 1991;7:292-302.
11. Milner CE, Ferber R, Pollard CD, et al. Biomechanical factors associated with tibial stress fracture in female runners. Med Sci Sports Exerc 2006;38:323-328.
12. Bennell K, Crossley K, Jayarajan J, et al. Ground reaction forces and bone parameters in females with tibial stress fracture. Med Sci Sports Exerc 2004;36:397-404.
13. Valimaki VV, Alfthan H, Lehmuskallio E, et al. Risk factors for clinical stress fractures in male military recruits: a prospective cohort study. Bone 2005;37:267-273.
14. Rome K, Handoll HH, Ashford R. Interventions for preventing and treating stress fractures and stress reactions of bone of the lower limbs in young adults. Cochrane Database Syst Rev 2005;2:CD000450.
15. Barrow G, Saha S. Menstrual irregularity and stress fracture in collegiate female distance runners. Am J Sports Med 1988;16: 209-216.
16. Lloyd T, Triantafyllou SJ, Baker ER, et al. Women athletes with menstrual irregularity have increased musculoskeletal injuries. Med Sci Sports Exerc 1986;18:374-379.
17. Marcus R, Cann C, Madvig P, et al. Menstrual function and bone mass in elite women distance runners: endocrine and metabolic factors. Ann Intern Med 1985;102:158-163.

18. Myburgh KH, Bachrach LK, Lewis B, et al. Low bone mineral density at axial and appendicular sites in amenorrheic athletes. Med Sci Sports Exerc 1993;25:1197-1202.
19. Keats TE. Radiology of Musculoskeletal Stress Injury. Chicago, Year Book, 1990.
20. Beaupre GS, Lew HL. Bone-density changes after stroke. Am J Phys Med Rehabil 2006;85:464-472.
21. Jiang SD, Dai LY, Jiang LS. Osteoporosis after spinal cord injury. Osteoporosis Int 2006;17:180-192.
22. Young JL, Press JM. Rehabilitation of running injuries. In Buschbacher R, Braddom R, eds. Sports Medicine and Rehabilitation: A Sport-Specific Approach. Philadelphia, Hanley & Belfus, 1994:123-134.
23. Hersman EB, Mally T. Stress fractures. Clin Sports Med 1990;9:183-214.
24. Pavlov H, Torg JS, Freiberger JH. Tarsal navicular stress fractures: radiographic evaluation. Radiology 1983;148:641-645.
25. Ruohola JP, Kiuru MJ, Pihlajamaki HK. Fatigue bone injuries causing anterior lower leg pain. Clin Orthop Relat Res 2006;444:216-223.
26. Major NM. Role of MRI in prevention of metatarsal stress fractures in collegiate basketball players. AJR Am J Roentgenol 2006;186:255-258.
27. Arendt EA, Griffith HJ. The use of MR imaging in the assessment and clinical management of stress reactions of bone in high-performance athletes. Clin Sports Med 1997;16:291-306.
28. Fredericson M, Bergman AG, Hoffman KL, et al. Tibial stress reaction in runners. Correlation of clinical symptoms and scintigraphy with a new magnetic resonance imaging grading system. Am J Sports Med 1995;23:472-481.
29. Snider RK, ed. Essentials of Musculoskeletal Care. Rosemont, Ill, American Academy of Orthopaedic Surgery, 1997:485-486.
30. Stovitz SD, Arendt EA. NSAIDs should not be used in treatment of stress fractures [comment]. Am Fam Physician 2004;70:1452-1454.
31. Ho ML, Chang JK, Chuang LY, et al. Effects of nonsteroidal anti-inflammatory drugs and prostaglandins on osteoblastic functions. Biochem Pharmacol 1999;58:983-990.
32. Wheeler P, Batt ME. Do non-steroidal anti-inflammatory drugs adversely affect stress fracture healing? A short review. Br J Sports Med 2005;39:65-69.
33. Arendt E, Agel J, Heikes C, Griffith H. Stress injuries to bone in college athletes: a retrospective review of experience at a single institution. Am J Sports Med 2003;31:959-968.
34. Windsor RE, Chambers K. Overuse injuries of the leg. In Kibler WB, Herring SA, Press JM, eds. Functional Rehabilitation of Sports and Musculoskeletal Injuries. Gaithersburg, Md., Aspen, 1998:186-187.
35. Myburgh KH, Hutchins J, Fataar AB, et al. Low bone density is an etiologic factor for stress fracture in athletes. Ann Intern Med 1990;113:754-759.
36. Carbon R, Sambrook PN, Deakin V, et al. Bone density of elite female athletes with stress fractures. Med J Aust 1990;153:373-376.
37. Brody DM. Techniques in the evaluation and treatment of the injured runner. Orthop Clin North Am 1982;13:541.
38. Kaeding CC, Yu JR, Wright R, et al. Management and return to play of stress fractures. Clin J Sports Med 2005;15:442-447.
39. Brukner P, Khan K. Clinical Sports Medicine. New York, McGraw-Hill, 1997:412.
40. Whitelaw GP, Wetzler MJ, Levy AS, et al. A pneumatic leg brace for the treatment of tibial stress fractures. Clin Orthop 1991;207:301-305.
41. Coris EE, Lombardo JA. Tarsal navicular stress fractures. Am Fam Physician 2003;67:85-90.
42. Potter N, Brukner P, Makdissi M, et al. Navicular stress fractures: outcomes of surgical and conservative management. Br J Sports Med 2006;40:692-695.
43. Van Staa TP, Leufkens HG, Cooper C. Use of nonsteroidal anti-inflammatory drugs and risk of fractures. Bone 2000;27:563-568.

Total Knee Replacement 71

Robert J. Kaplan, MD

Synonyms

Total knee arthroplasty
Total knee implant
Unicompartmental knee arthroplasty
Revision knee arthroplasty

ICD-9 Codes

715.16 Osteoarthrosis, localized, primary, lower leg
715.26 Osteoarthrosis, localized, secondary, lower leg

DEFINITION

Arthroplasty involves the reconstruction by natural modification or artificial replacement of a diseased, damaged, or ankylosed joint.

There are three basic types of total knee arthroplasty (TKA): totally constrained, semiconstrained, and totally unconstrained. The amount of constraint built into an artificial joint reflects the amount of stability the hardware provides. As such, a totally constrained joint has the femoral portion physically attached to the tibial component and requires no ligamentous or soft tissue support. The semiconstrained TKA has two separate components that glide on each other, but the physical characteristics of the tibial component prevent excessive femoral glide. The totally unconstrained device relies completely on the body's ligaments and soft tissues to maintain the stability of the joint.

The semiconstrained and totally unconstrained knee implants are most often used. In general, the totally unconstrained implants afford the most normal range of motion and gait.

In unicompartmental knee arthroplasty, only the joint surfaces on one side of the knee (usually the medial compartment) are replaced. Unicompartmental knee arthroplasty provides better relief than does a tibial osteotomy and greater range of motion than does a TKA, as well as improved ambulation velocity.

More recently, the concept of minimally invasive TKA has evolved from the procedures and investigations of unicompartmental knee arthroplasty. The distinctive features may be summarized as follows:

- Decreased skin incision length. The incision has been reduced to approximately twice the length of the patella, ranging between 6 and 11 cm.
- Flexion and extension of the lower limb for exposure. The surgeon should realize that flexing the knee exposes the posterior structures of the knee and extending it exposes the anterior structures of the knee. Repeated positioning can be facilitated by having an adjustable leg holder in the operating room to avoid the need for extra assistance.
- Symbiotic use of retractors. Relaxation of some retractors allows exposure of other parts of the knee.
- Quadriceps muscle-sparing approach. The method presently used is similar to the midvastus approach with a vastus medialis obliquus snip of approximately 1.5 to 3 cm.
- Inferior and superior patellar capsular releases. This step is very important to gain exposure of the entire joint as well as to be able to mobilize the patella, both medially and laterally.
- Lack of patellar eversion. There may be increased muscle tension increases when the patella is everted. This eversion strain on the extensor mechanism may also be exacerbated by the tethering of the quadriceps mechanism by the inflated tourniquet proximally. Thus, patellar eversion for up to an hour at a time or more may cause permanent dysfunction of the quadriceps muscle, as evidenced by postoperative weakness. In the minimally invasive technique, the patella is simply retracted out of the way after the vastus medialis obliquus snip.
- No joint dislocation. In this approach, the tibia and femur are cut in situ, thus avoiding dislocation of the tibiofemoral joint. This may minimize capsular damage and postoperative pain.
- Downsized instrumentation. New instruments that are roughly half the size of traditional instruments have been developed to facilitate minimally invasive total knee procedures.
- Use of cut bone surfaces as guides. Instead of using only instruments to guide cuts, after the initial

bone cuts are made, the surgeon can use the bone surface itself as a guide to complete the cuts. Bone can be excised in a piecemeal fashion if needed.

- Suspended-leg technique. This step has been borrowed from general knee arthroscopy techniques. Gravity is used to naturally expose the knee joint and to avoid the use of lamina spreaders to distract the joint.

TKA is a procedure that is widely performed for advanced arthropathies of the knee; it consistently alleviates pain, improves function, and enhances quality of life.[1] As the elderly population in the United States grows and indications for the procedure broaden, it is projected that an increasing number of patients will undergo TKA. The principal diagnoses most commonly associated with total knee replacement procedures are osteoarthrosis and allied disorders (90.9%), followed by rheumatoid arthritis and other inflammatory polyarthropathies (3.4%).[2] The knee is the joint most often replaced in arthroplasty procedures. The most common age group for total knee replacements is 65 to 84 years. Women in this age range are more likely to undergo TKA than are their male counterparts.

The increasing use of TKA has raised several public and clinical policy issues, including apparent racial and ethnic disparities in TKA use,[3] broadening indications for TKA to include younger and older patients, and evidence that outcomes are better when TKA is performed in higher volume centers.[4] These issues were partially addressed in the Agency for Healthcare Research and Quality report.[5] The major findings were summarized as follows:

> There is no evidence that age, gender, or obesity is a strong predictor of functional outcomes. Patients with rheumatoid arthritis show more improvement than those with osteoarthritis, but this may be related to their poorer functional scores at the time of treatment and hence the potential for more improvement. The underlying indication though is consistent across all these groups. Namely, that advanced osteoarthrosis of the knee compromises functional activities as the patient's knee pain becomes recalcitrant and unresponsive to conservative therapeutic interventions.

SYMPTOMS

Refractory knee pain is the most common symptom among patients who undergo TKA. Stiffness, deformity, and instability are symptoms also commonly seen in advanced osteoarthrosis or inflammatory polyarthropathy. In the postoperative period, acute surgical pain is manifested and is most intense during the first 2 weeks. Disruption and inflammation of the periarticular soft tissues present as a soft tissue stiffness pattern that differs from the preoperative rigid stiffness of advanced arthrosis. Joint proprioception impairment may give rise to a sense of mild knee instability in the postoperative period. Uncommonly, debris may generate a sense of cracking, popping, or locking.

PHYSICAL EXAMINATION

The findings of advanced arthrosis on examination are joint hypertrophy, joint line tenderness, and reduced passive and active range of motion associated with crepitus. Valgus deformity is common in osteoarthrosis. Varus deformity is more common in rheumatoid arthritis. Ligamentous laxity is more commonly encountered in rheumatoid arthritis compared with osteoarthritis. Additional findings include joint effusion and concomitant suprapatellar or pes anserine bursitis. In the postoperative period, staples or sutures appose the incision margins. A serosanguineous discharge may be present during the first week postoperatively. There is marked effusion of the knee joint. Increased warmth and erythema are prominent features along with hyperpathia or allodynia. Muscle inhibition of the quadriceps and hamstrings interferes with manual muscle testing. Range of motion is most often guarded secondary to pain.

FUNCTIONAL LIMITATIONS

The preoperative profile of a patient at risk for poor postoperative locomotor recovery is a woman with a high body mass index, many comorbidities, high intensity of knee pain, restriction in flexion amplitude, deficits in knee strength, and poor preoperative locomotor ability as measured by the 6-minute gait test. In addition, the preoperative gait power profiles, on the nonsurgical side, are characterized by low concentric push-off work by the plantar flexors and low concentric action of the hip flexors during early swing.[6] Postoperative pain scores and their associated psychological profiles ostensibly affect functional outcomes also.[7]

Subsequent studies have further identified factors associated with a suboptimal postoperative functional outcome. Patients who have marked functional limitation, severe pain, low mental health score, and other comorbid conditions before TKA are more likely to have a worse outcome at 1 year and 2 years postoperatively.[8] One consistent finding is that preoperative joint function is a predictor of function at 6 months after TKA. Those patients who had lower preoperative functional status related to knee arthritis functioned at a lower level at 6 months than did patients with a higher preoperative functional status.[9] Studies have focused on quadriceps strength as a significant contributing factor. Functional measures underwent an expected decline early after TKA, but recovery was more rapid than anticipated, and long-term outcomes were better than previously reported in the literature. The high correlation between quadriceps strength and functional performance suggests that improved postoperative quadriceps strengthening could be important to enhance the potential benefits of TKA.[10] However, preoperative quadriceps strength training exercise does not appear necessarily to enhance functional outcomes.[11]

DIAGNOSTIC STUDIES

Diagnostic studies are necessary to address preparatory assessment as well as potential complications of TKA.

Preoperative diagnostic testing appropriate for the evaluation of the patient with end-stage arthropathy of the knee includes standing anteroposterior and lateral radiographs to assess joint space compromise and valgus or varus deformity. If infection is suspected, arthrocentesis should be performed with synovial fluid analysis for Gram stain and culture sensitivity studies.

Postoperative diagnostic testing initially includes non–weight-bearing posteroanterior and lateral radiographs. During follow-up at 8 to 12 weeks, standing radiographs should be obtained to assess component and alignment integrity.

Diagnostic testing for suspected prosthetic loosening includes plain radiographs of the knee. If infection is suspected, joint fluid can be analyzed.

Differential Diagnosis of the Symptomatic Total Knee Arthroplasty

Prosthetic loosening

Infection

Periprosthetic fracture

Component failure

TREATMENT

Initial

Medical therapeutic interventions address the following.

Prophylaxis for Deep Venous Thrombosis

Warfarin, low-molecular-weight heparinoids, factor X, and thrombin inhibitors as well as sequential pneumatic compression devices for the lower limb are the most common and efficacious agents for deep venous thrombosis prophylaxis in the postoperative period after TKA.[12-19]

Postoperative Pain Management

During the first 48 to 72 hours, patients often receive controlled analgesia therapy administered through the intravenous or epidural route. Some anesthesiologists employ a perioperative femoral nerve block. Subsequently, patients are given oral opioids. Controlled-release and short-acting opioids may be used. Depending on the clinician's and patient's preferences, fixed or rescue dose opioid medications are selected. The opioids can be titrated to achieve balance of analgesia versus emerging side effects.[20-23]

Incision Site Care

Dry, sterile gauze dressings are applied as long as drainage is present. Staples and sutures can safely be removed 10 to 14 days after surgery.[24,25]

Postoperative Swelling

Properly fitting, thigh-high elastic compression stockings, a continuous passive motion (CPM) machine, and possibly local cryotherapy are used to manage swelling.[26-29]

Postoperative Anemia

The overall blood lost after unilateral TKA has been estimated at 2.2 units. Blood loss is greater for uncemented than for cemented prostheses. Patients are often advised before surgery to donate 1 to 3 units of packed red blood cells for autotransfusion, although this practice has recently been questioned.[30] In addition, postoperative blood collection and reinfusion through the surgical drain have been shown to be effective in reducing the need for bank blood and have a low morbidity rate when used with current techniques. Some patients are advised to commence a course of recombinant erythropoietin in conjunction with iron supplementation before surgery.[31] If the patient is receiving oral anticoagulation therapy, bridging therapy with a low-molecular-weight heparin compound may be considered by the patient's primary care physician or medical consultant.[32] If the perioperative red blood cell count reveals a macrocytic anemia, vitamin B_{12} and folic acid levels should be obtained. If the anemia is microcytic, serum iron level, total iron-binding capacity, or transferrin concentration should be determined along with a reticulocyte count.

Rehabilitation

Rehabilitation programs that use clinical pathways enhance the efficiency of postoperative rehabilitation for the patient with TKA. The rehabilitation program can be conceptualized as occurring in stages or phases. The first stage commences in the immediate postoperative period. The final stage concludes when the patient returns to the community and pursues optimal independent functional living. See Table 71-1 for an example of a clinical pathway that addresses the schedule of progression during the first phase.

Note that there are numerous protocols for the use of CPM machines during the first phase of TKA rehabilitation. Flexion can be increased approximately 5 to 10 degrees each day according to the patient's tolerance, unless otherwise indicated. CPM intervention demonstrates significant improvements in active knee flexion, reduces analgesic use 2 weeks postoperatively, and enhances physiotherapy goal achievement compared with physiotherapy alone.

In addition, length of hospital stay and need for knee manipulations were significantly decreased with CPM. However, it is unclear whether it is the degree of knee flexion applied or the number of hours of application of CPM that is clinically significant. There is no evidence that short-term CPM application versus long-term CPM application influences outcome. There is no substantial evidence that CPM influences the degree of swelling, risk of venous thromboembolism, or incidence of wound infection or incision site complications.[34]

TABLE 71-1 Clinical Pathway for First-Phase Rehabilitation[33]

Postoperative Day	Exercise	Mobility	Ambulation	Activities of Daily Living
0	Deep breathing	Sits to chair transfer		
	Incentive spirometer			
	Quadriceps and gluteal sets	Education on continuous passive motion machine		
	Straight-leg raise			
	Hip abduction			
	Ankle pumps			
1	Deep breathing	Bed mobility		Assess adaptive equipment: reachers, long-handled sponges, and shoehorns
	Lower extremity static resistance exercises	Bed to chair transfers with knee immobilizer		
	Ankle pumps and circles			
	Continuous passive motion			
2	Continue previously described exercises	Continue bed mobility and transfers	Assisted ambulation in room, partial weight bearing or weight bearing as tolerated with knee immobilizer	Raised toilet seat
	Short arc quads			Grooming and dressing well while seated
	Straight-leg raise with knee immobilizer	Begin toilet transfers		
	Upper extremity strengthening			
3	Continue previously described exercises	Decreased assistance in basic transfers	Independent ambulation with walker or crutches in room, partial weight bearing or weight bearing as tolerated with knee immobilizer	Independent toileting and grooming
	Sitting full arc motion flexion and extension in conjunction with supine passive flexion and extension		Trial of ambulation in corridor, possibly practice negotiating 2-4 stairs	Education on joint protection and energy conservation techniques
	Depending on community resources and home safety and support availability, the patient may be ready for hospital discharge and post–acute care rehabilitation at this time.			
4	Continue previously described exercises with increased intensity	Independent in basic transfers	Gait training to improve pattern and endurance	Continue previously described activities of daily living
			Discontinue knee immobilizer (if quadriceps strength is greater than 3/5)	
	Initiate active assistive range of motion exercises and quadriceps and hamstrings self-stretch			
5-6	Continue previously described exercises		Independent ambulation with assistive device	Independent dressing with tapered use of adaptive equipment
	Transition from passive to active assistive range of motion exercises		Begin stairs with railing, cane as needed	

In the immediate postoperative period, the inhibited quadriceps and hamstrings may not adequately stabilize the knee. The patient may require a knee immobilizer for transfers and walking.

The patient will often require a two-handed assistive device (e.g., walker or axillary crutches) for gait training initially. Adaptive equipment for bathing and dressing (e.g., tub or shower seat, grab bars, dressing sticks, sock aid) is generally necessary. Some patients may not have sufficient range of motion during the first week postoperatively to negotiate stairs. The motor reactions normalize by the third week; therefore, patients may return to driving activities if they can perform car transfers independently and can tolerate sitting for prolonged periods.[35]

During the second stage of TKA rehabilitation (weeks 1 to 4), the patient progresses to low-resistance dynamic exercise therapy for the involved lower extremity. This can be carried out with a stationary bicycle. Some patients may prefer aquatic-based exercise regimens during this period. Patients should be independent in ambulating with a two-handed or single-handed device if they are fully weight bearing on level surfaces up to 500 feet. They should be supervised in negotiating stairs. Electrical stimulation of the quadriceps can be considered for patients who have inhibited recruitment.[36] Soft tissue mobilization can be introduced to facilitate patellar glide. Most patients have a strength ratio favoring the hamstrings. During this period, the patient should be independent in all basic activities of daily living. During the last 10 years, there has been a significant temporal shift in expediting home and outpatient (clinic) TKA rehabilitation. Presently, there are no reproducible and enforceable guidelines that may be uniformly applied.[37-39]

During the third stage of TKA rehabilitation (weeks 4 to 8), the available range of motion should reach 0 to 115 degrees. Patients are able to advance their dynamic resistance exercise regimens and more freely pursue both open and closed kinetic chain and dynamic balance exercises. Patients advance to a single-handed device or no device for ambulation and at different speeds and on different terrain. They should be independent in negotiating stairs. Patients advance to independence in instrumental activities of daily living.

In the final stage (weeks 8 to 12), patients may return to their preoperative exercise regimens and recreation activities and kneeling.

Most patients who participated in sports before surgery are able to return to low-impact sport activities and exercise regimens. Patients are able to return to sedentary, light, and medium work categories. Patients who are on sick leave for more than 6 months preoperatively are less likely to return to work. There is published evidence that the degree of physical activity does not contribute to premature revision TKA.[40] However, younger patients may be at risk for earlier revision TKA, depending on their degree of physical activity.[41] Contact sports are advised against, and caution should be exercised with high-impact aerobic activities.[42-46]

Procedures

Manipulation

Some patients with unsatisfactory gains in knee range of motion may be candidates for manipulation. The role of manipulation for the patient with a TKA contracture remains controversial. Outcome studies are divided as to whether functional outcomes and quality of life are enhanced as a result of manipulation. When an orthopedic surgeon performs the procedure, it is carried out in an operating room with the use of general or epidural anesthesia. The goal is to overcome articular lesions with minimal force after quadriceps resistance is eliminated. Manipulation is most commonly performed during the second or third postoperative week if the range of motion of the involved knee is less than 75 degrees.[47,48]

Arthrocentesis

Aspiration of the knee for aerobic and anaerobic cultures and sensitivities is the most reliable method for diagnosis of infection. Strict sterile technique must be used throughout the aspiration procedure.[49]

Surgery

The most common materials presently used in replacement joints are cobalt-chromium and titanium on ultrahigh-molecular-weight polyethylene. In total knee arthroplasties, cobalt-chromium is always used on femoral weight-bearing surfaces because of its superior strength. Total knee arthroplasties can be stabilized with or without cement. In some cases, hybrid total knee arthroplasties are used.

There are three major surgical approaches for the standard TKA: the medial parapatellar retinacular approach, the midvastus approach, and the subvastus approach.[50] The medial parapatellar retinacular approach compromises the quadriceps tendon in its medial third, and this gives rise to more postoperative patellofemoral complications. The midvastus approach does not compromise the extensor mechanism of the knee joint. The subvastus approach also preserves the integrity of the extensor mechanism but does not expose the knee as well as the other two approaches do. The type of arthrotomy used will influence postoperative management. After a standard anteromedial arthrotomy between the vastus medialis and rectus tendons with eversion of the patella, active and passive range of motion may begin immediately. Protected ambulation with crutches or a walker is recommended for 4 to 6 weeks to allow healing of the arthrotomy repair and recovery of quadriceps strength. Although recovery after the subvastus approach may be more rapid than after the standard anteromedial approach, protected weight bearing with ambulatory aids for 3 to 6 weeks is still recommended to allow soft tissue healing. In the patient with limited preoperative range of motion, either tibial tubercle osteotomy or a V-Y quadricepsplasty needs to be performed. After tibial tubercle osteotomy, early range of motion and full weight bearing within 1 week of surgery is recommended. Variations of the conventional surgical exposures are also used in the minimally invasive TKA operative approaches.[51]

Weight-bearing status depends on the details of the surgical reconstruction and whether the components were inserted with or without cement. For the otherwise uncomplicated primary cemented TKA, the patient can tolerate weight bearing within the confines of safety. Protected weight bearing can be performed only after the patient demonstrates adequate control of the limb to prevent falling. The time to weight bearing after total arthroplasty depends on the use of cement or cementless fixation and whether large structural bone grafting was required. In cemented total knees, no differences in the incidence of radiolucent lines have been observed between immediate weight bearing and protected weight bearing for 12 weeks. Although weight bearing after cementless fixation might increase micromotion, many surgeons allow early weight bearing.[52]

The tibial and femoral components presently in use have a life expectancy of 10 to 20 years. This life span depends on the surgical technique, the components used, the bone stock, and the level of physical activity after TKA. Revision TKA is a surgical procedure that the patient with TKA may encounter several years after the original surgery.[53]

POTENTIAL DISEASE COMPLICATIONS

Potential disease complications of conditions involving the knee, such as osteoarthritis, rheumatoid arthritis, and osteonecrosis of the femoral epicondyle or tibial condyle, include intractable pain, swelling, stiffness, contracture, and valgus or varus deformity.

POTENTIAL TREATMENT COMPLICATIONS

Potential treatment complications include local complications, patellar complications, inadequate motion, instability, infection, and loosening:

Local complications include deep venous thrombosis and peroneal nerve palsy. The incidence of deep venous thrombosis after TKA is 40% to 80%. Distal deep venous thrombosis has a rate of occurrence of 50% to 70%, whereas proximal deep venous thrombosis has a rate of occurrence of 10% to 15%. Pulmonary embolism after TKA has an estimated rate of occurrence of 1.8% to 7%.[54] In the patient who does not receive anticoagulation therapy, the thrombus develops within the first 24 hours, and peak development is at 5 to 7 days after surgery. The growth ceases by day 10, and resolution of the thrombus (intrinsic thrombolysis) commences by day 14. Venography, Doppler ultrasound imaging, and impedance plethysmography are used to diagnose deep venous thrombosis. Doppler ultrasound studies are most commonly used in clinical practice. Currently, low-molecular-weight heparin or continuous intravenous heparin in conjunction with anticoagulation with warfarin is recommended for active deep venous thrombosis treatment.

The incidence of post-thrombotic syndrome is relatively low in the population of patients undergoing TKA.[55] Peroneal nerve injury occurs in less than 1% of patients in most series.[56] Most patients experience partial resolution of their nerve palsy within the first few months postoperatively. Few patients require use of a plastic or double metal upright ankle-foot orthosis.

Patellar complications include subluxation and dislocation. These are often due to excessive tracking of the patella, which is difficult to correct with conservative treatment after the initial surgery. These complications are often recognized during the initial operative procedure. When they are not recognized early, revision surgery is often needed.[57] Patella fractures can be traumatically induced or stress induced. These fractures are generally treated conservatively unless closed reduction is problematic.[58]

Inadequate motion may result in a flexion contracture of the knee. Aggressive pain management, early CPM, and mobilization of the patient can reduce the likelihood of contracture. A dynamic locking knee brace may help reduce small flexion contractures (less than 20 degrees). The need for manipulation depends on the available range of motion of the knee. The required range of motion for the knee during functional activities is shown in Table 71-2. Manipulation can be considered if the knee range of motion is less than 85 degrees.

Instability is usually due to surgical error and requires surgical revision rather than bracing.[59]

The overall infection rate for initial TKA is 1%.[60] This is higher in patients with advanced rheumatoid arthritis, revision TKA, and constrained prostheses. Deep infection can occur any time from days to months after surgery. Musculoskeletal infection usually presents as increase in pain with or without weight bearing, increase in swelling, and fever. Diagnosis is confirmed by joint fluid analysis, as described earlier. The patient requires a 6-week course of antibiotic treatment between the period of component removal and reimplantation. The most successful technique for treatment of the infected total knee replacement is a two-stage reimplantation of the TKA components. Infection must never be overlooked as a cause of implant loosening. Infection can occur early or late and can present with or without signs of systemic toxicity. The

TABLE 71-2 Flexor Tendon Injuries (Immediate Motion)	
Activity of Daily Living	**Extension-Flexion**
Walking in stance phase	15-40 degrees
Walking in swing phase	15-70 degrees
Stair climbing step over step	0-83 degrees
Standing up from a chair	0-93 degrees
Standing up from a toilet	0-105 degrees
Stooping to lift an object	0-117 degrees
Tying a shoelace	0-106 degrees

symptoms are commonly the same as those seen with aseptic loosening. A progressive radiolucency between the prosthesis and its adjacent bone almost always is considered an infection until proved otherwise. Negative aspirate from the knee, normal sedimentation rate and C-reactive protein level, and normal gallium or indium scans cannot rule out infection or prosthetic device. The patient should be advised that even in the presence of normal test results, infection of the prosthetic device may be discovered intraoperatively and necessitate the removal of the prosthetic device.

The most common reason for total arthroplasty failure has been loosening of the implant. Factors associated with loosening include infection, implant constraint, failure to achieve neutral mechanical alignment, instability, and cement technique. The prodromal features of impending loosening and failure of the components are an increase in pain and swelling with or without angular deformity of the knee.[61] The radiographic features include a widening radiolucent zone between the implant and the adjacent bone and subsidence of the implant. Loosening may occur at the component-cement interface or bone-cement interface. Implant loosening can be attributed to mechanical and biologic factors. The mechanical factors include limb alignment, ligamentous balance, and preservation of a contracted posterior cruciate ligament. Implant loosening can occur early or late. Early implant loosening usually occurs within the first 2 years and represents a mechanical failure of the interlock of the implant and host to bone. This early implant loosening is more appropriately called fixation failure and is often secondary to errors in judgment at the time of surgery or to problems with the technical aspects of the surgical procedure. Extremity malalignment, soft tissue imbalance, and poor cement technique individually or in combination contribute to loosening. Biologic factors are largely responsible for the phenomenon of late loosening. Late loosening of total knee implants is often secondary to the host biologic response to the implant's debris that weakens the mechanical bond of implant to bone established during surgery. Mechanical factors may contribute to late loosening, but they do not alone explain the loss of fixation device that has been stable for many years. The volume of particles generated from the articulation is influenced by the patient's weight and activity level, duration of implantation, polyethylene thickness, and contact stresses. Wear may be accelerated by malalignment, instability, and ligament imbalance, resulting in increased volume of particulate released into the joint.[62]

References

1. Lavernia CJ, Guzman JF, Gachupin-Garcia A. Cost effectiveness and quality of life in knee arthroplasty. Clin Orthop 1997;345:134-139.
2. American Academy of Orthopaedic Surgeons. Primary Total Hip and Total Knee Arthroplasty Projections to 2030 (Appendix C). Available at: http://www.aaos.org.ezproxy.galter.northwestern.edu/wordhtml/pdfs_r/tjr.pdf.
3. Dunlop DD, Song J, Manheim LM, Chang RW. Racial disparities in joint replacement use among older adults. Med Care 2003;41:288-298.
4. Hervey SL, Purves HR, Guller U, et al. Provider volume of total knee arthroplasties and patient outcomes in the HCUP-nationwide inpatient sample. J Bone Joint Surg Am 2003;85:1775-1783.
5. Kane RL, Saleh KJ, Wilt TJ, et al. Total Knee Replacement. Evidence Report/Technology Assessment No. 86. Rockville, Md, U.S. Dept. of Health and Human Services, Public Health Service, Agency for Healthcare Research and Quality, 2003. AHRQ publication 04-E006-2.
6. Parent E, Moffet H. Preoperative predictors of locomotor ability two months after total knee arthroplasty for severe osteoarthritis. Arthritis Rheum 2003;49:36-50.
7. Brander VA, Stulberg SD, Adams AD, et al. Predicting total knee replacement pain: a prospective, observational study. Clin Orthop Relat Res 2003;416:27-36.
8. Lingard EA, Katz JN, Wright EA, Sledge CB; Kinemax Outcomes Group. Predicting the outcome of total knee arthroplasty. J Bone Joint Surg Am 2004;86:2179-2186.
9. Jones CA, Voaklander DC, Suarez-Alma ME. Determinants of function after total knee arthroplasty. Phys Ther 2003;83:696-706.
10. Mizner RL, Petterson SC, Stevens JE, et al. Preoperative quadriceps strength predicts functional ability one year after total knee arthroplasty. J Rheumatol 2005;32:1533-1539.
11. Beaupre LA, Lier D, Davies DM, Johnston DB. The effect of a preoperative exercise and education program on functional recovery, health related quality of life, and health service utilization following primary total knee arthroplasty. J Rheumatol 2004;31:1166-1173.
12. Anderson FA Jr, Hirsh J, White K, Fitzgerald RH Jr. Temporal trends in prevention of venous thromboembolism following primary total hip or knee arthroplasty 1996-2001: findings from the Hip and Knee Registry. Chest 2003;124(Suppl):349S-356S.
13. Ragucci MV, Leali A, Moroz A, Fetto J. Comprehensive deep venous thrombosis prevention strategy after total-knee arthroplasty. Am J Phys Med Rehabil 2003;82:164-168.
14. Kim Y, Kim J. Incidence and natural history of deep-vein thrombosis after total knee arthroplasty: a prospective, randomised study. J Bone Joint Surg Br 2002;84:566-570.
15. Warwick D, Harrison J, Whitehouse S, et al. A randomised comparison of a foot pump and low-molecular-weight heparin in the prevention of deep-vein thrombosis after total knee replacement. J Bone Joint Surg Br 2002;84:344-350.
16. Francis CW, Berkowitz SD, Comp PC, et al. Comparison of ximelagatran with warfarin for the prevention of venous thromboembolism after total knee replacement. N Engl J Med 2003;349:1703-1712.
17. Pulido PA, Copp SN, Walker RH, et al. The efficacy of a single daily dose of enoxaparin for deep vein thrombosis prophylaxis following total knee arthroplasty. Orthopedics 2004;27:1185-1187.
18. Spruill WJ, Wade WE, Leslie RB. A cost analysis of fondaparinux versus enoxaparin in total knee arthroplasty. Am J Ther 2004;11:3-8.
19. Wang H, Boctor B, Verner J. The effect of single-injection femoral nerve block on rehabilitation and length of hospital stay after total knee replacement. Reg Anesth Pain Med 2002;27:139-144.
20. Farag E, Dilger J, Brooks P, Tetzlaff JE. Epidural analgesia improves early rehabilitation after total knee replacement. J Clin Anesth 2005;17:281-285.
21. Bourne MH. Analgesics for orthopedic postoperative pain. Am J Orthop 2004;33:128-135.
22. Cheville A, Chen A, Oster G, et al. A randomized trial of controlled-release oxycodone during inpatient rehabilitation following unilateral total knee arthroplasty. J Bone Joint Surg Am 2001;83:572-576.
23. Huenger F, Schmachtenberg A, Haefner H, et al. Evaluation of postdischarge surveillance of surgical site infections after total hip and knee arthroplasty. Am J Infect Control 2005;33:455-462.
24. Lucas B. Nursing management issues in hip and knee replacement surgery. Br J Nurs 2004;13:782-787.
25. Engel C, Hamilton NA, Potter PT, Zautra AJ. Comparing compression bandaging and cold therapy in postoperative total knee replacement surgery. Perianesth Ambulatory Surg Nurs Update 2002;10:51.

26. Esler CAN, Blakeway C, Fiddian NJ. The use of a closed-suction drain in total knee arthroplasty: a prospective, randomised study. J Bone Joint Surg Br 2003;85:215-217.

27. Smith J, Stevens J, Taylor M, Tibbey J. A randomized, controlled trial comparing compression bandaging and cold therapy in postoperative total knee replacement surgery. Orthop Nurs 2002;21:61-66.

28. Lieberman JR. A closed-suction drain was not beneficial in knee arthroplasty with cement. J Bone Joint Surg Am 2003;85:2257.

29. Brosseau L, Milne S, Wells G, et al. Efficacy of continuous passive motion following total knee arthroplasty: a metaanalysis. J Rheumatol 2004;31:2251-2264.

30. Muller U, Roder C, Pisan M, et al. Autologous blood donation in total knee arthroplasties is not necessary. Acta Orthop Scand 2004;75:66-70.

31. Rauh MA, Bayers-Thering M, LaButti RS, Krackow KA. Preoperative administration of epoetin alfa to total joint arthroplasty patients. Orthopedics 2002;25:317-320.

32. Dunn AS, Wisnivesky J, Ho W, et al. Perioperative management of patients on oral anticoagulants: a decision analysis. Med Decis Making 2005;25:387-397.

33. Thomas K. Clinical pathway for hip and knee arthroplasty. Physiotherapy 2003;89:603-609.

34. Lenssen AF, de Bie RA, Bulstra SK, van Steyn MJA. Continuous passive motion (CPM) in rehabilitation following total knee arthroplasty: a randomised controlled trial. Phys Ther Rev 2003;8:123-129.

35. Pierson JL, Earles DR, Wood K. Brake response time after total knee arthroplasty: when is it safe for patients to drive? J Arthroplasty 2003;18:840-843.

36. Avramidis K, Strike PW, Taylor PN, Swain ID. Effectiveness of electric stimulation of the vastus medialis muscle in the rehabilitation of patients after total knee arthroplasty. Arch Phys Med Rehabil 2003;84:1850-1853.

37. Epps CD. Length of stay, discharge disposition, and hospital charge predictors. AORN J 2004;79:975-976, 979-981, 984-988 passim.

38. Weaver FM, Hughes SL, Almagor O, et al. Comparison of two home care protocols for total joint replacement. J Am Geriatr Soc 2003;51:523-528.

39. Kramer JF, Speechley M, Bourne R, et al. Comparison of clinic- and home-based rehabilitation programs after total knee arthroplasty. Clin Orthop Relat Res 2003;410:225-234.

40. Jones DL, Cauley JA, Kriska AM, et al. Physical activity and risk of revision total knee arthroplasty in individuals with knee osteoarthritis: a matched case-control study. J Rheumatol 2004;31:1384-1390.

41. Harrysson OL, Robertsson O, Nayfeh JF. Higher cumulative revision rate of knee arthroplasties in younger patients with osteoarthritis. Clin Orthop Relat Res 2004;421:162-168.

42. Chatterji U, Ashworth MJ, Lewis PL, Dobson PJ. Effect of total knee arthroplasty on recreational and sporting activity. ANZ J Surg 2005;75:405-408.

43. Kuster MS. Exercise recommendations after total joint replacement: a review of the current literature and proposal of scientifically based guidelines. Sports Med 2002;32:433-445.

44. Lamb SE, Frost H. Recovery of mobility after knee arthroplasty: expected rates and influencing factors. J Arthroplasty 2003;18:575-582.

45. Hassaballa MA, Porteous AJ, Newman JH, Rogers CA. Can knees kneel? Kneeling ability after total, unicompartmental and patellofemoral knee arthroplasty. Knee 2003;10:155-160.

46. Clifford PE, Mallon WJ. Sports after total joint replacement. Clin Sports Med 2005;24:175-186.

47. Bong MR, Di Cesare PE. Stiffness after total knee arthroplasty. J Am Acad Orthop Surg 2004;12:164-171.

48. Ellis TJ, Beshires E, Brindley GW, et al. Knee manipulation after total knee arthroplasty. J South Orthop Assoc 1999;8:73-79.

49. Lonner JH, Siliski JM, Della Valle C, et al. Role of knee aspiration after resection of the infected total knee arthroplasty. Am J Orthop 2001;30:305-309.

50. Younger AS, Duncan CP, Masri BA. Surgical exposures in revision total knee arthroplasty. J Am Acad Orthop Surg 1998;6:55-64.

51. Scuderi GR, Tenholder M, Capeci C. Surgical approaches in mini-incision total knee arthroplasty. Clin Orthop Relat Res 2004;428:61-67.

52. Youm T, Maurer SG, Stuchin SA. Postoperative management after total hip and knee arthroplasty. J Arthroplasty 2005;20:322-324.

53. Mehrotra C, Remington PL, Naimi TS, et al. Trends in total knee replacement surgeries and implications for public health, 1990-2000. Public Health Rep 2005;120:278-282.

54. White RH, Henderson MC. Risk factors for venous thromboembolism after total hip and knee replacement surgery. Curr Opin Pulm Med 2002;8:365-371.

55. Deehan DJ, Siddique M, Weir DJ, et al. Postphlebitic syndrome after total knee arthroplasty: 405 patients examined 2-10 years after surgery. Acta Orthop Scand 2001;72:42-45.

56. Schinsky MF, Macaulay W, Parks ML, et al. Nerve injury after primary total knee arthroplasty. J Arthroplasty 2001;16:1048-1054.

57. Kelly MA. Extensor mechanism complications in total knee arthroplasty. Instr Course Lect 2004;53:193-199.

58. Chun KA, Ohashi K, Bennett DL, El-Khoury GY. Patellar fractures after total knee replacement. AJR Am J Roentgenol 2005;185:655-660.

59. Stiehl JB. Patellar instability in total knee arthroplasty. J Knee Surg 2003;16:229-235.

60. Leone JM, Hanssen AD. Management of infection at the site of a total knee arthroplasty. J Bone Joint Surg Am 2005;87:2335-2348.

61. Dennis DA. Evaluation of painful total knee arthroplasty. J Arthroplasty 2004;19(Suppl 1):35-40.

62. Callaghan JJ, O'Rourke MR, Saleh KJ. Why knees fail: lessons learned. J Arthroplasty 2004;19(Suppl 1):31-34.

Achilles Tendinitis 72

Michael F. Stretanski, DO

DEFINITION

Achilles tendinitis exists along the spectrum of peritendinitis to tendinosis or tendinopathy. This is a painful, swollen, and tender area of the Achilles tendon and peritenon usually secondary to repetitive activity or overuse. Athletes with particularly tight heel cords are predisposed to injury. This condition commonly affects middle-aged men who play tennis, basketball, or other quick start-and-stop sports. Collagen vascular disease and diabetes may also be risk factors. The dogma has been that the relative avascularity of the region 5 to 7 cm proximal to the calcaneus insertion is the primary predisposing risk factor; however, there is some question as to the role of thinning and twisting of the tendon at this midsection and whether vascularity is the primary factor.[1] Ongoing studies, such as profiling of metalloproteinases[2] and mRNA expression,[3] seem to question this dogma and are similar to research being done on other regions of the body (see Chapter 25); the classic perspective has been restricted to a structural pathologic process, yet there seems to be a growing understanding of the cellular molecular basis of the clinical presentation. The histopathologic feature is angiofibroblastic hyperplasia (tendinosis) of the body of the tendon (a degenerative process) with a concomitant and potentially secondary inflammatory response in the peritenon.[4,5] The maladies often occur simultaneously but may occur individually. An association with chronic quinolone exposure is well documented.[6-8]

SYMPTOMS

Pain and tenderness in the Achilles tendon are predominant symptoms, usually in association with running sports and fitness activities.[9] Activities with rapid starting and stopping or rapid eccentric contraction, such as classical ballet,[10] increase the risk. An athlete with this injury has a 200-fold risk of sustaining a contralateral rupture of the Achilles tendon.[11] In some patients, the pain actually improves with lower extremity exercise. Typically, the pain occurs with a change in the athletic training schedule. The most common location for tendinosis symptoms is at the apex of the Achilles tendon curvature. Different activities can lead to pathologic change in other regions of the tendon, namely, at the calcaneal insertion with or without a Haglund deformity or at the myotendinous junction. A history of an acute traumatic event in which the patient reports a "pop" should suggest an Achilles tendon partial or complete rupture, although a similar pop can occur with tear or rupture of the plantaris, peroneus, or posterior tibial tendon.

PHYSICAL EXAMINATION

The essential element in the physical examination is the localization of swelling and tenderness in the critical zone of the Achilles tendon, at the apex of the Achilles curve approximately 2½ inches proximal to the os calcis insertion. Exquisite tenderness to palpation is a classic examination finding. The degree of ankle plantar force generated has been shown to have a strong negative relationship with pain, and a standardized strength testing system has been suggested and shown to be reliable on a small sample.[12] Palpable heat is usually not evident unless peritendinitis is a major component. The Achilles is usually tight, with ankle dorsiflexion rarely extending beyond 90 degrees. Associated findings may include abnormal foot posture (pes planus or cavus), tight hamstrings, and muscle weakness of the entire hip and leg. Heels may not move into a normal varus position when standing on toes. Neurologic evaluation, including strength, sensation, and deep tendon reflexes, is normal. History of quinolone exposure, collagen vascular disease, anabolic steroid use, or smoking should be noted.

The examination should also include observation for a palpable defect and the Thompson test (squeezing the calf, which should result in plantar flexion in an attached tendon) to rule out rupture of the Achilles tendon (Fig. 72-1).

FUNCTIONAL LIMITATIONS

Impact weight-bearing activities, such as jogging, fast walking, and running, are usually limited. Dance or cutting "moves" typical of field sports are virtually impossible. Nonimpact fitness activities, such as cycling and using an elliptical trainer, may also result in symptoms. Patients may complain of pain with daily ambulatory activities, such as walking at work or climbing stairs. Whereas individual differences exist, early recovery of plantar flexion may be seen with little functional change, usually because of flexor hallucis longus compensation.[13]

DIAGNOSTIC STUDIES

Unless a special form of calcified Achilles tendinosis occurs at the os calcis insertion, regular radiographs are usually normal. Diagnostic ultrasonography or magnetic resonance imaging is capable of defining the extent of both tendinosis and peritendinitis, but serial magnetic resonance examinations, especially postoperatively, are not indicated and do not correlate with functional outcome.[14] Partial rupture is a diagnostic dilemma for diagnostic ultrasonography,[15] and if it is suspected, magnetic resonance imaging should still be considered the standard of care. Magnetic resonance imaging is also more useful in documenting a complete tear's distance and location as well as the existence of partial tear that may appear normal or questionable on diagnostic ultrasound examination. An evolving role of positron emission tomography may exist.[16] These studies are generally recommended only to help define the prognosis or in patients who are unresponsive to rehabilitation and for whom surgery is being considered.

Differential Diagnosis

Haglund deformity

Retrocalcaneal bursitis

Adventitial bursitis

Achilles tendon rupture

Tibial stress fracture

Medial gastrocnemius tear

TREATMENT

Initial

The initial treatment goal is to decrease pain and to reduce inflammation. Therefore, rest from aggravating activities is critical. Icing (20 minutes, two or three times daily) and nonsteroidal anti-inflammatory drugs or analgesics can be used for pain and inflammation. Counterforce bracing is often helpful. A simple heel lift (1/8 to 1/2 inch) can decrease some of the stress on the tendon. Warm-up before any weight-bearing activity and cooling with ice afterward are recommended. Good functional results can usually be achieved in about 75% of cases at 3 months with nonoperative treatment in compliant patients with a tendon separation distance of 10 mm or less apparent on diagnostic ultrasonography.[17]

Rehabilitation

The rehabilitative process focuses on biologic improvement of the damaged tendon and peritenon and restoration of function, rather than the comfort efforts of the initial treatment phase. Rehabilitation is best initiated in a structured physical therapy program followed by home therapeutic exercise. Modalities including ultrasound, iontophoresis, and phonophoresis often comfort and may enhance the rehabilitation goals and enable the rehabilitation program. Electrical stimulation should

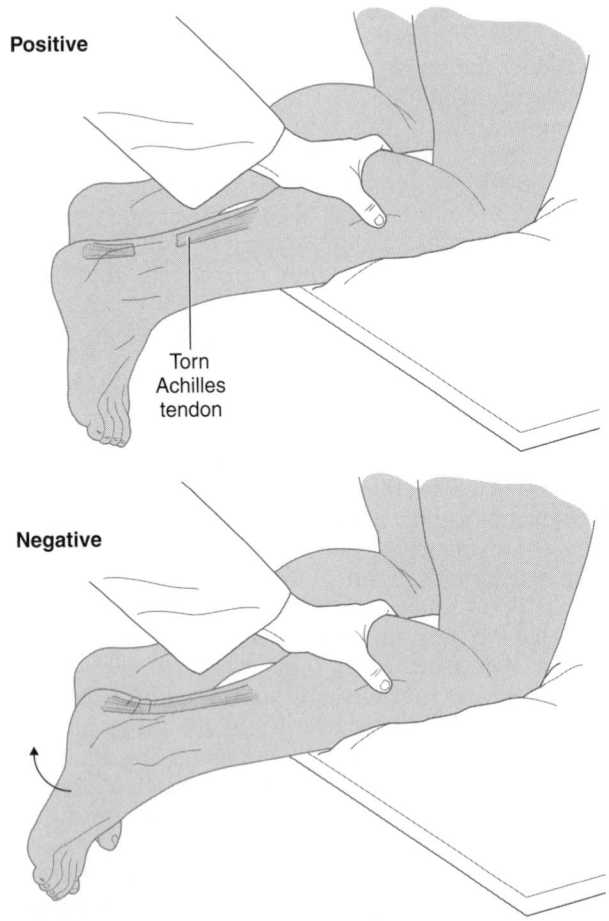

Positive

Torn Achilles tendon

Negative

FIGURE 72-1. The Thompson test is a reliable clinical test to identify a complete tear in the Achilles tendon. When the Achilles tendon is torn, a positive test result is elicited by squeezing the calf and seeing no plantar flexion of the foot. The test result is negative when the calf is squeezed and plantar flexion occurs in the foot.

probably be considered contraindicated in the face of the overuse etiology and counterphysiologic motor unit recruitment of muscle fibers.

Therapeutic exercise needs to be directed toward the entire kinetic chain because strength, endurance, and flexibility deficits are common, and most lower extremity sports activities occur as patterned motor engrams. Isokinetic strength and endurance testing usually aids in uncovering relative weakness and monitoring the rehabilitation progress. The postoperative goals of neovascularization, reduction of atrophy, fibroblastic infiltration, and collagen production and the restoration of strength, endurance, and flexibility are best served by early mobilization.[18]

Control of abusive force loads can be accomplished by counterforce bracing of the Achilles tendon or orthotics to minimize abnormal foot posture. Gradual, controlled return to running may be initiated through running in water programs. General fitness may be maintained by use of upper body land programs such as arm ergometry, resistance training, and water programs dedicated to the entire body. Return to sport or running is transitional, including plyometric and eccentric exercises. Full return generally requires normal strength, endurance, and flexibility. Repeated injury is not uncommon. Non–weight-bearing status and axillary crutches may have a role in the acute phase of treatment, with return to weight bearing as tolerated. A short leg cast or splint in 10 to 15 degrees of plantar flexion may also be used for no more than 2 weeks on the basis of the clinical picture. Return to normal activity, generally in 6 to 12 weeks, depends on level of participation (professional athlete versus weekend warrior), severity of the injury, and general medical condition.

Procedures

Control of pain by exogenous glucocorticoid injection is contraindicated as cellular death and tendon weakness with potential progression to tendon rupture are significant concerns in any region. Although there may be a developing role for hylan G-F 20,[19] this has been studied, to date, only in corticosteroid-induced Achilles tendinopathy in an animal model. Likewise, pulsed ultrasound,[20] indium-gallium-aluminum-phosphide diode laser irradiation,[21] and substance P injection[22] in an animal tenotomy model have shown promising early results.

Surgery

Rehabilitation failure may invite surgical intervention for ultimate problem resolution versus acceptance of the malady and alteration of activity level. Optimal surgical management strategy is controversial, but the relative avascularity of the region makes wound healing complications and deep infection ever-present threats. The concepts of surgery include removal of symptomatic peritendinitis tissue and resection of the abnormal tendinosis tissue in the body of the Achilles tendon with subsequent repair of the remaining adjacent normal tendon. This is usually accomplished with standard sutures or wires; however, fibrin sealant has been used,[23] and at least on the surface, it may seem a more biologic approach. Surgery is highly successful if all pathologic tissue is removed and appropriate postoperative rehabilitation is implemented.

In cases of suspected tendon rupture, a surgical consultation is warranted for consideration of other tendon ruptures. Endoscopic techniques have been proposed as an alternative to open surgery[24]; but with comparable re-rupture rates, there is some question as to whether the percutaneous repair, with an increased complication rate, should be done at all in lieu of a limited open technique.[25]

POTENTIAL DISEASE COMPLICATIONS

Chronic symptoms can result in weakening and subsequent complete rupture of the Achilles tendon. Chronic intractable pain and gait abnormality may develop.

POTENTIAL TREATMENT COMPLICATIONS

Side effects of nonsteroidal anti-inflammatory drugs include gastric, renal, and hepatic complications. Bracing for prolonged periods may lead to disuse weakness, atrophy, and poorly coordinated motor control when return to activity is attempted. Sural nerve injury can occur with open or percutaneous repair.[26] Significant alterations in gait can cause secondary knee, hip, forefoot, or low back pain. Overly aggressive physical therapy may cause tendon weakness and potential rupture. Surgical complications of bleeding, infection, and tibial or sural nerve injury are well known. Repeated tear may occur.

References

1. Theobald P, Benjamin M, Nokes L, Pugh N. Review of the vascularisation of the human Achilles tendon. Injury 2005;36:1267-1272.
2. Jones GC, Corps AN, Pennington CJ, et al. Expression profiling of metalloproteinases and tissue inhibitors of metalloproteinases in normal and degenerate human Achilles tendon. Arthritis Rheum 2006;54:832-842.
3. Corps AN, Robinson AH, Movin T, et al. Increased expression of aggrecan and biglycan mRNA in Achilles tendinopathy. Rheumatology 2006;45:291-294.
4. Kraushaar B, Nirschl R. Tendinosis of the elbow (tennis elbow). Clinical features and findings of histological, immunohistochemical, and electron microscopy studies. J Bone Joint Surg Am 1999;81:259-278.
5. Puddu G, Ippolito E, Postacchini F. A classification of Achilles tendon disease. Am J Sports Med 1976;4:145-150.
6. Lado Lado FL, Rodriguez MC, Velasco GM, et al. Partial bilateral rupture of the Achilles tendon associated with levofloxacin. An Med Interna 2005;22:28-30.
7. Chhajed PN, Plit ML, Hopkins PM, et al. Achilles tendon disease in lung transplant recipients: association with ciprofloxacin. Eur Respir J 2002;19:469-471.
8. McGarvey WC, Singh D, Trevino SG. Partial Achilles tendon ruptures associated with fluoroquinolone antibiotics: a case report and literature review. Foot Ankle Int 1996;17:494-498.
9. Nirschl R. Surgical considerations of ankle injuries. In O'Connor F, Wilder R, eds. The Complete Book of Running Medicine. New York, McGraw-Hill, 2001.

10. Stretanski MF, Weber GJ. Medical and rehabilitation issues in classical ballet. Am J Phys Med 2002;81:383-391.

11. Kongsgaard M, Aagaard P, Kjaer M, Magnusson SP. Structural Achilles tendon properties in athletes subjected to different exercise modes and in Achilles tendon rupture patients. J Appl Physiol 2005;99:1965-1971.

12. Paoloni JA, Appleyard RC, Murrell GA. The Orthopaedics Research Institute-Ankle Strength Testing System: inter-rater and intra-rater reliability testing. Foot Ankle Int 2002;23:112-117.

13. Finni T, Hodgson JA, Lai AM, et al. Muscle synergism during isometric plantarflexion in Achilles tendon rupture patients and in normal subjects revealed by velocity-encoded cine phase-contrast MRI. Clin Biomech 2006;21:67-74.

14. Wagnon R, Akayi M. Post-surgical Achilles tendon and correlation with functional outcome: a review of 40 cases. J Radiol 2005;86 (pt 1):1783-1787.

15. Kayser R, Mahlfeld K, Heyde CE. Partial rupture of the proximal Achilles tendon: a differential diagnostic problem in ultrasound imaging. Br J Sports Med 2005;39:838-842; discussion 838-842.

16. Huang SS, Yu JQ, Chamroonrat W, et al. Achilles tendonitis detected by PDG-PET. Clin Nucl Med 2006;31:147-148.

17. Hufner TM, Brandes DB, Thermann H, et al. Long-term results after functional nonoperative treatment of Achilles tendon rupture. Foot Ankle Int 2006;27:167-171.

18. Sorrenti SJ. Achilles tendon rupture: effect of early mobilization in rehabilitation after surgical repair. Foot Ankle Int 2006;27:407-410.

19. Tatari H, Skiak E, Destan H, et al. Effect of hylan G-F 20 in Achilles' tendonitis: an experimental study in rats. Arch Phys Med Rehabil 2004;85:1470-1474.

20. Yeung CK, Guo X, Ng YF. Pulsed ultrasound treatment accelerates the repair of Achilles tendon rupture in rats. J Orthop Res 2006;24: 193-201.

21. Salate AC, Barbosa G, Gaspar P, et al. Effect of In-Ga-Al-P diode laser irradiation on angiogenesis in partial ruptures of Achilles tendon in rats. Photomed Laser Surg 2005;23:470-475.

22. Steyaert AE, Burssens PJ, Vercruysse CW, et al. The effects of substance P on the biomechanic properties of ruptured rat Achilles' tendon. Arch Phys Med Rehabil 2006;87:254-258.

23. Kuskucu M, Mahirogullari M, Solakoglu C, et al. Treatment of rupture of the Achilles tendon with fibrin sealant. Foot Ankle Int 2005;26:826-831.

24. Morag G, Maman E, Arbel R. Endoscopic treatment of hind foot pathology. Arthroscopy 2003;19:E13.

25. Maes R, Copin G, Averous C. Is percutaneous repair of the Achilles tendon a safe technique? A study of 124 cases. Acta Orthop Belg 2006;72:179-183.

26. Majewski M, Rohrbach M, Czaja S, Ochsner P. Avoiding sural nerve injuries during percutaneous Achilles tendon repair. Am J Sports Med 2006;34:793-798.

Ankle Arthritis 73

David Wexler, MD, FRCS (Tr, Orth), Dawn M. Grosser, MD, and Todd A. Kile, MD

Synonym

Degenerative joint disease of the ankle

ICD-9 Codes

715.17   Osteoarthritis, localized, primary, ankle and foot
715.27   Osteoarthritis, localized, secondary, ankle and foot
716.17   Traumatic arthropathy, ankle and foot

DEFINITION

Ankle arthritis is degeneration of the cartilage within the tibiotalar joint; it can result from a wide range of causes, most commonly post-traumatic degenerative joint disease. An acute injury or trauma sustained a number of years before presentation or less severe, repetitive, minor injuries sustained during a longer period can lead to a slow but progressive destruction of the articular cartilage, resulting in degenerative joint disease.[1] Other common types of arthritis are osteoarthritis, rheumatoid arthritis, and septic arthritis. Osteoarthritis is usually less inflammatory than rheumatoid arthritis but can also involve many joints simultaneously.

SYMPTOMS

As with arthritis of any joint, the presenting symptoms are pain (which may be variable at different times of the day and exacerbated by weight bearing), swelling, stiffness, and progressive deformity.[1] Pieces of the cartilage can break off, forming a loose body, and the joint can "lock" or "catch," sticking in one position and causing acute, excruciating pain until the loose body moves from between the two irregular joint surfaces. Another symptom is that of "giving way" or instability of the joint, which may be a result of surrounding muscle weakness or ligamentous laxity. With progression of the arthritis, night pain can become a major complaint.

PHYSICAL EXAMINATION

Swelling, pain, and possibly increased temperature on palpation may be present. The pain is usually maximal along the anterior talocrural joint line and typically chronic and progressive. The ankle may be stiff on initial weight bearing; this improves after walking a while but then worsens with too much ambulatory activity. The pain is relieved with rest. If the patient's other ankle is normal, it is important to compare the two. Deformity and reduced range of motion in plantar flexion and dorsiflexion (normal: up to 20 degrees of dorsiflexion and 45 degrees of plantar flexion) may be seen. The patient may exhibit an antalgic gait or a limp. Septic arthritis presents very differently. It is acute in onset, warm, erythematous, swollen, and severely painful with passive range of motion and may be accompanied by constitutional symptoms.

FUNCTIONAL LIMITATIONS

Pain with walking distances and difficulty in negotiating stairs or inclines are particular functional disabilities. Even prolonged standing can become intolerable with advanced joint deterioration. Night pain can lead to difficulties with sleep. Patients will typically adjust their activities or eliminate many of them, particularly exercising, because of pain.

DIAGNOSTIC STUDIES

Plain anteroposterior and lateral standing radiographs provide sufficient information in the later stages of the disease (Figs. 73-1 and 73-2). Magnetic resonance imaging may show damage to articular cartilage and a joint effusion earlier in the course of the disease. In assessment of the radiographs, attention should also be paid to the other joints in the hindfoot because these will affect management options. Generalized bone density and alignment should also be noted.

In some cases, patients present with varying degrees of degeneration of other, adjacent joints. By performing

411

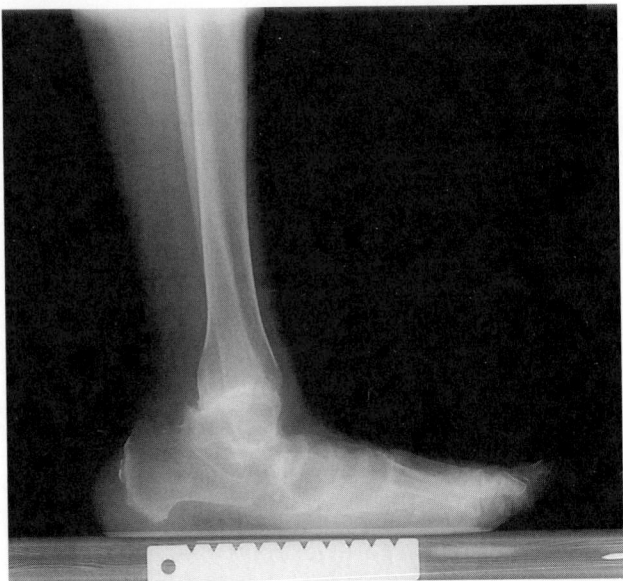

FIGURE 73-1. Lateral standing radiograph of the ankle in a patient with rheumatoid arthritis. This demonstrates loss of joint space and bone destruction of the ankle joint.

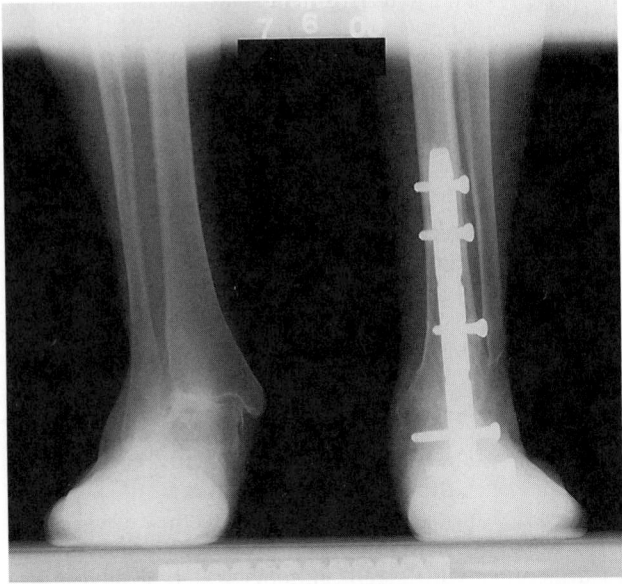

FIGURE 73-2. Anteroposterior standing radiograph of bilateral ankles in a patient with rheumatoid arthritis. This demonstrates the degenerative, destroyed joint on the left and one method of fusion with an intramedullary nail on the right.

differential blocks (i.e., isolated ankle block or subtalar block) with local anesthetic under radiographic control, the clinician may determine which of these joints are symptomatic.

TREATMENT

Initial

Initial treatment focuses on pain relief and minimizing inflammation. Nonsteroidal anti-inflammatory drugs or simple analgesics are used to alleviate the

Differential Diagnosis

Edema (e.g., edema secondary to congestive cardiac failure)

Subtalar joint degenerative disease

Posterior tibial tenosynovitis

Osteochondral defect

Fracture

Osteonecrosis

pain. Prefabricated orthoses ranging from flexible neoprene braces and lace-up or wraparound ankle supports to more rigid braces or walking boots can be prescribed to enhance stability and to reduce movement in the ankle joint, thus reducing pain levels.

Rehabilitation

A custom-molded rigid ankle-foot orthosis (AFO) fabricated by a skilled orthotist along with a rocker-bottom modification to the shoe (which can be accomplished by most cobblers) can provide dramatic pain relief for most patients with ankle arthritis. A physical therapist can instruct a patient in the proper technique for use of a walking stick or cane in the opposite hand. This is a simple but effective aid in reducing the forces across the ankle joint when the patient is ambulatory.

Mobilization, stretching techniques, and range of movement exercises may help alleviate pain and stiffness. Non–weight-bearing exercises are important, and if it is accessible, hydrotherapy has been shown to be an extremely useful and productive adjunct. Distraction and gliding mobilization techniques improve range of movement. Strengthening of surrounding muscle groups and proprioceptive rehabilitation will enhance stability.

Procedures

Other than the blocks that are performed to determine the location of the pathologic changes in confusing cases, injections are not typically done for ankle arthritis. Corticosteroid injection is generally of only limited duration, and steroids are chondrotoxic (cause cartilage damage). However, they can provide excellent temporary pain relief in patients with joints at end-stage disease.

Surgery

Surgery is indicated in patients who fail to respond to nonoperative management and especially in those with unremitting pain. In the earlier stages of arthritis, an arthroscopic washout and cartilage débridement of the ankle joint may provide significant improvement in pain levels. As the disease progresses, more extensive surgery is required. Many different variations and techniques of fusion have been described, ranging from minimally invasive arthroscopic arthrodesis to open fusion with hardware.[1-6] Total ankle joint replacement (arthroplasty) has been an alternative to ankle fusion since the 1970s in certain select populations of patients. It has undergone a series of alterations because the earlier generation models were more prone to failure and unpredictable results.[7] To date, there are no level I studies showing better cost-effectiveness[8] or better performance than the "gold standard," ankle fusion.[9] Selection of patients is of paramount importance; those with high demands (hiking, tennis, running) may be better served with a more predictable, stable fusion than with a replacement that has a high likelihood of failure and need of revision.

POTENTIAL DISEASE COMPLICATIONS

Progressive immobility, permanent loss of motion of the ankle joint, bone collapse leading to leg length discrepancy, and chronic intractable pain can result from ankle arthritis.

POTENTIAL TREATMENT COMPLICATIONS

Analgesics and nonsteroidal anti-inflammatory drugs have well-known side effects that most commonly affect the gastric, hepatic, and renal systems. Arthroscopy can be complicated by nerve damage or, rarely, septic arthritis. On occasion, with arthrodesis, fusion can fail to occur.[10] An alteration in gait is common.[11] Arthroplasty complications include infection, thromboembolism, bone collapse, and implant migration.

References

1. Richardson EG. Arthrodesis of ankle, knee and hip. In Canale ST, ed. Campbell's Operative Orthopaedics, 9th ed. St. Louis, Mosby, 1988:165-182.
2. Thordarson DB. Ankle and hindfoot arthritis: fusion techniques. In Craig EV, ed. Clinical Orthopaedics. Philadelphia, Lippincott Williams & Wilkins, 1999:883-890.
3. Mann RA, Van Manen JW, Wapner K, Martin J. Ankle fusion. Clin Orthop 1991;268:49-55.
4. Morgan CD, Henke JA, Bailey RW, Kaufer H. Long-term results of tibiotalar arthrodesis. J Bone Joint Surg Am 1985;67:546-550.
5. Kile TA. Ankle arthrodesis. In Morrey B, ed. Reconstructive Surgery of the Joints, 2nd ed. New York, Churchill Livingstone, 1996: 1771-1787.
6. Kile TA, Donnelly RE, Gehrke JC, et al. Tibiotalocalcaneal arthrodesis with an intramedullary device. Foot Ankle 1994;15: 669-673.
7. McGuire MR, Kyle RF, Gustilo RB, Premer RF. Comparative analysis of ankle arthroplasty versus ankle arthrodesis. Clin Orthop Relat Res 1988;226:174-181.
8. SooHoo NF, Kominski G. Cost-effectiveness analysis of total ankle arthroplasty. J Bone Joint Surg Am 2004;86:2446-2455.
9. Stengel D, Bauwens K, Ekkernkamp A, Cramer J. Efficacy of total ankle replacements with meniscal bearing devices: a systematic review and meta-analysis. Arch Orthop Trauma Surg 2005;125: 109-119.
10. Smith RW. Ankle arthrodesis. In Thompson RC, Johnson KA, eds. Master Techniques in Orthopaedic Surgery. The Foot and Ankle. Philadelphia, Raven Press, 1994:467-482.
11. Mazur JM, Schwartz E, Simon SR. Ankle arthrodesis: long-term follow-up with gait analysis. J Bone Joint Surg Am 1979;61: 964-975.

Foot and Ankle Bursitis 74

Allen N. Wilkins, MD, Daniel Sipple, DO, and Thomas H. Hudgins, MD

Synonyms

Fluid-filled sac of fibrous tissue
Glandular sac (a pouch at a joint to lessen friction)
Haglund deformity
Albert disease
Calcaneus altus
Cucumber heel
High-prow heel
Knobby heel
Prow beak deformity
Pump bump
Retrocalcaneal bursitis
Tendo Achilles bursitis
Winter heel
Hatchet-shaped heel
Achillodynia

ICD-9 Codes

726.71   Achilles bursitis or tendinitis
726.79   Retrocalcaneal bursitis
727.2   Specific bursitis often of occupational origin
727.3   Other bursitis disorders

DEFINITION

Bursae are closed sacs lined by a synovium-like membrane; they contain synovial fluid and are usually located in areas that are subject to friction. Their purpose is to mitigate friction and thus to facilitate the motion that occurs between bones and tendons, bones and skin, or tendons and ligaments.[1]

Bursae are classified according to their location, as shown in Table 74-1.[1,2]

Symptomatic malleolar bursae most likely result from abnormal contact pressures. They may also be secondary to shear forces that arise between the bony malleoli and the patient's footwear, particularly boots or athletic shoes that surround the ankle. These may occur either medially or laterally. However, medial bursae are more common.[1] The bone prominences of the malleoli have little inherent soft tissue to protect them from these excessive pressures. The body responds to this abnormal stress by developing an adventitious bursa at this site.

The skin and subcutaneous tissues are then able to glide over the bone prominences and thus dissipate these excessive forces. Eventually, these bursae may become inflamed, resulting in bursitis.

The posterior heel includes the retrocalcaneal bursa, which is located between the calcaneus and the Achilles tendon insertion site, and the retroachilles bursa, which is located between the Achilles tendon and the skin. Each bursa is a potential site of inflammation. The most common cause of posterior heel bursitis is ill-fitting footwear with a stiff posterior edge that abrades the area of the Achilles tendon insertion.

Retrocalcaneal inflammation may also be associated with a prominence of the posterosuperior lateral aspect of the calcaneus, causing irritation of the bursa, particularly from a poor-fitting shoe. This condition is called Haglund deformity. This entity often goes hand-in-hand with retrocalcaneal bursitis, and frequently there is an element of insertional tendinitis as well. The term *pump bump* has also been used to describe this condition.

Although Haglund deformity is more commonly found in women who wear high-heeled shoes, it is sometimes found in hockey players who wear a rigid heel counter that causes irritation. The population of patients that has this superolateral bone prominence tends to be younger than the patients with retrocalcaneal bursitis.[3]

Numerous biomechanical risk factors have been associated with Haglund deformity. These include a high-arched cavus foot, rearfoot varus, rearfoot equinus, and trauma to the apophysis in childhood[4-6] (Fig. 74-1).

Bursitis can also occur in the forefoot and may involve the intermetatarsal bursae or the adventitial bursae beneath the metatarsal heads.[2]

Risk factors for foot and ankle bursitis are outlined in Table 74-2. Runners, especially those who train uphill, sustain repeated ankle dorsiflexion. The retrocalcaneal bursa lies between the Achilles tendon and calcaneus and is compressed with each motion. Repetitive stress through this motion can lead to bursitis. Also, runners and recreational walkers with sudden increase in mileage are at risk for acquiring symptoms of tenderness, swelling, redness, and pain near the insertion of the Achilles tendon.

415

TABLE 74-1 Classification of Bursae According to Location

Bursal Type	Examples	Description
Deep	Retrocalcaneal	Found beneath the fibrous investing fascia Develop in utero Often communicate with joints
Subcutaneous	Olecranon, prepatellar	Develop during childhood Do not normally communicate with the adjacent joint
Adventitious	Malleolar, metatarsal head	Often have a thick, fibrous wall Are susceptible to inflammatory changes

TABLE 74-2 Risk Factors for Foot and Ankle Bursitis

Type of Bursitis	Risk Factors
Malleolar	Commonly found in repetitive overactivity in boot-wearing athletes, such as ice skaters
Retrocalcaneal	Athletic overactivity associated with repetitive trauma Most common in long-distance runners who run uphill as a training method Hindfoot varus Rigid plantar-flexed first ray
Retroachilles	Commonly found in women who wear high-heeled shoes In the athletic population, it is often found in hockey players who wear a rigid heel counter that causes irritation Retrocalcaneal bursitis Achilles tendinitis High-arched cavus foot Hindfoot varus Hindfoot equinus Trauma to the apophysis in childhood
Metatarsal	First metatarsal: dancers, squash players, or skiers Second to fourth metatarsals: chronic inflammatory arthritis

The most common cause of ankle bursitis is tight-fitting shoes with a firm heel counter. Women wearing high-heeled shoes, runners with improper shoe fit or overworn footwear, skaters, and patients with lower extremity edema are susceptible.

Other important causes of bursitis, in general, are trauma, infection, rheumatoid arthritis, and gout.

SYMPTOMS

The symptoms of bursitis are described in Table 74-3.

With malleolar bursitis, there may be exquisite tenderness surrounding the inflamed bursa, a fluctuant mass over the medial malleolus, and decreased range of motion of the ankle.

Retrocalcaneal bursitis is hallmarked by pain that is anterior to the Achilles tendon and just superior to its insertion on the os calcis. Compression of the bursa between the calcaneus and the Achilles tendon occurs every time the ankle is dorsiflexed; in a runner, the repetitions are countless, particularly with uphill running, when ankle dorsiflexion is increased. Patients often develop a limp, and wearing of shoes may eventually become increasingly painful. Thus, it is not surprising that long-distance runners who use uphill running as a training method frequently develop retrocalcaneal bursitis.

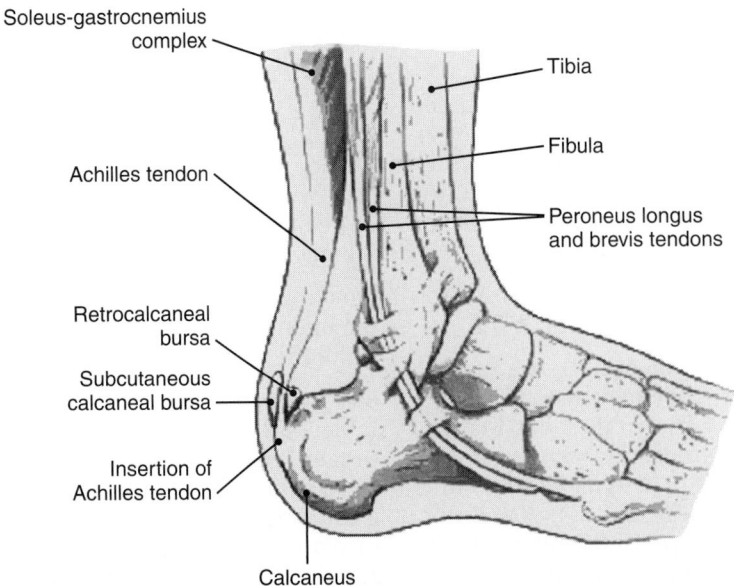

FIGURE 74-1. The anatomy of the structures around the ankle joint. (Reprinted with permission from Morelli V, James E. Achilles tendonopathy and tendon rupture: conservative versus surgical management. Prim Care 2004;31:1039-1054.)

TABLE 74-3 Bursitis—Symptoms

Type of Bursitis	Symptoms
Malleolar	Tender swelling at the malleolus
Retrocalcaneal	Posterior heel pain that is anterior to the Achilles tendon, just superior to Achilles insertion, and made worse by ankle dorsiflexion Tender swelling behind the ankle
Retroachilles	Often asymptomatic Tender swelling behind the ankle
Metatarsal	Throbbing pain under a metatarsal head that usually persists at rest and is exacerbated when the area is first loaded

Patients with retroachilles bursitis are often asymptomatic. However, when symptoms occur, the patient usually presents with a painful, tender subcutaneous swelling overlying the Achilles tendon, usually at the level of the shoe counter. The overlying skin may be hyperkeratotic or reddened.

Patients with metatarsal bursitis usually have exquisite tenderness surrounding the inflamed bursa, swelling over the metatarsal head, and decreased range of motion of the metatarsophalangeal joint.

PHYSICAL EXAMINATION

The physical examination findings in bursitis are described in Table 74-4.

The physical examination includes inspection of the patient's foot at rest and in a weight-bearing position. A visual survey of the foot may reveal swelling, bone deformities, bruising, or skin breaks. The physician should palpate bone prominences and tendinous insertions near the heel and midfoot, noting any tenderness or palpable defects. Passive range of motion of the foot

and ankle joints is assessed for indications of restricted movement. Foot posture and arch formation are visually examined while the patient is bearing weight; the physician is looking for abnormal pronation or other biomechanical irregularities.

In general, the site of the inflamed bursa is fluctuant and may have some mild associated tenderness and warmth. The patient should be examined closely for any erythema, edema, hypersensitivity, fever, or swollen lymph nodes to rule out septic bursitis.

Insertional tendinosis involves degeneration, not inflammation, of the most distal portion of the Achilles tendon and its attachment on the calcaneal tuberosity. Distinguishing insertional Achilles tendinosis from retrocalcaneal bursitis or osseous impingement, although desirable, is difficult because both may be a continuum of the same disease process and can coexist.

FUNCTIONAL LIMITATIONS

Adhesions of the surface of a bursa limit the degree of movement of the associated joint. Pain is a common cause of decreased function. The patient may be limited in ambulation, climbing stairs, and sports activity. The patient also may be limited in footwear, such as protective boots for work.

DIAGNOSTIC STUDIES

Careful physical examination will often yield the cause of most heel pain. Nonetheless, physicians often order radiographs to aid in the diagnostic workup and to exclude osseous causes of the pain. The radiographic findings of bursitis are listed in Table 74-5.

Levy and colleagues[7] demonstrated that routine radiographs are of limited value in the initial evaluation of nontraumatic plantar heel pain in adults and are not necessary in the initial evaluation. They suggested that radiographs should be reserved for patients who do not

TABLE 74-4 Bursitis—Physical Findings

Type of Bursitis	Physical Findings
Malleolar	Painful, tender subcutaneous swelling overlying the malleolus Overlying skin may be hyperkeratotic or reddened.
Retrocalcaneal	Tenderness and bogginess along the medial and lateral aspects of the Achilles tendon at its insertion Posterior heel pain with passive ankle dorsiflexion Posterior heel pain with active resisted plantar flexion A positive two-finger squeeze test result: pain elicited by application of pressure both medially and laterally with two fingers just superior and anterior to the Achilles insertion
Retroachilles	Painful, tender subcutaneous swelling overlying the Achilles tendon, usually at the level of the shoe counter, and on lateral side of Achilles tendon Overlying skin may be hyperkeratotic or reddened.
Metatarsal	If a superficial bursa is affected, there will be signs of acute inflammation, with fluctuant swelling and warmth. If a deep bursa is affected, tissues are tight and congested. Pain with direct pressure, compression, or dorsiflexion of the associated digit An overlying callus may suggest that this is a high-pressure site during normal gait.

TABLE 74-5 Bursitis—Radiographic Findings

Type of Bursitis	Radiographic Findings
Malleolar	Diagnosis is essentially clinical, and further evaluation is not required.
Retrocalcaneal	Magnetic resonance imaging shows a bursal fluid collection with low signal intensity on T1-weighted images and high signal intensity on T2-weighted and STIR images. A bursa larger than 1 mm anteroposteriorly, 7 mm craniocaudally, or 11 mm transversely is considered abnormal.[14]
Retroachilles	Diagnosis is essentially clinical, and further evaluation is not required. It may be discovered incidentally at magnetic resonance imaging performed to evaluate other heel injuries. Its appearance is similar to that of retrocalcaneal bursitis and consists of a bursal fluid collection just posterior to the distal Achilles tendon.
Metatarsal	Magnetic resonance imaging shows a well-defined fluid collection at a pressure point and demonstrates low signal intensity on T1-weighted images and high signal intensity on T2-weighted and STIR images. Small fluid collections with a transverse diameter of 3 mm or less in the first three intermetatarsal bursae may be physiologic. Peripheral enhancement is with gadopentetate dimeglumine.[15]

improve as expected or present with an unusual history or confounding physical findings.

Multiple studies have attempted to delineate Haglund deformity radiographically by looking at the height, length, and angular relationships of the calcaneus. Most authors cannot recommend one particular radiographic view as being consistently helpful in demonstrating this bone prominence or in making a diagnosis or planning treatment.

Differential Diagnosis

Metatarsal Bursitis
Trauma

Freiberg infarction

Infection

Arthritis

Tendon disorders

Non-neoplastic masses

Neoplasms

Ankle or Heel Bursitis
Achilles tendinitis

Calcaneus stress fracture

Rheumatoid arthritis

Gout

Seronegative spondyloarthropathies

Sural neuritis

TREATMENT

The treatment of bursitis is summarized in Table 74-6.

Initial

In general, nonoperative treatment of foot and ankle bursitis is always recommended first. Conservative treatment of heel pain, in general, includes use of nonsteroidal anti-inflammatory agents, physical therapy, and avoidance of repetitive high-impact activities.[8] If there is some associated Achilles tendon or plantar fascia disease present, a night splint may help relieve the acute pain many patients experience when they first get up in the morning.

Conservative treatment of general heel pain also includes use of heel lifts and open-back shoes. A portion of the heel counter can be cut away and replaced with a soft leather insert to cause less friction at the site where the heel counter meets the skin. Shoes without laces are to be avoided because they inherently fit close to the heel. Insertion of a heel cup in the shoe may help raise the inflamed region slightly above the restricting heel counter of the shoe. A heel cup also should be placed in the other shoe to avoid introducing leg length discrepancy. Pressure-off silicone sheet pads can be used long term when shoes with counters are worn. Custom orthotics are prescribed for those who have underlying structural abnormalities causing the symptoms.

Rehabilitation

The rehabilitation of bursitis is described in Table 74-7.

The patient is allowed weight bearing as tolerated and should be instructed to elevate the foot when not walking. If the patient has had surgery, the dressing is removed 3 days postoperatively, and the patient is allowed to shower. The patient is encouraged to perform active range of motion exercises at least three times a day for 10 minutes each time. The patient is allowed to wear regular shoes as soon as this is tolerated.

Physical therapy is used to teach stretching exercises of the Achilles tendon and plantar fascia to preserve range of motion. This gradual progressive stretching of the Achilles tendon may help relieve impingement on the subtendinous bursa. Stretching of the Achilles tendon can be performed in the following manner: place

TABLE 74-6 Bursitis—Treatment

Type of Bursitis	Treatment
Malleolar	Boot modification or change of footwear Doughnut-shaped cushion made to fit over malleoli Rest and activity modification
Retrocalcaneal	Rest and activity modification (e.g., avoidance of running and walking up hills and stairs) Encourage athletes to change running shoes on a regular basis Biomechanical control in the form of temporary heel lifts, tape immobilization, and, if abnormal pronation is present, custom foot orthotics Slight heel elevation with a felt heel pad A night splint to help keep the Achilles tendon and plantar fascia stretched to relieve acute morning pain and stiffness
Retroachilles	Rest and activity modification Heat application Padding Wearing a soft, nonrestrictive shoe without a counter (e.g., clogs, sandals)
Metatarsal	Rest and activity modification Protective padding Assess for any underlying deformity or foot type with abnormal function

TABLE 74-7 Bursitis—Rehabilitation

Type of Bursitis	Rehabilitation
Malleolar	Physical therapy is usually not necessary unless joint range of motion is affected. Physical therapy is then necessary to maintain ankle range of motion.
Retrocalcaneal	Physical therapy to teach stretching exercises of the Achilles tendon and plantar fascia Ice can be applied for 15 to 20 minutes, several times a day, during the acute period. Some clinicians also advocate use of contrast baths. Alternative means of maintaining strength and cardiovascular fitness include swimming, water aerobics, and other aquatic exercises.
Retroachilles	Physical therapy to teach stretching exercises of the Achilles tendon

the affected foot flat on the floor and lean forward toward the wall until a gentle stretch is felt within the ipsilateral Achilles tendon; maintain the stretch for 20 to 60 seconds and then relax. These stretches should be performed with the knee extended and repeated with the knee flexed. To maximize the benefit of the stretching program, repeat for several stretches per set, several times per day. Avoid ballistic (abrupt, jerking) stretches.

Contrast baths and ice massage are also used in the acute management. Icing can be performed for 15 to 20 minutes, several times a day, during the acute period.

The athlete may be expected to return to play without restrictions after demonstrating resolution of symptoms, resolution of physical examination findings (e.g., limping,

tenderness on palpation), and adequate performance of sports-specific practice drills without recurrence of symptoms or physical examination findings.

Procedures

If the patient remains symptomatic or finds the bursa to be aesthetically displeasing, the bursa can be aspirated and injected with a 1- to 2-mL solution of a corticosteroid, such as betamethasone. Many clinicians prefer not to repeat this injection more than once, resulting in a maximum of two injections. This stems from the belief that the risk of tendon rupture is not worth the limited benefits offered by corticosteroid injection. However, tendon rupture is a known complication when corticosteroids are injected directly into the tendon substance.[9,10] There is no available evidence-based literature suggesting an association between corticosteroid injections of ankle bursae and Achilles tendon rupture.

Surgery

About 10% of patients with retrocalcaneal or supracalcaneal bursitis do not respond to conservative treatment and seek a surgical solution. Open surgical techniques focus on resection of the posterosuperior portion of the calcaneus or performance of a calcaneal wedge osteotomy with or without débridement of diseased Achilles tendon. Endoscopic techniques provide visualization of the tendon-bone relationship with endoscopic inspection and allow precise débridement and evaluation for residual impingement. The smaller access allows easier closure and less extensive postoperative care. The small incision minimizes the potential for wound dehiscence, a painful scar, and nerve entrapment in scar tissue, and it provides a cosmetically superior result. The level of postoperative pain and the time to recovery are similar to those after the open procedure.

POTENTIAL DISEASE COMPLICATIONS

The primary disease complication is chronic bursitis with intractable pain that may limit footwear and joint mobility. Adhesive bursitis is another potential disease complication that may occur with chronic bursitis. In adhesive bursitis, two adjacent layers of the bursa may adhere and significantly decrease joint range of motion.

The course of bursitis may also be complicated by infection. Septic bursitis occurs when a bursa becomes infected. In this case, immediate surgical débridement and intravenous antibiotics are indicated. A *Staphylococcus aureus* organism is most often responsible and should be treated with appropriate antibiotics.

POTENTIAL TREATMENT COMPLICATIONS

Complications of open, endoscopic, and fluoroscopic surgical procedures include skin breakdown, avulsion of the Achilles tendon, inadequate decompression with recurrent pain, sensitive and disfiguring scars, altered sensation, and stiffness. In one series, open treatment was associated with a 14% rate of infection, a 17% rate of wound breakdown, a 23% rate of scar tenderness, and a 38% rate of altered sensation.[11]

The role of corticosteroid injections in the treatment of retrocalcaneal bursitis is controversial. There have been numerous case reports of patients who have sustained a tendon rupture after peritendinous injections of corticosteroids for the treatment of tendinitis or tendinosis. Little has been reported, however, on retrocalcaneal intrabursal injections for the treatment of bursitis. Martin and associates[12] investigated the mechanical properties and histologic changes in rabbit Achilles tendons after peritendinous steroid injection. They found that local injections of corticosteroid, both within the tendon substance and into the retrocalcaneal bursa, adversely affected the biomechanical properties of rabbit Achilles tendons. Another animal study also showed adverse effects of local injections of corticosteroid (within the tendon substance and into the retrocalcaneal bursa) on the biomechanical properties of Achilles tendons.[13]

Prolonged immobilization may result in adhesions and subsequent joint stiffening.

References

1. Brown TD, Varney TE, Micheli LJ. Malleolar bursitis in figure skaters: indications for operative and nonoperative treatment. Am J Sports Med 2000;28:109-111.
2. Ashman CJ, Klecker RJ, Yu JS. Forefoot pain involving the metatarsal region: differential diagnosis with MR imaging. Radiographics 2001;21:1425-1440.
3. Schepsis AA, Jones H, Hass AL. Achilles tendon disorders in athletes. Am J Sports Med 2002;30:287-305.
4. Clement DB, Taunton JE, Smart GW, et al. A survey of overuse running injuries. Physician Sportsmed 1981;9:47-58.
5. James SL, Bates BT, Osternig LR. Injuries to runners. Am J Sports Med 1978;6:40-50.
6. Krissoff WB, Ferris WD. Runners' injuries. Physician Sportsmed 1979;7:54-64.
7. Levy JC, Mizel MS, Clifford PD, Temple HT. Value of radiographs in the initial evaluation of nontraumatic adult heel pain. Foot Ankle Int 2006;27:427-430.
8. Mazzone MF, McCue T. Common conditions of the Achilles tendon. Am Fam Physician 2002;65:1805-1810.
9. Morelli V, James E. Achilles tendonopathy and tendon rupture: conservative versus surgical management. Prim Care 2004;31:1039-1054.
10. Wilson JJ, Best TM. Common overuse tendon problems: a review and recommendations for treatment. Am Fam Physician 2005;72:811-818.
11. Taylor GJ. Prominence of the calcaneus: is operation justified? J Bone Joint Surg Br 1986;68:467-470.
12. Martin DF, Carlson CS, Berry J, et al. Effect of injected versus iontophoretic corticosteroid on the rabbit tendon. South Med J 1999;92:600-608.
13. Hugate R, Pennypacker J, Saunders M, Juliano P. The effects of corticosteroids on biomechanical properties of rabbit Achilles tendons. J Bone Joint Surg Am 2004;86:794-801.
14. Narváez JA, Narváez J, Ortega R, et al. Painful heel: MR imaging findings. Radiographics 2000;20:333-352.
15. West SG, Woodburn J. ABC of rheumatology: pain in the foot. BMJ 1995;310:860-864.

Ankle Sprain 75

Brian J. Krabak, MD, MBA, and Jennifer Baima, MD

Synonym

Inversion sprain

ICD-9 Code

845.00   Sprains and strains of the ankle and foot

DEFINITION

Ankle sprain involves stretching or tearing of the ligaments of the ankle. According to O'Donoghue,[1] there are three grades of ankle sprain as determined by the extent of ligamentous injury. This injury is a common cause of morbidity in the general population, and the ankle is the most commonly injured joint complex among athletes.[2] Patients who play sports experience approximately one ankle sprain for every 1000 person-days of competition.[3] It is estimated that more than 23,000 ankle sprains require medical care in the United States per day.[4] Eighty-five percent of all ankle sprains occur on the lateral aspect of the ankle, involving the anterior talofibular ligament and calcaneofibular ligament (Fig. 75-1). Another 5% to 10% are syndesmotic injuries or high ankle sprains, which involve a partial tear of the distal anterior tibiofibular ligament. Identification of syndesmotic sprains is important; they may have a prolonged recovery compared with milder lateral ankle sprains and are more likely to require surgery. Only 5% of all ankle sprains involve the medial aspect of the ankle, as the strong medial deltoid ligament is quite resistant to tear. Most ankle sprains will recover during several weeks to months; only 20% to 40% result in chronic sequelae.[5] An ankle sprain that does not heal may be caused by injuries to other structures and will necessitate further investigation for other causes.[6]

Ligamentous injuries are categorized into three gradations:

- Grade I is a partial tear without laxity and only mild edema.
- Grade II is a partial tear with mild laxity and moderate pain, tenderness, and instability.
- Grade III is a complete rupture resulting in considerable swelling, increased pain, significant laxity, and often an unstable joint (Fig. 75-2).

Sprains and strains are the most common lower extremity injuries sustained during recreation. Patients aged 5 to 24 years have the highest incidence of injuries. Overall, basketball is the most common activity during which sports- and recreation-related injuries occur.[7] Female basketball players are 25% more likely than their male counterparts to suffer mild ankle sprains. However, there is no known increased risk for moderate to severe ankle sprain in female athletes.[8] The prognosis is overall worse in younger patients, presumably because of resultant ligamentous laxity.[9]

SYMPTOMS

Acutely, the injured patient will report pain and tenderness over the injured ligaments. Some patients hear an initial "pop" at the time of injury. Initially, they may have difficulty weight bearing on the injured ankle and with subsequent ambulation. Usually, the patient notes swelling around the area of injury and may report some ecchymosis after several days. Decreased function and range of motion along with instability are seen more often in grade II and grade III injuries. There may be sensory symptoms in the superficial or deep peroneal nerve territory.

PHYSICAL EXAMINATION

Inspection of the ankle will reveal edema and sometimes ecchymoses around the area of injury. Range of motion of the ankle joint may be limited by associated swelling and pain. Palpation should include the anterior talofibular and calcaneofibular ligaments, syndesmotic area, and medial deltoid ligament. In addition, the examiner should palpate the distal fibula, medial malleolus, base of the fifth metatarsal, cuboid, lateral process of the talus (snowboarder's fracture), and epiphyseal areas to assess for any potential fractures.[10] Although it is uncommon, ankle inversion injuries are associated with peroneal nerve injury and may result in sensory changes on the dorsum of the foot (superficial peroneal nerve) or the first web space (deep peroneal nerve). Deep peroneal nerve injury could result in decreased strength in dorsiflexion and eversion.

421

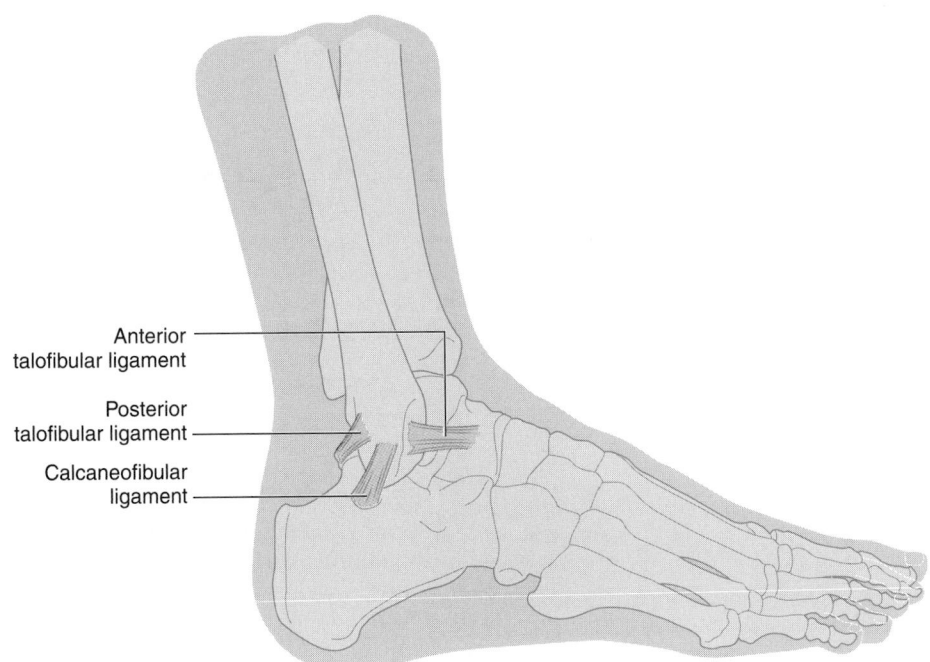

Anterior talofibular ligament

Posterior talofibular ligament

Calcaneofibular ligament

FIGURE 75-1. Ligaments of the lateral ankle.

Ankle stability should be examined through a variety of tests and compared with the noninjured side to assess the amount of abnormal translation in the joint.[11,12] The anterior drawer test of the ankle will assess the integrity of the anterior talofibular ligament. It is performed by plantar flexing the ankle to approximately 30 degrees and applying an anterior force to the calcaneus while stabilizing the tibia with the other hand. Increased translation compared with the other side implies injury to the anterior talofibular ligament. The talar tilt test (Fig. 75-3) is done with the ankle in neutral and assesses the integrity of the calcaneofibular ligament. The squeeze test (Fig. 75-4) is used to diagnose a syndesmotic injury. It is performed by squeezing the proximal fibula and tibia at the midcalf and causes pain over the syndesmotic area. Similarly, the external rotation stress test is performed by placing the ankle in a neutral position and externally rotating the tibia, leading to pain in the syndesmotic region. However, some cadaver studies have demonstrated poor correlation between clinical stress test results and the degree of ligamentous disruption.[11,13]

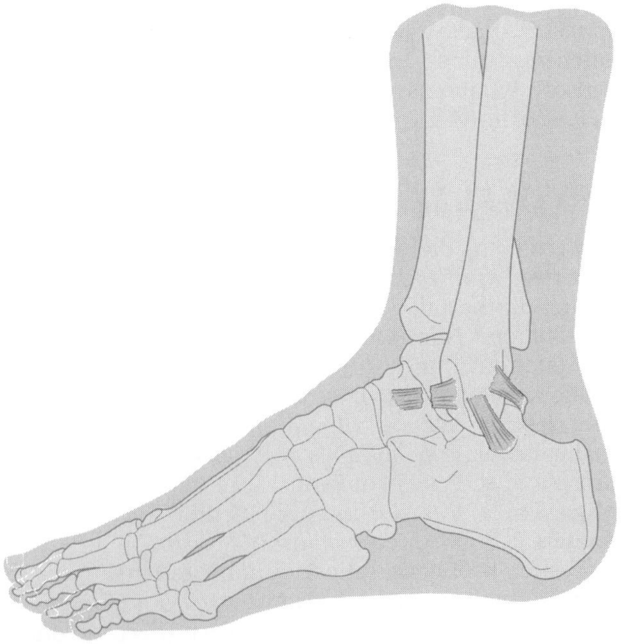

The patient should be examined for decreased range of motion, strength deficits, or reflex abnormalities, which could reveal concurrent injury. Reduced dorsiflexion range of motion may predispose the joint to an ankle sprain.[14] Low lumbar radiculopathy can present with isolated ankle pain, although there will not be associated soft tissue edema with this condition. Although pes planus may predispose to stress fractures, there is no association of pes planus with increased incidence of ankle sprain.[15]

FUNCTIONAL LIMITATIONS

The patient may have difficulty in walking secondary to pain and swelling. Proprioception and balance on the injured ankle will be abnormal as noted by greater difficulty with single-leg standing on the injured leg.[16] The athlete will have difficulty with return to play until swelling and pain have diminished and rehabilitation is nearly completed. Incomplete recovery or inadequate rehabilitation may predispose the patient to reinjury.[17]

FIGURE 75-2. Grade III ankle sprain with a complete tear of the anterior talofibular ligament.

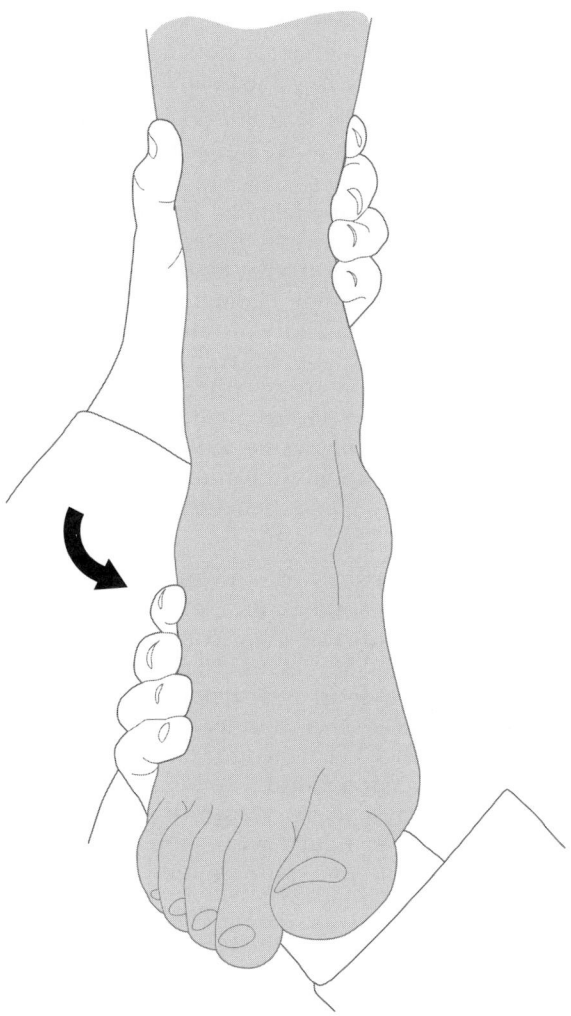

FIGURE 75-3. The talar tilt (inversion stress) test of the ankle.

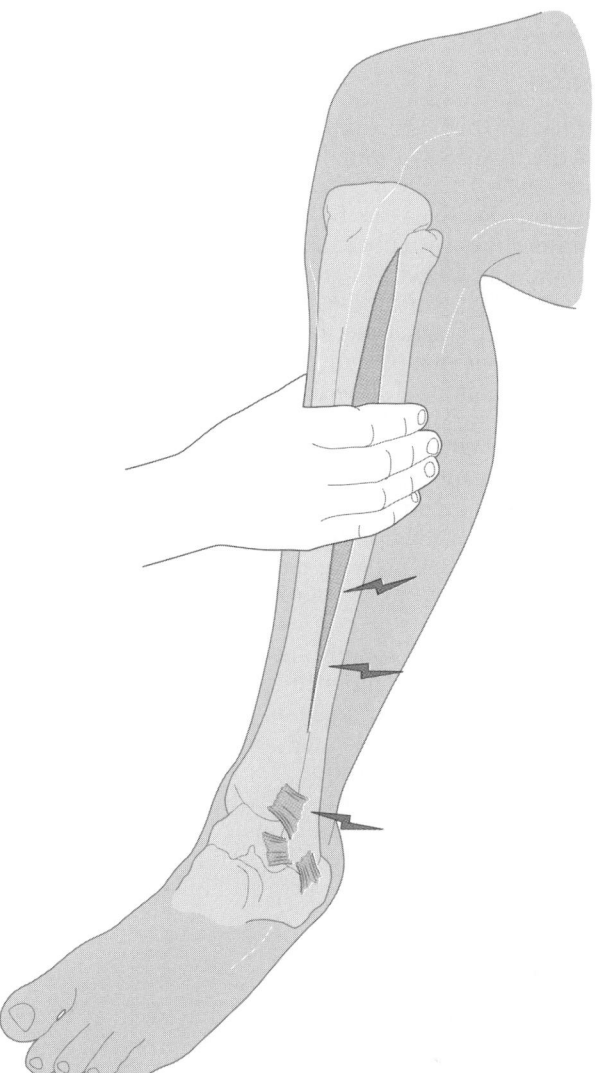

FIGURE 75-4. The squeeze test detects tears of the syndesmosis. The test result is positive when squeezing of the midcalf produces pain in the distal interosseous membrane and syndesmosis.

Of note, the single-leg balance test can be helpful in predicting which athletes may sustain an ankle injury.[18] Chronic ankle sprains can result in mechanical instability, with objective instability or laxity noted on examination in all patients.[19]

DIAGNOSTIC STUDIES

Standard anteroposterior, mortise, and lateral radiographs should be considered in cases in which there is tenderness over the lateral malleolus, ankle joint, syndesmosis, or other bony structure to rule out an underlying fracture.[10] In addition, radiographs should be considered when the athlete is unable to bear weight immediately and on subsequent evaluation. At 4 to 6 weeks, a slowly healing lateral ankle injury without significant pain resolution or improvement should be evaluated radiographically if an initial radiograph was not obtained. A magnetic resonance imaging scan can help identify the soft tissue disease as well as evaluate the osteochondral joint surface when the ankle does not heal despite adequate rehabilitation. Stress radiographs are optional and have questionable reliability because of the great spectrum of normal.[20]

Differential Diagnosis

High ankle sprain, syndesmotic sprain

Osteochondral fracture of the talar dome

Neurapraxia of the common, superficial, or deep peroneal nerve

Fracture of the lateral process of the talus (snowboarder's fracture)

Avulsion or fracture of the tip of the fibula

Fracture of the base of the fifth metatarsal

Peroneal tendon injury

Subtalar joint instability[12]

Posterior impingement or fracture of the os trigonum

TREATMENT

Initial

Protection, rest, ice, compression, and elevation (PRICE) are the mainstay of initial treatment and are introduced immediately. Crutches should be used if weight bearing causes pain; they can be discontinued as ambulatory pain declines (usually in 2 to 3 days). Grade III sprains may require longer use of assistive devices. The duration of disability with these sprains ranges from $4^{1}/_{2}$ to 26 weeks.[21] Patients should be cautioned to avoid hanging the ankle in a plantar flexed position because it may stretch the injured anterior talofibular ligament. Positioning in maximum dorsiflexion also minimizes resultant joint effusion.[22] Plastic removable walking cast boots or air splints are occasionally used in higher grade injuries until pain-free weight bearing is achieved. This can be weeks to months, depending on the extent of injury. Most patients have returned to prior activities by 6 weeks but may prefer to use bracing for persistent disability. Regardless of severity of ankle sprain, patients with syndesmosis sprains are most likely to experience prolonged functional deficit up to 6 months.[23] The use of an air stirrup brace together with an elastic wrap has been shown to decrease the interval to preinjury function.[24] Local ice applications for 20 to 30 minutes three or four times daily combined with compression immediately after injury is effective in decreasing edema, pain, and dysfunction. Nonsteroidal anti-inflammatory drugs are employed to decrease pain and inflammation.[25]

Rehabilitation

Rehabilitation is aimed at minimizing swelling, decreasing pain, and preventing chronic ankle problems. Various modalities, such as ultrasound and electrical stimulation, are used as needed during the rehabilitative phase to decrease pain and edema starting 24 to 48 hours after injury. Achilles stretching is begun to avoid disuse contracture. Active range of motion is initially performed without resistance. Dorsiflexion and eversion strengthening can be started with static exercises and progress to concentric and eccentric exercises with tubing when the patient tolerates pain-free weight bearing. These muscles are responsible for actively resisting an inversion–plantar flexion injury.[24] Double-leg toe raises should progress to single-leg and can be done in water if they are not tolerated on land. Endurance and lower extremity strengthening are incorporated and increased as functional exercises are begun. Proprioception training can start in a seated position and then advance to standing balance exercises. Standing exercises begin with single-leg stance while swinging the raised leg. Then, single-leg squats are required. Finally, exercises progress to single-leg stance and functional or sport-specific activity, such as dribbling, catching, or kicking. Poor proprioception is a major cause of repeated sprain and chronic functional instability.[18,26,27] In athletes, when forward running is pain free, agility drills that mimic their sport or activity are added. Skipping rope may be beneficial in the later stages of rehabilitation. There is evidence that patients with chronic ankle instability have decreased hip abduction strength.[28] In general, functional skills that gradually stress the lower extremity will be added as strength and range of motion are obtained and balance is improved.

The use of orthotic bracing is somewhat controversial. Bracing and taping may decrease recurrent injury rates in the previously injured ankle, but they have not been shown to be effective in athletes without a prior injury.[29,30] A study suggests that treatment of first-time grade I and grade II ankle ligament sprains with the air stirrup brace combined with an elastic wrap provides earlier return to preinjury function than with use of the air stirrup brace alone, an elastic wrap alone, or a walking cast for 10 days.[24] Bracing and proprioception training along with peroneal muscle strengthening are strongly recommended to decrease reinjury. These may play a beneficial role in preventing first-time injuries as well.

Orthotic shoe inserts, with the exception of ankle braces, do not have a role in preventing ankle sprain.[15] Athletes should purchase new competitive footwear every 12 months or 500 miles. The main function of ankle braces is to restrict inversion.[31] Consequently, shoes with a raised heel counter may predispose to ankle sprain as they place the foot in increased plantar flexion and inversion during ambulation. Heat and contrast baths have been shown to increase ankle edema after acute injury and should be avoided acutely.[32] As such, cryotherapy should be the standard of care for these injuries.

Procedures

Procedures are generally not done in ankle sprains.

Surgery

Surgery is rare for ankle sprains. Most grade III ankle sprains with complete tears of the anterior talofibular ligament and instability are *not* treated surgically. If necessary, surgical repair may be completed after the sports season and is usually successful. Reconstruction of the lateral ankle ligaments involves anatomic reconstruction of the ligament (modified Brostrom) and tendon weaving through the fibula (Watson-Jones, Chrisman-Snook).[33] The direct repair of the ligament, even years after the injury, can be highly successful.

On occasion, the patient with an ankle sprain that does not heal with proper time and rehabilitation may undergo arthroscopic evaluation for other sources of disease.

POTENTIAL DISEASE COMPLICATIONS

Recurrent sprains may lead to both mechanical (gross laxity) and functional (giving way) instability. The patient may present with undiagnosed secondary sources of pain, and these must be sought (see the section on differential diagnosis). Chronic intractable pain is another potential complication.

POTENTIAL TREATMENT COMPLICATIONS

Lack of recognition of and the prevalence of subacute sequelae in ankle sprains may lead to undertreatment and subsequent chronic pain or instability. Nonsteroidal anti-inflammatory drugs may cause gastric, hepatic, or renal complications. Return to work, sport, or activity before adequate healing and rehabilitation may result in chronic pain and giving way (functional instability) and gross laxity (mechanical instability). As noted, the heat and contrast baths should be avoided during the acute stage of injury as these modalities could promote swelling and bleeding.

References

1. O'Donoghue DH. Treatment of Injuries to Athletes. Philadelphia, WB Saunders, 1976:698-746.
2. Braun B. Effects of ankle sprain in a general clinic population 6 to 18 months after medical evaluation. Arch Fam Med 1999;8:143-148.
3. Beynnon BD, Vacek PM, Murphy D, et al. First-time inversion ankle ligament trauma: the effects of sex, level of competition, and sport on incidence of injury. Am J Sports Med 2005;33:1485-1491.
4. Garrick JG, Regina RK. The epidemiology of foot and ankle injuries in sports. Clin Sports Med 1988;17:29-36.
5. Safran MR, Benedetti RS, Bartolozzi AR 3rd, Mandelbaum BR. Lateral ankle sprains: a comprehensive review. Part 1: etiology, pathoanatomy, histopathogenesis, and diagnosis. Med Sci Sports Exerc 1999;31(Suppl 7):S429-S437.
6. Renstrom PA. Persistently painful sprained ankle. J Am Acad Orthop Surg 1994;2:270-280.
7. Conn JM, Annest JL, Gilchrist J. Sports and recreation related injury episodes in the US population, 1997-99. Inj Prev 2003;9:117-123.
8. Hosea TM, Carey CC, and Harrer MF. The gender issue: epidemiology of ankle injuries in athletes who participate in basketball. Clin Orthop Relat Res 2000;372:45-49.
9. Brostrom L. Sprained ankles. V. Treatment and prognosis in recent ligament ruptures. Acta Chir Scand 1966;132:537-550.
10. Bachmann LM, Kolb E, Koller MT, et al. Accuracy of Ottawa ankle rules to exclude fractures of the ankle and mid-foot: systematic review. BMJ 2003;326:417.
11. Bahr R, Pena F, Shine J, et al. Mechanics of the anterior drawer and talar tilt tests. A cadaveric study of lateral ligament injuries of the ankle. Acta Orthop Scand 1997;68:435-441.
12. Hertel J, Denegar C, Monroe M, Stokes W. Talocrural and subtalar joint instability after lateral ankle sprain. Med Sci Sports Exerc 1999;31:1501-1507.
13. Fujii T, Luo ZP, Kitaoka HB, An KN. The manual stress test may not be sufficient to differentiate ankle ligament injuries. Clin Biomech (Bristol, Avon) 2000;15:619-623.
14. de Noronha M, Refshauge KM, Herbert RD, et al. Do voluntary strength, range of motion, or postural sway predict occurrence of lateral ankle sprain? Br J Sports Med 2006;40:824-828.
15. Michelson JD, Durant DM, McFarland E. The injury risk associated with pes planus in athletes. Foot Ankle Int 2002;23:629-633.
16. Docherty CL, Valovich McLeod TC, Shultz SJ. Postural control deficits in participants with functional ankle instability as measured by the balance error scoring system. Clin J Sport Med 2006;16:203-208.
17. Ross SE, Guskiewicz KM. Examination of static and dynamic postural stability in individuals with functionally stable and unstable ankles. Clin J Sport Med 2004;14:332-338.
18. Trojian TH, McKeag DB. Single leg balance test to identify risk of ankle sprains. Br J Sports Med 2006;40:610-613.
19. Hubbard TJ, Hertel J. Mechanical contributions to chronic lateral ankle instability. Sports Med 2006;36:263-277.
20. Hubbard TJ, Kaminski TW, Vander Griend RA, Kovaleski JE. Quantitative assessment of mechanical laxity in the functionally unstable ankle. Med Sci Sports Exerc 2004;36:760-766.
21. Iversen LD, Clawson DK. Manual of Acute Orthopedics. Boston, Little, Brown, 1982:231-236.
22. Kessler RM, Hertling D. Management of Common Musculoskeletal Disorders. Philadelphia, Harper & Row, 1983:379-443.
23. Gerber JP, Williams GN, Scoville CR, et al. Persistent disability associated with ankle sprains: a prospective examination of an athletic population. Foot Ankle Int 1998;19:653-660.
24. Beynnon BD, Renstrom PA, Haugh L, et al. A prospective, randomized clinical investigation of the treatment of first-time ankle sprains. Am J Sports Med 2006;34:1401-1412.
25. Brotzman SB, Brasel J. Foot and ankle rehabilitation. In Brotzman SB, ed. Clinical Orthopaedic Rehabilitation. St. Louis, Mosby, 1996:250-252.
26. Hurwitz S, Ernst G, Yi S. The foot and ankle. In Canavan P, ed. Rehabilitation and Sports Medicine. Stamford, Conn, Appleton & Lange, 1998:346-347.
27. McGuine TA, Keene JS. The effect of a balance-training program on the risk of ankle sprains in high school athletes. Am J Sports Med 2006;34:1103-1111.
28. Friel K, McLean N, Myers C, Caceres M. Ipsilateral hip abductor weakness after inversion ankle sprain. J Athl Train 2006;41:74-78.
29. Gross MT, Liu HY. The role of ankle bracing for prevention of ankle sprain injuries. J Orthop Sports Phys Ther 2003;33:572-577.
30. Olmsted LC, Vela LI, Denegar CR, Hertel J. Prophylactic ankle taping and bracing: a numbers-needed-to-treat and cost-benefit analysis. J Athl Train 2004;39:95-100.
31. Eils E, Rosenbaum D. The main function of ankle braces is to control the joint position before landing. Foot Ankle Int 2003;24:263-268.
32. Cote DJ, Prentice WE Jr, Hooker DN, Shields EW. Comparison of three treatment procedures for minimizing ankle sprain swelling. Phys Ther 1988;68:1072-1076.
33. Liu SH, Baker CL. Comparison of lateral ankle ligamentous reconstruction procedures. Am J Sports Med 1992;20:594-600.

Bunion and Bunionette 76

David Wexler, MD, FRCS (Tr, Orth), Dawn M. Grosser, MD, and Todd A. Kile, MD

David Wexler, MD, FRCS (Tr, Orth), Dawn M. Grosser, MD, and Todd A. Kile, MD

Synonyms

Hallux valgus
Lateral deviation of the great toe

ICD-9 Codes

727.1 Bunion
735.0 Hallux valgus (acquired)

BUNION

DEFINITION

The term *bunion* stems from the Latin word *bunio*, which means "turnip," an image suggestive of an apparent growth or enlargement around the joint. The medical term for this is hallux valgus. Hallux valgus is a common deformity of the forefoot and the most common deformity of the first metatarsophalangeal joint (MTP), often causing pain (Figs. 76-1 and 76-2). The pathophysiologic process stems from both the proximal phalanx and the metatarsal. The proximal phalanx deviates laterally on the head of the first metatarsal, exacerbated by the pull of the adductor hallucis muscle. The lateral capsule becomes contracted, and the medial structures are attenuated. The metatarsal deviates medially, but the underlying sesamoids remain in their relationship to the second metatarsal, thus creating dissociation of the metatarsal-sesamoid complex. As these two processes occur together, the pull of the abductor hallucis moves more plantarly and the pull of the extensor tendon moves laterally, causing pronation and further lateral deviation of the great toe, respectively. As the metatarsal head becomes more uncovered, a prominent medial eminence or bunion is apparent. There is a bursa between the metatarsal head and the skin that may become inflamed and painful. Depending on the amount of axial rotation of the first metatarsal and pronation of the toe, the first ray becomes dysfunctional, leading to increased weight bearing on the more lateral metatarsal heads and "transfer metatarsalgia," causing pain under the plantar aspect of the forefoot.[1]

The etiology of hallux valgus is multifactorial and can be either intrinsic or extrinsic.[2] The intrinsic causes are essentially genetic and are related to hypermobility of the first ray (hallux metatarsal) at its articulation with the medial cuneiform. Ligamentous laxity (e.g., Marfan syndrome, Ehlers-Danlos syndrome) can lead to this deformity as well as to variations in the shape of the metatarsal head (i.e., a rounder head is less stable than a flat one). Another contributing factor is metatarsus primus varus, or medial deviation of the first metatarsal, which is thought to be associated with a juvenile bunion.[3] Pes planus and first metatarsal length have also been evaluated for their contribution to hallux valgus, but findings were equivocal.[4]

The principal extrinsic cause is inappropriate, nonconforming footwear, with abnormal valgus forces creating deformity.[5] This is particularly notable in women who wear high-heeled shoes with narrow toe boxes. The ratio of hallux valgus between women and men has been reported to be 15:1.[6]

SYMPTOMS

Presenting symptoms can vary. The patient may complain only of a painless prominent medial eminence. However, more commonly, there will be pain that is worse when constrictive shoes are worn and relieved by walking barefoot or with open-toed shoes. If there is significant arthritis, patients may have pain throughout range of motion of the MTP joint while walking. The bunion may become red and inflamed as the bursa enlarges and overlying skin becomes abraded by the shoe. The patient will have difficulty finding comfortable shoes. As the hallux deviates into increased valgus, it tends to impinge on the medial aspect of the pulp of the second toe, causing pressure and soreness.[7]

PHYSICAL EXAMINATION

There is generally an obvious medial enlargement overlying the metatarsal head, with occasional signs of inflammation (bursitis). The great toe will be laterally

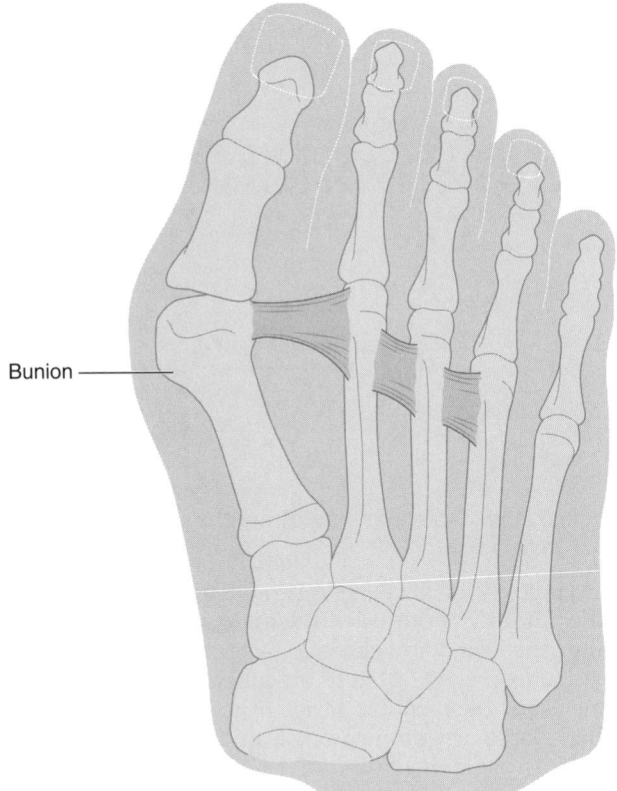

Bunion —

FIGURE 76-1. Anatomy of a bunion.

deviated, and with progression of deformity, it will be pronated (axially rotated). There may be splaying of the forefoot and callosities visible under the metatarsal heads of the lesser toes. Passive extension of the hallux MTP joint will reveal any limitation of range of motion (normally approximately 70 degrees). This may indicate concomitant degenerative joint disease of the MTP joint. Mobility of the hallux at the first metatarsal-medial cuneiform joint is assessed in relation to the second ray.

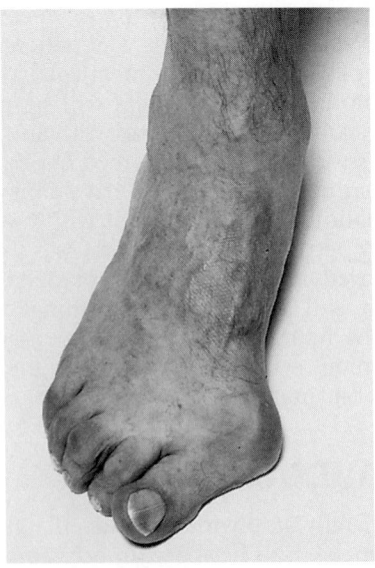

FIGURE 76-2. Clinical photograph demonstrating a bunion or hallux valgus deformity. Note also the pronation of the digit.

Hammer toes are commonly noted as a consequence of the crowding in the shoe by the great toe.

FUNCTIONAL LIMITATIONS

Limitations are principally in walking long distances and wearing shoes with a narrow toe box or high heels for prolonged periods. As hallux valgus progresses, arthritis may become a component and lead to stiffness and pain with any activity (biking, hiking, walking short distances, or even standing).

DIAGNOSTIC STUDIES

Weight-bearing plain radiographs will provide most of the necessary information. The anteroposterior view (Fig. 76-3) demonstrates the angle (Fig. 76-4) between the first and second metatarsals (intermetatarsal angle). The congruency of the first MTP joint can also be assessed for any evidence of arthritis. These all have a bearing on any proposed surgery.[8,9]

Differential Diagnosis
Gout
Hallux rigidus
Rheumatoid arthritis
Infection

TREATMENT

Initial

Nonsteroidal anti-inflammatory medications and analgesics may be used to alleviate pain. However, key measures include education about footwear, namely, shoes with low heels, well-cushioned soles, extra depth, and broad toe boxes. Many orthoses are available of varying efficacy. These include sponge wedges to be placed in the first web space, more formal braces that attempt to pull the hallux into a more neutral position, and custom-molded orthotic appliances to resist foot pronation and to encourage larger shoes. A study showed promising results of a total-contact insole with a fixed toe separator that improved pain, walking ability, and the radiographic hallux valgus angle in patients with painful hallux valgus treated nonoperatively.[10]

Rehabilitation

Once the structural deformity has progressed, physical therapy has a limited role. This includes mobilization of the first MTP joint and strengthening of the intrinsic muscles of the foot, which may improve symptoms. Distraction techniques like varus stretching or toe spacers may also be useful.

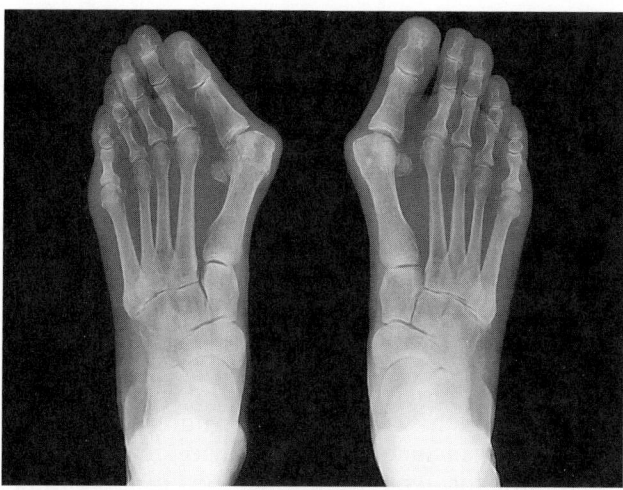

FIGURE 76-3. Standing anteroposterior radiograph of both feet in a patient with bilateral hallux valgus. This is more pronounced on the left. Note also the lateral deviation of the sesamoid bones.

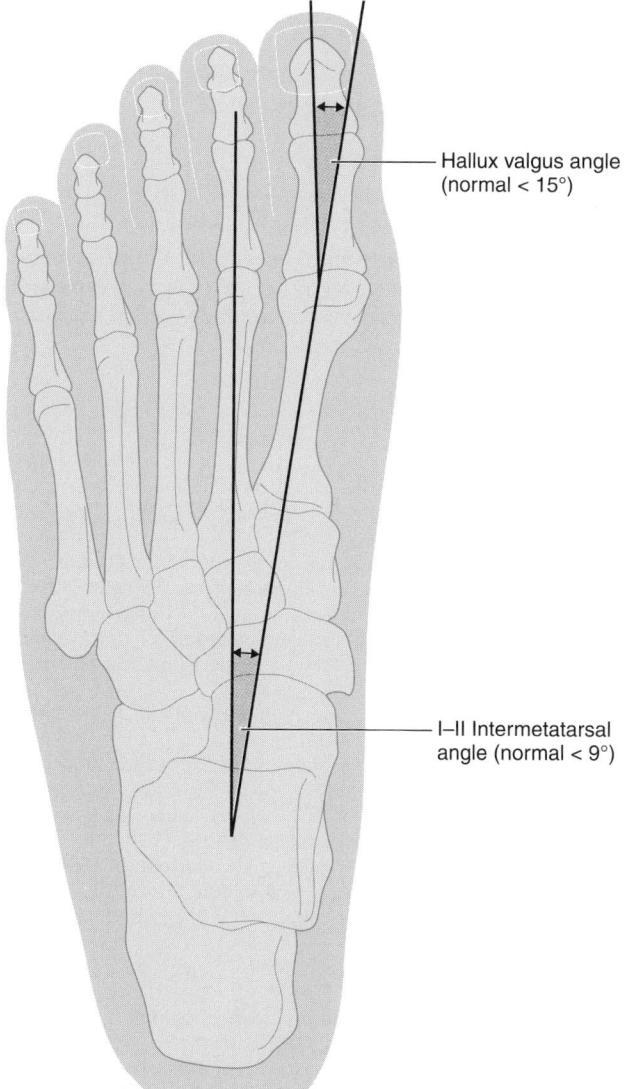

Hallux valgus angle (normal < 15°)

I–II Intermetatarsal angle (normal < 9°)

FIGURE 76-4. The hallux valgus angle and the intermetatarsal angle are measured from the patient's standing anteroposterior radiograph.

Procedures

Local anesthetic and steroid injection into the first MTP joint may provide short-term pain relief but is certainly not curative and generally not recommended.

Surgery

After conservative management has failed, surgery is a consideration. Over the years, a vast array of different surgical procedures have been described.[3,11] Furthermore, no single procedure has provided sufficient evidence of being superior to any other. The complication and recurrence rates can be relatively high, and satisfaction of the patient is difficult to achieve. A study reported that the desired outcome of surgery for patients is threefold: a painless great toe that "when wearing conventional shoes, gives no problems," an improvement in the bursitis and appearance of the bunion, and the ability to walk as much as they wish.[12] These are not unreasonable goals, but it is very important to counsel patients preoperatively, explaining the complications and that there are no guarantees they will be able to return to wearing high-heeled fashionable footwear.[13] The principal goals of surgery are to relieve pain and to provide a foot capable of wearing a shoe.

The type of surgery, whether it is a distal soft tissue procedure[14] combined with a proximal metatarsal osteotomy, a distal osteotomy alone, or even an MTP arthrodesis, depends on the presenting anatomic deformity and its complexity.

POTENTIAL DISEASE COMPLICATIONS

Disease complications include ulceration of the medial eminence, metatarsalgia, callosities, hammer toe deformity, and stress fractures of the lesser toes.

POTENTIAL TREATMENT COMPLICATIONS

Analgesics and nonsteroidal anti-inflammatory drugs have well-known side effects that most commonly affect the gastric, hepatic, and renal systems. Treatment can result in recurrent hallux valgus deformity, hallux varus from surgical overcorrection,[15] and hallux extensus (cock-up toe). Procedures in which the first metatarsal is excessively shortened may result in transfer metatarsalgia. Osteonecrosis of the first metatarsal head can occur if the blood supply is disrupted significantly. Nonunion can occur with the osteotomies and MTP arthrodesis.

BUNIONETTE

DEFINITION

A bunionette is similar to a bunion as a painful bone prominence of a metatarsal head and overlying bursa, but it involves the fifth metatarsal. The fifth metatarsal deviates laterally and the fifth toe medially. It has also been called a tailor's bunion as a cross-legged sitting position, often associated with a tailor, can cause pressure over the fifth toe and potentially encourage this deformity. Like the bunion, a bunionette has a high association with constrictive shoes and is much more common in women than in men (4:1).[4]

SYMPTOMS

Patients may be asymptomatic or complain of irritation over the lateral eminence with tight or stiff shoe wear. Typically, when they wear open shoes without pressure over the bunionette, they have no discomfort. However, they occasionally have an inflamed bursa that is acutely painful and red. If patients adjust their shoe wear, the pain can resolve.

PHYSICAL EXAMINATION

A prominent fifth metatarsal head with a widened appearance of the forefoot is often seen. Patients may develop lateral or plantar callosities over the bone prominence. Hallux valgus may be a concomitant finding, and the foot is considered a "splay foot" if both diagnoses are present.[4]

FUNCTIONAL LIMITATIONS

Patients typically have pain with restrictive shoe wear that is improved or absent when they are barefoot or wearing open shoes, like flip-flops, that do not put pressure over the fifth metatarsal head. Their walking tolerance may be affected when inappropriate shoes are worn.

DIAGNOSTIC STUDIES

Three radiographic views of the foot are obtained: anteroposterior, lateral, and oblique. Anatomic differences that can be appreciated radiographically may influence the surgical approach. These are of three types: type I, an enlarged fifth metatarsal head; type II, an abnormal lateral bowing of the fifth metatarsal shaft; and type III, a wide intermetatarsal 4-5 angle.

TREATMENT

Initial

Addressing the constrictive shoe wear is the first approach. Wide, extra-depth shoes or tennis shoes may help decrease the irritation and bursitis. On occasion, pronation can exacerbate the pressure of the lateral eminence against the shoe, and an orthotic can unload or change the position enough to relieve this. Patients may also take their leather shoes to a shoemaker, who can create a focal stretch over the pressure area of the shoe.

Procedures

If a callus develops, it may be débrided, or patients can be advised to use a pumice stone after daily showers to gently buff the hypertrophic tissue that accumulates laterally or plantarly. Because the discomfort from the bunionette is a pressure phenomenon, injections are not helpful. The bursitis that occasionally accompanies this deformity will improve with appropriate shoe wear and keeping the callus thin.

Surgery

More than 20 different surgical procedures have been described for the correction of a bunionette deformity. These include lateral condylectomy or distal osteotomy for type I, midshaft or distal oblique osteotomy for type II, and proximal osteotomy for type III.[4]

POTENTIAL DISEASE COMPLICATIONS

Ulcerations and callosities may develop if patients continue to wear restrictive shoes.

POTENTIAL TREATMENT COMPLICATIONS

Treatment can result in recurrence of deformity, particularly with an isolated lateral condylectomy; flail toe with metatarsal head resection; malunion or nonunion of osteotomies; and vascular compromise leading to osteonecrosis, particularly with proximal osteotomies.

References

1. Richardson EG, Donley BG. Disorders of the hallux. In Canale ST, ed. Campbell's Operative Orthopaedics, vol 2, 9th ed. St. Louis, Mosby, 1998:1621-1711.
2. Pedowitz W. Hallux valgus. In Craig EV, ed. Clinical Orthopaedics. Philadelphia, Lippincott Williams & Wilkins, 1999:904-912.
3. Austin D, Leventen E. A new osteotomy for hallux valgus: a horizontally directed V displacement osteotomy of the metatarsal head for hallux valgus and primus varus. Clin Orthop Relat Res 1981;157:25-30.
4. Coughlin MJ, Mann RA. Surgery of the Foot and Ankle, 7th ed. St. Louis, Mosby, 1999:150-178.
5. Seale KS. Women and their shoes: unrealistic expectations? Instr Course Lect 1995;44:379-384.
6. Hardy RH, Clapham JC. Observations on hallux valgus; based on a controlled series. J Bone Joint Surg Br 1951;33:376-391.
7. Hertling D, Kessler RM. The leg, ankle and foot. In Hertling D, Kessler RM, eds. Management of Common Musculoskeletal Disorders, 3rd ed. Philadelphia, Lippincott Williams & Wilkins, 1996:435-438.
8. Mann RA. Decision making in bunion surgery. Instr Course Lect 1990;39:3-13.
9. Bordelon RL. Evaluation and operative procedures for hallux valgus deformity. Orthopaedics 1987;10:38-44.
10. Torkki M, Malmivaara A, Seitsalo S, et al. Hallux valgus: immediate operation versus 1 year of waiting with or without orthoses: a randomized controlled trial of 209 patients. Acta Orthop Scand 2003;74:209-215.

11. Donnelly RE, Saltzman CL, Kile TA, Johnson KA. Modified osteotomy for hallux valgus. Foot Ankle 1994;15:642-645.

12. Schneider W, Knahr K. Surgery for hallux valgus. The expectations of patients and surgeons. Int Orthop 2001;25:382-385.

13. Hattrup SJ, Johnson KA. Chevron osteotomy: analysis of factors in patients' dissatisfaction. Foot Ankle 1985;5:327-332.

14. Mann RA, Rudicel S, Graves SC. Repair of hallux valgus with a distal soft-tissue procedure and proximal metatarsal osteotomy. J Bone Joint Surg Am 1992;74:124-129.

15. Tourne Y, Saragaglia D, Picard F, et al. Iatrogenic hallux varus surgical procedure: a study of 14 cases. Foot Ankle Int 1995;16:457-463.

Chronic Ankle Instability 77

Michael D. Osborne, MD

DEFINITION

Chronic ankle instability is a condition characterized by a constellation of symptoms (typically including pain, weakness, and a feeling that the ankle episodically gives way) that persist after an acute lateral ankle sprain. Although chronic ankle instability may occur after a single ankle sprain, it is more commonly a sequela of repeated sprains. It has been reported to occur in up to 40% of individuals with a history of ankle sprain and as late as $6\frac{1}{2}$ years after an initial injury.[1] Anatomic lateral ankle ligament laxity (mechanical instability), peroneal muscle weakness, and ankle proprioceptive deficits are three primary factors classically thought to cause and to perpetuate symptoms. Arthrogenic muscle inhibition of the peroneal and soleus muscles has also been implicated as a possible contributing factor.[2] These causative factors may coexist with other pathologic processes of the ankle (such as those listed in the differential diagnosis section), which may serve to amplify and to perpetuate symptoms of functional instability. The establishment of additional diagnoses does not preclude a diagnosis of chronic ankle instability.

SYMPTOMS

Usual symptoms are ankle pain, swelling around the lateral malleolus, weakness of the ankle evertors, and a feeling that the ankle is episodically unstable. The term *functional instability* describes the subjective sensation of "giving way" that often persists after ankle sprains.[3] Functional instability may occur in the absence of true mechanical ligament laxity and vice versa. Symptoms can continue for months or years after the original injury, range from mild to severe, and often are manifested as recurrent acute lateral ankle sprains.

PHYSICAL EXAMINATION

Objective findings are variable and can often be minimal. Potential examination findings in patients with chronic ankle instability may include reduced passive or active ankle range of motion, lateral ankle swelling, ecchymosis, lateral ankle tenderness (typically over the lateral ligament complex or peroneal tendons), weakness of the peroneal muscles, proprioceptive deficits (manifested by decreased ability to perform a single-leg stance), and mechanical laxity (demonstrated by increased motion on anterior drawer or talar tilt test compared with the contralateral ankle). Abnormal alignment, such as calcaneal varus, calcaneal valgus, or pes planus, may be evident. A limp may also be observed. Examination of the affected ankle should always be compared with the contralateral unaffected ankle.

Findings of the neurologic examination, including sensation and deep tendon reflexes, are commonly normal. Results of manual muscle testing should also be normal, with the exception of muscles surrounding the ankle that may exhibit weakness from disuse or because of pain.

FUNCTIONAL LIMITATIONS

Affected persons may have difficulty participating in sports, particularly high-demand sports that require quick starts and stops, cutting, and jumping (such as soccer, football, and basketball) as well as sports that involve a lot of lateral movement (such as tennis). When symptoms are severe, limitations can include difficulty with climbing steps, ambulation, and activities that require prolonged standing.

DIAGNOSTIC STUDIES

Diagnosis is made by confirming a history of prior sprain with subsequent development of typical symptoms of functional instability in conjunction with consistent examination findings. Adjunctive diagnostic testing can be helpful in establishing the diagnosis, particularly by identifying pathologic changes and conditions that may produce similar symptoms. Testing that may be useful when the diagnosis of chronic ankle instability is being considered includes routine radiography, stress radiography, computed tomography, bone scan, magnetic resonance imaging, ankle arthrography, and magnetic resonance arthrography.

Routine radiographs are useful to rule out old or chronic fractures (most commonly of the fibula, tibia, talus, and fifth metatarsal), to assess the integrity of the ankle mortise, and to assess for ankle arthritis. A routine radiographic series should include anteroposterior, lateral, and mortise views. Widening of the ankle mortise may indicate a syndesmotic disruption or significant deltoid ligament tear. Radiographs should be obtained in all cases with a history of significant trauma at initial injury.

Stress radiographs may be helpful in determining the presence of chronic mechanical instability. Although the routine use of stress radiographs remains controversial, a finding of more than 5 mm of anterior displacement of the talus during anterior drawer testing is typically considered to be abnormal.[4] Inversion stress radiographs are considered abnormal with a finding of more than 5 degrees of side-to-side difference in tibiotalar tilt.[4] However, a review found the published data regarding stress radiographs too variable to determine accepted normal values for acute and chronic sprains.[5] The sensitivity of stress radiographs in diagnosis of chronic lateral ligament tears (surgically confirmed) is low, although specificity is high.[5]

Computed tomography can identify subtle talus fractures and other bone disease, such as tumors. Bone scans are particularly helpful in identifying stress fractures and can be a useful screening tool to evaluate for ongoing ankle disease, such as significant arthritis, infection, tumors, and reflex sympathetic dystrophy. Magnetic resonance imaging and magnetic resonance arthrography generally give the most information about soft tissue injury, although they also can be helpful in identifying fractures (such as osteochondral fractures), tumors, and chronic infections. Magnetic resonance imaging and magnetic resonance arthrography both have high specificity for identification of chronic ligament tears, but magnetic resonance arthrography has higher sensitivity.[6] The appropriate timing of advanced imaging is variable; it is typically governed by the clinical suspicion of further injury or pathologic change not evident on routine radiographs or persistent symptoms despite appropriate treatment. Figures 77-1 and 77-2 demonstrate anterior talofibular and calcaneofibular ligament tears as observed with ankle arthrography.

TREATMENT

Initial

The initial treatment regimen depends, in part, on symptom acuity and whether a recent sprain has occurred. Initial treatment options include ice massage,

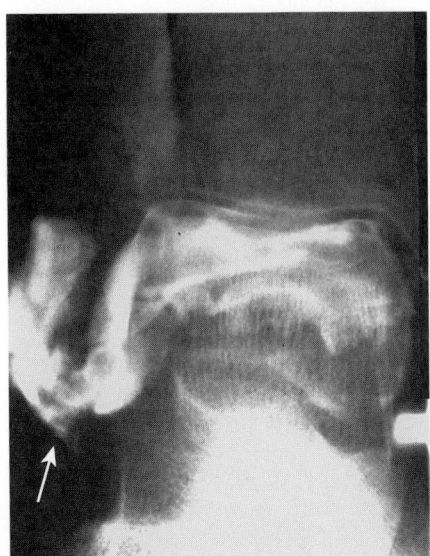

FIGURE 77-1. Ankle arthrogram. Anteroposterior view after ankle injection demonstrates extravasation laterally *(arrow)* resulting from anterior talofibular ligament tear. There is no filling of the peroneal tendon sheath. (Reprinted with permission from Berquist TH. Radiology of the Foot and Ankle, 2nd ed. Philadelphia, Lippincott Williams & Wilkins, 2000. © Mayo Foundation, 2000.)

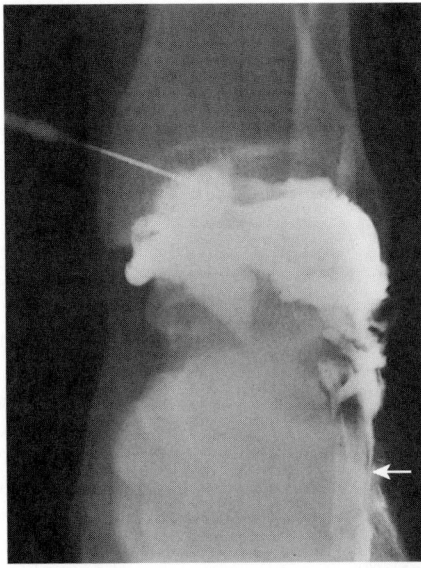

FIGURE 77-2. Ankle arthrogram. Anteroposterior view taken during ankle injection demonstrates filling of the peroneal tendon sheaths *(arrow)* resulting from calcaneofibular ligament disruption. (Reprinted with permission from Berquist TH. Radiology of the Foot and Ankle, 2nd ed. Philadelphia, Lippincott Williams & Wilkins, 2000. © Mayo Foundation, 2000.)

compression, elevation, taping or bracing, and nonsteroidal anti-inflammatory drugs or analgesics. The goal with bracing at this juncture is to prevent recurrent sprains and further tissue trauma. Comprehensive literature reviews indeed validate the use of ankle supports to prevent reinjury.[7,8] Many patients can successfully be weaned from the brace after rehabilitation. However, high-demand athletes may choose to brace or to tape during athletic participation indefinitely. High-top sneakers may help reduce symptoms as well.

Differential Diagnosis

Peroneal tendinopathy: subluxation, tear, chronic tendinitis

Ankle impingement syndrome

Sinus tarsi syndrome

Subtalar instability

Sprain: midfoot, subtalar

Fracture: distal tibia-fibula, talar, osteochondral, stress fracture, fifth metatarsal, physeal

Arthropathy: degenerative, inflammatory, crystalline, infectious

A thin lateral heel wedge will put the ankle in slight valgus alignment and potentially diminish symptoms of instability and the tendency for spontaneous ankle inversion with activity. This can be considered in patients with normal alignment for short-term symptom management. Eventually, restoration of neutral foot and ankle alignment should be pursued through orthotic prescription. A three-quarter-length rigid medial longitudinal arch support is recommended in patients with pes planus. In patients with varus or valgus alignment of the ankle, wearing of a shoe that has a firm heel counter is recommended.

Rehabilitation

Rehabilitation first starts by normalizing ankle range of motion, with primary emphasis on restoring ankle dorsiflexion and eversion. This typically includes Achilles tendon stretching with the knee straight (to stretch the gastrocnemius) and flexed 30 degrees (to stretch the soleus) as well as eversion (posterior tibialis) stretching. Care must be taken to avoid recurrent inversion stress to the ankle, which can perpetuate lateral capsuloligamentous laxity.

As symptoms allow, the patient begins an ankle group strengthening program with an emphasis on ankle evertor strengthening. Resistance exercises can begin when there is no pain through the available range of motion, with full weight bearing.[9] The rehabilitation program may start with low-level strengthening, such as submaximal static exercises, and progress in a pain-free fashion to dynamic and isokinetic strengthening. Typically, a combination of open and closed kinetic chain strengthening is employed in the rehabilitation process.[10] Open kinetic chain exercises include the use of ankle weights and resistance tubing. Closed kinetic chain exercises are more functionally based; the foot is planted on the ground, and the patient engages in an activity that requires the activation of antagonistic muscles that stabilize the ankle. Because eccentric muscle contractions place the greatest force on the muscle, this mode of strengthening should be reserved for the final stages of the rehabilitation program.

Balance challenge and proprioceptive exercises are an important part of chronic ankle instability rehabilitation and have been found to decrease symptoms of functional instability as well as to reduce the rate of re-injury.[11,12] Ankle disks or wobble boards are devices that facilitate proprioceptive training. These exercises can be started without specialized equipment by having the patient perform a single-leg stance on the affected ankle; the skill level is then increased by having the patient close the eyes or stand on a pillow.

Functional exercises and sport-specific drills can begin when the patient has full range of motion, no pain, and at least 85% peroneal strength compared with the contralateral ankle.[13] These exercises add progressively difficult challenges and facilitate the attainment of dynamic strength and balance. Examples of these exercises are jogging, running, double-leg jumping, single-leg hopping, skipping rope, figure-eight drills, lateral cutting drills, and plyometrics. Patients should start at a low level of intensity and progress with increased intensity and difficulty only if they remain pain free while performing the exercise and have no pain or swelling after the training session.

Adjunctive modalities may be helpful throughout the rehabilitation process. These may include regular ice application (ice massage, ice pack, ankle Cryo/Cuff) after therapy sessions or heat application (superficial heat or ultrasound) to facilitate range of motion of a stiff joint. Electrical stimulation may be helpful for pain and edema control.

Procedures

Corticosteroid injections around the ankle ligaments are not advised and may further weaken the ligaments, accelerating mechanical instability. Prolotherapy, the injection of an irritant solution around the capsuloligamentous structures of the ankle, can be considered. The injectate (typically a low-concentration dextrose solution or a combination of phenol, glycerin, and glucose) acts as a local tissue irritant and activates the inflammatory cascade.[14] Given its mechanism of action, it can sometimes be a painful treatment. The purported result of this treatment is ligament and capsular hypertrophy causing reduction in laxity and thereby decreased pain.[14] Although no randomized controls or large case series exist for the use of prolotherapy as a treatment of chronic ankle instability, it has been used for the treatment of knee pain due to osteoarthritis and knee laxity with promising results.[15]

Surgery

Surgery should be considered for patients who sustain recurrent lateral ankle sprains or exhibit significant symptoms of functional instability despite appropriate rehabilitation interventions. The goal of surgery is to restore mechanical stability to the ankle and thereby significantly reduce or eliminate chronic symptoms of instability. Late ankle reconstruction for chronic lateral instability is successful in approximately 85% of patients, regardless of the type of surgical procedure performed.[16] Primary anatomic repair of the anterior talofibular and calcaneofibular ligaments is the preferred method of ankle ligament reconstruction.[16] However, in cases in which there is excessive joint laxity or insufficient capsular tissue is available, reconstructions such as the Chrisman-Snook procedure with use of the split peroneal brevis tendon, the semitendinosus, or an allograft may be preferred.[16-18] If the patient has significant varus predisposing to ankle instability, a Dwyer calcaneal closing wedge or lateral calcaneal slide may be appropriate.

POTENTIAL DISEASE COMPLICATIONS

Potential long-term sequelae of chronic ankle instability include the development of ankle impingement syndrome; chronic peroneal tendinopathy or subluxation; tibiotalar osteochondral injury; degenerative arthritis; superficial peroneal neuropathy; and chronic pain syndromes, such as complex regional pain syndrome type I (reflex sympathetic dystrophy).

POTENTIAL TREATMENT COMPLICATIONS

Potential treatment complications include frostbite from overly aggressive use of ice; exacerbation of edema from inappropriate ankle taping, wrapping, or bracing; and pain exacerbation or reinjury during physical therapy. Analgesics and nonsteroidal anti-inflammatory drugs have well-known side effects that most commonly affect the gastric, hepatic, and renal systems. Surgical complications include failed repair, wound or bone infection, loss of ankle range of motion from an aggressive reconstruction, and persistent ankle pain despite appropriate rehabilitation or surgical repair or reconstruction.

References

1. Verhagen R, de Keizer G, van Dijk CN. Long term follow-up of inversion trauma of the ankle. Arch Orthop Trauma Surg 1995;114:92-96.
2. McVey ED, Palmieri RM, Docherty CL, et al. Arthrogenic muscle inhibition in the leg muscles of subjects exhibiting functional ankle instability. Foot Ankle Int 2005;26:1055-1061.
3. Freeman M. Instability of the foot after injuries to the lateral ligaments of the foot. J Bone Joint Surg Br 1965;47:669-677.
4. Miller MD, Cooper DE, Warner JP. Review of Sports Medicine and Arthroscopy. Philadelphia, WB Saunders, 1995:90.
5. Frost SC, Amendola A. Is stress radiography necessary in the diagnosis of acute or chronic ankle instability? Clin J Sport Med 1999;9:40-45.
6. Chandnani VP, Harper MT, Ficke JR, et al. Chronic ankle instability: evaluation with MR arthrography, MR imaging, and stress radiography. Radiology 1994;192:189-194.
7. Handoll HH, Rowe BH, Quinn KM, de Bie R. Interventions for preventing ankle ligament injuries. Cochrane Database Syst Rev 2001;3:CD000018.
8. Hume PA, Gerrard DF. Effectiveness of external ankle support: bracing and taping in rugby union. Sports Med 1998;25:285-312.
9. Demaio M, Paine R, Drez D. Chronic lateral ankle instability-inversion sprains: part I. Orthopedics 1992;15:87-96.
10. Osborne MD, Rizzo TD. Prevention and treatment of ankle sprain in athletes. Sports Med 2003;33:1145-1150.
11. Gauffin H, Tropp H, Odenrick P. Effect of ankle disk training on postural control in patients with functional instability of the ankle joint. Int J Sports Med 1988;9:141-148.
12. Tropp H, Askling C, Gillquist J. Prevention of ankle sprains. Am J Sports Med 1985;13:259-262.
13. Demaio M, Paine R, Drez D. Chronic lateral ankle instability-inversion sprains: part II. Orthopedics 1992;15:241-248.
14. Rabago D, Best TM, Beamsley M, Patterson J. A systematic review of prolotherapy for chronic musculoskeletal pain. Clin J Sport Med 2005;15:376.
15. Reeves KD, Hassanein KM. Long-term effects of dextrose prolotherapy for anterior cruciate ligament therapy. Altern Ther Health Med 2003;9:58-62.
16. Colville MR. Surgical treatment of the unstable ankle. J Am Acad Orthop Surg 1998;6:368-377.
17. Peters JW, Trevio SG, Renstrom PA. Chronic lateral ankle instability. Foot Ankle 1991;12:182-191.
18. Marsh JS, Daigneault JP, Polzhofer GK. Treatment of ankle instability in children and adolescents with a modified Chrisman-Snook repair: a clinical and patient-based outcome study. J Pediatr Orthop 2006;26:94-99.

Claw Toe 78

David Wang, DO

Synonyms

Claw toe
Clawed hallux (great toe only)

ICD-9 Codes

735.5   Claw toe (acquired)
735.8   Other acquired deformities of toe

DEFINITION

Claw toe is defined as hyperextension of the metatarsophalangeal (MTP) joint and flexion of the proximal interphalangeal joint with or without flexion of the distal interphalangeal joint (Fig. 78-1). This hyperextension at the MTP joint specifically differentiates this condition from hammer toe and mallet toe.[1] The deformity may affect any toe, and often all toes are involved.[2] The term *clawed hallux* describes clawing of only the great toe while the lesser toes are unaffected.[3] Claw toe can be either a flexible deformity, in which the toes can be passively reduced to neutral position, or a fixed deformity, in which there is contracture at any or all of the joints that cannot be passively corrected.[2] Claw toe has been associated with a number of conditions in the medical literature, including diabetes mellitus,[4] rheumatoid arthritis,[5] stroke,[6,7] spinal cord injury,[8] myelodysplasia,[9] lipomeningocele,[7] post-poliomyelitis syndrome,[10] deep posterior compartment syndrome,[11] ankle or tibial fracture,[12,13] ankle surgery,[14] spasticity or contraction of the peroneus longus muscle, hereditary sensorimotor neuropathy type I (Charcot-Marie-Tooth disease),[7,15] intrinsic muscle weakness, paralysis of the lateral plantar nerve, congenital syphilis, peripheral vascular disease,[3] idiopathic pes cavus, spina bifida occulta, cerebral palsy, head injury, brain abscess, and tethered spinal cord.[7,16] Although data are not readily available on incidence or prevalence of claw toe, one study by Badlissi and colleagues[17] found that of 784 community-dwelling adults older than 65 years with foot disorders, 8.7% had claw toe deformity.

From a biomechanical standpoint, clawing of the toes results from the relative dominance of the extrinsic muscles of the foot over the intrinsic muscles, particularly the interossei. The dominant extrinsic muscles of the foot include the peroneus longus, extensor digitorum longus, extensor hallucis longus, and flexor hallucis longus. This extrinsic overpowering may be due to increased extensor activity (e.g., peroneus longus spasticity), shortening of the extrinsic flexor muscles (flexor hallucis longus and flexor digitorum longus; e.g., compartment syndrome), or intrinsic muscle weakness (e.g., motor neuron disease). Extrinsic flexor shortening can be secondary to contracture after deep posterior compartment syndrome[11] or tethering of the flexor hallucis longus tendon (known as a checkrein deformity) after ankle-tibial trauma from fracture or surgery.[12,14] With intrinsic muscle weakness, there is loss of the interossei, which act as flexors at the MTP joint because they run plantar to the MTP axis of rotation. This results in unopposed extension at the MTP joints by the extensor digitorum longus and extensor hallucis longus muscles as well as by the extensor hallucis brevis. Furthermore, in normal anatomy, when the MTP joints are in neutral position, the extrinsic extensors counterbalance flexion at the interphalangeal joints by the flexor hallucis longus and flexor digitorum longus. However, once the MTP joint is hyperextended, the extensor muscles lose their excursion and become slack, resulting in unopposed flexion of the proximal interphalangeal and distal interphalangeal joints by the long flexors, creating the clawed deformity.[2] Olson and associates[3] quantitatively demonstrated by fresh-frozen human cadaver foot studies that with respect to clawed hallux, the peroneus longus contributed the most to increased plantar pressure under the first metatarsal, and extensor hallucis longus and flexor hallucis longus overpull contributed the most to angular changes resulting in the hallux clawing itself. Hyperextension of the MTP joint causes plantar displacement of the metatarsal heads, predisposing them to increased pressure during gait, which has been quantified in biomechanical studies of patients with diabetic peripheral neuropathy.[18,19]

SYMPTOMS

Patients who are symptomatic usually complain of pain and callus formation on the dorsum of the proximal interphalangeal joint due to increased contact pressure

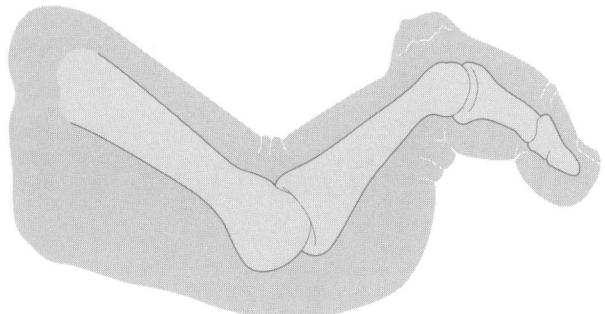

FIGURE 78-1. Diagrammatic representation of claw toe.

with footwear. Increased pressure at the metatarsal heads from marked dorsiflexion of the MTP joint can also cause callus formation and pain.[20] This pain often causes difficulty with wearing of shoes.[21] Individuals with contracture or tethering of the extrinsic toe flexors may complain of increased toe pain during dorsiflexion.[11] Patients often do not complain of pain, however,[17] and the deformity in these cases may present solely cosmetic issues.

PHYSICAL EXAMINATION

Inspection of the foot at rest reveals hyperextension of the MTP joint and increased flexion of the proximal interphalangeal or distal interphalangeal joint. Single or multiple toes may be affected. Calluses, ulcerations, or other signs of skin irritation and breakdown may correlate with clinical symptoms of localized pain. Passive and active range of motion of each joint for each toe should be noted. Correction of the claw toe with passive ankle plantar flexion indicates a flexible as opposed to a fixed deformity,[11] which has important treatment implications. Testing of sensation and proprioception in the lower extremities can detect possible neuropathy; manual muscle testing of the toe flexors and extensors can reveal muscle imbalance and weakness. A complete neuromuscular examination should be performed; the coexistence of other lower extremity problems, such as peripheral neuropathy, pes cavus, hammer toe, inflamed joints, or previous ankle trauma, may provide evidence for an underlying structural or neuromuscular cause.

FUNCTIONAL LIMITATIONS

The degree of limitation seems to depend on whether the claw toe deformity is causing pain. Various studies have shown that painful foot conditions cause increased difficulty with walking, activities of daily living, and instrumental activities of daily living.[22,23] However, Badlissi and colleagues[17] reported that lesser toe deformities, including claw toe, are generally not painful, and they concluded that hallux valgus, lesser digit deformities, and bunionette, when asymptomatic, may not be of great clinical importance.

DIAGNOSTIC STUDIES

Radiologic studies are not necessary for diagnosis. However, they can evaluate for potential osteomyelitis with advanced toe ulcerations and are important for surgical planning.[7,21] Magnetic resonance imaging has been used to assess fat pad geometry at the submetatarsal heads in patients with diabetic peripheral neuropathy,[24] but this is not done as part of a routine clinical workup.

Differential Diagnosis

Hammer toes

Mallet toes

Interdigital (Morton) neuroma

Nonspecific synovitis of the metatarsophalangeal joint

Triggering of the toes (lower limb analogue of trigger finger)

Fracture-dislocation of the toes

Hallux valgus

Plantar fasciitis

TREATMENT

Initial

Patients should be educated about proper shoe wear, foot care, and hygiene to minimize symptomatic callus and ulcer formation. High-heeled shoes and shoes with narrow or flat toe boxes should be avoided.[21] The clinician may prescribe shoes with extra-depth toe boxes to minimize contact pressure at the joints. Alternatively, standard shoes can be modified by cutting off the front of the soft insole just distal to the MTP joint. This maintains the cushioning for the metatarsal heads while providing increased room for the clawed toes.[25] Pressure-unloading and custom-molded orthotics can be used to reduce contact pressure. Toe props have been shown to significantly decrease pressure under the lesser toes and metatarsal heads by redistributing it to the area of the third toe sulcus.[26] Bus and coworkers[27] found that although custom-made orthotic insoles were either moderately or very successful in reducing pressure at the first metatarsal head in 14 of 21 feet, there was significant variability among subjects, and they concluded that a comprehensive evaluation including in-shoe pressure measurements should be done to design the most effective insole for patients with diabetic peripheral neuropathy. In addition, nonsteroidal anti-inflammatory drugs can be used for management of pain and inflammation.[28]

Rehabilitation

For mild cases of flexible claw toe deformity, stretching of the ankle dorsiflexors and toes can help prevent fixed joint contractures.[21] After stretching, commercially available straps or over-and-under taping can be applied to passively hold the toes in neutral position (Fig. 78-2).[21,29] Strengthening of the intrinsic foot muscles through exercises such as towel rolling or picking up small objects (e.g., marbles) with the toes can maintain proper muscle balance.[25]

Procedures

Nonsurgical procedures are not typically done in treating claw toe. However, if synovitis develops, this may benefit from corticosteroid injection.[28]

Surgery

Surgical correction should be considered only if conservative measures are ineffective in improving symptoms or functional deficits. Flexible and fixed claw toe deformities warrant different surgical approaches. For flexible clawed hallux, the classic operation has been the Robert Jones procedure, which involves transfer of the extensor hallucis longus tendon to the neck of the first metatarsal with release of the plantar fascia.[30] An alternative technique entails the transfer of the flexor hallucis longus tendon to the proximal phalanx of the great toe. Steensma and colleagues[28] reported significant improvement in joint alignment, first metatarsal head pain, and shoe comfort as well as good overall satisfaction of patients at an average follow-up time of 24 months for all six subjects with flexible clawed hallux. A series by Kadel and associates[7] described 19 patients with either flexible or fixed clawed hallux who underwent flexor hallucis longus tendon transfer with or without arthrodesis. At an average of 51 months postoperatively, 13 patients were fully satisfied and six were somewhat satisfied with the overall result of the surgery. With clawing of the lesser toes, the Girdlestone flexor tendon transfer, whereby the flexor digitorum longus tendon is transposed to the dorsal aspect of the proximal phalanx, provides increased plantar flexion pull at the MTP joint.[20] For patients with flexible claw toes secondary to extrinsic muscle contracture from closed tibial fractures or deep posterior compartment syndromes, Feeney and colleagues[11] reported promising results with lengthening of the flexor digitorum longus or flexor hallucis longus at a retromalleolar level. In their series of 10 subjects, all reported adequate pain relief, ease of shoe fitting, and improved gait with no recurrence of clawing at 12 to 20 months of follow-up.

For fixed clawed hallux, a modified Jones procedure, which incorporates fusion of the interphalangeal joint with temporary Kirschner wire fixation in addition to the extensor hallucis longus tendon transfer, has been the traditional approach.[7,30] One series reported correction of clawed hallux in 80 of 81 feet with an overall rate of satisfaction of patients of 86%.[30] Another study found that the modified Jones tendon transfer relieved overall symptoms in 90% of patients but cured pain at the first metatarsal head in only 43%.[16] Additional surgical management of fixed claw toe deformities may include extensor hallucis longus and extensor digitorum longus lengthening, extensor hallucis brevis and extensor digitorum brevis tenotomy, MTP dorsal capsulotomy, resection of the head and neck of the proximal phalanges, and plantar fascia release.[2] More recently, an arthroscopic technique has been developed in which the dorsal capsule of the MTP joint is released and the plantar plate is then anchored and sutured to the extensor digitorum longus tendon, thereby stabilizing the plantar plate and reducing the MTP joint.[1] Postoperative care may include protected or no weight bearing for approximately 6 weeks,[7,28] followed by temporary protective orthopedic shoes and physical therapy.[30]

POTENTIAL DISEASE COMPLICATIONS

Skin ulcerations at the plantar metatarsal heads and the dorsal proximal and distal interphalangeal joints can lead to infection and osteomyelitis,[21] especially in patients with peripheral neuropathy. Interestingly, in a prospective study of 749 diabetic veterans, Boyko and colleagues[4] found that hammer or claw toes were associated with an increased relative risk of foot ulcers only in patients who did not report prior histories of foot or leg ulcers. Additional complications of claw toe deformity include synovitis due to vertical instability of the involved joints[28] and posteromedial middle-third tibial pain secondary to overactivity of the flexor digitorum longus muscle.[31]

POTENTIAL TREATMENT COMPLICATIONS

Complications from use of nonsteroidal anti-inflammatory drugs include gastritis, gastrointestinal bleeding, renal toxicity, and platelet inhibition as well as the possible increased risk of cardiovascular events with cyclooxygenase 2 inhibitors.[32] Adverse gastrointestinal events related to nonsteroidal anti-inflammatory drugs can be minimized with the use of a cyclooxygenase 2 inhibitor or concomitant use of a

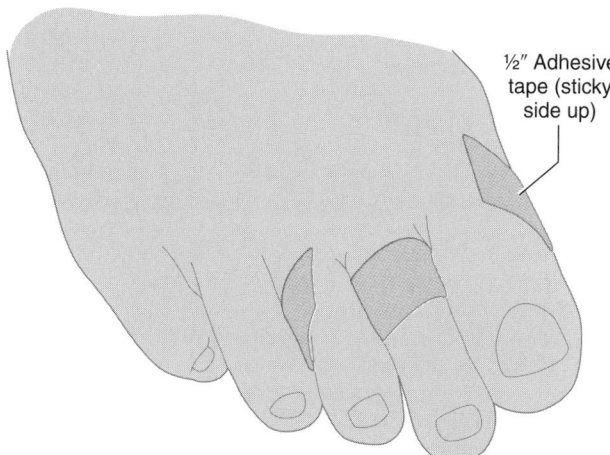

½" Adhesive tape (sticky side up)

FIGURE 78-2. Over-and-under taping method for reducing flexible claw toe deformity. (Reprinted with permission from Mercier LR. Practical Orthopedics, 5th ed. St. Louis, Mosby, 2000:215.)

gastroprotective agent, such as a proton pump inhibitor or H_2 blocker. Complications resulting from surgical correction include catching of the great toe when walking barefoot, metatarsalgia, hallux flexus, hallux limitus, asymptomatic nonunion of the interphalangeal joint, and recurrence of clawing.[16,28,30,33]

References

1. Lui TH. Arthroscopic-assisted correction of claw toe or overriding toe deformity: plantar plate tenodesis. Arch Orthop Trauma Surg 2006 Sep 27; [Epub ahead of print].
2. Canale ST. Campbell's Operative Orthopaedics, 9th ed. St. Louis, Mosby–Year Book, 1998:1750-1751.
3. Olson SL, Ledoux WR, Ching RP, Sangeorzan BJ. Muscular imbalances resulting in a clawed hallux. Foot Ankle Int 2003;24: 477-485.
4. Boyko EJ, Ahroni JH, Stensel V, et al. A prospective study of risk factors for diabetic foot ulcer. The Seattle Diabetic Foot Study. Diabetes Care 1999;22:1036-1042.
5. Fuhrmann RA. The treatment of rheumatoid foot deformities [in German]. Orthopade 2002;31:1187-1197.
6. Yelnik AP, Bonan IV. Post stroke hemiplegia: lower limb benefit from botulinum toxin (review) [in French]. Ann Readapt Med Phys 2003;46:281-285.
7. Kadel NJ, Donaldson-Fletcher EA, Hansen ST, Sangeorzan BJ. Alternative to the modified Jones procedure: outcomes of the flexor hallucis longus (FHL) tendon transfer procedure for correction of clawed hallux. Foot Ankle Int 2005;26:1021-1026.
8. Ozdolop S, Mathew KM, McClelland M, Ravichandran G. Modified Girdlestone-Taylor procedure for claw toes in spinal cord injury. Spinal Cord 2006;44:787-790.
9. Cyphers SM, Feiwell E. Review of the Girdlestone-Taylor procedure for clawtoes in myelodysplasia. Foot Ankle 1988;8:229-233.
10. Faraj AA. Modified Jones procedure for post-polio claw hallux deformity. J Foot Ankle Surg 1997;36:356-359.
11. Feeney MS, Williams RL, Stephens MM. Selective lengthening of the proximal flexor tendon in the management of acquired claw toes. J Bone Joint Surg Br 2001;83:335-338.
12. Rosenberg GA, Sferra JJ. Checkrein deformity—an unusual complication associated with a closed Salter-Harris type II ankle fracture: a case report. Foot Ankle Int 1999;20:591-594.
13. Clawson DK. Claw toes following tibial fracture. Clin Orthop Relat Res 1974;103:47-48.
14. Sanhudo JA, Lompa PA. Checkrein deformity—flexor hallucis tethering: two case reports. Foot Ankle Int 2002;23:799-800.
15. Gravante G, Pomara F, Russo G, et al. Plantar pressure distribution analysis in normal weight young women and men with normal and claw feet: a cross-sectional study. Clin Anat 2005;18:245-250.
16. Tynan MC, Klenerman L. The modified Robert Jones tendon transfer in cases of pes cavus and clawed hallux. Foot Ankle Int 1994;15: 68-71.
17. Badlissi F, Dunn JE, Link CL, et al. Foot musculoskeletal disorders, pain, and foot-related functional limitation in older persons. J Am Geriatr Soc 2005;53:1029-1033.
18. Mueller MJ, Hastings M, Commean PK, et al. Forefoot structural predictors of plantar pressures during walking in people with diabetes and peripheral neuropathy. J Biomech 2003;36:1009-1017.
19. Bus SA, Maas M, de Lange A, et al. Elevated plantar pressures in neuropathic diabetic patients with claw/hammer toe deformity. J Biomech 2005;38:1918-1925.
20. Weinstein SL. Turek's Orthopaedics Principles and Their Application, 6th ed. Philadelphia, Lippincott Williams & Wilkins, 2005: 681-683.
21. Green WB. Essentials of Musculoskeletal Care, 2nd ed. Rosemont, Ill, American Academy of Orthopedic Surgeons, 2001:513-515.
22. Benvenuti F, Ferrucci L, Guralnik JM, et al. Foot pain and disability in older persons: an epidemiologic survey. J Am Geriatr Soc 1995;43:479-484.
23. Leveille SG, Guralnik JM, Ferrucci L, et al. Foot pain and disability in older women. Am J Epidemiol 1998;148:657-665.
24. Bus SA, Maas M, Cavanagh PR, et al. Plantar fat-pad displacement in neuropathic diabetic patients with toe deformity: a magnetic resonance imaging study. Diabetes Care 2004;27:2376-2381.
25. Hunt GC. Physical Therapy of the Foot and Ankle, 2nd ed. New York, Churchill Livingstone, 1995:231.
26. Claisse PJ, Binning J, Potter J. Effect of orthotic therapy on claw toe loading: results of significance testing at pressure sensor units. J Am Podiatr Med Assoc 2004;94:246-254.
27. Bus SA, Ulbrecht JS, Cavanagh PR. Pressure relief and load redistribution by custom-made insoles in diabetic patients with neuropathy and foot deformity. Clin Biomech (Bristol, Avon) 2004;19: 629-638.
28. Steensma MR, Jabara M, Anderson JG, Bohay DR. Flexor hallucis longus tendon transfer for hallux claw toe deformity and vertical instability of the metatarsophalangeal joint. Foot Ankle Int 2006;27:689-692.
29. Mercier LR. Practical Orthopedics, 5th ed. St. Louis, Mosby, 2000:215.
30. Breusch SJ, Wenz W, Doderlein L. Function after correction of a clawed great toe by a modified Robert Jones transfer. J Bone Joint Surg Br 2000;82:250-254.
31. Garth WP Jr, Miller ST. Evaluation of claw toe deformity, weakness of the foot intrinsics, and posteromedial shin pain. Am J Sports Med 1989;17:821-827.
32. Walsh P. Physicians' Desk Reference, 59th ed. Montvale, NJ, Thomson Healthcare, 2005:3130.
33. de Palma L, Colonna E, Travasi M. The modified Jones procedure for pes cavovarus with claw hallux. J Foot Ankle Surg 1997;36: 279-283.

Corns 79

Robert J. Scardina, DPM, and Sammy M. Lee, DPM

Synonyms

Clavus
Heloma
Helomata
Callosity
Callositas
Hyperkeratosis

ICD-9 Code

700   Corns and calluses

DEFINITION

A corn is a circumscribed, focal thickening of epidermis composed of impacted, dead keratinocytes,[1] usually located over dorsally prominent digital interphalangeal joints of the foot. These cutaneous lesions form in response to excessive and repetitive pressure or friction from shoe gear. They are usually hard and ovoid or circular with a polished or translucent center, like a kernel of corn (from which they take their name), and they may become painfully inflamed or ulcerated.[2] They develop as a normal protective response of the skin and become pathologic when the lesion grows so large as to become a source of symptoms.[3]

There are two general types of corns, hard and soft. Heloma durum (hard corn), the most common (Fig. 79-1), develops dorsally over digital interphalangeal joints and distally on toes; it is caused primarily by toe deformity and may be accentuated by improper or ill-fitting shoes. The second type (Fig. 79-2), known as heloma molle (soft corn), occurs primarily interdigitally and most commonly in the web space between toes four and five; it is usually the result of wearing tight-fitting shoes or excessive pressure from adjacent bone (phalangeal) abnormalities, including exostoses.[4] Both of these lesions develop as the body attempts to protect the irritated skin by accumulation of the horny layer of the epithelium. This epithelial accumulation itself causes an additional prominence, which increases the local pressure in a tight shoe. Thus, a vicious circle is generated that may ultimately lead to the keratin plug's pressing into the dermis and causing pain.[5]

SYMPTOMS

Symptoms range from sharp, shooting pain to dull, aching soreness, aggravated by wearing closed shoe gear. If secondary ulceration develops, infection may ensue with subsequent local and systemic manifestations.

PHYSICAL EXAMINATION

On inspection, these cutaneous lesions are typically hard (or in the case of heloma molle, soft or macerated), with thickened skin and a yellowish or translucent nidus or center. In contrast to warts (verrucae), which are spongy in appearance with dark pinpoint areas (capillary bleeding points) and typically painful with lateral compression, corns are more painful to direct pressure. Bones of the foot have many projections, especially on the condyles of the phalangeal heads or bases. Pressure and friction are generated on the skin overlying those bone projections, either from a tight shoe or from digital movement during walking. Corns are usually associated with digital deformities, including hammer toes, claw toes, and mallet toes, or combined interphalangeal joint deformities.[6] Hammer toe or claw toe deformities may contribute to "retrograde" metatarsalgia, with plantarly prominent lesser metatarsal heads. Other forefoot deformities associated with hammer toes include bunion and hallux valgus.

FUNCTIONAL LIMITATIONS

Corns can result in difficulty walking (primarily in closed shoe gear), pain associated with running or athletic activities, and residual non–weight-bearing or nocturnal pain.

DIAGNOSTIC STUDIES

The diagnosis of a corn (or clavus) is made primarily on a clinical basis. However, plain radiographic analysis may be helpful in identifying underlying bone abnormality (e.g., exostosis), primary structural digital deformity (e.g., hammer toe), associated or contributing forefoot deformities (e.g., hallux abductus and bunion), or in the case of ulceration with infection, evidence of osteomyelitis.

441

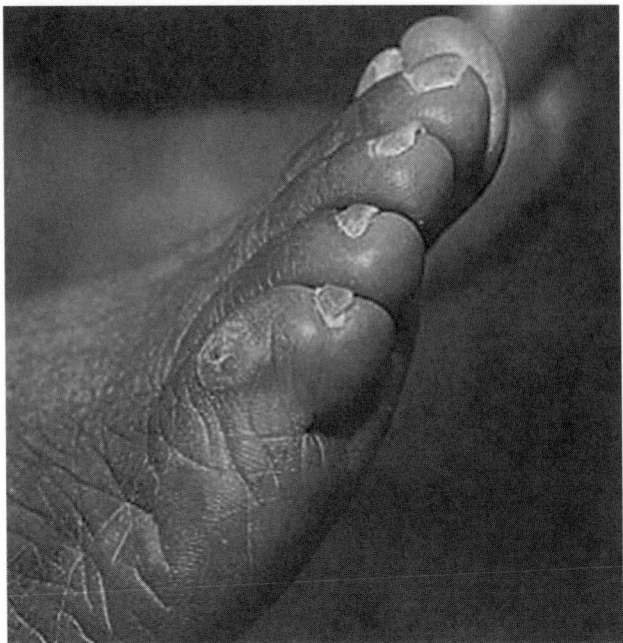

FIGURE 79-1. Hard corn at the lateral aspect of the proximal interphalangeal joint of the small toe.

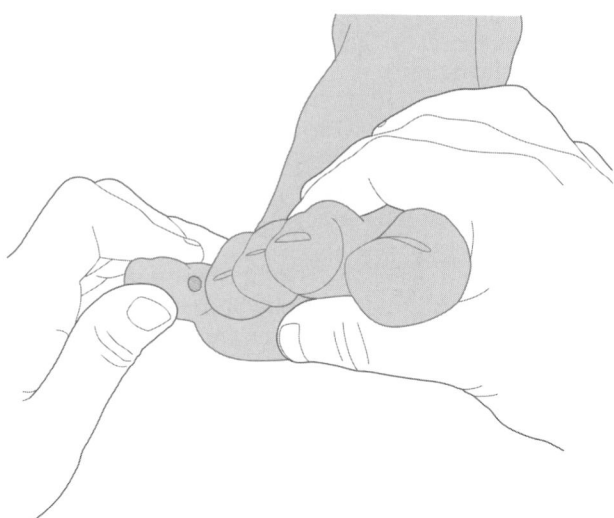

FIGURE 79-2. Soft corn on the medial aspect of the small toe.

Differential Diagnosis

Verruca (wart)

Subcutaneous bursa

Benign or malignant cutaneous neoplasm

Superficial foreign body

Tinea pedis (fourth web space lesions)

Keratoderma

Porokeratoma

TREATMENT

Initial

Conservative measures for symptomatic relief include efforts to reduce or to eliminate direct friction or pressure at the involved site by use of various padding or shielding methods (e.g., moleskin pads, aperture pads, silicone sleeves; Fig. 79-3), orthodigital (toe-straightening) devices for reducible deformity only (Fig. 79-4), and proper shoe gear allowing adequate toe box room.[7] Patients should be counseled to avoid wearing improper footwear, such as narrow shoes and high heels.

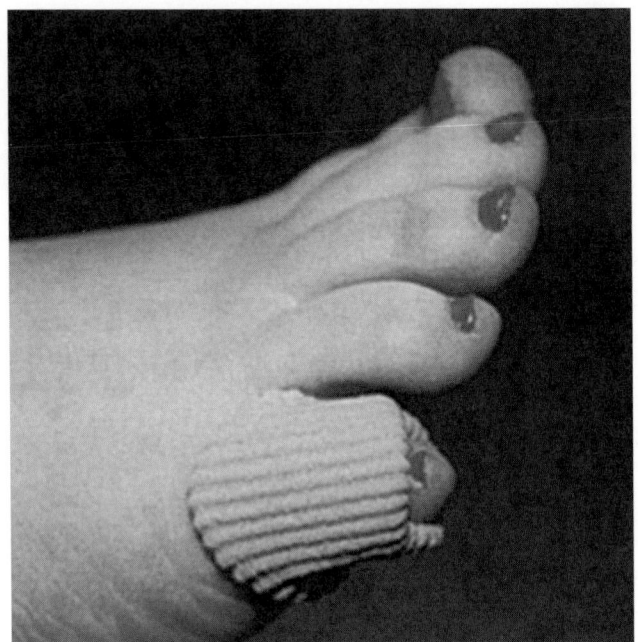

FIGURE 79-3. Silicone sleeve on fifth toe.

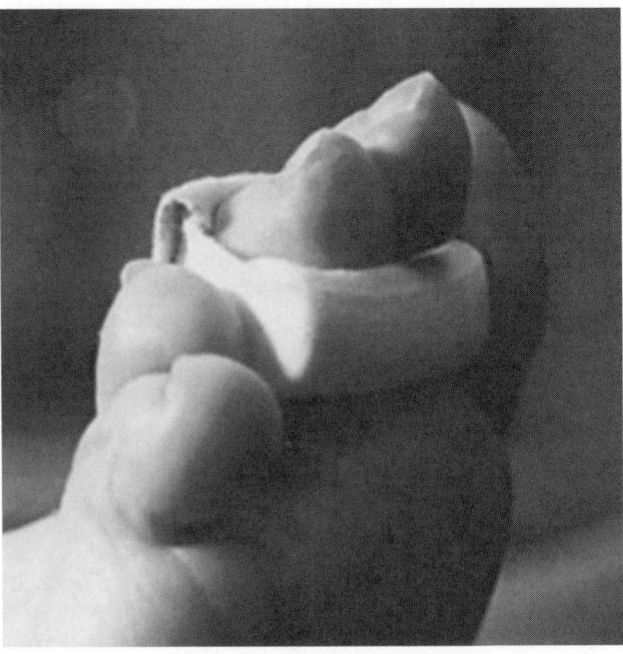

FIGURE 79-4. Lateral view of crest pad beneath second and third toes.

Use of over-the-counter keratolytic agents (e.g., salicylic acid) is a common self-care measure. However, these should be discouraged because of potential for ulceration or infection, especially in the diabetic, neuropathic, or dysvascular patient. Skin breakdown and ulceration with infection may occur, requiring débridement, local wound care, and systemic antibiotics.

Oral analgesics and nonsteroidal anti-inflammatory drugs may be used in the short term to treat acute pain.

Rehabilitation

There are no true "rehabilitative" modalities for corns. However, should these cutaneous lesions respond to initial conservative measures, one may consider continued use of custom shoe gear (e.g., extra depth, molded), orthodigital devices, and custom orthoses to improve foot biomechanics.

Procedures

Trimming or paring of a corn should be done under aseptic technique, to a proper level, and with appropriate instrumentation (Fig. 79-5). This type of palliative treatment is usually provided to patients who are not surgical candidates, either by individual choice or because of medical contraindication. The interval for this type of ongoing care generally ranges from every 6 to 12 weeks, depending on the nature and extent of the lesions as well as the patient's activity level and compliance with other conservative (including self-care) measures.

Other invasive, nonsurgical procedures include subcutaneous injection of a local anesthetic and soluble corticosteroid preparation for *acutely* painful lesions with bursitis.[8] These injections should not be performed more than a few times as they may lead to dermal atrophy.

Surgery

Surgical treatment may involve exostectomy (condylectomy) or correction of the underlying structural deformity (hammer toe, claw toe, or mallet toe) by interphalangeal joint resection or arthrodesis, with or without flexor or extensor tenoplasty.[9-12]

POTENTIAL DISEASE COMPLICATIONS

Potential disease complications include refractory or intractable pain, cutaneous nerve entrapment, secondary functional limitation, superficial or deep skin ulceration, infection, and shoe gear restrictions.

POTENTIAL TREATMENT COMPLICATIONS

Analgesics and nonsteroidal anti-inflammatory drugs have well-known side effects that most commonly affect the gastric, hepatic, and renal organ systems. Treatment complications from local conservative care include skin ulceration and infection due to overly aggressive sharp débridement or use of keratolytic agents. Postsurgical complications include infection, wound problems, nerve injury or numbness, chronic digital edema, nonunion (in arthrodesis), and recurrent deformity.

References

1. DeLauro TM. Keratotic lesions of the foot. Clin Podiatr Med Surg 1996;13:73-84.
2. Neale D. Common Foot Disorders: Diagnosis and Management. New York, Churchill Livingstone, 1981:77-81.
3. Freeman DB. Corns and calluses resulting from mechanical hyperkeratosis. Am Fam Physician 2002;65:2277-2280.
4. Birrer RB, DellaCorte MP, Grisafi PJ. Common Foot Problems in Primary Care. Philadelphia, Hanley & Belfus, 1998:48-49.
5. Singh D, Bentley G, Trevino SG. Fortnightly review: callosities, corns and calluses. BMJ 1996;312:1403-1406.
6. Oliver TP, Armstrong DG, Harkless LB, Krych SM. The combined hammer toe–mallet toe deformity with associated double corns: a retrospective review. Clin Podiatr Med Surg 1996;13:263-268.
7. Gould JS. The Foot Book. Baltimore, Williams & Wilkins, 1988: 73-76.
8. Yale YR. Yale's Podiatric Medicine. Baltimore, Williams & Wilkins, 1987:134-153.
9. Boderlon RL. Surgical and Conservative Foot Care. Thorofare, NJ, Slack, 1988:92-94.
10. Day RD, Reyzelman AM, Harkless LB. Evaluation and management of the interdigital corn: a literature review. Clin Podiatr Med Surg 1996;13:201-206.
11. O'Kane C, Kilmartin T. Review of proximal interphalangeal joint excisional arthroplasty for the correction of second hammer toe deformity in 100 cases. Foot Ankle Int 2005;26:320-325.
12. Caterini R, Farsetti P, Tarantino U, et al. Arthrodesis of the toe joints with an intramedullary cannulated screw for correction of hammertoe deformity. Foot Ankle Int 2004;25:256-261.

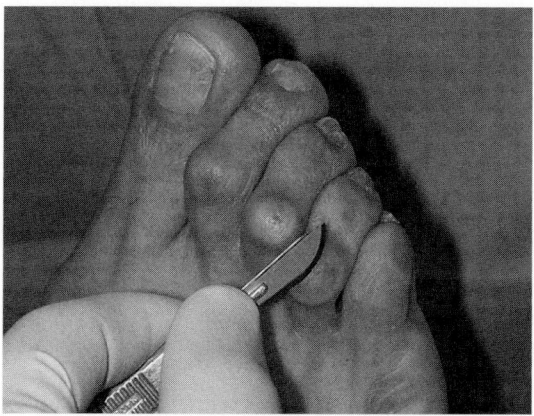

FIGURE 79-5. Trimming of hard corn on hammer toe.

Foot and Ankle Ganglia 80

Robert J. Krug, MD, Elliot Pollack, DPM, and Jeffrey T. Brodie, MD

Synonyms

Cyst of joint capsule
Cyst of tendon
Cyst of tendon sheath
Myxomatous cyst
Mucoid cyst

ICD-9 Code

727.43   Ganglion and cyst of synovium, tendon, and bursa, unspecified

DEFINITION

Ganglia are benign cystic fibrous lesions that are contained by thin walls of connective tissue; they are often multilocular and contain relatively colorless fluid that is thickened and gelatinous.[1] Many authors believe that ganglion cysts are due to myxoid degeneration of surrounding connective tissue.[2,3] They are most commonly found in the hand; however, the foot and ankle are also common sites for these benign lesions, especially on the dorsolateral surface.[3] They are most commonly seen in the soft tissues of young and middle-aged adults and have a preponderance in women. Ganglia can connect with a joint through a stalk and can be seen within tendons and bone.[4] Rarely, they can form in the epineurium of nerves, known as intraneural ganglion.[5]

SYMPTOMS

Whereas the majority of patients present with a painful mass in the soft tissues of the foot or ankle, a small percentage of patients are asymptomatic and are more concerned about the possibility of malignant transformation or simply cosmesis. The symptoms are often brought about only by certain types of shoe gear that may cause direct compression of the mass or indirectly through traction of the adjacent skin. If the mass is compressing a sensory nerve, it is called an extraneural ganglion. It can lead to burning, radiating neuritic pain.[6] If this occurs in the posteromedial aspect of the ankle, it can cause symptoms consistent with tarsal tunnel syndrome by compression of the posterior tibial nerve.[7]

PHYSICAL EXAMINATION

Evaluation of a soft tissue mass on the foot and ankle should include a complete history, careful physical examination, and radiographic studies. These lesions are generally less than 2 cm in diameter but can be larger. They can be soft, firm, or hard, depending on their size and location. Although they may be found on the plantar aspect of the foot, they are most commonly seen on the dorsal aspect.[4,8] If they are compressing a nerve, Tinel sign may be present, or there may be a region of dysesthesia or anesthesia.[9] Transillumination may be possible if the ganglion is close to the skin surface. These lesions are not associated with a particular foot type; however, foot abnormalities should be noted (e.g., pes planus or flat feet).

FUNCTIONAL LIMITATIONS

Because these lesions are rarely symptomatic outside of shoe gear, the only significant limitations are due to inability to tolerate certain types of shoes. This could limit walking, running, or sports that involve kicking, such as soccer. They can be symptomatic if the ganglia are from joints of the rearfoot or ankle.

DIAGNOSTIC STUDIES

Plain radiographs are typically normal, but anteroposterior and lateral views should be obtained to rule out bone exostoses or soft tissue calcification. In most cases, the diagnosis is confirmed with aspiration of the lesion, which will reveal the classic clear, gelatinous fluid and provide definitive diagnosis. However, if the lesion is too small or if the fluid is too thick to be aspirated, magnetic resonance imaging can provide useful and often diagnostic information about these masses.[10] Ganglia visualized on magnetic resonance imaging will demonstrate low to intermediate signal intensity on T1-weighted images and high signal intensity on T2-weighted images (Fig. 80-1). They are commonly septated or lobulated in appearance.[9,11] Also, sonography is used, particularly with ankle ganglia; sonographic appearance is both hypoechoic and

445

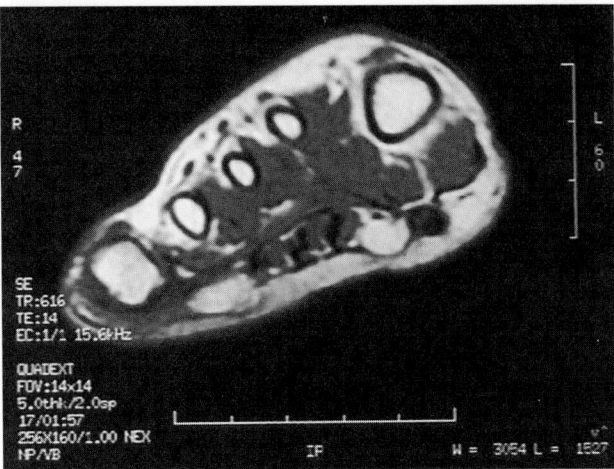

FIGURE 80-1. Magnetic resonance image of a ganglion cyst below the skin, inferior and lateral to the fibular sesamoid.

anechoic.[12] Communication with specific joints or tendon sheaths may be noted.[13]

Differential Diagnosis

Giant cell tumor of tendon sheath

Hypertrophic synovial cysts

Lipoma

Pigmented villonodular synovitis

Soft tissue calcifications

Malignant sarcoma

Benign synoviomas

Bone exostoses

TREATMENT

Initial

Shoe gear modification can alleviate the pressure exerted on many of these lesions. Many times, alteration of lacing patterns in athletic shoes can eliminate these symptoms. Oral medications have not been demonstrated to be of benefit in the treatment of ganglion cysts; however, if pain is acute, traditional analgesics or nonsteroidal anti-inflammatory drugs can be used.

Rehabilitation

No formal rehabilitative techniques have been demonstrated as effective treatment options for ganglia. However, for the rare mass on the plantar aspect of the foot, biomechanical unloading can be accomplished with custom orthoses.

Procedures

Simple aspiration of ganglion cysts has resulted in recurrence rates as high as 60% to 100%.[4,6,8,14] The addition of steroid injection after aspiration can reduce the rate of recurrence to 33% to 50%.[6,15]

After preparation of the skin, ethyl chloride spray can be used as a local anesthetic. Then, under sterile conditions, a large-bore needle (e.g., 18-gauge) is used with a 5- or 10-mL syringe to apply sufficient suction to allow the thick material to pass into the syringe. Without removal of the needle, usually less than 0.5 to 1.0 mL of a local corticosteroid (e.g., triamcinolone) is injected into the evacuated cyst. Compression and ice can be applied after this procedure. This process can be repeated a second time after at least 2 to 4 weeks, if necessary. If no fluid can be aspirated, a solid tumor should be considered, and further workup may include computed tomography, magnetic resonance imaging, or possibly biopsy.[2]

Surgery

If conservative treatment of ganglia has failed, surgical excision can be curative (Fig. 80-2). Because there is a high rate of failure of conservative treatment, approximately one third to one half of symptomatic ganglia go on to require surgery. Unfortunately, recurrence rates can still run as high as 10% to 27% after excision; therefore, it is imperative that careful, meticulous dissection of the entire mass be performed to minimize this risk,[1,8,14] along with tying off of any stalks that may be present, particularly in ganglia coming out of joints.

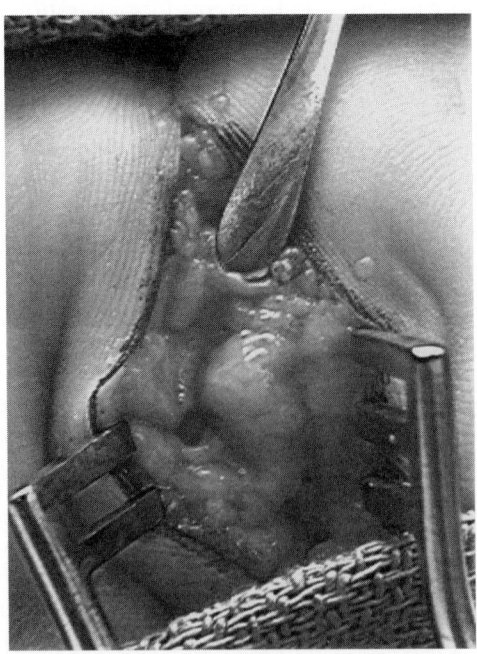

FIGURE 80-2. Surgical exposure of the lesion seen in Figure 80-1. Note the round mass in the center of the surgical field just below the surgical instrument. This cyst was compressing the plantar digital nerve in this web space.

POTENTIAL DISEASE COMPLICATIONS

The main disease complication is chronic pain. This may lead to an inability to wear certain types of shoes.

POTENTIAL TREATMENT COMPLICATIONS

Analgesics and nonsteroidal anti-inflammatory drugs have well-known side effects that most commonly affect the gastric, hepatic, and renal systems. As previously noted, recurrence of the cyst is the most common complication from surgical excision. Painful scars and keloids can occur, as with any surgical procedure. If the cyst is in the vicinity of a motor or sensory nerve, injury to the nerve is possible. In addition, incisions near the anterior aspect of the ankle can lead to joint stiffness from scar contracture.[1,4,8] Care must be taken with cortisone injections to reduce the risk of fat necrosis in the subcutaneous tissues. Small amounts of cortisone should be used (less than 1 mL), and an attempt should be made to keep the needle within the potential space of the evacuated cyst.

References

1. Rozbruch SR, Chang V, Bohne WH, Deland JT. Ganglion cysts of the lower extremity: an analysis of 54 cases and review of the literature. Orthopedics 1998;21:141-148.
2. Walling AK, Gasser SI. Soft-tissue and bone tumors about the foot and ankle. Clin Sports Med 1994;13:909-938.
3. Carnesale PG. Soft tissue tumors and nonneoplastic conditions simulating bone tumors. In Crenshaw AH, ed. Campbell's Operative Orthopaedics, 8th ed. St. Louis, Mosby, 1992:299-300.
4. Kliman ME, Freiberg A. Ganglia of the foot and ankle. Foot Ankle 1982;3:45-46.
5. Spinner RJ, Dellon AL, Rosson GD, et al. Tibial intraneural ganglia in the tarsal tunnel: is there a joint connection? J Foot Ankle Surg 2007;46:27-31.
6. Slavitt JA, Beheshti F, Lenet M, Sherman M. Ganglions of the foot: a six-year retrospective study and a review of the literature. J Am Podiatry Assoc 1980;70:459-465.
7. Takakura Y, Kitada C, Sugimoto K, et al. Tarsal tunnel syndrome: causes and results of operative treatment. J Bone Joint Surg Br 1991; 73:125-128.
8. Pontious J, Good J, Maxian SH. Ganglions of the foot and ankle: a retrospective analysis of 63 procedures. J Am Podiatr Med Assoc 1999;89:163-168.
9. Steiner E, Steinbach LS, Schnarkowski P, et al. Ganglia and cysts around joints. Radiol Clin North Am 1996;34:395-425.
10. Woertler K. Soft tissue masses in the foot and ankle: characteristics on MR imaging. Semin Musculoskelet Radiol 2005;9:227-242.
11. Wetzel LH, Levine E. Soft-tissue tumors of the foot: value of MR imaging for specific diagnosis. AJR Am J Roentgenol 1990;155: 1025-1030.
12. Ortega R, Fessell DP, Jacobson JA, et al. Sonography of ankle ganglia with pathologic correlation in 10 pediatric and adult patients. AJR Am J Roentgenol 2002;178:1445-1449.
13. Desy NM, Amrami KK, Spinner RJ. Ganglion cysts and nerves. Neurosurg Q 2006;16:187-194.
14. Johnston JO. Tumors and metabolic diseases of the foot. In Mann RA, Coughlin MJ, eds. Surgery of the Foot and Ankle, 6th ed. St. Louis, Mosby, 1993:997.
15. Derbyshire RC. Observations on the treatment of ganglia: with a report on hydrocortisone. Am J Surg 1966;112:635-636.

Hallux Rigidus 81

David Wexler, MD, FRCS (Tr, Orth), Dawn M. Grosser, MD, and Todd A. Kile, MD

Synonyms

Osteoarthritis or degenerative joint disease of the first metatarsophalangeal joint
Osteoarthritis of the great toe[1]

ICD-9 Code

735.2   Hallux rigidus

DEFINITION

Degenerative joint disease or loss of articular cartilage from the first metatarsophalangeal (MTP) joint leading to painful restriction of motion is called hallux rigidus. The normal range is 30 to 45 degrees of plantar flexion to almost 90 degrees of dorsiflexion. The limited range of motion and pain with hallux rigidus are exacerbated by overgrowth of bone (osteophytes or "bone spurs") on the dorsal aspects of the base of the proximal phalanx and the head of the metatarsal, which impinge on one another as the great toe dorsiflexes.[2] Hallux rigidus is the second most common problem in the first MTP joint, after hallux valgus; 1 in 40 people older than 50 years will develop hallux rigidus.[3]

In general, the cause is unknown, although it is associated with generalized osteoarthritis of other joints and repeated microtrauma (e.g., in soccer players). Sustaining repetitive turf toe–type injuries may lead to this form of early joint degeneration.[4] As the plantar capsuloligamentous complex of the first MTP joint is injured by hyperflexion of the great toe, it may acutely compress the articular surfaces of the joint, causing articular damage, or become chronically unstable, predisposing the MTP joint to hallux rigidus.[5]

SYMPTOMS

Patients typically report pain, either intermittent or constant, that occurs with walking and is relieved by rest. It is insidious in onset and may be associated with stiffness, swelling, and sometimes inflammation. On occasion, there can be locking due to a cartilaginous loose body. Patients may notice that they are walking on the outside of the foot to avoid pushing off with the great toe during the terminal stance and toe-off phases of the gait cycle. As the degeneration increases, the pain may intensify and result in a limp.

PHYSICAL EXAMINATION

On inspection, there will usually be swelling around the MTP joint with tenderness of the joint line. Dorsal osteophytes may be palpable and may cause irritation of overlying skin with shoe wear abrasion. Pain is reproduced with forcible dorsiflexion of the great toe, which is also restricted in range. Plantar flexion may also be affected. Patients may have an antalgic (painful) gait, and single-stance toe raise may be difficult secondary to a painful MTP joint, as opposed to posterior tibial tendon deficiency. Findings of the neurologic examination, including strength, sensation, and reflexes, are typically normal.

FUNCTIONAL LIMITATIONS

Functional limitations include walking long distances, running any distance, and ascending stairs. As the severity increases, walking even short distances, daily errands, and standing for long periods may be difficult. Flexible shoes as well as shoes with a tight toe box may prove to be uncomfortable. This may lead to pressure areas dorsally over the osteophytes.

DIAGNOSTIC STUDIES

Plain anteroposterior and lateral standing radiographs will usually suffice in confirming the diagnosis (Fig. 81-1). The signs are consistent with degenerative joint disease, namely, loss of joint space and congruency, large dorsal osteophytes (bone spurs), sclerosis (increased density of bone), and subchondral cysts. There may be evidence of a loose body. This disease process has been divided into three grades on the basis of the severity of radiographic and clinical findings, which help guide surgical treatment.

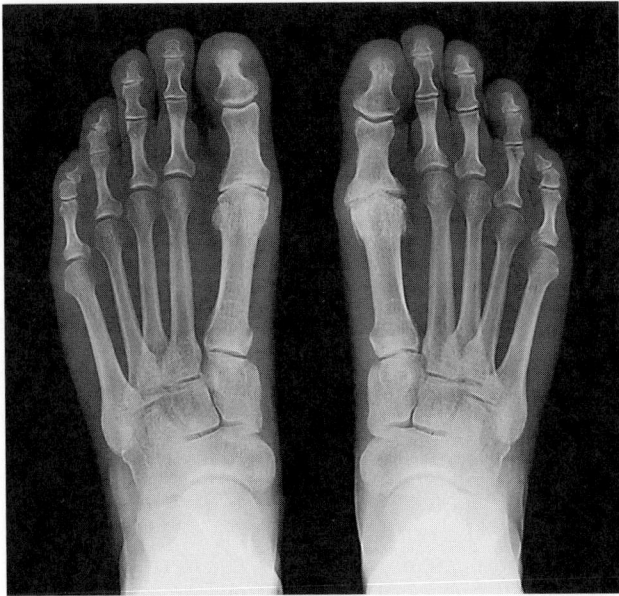

FIGURE 81-1. Standing anteroposterior radiograph of both feet. This demonstrates bilateral hallux rigidus or degenerative joint disease of the hallux MTP joints. The signs are narrowing of the joint space, osteophyte formation, and sclerosis. This is more pronounced on the right.

Grade I demonstrates mild dorsal osteophytes with preservation of the MTP joint space on radiographic examination and typically intermittent pain with ambulation. Grade II demonstrates moderate dorsal osteophyte formation and asymmetric joint space narrowing radiographically and often constant pain with ambulation. Grade III has extensive osteophytes and severe dorsal and plantar joint space narrowing, often with noticeable loose bodies; clinically, patients will have constant pain with ambulation and significant limitation of motion.[6]

TREATMENT

Initial

Nonsteroidal anti-inflammatory drugs may provide symptomatic relief. Footwear modifications and orthoses to limit stresses at the MTP joint (carbon fiber inserts or Morton's extension orthotic devices), as well as avoidance of high heels or shoes with very flexible soles, may be useful conservative treatment options.[7]

Differential Diagnosis

Gout

Hallux valgus

Turf toe

Fracture

Rehabilitation

More advanced shoe modifications can be made by a certified pedorthist. These include a steel shank and possibly a rocker-bottom that may be applied to the soles of many different types of shoes, including athletic shoes. Anecdotally, many patients prefer first to try a steel shank because there is no cosmetic change to the shoe. With a rocker-bottom, the sole is altered, and this is sometimes less cosmetically acceptable to patients.

If there is evidence of other foot deformities, such as pes planus (flatfoot), orthotic inserts may provide correction and help with gait biomechanics.

Physical therapy is not generally indicated but may include basic mobilization and distraction techniques as well as strengthening exercises of the flexor and extensor hallucis muscles to enhance joint stability. Modalities such as contrast baths and ice may help with pain control.

Procedures

Intra-articular injection of the MTP joint with local anesthetic and steroid may provide short-term relief.

Surgery

The principal indications for surgery are continuing pain and failed nonoperative management. Depending on the severity of the degeneration, there are two broad approaches to surgery. For grade I and grade II, the appropriate treatment is joint preserving; the impinging dorsal osteophytes are excised and the joint is debulked, thus improving dorsiflexion.[8-10] A phalangeal osteotomy (i.e., Moberg procedure) may also be used to improve dorsiflexion. The second approach is joint sacrificing for grade III disease. These procedures range from resection arthroplasty, resulting in a floppy or flail shortened toe, to arthrodesis (Fig. 81-2), resulting in a stiff, rigidly fixed toe.[6,11,12] A number of manufacturers have tried to produce artificial great toe joints, made of Silastic, metal, and polyethylene or ceramic,[13,14] but the long-term results of these have not lived up to expectations. A randomized controlled trial comparing arthrodesis to arthroplasty found better improvement in pain, satisfaction of patients, and cost ratio with arthrodesis. Patients receiving arthroplasty had minimal improvement in range of motion, had continued altered gait mechanics, and required removal secondary to loosening in a significant number.[15] Interposition arthroplasty (with use of autologous tissue attached between the two joint surfaces) has also been advocated as a reasonable option instead of fusing the joint for grade III disease.[16] Arthroscopic surgery has also been attempted.

POTENTIAL DISEASE COMPLICATIONS

Hallux rigidus may produce intractable pain and reduced mobility.

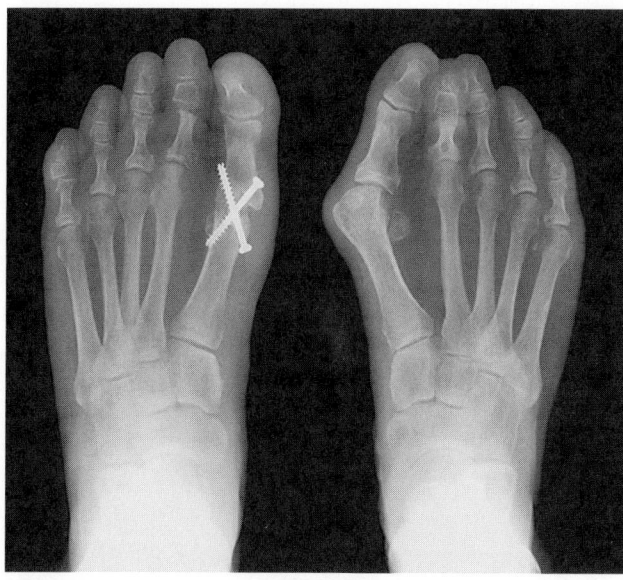

FIGURE 81-2. Standing anteroposterior radiograph of both feet. This demonstrates, on the left foot, one of the techniques for fusing the MTP joint, with crossed cannulated screws. The right foot shows a hallux valgus deformity.

POTENTIAL TREATMENT COMPLICATIONS

Analgesics and nonsteroidal anti-inflammatory drugs have well-known side effects that most commonly affect the gastric, hepatic, and renal systems. Steroid injection can rarely introduce infection.

Complications of surgery can range from failure of improvement with insufficient osteophyte resection to toe shortening with subsequent transfer metatarsalgia (pain under the metatarsal heads of the lesser toes). Arthroplasty complications include implant failure, silicone wear, foreign body reaction, and osteolysis. Arthrodesis complications include malunion and nonunion.

References

1. O'Malley MJ. Hallux rigidus. In Craig EV, ed. Clinical Orthopaedics. Philadelphia, Lippincott Williams & Wilkins, 1999:913-919.
2. Richardson EG, Donley BG. Disorders of hallux. In Canale ST, ed. Campbell's Operative Orthopaedics, vol 2, 9th ed. St. Louis, Mosby, 1998:1621-1711.
3. Coughlin MJ, Mann RA. Surgery of the Foot and Ankle, 7th ed. St. Louis, Mosby, 1999:605-632.
4. Mann RA. Disorders of the first metatarsophalangeal joint. J Am Acad Orthop Surg 1995;3:34-40.
5. Sammarco GJ. Biomechanics of the foot. In Frankel VH, Nordin M, eds. Biomechanics of the Skeletal System. Philadelphia, Lea & Febiger, 1980:193-219.
6. Alexander IA. Hallux metatarsophalangeal arthrodesis. In Thompson RC, Johnson KA, eds. Master Techniques in Orthopaedic Surgery. The Foot and Ankle. Philadelphia, Raven Press, 1994:49-64.
7. Hertling D, Kessler RM. The leg, ankle and foot. In Hertling D, Kessler RM, eds. Management of Common Musculoskeletal Disorders, 3rd ed. Philadelphia, Lippincott Williams & Wilkins, 1996:435-438.
8. Geldwert JJ, Rock GD, McGrath MP, Mancuso JE. Cheilectomy: still a useful technique for grade I and grade II hallux limitus/rigidus. J Foot Surg 1992;31:154-159.
9. Hattrup SJ, Johnson KA. Subjective results of hallux rigidus following treatment with cheilectomy. Clin Orthop 1988;226:182-189.
10. Pfeffer GB. Cheilectomy. In Thompson RC, Johnson KA, eds. Master Techniques in Orthopaedic Surgery. The Foot and Ankle. Philadelphia, Raven Press, 1994:119-133.
11. Coughlin MJ. Arthrodesis of first metatarsophalangeal joint. Orthop Rev 1990;19:177-186.
12. Curtis MJ, Myerson M, Jinnah RH, et al. Arthrodesis of the first metatarsophalangeal joint: a biomechanical study of internal fixation techniques. Foot Ankle 1993;14:395-399.
13. Wenger RJ, Whalley RC. Total replacement of the first MTP joint. J Bone Joint Surg Br 1978;60:88-92.
14. Townley CO, Taranow WS. A metallic hemiarthroplasty resurfacing prosthesis for the hallux metatarsophalangeal joint. Foot Ankle Int 1994;15:575-580.
15. Gibson JN, Thomson CE. Arthrodesis or total replacement arthroplasty for hallux rigidus: a randomized controlled trial. Foot Ankle Int 2005;26:680-690.
16. Kennedy JG, Chow FY, Dines J, et al. Outcomes after interposition arthroplasty for treatment of hallux rigidus. Clin Orthop Relat Res 2006;445:210-215.

Hammer Toe 82

Robert J. Krug, MD, Elise H. Lee, MD, Sheila Dugan, MD, and Katherine Mashey, DPM

Synonyms

Flexion contracture of the proximal interphalangeal joint
Lesser toe deformity
Hammer toe syndrome

ICD-9 Codes

735.4   Hammer toe (acquired)
735.8   Other acquired deformities of toe

DEFINITION

Hammer toe refers to an abnormal flexion posture at the proximal interphalangeal (PIP) joint of one or more of the lesser four toes. A hammer toe involves hyperextension of the metatarsophalangeal (MTP) joint, flexion of the PIP joint, and extension of the distal interphalangeal joint (Fig. 82-1). In contrast to clawing, which tends to involve all toes, hammer toe deformity usually affects only one or two toes.[1] Hammer toes are classified as either flexible or rigid. The most commonly affected toe is the second, although multiple digits can be involved.[2]

Hammer toe is the most common of the lesser toe deformities and occurs primarily in the sagittal plane. It is arguably the most common toe disorder presented to the foot and ankle surgeon. Women are more commonly affected, and the incidence of hammer toe increases with age.[3]

The most common cause of hammer toe deformity is flexor stabilization in a pronated foot. The pronated foot requires more effort from the intrinsic muscles of the toes to stabilize the foot during toe-off.[4] Hammer toe deformities progress from flexible to rigid over time. Contributing factors include long-term wear of poorly fitting shoes, especially those with tight, narrow toe boxes. Crowding and overlapping from hallux valgus are other causes. A long second ray with subsequent buckling of the toe may also lead to the deformity. Other predisposing factors are diabetes, connective tissue disease, and trauma.[3] Importantly, unlike with claw toes, there is no imbalance of the intrinsic muscles of

the foot or association with neuromuscular disease.[1] Contracture of the flexor digitorum longus, however, may be present in some cases.

SYMPTOMS

Patients commonly complain of pain or tenderness in the area of the PIP joint, especially when shoes are worn or during weight-bearing activities. Patients also commonly present with cosmetic complaints. Pain may be the result of clavus formation over the dorsal aspect of the PIP joint from shoe compression. In cases in which hyperextension of the MTP joint has occurred, there is also increased pressure under the metatarsal heads. Metatarsalgia with subsequent callus formation underneath the metatarsal heads may occur secondary to their plantar displacement,[1] with distal displacement of the plantar fat pad.

PHYSICAL EXAMINATION

The diagnosis is confirmed by MTP joint hyperextension, PIP joint flexion, and distal interphalangeal joint extension in the affected toe. Palpation of the PIP joint usually causes tenderness, with the plantar aspect more commonly affected.

On inspection, determine the degree of PIP joint flexion. Also note accompanying foot deformities, such as ulcerations and callus formation over the PIP joint and tip of the toe. Hammer toe deformities become more prominent in stance phase. Stance phase is 40% of the normal gait cycle, and 75% of stance stage is spent on forefoot, where intrinsic muscles are functioning.

Next, determine whether the hammer toe deformity is fixed or flexible. Flexor digitorum longus contracture is assessed with the ankle in dorsiflexion and plantar flexion. Correction of the deformity on plantar flexion signifies a flexible hammer toe. Dorsiflexion, in turn, accentuates the deformity.[5]

Perform a joint range of motion examination of the affected toe to determine flexibility and presence or absence of crepitus. The Kelikian push-up test is used to assess the degree of flexibility. Press upward on the

453

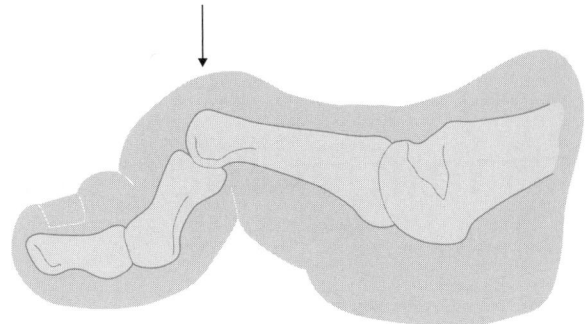

FIGURE 82-1. Diagrammatic representation of hammer toe.

plantar aspect of the metatarsal head; in flexible deformities, the MTP joint will align and the proximal phalanx will assume a more normal position.

Also assess for signs of swelling, temperature change, or erythema that might indicate the presence of an infectious or rheumatic process responsible for the deformity.

Inspection of the patient's footwear is necessary to determine the ability of the toe box to accommodate the forefoot. The presence of clavi or corns over the PIP joint, which may ulcerate, is often indicative of poorly fitting footwear.

Standard neurologic and vascular examinations will reveal no abnormal findings in uncomplicated hammer toe deformities. If there is a superficial peroneal nerve injury causing a dropfoot deformity, hammer toes will result because of extensor substitution. Likewise, a weakness of the gastrocnemius can lead to flexor substitution, causing a hammer toe.

If the patient has peripheral vascular disease or atherosclerosis, ulceration over a PIP joint may lead to toe loss unless the toe is revascularized.

FUNCTIONAL LIMITATIONS

Functional limitations mostly result from pain incurred by clavus and callus formation. Walking and other weight-bearing activities can be painful. The ability to tolerate footwear with a narrow toe box is also impaired.

DIAGNOSTIC STUDIES

The diagnosis is primarily a clinical one. However, radiographs can be useful in assessing a rigid hammer toe; weight-bearing views are preferred. An apparent joint space narrowing corresponds to subluxation of the proximal phalanx on the metatarsal head at the MTP joint.[3,5]

TREATMENT

Initial

Education of the patient is critical. The first step involves fitting for shoes with an adequate toe box to accommodate the dorsiflexed position of the proximal phalanx.

High heels should be avoided as much as possible. A soft insole is useful for pressure relief.[7] Nonsteroidal anti-inflammatory drugs can help with pain and inflammation, if present. Analgesic medications may be taken for pain relief. Ulcer and callus management may be necessary, and patients should be educated about monitoring the skin for breakdown, especially in the setting of peripheral neuropathy.

Local icing may also help with acute pain (10 minutes, two or three times a day). However, ice should be avoided in patients with significant peripheral vascular disease because of its vasoconstrictive properties and in individuals with impaired sensation because of the risk of frostbite.

Initial treatment is palliative rather than corrective and predominantly consists of attempts to accommodate the toe deformity by changing the patient's footwear and débridement of clavi if present. This may include stretching the shoes or switching to shoes with a deeper toe box or to extra-depth shoes. Padding, such as toe crest pads or custom or premade hammer toe regulators, may relieve pressure over the involved joints. Patients with clavi on the PIP joint may benefit from digital caps or silicone cushions.

Rehabilitation

Formal physical therapy is usually not required, although some patients might benefit from a supervised paraffin treatment, which should be followed by stretching exercises. Paraffin baths are contraindicated if ulcers or sensory deficits are present.

Stretching exercises can relieve the "tight" sensation in patients with a flexible or semiflexible deformity. Exercises such as picking up a towel with the toes are recommended for both stretching and strengthening of the intrinsic foot muscles.

Functional orthotics will provide flexor stabilization and, in some instances, symptomatic relief to overpronators with a flexible hammer toe deformity. Orthotics may slow the progression of the deformity by improving the biomechanics of feet.

The clinician may prescribe shoes with deep, wide toe boxes. Alternatively, extra depth can be achieved in a standard shoe by trimming the existing shoe insert just distal to the metatarsal heads.[8] Lamb's wool or felt around the toes provides extra padding. An external metatarsal bar and rocker-bottom shoes may provide additional comfort-enhancing options. Specific strapping devices and hammer toe straightening orthoses are available.

Procedures

Steroid injections may be indicated for patients with painful PIP joint capsulitis or arthritic flare secondary to a hammer toe deformity. Combine steroid injections with padding or splinting for optimal relief. By use of a 27-gauge needle and corticosteroid with local anesthetic mixture, introduce the solution into the joint capsule through the dorsomedial or dorsolateral aspect of the joint. Surgical preparation before injection of the joint is recommended. The patient should be advised about the possibility of a steroid flare.

Surgery

Operative treatment should be pursued when conservative treatment fails. Cosmesis alone is not a good indication for surgery. Associated deformities must also be corrected for optimal surgical outcome (e.g., hallux valgus).[5]

For a mild deformity in which contractures are mild, soft tissue procedures are preferred. Flexor digitorum longus tenotomy in isolation is one such option.[9] The Girdlestone-Taylor flexor tendon transfer, involving transposition of the flexor digitorum longus to the dorsal extensor hood of the proximal phalanx, provides increased plantar flexion pull at the joint.[10] This can be done by passing the split flexor digitorum longus around the proximal phalanx or by using a drill hole through the head of the proximal phalanx to pass through the tendon.

For the more severe deformity, bone and joint procedures are used. Resection arthroplasty of the distal third of the proximal phalanx is a common option. Intramedullary Kirschner wire fixation is necessary for a dislocated metatarsal head. Extensor digitorum longus and brevis tendon lengthening with dorsal MTP joint capsulotomy and collateral ligament sectioning can be performed to reduce flexible MTP joint hyperextension. Flexor digitorum longus split tendon transfer can be an additional option. Some or all of these procedures are performed until correction is obtained.[1,2] Proper correction should result in slight plantar flexion of the PIP joint. Full weight-bearing status in a postoperative shoe or an appropriate pedal splint device is generally permissible immediately after the surgery.[3]

Arthroplasty of the PIP joint is the usual surgical treatment of digits with flexible or semiflexible deformities.[9] Shortening the toe lessens the extensor and flexor tension. The soft tissue and head of the proximal phalanx are resected, enough tissue and bone are removed to relieve tension, and the length of the neighboring toes is approximated. Because the toe retains flexibility, this may provide better functional and cosmetic results for some patients. Recognize that if the cause of the deformity is still present or continues after the surgical correction, the deformity is likely to recur. Postsurgical treatment should include use of a Darco device or splinting to prevent complications.

For patients in need of additional joint stability or in instances of a rigid deformity, an arthrodesis procedure may be a better choice.[9] In severe deformities, an arthrodesis may be combined with a Girdlestone-Taylor flexor-extensor tendon transfer. The arthrodesis may be either an end-to-end type, a peg-in-hole arthrodesis, or a StayFuse implant arthrodesis.[11] The peg-in-hole technique has the advantage of shortening the toe to reduce tension on the joint. Postsurgical treatment for arthrodesis should also include use of a Darco device or splinting to prevent complications.

POTENTIAL DISEASE COMPLICATIONS

A potential disease complication is chronic intractable pain that limits all mobility. Other complications may include metatarsalgia, plantar and point of contact ulcerations in the insensate foot, arthralgia and joint stiffness if subluxation has occurred, toenail deformities, and bursitis or synovitis.[3] Gait abnormalities may contribute to more proximal pain symptoms (e.g., low back and hip pain).

Diabetic neuropathy and advanced peripheral vascular disease are relative contraindications to splinting.[9] Correction is nonsurgical.

Common potential complications include PIP joint ulceration due to excessive pressure, fixed foot deformity, and postural changes resulting from pain-induced gait deviations.

POTENTIAL TREATMENT COMPLICATIONS

Local icing can cause vasoconstriction and frostbite. Analgesics, nonsteroidal anti-inflammatory drugs, and cyclooxygenase 2 inhibitors have well-known side effects that most commonly affect the gastric, hepatic, and renal systems. Postsurgical complications include toe ischemia, digital nerve palsy, nonunion, malalignment, reduced toe range of motion, rigid and excessively straight toe, persistent edema, flail toe, and osseous regrowth. Potential complications of surgical correction include flail or "floppy" toes, which can be repaired by collateral ligament repair or arthrodesis. Infection and, in severe cases, osteomyelitis can occur either before or as a complication of surgery. If intravenous antibiotic treatment is unsuccessful, partial or total toe amputation may be required.

References

1. Canale ST, ed. Campbell's Operative Orthopaedics, vol 2, 9th ed. St. Louis, Mosby, 1998.
2. Myerson MS, Sherefff MJ. The pathological anatomy of claw and hammer toes. J Bone Joint Surg Am 1989;71:45-49.
3. Preferred Practice Guidelines. Hammer toe syndrome. J Foot Ankle Surg 1999;38:1067-2516.
4. Mann R, Inman VT. Phasic activity of the intrinsic muscles of the foot. J Bone Joint Surg Am 1964;46:469.
5. Wheeless CR. Wheeless' Textbook of Orthopaedics. Available at: www.wheelessonline.com.
6. Martin MG, Masear VR. Triggering of the lesser toes at a previously undescribed distal pulley system. Foot Ankle Int 1998;19:113-117.
7. Hunt GC, McPoil TG, eds. Physical Therapy of the Foot and Ankle, 2nd ed. New York, Churchill Livingstone, 1995.
8. Kaye RA. The extra-depth toe box: a rational approach. Foot Ankle Int 1994;15:146-150.
9. McGlamry ED, Banks AS, Downey MS, eds. Comprehensive Textbook of Foot Surgery. Baltimore, Williams & Wilkins, 1992:341.
10. Padanilam TG. The flexible hammertoe: flexor-to-extensor transfer. Foot Ankle Clin 1998;3:259.
11. Briggs L. Proximal interphalangeal joint arthrodesis using the StayFuse implant. Tech Foot Ankle Surg 2004.
12. Siffri P, Anderson R, Daus W, Cohen B. Partial syndactylization for the painful interdigital clavus. Tech Foot Ankle Surg 2004;3:113-117.
13. Femino J, Mueller K. Complications of lesser toe surgery. Clin Orthop Relat Res 2001;381:72-88.
14. Kirchner J, Wagner E. Girdlestone-Taylor flexor extensor tendon transfer. Tech Foot Ankle Surg 2004;3:91-99.
15. Steensma MR, Jabara M, Anderson JG, Bohay DR. Flexor hallucis longus tendon transfer for hallux claw toe deformity and vertical instability of the metatarsophalangeal joint. Foot Ankle Int 2006;27:689-692.
16. Pietrazak WS, Lessek TP, Perns SV. A bioabsorbable fixation implant for use in proximal interphalangeal joint arthrodesis: biomechanical testing in a synthetic bone substrate. J Foot Ankle Surg 2006;45:288-294.
17. O'Kane C, Kilmartin T. Review of proximal interphalangeal joint excisional arthroplasty for the correction of second hammer toe deformity in 100 cases. Foot Ankle Int 2005;26:320-325.
18. Gallentine JW, DeOrio JK. Removal of the second toe for severe hammertoe in elderly patients. Foot Ankle Int 2005;26:353-358.
19. Hofbauer M, Reeves A. Lesser digital surgery. In Chang T, ed. Master Techniques in Podiatric Surgery. The Foot and Ankle. Philadelphia, Lippincott Williams & Wilkins, 2005.

Mallet Toe 83

Sandra Maguire, MD

DEFINITION

Mallet toe refers to an abnormal flexion deformity at the distal interphalangeal (DIP) joint (Fig. 83-1). Typically, there is normal alignment of the metatarsophalangeal and proximal interphalangeal joints. The most commonly affected toe is the second, although multiple digits can be involved. The third and fourth toes are also commonly involved. The deformity may be fixed (rigid) or flexible, and the condition may occur in both feet. High-heeled shoes and shoes with a narrow toe box aggravate the deformity.[1] There is some observational evidence to suggest that a toe longer than adjacent toes is at increased risk for development of lesser toe deformities.[2] Incidence of lesser toe deformities at the distal interphalangeal (mallet toe) and proximal interphalangeal (hammer toe) joints is between 2% and 20%.[3]

SYMPTOMS

Patients typically complain of pain or tenderness in the area of the DIP joint. This is often most prominent in wearing shoes, particularly shoes with high heels or a narrow toe box. The symptoms are also worse during weight bearing, and activities such as running may promote symptoms. Patients also have cosmetic complaints, such as toenail deformities. Pain may be the result of corn formation over the dorsal aspect of the DIP joint from shoe compression.

PHYSICAL EXAMINATION

On inspection, the degree of DIP joint flexion should be determined. Accompanying foot deformities, such as ulcerations and callus formation, may also be present.

Note whether the deformity changes with standing and whether it is fixed (rigid) or flexible.

A joint range of motion examination of the affected toe must be performed to determine flexibility and the presence of crepitus. Swelling, temperature change, or erythema might indicate an infectious or rheumatic process as the underlying cause of the deformity.

Inspection of the patient's footwear is necessary to determine the ability of the toe box to accommodate the forefoot. The presence of clavi or corns, which may ulcerate, is often indicative of poorly fitting footwear.

Standard neurologic and vascular examinations will reveal no abnormal findings in uncomplicated mallet toe deformities. If the patient has peripheral vascular disease or atherosclerosis, ulceration over a joint may lead to toe loss unless the toe is revascularized.

FUNCTIONAL LIMITATIONS

Functional limitations mostly result from pain, particularly with weight-bearing activities. Thus, walking may be limited, and high-impact activities such as running may be altogether too painful. Women may complain that they are unable to dress appropriately for work because high heels are uncomfortable. Mallet toe commonly occurs without pain and in such cases does not generally cause functional limitations and does not require treatment.[4]

DIAGNOSTIC STUDIES

The diagnosis is clinical. However, radiographs can be useful in assessing a fixed or rigid mallet toe; weight-bearing views are preferred.

TREATMENT

Initial

Education of the patient is critical. The first step involves fitting for shoes with an adequate toe box to accommodate the deformity. High heels should be avoided as much as possible. A soft insole, particularly

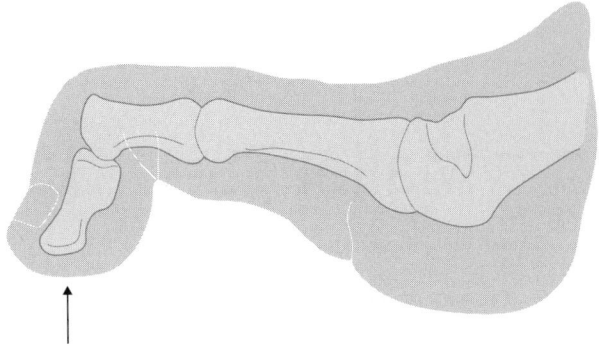

FIGURE 83-1. Mallet toe (*arrow* indicates usual area of callus formation).

Differential Diagnosis

Claw toe

Hammer toe

Interdigital neuroma

Nonspecific synovitis of the metatarsophalangeal joint

Triggering of the lesser toes (lower limb analogue of trigger finger)[5]

Rheumatoid or psoriatic arthritis

Plantar plate rupture

a soft metatarsal pad or bar placed just proximal to the metatarsal head, is useful for pressure relief.[6,7] Nonsteroidal anti-inflammatory drugs can help with pain and inflammation, if present. Analgesic medications may be taken for pain relief.

Local icing may also help with acute pain (20 minutes, two or three times a day). However, ice should be avoided in patients with significant peripheral vascular disease because of its vasoconstrictive properties and in individuals with impaired sensation because of the risk of frostbite.

Initial treatment is palliative rather than corrective. This predominantly consists of attempts to accommodate the toe deformity by changing the patient's footwear. This may include stretching the shoes or switching to shoes with a deeper toe box or to extra-depth shoes. Padding, such as toe crest pads or custom or premade mallet toe regulators, may relieve pressure over the involved joints. Patients with clavi may benefit from digital caps or silicone cushions. Ulcer and callus management may be required, and patients should be educated about monitoring the skin for breakdown, especially in the setting of peripheral neuropathy.

Rehabilitation

Formal physical therapy is usually not required, although some patients might benefit from a supervised paraffin treatment, which should be followed by stretching exercises. Paraffin baths are contraindicated if ulcers or sensory deficits are present.

Stretching exercises can relieve the "tight" sensation in patients with a more flexible or semiflexible deformity but may do little if the DIP joint is rigid. Exercises such as picking up a towel with the toes are recommended for both stretching and strengthening of the intrinsic foot muscles, regardless of degree of flexibility of the deformity.

Functional orthoses will provide flexor stabilization and, in some instances, symptomatic relief to overpronators with a flexible mallet toe deformity. Orthoses have not, however, been found to alter the progression of the deformity.

The clinician may prescribe shoes with deep, wide toe boxes. Alternatively, extra depth can be achieved in a standard shoe by trimming the existing shoe insert just distal to the metatarsal heads.[8] Lamb's wool or felt around the toes provides extra padding. An external metatarsal bar or rocker-bottom shoe is an additional comfort-enhancing option.

Procedures

Steroid injections may be indicated for patients with a painful mallet toe deformity. Combine steroid injections with padding or splinting for optimal relief. By use of a 27-gauge needle and corticosteroid with local anesthetic mixture, introduce the steroid into the joint capsule through the dorsomedial or dorsolateral aspect of the joint. Surgical preparation before injection of the joint is recommended. The patient should be advised about the possibility of a steroid flare.

Surgery

Operative treatment should be pursued only if conservative treatment fails. Cosmesis alone is not a good indication for surgery. Associated deformities must also be fixed for optimal surgical outcome (e.g., hallux valgus). In some instances, surgical management will need to address a combined mallet toe–hammer toe deformity.

For a mild deformity in which contractures do not exist, soft tissue procedures are the procedures of choice. For the more severe deformity, bone and joint procedures are used. Full weight-bearing status in a postoperative shoe or an appropriate pedal splint device is generally permissible immediately after the outpatient surgery.

Because of the progressive nature of this deformity, most patients eventually are treated with surgical options. Surgical treatment depends on the etiology, extent, and severity of the deformity.

In younger patients, a flexor tenotomy alone is often sufficient to treat the mallet toe deformity. For patients in need of additional joint stability or in instances of a rigid deformity, an arthrodesis may be a better choice. In severe deformities, an arthrodesis is sometimes combined with a flexor tendon release. Retrospective studies have shown that an excisional arthroplasty of the DIP joint that achieves DIP fusion, with a simultaneous flexor tenotomy, optimizes the chance for a good outcome.[9] Postoperative anteroposterior and lateral weight-bearing radiographs can illustrate whether an actual fusion of the DIP joint has been achieved. In the setting of a stiff joint without actual fusion, the outcome is still usually satisfactory. The arthrodesis may be an end-to-end type, or the joint may be remodeled into a peg-in-hole arthrodesis. The peg-in-hole technique has advantages in which shortening of the toe can reduce tension on the joint. Postsurgical treatment for arthrodesis should also include use of a Darco device or splinting to prevent complications.

POTENTIAL DISEASE COMPLICATIONS

A potential disease complication is chronic intractable pain that limits all mobility. Other complications may include metatarsalgia, plantar and point of contact ulcerations in the insensate foot, arthralgia and joint stiffness if subluxation has occurred, toenail deformities, and bursitis or synovitis. Gait abnormalities may contribute to more proximal pain symptoms (e.g., low back and hip pain).

Potential complications of nonsurgical treatment also include deviation of the toes, especially overlapping second toes. This may be prevented by splinting or use of a Darco device. Diabetic neuropathy and advanced peripheral vascular disease are relative contraindications to splinting.

Common potential complications include DIP joint ulceration due to excessive pressure, fixed foot deformity, and postural changes resulting from pain-induced gait deviations.

POTENTIAL TREATMENT COMPLICATIONS

Local icing can cause vasoconstriction and frostbite. Analgesics and nonsteroidal anti-inflammatory drugs have well-known side effects that most commonly affect the gastric, hepatic, and renal systems. Postsurgical complications include toe ischemia, digital nerve palsy, nonunion, malalignment, reduced range of motion, rigid and excessively straight toe, persistent edema, flail toe, and osseous regrowth. Potential complications of surgical correction include flail or "floppy" toes, which can be repaired by collateral ligament repair, and hyperextension of the DIP joint. Infection and, in severe cases, osteomyelitis can occur either before or as a complication of surgery. If intravenous antibiotic treatment is unsuccessful, partial or total toe amputation may be required.

References

1. Birrer RB, DellaCorte MP, Grisafi PJ, eds. Common Foot Problems in Primary Care. Philadelphia, Hanley & Belfus, 1992.
2. Coughlin MJ, Mann RA. Lesser toe deformities. In Coughlin MJ, Mann RA. Surgery of the Foot, 6th ed. St. Louis, Mosby, 1993: 341-412.
3. Caselli MA, George DH. Foot deformities: biomechanical and pathomechanical changes associated with aging, part I. Clin Podiatr Med Surg 2003;20:487-509.
4. Badlissi, F, Dunn, JE, Link CL, et al. Foot musculoskeletal disorders, pain, and foot-related functional limitation in older persons. J Am Geriatr Soc 2005;53:1029-1033.
5. Martin MG, Masear VR. Triggering of the lesser toes at a previously undescribed distal pulley system. Foot Ankle Int 1998;19: 113-117.
6. Hunt GC, McPoil TG, eds. Physical Therapy of the Foot and Ankle, 2nd ed. New York, Churchill Livingstone, 1995.
7. Guldemond NA, Leffers P, Schaper NC, et al. Comparison of foot orthoses made by podiatrists, pedorthists and orthotists regarding plantar pressure reduction in The Netherlands. BMC Musculoskelet Disord 2005;6:61-67.
8. Kaye RA. The extra-depth toe box: a rational approach. Foot Ankle Int 1994;15:146-150.
9. Coughlin MJ. Operative repair of the mallet toe deformity. Foot Ankle Int 1995;16:109-116.

Metatarsalgia 84

Sandra Maguire, MD

Synonyms

Pain in the metatarsal heads
Forefoot pain

ICD-9 Code

726.70   Enthesopathy of ankle and tarsus, unspecified metatarsalgia

DEFINITION

Metatarsalgia refers to pain in the plantar aspect of the foot in the region of the metatarsal heads. It may be a primary or secondary condition and cause acute or chronic pain. Intrinsic or extrinsic biomechanical conditions that increase stress on the metatarsal heads may result in metatarsalgia.[1] Primary metatarsalgia is usually due to biomechanical reasons, such as excessive foot pronation (flatfoot), wearing of high-heeled or pointed shoes, wearing of shoes with poor padding, obesity, or pes planus (splayed foot with loss of metatarsal arch).[2] Primary metatarsalgia can also be congenital or may be due to recent surgery for other foot conditions. Secondary metatarsalgia may be due to conditions such as gout, rheumatoid arthritis, sesamoiditis, trauma, and stress fractures.

SYMPTOMS

Metatarsalgia is pain in the forefoot that occurs with weight bearing. Patients typically report severe pain in the metatarsophalangeal region of the foot during prolonged weight-bearing activities and ambulation; however, in severe metatarsalgia, pain can be present with initial weight bearing. Pain is often described "like walking with a pebble in the shoe." The patient usually cannot describe a precipitating cause but rather recounts the pain as gradual in onset.

PHYSICAL EXAMINATION

The clinician should evaluate the foot in both weight-bearing (functional position) and non–weight-bearing positions. In a non–weight-bearing position, the clinician inspects for swelling, masses, and calluses. Calluses develop in response to abnormal weight bearing and are good indicants of stress and pressure. The clinician should observe the toes. A relative long second metatarsal with a short first metatarsal (Morton foot) may result in increased loading of the second metatarsal head. Hammer or claw toes may be indicative of a collapsed transverse arch. With the patient standing, the foot is examined for collapse of the arches, especially the transverse (or metatarsal) one. The hindfoot is examined for varus and valgus deformities that will affect placement of the forefoot. The physical examination should include an evaluation of the lower limb for rotational deformities that may affect placement of the forefoot. The foot should be palpated for calluses (that may not be obvious to inspection), swelling, and masses (Fig. 84-1). Pain with palpation between metatarsal head and metatarsal neck may be indicative of an intermetatarsal bursitis. Pain with the metatarsal compression test may indicate irritation of a Morton neuroma. Pain with palpation under the first metatarsal head may be due to sesamoiditis. Laxity in the first metatarsal–cuneiform joints, resulting in a hypermobile first ray, will increase weight bearing under the second and third metatarsals and predispose the patient to metatarsalgia. A tight Achilles tendon will increase forefoot load in the late stance phase and increase the biomechanical stress on the forefoot.

Diffuse pain and swelling along with stiffness of the metatarsophalangeal joint may be due to an inflammatory arthropathy, such as rheumatoid arthritis and gout. Because of destruction of the joint capsule and stretching of the plantar intertarsal ligaments, rheumatoid arthritis–induced synovitis of metatarsophalangeal joints is associated with volar subluxation of metatarsal heads. In this condition, the shortening of the long toe extensors and the excess tension of the long toe flexors may lead to hammer toes.[3]

In metatarsalgia, the neurologic portion of the overall evaluation is normal (e.g., normal strength, sensation, and deep tendon reflexes). If there are paresthesias within the adjacent border of the affected toes (in the digital nerve distribution), the clinician should suspect

At foot flat and heel rise, there is rapid acceleration of pressure initially located in the central heel, then across the midfoot to the forefoot, where the pressure center is under the second metatarsal head. This is the moment of most intense discomfort. The center of pressure then shifts to the hallux at toe-off.[1,5]

FUNCTIONAL LIMITATIONS

Metatarsalgia may severely restrict ambulation. This may affect patients' ability to perform activities of daily living and recreational and vocational activities. This condition may also affect the ability to exercise or to compete in athletic events.

DIAGNOSTIC STUDIES

Metatarsalgia remains a diagnosis made by clinical evaluation. If, however, the history and physical examination suggest a fracture, radiographs may be indicated. If stress fracture is suspected, a technetium bone scan may prove useful. Electromyography and nerve conduction studies may provide diagnostic clarity if tarsal tunnel syndrome or S1 radiculopathy is in the differential diagnosis.

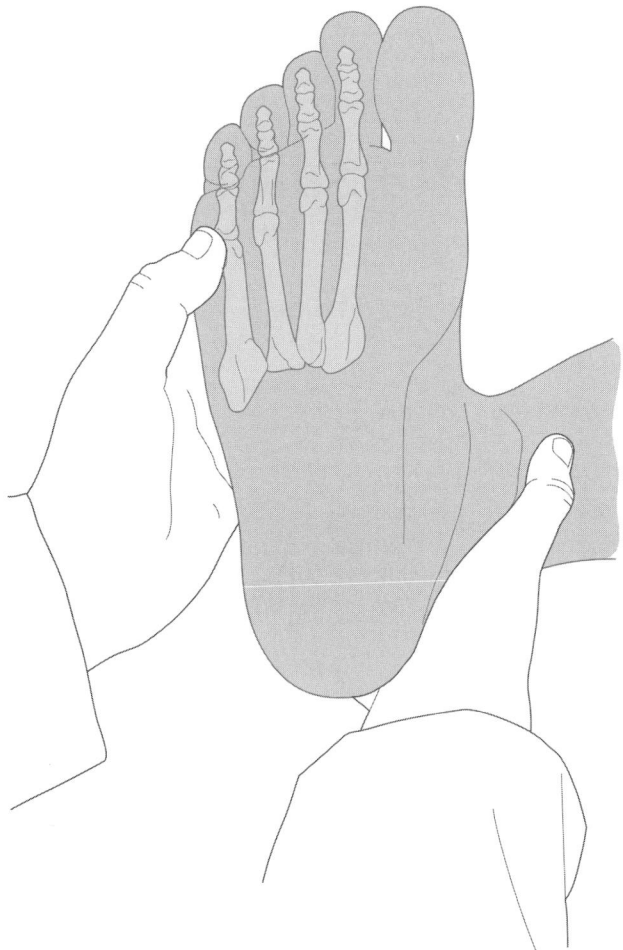

FIGURE 84-1. The metatarsal heads should be palpated with the thumb on the plantar surface and the forefinger on the dorsal surface. Palpate each head individually.

Morton neuroma or lateral or medial plantar neuropathy if paresthesias radiate proximally.

The patient with metatarsalgia requires evaluation for any postural abnormalities or asymmetries that may be extrinsic biomechanical causes of the condition. These abnormalities or asymmetries include pelvic obliquity; leg length discrepancy; scoliosis; rotation of hip, femur, knee, and tibia; and valgus and varus deformities of the knee and ankle. These may lead to displacement of the forefoot and contribute to metatarsalgia.[3,4]

During ambulation, the patient with extrinsic biomechanical causes of metatarsalgia may have increased abduction of forefoot at toe-off. The foot is in its maximum position of flexibility at flatfoot and then becomes rigid at heel rise as the subtalar joint inverts and the transverse tarsal joint becomes locked. It is during this period of forefoot rigidity in late stance phase that the forefoot experiences most of its stresses. During heel rise and toe-off, the hallux and lesser toes reach their maximum dorsiflexion. Toe dorsiflexion places traction on the plantar fascia and helps elevate the medial longitudinal arch through the windlass mechanism of the plantar fascia.[1]

Differential Diagnosis

Intermetatarsal ligament strain

Intermetatarsal bursitis

Morton neuroma

Stress fracture

Metatarsal head avascular necrosis (Freiberg infarction)

Sesamoiditis

Tarsal tunnel syndrome

S1 radiculopathy

TREATMENT

Initial

Initial treatment of metatarsalgia includes analgesics, nonsteroidal anti-inflammatory drugs, orthotic devices for correction of pronated feet (if present), and posting of the metatarsal arch with a metatarsal pad proximal to metatarsal heads.[6,7] It is also important to include modification of activities (avoidance of running and jumping activities) and change of footwear (e.g., avoidance of high-heeled shoes and promotion of shoes with proper cushioning and extra depth). Rocker-bottom soles or steel shanks to increase the rigidity of the shoe can be considered if hallux rigidus is present.

Rehabilitation

The goal of rehabilitation is the correction of postural dysfunction that may be contributing to the metatarsalgia. Postural problems that can affect the forefoot include pelvic obliquity due to leg length discrepancy, which can be corrected with manual therapies, stretching, strengthening, or heel lifts, if necessary. Correction of pronated feet by detailed evaluation of rearfoot and forefoot deformities followed by appropriate design of orthotic devices to improve foot biomechanics will relieve pain and prevent progression. Correct orthotic treatment with physical therapy, when indicated, may help reduce functional rotational deformities of the hip and knee as well as correct the position of the foot.

Realignment by strengthening alone is of limited value and needs to be done in conjunction with biomechanical correction, appropriate stretching, orthotics, and surgery (in extreme cases) to improve alignment. Strengthening exercises for the intrinsic muscles of the foot include using the toes to pick up small objects and transfer them to a container and rolling a tennis ball under the feet.[3] Instruct the patient to perform the exercises to fatigue. Strengthening exercises need to be progressed to closed chain activities because most of the symptoms of metatarsalgia and most of the functional demands of the foot are during weight-bearing activities.[3] The patient should be instructed in stretching exercises to include the Achilles tendon, digits, and other lower extremity muscles, as needed, to improve posture.

Modalities such as ultrasound and iontophoresis may have some limited value.

Procedures

Procedures are generally not indicated in metatarsalgia.

Surgery

Surgery may be indicated when conservative management fails to relieve the pain with ambulation. Several procedures can be performed for resection of the involved metatarsal heads and proximal phalanges, which are beyond the scope of this chapter.[3,8-10]

POTENTIAL DISEASE COMPLICATIONS

Disease-related complications might include deconditioning due to the patient's difficulty with ambulation and chronic intractable pain. Patients who are diabetic or who have metatarsalgia due to faulty foot mechanics are at higher risk for skin ulcerations.[11,12]

POTENTIAL TREATMENT COMPLICATIONS

Analgesics and nonsteroidal anti-inflammatory drugs have well-known side effects that most commonly affect the gastric, hepatic, and renal systems. Orthotic devices are generally well tolerated but may cause skin breakdown. Additional musculoskeletal issues may arise when the kinetic chain is altered.

References

1. Hockenbury RT. Forefoot problems in athletes. Med Sci Sports Exerc 1999;31:S448-S458.
2. Pyasta RT, Panush RS. Common painful foot syndromes. Bull Rheum Dis 1999;48:1-4.
3. Kisner C, Colby LA. The ankle and foot. In Kisner C, Colby LA, eds. Therapeutic Exercise: Foundations and Techniques, 2nd ed. Philadelphia, FA Davis, 1990:385-408.
4. Donatelli RA. Abnormal biomechanics. In Donatelli RA, ed. The Biomechanics of the Foot and Ankle, 2nd ed. Philadelphia, FA Davis, 1996:34-72.
5. Hsi W, Kang J, Lee X. Optimum position of metatarsal pad in metatarsalgia for pressure relief. Am J Phys Med Rehabil 2005;84:514-520.
6. Kelly A, Winson I. Use of ready-made insoles in treatment of lesser metatarsalgia: prospective randomized controlled trial. Foot Ankle Int 1998;19:217-220.
7. Hodge MC, Bach TM, Carter GM. Orthotic management of plantar pressure and pain in rheumatoid arthritis. Clin Biomech 1999;14:567-575.
8. Fuhrmann RA, Roth A, Venbrocks RA. Metatarsalgia. Differential diagnosis and therapeutic algorithm. Orthopade 2005;34:767-768, 769-772, 774-775.
9. Hofstaetter SG, Hofstaetter JG, Petroutsas JA, et al. The Weil osteotomy: a seven year follow-up. J Bone Joint Surg Br 2005;87:1507-1511.
10. Snyder J, Owen J, Wayne J, Adelaar R. Plantar pressure and load in cadaver feet after a Weil or chevron osteotomy. Foot Ankle Int 2005;26:158-165.
11. Mueller MJ, Minor SD, Diamond JE, Clair VP. Relationship of foot deformity to ulcer location in patients with diabetes mellitus. Phys Ther 1990;70:356-362.
12. Wu KK. Morton neuroma and metatarsalgia. Curr Opin Rheumatol 2000;12:131-142.

Morton Neuroma 85

Robert J. Scardina, DPM, and Sammy M. Lee, DPM

Synonyms

Metatarsal neuralgia
Perineural fibroma
Plantar neuralgia
Morton neuralgia
Intermetatarsal neuroma
Pseudoneuroma
Metatarsal neuroma
Interdigital neuroma
Morton toe syndrome
Morton entrapment

ICD-9 Code

355.6   Mononeuritis of lower limb; lesion of plantar nerve

DEFINITION

Morton neuroma is not a true neoplasm but rather an enlargement of the third plantar intermetatarsal nerve with associated perineural fibrosis[1] caused by an accumulation of collagenous material within the sheath of Schwann, usually the result of repetitive trauma (Fig. 85-1). As such, it is more accurately referred to as an intermetatarsal nerve entrapment.[2] The exact etiology has not been clearly identified or proved conclusively, but the following have been postulated as contributing factors: flatfoot (pes planus); anterior splay foot; high arch foot (pes cavus); equinus deformity[3]; ill-fitting (tight or high-heeled) shoe gear; abnormal proximity of neighboring metatarsal heads[4]; and associated forefoot deformities, including hallux abductus, bunion, and hammer toes.

Plantar intermetatarsal nerves of the foot are purely sensory at and distal to the level of the metatarsophalangeal joints, as they course through a fibro-osseous canal composed of neighboring metatarsal heads and the overlying deep transverse intermetatarsal ligament.[5] Anatomic (cadaver) studies have identified the third intermetatarsal nerve as most commonly receiving proximal branches from both the medial plantar and lateral plantar nerves, each arising from the common posterior tibial nerve. Therefore, anatomically, the third intermetatarsal nerve is usually enlarged to some degree when it develops from proximal trunks of two separate nerve branches. This anatomic configuration may or may not be a causative factor.

The classic Morton neuroma occurs in the third intermetatarsal space. Similar nerve disease occurs less commonly in the second intermetatarsal space (Hauser neuroma) and rarely in the first (Heuter neuroma) and fourth (Iselin neuroma) intermetatarsal spaces.[2] They are all treated in a similar fashion.

SYMPTOMS

Morton neuroma may present symptomatically in a variety of ways: localized sharp, lancinating, or burning pain; paresthesias and dysesthesias; numbness and tingling; and toe cramping. Symptoms typically radiate distally, involving the opposing sides of the third and fourth toes, but pain exclusively in the fourth toe is not uncommon.

Unilateral presentation is most common, whereas bilateral occurrence is less so. Symptoms occur predominantly during weight-bearing activities, but residual non–weight-bearing or nocturnal pain is sometimes present. Not uncommonly, patients may experience symptoms while driving an automobile with the foot held in a slightly dorsiflexed position. A characteristic patient maneuver is to remove a shoe and massage or manipulate the forefoot, producing transient relief of symptoms.[6]

PHYSICAL EXAMINATION

On inspection, the foot may appear normal or may demonstrate a subtle divergence of the third and fourth toes, enhanced with weight bearing. When present, palpable pain about the site is usually plantar. The lateral forefoot squeeze test may mimic a tight shoe, thereby reproducing symptoms. In long-standing cases, hypoesthesia or anesthesia may be noted in the third interdigital web space, on the opposing sides of the involved toes or plantar area just distal to the metatarsal heads.

The most diagnostic and reliable clinical maneuver is the Mulder test,[7] performed by alternating lateral

465

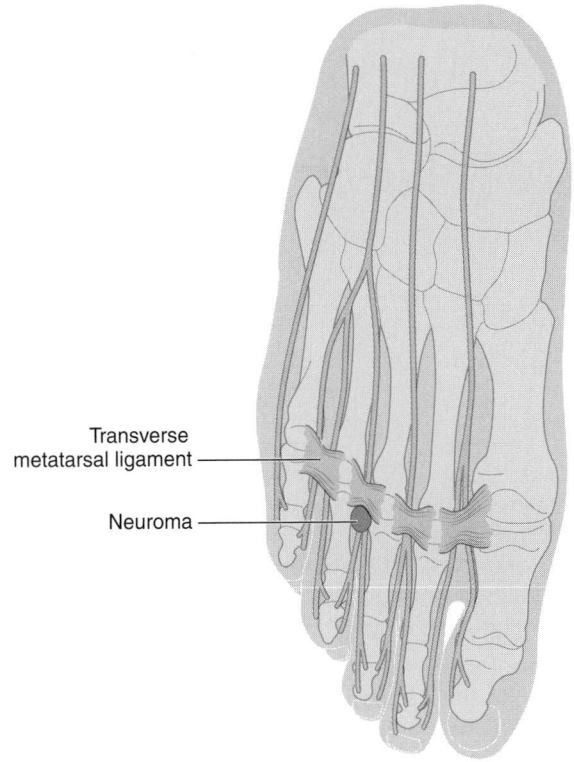

FIGURE 85-1. Morton neuroma.

Transverse metatarsal ligament

Neuroma

is usually pain free without crepitus. Unilateral antalgic (pain-avoidance) gait may also be observed.

FUNCTIONAL LIMITATIONS

Functional limitations include difficulty with walking or running any significant distance and in performing other weight-bearing physical activities, as well as the inability to wear dress shoes comfortably (particularly women's high heels).

DIAGNOSTIC STUDIES

The diagnosis of Morton neuroma is generally made from history and clinical examination. However, other supportive diagnostic studies may be helpful in establishing a diagnosis, especially when surgical intervention is being considered or in the event of failed conservative measures.

Ultrasonography is a relatively simple, inexpensive, and helpful diagnostic tool.[8,9] In the evaluation of a primary neuroma, a 5.0-mm or greater hypoechoic mass, visualized in the coronal (frontal) plane projection between the neighboring metatarsal heads, is considered a positive finding.[10,11] Magnetic resonance imaging, although generally not recommended in the initial evaluation, may also be used, particularly in the presence of equivocal or negative ultrasonographic findings (e.g., small lesions) and when surgical excision is being considered.[12-14] Both ultrasonography and magnetic resonance imaging are used in the diagnosis of postsurgical recurrent or "stump" neuroma.[15-17] Performance of the Mulder test during sonography is a newly described real-time imaging method, helpful in assessing the dimensions of the nerve as well as the local "dynamics" of the pathologic process (Fig. 85-3).[10] New high-resolution, high-frequency ultrasound scanning may provide a means of differentiating a neuroma from disease of neighboring soft tissue structures, including the plantar plate and flexor tendons.[11]

compression of the forefoot with one hand and dorsal-plantar compression of the involved distal intermetatarsal space with the opposite forefinger and thumb (Fig. 85-2).[6] A Mulder sign is considered present when symptoms are reproduced, along with a palpable and sometimes audible click.

In general, there are no signs of proximal nerve involvement (e.g., tarsal tunnel syndrome), vasomotor instability, or arterial insufficiency. Predisposing foot types (pes planus or pes cavus) or a tight heel cord (equinus)[3] may be evident on clinical examination. Passive range of motion of the neighboring metatarsophalangeal joints

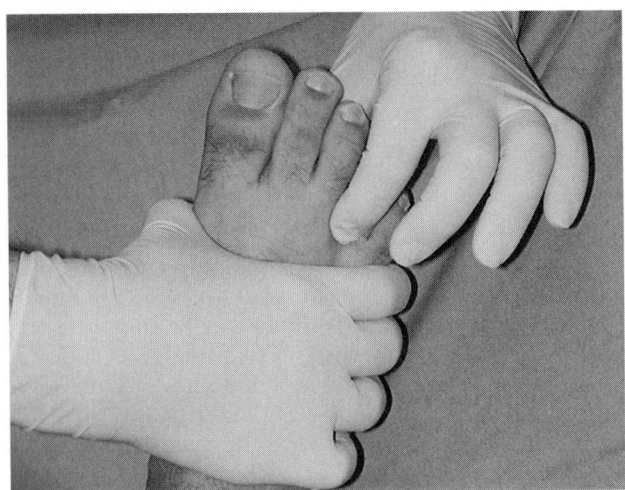

FIGURE 85-2. Technique to elicit Mulder sign.

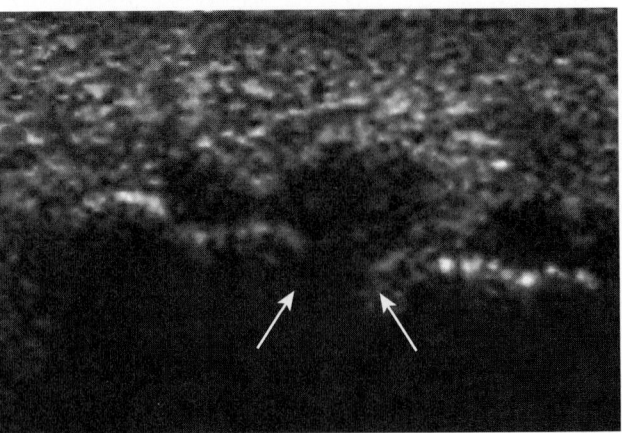

FIGURE 85-3. Dynamic frontal plane ultrasound image demonstrating plantar displacement of neuroma. *Arrows* indicate plantar displacement of neuroma beneath metatarsal heads. (From Torriani M, Kattapuram S. Dynamic sonography of the forefoot: the sonographic Mulder sign. AJR Am J Roentgenol 2003;180:1121-1123.)

The neuroma itself is not visible by plain radiographic imaging, but radiographs may be obtained to rule out metatarsal stress fracture, metatarsophalangeal joint disease (degenerative or inflammatory), or contributing abnormality of the neighboring metatarsal heads. Sensory nerve conduction studies can be used, but because of the difficulty in isolating individual nerve trunks or branches, results are not consistently accurate or helpful. Last, a local anesthetic intermetatarsal space injection can be a useful minimally invasive diagnostic maneuver to support the diagnosis.

Differential Diagnosis

Metatarsal stress fracture

Metatarsal head avascular necrosis (Freiberg infarction)

Osseous neoplasm

Soft tissue neoplasm

Localized metatarsophalangeal joint synovitis

Metatarsophalangeal joint capsulitis

Metatarsophalangeal joint plantar plate rupture or tear

Oligoarticular systemic synovitis (e.g., rheumatoid)

Metatarsophalangeal joint arthritis (e.g., degenerative, rheumatoid, post-traumatic)

Submetatarsal head bursitis

Localized ischemia

Tarsal tunnel syndrome

Proximal nerve root syndrome (e.g., radiculopathy)

Peripheral neuritis

Peripheral neuropathy (e.g., diabetic, alcoholic)

TREATMENT

Initial

Conservative treatment modalities include shoe gear modifications (e.g., wider toe box), adhesive tape strapping or padding of the foot, and use of foot orthoses. Nonsteroidal anti-inflammatory drugs and oral analgesics may provide some relief from acute symptoms but are not recommended for long-term treatment. Posterior lower leg stretching exercises may be helpful in the presence of gastrocnemius equinus.

Rehabilitation

Physiotherapy modalities, including both iontophoresis and phonophoresis, may help manage acute pain. If symptoms respond to initial conservative "mechanical" measures, more individualized therapies such as custom foot orthoses may provide additional symptomatic relief; these usually require referral to a podiatrist or pedorthist for fabrication.

Procedures

Injections with sclerosing agents, such as alcohol,[18,19] phenol, and vitamin B_{12}, may be used if initial conservative noninvasive treatments fail. Local anesthetic-corticosteroid injections,[14,20] however, are more commonly used and may provide transient (but rarely long-term) relief of symptoms (Fig.85-4). These injections are limited to no more than three within a 3- to 6-month period because of the potential for plantar fat pad atrophy. Cryoablation and radiofrequency lesioning have been used with mixed results and with a potential for iatrogenic injury to neighboring soft tissue structures.

Surgery

Conservative measures do not always result in symptomatic improvement.[21] The neuroma as well as the distal digital branches and proximal nerve trunk may be too large for their confined space. In these cases, surgical excision may be necessary.[22] The success rate of surgical excision is approximately 85% to 90%, and surgical revision or reexploration generally carries a poor prognosis.[23]

Less traditional surgical techniques include neurolysis, decompression with dorsal nerve transposition,[24] transection of the deep transverse intermetatarsal ligament (open or endoscopic), laser treatment (vaporization), distal lesser metatarsal osteotomies, and gastrocnemius recession (in the presence of equinus deformity).[25-28]

POTENTIAL DISEASE COMPLICATIONS

Potential disease complications include persistent refractory or intractable nerve pain, reduced mobility, functional limitation, and shoe gear restrictions.

POTENTIAL TREATMENT COMPLICATIONS

Few complications may arise from conservative measures, such as padding, strapping, orthoses, and shoe modifications. On occasion, ipsilateral or contralateral

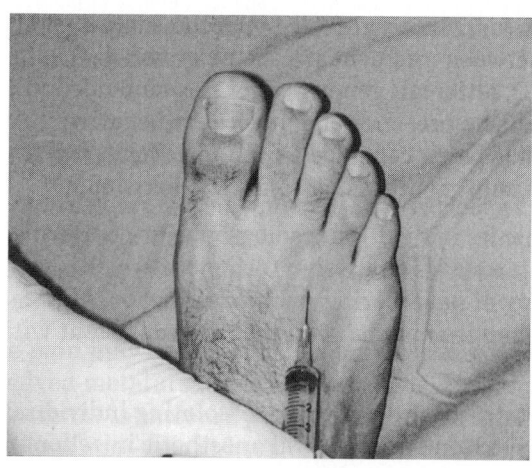

FIGURE 85-4. Technique of injection of a Morton neuroma.

knee, ankle, hip, or even low back pain may be encountered, but these respond rapidly after discontinuation of treatment. Likewise, there are no significant treatment complications from physiotherapy measures when they are used and applied properly. Long-term use of nonsteroidal anti-inflammatory drugs may lead to gastrointestinal irritation.

Injection therapy with corticosteroids may result in plantar fat pad atrophy and secondary metatarsalgia or metatarsophalangeal joint plantar plate or collateral ligament rupture and subsequent digital deformity. Injection therapy with sclerosing agents may result in perineural irritation, inflammation, and pain.

Postsurgical complications include infection, hematoma, vascular compromise, dorsal cutaneous nerve injury, incomplete resection, recurrence,[29,30] stump neuroma,[31] plantar fat pad atrophy, painful hypertrophic scar formation (especially with plantar incision approach), and reflex sympathetic dystrophy.[29,30]

References

1. Addante JB, Peicott PS, Wong KY, Brooks DL. Interdigital neuromas: results of surgical excision of 152 neuromas. J Am Podiatr Med Assoc 1986;76:493-495.
2. Larson EE, Barrett SL, Battiston B, et al. Accurate nomenclature for forefoot nerve entrapment: a historical perspective. J Am Podiatr Med Assoc 2005;95:298-306.
3. Barrett SL, Jarvis J. Equinus deformity as a factor in forefoot nerve entrapment: treatment with endoscopic gastrocnemius recession. J Am Podiatr Med Assoc 2005;95:464-468.
4. Levitsky KA, Alman BA, Jevsevar DS, Morehead J. Digital nerves of the foot: anatomic variations and implications regarding the pathogenesis of interdigital neuroma. Foot Ankle 1993;14:208-214.
5. McMinn RM, Hutchings RT, Logan BM. Foot and Ankle Anatomy. London, Mosby-Wolfe, 1996:71.
6. Wu KK. Morton's interdigital neuroma. A clinical review of its etiology, treatment, and results. J Foot Ankle Surg 1996;35:112-119.
7. Mulder JD. The causative mechanism in Morton's metatarsalgia. J Bone Joint Surg Br 1951;33:94-95.
8. Pollak RA, Bellacosa RA, Dornbluth NC, et al. Sonographic analysis of Morton's neuroma. J Foot Surg 1992;31:534-537.
9. Read JW, Noakes JB, Kerr D, et al. Morton's metatarsalgia: sonographic findings and correlated histopathology. Foot Ankle Int 1999;20:153-161.
10. Torriani M, Kattapuram S. Dynamic sonography of the forefoot: the sonographic Mulder sign. AJR Am J Roentgenol 2003;180: 1121-1123.
11. Kincaid BR, Barrett SL. Use of high-resolution ultrasound in evaluation of the forefoot to differentiate forefoot nerve entrapments. J Am Podiatr Med Assoc 2005;95:429-432.
12. Biasca N, Zanetti M, Zollinger H. Outcomes after partial neurectomy of Morton's neuroma related to preoperative case histories, clinical findings, and findings on magnetic resonance imaging scans. Foot Ankle Int 1999;20:568-575.
13. Waldt S, Rechl H, Rummeny EJ, Woertler K. Imaging of benign and malignant soft tissue masses of the foot. Eur Radiol 2003; 1125-1136.
14. Tallia AF, Cardone DA. Diagnostic and therapeutic injection of the ankle and foot. Am Fam Physician 2003;1356-1362.
15. Levine SE, Myerson MS, Shapiro PP, Shapiro SL. Ultrasonographic diagnosis of recurrence after excision of an interdigital neuroma. Foot Ankle Int 1998;19:79-84.
16. Resch S, Stenstrom A, Jonnsson K. The diagnostic efficacy of magnetic resonance imaging and ultrasonography in Morton's neuroma: a radiological-surgical correlation. Foot Ankle Int 1994;15:88-92.
17. Terk MR, Kwong PK, Suthar M, et al. Morton's neuroma: evaluation with MR imaging performed with contrast enhancement and fat suppression. Radiology 1993;189:239-241.
18. Dockery GL. The treatment of intermetatarsal neuromas with 4% alcohol sclerosing injections. J Foot Ankle Surg 1999;38:403-408.
19. Fanucci E, Masala S, Fabiano S, et al. Treatment of intermetatarsal Morton's neuroma with alcohol injection under US guide: 10-month follow-up. Eur Radiol 2004;14:514-518.
20. Greenfield J, Read J, Lifeld FW. Morton's interdigital neuroma: indication for treatment by local injections versus surgery. Clin Orthop 1984;185:142-144.
21. Bennett GL, Graham CE, Mauldin DM. Morton's interdigital neuroma: a comprehensive treatment protocol. Foot Ankle Int 1995;16: 760-763.
22. Miller SJ. Intermetatarsal neuromas and associated nerve problems. In Butterworth R, Dockery GL, eds. Color Atlas and Text of Forefoot Surgery. London, Mosby-Wolfe, 1996:159-182.
23. Mann RA, ed. Surgery of the Foot. St. Louis, Mosby, 1986:204.
24. Vito GR, Talarico LM. A modified technique for Morton's neuroma. Decompression with relocation. J Am Podiatr Med Assoc 2003;93:190-194.
25. Delon AL. Treatment of Morton's neuroma as a nerve compression. The role for neurolysis. J Am Podiatr Med Assoc 1992;82:389-402.
26. Diebold PF, Daum B, Dang-Vu V, Litchinko M. True epineural neurolysis in Morton's neuroma: a 5-year follow up. Orthopedics 1996;19:397-400.
27. Gauthier G. Thomas Morton's disease: a nerve entrapment syndrome. A new surgical technique. Clin Orthop 1979;142:90-92.
28. Sharp RJ, Wade CM, Hennessy MS, Saxby TS. The role of MRI and ultrasound imaging in Morton's neuroma and the effect of size of lesion on symptoms. J Bone Joint Surg Br 2003;85:999-1005.
29. Amis JA, Siverhus SW, Liwnicz BH. An anatomic basis for recurrence after Morton's neuroma excision. Foot Ankle 1992;12:153-156.
30. Banks AS, Vito GR, Giorgini TL. Recurrent intermetatarsal neuroma. A follow-up study. J Am Podiatr Med Assoc 1996;86:299-306.
31. Ernberg LA, Adler RS, Lane J. Ultrasound in the detection and treatment of a painful stump neuroma. Skeletal Radiol 2003;32: 306-309.

Plantar Fasciitis 86

Paul F. Pasquina, MD, and Leslie S. Foster, DO

DEFINITION

The plantar fascia is a multilayered fibrous aponeurosis that originates from the medial calcaneal tuberosity and extends distally, both wider and thinner, splitting into five bands. Each band then divides into a superficial and deep layer to insert onto the transverse tarsal ligament, flexor sheath, volar plate, and periosteum of the base of the proximal phalanges of the toes[1] (Fig. 86-1).

Plantar fasciitis is an overuse injury resulting from repetitive microtears of the plantar fascia at its origin at the tuberosity of the os calcis deep to the distal medial heel pad.[2] It is classically described as a local inflammatory reaction, although recent research has demonstrated the relative absence of inflammatory cells in the injured tissue, suggesting more of a degenerative process; therefore, the terms *tendinosis* and *fasciosis* are advocated.[3]

Plantar fasciitis is one of the most common injuries of runners. This condition occurs equally in both sexes in young people; some studies show that a peak incidence may occur in women 40 to 60 years of age.[4] The condition is typically precipitated by a change in the athlete's training program. Such changes may include an increase in intensity or frequency, a decrease in recovery time, or a change in terrain or running surface. In the nonathlete, an increase in the amount of walking, standing, or stair climbing may also precipitate symptoms. There is a correlation of plantar fasciitis with professions requiring prolonged standing (e.g., police officers and hairdressers).

Risk factors such as pes planus (flat feet), pes cavus with rigid high arches, excessive pronation, obesity, Achilles tendon contracture, and poor footwear (usually a loose heel counter and inadequate arch support) may contribute to the development of this condition. Multiple authors have demonstrated that the successful treatment of plantar fasciitis is not contingent on the surgical removal of a heel spur. Prior studies have shown that only 50% of patients with plantar heel pain had a heel spur and that only 10% of patients with a heel spur were symptomatic.[5]

SYMPTOMS

Patients typically complain of sharp, knife-like pain in the plantar aspect of the heel at the base of the fascial insertion to the calcaneus. Pain is generally worse with standing or during the initial steps on awakening or after prolonged sitting. Patients will often complain of the classic "pain with the first steps in the morning" that eases after being up and about for a while. Pain also typically worsens at the beginning of a workout but decreases during exercise. The athlete may describe being able to "run through" the pain. Complaints of numbness, paresthesias, or weakness are atypical for plantar fasciitis; therefore, if these complaints are present, the clinician should suspect an underlying nerve injury.

PHYSICAL EXAMINATION

Palpation reveals tenderness at the origin of the fascia of the medial calcaneal tubercle, but there may be tenderness along the majority of the fascia. Range of motion often reveals limited great toe dorsiflexion from a tight plantar fascia as well as decreased ankle dorsiflexion from a tight Achilles tendon. Dorsiflexion should be tested with the knee straight (gastrocnemius on stretch) and with the knee bent (gastrocnemius relaxed, soleus on stretch) to better differentiate tightness of the gastrocnemius and soleus muscles. The neurologic examination should reveal normal muscle strength, sensation, and deep tendon reflexes, unless a concomitant neuropathy is present.

FUNCTIONAL LIMITATIONS

Depending on the severity of disease, patients may complain of symptoms only when they try to increase running intensity or distance. More severe cases may

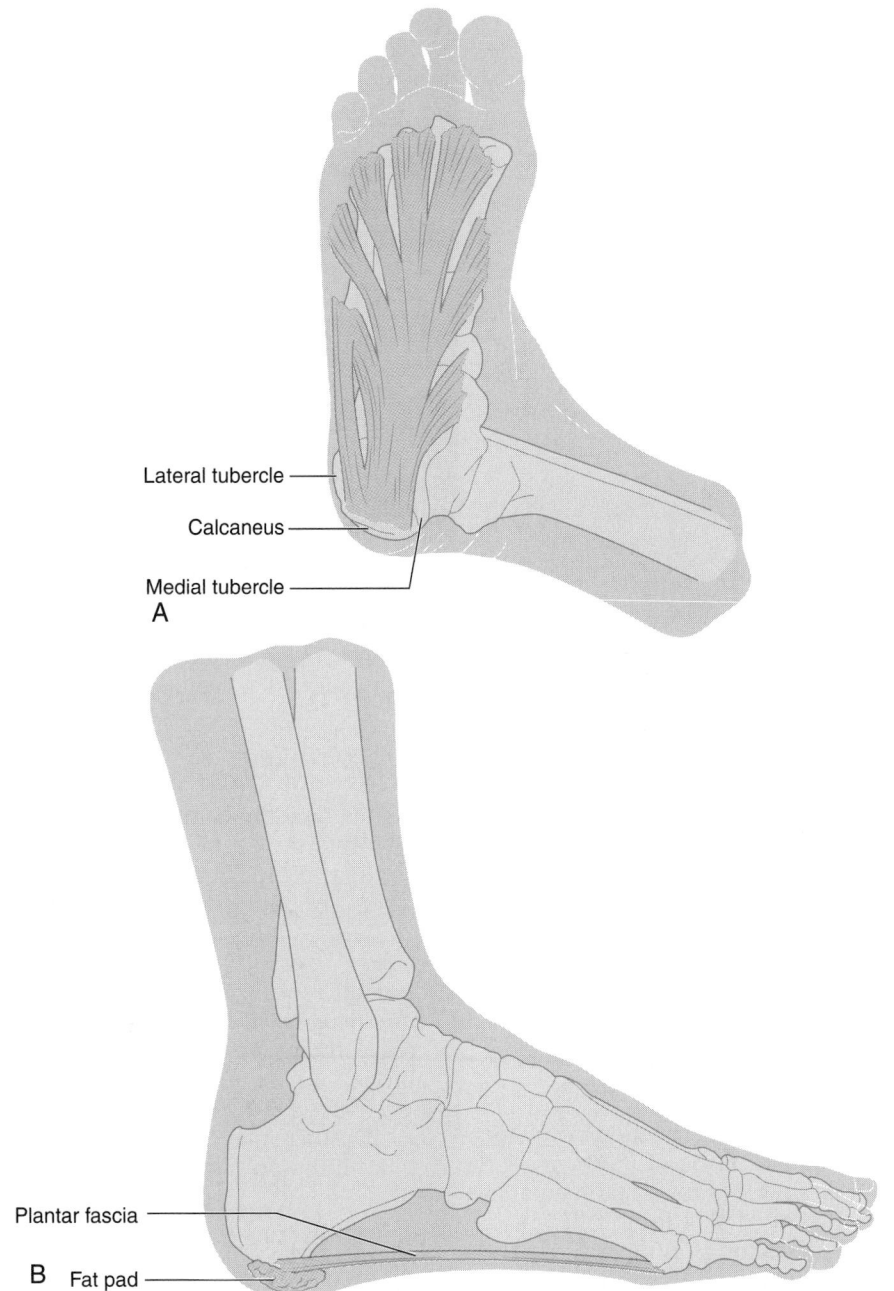

Lateral tubercle

Calcaneus

Medial tubercle

A

Plantar fascia

B   Fat pad

FIGURE 86-1. **A,** Plantar view of origin and insertion of plantar fascia. **B,** Bowstring effect of plantar fascia.

significantly limit a patient's ability to ambulate during daily activities or climbing stairs. Professions requiring extensive walking or standing (e.g., postal workers, nurses, or waitresses) may require job modification as well as more aggressive splinting or even casting during the initial phase of treatment.

DIAGNOSTIC TESTING

Plantar fasciitis is usually a clinical diagnosis. However, radiographs of the foot may be helpful in ruling out other potential causes of heel or foot pain. It is a common misconception that the pain of plantar fasciitis is the direct result of the often (50%) associated anterior

calcaneal spur (heel spur). In fact, a study of 461 asymptomatic patients showed radiographic evidence of heel spurs in 27% of those studied.[5]

Electrodiagnostic testing (electromyography) may be helpful in ruling out the possibility of a nerve entrapment.

Ultrasound and magnetic resonance imaging studies may be helpful before surgical intervention is considered; these studies may demonstrate signal changes or swelling within the fascia. Magnetic resonance imaging usually demonstrates edematous involvement of the calcaneal insertion of the plantar aponeurosis, with marked thickening of the central cord of the plantar fascia.

Differential Diagnosis

The differential diagnosis of heel pain[6] includes the following inflammatory, metabolic, degenerative, and nerve entrapment conditions.

Inflammatory
Juvenile rheumatoid arthritis

Rheumatoid arthritis

Ankylosing spondylitis

Reiter syndrome

Gout

Diffuse idiopathic skeletal hyperostosis

Psoriatic arthritis

Metabolic
Migratory osteoporosis

Osteomalacia

Degenerative
Osteoarthritis

Atrophy of the heel fat pad

Nerve Entrapment
Tarsal tunnel syndrome

Entrapment of the medial calcaneal branch of the posterior tibial nerve

Other
Tumors

Vascular compromise

Infection

TREATMENT

Initial

As with most overuse injuries, initial treatment should follow the PRICEMM principles: protection, rest, ice, compression, elevation, medications, and modalities. Protection and rest usually involve "relative rest"; the patient avoids aggravating activities while maintaining cardiovascular and muscular fitness by participating in low-impact activities such as swimming, bicycling, and weightlifting. Ice massage to the plantar fascia can easily be performed by the patient at home. Have the patient put a Styrofoam or paper cup full of water into the freezer. Once the water becomes ice, the patient may massage the block of ice along the origin of the plantar fascia for approximately 10 to 15 minutes. Icing is most helpful after activities or at the end of the day. Compression by way of taping the sole of

the foot or applying an elastic wrap around the foot may offer comfort to the patient, as may soft gel heel cups, which may be placed in the patient's shoes. Casting in neutral helps in difficult cases. Keeping the foot elevated while sitting or lying may also help reduce any local inflammation and swelling. Nonsteroidal anti-inflammatory drugs are often used to treat pain and any inflammatory component to the disease process. No studies have specifically examined the effectiveness of nonsteroidal anti-inflammatory drugs alone. More than 90% of patients with plantar fasciitis are cured with conservative measures.[6] Patients are often advised to obtain "stress mats" for prolonged standing on hard floors. Modalities are addressed in the following section.

Rehabilitation

The key elements of rehabilitation include stretching and strength training of not only the lower leg and foot but also the thigh, hip, and back. These include the plantar fascia, gastrocnemius-soleus complex, quadriceps, hamstrings, and hip flexors and extensors.[7]

Increased flexibility is achieved through frequent stretching during the day. Each stretch should be held for 30 seconds. It is beneficial to tell patients that muscles need to be reminded to stay elongated; therefore, it is better to stretch for 30 seconds 10 times per day than to dedicate an hour once a day to perform stretches. This also helps achieve the patient's compliance.

Strengthening of the foot intrinsic muscles may be achieved by placing a towel on the floor and having the patient crunch up the towel into a ball and then spread it back out by flexing and extending the toes. Alternative aerobic exercises or "cross-training" should be prescribed to minimize the effects of deconditioning. This can generally be achieved with running or swimming in the pool as well as by low-resistance cycling.

Modalities often prescribed include local ultrasound, iontophoresis, and phonophoresis. Although there is little evidence in the literature to suggest that these modalities hasten the resolution of the underlying problem, they may be helpful in controlling the patient's pain symptoms, thus allowing better participation in a rehabilitation exercise program. As symptoms resolve and the patient has achieved good flexibility as well as normal peroneal and posterior tibial muscle strength, a gradual return to running is attempted. An appropriate return to running program should be established by the provider together with the patient. This can generally be achieved by having the patient start at half of the time or distance and intensity that he or she was running before the injury, divided into equal walk and jog intervals. For example, if a patient was running up to 30 minutes before the injury, an appropriate return to running schedule might be as follows: Alternate 4 minutes of walking with 1 minute of jogging for a total of 15 minutes. Increase by 5 minutes every week until 30 minutes is reached. Next, decrease the walk time intervals to 3 minutes each and increase the jog time intervals to 2 minutes. Each week, diminish walk time intervals by 1 minute and add 1 minute to the jog interval. Walk-jog sessions should be performed three times per week, allowing 24 hours of rest between workouts. If at any time the symptoms begin to reappear, return to the walk-jog intensity of the previous week for another week until advancing again. It is generally recommended to start on level surfaces before introducing hills. Patients must be cautioned to not "overdo it" and to stay within a structured rehabilitation program because reinjury is common.

Management of excessive foot pronation is essential to correction of a common contributing biomechanical factor.[8] This may be achieved simply by stretching the Achilles tendon; however, a change in footwear is often indicated. Numerous running shoes are on the market, and a good running shoe store with a knowledgeable staff may be helpful in finding the appropriate shoe for a particular type of foot. Essential components include a good heel counter and reasonable midfoot flexibility. Patients who demonstrate excessive hindfoot and forefoot varus deformities typically benefit from custom-made orthotics that incorporate medial side wedging. Patients should be cautioned about wearing high-heeled shoes, especially those with hard soles, as this will increase the forces across the plantar fascia as well as promote Achilles tendon shortening.

Procedures

Posterior night splinting may prove effective in resistant cases. Off-the-shelf devices are available, or fabrication of a posterior splint is simple with use of fiberglass casting tape. The patient's foot should be splinted in maximum dorsiflexion to allow maximum lengthening of the plantar fascia and to prevent the stiffening and contraction that normally occur during sleep. The splint should be applied every evening and worn throughout the night for 2 to 3 weeks. If the patient finds wearing the splints uncomfortable at first, a gradual "break-in" period may be necessary, with the goal of wearing the splints throughout the night in 1 to 2 weeks. A study demonstrated that about 90% of patients with refractory symptoms improved after only 1 month of treatment.[9]

Corticosteroid injections can often be avoided if an effective treatment plan is adhered to. In refractory cases, however, a local steroid injection may allow the patient to be more compliant with the established rehabilitation program.[10] We prefer to inject a combination of 10-20 mg of triamcinolone (Kenalog) and 4 mL of 1% lidocaine with a 25-gauge 1½-inch needle. A medial approach is used as it is generally better tolerated by the patient. The needle is aimed toward the medial tubercle of the calcaneus or most tender point, ensuring that the injection is above the fat pad to avoid potential fat pad atrophy (Fig. 86-2).

Extracorporeal shock wave therapy is a treatment that generates shock waves by electrohydraulic, piezoelectric, and electromagnetic methods. A meta-analysis evaluated 20 published studies that clinically supported this

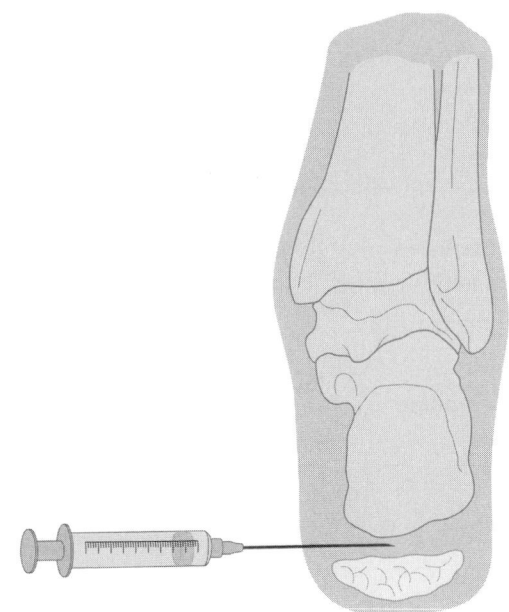

FIGURE 86-2. Proper approach for injection of plantar fascia.

treatment method as effective for plantar fasciitis. Two mechanisms are hypothesized for this treatment's efficacy. First, it is thought that the transmitted waves have an effect on pain receptor physiology. Second, the transmitted waves initiate fascial tissue healing through microtrauma and a subsequent healing response by the release of molecular agents and growth factors. An advantage to this treatment method is immediate weight bearing and return to most activities in 1 to 2 weeks.[11]

Autologous blood injections have shown promise for recalcitrant plantar fasciitis. Martin[12] injected 1 mL of lidocaine and 2 mL of autologous blood where the plantar fascia was most tender. This treatment has been shown to decrease pain severity and to increase functional activity.

Babcock and Foster[13] investigated the effect of botulinum toxin in refractory plantar fasciitis. This randomized, double-blind, placebo-controlled study yielded significant improvements in pain relief and overall foot function at both 3 and 8 weeks after treatment.

Surgery

Surgery may be indicated in patients with significant disability and persistent pain when conservative measures have failed. The two most common surgical options are open and endoscopic release. Overall successful outcomes range from 48% to 90%.[14] A successful outcome could be expected for most patients who are treated for recalcitrant plantar fasciitis.

POTENTIAL DISEASE COMPLICATIONS

Patients who continue untreated and "run through" their pain typically have progressive symptoms, which begin to interfere with their activities of daily living and may lead to irreversible fascial degeneration and damage.

POTENTIAL TREATMENT COMPLICATIONS

Although corticosteroid injections may help selected patients to participate in a more effective rehabilitation program, this procedure should be performed with reservation because it may lead to heel fat pad atrophy or even plantar fascia rupture.[15] For this reason, it may be helpful to apply a walking splint or cast for several days after an injection.

Because of the risk of gastrointestinal bleeding, long-term use of nonsteroidal anti-inflammatory drugs should be avoided, and they should be used with caution in elderly patients or those with a prior history of gastrointestinal or bleeding disorders. The use of nonsteroidal anti-inflammatory drugs is contraindicated in patients with a known hypersensitivity to them.

Surgery, whether endoscopic or open, is associated with several risks (infection, complete rupture). Postoperative rehabilitation may require several weeks of limited or no weight bearing on the affected extremity.

References

1. Karr SD. Subcalcaneal heel pain. Orthop Clin North Am 1994;25:161-174.
2. McBryde AM, Hoffman JL. Injuries to the foot and ankle in athletes. South Med J 2004;97:738-741.
3. Dyck DD, Boyajian-O'Neill LA. Plantar fasciitis. Clin J Sport Med 2004;14:305-309.
4. Gill LH, Kiebzak GM. Outcome of nonsurgical treatment for plantar fasciitis. Foot Ankle Int 1996;17:527-532.
5. Rubin G, Witten M. Plantar calcaneal spurs. Am J Orthop 1963;5:38-41.
6. Chacko K. Heel pain: diagnosis and treatment. Primary Care Case Reviews 2003;6:50-56.
7. DiGiovanni BF, Nawoczenski DA. Plantar fascia–specific stretching exercise improves outcomes in patients with chronic plantar fasciitis: a prospective clinical trial with two-year follow-up. J Bone Joint Surg Am 2006;88:1775-1781.
8. Riddle DL, Pulisic M. Risk factors for plantar fasciitis: a matched case-control study. J Bone Joint Surg Am 2003;85:872-877.
9. Powell M, Post WR. Effective treatment of plantar fasciitis with dorsiflexion night splints. Foot Ankle Int 1998;19:10-18.
10. Borchers JR, Best TM. Corticosteroid injection compared with extracorporeal shockwave therapy for plantar fasciopathy. Clin J Sport Med 2006;16:452-453.
11. Ogden JA, Alvarez R. Shock wave therapy for chronic proximal plantar fasciitis. Clin Orthop Relat Res 2001;387:47-59.
12. Kline, A. Autologous Blood Injection in the Treatment of Plantar Fasciitis. The Foot Blog, Nov. 29, 2006. http://thefootblog.org.
13. Babcock MS, Foster LS. Treatment of pain attributed to plantar fasciitis with botulinum toxin A: a short-term, randomized, placebo-controlled, double-blind study. Am J Phys Med Rehabil 2005;84:649-654.
14. Davies MS, Weiss GA. Plantar fasciitis: how successful is surgical intervention? Foot Ankle Int 1999;20:803-807.
15. Dimeff RJ. Complications of corticosteroid therapy in athletic injuries: a review. Clin J Sport Med 2006;16:279-280.

Posterior Tibial Tendon Dysfunction 87

David Wexler, MD, FRCS (Tr, Orth), Todd A. Kile, MD, and Dawn M. Grosser, MD

Synonyms

Chronic tenosynovitis
Tibialis posterior tendon insufficiency
Asymmetric pes planus
Adult acquired flatfoot deformity[1]

ICD-9 Code

726.72   Tibialis tendinitis (posterior)

DEFINITION

The posterior tibial tendon, originating from the upper tibia and fibula with a broad insertion plantarly on the navicular, cuneiform, cuboid, and metatarsal bases, normally functions to invert the subtalar joint and to adduct the forefoot. Its principal antagonist is the peroneus brevis, which normally everts the subtalar joint and abducts the forefoot. Posterior tibial tendon dysfunction is a condition, as its name suggests, that is characterized by the loss of function of the posterior tibial tendon. This disabling problem may be caused by trauma, degeneration, or inflammatory arthritides and is most commonly seen in the sixth to seventh decades of life.[2] These pathologic processes can lead to reduction of effective excursion of the tendon or even rupture, resulting in progressive loss of the medial arch, midfoot abduction, and forefoot pronation. Posterior tibial tendon dysfunction is the most common cause of acquired flatfoot in the adult. Typically, posterior tibial tendon dysfunction occurs during a prolonged period, but spontaneous rupture can occur in patients receiving long-term steroid therapy or from trauma.

In regard to pathophysiology, the posterior tibial tendon functions in concert with the gastrocnemius-soleus complex to stabilize the hindfoot. The longitudinal arch is stabilized primarily by bone articulations and ligamentous structures (spring ligament, talocalcaneal interosseous ligament, superficial deltoid) and only secondarily supported by the posterior tibial tendon. The initial pathologic change is typically tendinosis of the posterior tibial tendon with maintenance of the longitudinal arch. As the tendon becomes less effective, more stress is placed on the medial ligamentous structures, which attenuate, leading to progressive loss of the arch and abduction of the midfoot.[3] The posterior tibial tendon begins to atrophy while the flexor digitorum longus hypertrophies, attempting to compensate.[4] Next, the calcaneus will drift into a valgus posture, changing the lever arm of the Achilles and causing a contracture. The peroneus brevis becomes an unopposed antagonist and contributes to the deformity.

SYMPTOMS

Patients, most commonly middle-aged women, primarily complain of pain on the inner or medial aspect of the ankle and the hindfoot. As the insufficiency progresses, pronation increases, leading to pain over the dorsolateral aspect of the midfoot.[5,6] Typically, this results in a gradual loss of the arch associated with a gradual increase in pain.

Rarely, there is a history of a rapid collapse from rupture after an acute injury.[7,8] There have been only six reported cases in the literature of athletes (basketball players and runners) younger than 30 years with acute posterior tibial tendon ruptures.[9-12]

PHYSICAL EXAMINATION

The physical examination reveals swelling confined to the area around the medial malleolus. In general, there is tenderness along the course of the tendon, and there may be exquisite tenderness just distal to the medial malleolus where the tendon most commonly tears.[13,14]

Assessment of the lower extremity in the weight-bearing position best demonstrates the essential elements of the deformity: valgus hindfoot (calcaneovalgus), midfoot abduction, and forefoot pronation. This complex deformity clinically demonstrates a "too many toes" sign, that is, when the feet are viewed from behind, there appear to be more toes on the affected side than on the unaffected side. The severity of the patient's presentation depends on the chronicity of the insufficiency and the magnitude of the tendon dysfunction. The medial longitudinal arch of the foot may be entirely lost.

The anterior tibial tendon may become more visible than on the normal side as the patient, subconsciously, tries to regain the arch. Patients may have difficulty walking on their tiptoes or have difficulty performing a one-sided toe-stand while holding onto the clinician's hands. The heel fails to invert into a varus position. Asking the patient to invert the plantar-flexed foot against resistance can be overcome by the clinician's hand. Assessment of the patient on the couch reveals altered posture of the foot due to the unopposed action of the peroneus brevis. A callosity can be seen in the region of the medial, plantar aspect of the midfoot.

Posterior tibial tendon dysfunction can be classified in three stages that are correlated to the treatment. Stage I is a tenosynovitis, normal tendon function, and no deformity. Stage II is a spectrum of disease that includes tendinosis but also posterior tibial tendon dysfunction and weakness. Loss of the medial arch and progressive valgus of the heel with mild lateral impingement can be seen. Early in stage II, the patient may be able to perform a single heel raise, but as this stage progresses, this function is lost. Most important, the flexibility of the foot is maintained with nearly normal subtalar, midtarsal, and forefoot motion. This continuum of disease may progress to stage III as the deformity becomes more rigid and subtalar degeneration occurs with subsequent decreased motion. An Achilles tendon contracture is typically present.

FUNCTIONAL LIMITATIONS

Patients may experience fatigue after only limited activity as their gait mechanics change with progressive pronation. They may have difficulty finding well-fitting footwear. Pain is usually the greatest complaint and also limits walking and sports-related activities.[15]

DIAGNOSTIC STUDIES

Weight-bearing foot and ankle radiographs are usually helpful, depending on the severity of the clinical findings. In the earlier stages of tenosynovitis, the radiographs are usually normal, even if there is some mild clinical flattening of the medial longitudinal arch. As the problem progresses, radiographic changes occur (Figs. 87-1 and 87-2). These include, on the anteroposterior view, uncovering of the head of the talus (as the navicular moves laterally) and increase of the angle between the bodies of the talus and the calcaneus; on the lateral view, plantar flexion of the talus, collapse of the navicular-cuneiform joint, and overlapping of the four medial metatarsals are noted.

Ultrasonography has been used in the past to visualize the posterior tibial tendon both statically and dynamically and to demonstrate the tendon's excursion. Currently, the "gold standard" is magnetic resonance imaging to evaluate the continuity of the tendon. This provides a reasonably accurate view of the degree of inflammation and synovial fluid present within the tendon sheath as well as determines whether a tear of the tendon is present.

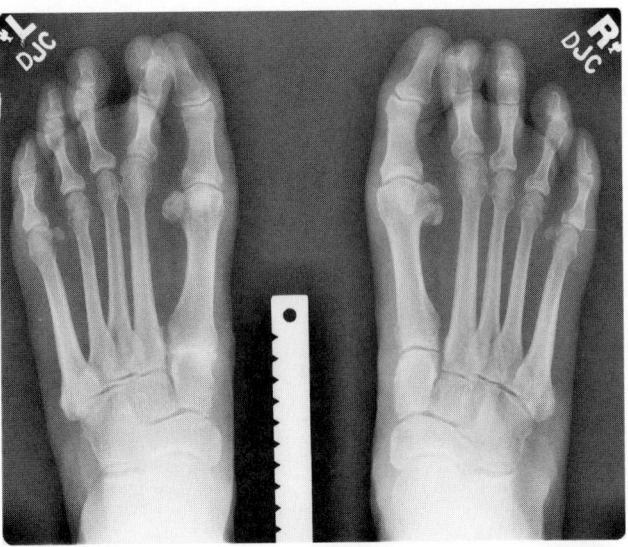

FIGURE 87-1. Anteroposterior view of the foot. Stage II with uncovering of the talar head.

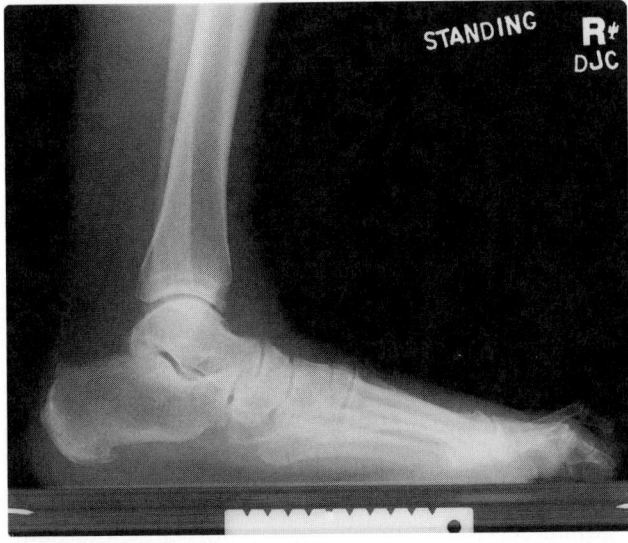

FIGURE 87-2. Lateral view of the foot. Stage II with decreased calcaneal height and talo-1st metatarsal angle.

Differential Diagnosis

Tarsal coalition–spastic flatfoot

Degenerative arthritic deformity

Idiopathic flexible pes planus

Neuropathic arthropathy (e.g., secondary to diabetes mellitus)

Midtarsal collapse

Congenital pes planus

Lisfranc dislocation

Generalized dysplasia (ligamentous laxity)

TREATMENT

Initial

The first line of management, in stage I of posterior tibial tendon insufficiency, is with orthoses. Custom orthotic devices with longitudinal arch support and medial heel lift to insert into the shoes, UCBL (University of California Biomechanics Laboratory) inserts, rigid ankle-foot orthoses, and even double upright braces may be necessary. Unfortunately, there is no proof that any orthotic device can halt progression of the disorder, and if the deformity is less flexible, orthoses may be poorly tolerated. On occasion, a short leg cast is applied for 4 to 6 weeks for rest. Patients who have enough pain to require a boot or cast are also given a prescription for a wheelchair and walker. They are advised to be minimally weight bearing for at least 2 weeks. If the pain improves, they may gradually progress weight bearing in the boot. When they are pain free with weight bearing in the boot, they progress to a cushioned lace-up shoe and arch support. Pain should be the guide as to how fast patients may progress weight bearing. Anti-inflammatory medication may help alleviate some of the pain from the tenosynovitis. In obese individuals, weight loss can be critical.

Rehabilitation

Once the acute inflammation has settled, an exercise program may be started to strengthen the posterior tibial tendon. This can include active-resisted exercise routines with elastic materials (such as Cliniband or Thera-Band) and an exercise akin to trying to "pick up carpet with the sole of the foot" or "grasping a towel." Further methods include muscle stretching and strengthening techniques, particularly aimed at the Achilles tendon. Proprioceptive drills on the wobble board and gait reeducation are also important.

Postoperative rehabilitation can include therapy for range of motion exercises after tenosynovectomy and most certainly after tendon transfer surgery to strengthen the muscle-tendon complex. After a subtalar or triple arthrodesis, the patient will have had a lengthy period of cast immobilization, and therefore gait reeducation can be beneficial.

Procedures

Injection of local anesthetic and steroid into the tendon sheath is a contentious subject and is not recommended because of the possibility of tendon rupture.

Surgery

Different surgical procedures are recommended, depending on the stage of the disease. Continuing pain and failure of nonoperative management of tenosynovitis (stage I) are the main indications for tenosynovectomy to remove all the inflamed synovium. This is followed by a period of cast immobilization. Repair of incomplete tears of the tendon may also be indicated and can be augmented by tendon transfers.

Complete tendon disruption, in the absence of bone collapse (stage II), can be treated with tendon transfers, combining a flexor digitorum longus transfer with a calcaneal medial slide osteotomy. Subtalar or triple arthrodesis may be indicated for patients with progressively worsening deformity and lateral hindfoot pain (stage III).[16,17]

Postoperative gait analysis of patients after tendon transfer and osteotomy shows improvements compared with the preoperative analysis in ankle push-off power, step length, velocity, and cadence.[18] Long-term satisfaction with this procedure is high: 97% improvement in pain, 94% improvement in function, and 84% ability to wear shoes without modification or orthotic device.[19]

POTENTIAL DISEASE COMPLICATIONS

Posterior tibial dysfunction can result in progressive pain and deformity, restriction of mobility, valgus deformity of the knee, and medial longitudinal arch ulceration as the medial midfoot collapses, causing increased pressure with weight bearing in this region.

POTENTIAL TREATMENT COMPLICATIONS

Analgesics and nonsteroidal anti-inflammatory drugs have well-known side effects that most commonly affect the gastric, hepatic, and renal systems. Steroid injection can cause tendon rupture. Complications of surgery include wound infection (in an area that can be notoriously slow to heal) and nonunion or failure of fusion in attempted arthrodesis.

References

1. Deland JT. Posterior tibial tendon dysfunction. In Craig EV, ed. Clinical Orthopaedics. Philadelphia, Lippincott Williams & Wilkins, 1999:883-890.
2. Richardson EG. Disorders of tendons and fascia. In Canale ST, ed. Campbell's Operative Orthopaedics, vol 2, 9th ed. St. Louis, Mosby, 1998:1889-1923.
3. Mann RA. Surgery of the Foot and Ankle, 7th ed. St. Louis, Mosby, 1999:745-767.
4. Wacker J, Calder JD, Engstrom CM, Saxby TS. MR morphometry of posterior tibial muscle in adult acquired flatfoot. Foot Ankle Int 2003;24:354-357.
5. Hertling D, Kessler RM. The leg, ankle and foot. In Hertling D, Kessler RM, eds. Management of Common Musculoskeletal Disorders, 3rd ed. Philadelphia, Lippincott Williams & Wilkins, 1996:435-438.
6. Mann RA. Biomechanics of the foot and ankle. In Mann RA, Coughlin MJ, eds. Surgery of the Foot and Ankle, 6th ed. St. Louis, Mosby, 1993:3-44.
7. Myerson MS. Adult acquired flatfoot deformity. J Bone Joint Surg Am 1996;78:780-792.
8. Mann RA, Thompson FM. Rupture of the posterior tibial tendon causing flat foot. Surgical treatment. J Bone Joint Surg Am 1985;67:556-561.
9. Henceroth WD 2nd, Deyerle WM. The acquired unilateral flatfoot in the adult: some causative factors. Foot Ankle 1982;2:304-308.

10. Woods L, Leach RE. Posterior tibial tendon rupture in athletic people. Am J Sports Med 1991;19:495-498.

11. Trevino S, Gould N, Korson R. Surgical treatment of stenosing tenosynovitis at the ankle. Foot Ankle 1981;2:37-45.

12. Kettelkamp DB, Alexander HH. Spontaneous rupture of the posterior tibial tendon. J Bone Joint Surg Am 1969;51:759-764.

13. Johnson KA, Strom DE. Tibialis posterior tendon dysfunction. Clin Orthop Relat Res 1989;239:196-206.

14. Johnson KA. Tibialis posterior tendon rupture. Clin Orthop 1983;177:140-147.

15. Pedowitz WJ, Jovatis P. Flatfoot in the adult. J Am Acad Orthop Surg 1995;3:293-302.

16. Myerson MS, Corrigan J. Treatment of posterior tibial tendon dysfunction with flexor digitorum longus tendon transfer and calcaneal osteotomy. Orthopaedics 1996;19:383-388.

17. Johnson KA. Tibialis posterior tendon release-substitution. In Thompson RC, Johnson KA, eds. Master Techniques in Orthopaedic Surgery. The Foot and Ankle. Philadelphia, Raven Press, 1994:271-283.

18. Brodsky JW. Preliminary gait analysis results after posterior tibial tendon reconstruction—a prospective study. Foot Ankle Int 2004;25:96-100.

19. Myerson MS, Badekas A, Schon LC. Treatment of stage II posterior tibial tendon deficiency with FDL transfer and calcaneal osteotomy. Foot Ankle Int 2004;25:445-450.

Tibial Neuropathy (Tarsal Tunnel Syndrome) 88

David R. Del Toro, MD

Synonyms

Tibial neuropathy at the ankle
Compression or entrapment neuropathy of the tibial nerve
Posterior tarsal tunnel syndrome
Posterior tibial nerve entrapment

ICD-9 Code

355.5   Tarsal tunnel syndrome

DEFINITION

Tarsal tunnel syndrome may be described as a constellation of signs and symptoms caused by entrapment or compression of the tibial nerve or any of its branches in the region beneath the flexor retinaculum in the medial aspect of the ankle (Fig. 88-1). The tibial nerve branches that may be involved deep to the tarsal tunnel include the medial plantar nerve, lateral plantar nerve, Baxter nerve (also called the first branch of the lateral plantar nerve or inferior calcaneal nerve), and medial calcaneal nerve.[1] Anatomically, the tarsal tunnel is a fibro-osseous structure that begins just posterior to the medial malleolus; the roof is the flexor retinaculum (also called the laciniate ligament), and the floor is formed by the tendons of the posterior tibialis, flexor digitorum longus, and flexor hallucis longus muscles. The tibial nerve usually divides into three branches at the level of the ankle: the medial plantar nerve, the lateral plantar nerve, and the medial calcaneal nerve. However, the Baxter nerve (i.e., the first branch of the lateral plantar nerve) usually branches from the lateral plantar nerve (but can branch off the tibial nerve) just distal to the origin of the medial calcaneal nerve at the level of the tarsal tunnel.[2,3] Then it traverses laterally across the anterior aspect of the heel and terminates with motor branches to the abductor digiti quinti pedis muscle.[2] It is likely that true tarsal tunnel syndrome occurs infrequently compared with other focal entrapment neuropathies, such as carpal tunnel syndrome, ulnar neuropathy at the elbow, and peroneal neuropathy. In fact, in a retrospective review of isolated tibial neuropathies in the foot, the incidence of Baxter neuropathy (17%) was much greater than that of true tarsal tunnel syndrome (5%).[4]

There are generally considered to be five basic categories that account for the etiology of tarsal tunnel syndrome: trauma and post-traumatic changes, space-occupying lesions causing compression, systemic diseases, biomechanical causes related to joint structure or deformity, and idiopathic causes. In addition, the underlying pathophysiologic mechanism of tarsal tunnel syndrome remains elusive; a portion of the literature supports the process of demyelination, whereas other case reports implicate axonal degeneration as the primary process.[5,6] It is believed that the tibial nerve may be entrapped proximally within the tarsal tunnel, or one of its branches (e.g., the medial plantar nerve) may be entrapped distally in its own calcaneal chamber.[1] Also, entrapment of the first branch of the lateral plantar nerve (Baxter nerve) has been described as a cause of heel pain.[7-10] Therefore, in a case of suspected tarsal tunnel syndrome, the tibial nerve and its major terminal branches (including the medial plantar nerve, lateral plantar nerve, and Baxter nerve) should be thoroughly evaluated.[4]

In the current literature, there is no mention of an age or gender preference in patients with tarsal tunnel syndrome. One possible explanation for this is the relatively low incidence and various causes of tarsal tunnel syndrome.

SYMPTOMS

The patient usually presents with pain or paresthesias along with numbness over the sole of the foot.[11] The pain is typically described as burning or a dull ache, but it may also be expressed as throbbing, cramping, or even tightness and may radiate proximally up to the medial calf. Symptoms are often exacerbated by prolonged standing or walking and may be worse at night but may not be well localized. However, if the distribution is limited to a particular region of the foot, symptoms might correspond to a specific tibial nerve branch that is involved (e.g., medial sole of foot due to medial plantar nerve involvement). Obvious weakness of the

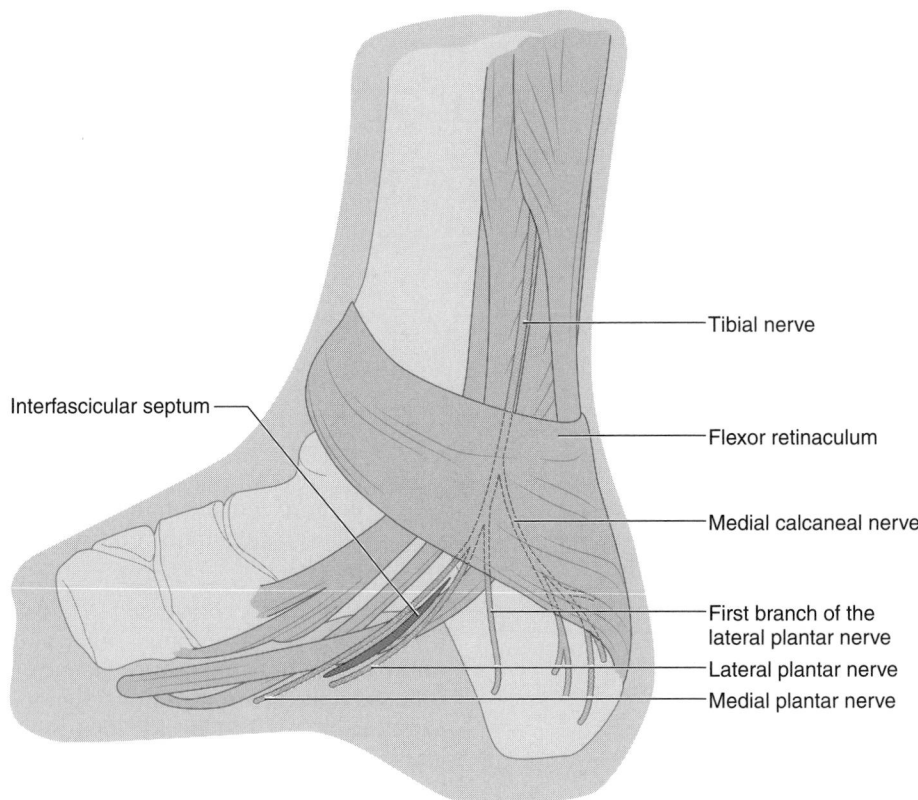

FIGURE 88-1. The medial aspect of a right foot. Note that the medial calcaneal nerve branches pierce the flexor retinaculum as they course toward the medial plantar aspect of the heel.

intrinsic foot muscles is uncommon and may be manifested only if the resulting foot deformity is grossly noticeable or so severe that it causes an unstable gait pattern. Patients with true tarsal tunnel syndrome generally present with unilateral symptoms.

PHYSICAL EXAMINATION

A patient with tarsal tunnel syndrome often has a Tinel sign over the tibial nerve or one of its branches in the tarsal tunnel (Fig. 88-2). On occasion, percussion over the tibial nerve at the ankle will elicit pain extending proximally along the course of the tibial nerve; this sign is called the Valleix phenomenon. There may also be palpable tenderness over the tibial nerve in the tarsal tunnel. Two other provocative maneuvers that may reproduce symptoms in the foot or ankle are extension of the great toe and sustained passive eversion of the ankle.[1] Sensory examination should reveal decreased light touch or pinprick over the plantar aspect of the foot corresponding to the distribution of one or all of the tibial nerve branches involved (Fig. 88-3). Motor examination of the intrinsic foot muscles is challenging because it is often difficult for patients to selectively activate these muscles. However, one may be able to appreciate muscle atrophy around the foot that is asymmetrical compared with the other side.[1] Muscle stretch reflexes in the lower extremity (including patellar, medial hamstring, and Achilles) should be normal and symmetrical compared with the unaffected side. Peripheral pulses

(posterior tibial and dorsalis pedis) are usually palpable and full. Also, if the biomechanical configuration of the foot is altered severely enough, gait deviations could be observed.

FUNCTIONAL LIMITATIONS

Impaired balance or a perception of instability due to diminished sensation or pain on the sole of the foot may be the only functional impairment that is noted by the patient. As a consequence, limited walking tolerance or distance, stumbling, or falls may be reported by the patient.

DIAGNOSTIC STUDIES

Electrodiagnostic testing should be performed for any patient with suspected tarsal tunnel syndrome; this is the only diagnostic study that evaluates the electrophysiologic function of the tibial nerve and its major terminal branches. Both needle electromyography and nerve conduction studies (i.e., motor, sensory, or mixed nerve studies) should be done. Furthermore, it is imperative that the tibial nerve be thoroughly evaluated from an electrophysiologic standpoint because either the tibial nerve or only one of its branches may be involved in a case of suspected tarsal tunnel syndrome.[4] A magnetic resonance imaging study may be useful in detecting a space-occupying mass or lesion that is impinging on or compressing the tibial nerve within the

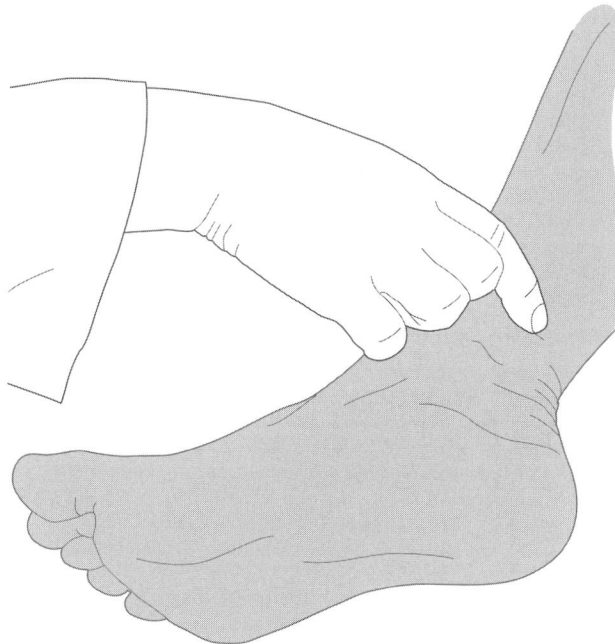

FIGURE 88-2. Tinel sign over the tibial nerve at the medial ankle.

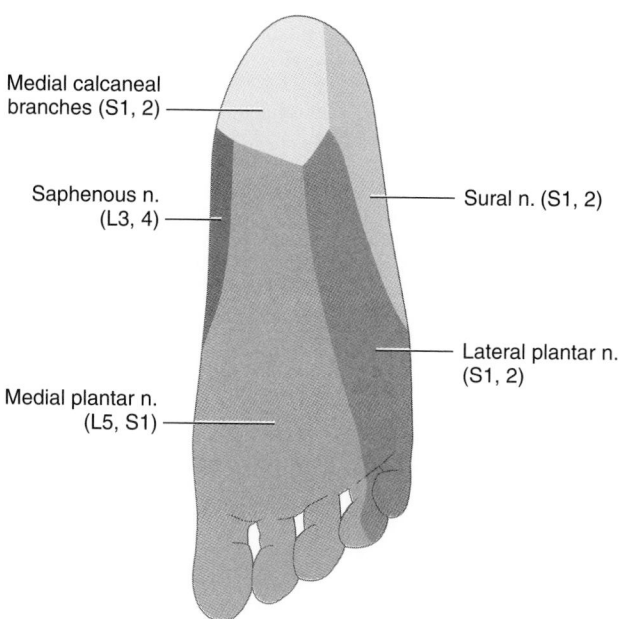

Medial calcaneal branches (S1, 2)

Saphenous n. (L3, 4)

Sural n. (S1, 2)

Lateral plantar n. (S1, 2)

Medial plantar n. (L5, S1)

FIGURE 88-3. Cutaneous innervation of the sole of the foot.

tarsal tunnel. The magnetic resonance imaging study can also provide a "road map" for surgical exploration of the tarsal tunnel and then direct the procedure toward suitable anatomic decompression of the nerve.[12] Also, recent literature indicates that ultrasonography could be a promising diagnostic imaging technique for cases of suspected tarsal tunnel syndrome by identifying space-occupying lesions such as ganglia.[13] Plain radiographs and a bone scan may be needed to rule out a possible fracture or other bone lesion.

Differential Diagnosis

Plantar fasciitis

Peripheral neuropathy

Sciatic neuropathy

Lumbosacral plexopathy

Posterior tibialis dysfunction

Lumbosacral radiculopathy

TREATMENT

Initial

Conservative measures are often effective in the majority of tarsal tunnel syndrome cases, and therefore most patients should be given an adequate trial, which is generally at least 3 to 6 months. Initial management usually includes nonsteroidal anti-inflammatory drugs and possibly a neuropathic pain medication (such as gabapentin). If there is a biomechanical foot condition that can be corrected or supported, the patient could benefit from a medial arch support (for a pronated foot) or a foot orthosis (for hindfoot valgus).[7] Also, a short leg walking cast or boot brace in some patients can provide symptomatic relief.[14]

Rehabilitation

Physical therapy can be useful in certain cases, most typically with modalities such as iontophoresis to reduce symptoms of inflammation, deep massage to mobilize scar tissue, desensitization, and various exercises—specifically, stretching exercises of the toe flexors, both active and passive, and of the ankle muscle groups (i.e., dorsiflexors, plantar flexors, inverters, and everters) if ankle range of motion is affected. Strengthening exercises for the toe flexors and extensors and for these ankle muscle groups may also be prescribed for distinct motor deficits with a goal of equalizing any muscle imbalance. In addition, gait training along with balance training, both static and dynamic, may be necessary. The patient may require extra-depth shoes to accommodate a medial arch support or a custom-made foot orthosis. Therefore, an orthotist or pedorthist may need to manufacture custom orthotics or footwear.

Procedures

For diagnostic and therapeutic purposes, a local anesthetic-steroid injection into the tarsal tunnel can give relatively immediate relief of local swelling and inflammation surrounding the tibial nerve.

Surgery

Surgical management consists of release of the flexor retinaculum and possibly exploration for a mass or space-occupying lesion and neurolysis of the tibial nerve, depending on the surgeon.[1] In addition, some surgeons advocate release of the superficial and deep fascia of the abductor hallucis to more completely decompress the tibial nerve and its branches. The success rate (good to excellent outcome) for tarsal tunnel release is variable and reported to be 44% to 78%, depending on the study.[12] Endoscopic release of the tarsal tunnel may be a potential surgical option in some cases.[12,15]

POTENTIAL DISEASE COMPLICATIONS

Several potential disease complications may be a consequence of tarsal tunnel syndrome. Skin breakdown, including ulcerations, can occur over the plantar aspect of the foot as a result of impaired sensation. An altered gait pattern may develop with decreased balance or a "feeling of unsteadiness" from impaired sensation, particularly with respect to proprioception and light touch or pressure in the foot, or because the biomechanical configuration of the foot is distorted. Also, low back pain or lower extremity joint pain (probably hip or knee) may arise as a consequence of the gait deviation.

POTENTIAL TREATMENT COMPLICATIONS

Nonsteroidal anti-inflammatory drugs may cause, most commonly, gastric or renal complications. Skin breakdown can develop over the foot or ankle from a poorly fitting orthotic device. Tendon rupture may occur after steroid injection into the incorrect location (e.g., flexor tendon sheath). In addition, the symptoms of pain, numbness, and paresthesias in the foot can be exacerbated after a local anesthetic-steroid injection or after surgical decompression of the tarsal tunnel.

References

1. Park TA, Del Toro DR. Electrodiagnostic evaluation of the foot. Phys Med Rehabil Clin North Am 1998;9:871-896.
2. Sarrafian SK. Anatomy of the Foot and Ankle. Philadelphia, JB Lippincott, 1983:356-390.
3. Govsa F, Bilge O, Ozer MA. Variations in the origin of the medial and inferior calcaneal nerves. Arch Orthop Trauma Surg 2006;126:6-14.
4. Zaza DI, Del Toro DR, White KT. A retrospective review of isolated tibial neuropathies in the foot. Muscle Nerve 2006;34:517.
5. Kraft GH. Tarsal tunnel entrapment. Course E: Entrapment Neuropathies. Boston, AAEE Ninth Annual Continuing Education Course, 1986:13-18.
6. Spindler HA, Reischer MA, Felsenthal G. Electrodiagnostic assessment in suspected tarsal tunnel syndrome. Phys Med Rehabil Clin North Am 1994;5:595-612.
7. Przylucki H, Jones CL. Entrapment neuropathy of muscle branch of lateral plantar nerve. J Am Podiatr Med Assoc 1981;71:119-124.
8. Schon LC, Baxter DE. Heel pain syndrome and entrapment neuropathies about the foot and ankle. In Gould JS, ed. Operative Foot Surgery. Philadelphia, WB Saunders, 1994:192-208.
9. Park TA, Del Toro DR. Isolated inferior calcaneal neuropathy. Muscle Nerve 1996;19:106-108.
10. Del Toro DR, Dei RL, Marquardt T. Electrodiagnostic findings and surgical outcome in isolated first branch lateral plantar neuropathy: a case series. Arch Phys Med Rehabil 2002;83:1657.
11. Patel AT, Gaines K, Malamut R, et al; American Association of Neuromuscular and Electrodiagnostic Medicine. Usefulness of electrodiagnostic techniques in the evaluation of suspected tarsal tunnel syndrome: an evidence-based review. Muscle Nerve 2005;32:236-240.
12. Haddad SL. Compressive neuropathies of the foot and ankle. In Myerson MS, ed. Foot and Ankle Disorders. Philadelphia, WB Saunders, 2000:808-833.
13. Nagaoka M, Matsuzaki H. Ultrasonography in tarsal tunnel syndrome. J Ultrasound Med 2005;24:1035-1040.
14. Mann RA. Diseases of the nerves. In Coughlin MJ, Mann RA, eds. Surgery of the Foot and Ankle. St. Louis, Mosby, 1999:502-524.
15. Krishnan KG, Pinzer T, Schackert G. A novel endoscopic technique in treating single nerve entrapment syndromes with special attention to ulnar nerve transposition and tarsal tunnel release: clinical application. Neurosurgery 2006;59(Suppl 1):ONS89-100.

PAIN

Occipital Neuralgia 89

Aneesh Singla, MD, MPH

DEFINITION

Occipital neuralgia is one type of cervicogenic headache described as pain in the distribution of the greater and lesser occipital nerves (Fig. 89-1), associated with posterior scalp dysesthesia or hyperalgesia. The pain is described as a lancinating, sharp, throbbing, electric shock–like pain.[1-3] Two broad categories of patients with occipital neuralgia are those with structural pathologic changes and those without an apparent cause.[4] Proposed causes include myofascial tightening, trauma of C2 nerve root (whiplash injury), prior skull or suboccipital surgery, other type of nerve entrapment, idiopathic causes, hypertrophied atlantoepistrophic (C1-2) ligament, sustained neck muscle contractions, and spondylosis of the cervical facet joints.[1,3,5-8] Most patients with occipital neuropathy do not have discernible lesions.[4]

The greater occipital nerve innervates the posterior skull from the suboccipital area to the vertex. It is formed from the medial (sensory) branch of the posterior division of the second cervical nerve.[4] It emerges between the atlas and lamina of the axis below the oblique inferior muscle and then ascends obliquely on this muscle between it and the semispinalis muscle.[4] The course of the greater occipital nerve does not appear to differ in males and females.[9]

The lesser occipital nerve forms from the medial (sensory) branch of the posterior division of the third cervical nerve, ascends like the greater occipital nerve, and pierces the splenius capitis and trapezius muscles just medial to the greater occipital nerve.[4] It ascends along the scalp to reach the vertex, where it provides sensory fibers to the area of the scalp lateral to the greater occipital nerve.

The condition appears to be more common in females.[10]

SYMPTOMS

Occipital neuralgia may occur as an intermittent (paroxysmal) or a continuous headache. In continuous occipital neuralgia, the headaches may be further classified as acute or chronic.

Paroxysmal occipital neuralgia describes pain occurring only in the distribution of the greater occipital nerve. The attacks are unilateral, and the pain is sudden and severe. The patient may describe the pain as sharp, twisting, a dagger thrust, or an electric shock. The pain rarely demonstrates a burning characteristic. Although single flashes of pain may occur, multiple attacks are more frequent. The attacks may occur spontaneously or be provoked by specific maneuvers applied to the back of the scalp or neck regions, such as brushing the hair or moving the neck.[11]

Acute continuous occipital neuralgia often has an underlying cause. The attacks last for many hours and are typically devoid of radiating symptoms (e.g., trigger zones to the face). The entire episode of neuralgia will continue up to 2 weeks before remission. Exposure to cold is a common trigger.[11]

In chronic continuous occipital neuralgia, the patient may experience painful attacks that last for days to weeks. These attacks are generally accompanied by localized spasm of the cervical or occipital muscles. The reported pain originates in the suboccipital region up to the vertex and radiates to the frontotemporal region. Radiation to the orbital region is also common. Sensory triggers to the face or skull can initiate a painful episode. Similarly, pain may increase with pressure of

485

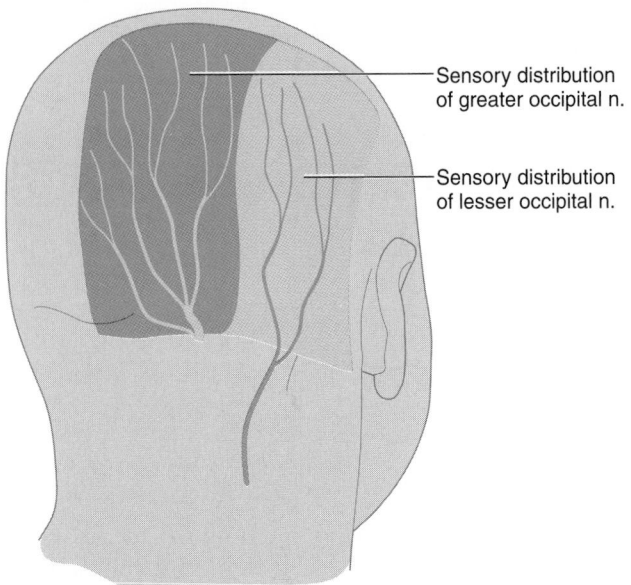

——— Sensory distribution of greater occipital n.

——— Sensory distribution of lesser occipital n.

FIGURE 89-1. Occipital nerve anatomy. The greater occipital nerve pierces the fascia just below the superior nuchal ridge along with the artery. It supplies the medial portion of the posterior scalp. The lesser occipital nerve passes superiorly along the posterior border of the sternocleidomastoid muscle, dividing into the cutaneous branches that innervate the lateral portion of the posterior scalp and the cranial surface of the pinna. (Reprinted with permission from Waldman SD. Greater and lesser occipital nerve block. In Waldman SD, ed. Atlas of Interventional Pain Management, 2nd ed. Philadelphia, WB Saunders, 2004:23-26.)

the head on a pillow. Prolonged abnormal fixed postures that occur in reading or sleeping positions and hyperextension or rotation of the head to the involved side may provoke the pain. The pain may be bilateral, although the unilateral pattern is more common. Often, a previous history of cervical or occipital trauma or of arthritic disease of the cervical spine is obtained. On occasion, patients may report other autonomic symptoms concurrently, such as nausea, vomiting, photophobia, diplopia, ocular and nasal congestion, tinnitus, and vertigo.[11] Severe ocular pain has also been described, as have symptoms in other distributions of the trigeminal nerve.[5,12-14] Convergence of sensory input from the upper cervical nerve roots into the trigeminal nucleus may explain this phenomenon.[8]

PHYSICAL EXAMINATION

On examination, pain is generally reproduced by palpation of the greater and lesser occipital nerves. Allodynia or hyperalgesia may be present in the nerve distribution. Myofascial pain may be present in the neck or shoulders. Pain may limit cervical range of motion. Neurologic examination findings of the head, neck, and upper extremities are generally normal.

Entrapment of the nerve near the cervical spine may result in increased symptoms during flexion, extension, or rotation of the head and neck. Compression of the skull on the neck (Spurling maneuver), especially with extension and rotation of the neck to the affected side,

may reproduce or increase the patient's pain if cervical degenerative disease is the cause of the neuralgia.[11] Pressure over both the occipital nerves along their course in the neck and occiput or pressure on the C2-3 facet joints should cause an exacerbation of pain in such patients, at least when the headache is present. Even if the actual pathologic process is in the cervical spine, tenderness over the occipital nerve at the superior nuchal line is usually present.

FUNCTIONAL LIMITATIONS

In general, there are no neurologic deficits from occipital neuralgia. However, the pain from this entity may result in significant limitations in activities of daily living. During exacerbations, patients may have significant functional limitations, including insomnia, loss of work time, and inability to perform physical activity or to drive a vehicle. Tasks that involve the cervical spine or upper extremities, such as talking on the telephone, working at the computer, reading a book, cooking, gardening, and driving, may be painful and limited.

DIAGNOSTIC STUDIES

The diagnosis of occipital neuralgia is generally made clinically on the basis of history and physical examination. Imaging may help confirm the diagnosis when there is an anatomic cause. Diagnostic local anesthetic nerve blocks may be required for a definitive diagnosis to be obtained; these blocks are done with or without the addition of corticosteroid.[1,4,8] The relief of pain after a diagnostic local anesthetic block of the greater and lesser occipital nerves is generally confirmatory of the diagnosis of occipital neuralgia.

In addition, magnetic resonance imaging or computed tomography of the cervical spine should be performed to rule out an anatomic cause, such as tumor, vascular malformation, infection, or spondylotic arthritis, that may be compressing the medial (sensory) branches of C2-3.[15] Radiographs may be obtained to rule out gross abnormalities as an initial screening test but will not generally provide the level of detail needed for diagnostic purposes. Single-photon emission computed tomography and positron emission tomography are being increasingly used for diagnosis and treatment of certain headache syndromes and may be useful in occipital neuralgia if there is functional pathologic change involved or in trying to distinguish between occipital neuralgia and cluster or migraine headache.[8] Radiologic degenerative changes of the cervical spine do not necessarily correlate with the patient's symptoms and examination findings, but C2-3 arthritic changes in the absence of other gross or radiographic abnormalities may explain the etiology. Other rare causes of occipital neuralgia reported in the literature include upper respiratory tract infection,[16] herpes zoster infection or postherpetic neuralgia,[17] myelitis,[18] hypermobile C1 vertebrae,[19] and giant cell arteritis.[20,21]

Differential Diagnosis

C2-3 subluxation or arthropathy

C2-3 radiculopathy

Migraine headache

Cluster headache

Tension-type headache

Tumor (e.g., posterior fossa)

Congenital or acquired abnormalities at the craniocervical junction (e.g., Arnold-Chiari malformation or basilar invagination)

Rheumatoid arthritis

Atlantoaxial subluxation

Cervical myelopathy

Pott disease–osteomyelitis

Paget disease

Vascular abnormalities

Herpes zoster or postherpetic neuralgia

Giant cell arteritis

Trauma

Whiplash injury

TREATMENT

Initial

Treatments that may help with pain from occipital neuralgia include heat or cold therapy, massage, avoidance of excessive cervical spine flexion-extension or rotation, acupuncture, and application of transcutaneous electrical nerve stimulation.

Pharmacologic therapy with nonsteroidal anti-inflammatory drugs or acetaminophen as well as other analgesics may be used. Tricyclic antidepressants, anticonvulsants, and muscle relaxants may also prove useful. Anticonvulsants such as carbamazepine, gabapentin, and pregabalin have been used for neuropathic pain with good results. Certain patients with comorbid psychological stressors may have pain complaints out of proportion to physical examination findings and should have their psychological symptoms treated with appropriate medications and psychological or cognitive-behavioral therapy.

Patients will often benefit from adaptive equipment at home and work, such as a telephone earset or bookstand. It is also important to determine whether patients are using bifocal glasses and whether adjusting the neck to use these glasses is contributing to the condition.

Rehabilitation

The incorporation of stretching and strengthening exercises for the paracervical and periscapular muscles may be appropriate for the patient with subacute or chronic occipital neuralgia, particularly if the condition is provoked by cervical spine or trunk movement. Postural training and relaxation exercises should be incorporated into the exercise regimen. Principles of ergonomics should be addressed if work site activity is limited by pain exacerbations (e.g., use of a telephone headset, document holder).[11] An ergonomic workstation evaluation may be beneficial.

Manual therapy, including spinal manipulation and spinal mobilization, has been used to treat patients with cervicogenic headaches. A review of trials done with spinal manipulation for cervicogenic headache revealed two with positive results regarding headache intensity, headache duration, and medication intake.[22] Only one trial showed a decrease in headache frequency.[22] There is clearly a need for more well-designed randomized controlled trials to evaluate these therapies.[23] Any spinal manipulation should be done with caution because there are serious risks if it is improperly performed.[24] Anecdotal reports support a trial of cervical traction in some cases.[11]

Procedures

Blockade of the greater or lesser occipital nerve with a local anesthetic is diagnostic and therapeutic (Fig. 89-2). Pain relief can vary from hours to months. In general, at least 50% of patients will experience more than 1 week of relief after one injection. Isolated pain relief for more than 17 months has been reported after a series of five blocks.[3] The addition of a cortisone preparation is controversial, but it may provide additional benefit.[10]

Dorsal rhizotomy of C1, C2, C3, and C4 has been described; about 71% to 77% of patients report significant benefit.[3,25-27] Before dorsal rhizotomy, local anesthetic blockade of the suspected medial (sensory) branches should be performed for diagnostic purposes. Botulinum toxin A injection into the greater occipital nerve has also been described.[10,28]

Surgery

Surgical release of the inferior oblique muscles has been described as a potential treatment of occipital neuralgia, particularly when compression of the nerve by this muscle is suspected. In a small, retrospective study of 10 patients, the average visual analogue score for pain decreased from 8 of 10 to 2 of 10 after the procedure.[29] Dorsal root entry zone lesioning has also been reported for occipital neuralgia.[30] In cases in which there is a clear anatomic abnormality, surgery may be a therapeutic option. In addition, neurostimulation is a new technique that appears to be effective in small groups of patients and in case reports.[2] This is performed by subcutaneous implantation of electrical leads in the suboccipital region, which can modulate afferent pain nociceptive fibers to decrease the transmission of painful impulses. This is thought to occur through the gate control theory of pain or possibly through modulation of neurotransmitters in the central nervous system[31] (Fig. 89-3). One should consider surgical treatment after conservative therapy has

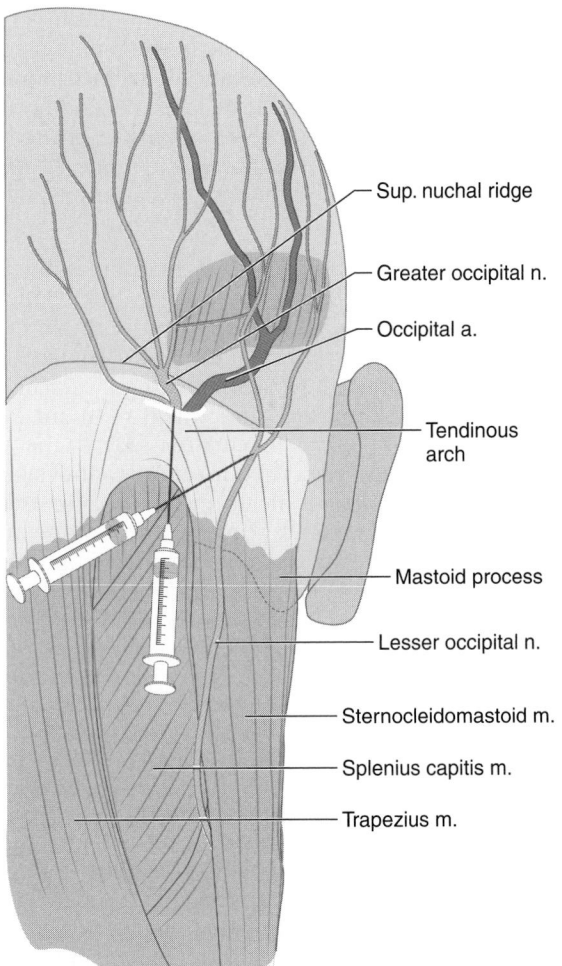

FIGURE 89-2. Occipital nerve block. The patient is placed in a sitting position with the cervical spine flexed and the forehead on a padded bedside table. A total of 8 mL of local anesthetic is drawn up in a 12-mL sterile syringe. A total of 80 mg of depot steroid is added to the local anesthetic with the first block and 40 mg with subsequent blocks. The occipital artery is palpated at the level of the superior nuchal ridge. After preparation of the skin with antiseptic solution, a 22- or 25-gauge, 1¹⁄₂-inch needle is inserted just medial to the artery and advanced perpendicularly until the needle approaches the periosteum of the underlying occipital bone. A paresthesia may be encountered. The needle is then redirected superiorly, and after gentle aspiration, 5 mL of solution is injected in a fan-like distribution, with care being taken to avoid the foramen magnum. (Reprinted with permission from Waldman SD. Greater and lesser occipital nerve block. In Waldman SD, ed. Atlas of Interventional Pain Management, 2nd ed. Philadelphia, WB Saunders, 2004:23-26.)

failed, including but not limited to membrane stabilizers, tricyclic antidepressants, opioids, spinal manipulation, occipital nerve or cervical medial branch blocks, and partial posterior rhizotomy of C1-3.[2]

POTENTIAL DISEASE COMPLICATIONS

Occipital neuralgia is generally a self-limited disease, but it may progress in some cases to a chronic intractable pain syndrome. In refractory cases, it is critical to rule out more ominous conditions. Patients involved in

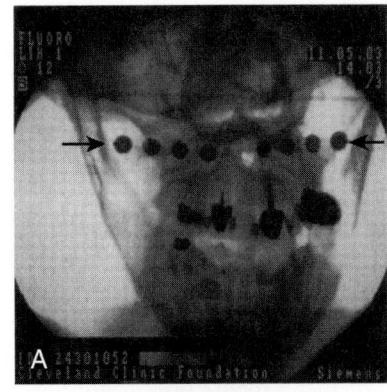

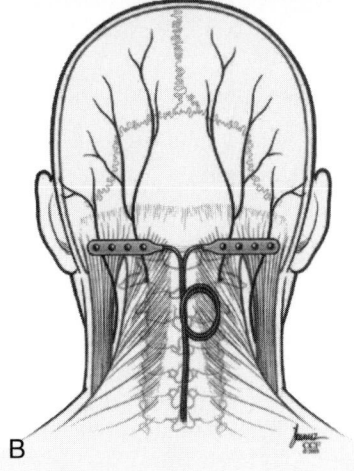

FIGURE 89-3. Occipital nerve stimulation. Radiograph **(A)** and schematic **(B)** of the midline subcutaneous approach in surgical lead positioning for electrical stimulation of the occipital nerve. **A,** Bilateral position of subcutaneous leads *(arrows)* after initial adjustment and just before intraoperative stimulation testing. Note that both leads are at the level of C1-2 dens and aimed laterally. **B,** Schematic of the lead positioning in the subcutaneous occipital area. Note that the lead cable extensions form the loop just below the implant's position and through the same midline incision. (Reprinted with permission from Kapural L, Mekhail N, Hayek SM, et al. Occipital nerve electrical stimulation via the midline approach and subcutaneous surgical leads for treatment of severe occipital neuralgia: a pilot study. Anesth Analg 2005;101:171-174.)

litigation or who have psychosocial stresses or vocational disputes may have a poorer outcome.

POTENTIAL TREATMENT COMPLICATIONS

Nonsteroidal anti-inflammatory drugs have a number of well-established side effects, as do tricyclic antidepressants (Table 89-1). The anesthetic block of the greater or lesser occipital nerve is considered relatively safe.[32] Contraindications to this block include coagulopathy and current infection. Potential complications include bleeding, infection, nerve injury, seizure from intravascular injection of local anesthetic, and headache exacerbation. Care must be taken not to puncture the posterior occipital artery. If the artery is punctured, pressure should be applied vigorously.

TABLE 89-1 Pharmacologic Treatment of Occipital Neuralgia

Medication	Dosage	Common Side Effects
Nonsteroidal anti-inflammatory drugs	Variable	Gastrointestinal bleed, dyspepsia, nausea, headache, dizziness, rash, fluid retention, urticaria, hepatotoxicity, acute renal failure
Cyclooxygenase 2 inhibitors Celecoxib (Celebrex)	Celecoxib: 100 mg bid or 200 mg qd	Dyspepsia, nausea, abdominal pain, constipation, anorexia, elevated liver enzymes, acute renal failure, anaphylaxis, agranulocytosis

Tricyclic antidepressants
  Amitriptyline
  Nortriptyline
  Imipramine
	Start at 10 mg qhs and titrate to 75 mg qhs or until clinical response	Dry mouth, constipation, urinary obstruction, sedation, postural hypertension, decreased seizure threshold

Carbamazepine (Tegretol)	Start at 100 mg bid; titrate to 400 mg bid	Sedation, unsteadiness, nausea, blurred vision, seizures, hepatitis, aplastic anemia
Gabapentin (Neurontin)	Start at 300 mg qd; titrate to 1200 mg tid	Dyspepsia, dizziness, tremor, coordination problems, insomnia, diarrhea, palpitations, nervousness, headache, tinnitus, depression, rash, dyspepsia, dry mouth, anorexia, fatigue, arrhythmia
Mexiletine	Start at 150 mg qd × 3 d, then 300 mg qd × 3 d, then 10 mg/kg qd	Somnolence, dizziness, ataxia, fatigue, nystagmus, tremor, blurred vision, myalgia, weight gain, nausea, amnesia, leukopenia

References

1. Slavin KV, Nersesyan H, Wess C. Peripheral neurostimulation for treatment of intractable occipital neuralgia. Neurosurgery 2006;58:112-119.
2. Kapural L, Mekhail N, Hayek SM, et al. Occipital nerve electrical stimulation via the midline approach and subcutaneous surgical leads for treatment of severe occipital neuralgia: a pilot study. Anesth Analg 2005;101:171-174.
3. Kapoor V, Rothfus WE, Grahovac SZ, et al. Refractory occipital neuralgia: preoperative assessment with CT-guided nerve block prior to dorsal cervical rhizotomy. AJNR Am J Neuroradiol 2003;24:2105-2110.
4. Loeser JD, et al. Bonica's Management of Pain, 3rd ed. Philadelphia, Lippincott Williams & Wilkins, 2001:979.
5. Hammond SR, Danta G. Occipital neuralgia. Clin Exp Neurol 1978;15:258-270.
6. Star MJ, Curd JG, Thorne RP. Atlantoaxial lateral mass osteoarthritis. A frequently overlooked cause of severe occipitocervical pain. Spine 1992;17(Suppl):S71-S76.
7. Kuhn WF, Kuhn SC, Gilberstadt H. Occipital neuralgias: clinical recognition of a complicated headache. A case series and literature review. J Orofac Pain 1997;11:158-165.
8. Hecht JS. Occipital nerve blocks in postconcussive headaches: a retrospective review and report of ten patients. J Head Trauma Rehabil 2004;19:58-71.
9. Natsis K, Baraliakos X, Appell HJ, et al. The course of the greater occipital nerve in the suboccipital region: a proposal for setting landmarks for local anesthesia in patients with occipital neuralgia. Clin Anat 2006;19:332-336.
10. Volcy M, Tepper SJ, Rapoport AM, et al. Botulinum toxin A for the treatment of greater occipital neuralgia and trigeminal neuralgia: a case report with pathophysiological considerations. Cephalalgia 2006;26:336-340.
11. Handel TE, Kaplan RJ. Occipital neuralgia. In Frontera WR, Silver JK, eds. Essentials of Physical Medicine and Rehabilitation. Philadelphia, Hanley & Belfus, 2001:38-43.
12. Mason JO 3rd, Katz B, Greene HH. Severe ocular pain secondary to occipital neuralgia following vitrectomy surgery. Retina 2004;24:458-459.
13. Knox DL, Mustonen E. Greater occipital neuralgia: an ocular pain syndrome with multiple etiologies. Trans Sect Ophthalmol Am Acad Ophthalmol Otolaryngol 1975;79(pt 2):OP513-519.
14. Fredriksen TA, Hovdal H, Sjaastad O. "Cervicogenic headache": clinical manifestation. Cephalalgia 1987;7:147-160.
15. Cerrato P, Bergui M, Imperiale D, et al. Occipital neuralgia as isolated symptom of an upper cervical cavernous angioma. J Neurol 2002;249:1464-1465.
16. Mourouzis C, Saranteas T, Rallis G, et al. Occipital neuralgia secondary to respiratory tract infection. J Orofac Pain 2005;19:261-264.
17. Hardy D. Relief of pain in acute herpes zoster by nerve blocks and possible prevention of post-herpetic neuralgia. Can J Anaesth 2005;52:186-190.
18. Boes CJ. C2 myelitis presenting with neuralgiform occipital pain. Neurology 2005;64:1093-1094.
19. Post AF, Narayan P, Haid RW Jr. Occipital neuralgia secondary to hypermobile posterior arch of atlas. Case report. J Neurosurg 2001;94(Suppl):276-278.
20. Gonzalez-Gay MA, Garcia-Porrua C, Branas F, Alba-Losada J. Giant cell arteritis presenting as occipital neuralgia. Clin Exp Rheumatol 2001;19:479.
21. Jundt JW, Mock D. Temporal arteritis with normal erythrocyte sedimentation rates presenting as occipital neuralgia. Arthritis Rheum 1991;34:217-219.
22. Fernandez-de-las-Penas C, Alonso-Blanco C, Cuadrado ML, Pareja JA. Spinal manipulative therapy in the management of cervicogenic headache. Headache 2005;45:1260-1263.
23. Fernandez-de-las-Penas C, Alonso-Blanco C, San-Roman J, Miangolarra-Page JC. Methodological quality of randomized controlled trials of spinal manipulation and mobilization in tension-type headache, migraine, and cervicogenic headache. J Orthop Sports Phys Ther 2006;36:160-169.
24. Oppenheim JS, Spitzer DE, Segal DH. Nonvascular complications following spinal manipulation. Spine J 2005;5:660-666; discussion 666-667.
25. Koch D, Wakhloo AK. CT-guided chemical rhizotomy of the C1 root for occipital neuralgia. Neuroradiology 1992;34:451-452.
26. Ehni G, Benner B. Occipital neuralgia and the C1-2 arthrosis syndrome. J Neurosurg 1984;61:961-965.
27. Dubuisson D. Treatment of occipital neuralgia by partial posterior rhizotomy at C1-3. J Neurosurg 1995;82:581-586.
28. Martelletti P, van Suijlekom H. Cervicogenic headache: practical approaches to therapy. CNS Drugs 2004;18:793-805.

29. Gille O, Lavignolle B, Vital JM. Surgical treatment of greater occipital neuralgia by neurolysis of the greater occipital nerve and sectioning of the inferior oblique muscle. Spine 2004;29:828-832.

30. Rasskazoff S, Kaufmann AM. Ventrolateral partial dorsal root entry zone rhizotomy for occipital neuralgia. Pain Res Manag 2005;10:43-45.

31. Stojanovic MP. Stimulation methods for neuropathic pain control. Curr Pain Headache Rep 2001;5:130-137.

32. Waldman SD. Greater and lesser occipital nerve block. In Waldman SD, ed. Atlas of Interventional Pain Management, 2nd ed. Philadelphia, WB Saunders, 2004:23-26.

Trigeminal Neuralgia 90

Aneesh Singla, MD, MPH

DEFINITION

Trigeminal neuralgia is defined as pain in the distribution of the trigeminal dermatomes. The pain is described as an electric shock–like, stabbing, unilateral pain having abrupt onset and termination. Intervals between attacks are pain free; non-noxious triggers occur in the same or different sensory areas of the face, and there is minimal or no sensory loss in the region of pain.[1-7] The incidence of trigeminal neuralgia is 4 or 5 per 100,000 people.[7-9]

Observations made by surgeons and reported in the literature suggest that the majority of patients with classic symptoms have mechanical compression of the trigeminal nerve as it leaves the pons and travels in the subarachnoid space toward Meckel cave.[10-12] Most commonly, the mechanism is by cross-compression by a major artery. Other proposed causes include demyelinating plaque from multiple sclerosis or by foci of abscess and bone resorption with irritation of the trigeminal nerve in the maxilla or mandible. Trigeminal neuralgia occurs in about 1% of patients with multiple sclerosis, and approximately 2% to 8% of patients with trigeminal neuralgia have multiple sclerosis.[7,8,13] Regardless of the etiology, it is likely that both peripheral and central mechanisms play a role in the pathogenesis of this syndrome. Trigeminal neuralgia has a prevalence of 0.1 to 0.2 per 1000 and an incidence ranging from about 4 or 5 per 100,000 per year up to 20 per 100,000 per year after the age of 60 years. The female-to-male ratio is about 3:2.[14]

The trigeminal nerve (cranial nerve V) is the largest of the cranial nerves. It begins in the brainstem at the trigeminal nucleus and travels along the ventrolateral surface of the pons and through the subarachnoid space until it enters the temporal bone, where it forms into the gasserian ganglion located in Meckel cave.[10] The divisions are the ophthalmic or V1 branch, the maxillary or V2 branch, and the mandibular or V3 branch (Figs. 90-1 and 90-2). The relative distribution of pain in trigeminal neuralgia is as follows: V1, 20%; V2, 44%; V3, 36%.[10]

SYMPTOMS

Typical trigeminal neuralgia symptoms involve electric shock–like pain in the distribution of one or more branches of the trigeminal nerve. Pain is often intermittent, with pain-free intervals of months or even years.[10] The pain may last a few seconds to less than 2 minutes. The pain has at least four of the following five characteristics: distribution along one or more divisions of the trigeminal nerve; sudden intense, sharp, superficial, stabbing, or burning quality; severe intensity; precipitation from trigger areas or by certain daily activities, such as eating, talking, washing the face, or cleaning the teeth; and between paroxysms, the patient is completely asymptomatic.[6,15] In general, no neurologic deficit is present.

PHYSICAL EXAMINATION

The diagnosis of trigeminal neuralgia is made primarily by history. The Sweet criteria for this diagnosis are five pain descriptors. The diagnosis must be questioned if these criteria are not met,[5] as follows: the pain is paroxysmal; the pain may be provoked by light touch to the face (trigger zones); the pain is confined to the trigeminal distribution; the pain is unilateral; and the clinical sensory examination is normal.[5,16] When possible, physical examination of the oral cavity, dentition, and trigeminal nerve distribution should be performed to rule out obvious disease. A complete cranial nerve examination should be performed. In general, no sensory or motor deficits are present, but serial examinations may detect a change and identify a secondary cause of trigeminal neuralgia.[6]

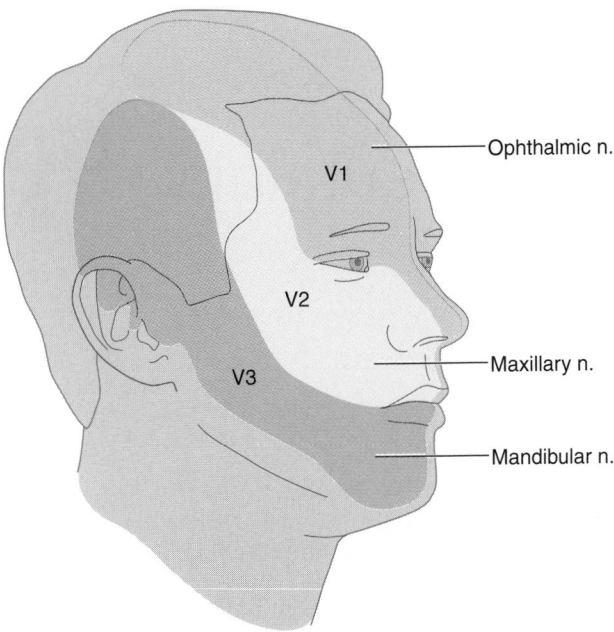

FIGURE 90-1. Dermatomes for trigeminal nerve. V1, ophthalmic nerve. V2, maxillary nerve. V3, mandibular nerve. (Reprinted with permission from Waldman SD. Trigeminal nerve block: coronoid approach. In Waldman SD, ed. Atlas of Interventional Pain Management, 2nd ed. Philadelphia, WB Saunders, 2004:33-37.)

FUNCTIONAL LIMITATIONS

In general, there are no neurologic deficits from trigeminal neuralgia. However, the pain from this entity may result in significant morbidity in activities of daily living. During exacerbations, patients may be functionally incapacitated because of pain; they may be unable to perform functions in the trigeminal nerve distribution, such as comb hair, chew food, or shave. Talking on the telephone may be painful. Wearing glasses or makeup may be precluded. The pain from trigeminal neuralgia is not continuous but paroxysmal, suggesting spontaneous discharges from specific neurons, and it frequently occurs by innocuous tactile stimuli.[4] Therefore, any activity that involves contact with the face may become difficult or impossible.

DIAGNOSTIC STUDIES

After a diagnosis of trigeminal neuralgia is suspected or confirmed, patients should have diagnostic brain imaging with computed tomography or magnetic resonance imaging. Magnetic resonance imaging may be better to rule out multiple sclerosis plaques and to see the anatomic relationships of the trigeminal root as well as to see subtle vascular abnormalities that may be causing compression.[5] Electromyography, nerve conduction studies, and quantitative sensory testing may provide sensitive, quantitative, and objective results for the diagnosis, localization, and accuracy of damage to the trigeminal nerve.[17]

Other studies that may have a role in diagnosis include intraoral, skull, and sinus radiographs and daily diaries of pain.

Differential Diagnosis

See Table 90-1.

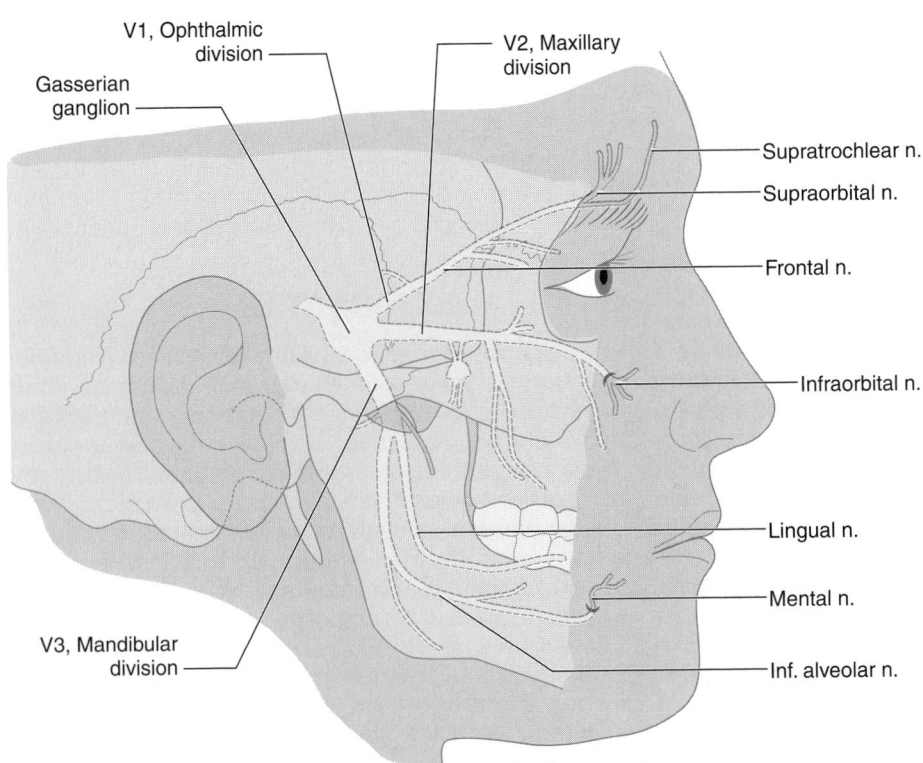

FIGURE 90-2. Anatomy of trigeminal nerve. The gasserian ganglion is formed from two roots that exit the ventral surface of the brainstem at the midpontine level. These roots pass in a forward and lateral direction in the posterior cranial fossa across the border of the petrous bone. They then enter Meckel cave. The gasserian ganglion has three sensory divisions, the ophthalmic (V1), the maxillary (V2), and the mandibular (V3). (Reprinted with permission from Waldman SD. Gasserian ganglion block. In Waldman SD, ed. Atlas of Interventional Pain Management, 2nd ed. Philadelphia, WB Saunders, 2004:27-32.)

TABLE 90-1 Differential Diagnosis of Trigeminal Neuralgia or Facial Pain

Condition	Prevalence	Major Location and Radiation	Timing	Character and Severity	Provoking Factors	Associated Factors
Dental						
Pulpal	Very common	Well localized to a tooth	Can last 10-20 minutes after sugary stimulus	Sharp, stabbing, throbbing, dull, moderate to severe	Hot, cold, or sweet foods provoke it, rarely spontaneous	Immediate relief on removal of stimulus
Fractured or cracked tooth	Fairly common	Localized to one or two teeth, but may be poorly localized, difficult to visualize	Very short lasting, seconds, intermittent	Sharp, moderate	Biting, never spontaneous, may be sensitive to heat	Rebound pain, worse after force removed, opposing natural tooth normally present
Pulpal—chronic pulpitis	Common	Poorly localized intraorally	Intermittent, hours	Mild, dull, throbbing	Occasionally heat	Often large restoration
Periodontal—chronic apical periodontitis	Common	Poorly localized, intraoral	Intermittent, minutes to hours	Mild, dull, throbbing	Large restoration	Sinus may be visible, bad taste
Bone pain–osteomyelitis	Rare	Most often mandible, widespread	Continuous	Throbbing, severe	Biting on mobile teeth	Pyrexia, malaise, trismus, swelling, may be paresthesia, pus, mobile teeth, sequestra
Denture pain, pressure on mental nerve, secondary trigeminal neuralgia	Rare	Localized intraoral	Intermittent, daily	Aching, may be sharp if over mental nerve	Eating with denture	Often redness, ulceration in area of pressure
Neurologic trigeminal neuralgia						
Classic, typical[15]	Rare	Intraoral or extraoral in trigeminal region	Each episode of pain lasts for seconds to minutes; refractory periods, and long periods of no pain	Sharp, shooting, moderate to very severe	Light touch provoked (e.g., eating, washing, talking)	Discrete trigger zones
Atypical trigeminal neuralgia[18]	Rare	Intraoral or extraoral in trigeminal region	Sharp attacks lasting seconds to minutes, more continuous-type background pain, less likely to have complete pain remission	Sharp, shooting, moderate to severe but also dull, burning, continuous mild background pain	Light touch provoked, but continuous-type pain not so clearly provoked	May have small trigger areas, variable pattern
Trigeminal neuropathy[19]	Very rare	Trigeminal area, but may radiate beyond	Continuous	Dull with sharp exacerbation	Areas of allodynia, light touch	Sensory loss, subjective-objective, progressive, vasodilation and swelling may occur
Glossopharyngeal neuralgia	Very rare	Intraoral in distribution of glossopharyngeal	Each episode lasts for seconds up to 2 minutes	Sharp, stabbing, burning, severe	Swallowing, chewing, talking	No neurologic deficit
Postherpetic neuralgia[20]	Rare	Most commonly first division of trigeminal	Continuous pain	Tingling, severity varies	Tactile allodynia	More than 6/12 after acute herpes zoster

Continued

TABLE 90-1   Differential Diagnosis of Trigeminal Neuralgia or Facial Pain—cont'd

Condition	Prevalence	Major Location and Radiation	Timing	Character and Severity	Provoking Factors	Associated Factors
Vascular						
Cluster head-ache, episodic pain-free periods, chronic, no remissions[15]	Rare	Orbital, supraor-bital, temporal	15-180 minutes to several hours, from 1 every other day to 8 per day	Hot, searing, punctuate, severe	Vasodilators (e.g., alcohol)	Conjunctival injection, lacrimation, nasal congestion, rhinor-rhea, sweating, mio-sis, ptosis, eyelid edema, restlessness
SUNCT[21]	Very rare	Ocular, periocular, but may radi-ate to fronto-temporal area, upper jaw, and palate	Each episode last up to 2 minutes; intermittent, sev-eral attacks per day and then may remit	Burning, electrical, stabbing, severe	Neck movements	Conjunctival injection, lacrimation, nasal stuffiness, rhinorrhea
Chronic paroxysmal hemicrania[21]	Very rare	Eye, forehead	Pain lasts 2-45 minutes, 5-10 daily	Stabbing, throb-bing, boring	Head movements, responds to indometha-cin	Autonomic symptoms as for SUNCT
Giant cell arteritis[21]	Rare	May be bilateral, mostly over temporal artery	Continuous	Aching, throb-bing, boring, sharp	Chewing	Jaw claudication, neck pain, anorexia, visual symptoms; temporal artery biopsy is "gold standard"
Temporoman-dibular disor-ders, idio-pathic orofacial pain, facial arthro-myalgia[20]	Relatively common	May be bilateral, periauricular, radiate to neck, temples	Intermittent, may last for hours, may have severe exacerbations	Throbbing, sharp, or dull aching	Clenching and grinding, opening wide, psy-chosocial factors, trauma	May be limitation in opening, tender-ness of muscles of mastication, altered occlusion, responds to relaxation
Atypical facial pain[22]	Relatively common	May be bilateral or unilateral, can radiate widely beyond trigemi-nal area, vari-able location	Intermittent or continuous, of-ten long history of pain	Nagging, throb-bing, aching, sharp (wide range of words used) and se-verity mild to moderate	Life events, stress, weather changes, movements	Dysesthesia, facial edema, headaches, depression
Atypical odon-talgia, phan-tom tooth[20]	Rare	Intraoral in a tooth or teeth, gingival, moves to another area	Continuous, few minutes to hours	Dull, throbbing, may be sharp, mild to moderate	Life events, emotional, teeth hyper-sensitive to temperature and pressure	Often history of tooth extraction

Reprinted with permission from Zakrzewska JM. Diagnosis and differential diagnosis of trigeminal neuralgia. Clin J Pain 2002;18:14-21.

TREATMENT

Initial

Treatments that may help with pain from trigeminal neu-ralgia include heat or cold therapy, massage, avoidance of triggers, and application of transcutaneous electrical nerve stimulation. Topical ointments such as lidocaine, ket-amine, and ketoprofen may help as well. Pharmacologic options are listed in Table 90-2. The anticonvulsant carba-mazepine has been efficacious in the management of trigeminal neuralgia as observed by several controlled trials.[23-26] Baclofen and lamotrigine have also been helpful in controlled trials.[23,27,28] Uncontrolled observa-tions, clinical practice, and the author's experience also suggest that phenytoin, clonazepam, topiramate, so-dium valproate, gabapentin, pregabalin, oxcarbazepine, zonisamide, levetiracetam, mexiletine, and lidocaine may be useful.[23] Pharmacologic therapy with nonsteroidal anti-inflammatories, acetaminophen, tricyclic antidepres-sants, serotonin-norepinephrine reuptake inhibitors, and muscle relaxants may also prove useful. A study showed that intranasal lidocaine 8% administered by a

TABLE 90-2 Pharmacologic Options for Trigeminal Neuralgia Reported in Literature

Drug	Daily Dose	NNT
*Carbamazepine	300-2400 mg	1.4-2.1 (1.1-3.9)
*Baclofen	60-80 mg	1.4 (1.0-2.6)
*Lamotrigine	400 mg	2.1 (1.3-6.1)
Phenytoin	300-400 mg	
Clonazepam	6-8 mg	
Valproate	1200 mg	
Oxcarbazepine	1200-1400 mg	
Gabapentin	600-2000 mg	
Intravenous lidocaine	2-5 mg/kg	
Mexiletine	10 mg/kg	

*Indicates data from placebo-controlled trials.
NNT is numbers needed to treat to obtain 1 patient with at least 50% pain relief.
From Sindrup SH, Jensen TS. Pharmacotherapy of trigeminal neuralgia. Clin J Pain 2002;18:22-27.

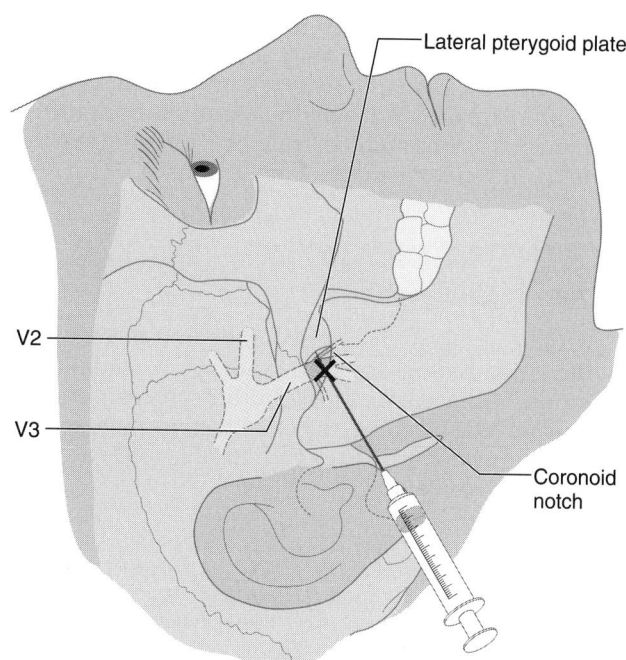

FIGURE 90-3. Technique of trigeminal nerve block. The patient is placed in the supine position with the cervical spine in the neutral position. The coronoid notch is identified by asking the patient to open and close the mouth several times and palpating the area just anterior and slightly inferior to the acoustic auditory meatus. After the notch is identified, the patient is asked to hold the mouth in neutral position. A total of 7 mL of local anesthetic is drawn up in a 12-mL sterile syringe. In treatment of trigeminal neuralgia, atypical facial pain, or other painful conditions involving the maxillary and mandibular nerves, a total of 80 mg of depot steroid is added to the local anesthetic with the first block and 40 mg with subsequent blocks. After the skin overlying the coronoid notch is prepared with antiseptic solution, a 22-gauge, 3½-inch styleted needle is inserted just below the zygomatic arch directly in the middle of the coronoid notch. The needle is advanced approximately 1½ to 2 inches in a plane perpendicular to the skull until the lateral pterygoid plate is encountered. At this point, if blockade of both the maxillary and mandibular nerves is desired, the needle is withdrawn slightly. After careful aspiration, 7 to 8 mL of solution is injected in incremental doses. During the injection procedure, the patient must be observed carefully for signs of local anesthetic toxicity. (Reprinted with permission from Waldman SD. Trigeminal nerve block: coronoid approach. In Waldman SD, ed. Atlas of Interventional Pain Management, 2nd ed. Philadelphia, WB Saunders, 2004:33-37.)

metered-dose spray produced prompt but temporary analgesia without serious adverse reactions in patients with second-division trigeminal neuralgia.[29]

In general, 80% of patients will respond to medical therapy.[7]

Rehabilitation

Modalities for pain control, such as electrical stimulation, ice massage, and hot packs, can play a role in rehabilitation and recovery from trigeminal neuralgia. Speech therapy may be indicated to help with oral motor deficits that affect speech or swallowing.

Adaptive equipment, such as a telephone earset, may be recommended. Some general chronic pain rehabilitation approaches may also be useful, such as improved sleep hygiene, low-intensity aerobic exercise, biofeedback, cognitive-behavioral therapy, and relaxation techniques.

Procedures

Trigeminal nerve blocks may reduce the intensity or the episodes of pain (Fig. 90-3). Local anesthetic nerve blocks may temporarily decrease the pain from trigeminal neuralgia. The pain may sometimes outlast the duration of the local anesthetic. If it is clinically warranted, nerve blocks can be repeated at intervals, but the clinician must carefully weigh the risks and benefits of these blocks. Nerve blocks may be used for diagnostic purposes and to show patients the effects of a planned neurectomy or rhizotomy.[3] Some have reported good short-term results with neurolytic blocks with alcohol or glycerol, but the consensus among most physicians is that the long-term results of neurolytic blocks are not favorable because of progressively lower success rates and higher morbidity.[3] Acupuncture may also have a role in the management of trigeminal neuralgia.[30]

Surgery

The mainstay of surgical therapy remains microvascular decompression, with excellent long-term outcomes; 70% have positive results.[31] Other therapies that may have a role include peripheral neurectomy, gasserian neurotomy, gangliolysis, trigeminal tractotomy, radiofrequency ablation, cryoneurolysis, and peripheral stimulation.[3,32]

POTENTIAL DISEASE COMPLICATIONS

Trigeminal neuralgia is generally amenable to surgical treatment or pharmacotherapy. However, it can progress to become a chronic intractable pain syndrome. In refractory cases, it is important to consider other diagnoses or facial pain syndromes. Care must be taken to treat and to manage the psychosocial effects of this chronic pain syndrome by appropriate adjunctive therapy, including biofeedback, cognitive-behavioral therapy, and stress management techniques.

POTENTIAL TREATMENT COMPLICATIONS

Care must be taken to understand the side effects of any of the pharmacologic options available. Potential complications from nerve blocks, other procedures, and surgery include bleeding, infection, nerve injury, seizure from intravascular injection of local anesthetic, and headache exacerbation.

References

1. Kitt CA, Gruber K, Davis M, et al. Trigeminal neuralgia: opportunities for research and treatment. Pain 2000;85:3-7.
2. Devor M, Amir R, Rappaport ZH. Pathophysiology of trigeminal neuralgia: the ignition hypothesis. Clin J Pain 2002;18:4-13.
3. Loeser J. Bonica's Management of Pain, 3rd ed. Philadelphia, Lippincott Williams & Wilkins, 2001:859-860.
4. Nurmikko TJ, Eldridge PR. Trigeminal neuralgia—pathophysiology, diagnosis and current treatment. Br J Anaesth 2001;87:117-132.
5. Scrivani SJ, Mathews ES, Maciewicz RJ. Trigeminal neuralgia. Oral Surg Oral Med Oral Pathol Oral Radiol Endod 2005;100:527-538.
6. Zakrzewska JM. Diagnosis and differential diagnosis of trigeminal neuralgia. Clin J Pain 2002;18:14-21.
7. Kapur N, Kamel IR, Herlich A. Oral and craniofacial pain: diagnosis, pathophysiology, and treatment. Int Anesthesiol Clin 2003;41:115-150.
8. Tenser RB. Trigeminal neuralgia: mechanisms of treatment. Neurology 1998;51:17-19.
9. Jackson EM, Bussard GM, Hoard MA, Edlich RF. Trigeminal neuralgia: a diagnostic challenge. Am J Emerg Med 1999;17:597-600.
10. Loeser JD. Bonica's Management of Pain, 3rd ed. Philadelphia, Lippincott Williams & Wilkins, 2001:833-866.
11. Dandy W. Concerning the cause of trigeminal neuralgia. Am J Surg 1934;204:447-455.
12. Jannetta PJ. Microsurgical approach to the trigeminal nerve for tic douloureux. Proc Neurosurg 1976;7:180-200.
13. Silberstein SD, Young WB. Headaches and facial pain. In Goetz CG, ed. Textbook of Clinical Neurology. Philadelphia, WB Saunders, 1999:1089-1105.
14. Manzoni GC, Torelli P. Epidemiology of typical and atypical craniofacial neuralgias. Neurol Sci 2005;26(Suppl 2):s65-s67.
15. Classification and diagnostic criteria for headache disorders, cranial neuralgias and facial pain. Headache Classification Committee of the International Headache Society. Cephalalgia 1988;8 (Suppl 7):1-96.
16. White J, Sweet WH. Pain and the Neurosurgeon. Springfield, Ill, Charles C Thomas, 1969.
17. Jaaskelainen SK. The utility of clinical neurophysiological and quantitative sensory testing for trigeminal neuropathy. J Orofac Pain 2004;18:355-359.
18. Zakrzewska JM, Jassim S, Bulman JS. A prospective, longitudinal study on patients with trigeminal neuralgia who underwent radiofrequency thermocoagulation of the Gasserian ganglion. Pain 1999;79:51-58.
19. Goadsby PJ, Lipton RB. A review of the paroxysmal hemicranias, SUNCT syndrome and other short-lasting headaches with autonomic feature, including new cases. Brain 1997;120:193-209.
20. Merskey H, Bogduk N. Classification of Chronic Pain. Descriptors of Chronic Pain Syndromes and Definitions of Pain Terms. Seattle, IASP Press, 1994:1.
21. Hayreh SS, Podhajsky PA, Raman R, Zimmerman B. Giant cell arteritis: validity and reliability of various diagnostic criteria. Am J Ophthalmol 1997;123:285-296.
22. Pfaffenrath V, Rath M, Pollmann W, Keeser W. Atypical facial pain: application of the IHS criteria in a clinical sample. Cephalalgia 1993;13(Suppl 12):84-88.
23. Sindrup SH, Jensen TS. Pharmacotherapy of trigeminal neuralgia. Clin J Pain 2002;18:22-27.
24. Campbell FG, Graham JG, Zilkha KJ. Clinical trial of carbamazepine (Tegretol) in trigeminal neuralgia. J Neurol Neurosurg Psychiatry 1966;29:265-267.
25. Killian JM, Fromm GH. Carbamazepine in the treatment of neuralgia. Use of side effects. Arch Neurol 1968;19:129-136.
26. Nicol CF. A four year double-blind study of Tegretol in facial pain. Headache 1969;9:54-57.
27. Fromm GH, Terrence CF, Chattha AS. Baclofen in the treatment of trigeminal neuralgia: double-blind study and long-term follow-up. Ann Neurol 1984;15:240-244.
28. Zakrzewska JM, Chaudhry Z, Nurmikko TJ, et al. Lamotrigine (Lamictal) in refractory trigeminal neuralgia: results from a double-blind placebo controlled crossover trial. Pain 1997;73:223-230.
29. Kanai A, Suzuki A, Kobayashi M, Hoka S. Intranasal lidocaine 8% spray for second-division trigeminal neuralgia. Br J Anaesth 2006;97:559-563.
30. Millan-Guerrero RO, Isais-Millan S. Acupuncture in trigeminal neuralgia management. Headache 2006;46:532.
31. Barker FG 2nd, Jannetta PJ, Babu RP, et al. Long-term outcome after operation for trigeminal neuralgia in patients with posterior fossa tumors. J Neurosurg 1996;84:818-825.
32. Lopez BC, Hamlyn PJ, Zakrzewska JM. Systematic review of ablative neurosurgical techniques for the treatment of trigeminal neuralgia. Neurosurgery 2004;54:973-982; discussion 82-83.
33. Waldman SD. Trigeminal nerve block: coronoid approach. In Waldman SD, ed. Atlas of Interventional Pain Management, 2nd ed. Philadelphia, WB Saunders, 2004:33-37.
34. Waldman SD. Gasserian ganglion block. In Waldman SD, ed. Atlas of Interventional Pain Management, 2nd ed. Philadelphia, WB Saunders, 2004:27-32.

Thoracic Outlet Syndrome 91

Karl-August Lindgren, MD, PhD

DEFINITION

Thoracic outlet syndrome is a symptom complex caused by compression or irritation of the neurovascular structures as they leave the thoracic cage through its narrow outlet. The thoracic outlet contains many structures in a confined space. The base of the thoracic outlet is formed by the first rib and the fascia of Sibson, which is attached to the transverse process of the seventh cervical vertebra, the pleura, and the first rib. The outlet is bounded superiorly by the subclavius muscle and the clavicle, anteriorly by the anterior scalene muscle, and posteriorly by the middle scalene muscle. The brachial plexus and the subclavian artery pass over the first rib between the anterior and middle scalene muscles (Fig. 91-1).

Neurovascular compression occurs most frequently at three levels:

- in the superior thoracic outlet, bordered posteriorly by the spine, anteriorly by the manubrium, and laterally by the first rib;
- in the costoscalene hiatus, bordered anteriorly by the anterior scalene muscle, posteriorly by the middle scalene muscle, and caudally by the first rib; and
- in the costoclavicular passage, bordered laterally by the clavicle, posteriorly by the scapula, and medially by the first rib.

The clinical symptoms of thoracic outlet syndrome are divided into categories according to the structures under pressure. True neurologic thoracic outlet syndrome is often caused by the distal C8-T1 roots or proximal fibers of the lower trunk of the plexus being stretched over a taut congenital band extending from the tip of a rudimentary cervical rib to the first rib. The most common form of thoracic outlet syndrome is the disputed neurologic thoracic outlet syndrome. The term *disputed* has been chosen because so many of the basic tenets of this syndrome are in dispute. Symptoms caused by pure venous compression (venous thoracic outlet syndrome) occur in 1.5% of patients and are manifested as axillary–subclavian vein thrombosis, usually in young patients engaged in vigorous physical activity that emphasizes upper limb and shoulder motion (such as cricket, tennis, and baseball). Arterial thoracic outlet syndrome is very rare and may be suspected if the patient presents with claudication of the arm, coldness, and ischemia of a finger or a hand. Individuals who have congenital bone or fibromuscular variations at these spaces and experience trauma are at risk for development of thoracic outlet syndrome. Anatomic variations and anomalies probably play a secondary role in the etiology. Congenital bands and ligaments are observed in a large majority of patients with thoracic outlet syndrome, and nine different types have been recognized.[1] In a human cadaver study, only 10% had a bilaterally normal anatomy, and it is suggested that fibrous bands confer a predisposition to symptoms of thoracic outlet syndrome after stress or injury.[2] Variation in the course of the brachial plexus that may predispose to symptoms of thoracic outlet syndrome has also been presented.[3] Cervical ribs are regarded as predisposing factors; however, cervical ribs are present since birth. In 80% of patients with cervical ribs, symptoms did not develop until after a neck injury.[4] Post-traumatic thoracic outlet syndrome has been presented in several articles.[5-7]

According to Roos,[8] anomalies are always the reason behind symptoms of thoracic outlet syndrome. However, only a few other surgeons have observed such anomalies.[9] In the case of the first rib, the costovertebral and costotransverse joints allow a fair amount of rotation to take place along the long axis of the rib. Moreover, this rib has attached to it the anterior and middle scalene muscles, which act either by raising the thorax or by flexing and rotating the cervical part of the spine. In consequence, this first rib bears more stresses and strains than any of the other ribs, and these are greatest at the costotransverse joint.[10] Osteoarthritic changes are found more frequently in the costotransverse joint of the first rib. The lack of a superior supporting ligament

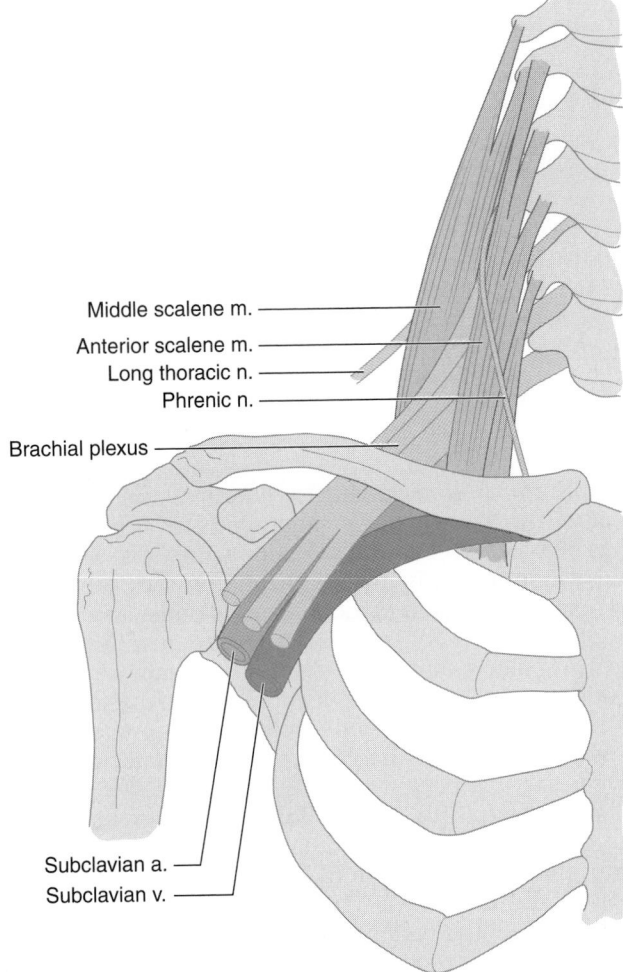

Middle scalene m.
Anterior scalene m.
Long thoracic n.
Phrenic n.
Brachial plexus

Subclavian a.
Subclavian v.

FIGURE 91-1. Anatomy of the thoracic outlet area. (Reprinted with permission from the Christine M. Kleinert Institute for Hand and Microsurgery, Inc.)

may explain why this joint of the first rib is relatively weaker than those of the other ribs.[10]

The elevation of the ribs during inspiration increases the anteroposterior diameter of the upper thorax. The range of this motion is reduced in older people. A disturbance of the function of the upper thoracic aperture will predispose to thoracic outlet syndrome symptoms. A subluxation of the first rib at the costotransverse joint causes a restricted movement of the first rib.[11,12] In patients with thoracic outlet syndrome, the C8 and T1 nerve roots are most commonly affected. These roots constitute the part of the brachial plexus closest to the costotransverse joint. The stellate ganglion is located in the immediate vicinity of the first costotransverse joint and has numerous connections to the C8 and T1 roots. Minimal trauma associated with static, repetitive work, especially in young women, can cause abnormal stress on the upper aperture, and the poorly stabilized first rib can subluxate at the costotransverse joint. A subluxation at the first costotransverse joint could irritate the nerve roots C8 and T1 emerging in front of this joint. This irritation could explain the predominantly subjective pain and sensory loss in the ulnar distribution. The

weakness of the hand and the various symptoms resembling complex regional pain syndrome may be explained by the irritation of the stellate ganglion.[13]

SYMPTOMS

True neurologic thoracic outlet syndrome presents with a long history of sensory symptoms mainly along the medial forearm, associated with hand weakness and wasting, particularly of the thenar muscles (Fig. 91-2). In the upper plexus type presented by Roos,[8] pain is felt over the brachial plexus radiating from the ear, through the anterior cervical region, over the clavicle into the upper part of the chest, posteriorly into the rhomboid and scapular areas, across the trapezius, and down the outer arm into the radial aspect of the forearm in a C5-6 distribution. In the lower plexus type, pain is felt in the supraclavicular and infraclavicular fossae, radiating into the upper part of the back and from the axilla down the inner arm along the ulnar nerve distribution.

In contrast, disputed neurologic thoracic outlet syndrome possesses none of these characteristics. The most common symptoms are pain and paresthesias in an ulnar distribution and numbness, tingling, weakness, or dysfunction of the hand. The list of symptoms attributed to disputed neurologic thoracic outlet syndrome is long. These patients are often told by their physicians that their symptoms are exaggerated or that their complaints are not real. Coldness, easy fatigability, ischemia of a finger or a hand, and pallor on elevation are considered to be symptoms of arterial origin. Swelling, discoloration, and a heavy feeling in the hand are considered to be symptoms of venous origin. Swelling, hyperesthesia, discoloration, and a feeling of alternate cold and warm could also be signs of complex regional pain syndrome. Traction on the stellate ganglion has also been considered a possible cause of pain in these patients.[10] In general, in the absence of peripheral emboli, most "vascular symptoms" or "Raynaud phenomena" probably result from irritation of the sympathetic nerves rather than from compression of the subclavian artery in the thoracic outlet. A common

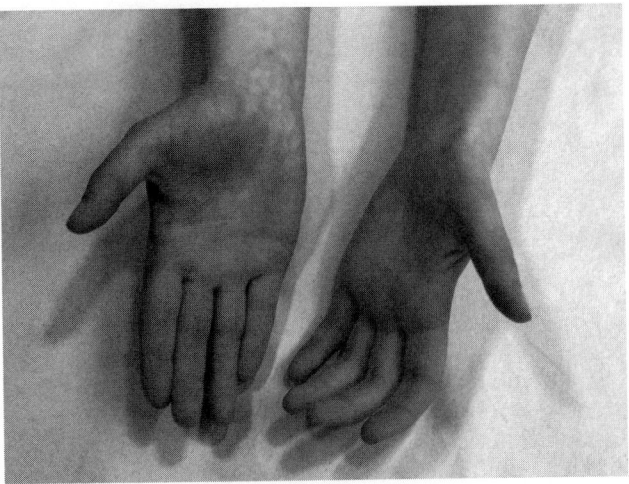

FIGURE 91-2. The hands of a patient with true neurologic thoracic outlet syndrome. Wasting of the muscles is clearly shown in the left hand.

feature of the symptoms is their intermittence and provocation by use of the arm above shoulder level. Aggravation of the symptoms often occurs after rather than during exercise.

PHYSICAL EXAMINATION

The diagnosis of thoracic outlet syndrome is a clinical one based on a detailed history and physical examination. This takes time and effort. Years of inappropriate diagnosis and ineffective therapy take a heavy toll on these patients. In the physical examination, the individual as a whole must be taken into consideration. One must remember that many of these patients have some psychological complaints. A thorough clinical examination including a logical explanation for the symptoms will often relieve the psychic burden.

The physical examination starts with an inspection of the neck, shoulders, and upper extremities. Color, muscle atrophy, edema, temperature, and nails are examined. This examination requires the patient to be examined with the shirt off. The cervical spine is then examined to exclude symptoms of cervical origin caused by a cervical disc or spondylarthrotic intervertebral foramen. A typical pain radiation in C5 to C8 distribution indicates that a nerve root irritation is present. A local distribution of pain with neck extension indicates a facet joint problem.

A neurologic examination is performed to include sensory testing, muscle strength testing (C5-8), and reflexes. Tinel sign is tested to exclude carpal tunnel syndrome. Palpation of the median, ulnar, and radial nerves from the axilla to the hand may reveal tenderness. This tenderness will vanish if a successful therapy is administered.[14]

Almost all clinical tests used in the examination of the patient with thoracic outlet syndrome aim to provoke the symptoms felt by the patient, presuming that the compressing structure may be provoked to irritate the neurovascular bundle in the area of the thoracic outlet during the test. These maneuvers are unreliable in general.[15] A clinical test in extensive use is the Adson test.[16] With the patient sitting, hands resting on the thighs, both radial pulses are simultaneously palpated. During forced inspiration, hyperextension of the neck, and turning of the head to the affected side, the radial pulse is palpated for obliteration, and auscultation is done for supraclavicular bruit. The test has changed during the years. In 1927, when Adson described his test, the vascular changes were considered to be pathognomonic of thoracic outlet syndrome. Later, neurologic changes occurred more frequently than vascular ones, and these can be detected better when the head is rotated to the contralateral rather than the ipsilateral side, as initially described.

Radial pulse obliteration or subclavian bruit is found in 69% of normal patients.[17] All studies clearly indicate that pulse obliteration with the arm and head in various positions is a normal finding and has no relation to thoracic outlet syndrome.

In the hyperabduction test, symptoms are reproduced by hyperabduction of the arm.[18] However, more than 80% of normal individuals experience obliteration of the radial pulse during this test.[18] In the exaggerated military maneuver, also called Eden test, symptoms are reproduced by pulling back the acromioclavicular joint in an exaggerated military "attention" position. The neurovascular structures could be compressed between the first rib and the clavicle, without any anatomic predisposing factors. This maneuver is also referred to as the costoclavicular test. Arterial compression is found in 60% of asymptomatic individuals by this test.[19]

In the abduction–external rotation test, also called Roos test or elevated arm stress test (EAST), the hands are in the "stick up" position and are then repeatedly opened and closed for 3 minutes. When Roos first described this procedure in 1966, he considered the symptoms to be due to both arterial and brachial plexus compression and referred to this procedure as a claudication test.[20] By 1974, Roos was convinced that thoracic outlet syndrome was neurologic rather than vascular in origin but claimed that the EAST procedure was the most reliable procedure. Roos has also claimed that the EAST procedure has great specificity, with a positive result in thoracic outlet syndrome but generally negative results in carpal tunnel syndrome and cervical radiculopathy. However, in a controlled study, it was found that the EAST procedure is an excellent test for carpal tunnel syndrome; the result is positive in 92% of patients with carpal tunnel syndrome and in 74% of normal controls.[21] Positional compression during all of these tests is a common phenomenon in normal subjects,[22] and diminishing of the pulse in Adson test, the costoclavicular maneuver, and the hyperabduction test is considered to be a normal finding rather than a pathologic one.[23] None of these tests unequivocally establishes the presence or absence of thoracic outlet syndrome. Ribbe and colleagues[23] used a "thoracic outlet syndrome index" to establish the diagnosis of thoracic outlet syndrome. According to these authors, a patient with thoracic outlet syndrome should have at least three of the following four symptoms or signs:

1. a history of aggravation of symptoms with the arm in the elevated position;
2. a history of paresthesia in the segments C8-T1;
3. tenderness over the brachial plexus supraclavicularly; and
4. a positive "hands-up" (abduction–external rotation) test result.

The function of the upper thoracic aperture should be analyzed with the cervical rotation–lateral flexion test.[24] The test is carried out as follows. The neutrally positioned cervical spine is first passively and maximally rotated away from the side being examined, and then, in this position, gently flexed as far as possible, moving the ear toward the chest. This is done in both directions. A restriction blocking the lateral flexion part of the movement indicates a positive test result; a free movement indicates a negative test result (Fig. 91-3).

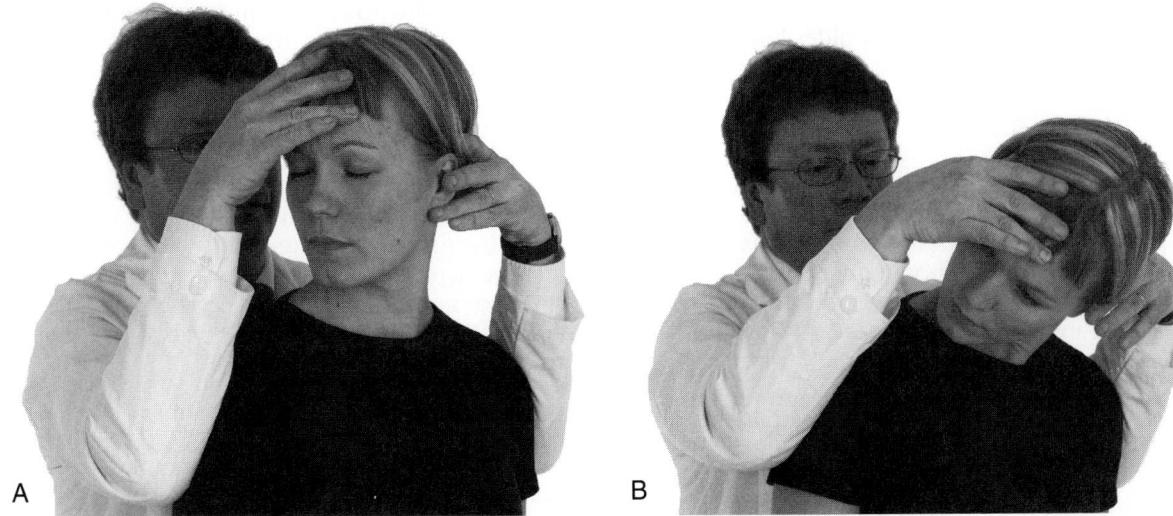

FIGURE 91-3. The performance of the cervical rotation–lateral flexion test. **A,** The head is rotated away from the side to be examined. **B,** In this position, the neck is tilted forward, bringing the ear toward the chest. If this movement is restricted, the test result is considered positive and is indicative of a malfunction of the first rib. A normal free movement indicates a negative test result. (Reproduced with permission of Kustannus Oy Duodecim.)

This test indicates an abnormal function of the upper thoracic aperture. The test is indicative of a subluxation of the first rib at the costotransverse joint. The test has been used to identify patients who did not gain from surgery[25,26] as well as in a 2-year follow-up study after conservative treatment.[14]

In the surgery series,[25,26] it was hypothesized that the remaining stump of the first rib was subluxated and that is why the symptoms persisted after surgery. The importance of the length of the remaining stump has also been stressed by other authors.[27-29] It is mandatory to analyze the function of the upper thoracic aperture and not only rely on provocative maneuvers that may lead to unnecessary surgical interventions.

FUNCTIONAL LIMITATIONS

The patients with symptoms of thoracic outlet syndrome have difficulty in working over the horizontal level, such as cleaning windows and putting up draperies. Static work, such as working with a keyboard, may be difficult because of paresthesias and difficulty in controlling the movements of the arm. Many patients cannot "rely" on the hand. Sleep is disturbed because of pain and tingling after exertion during the day.

DIAGNOSTIC STUDIES

Radiologic examination in the thoracic outlet syndrome can detect cervical ribs, bone anomalies of the first or second ribs, tumors, or the "droopy shoulder" syndrome. The incidence of arterial compression of clinical significance is extremely low, and arteriography should not be used in the diagnosis of thoracic outlet syndrome, except in patients with signs of pronounced compression or ischemia. Arterial compression inside the thoracic outlet can be detected with Doppler ultrasonography.[30]

Magnetic resonance imaging has been used to detect anomalies, but these may not correlate with symptoms.[31,32] Functional magnetic resonance imaging may show a smaller distance between the first rib and the clavicle,[33] but the significance remains to be shown. A kineradiographic study can detect abnormal movement of the structures of the upper aperture,[12] but this can be detected with clinical tests.[24]

Somatosensory evoked potentials can document the neurocompressive component of thoracic outlet syndrome and provide an objective assessment.[34] The theory of the "double-crush" syndrome suggests that nerve compression at one level makes the whole nerve more vulnerable to compression injury at another level.[35] Symptoms after an unsuccessful carpal tunnel operation disappeared after a first rib excision.[36] The double-crush phenomenon should be taken into account and neurophysiologic examination should be performed to exclude more distal sites of nerve compression than the thoracic outlet, such as nerve entrapment in the carpal tunnel.

Differential Diagnosis

Radiculopathy

Multiple sclerosis

Syringomyelia

Glenohumeral instability

Tumors of the cervical spine

Pancoast tumor

Myofascial pain syndrome in the cervical region

Trapezius strain

TREATMENT

Initial

After the thorough clinical examination and detailed history, what the examining physician suspects to be the origin of the symptoms must be explained to the patient. Good pain management, not only using pain-killers but also taking into account sleeping hygiene, is important. A multiprofessional team should be consulted so that all therapy modalities are taken into account. This includes physiatrists, physiotherapists, occupational therapists, social workers, and psychologists; also, there must be a possibility to consult specialists in neurology and psychiatry, thoracic surgeons, and neurosurgeons.

Rehabilitation

The outcome of conservative therapy varies among different studies. Sällström's and Celegin's program brought relief in 83% of patients with mild symptoms but in only 9% of those with severe symptoms.[37] Even a success rate of 100% has been reported (a supervised physiotherapy program of graduated resisted shoulder elevation exercises in eight patients).[38] Almost all authors have emphasized exercises to improve patients' posture as well as strengthening exercises of the shoulder girdle. However, it is very difficult to compare the different studies because the diagnostic criteria are seldom mentioned, the severity of the symptoms varies, and hardly ever is the type of therapy described.

Procedures

During the last 20 years, I have recommended and used a multidisciplinary approach. The therapy itself starts with shoulder exercises, the purpose of which is to restore the movement of the whole shoulder girdle and to provide more space for the neurovascular structures. Restoration of the movement and function of the cervical spine follows. The exercises that aim to activate the anterior, middle, and posterior scalene muscles are the most important part (Fig. 91-4). These exercises have been shown to correct any malfunction of the first ribs, thus normalizing the function of the upper thoracic aperture[39] and enabling normal movement of the first ribs. Stretching of the muscles of the shoulder girdle involves the upper part of the trapezius muscles, the sternocleidomastoid muscles, the levator scapulae, and the small pectoral muscle. Further stretching exercises should be administered as needed, depending on the clinical findings in the individual case. Strengthening exercises for the anterior serratus muscle should be included, thus enhancing the stability of the scapula. Nerve gliding exercises are used to restore the mobility of the nerves.[40] The patients should be observed for a long time because relapses are common. With use of

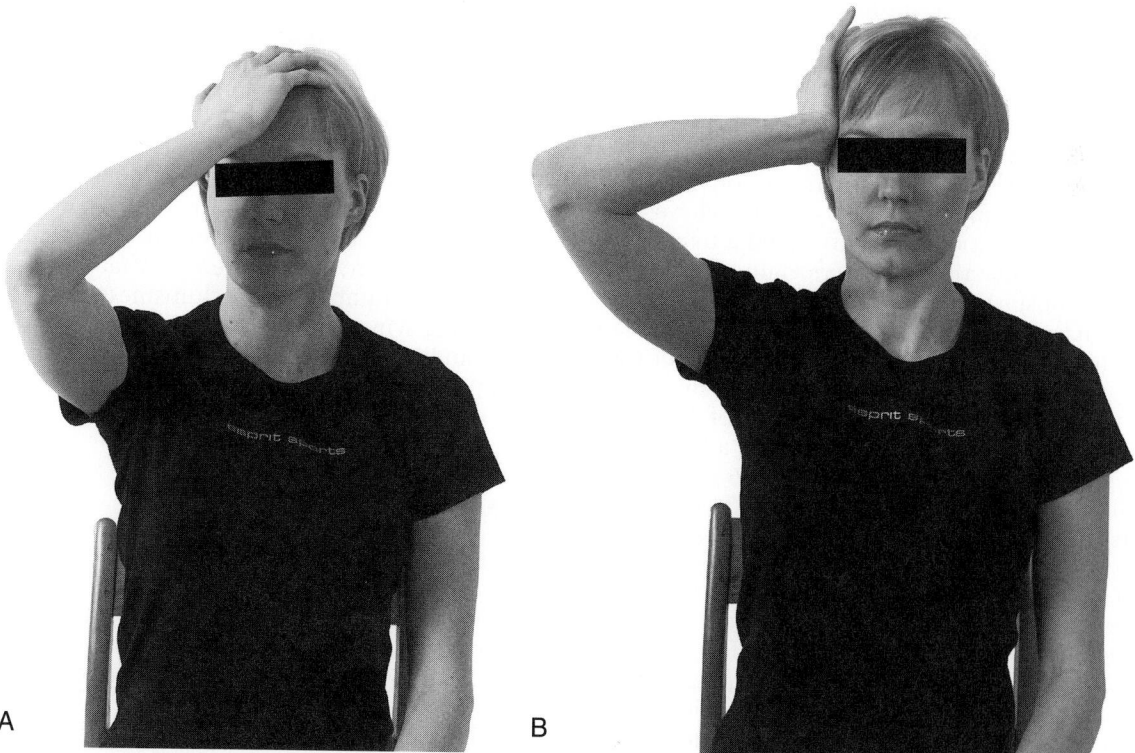

A   B

FIGURE 91-4. Normal function of the first ribs and the upper aperture can be achieved by activation of the scalene muscles by the patient. **A,** The patient first activates the anterior scalene muscles by pressing the forehead against the palm, with the cervical spine being all the time in a neutral position. **B,** The middle scalene muscles are activated by pressing sidewards against the palm. The exercises are done five or six times for a duration of 5 seconds each and with about 15 seconds between the exercises. The exercises are done on both sides. (Reproduced with permission of Kustannus Oy Duodecim.)

this program, I found that 88.1% of the patients were satisfied with the outcome, that is, their symptoms had either disappeared or were much abated, or the real cause of the symptoms had been diagnosed.

Recommendations were carried through during a 2-year follow-up period in 87.9% of cases. Of the patients who were advised to retire because of symptoms, the primary problem was found to be other than thoracic outlet syndrome (psychiatric causes, complex regional pain syndrome, polyneuropathy, multiple sclerosis, other).[41] This has also been stressed in a study.[42] Conservative therapy is the treatment of choice in thoracic outlet syndrome because it is safe and can be implemented as a self-treatment program.

If symptoms are not abated despite restored function, the differential diagnosis should be reviewed. The fact that conservative treatment is tedious and relapses are common should not be considered a reason for surgical intervention. Surgery is a viable option only if there are signs of significant motor loss, atrophy, or vascular thrombosis. Psychosocial aspects should always be taken into account. It is extremely important to evaluate the degree of disability that thoracic outlet syndrome symptoms cause in relation to the patient's life situation and psychosocial abilities.

Surgery

Cherington[43] stated already in 1991, "It is important for surgeons and primary care physicians to be aware of the rising tide of scepticism surrounding the diagnosis and treatment of the thoracic outlet syndrome." Scepticism is indeed justified for several reasons. The most often diagnosed and surgically treated form of thoracic outlet syndrome in the United States, disputed neurologic thoracic outlet syndrome, has no objective clinical, radiologic, or electrodiagnostic criteria. Adson introduced in 1927 scalenotomy as an approach to relieve structures from compression. Roos presented a transaxillary resection of the first rib, and this operation has perhaps been the most used approach. Supraclavicular approaches have also been presented. Some authors claim the results of surgical management to be good or excellent in more than 90% of patients. Different studies, however, are difficult to compare because of the various criteria used to assess the outcome. In addition, the numbers of patients have ranged from 26 to 1336 and the follow-up times from 1 month to 15 years. Some authors do not state the follow-up time at all. A combined surgical treatment using transaxillary first rib resection and transcervical scalenotomy is said to be more effective than either of these alone.[44] There have been only a couple of studies in which the follow-up examination was done by independent examiners not involved in the surgical procedure or selection of the patients. This seems to affect the results after surgery. Among the different operative procedures, scalenotomy seems to speed up patients' retirement.[45] Cuetter and Bartoszek[46] and Lindgren[47] have reevaluated patients treated unsuccessfully with surgery for thoracic outlet syndrome; they found that in each case, another disease or functional disturbance explained the patient's complaints.

Recurrence after unsuccessful procedures may be a disabling and difficult problem for patients. This is extremely tragic in patients who have been found to have pulse changes in provocative positions in the absence of any other symptoms. Even abnormal electrodiagnostic findings before an operation do not predict the outcome of surgery.[48,49] Long-term results of operation for thoracic outlet syndrome may be much worse than those initially achieved.[50] Patients who present with poorly systematized neurologic symptoms have poor results after surgery and should be denied surgery or at least informed that postoperative results may be disappointing.[51]

POTENTIAL DISEASE COMPLICATIONS

It is very important to detect those patients with posttraumatic thoracic outlet syndrome. These may present with worsening of the symptoms, such as a decrease in muscle strength, increase of pain, and tingling in the radicular territory, as well as unspecific disturbances, such as dizziness and face pain. In the case of these patients, one must consider surgical options.[6] It has been said that true neurogenic thoracic outlet syndrome is rare. Overdiagnosis of this syndrome results from a failure to realize that a wide range of symptoms occurs regularly in patients with carpal tunnel syndrome and that these are commonly outside the anatomic distribution of the median nerve. The failure to recognize this can reinforce abnormal behavior in patients, particularly when they are subjected to unnecessary brachial plexus or ulnar nerve surgery, undertaken without neurophysiologic identification of an appropriate neurogenic abnormality.[52] If not dealt with correctly, these patients will suffer for long periods of time with more than one symptom. These may include muscle atrophy, swelling in the supraclavicular fossa, abnormal posture, and tendency to faint with certain movements. Numbness and clumsiness of the hand is the leading symptom, but pain in the occiput-shoulder area is an important symptom too.[42] These may worsen without proper therapy.

POTENTIAL TREATMENT COMPLICATIONS

Surgery for thoracic outlet syndrome is not as innocuous as it was once thought. Dale[53] found that more than half of those who reported performing the surgery had encountered brachial plexus injuries severe enough to produce clinical weakness, nearly one fifth of which were permanent. Large numbers of failed thoracic outlet syndrome surgery have been reported during the last decades. Brachial plexus lesions, infections, and cases of life-threatening hemorrhage have been published. Even deaths have been reported. Franklin and colleagues[54] reported that 60% of workers were still work disabled 1 year after thoracic outlet syndrome decompression surgery.

References

1. Roos DB. Thoracic outlet and carpal tunnel syndromes. In Rutherford RB, ed. Vascular Surgery. Philadelphia, WB Saunders, 1984:708-724.

2. Juvonen T, Satta J, Laitala P, et al. Anomalies at the thoracic outlet are frequent in the general population. Am J Surg 1995;170:33-37.

3. Natsis K, Totlis T, Tsikaras P, et al. Variations of the course of the upper trunk of the brachial plexus and their clinical significance for the thoracic outlet syndrome: a study on 93 cadavers. Am Surg 2006;72:188-192.

4. Sanders RJ, Hammond SL. The significance and management of cervical ribs and anomalous first ribs. J Vasc Surg 2002;36:51-56.

5. Crotti FM, Carai A, Carai M, et al. Post-traumatic thoracic outlet syndrome (TOS). Acta Neurochir Suppl 2005;92:13-15.

6. Alexandre A, Corò L, Azuelos A, et al. Thoracic outlet syndrome due to hyperextension-hyperflexion cervical injury. Acta Neurochir Suppl 2005;92:21-24.

7. Casbas L, Chauffor X, Can J, et al. Post-traumatic thoracic outlet syndromes. Ann Vasc Surg 2005;19:25-28.

8. Roos DB. The thoracic outlet syndrome is underrated. Arch Neurol 1990;47:327-328.

9. Wilbourn AJ, Porter JM. Thoracic outlet syndromes .In Weiner MA, ed. Spine: State of the Art Reviews. Philadelphia, Hanley & Belfus, 1988:597-626.

10. Shulman J. Brachial neuralgia. Arch Phys Med Rehabil 1949;30:150-153.

11. Lindgren K-A, Leino E. Subluxation of the first rib: a possible thoracic outlet syndrome mechanism. Arch Phys Med Rehabil 1988;69:692-695.

12. Lindgren K-A, Leino E, Manninen H. Cineradiography of the hypomobile first rib. Arch Phys Med Rehabil 1989;70:408-409.

13. Lindgren K-A. The thoracic outlet syndrome and the first rib [dissertation]. Kuopio and Helsinki Universities, 1992.

14. Lindgren K-A. Conservative treatment of thoracic outlet syndrome: a 2-year follow-up. Arch Phys Med Rehabil 1997;78:373-378.

15. Plewa MC, Delinger M. The false-positive rate of thoracic outlet syndrome shoulder maneuvers in healthy subjects. Acad Emerg Med 1998;5:337-342.

16. Adson AW, Coffey JR. Cervical rib. A method of anterior approach for relief of symptoms by division of the scalene anticus. Ann Surg 1927;85:839-857.

17. Gilroy J, Meyer JS. Compression of the subclavian artery as a cause of ischaemic brachial neuropathy. Brain 1963;86:733-746.

18. Wright IS. The neurovascular syndrome produced by hyperabduction of the arms. Am Heart J 1945;29:1-19.

19. Falconer MA, Weddel G. Costoclavicular compression of the subclavian artery and vein. Lancet 1943;2:539-544.

20. Roos DB. Transaxillary approach for the first rib resection to relieve thoracic outlet syndrome. Ann Surg 1966;163:354-358.

21. Costigan DA, Wilbourn AJ. The elevated arm stress test: specificity in the diagnosis of the thoracic outlet syndrome. Neurology 1985;35(Suppl 1):74-75.

22. Sällström J, Gjöres JE. Surgical treatment of the thoracic outlet syndrome. Acta Chir Scand 1983;149:555-560.

23. Ribbe E, Lindgren SHS, Norgren L. Clinical diagnosis of thoracic outlet syndrome—evaluation of patients with cervicobrachial symptoms. Manual Med 1986;2:82-85.

24. Lindgren K-A, Leino E, Manninen H. Cervical rotation lateral flexion test in brachialgia. Arch Phys Med Rehabil 1992;73:735-737.

25. Lindgren K-A, Leino E, Lepäntalo M, et al. Recurrent thoracic outlet syndrome after first rib resection. Arch Phys Med Rehabil 1991;72:208-210.

26. Lindgren K-A. Reasons for failures in the surgical treatment of thoracic outlet syndrome. Muscle Nerve 1995;18:1984-1986.

27. Geven LI, Smit AJ, Ebels T. Vascular thoracic outlet syndrome. Longer posterior rib stump causes poor outcome. Eur J Cardiothorac Surg 2006;30:232-236.

28. Ambrad-Chalela E, Thomas GI, Johansen KH. Recurrent neurogenic thoracic outlet syndrome. Am J Surg 2004;187:505-510.

29. Mingoli A, Sapienza P, di Marzo L, et al. Role of first rib stump length in recurrent neurogenic thoracic outlet syndrome. Am J Surg 2005;190:156.

30. Demondion X, Vidal C, Herbinet P, et al. Ultrasonographic assessment of arterial cross-sectional area in the thoracic outlet on postural maneuvers measured with power Doppler ultrasonography in both asymptomatic and symptomatic populations. J Ultrasound Med 2006;25:217-224.

31. Panegyres PK, Moore N, Gibson R, et al. Thoracic outlet syndromes and magnetic resonance imaging. Brain 1993;116:823-841.

32. Cherington M, Wilbourn AJ, Shils J, et al. Thoracic outlet syndromes and MRI. Brain 1995;118:819-820.

33. Smedby Ö, Rostad H, Klaastad Ö, et al. Functional imaging of the thoracic outlet syndrome in an open MR scanner. Eur Radiol 2000;10:597-600.

34. Machleder HI, Moll F, Nuwer M, et al. Somatosensory evoked potentials in the assessment of thoracic outlet compression syndrome. J Vasc Surg 1987;6:177-184.

35. Lundborg G. The "double crush" and "reversal double crush" syndrome. In Lundborg G, ed. Nerve Injury and Repair. New York, Churchill Livingstone, 1988:142-143.

36. Wilhelm A, Wilhelm F. The thoracic outlet syndrome and its importance for hand surgery. Handchir Mikrochir Plast Chir 1985;17:173-187.

37. Sällström J, Celegin Z. Physiotherapy in patients with thoracic outlet syndrome. Vasa 1983;12:257-261.

38. Kenny RA, Traynor GB, Withington D, et al. Thoracic outlet syndrome: a useful exercise treatment option. Am J Surg 1993;165:282-284.

39. Lindgren K-A, Manninen H, Rytkönen H. Thoracic outlet syndrome—a functional disturbance of the thoracic upper aperture? Muscle Nerve 1995;18:526-530.

40. Wehbé MA, Schlegel JM. Nerve gliding exercises for thoracic outlet syndrome. Hand Clin 2004;20:51-55.

41. Lindgren K-A. Conservative treatment of thoracic outlet syndrome: a 2-year follow-up. Arch Phys Med Rehabil 1997;78:373-378.

42. Muizelaar JP, Zwienenberg-Lee M. When it is not cervical radiculopathy: thoracic outlet syndrome—a prospective study on diagnosis and treatment. Clin Neurosurg 2005;52:243-249.

43. Cherington M. Thoracic outlet syndrome: rise of the conservative viewpoint. Am Fam Physician 1991;43:1998-1999.

44. Atasoy E. Combined surgical treatment of thoracic outlet syndrome: transaxillary first rib resection and transcervical scalenotomy. Handchir Mikrochir Plast Chir 2006;38:20-28.

45. Gockel M, Vastamäki M, Alaranta H. Long-term results of primary scalenotomy in the treatment of thoracic outlet syndrome. J Hand Surg Br 1994;19:229-233.

46. Cuetter AC, Bartoszek DM. Thoracic outlet syndrome: controversies, overdiagnosis, overtreatment and recommendations for management. Muscle Nerve 1989;12:410-419.

47. Lindgren K-A. Reasons for failures in the surgical treatment of thoracic outlet syndrome. Muscle Nerve 1995;18:1484-1486.

48. Colli BO, Carlotti CG, Assirati JA, et al. Neurogenic thoracic outlet syndromes: a comparison of true and nonspecific syndromes after surgical treatment. Surg Neurol 2006;65:262-272.

49. Lepäntalo M, Lindgren K-A, Leino E, et al. Long-term outcome after resection of the first rib for thoracic outlet syndrome. Br J Surg 1989;76:1255-1256.

50. Altobelli GG, Kudo T, Haas BT, et al. Thoracic outlet syndrome: pattern of clinical success after operative decompression. J Vasc Surg 2005;42:122-128.

51. Degeorges R, Reynaud C, Becquemin J-P. Thoracic outlet syndrome surgery: long term functional results. Ann Vasc Surg 2004;18:558-565.

52. Burke D. Symptoms of thoracic outlet syndrome in women with carpal tunnel syndrome. Clin Neurophysiol 2006;117:928-931.

53. Dale WA. Thoracic outlet compression syndrome. Arch Surg 1982;117:1437-1445.

54. Franklin GM, Fulton-Kehoe D, Bradley C, et al. Outcome of surgery for thoracic outlet syndrome in Washington State workers' compensation. Neurology 2000;54:1252-1257.

Chronic Pain Syndrome 92

S. Ali Mostoufi, MD

S. Ali Mostoufi, MD

Synonyms

Chronic pain disorder
Intractable pain

ICD Code

338.4   Chronic pain syndrome

DEFINITION

"Pain is an unpleasant sensory and emotional experience associated with actual or potential tissue damage, or described in terms of tissue damage."[1] Chronic pain is defined as a pain status that persists beyond a reasonable expected healing period for the involved tissue. Most pain specialists consider a pain disorder to be chronic if it persists for 6 months or more despite active management. It is called a syndrome because a constellation of symptoms develops in those patients facing this chronic pain. This constellation of symptoms is listed in Table 92-1.

As many as 50 million Americans suffer from chronic pain and are disabled to a certain degree from this condition.[2] Chronic pain syndrome is more prevalent in women[3] by up to twofold in some diagnoses (e.g., fibromyalgia).[4] It is often a hidden problem and may be an issue that individuals are reluctant to mention to family or friends. This may have an impact on the awareness of chronic pain syndrome in the community at large. Some authors have reported a higher prevalence of chronic pain syndrome in individuals with a history of childhood abuse, personality disorder (borderline, narcissistic), and lower socioeconomic status.[5]

Criteria used by the government (Social Security Administration) to establish disability on the basis of chronic pain are listed in Table 92-2.

Given its unclear pathophysiology and the lack of a definitive diagnostic test or successful treatment, chronic pain syndrome imposes a challenge to health care providers. A majority of the patients are often unsatisfied with the treatment outcomes, leading to psychosocial stress, chronic pain behaviors, pain medication seeking, and disability.

The most common conditions leading to chronic pain syndromes include headaches, repetitive stress injuries, back pain, whiplash injury, degenerative joint disorders, cancer, complex regional pain syndrome, shingles, fibromyalgia, neuropathy, central pain, and multiple surgeries.[2]

SYMPTOMS

The primary symptom is pain that is seemingly out of proportion to the objective pathophysiologic process. The pain may be localized to a body segment, or it may be a generalized body pain. In general, pain is considered subjective, and it cannot be measured directly and is difficult to validate. The measurement of severity is therefore subjective and typically relies on the patient's report as well as functional ability (work, activity of daily living, hobbies). The numeric scale (0-10) or the visual analogue scale that is used to assess pain often does not correctly reflect the pain intensity, and despite adjustments to medical management, the reported pain level is unchanged. Because of this, specialists typically focus on functional gains, rather than on pain relief, as a measure of treatment success.

In chronic pain syndrome, there are often associated pain behaviors that help establish the diagnosis. This may include fear-avoidance behavior, which will result in deconditioning and decline in functional ability for simple day-to-day activities.[6] Deconditioning will result in increased pain experience by patients when they increase their level of activity. Other observable pain behaviors include poor posture, abnormal gait (limping), facial grimacing, stiff movements, and use of assistive devices that have not been medically prescribed (canes, wheelchairs, and electric scooters). If the abnormal pain behavior is reinforced by health care providers or the patient's family, it will result in chronicity of the symptoms.

Mood and affect disorders including depression, anxiety, emotional instability, and anger are the commonly associated symptoms in patients with chronic pain syndrome.[7] Some studies have reported up to fourfold

TABLE 92-1 Common Associated Symptoms and Signs in Chronic Pain Syndrome

Depression	Sleep disorders
Anxiety	Irritable bowel
Emotional lability	Cognitive difficulty (memory, concentration)
Chronic fatigue	Pain behaviors
Medication seeking	Dramatization of symptoms
"Doctor shopping"	Legal action—secondary gain

TABLE 92-2 Criteria for Disability Based on Chronic Pain*

Six months of intractable pain

Limited daily activities secondary to pain

Excessive use of medication and medical services

Behavioral changes including depression and anxiety

Lack of clear relationship of pain to organic disorder

History of multiple diagnostic tests, unsuccessful treatments, and surgeries

*Used by Office of Disability, Social Security Administration. All criteria must be met.

increased depression in patients with chronic back pain.[8] Chronicity of the pain, lack of clear etiology, and poor treatment outcomes contribute to the emotional aspect of this disorder. Pure management of the pain without addressing the psychosocial component often results in poor outcomes and further suffering. Part of the reasonable success associated with the multidisciplinary pain programs is related to management of the psychosocial component of the chronic pain syndrome. Associated symptoms and signs of chronic pain syndrome including emotional and psychosocial disorder components are listed in Table 92-1.

Insomnia is a common complaint of patients with chronic pain syndrome. Studies have shown that insomnia severity ratings contribute to the prediction of pain severity.[9] The insomnia associated with chronic pain needs to be anticipated and treated. As with any symptom of a chronic pain syndrome, one should attempt to treat the sleep disruption in conjunction with proper treatments of the chronic pain. Many behavioral and psychological approaches to chronic pain treatment will also help with the symptoms of sleep disorder. Sleep-inducing medications can be used if other types of treatment do not work. Hypnotics are commonly used for this purpose. Special attention needs to be paid to the elderly with chronic pain and insomnia. The increased risk of medication side effects is statistically significant and potentially clinically relevant in older people at risk for falls and cognitive impairment. In people older than 60 years, the benefits of these drugs may not justify the increased risk, particularly if the patient has additional risk factors for cognitive or psychomotor adverse events.[10]

PHYSICAL EXAMINATION

Because chronic pain syndrome is a diagnosis of exclusion, physical examination is directed toward identification of abnormalities that may be treatable.

One of the most important parts of the physical examination is the observation of body motion, gait, posture, and facial expression and documentation of abnormal pain behaviors. It is not uncommon to find pain behaviors that appear to be exaggerated compared with the pathophysiologic process and physical examination findings.

Regardless of the presentation or duration of pain, a systematic and detailed musculoskeletal and neurologic examination needs to be conducted. There are challenges specific to examination of painful limbs or body area; but with experience, results of the examination often will be satisfactory. If the chronic pain syndrome follows an injury, focused examination of the injured body part is needed.

On physical examination of the patient with chronic pain syndrome, if it is done repeatedly, inconsistencies may be found. Redirecting the patient's attention while repeating some of the examination may alter your findings and point to pain behaviors. For example, diffuse tender points may not be tender if the patient's focus is diverted. Another example is a negative result of the seated straight-leg test (patients are less knowledgeable about it) versus a positive result of the supine straight-leg test in the same patient. Often, give-away weakness is demonstrated in patients with chronic pain or a nondermatomal pain pattern, or numbness is identified on physical examination.

There are diagnosis-specific examination findings that may be noted. For example, chronic pain related to complex regional pain syndrome may be associated with allodynia to touch, hyperemia, decreased range of motion, and abnormal hair and nail growth, consistent with the diagnosis. This may be found in the area of the initial injury or in a different limb or body part. Depending on the complaint, examination of other systems, including gastrointestinal, urologic, and reproductive, may be indicated.

FUNCTIONAL LIMITATIONS

Typically, there is a disproportionate loss of function in patients with chronic pain syndrome when it is matched to the injury and the stated age. The fear-avoidance behavior may promote further loss of function. This results in patients' reducing their daily activities to avoid pain. This leads to further loss of function, hence deconditioning. Deconditioning in turn results in an increased perception of pain, reduced quality of life, and further psychosocial stress and disability.

DIAGNOSTIC STUDIES

Diagnostic studies performed in chronic pain syndrome are indicated to rule out undiagnosed causes that may be treatable. The results of such studies are often inconclusive or negative. Unless the presentation of symptoms has changed, repetition of previous testing is of no value. Diagnostic testing may include laboratory work, electrodiagnostics, and imaging studies. Equally important is psychological testing. The Minnesota Multiphasic Personality Inventory is the most common psychological test used in patients with chronic pain and has been shown to help understand the psychological impact on individuals with chronic pain.[11]

Differential Diagnosis

Somatoform disorders

Somatization disorder: in addition to pain, patients have gastrointestinal, pseudoneurologic, and sexual complaints

Conversion disorder: dramatic loss of voluntary motor or sensory function (e.g., inability to walk, sudden blindness, paralysis); no evidence that the symptom is feigned or intentionally produced; loss of function is not due to medical illness

Hypochondriasis

Malingering

TREATMENT

Initial

The initial treatment focuses on management of the pain and improvement of function. In review of the literature, numerous studies suggest a multidisciplinary approach for management of chronic pain syndrome.[12,13] These studies show that multidisciplinary treatments of chronic pain are superior to no treatment as well as to single-discipline treatments, such as medical treatment or physical therapy. The effects appeared to be stable over time, and the beneficial effects of multidisciplinary treatment were not limited to improvements in pain but also extended to variables such as return to work and use of the health care resources.

Members of the multidisciplinary treatment team include a pain specialist, a mental health team, a physical therapist, an occupational therapist, the primary care provider, and the patient. Ideally, the rehabilitation component is 2 to 3 hours each day, three times per week, for 6 to 12 weeks. In addition, patients will see mental health counselors weekly and are monitored every 2 weeks by the pain specialist who is overseeing the entire care. Components of a multidisciplinary management include the following.

Education of the Patient

It is crucial for the patients dealing with chronic pain syndrome to be educated in the complexity of the disorder and possible factors affecting its management. It is important for the patients to be clear about their role in

the treatment plan. Both patient and family should have a good understanding about the multifactorial nature of it and the benefits of a multidisciplinary management plan. Education of the patient should be done by all parties involved in care, including the primary care provider, pain specialist, pain interventionalist, rehabilitation team, and psychiatry or psychology team.

Mental Health Treatment

Psychological interventions help patients find ways to accept this chronic condition and to adjust to it. The focus of the mental health counseling is to work on pain behaviors and to educate patients about the adverse consequences of this atypical behavior. Patients need to understand that negative thoughts stemming from pain will influence mood, behavior, sleep, and the chronicity of the pain.

Individual or group treatment may include electromyographic biofeedback, relaxation training, coping mechanism, clinical hypnosis, and cognitive therapy techniques.[14] These may result in improved ability to manage pain.

Advanced psychological or psychiatric treatments may include pharmacologic interventions to address emotional problems, affect disorders, anxiety disorders, sleep disturbances, and panic attacks.[15] Common pharmacologic substances used to address psychological disorders in chronic pain syndrome are listed in Table 92-3.

If opioid management is being considered in chronic pain syndrome, a consultation with a pain psychologist is indicated to determine risk of future abuse.

Medications

In chronic pain syndrome, pain killers and adjunct medication are not able to eliminate pain, but the analgesic effect may lead to increased function, augmented rehabilitation outcomes, restored sleep, and improved mood. The most commonly used pain medications and adjunct pharmaceutical substances in chronic pain syndrome are listed in Table 92-4.

Use of these medications needs to be directed by pain specialists, monitored often and adjusted if necessary. Short-term use of medications for pain is rarely worrisome, but prolonged use may increase the possibility of adverse reactions, including gastrointestinal side effects,

---

TABLE 92-3 Common Medications Used to Address Psychological Issues in Chronic Pain Syndrome

Antidepressants	Amitriptyline, nortriptyline, clonazepam, venlafaxine, citalopram, fluoxetine, bupropion, escitalopram, sertraline
Anxiolytics	Lorazepam, clonazepam, oxazepam, diazepam, alprazolam, buspirone
Mood stabilizers	Divalproex, lithium, gabapentin

TABLE 92-4	Common Analgesics and Adjunct Medications Used in Chronic Pain Syndrome
Nonsteroidal analgesics	Salicylates: aspirin
	Arylalkanoic acids: diclofenac, etodolac, indomethacin, nabumetone
	Arylpropionic acids: ketoprofen, ibuprofen, naproxen
	Oxicams: piroxicam, meloxicam
	Coxibs: celecoxib
Opioid medications	Codeine, meperidine, propoxyphene, hydrocodone, hydromorphone, morphine (short and long acting), oxycodone (short and long acting), methadone, fentanyl
Partial mu-opioid agonist and kappa-opioid receptor antagonist	Buprenorphine
Adjunct medications	Antiseizure medications: pregabalin, gabapentin, lamotrigine, topiramate, clonazepam
	Antidepressants (see Table 92-3)
Sedatives	Benzodiazepines: temazepam, diazepam, lorazepam
	Nonbenzodiazepines: eszopiclone, zaleplon, zolpidem

internal organ damage, balance issues, and memory or concentration disturbances.

Use of opioid analgesics, although controversial, is fairly common. Opioid analgesics must be used with utmost caution and with understanding of the challenges related to chronic opioid management as well as all the social stigma attached to them. The author recommends an opioid contract and involvement of the primary care provider in decision-making.

Rehabilitation

A major component of the multidisciplinary approach to chronic pain syndrome is involvement of the rehabilitation team, including physiotherapy and occupational therapy. The rehabilitation team will work with the patient to establish a structured day, which includes daily exercises. The duration of treatment may be slightly longer than average for painful musculoskeletal issues (e.g., tennis elbow or degenerative joint disease). This population of patients starts from a lower functional level, which contributes to a prolonged rehabilitation care that may take as long as 12 weeks.

The basic exercise structure will include stretching activities, progressive strengthening (light weight training), and aerobic exercise training. The focus will be on body mechanics, postural corrections, restoration of function, modification of maladaptive behaviors, and provision of pain relief by incorporation of modalities (heat, ice, ultrasound) and relaxation techniques. Deep

tissue massage, myofascial release, Pilates, Tai Chi, and yoga may be helpful in symptomatic relief. Self-directed swimming is also of some value. The challenge for the rehabilitation team remains the fear-avoidance behavior.

Inpatient Rehabilitation Care

Inpatient care is rarely needed for management of chronic pain syndromes. The criteria commonly used for admission into an inpatient unit are listed in Table 92-5. In the managed care era, obtaining approval for this method of care is difficult.

Procedures

On occasion, specific procedures are helpful to patients with chronic pain syndrome. This is especially true if previous medical care has insufficiently addressed the need for a specific intervention. Once relative pain relief is achieved, tapering of the pain medications as well as advancement in the rehabilitation regimen is a must. Procedures that may be tried include neuraxial blocks, facet injections, radiofrequency ablation, sacroiliac blocks, paravertebral blocks, large joint injections, trigger point injections, and infiltration of inflamed bursa or tendons. Medical acupuncture may be considered among these interventions.

Surgery

There is a limited indication for surgery in chronic pain syndrome. If the pain generator is identifiable and modern surgical methods are available to treat it, this method may be indicated. There is a potential for continued pain despite surgical care.

POTENTIAL DISEASE COMPLICATIONS

Significant disability secondary to pain as well as suicidal ideation or attempt (secondary to psychosocial comorbidities) may complicate the clinical picture.

POTENTIAL TREATMENT COMPLICATIONS

Medication side effects are expected in a certain percentage of patients who take them. These side effects are specific to the class of medication. In the case of

TABLE 92-5	Criteria for Inpatient Care for Management of Chronic Pain Syndrome

Major functional disabilities secondary to pain

Extensive disruption in family functioning due to pain

Patient needs temporary removal from a detrimental home situation to refocus his or her life away from the pain

Need for extensive psychological or behavioral therapy

opioids, the potential for tolerance, dependency, and abuse exists.

Rehabilitation intensity disproportionate to the functional status of the patient may lead to dissatisfaction and poor compliance, which encourages fear-avoidance behavior.

References

1. LaRocca H. A taxonomy of chronic pain syndromes. Spine 1992;17(Suppl):S344-S355.
2. American Chronic Pain Association. Pain Fact Sheets. Available at www.theacpa.org/.
3. Unruh AM. Gender variations in clinical pain experience. Pain 1996;65:123-167.
4. Wolfe F, Ross K, Anderson J, et al. The prevalence and characteristics of fibromyalgia in the general population. Arthritis Rheum 1995;38:19-28.
5. Craig TK, Drake H. The South London somatisation study II. Br J Psychiatry 1994;165:248-258.
6. Pfingsten M, Leibing E, Harter W, et al. Fear-avoidance behavior and anticipation of pain in patients with chronic low back pain: a randomized controlled study. Pain Med 2001;2:259-266.
7. Currie SR, Wang J. Chronic back pain and major depression in the general Canadian population. Pain 2004;107:54-60.
8. Sullivan MJ, Reesor K, Mikail S, Fisher R. The treatment of depression in chronic low back pain: review and recommendations. Pain 1992;50:5-13.
9. Wilson KG, Eriksson MY, D'Eon JL, et al. Major depression and insomnia in chronic pain. Clin J Pain 2002;18:77-83.
10. Jennifer G, Krista L, Nathan H. Sedative hypnotics in older people with insomnia: meta-analysis of risks and benefits. BMJ 2005;331:1169-1173.
11. Deardorff WW, Chino AF, Scott DW. Characteristics of chronic pain patients: factor analysis of the MMPI-2. Pain 1993;54:153-158.
12. Flor H, Fydrich T, Turk DC. Efficacy of multidisciplinary pain treatment centers: a meta-analytic review. Pain 1992;49:221-230.
13. Lang E, Liebig K, Kastner S, et al. Multidisciplinary rehabilitation versus usual care for chronic low back pain in the community: effects on quality of life. Spine J 2003;3:270-276.
14. Weitz SE, Witt PH, Greenfield DP. Treatment of chronic pain syndrome. N J Med 2000;97:63-67.
15. National Institute of Mental Health. Medications. Available at: www.nimh.nih.gov/health/publications/medications/complete-publication.shtml.

Complex Regional Pain Syndrome **93**

Allison Bailey, MD, and Joseph F. Audette, MA, MD

Synonyms

Reflex sympathetic dystrophy
Post-traumatic dystrophy
Sudeck atrophy
Sudeck syndrome
Causalgia
Osteodystrophy
Neuroalgodystrophy
Post-traumatic osteoporosis
Shoulder-hand syndrome
Sympathetically maintained pain

ICD-9 Codes

337.21 Reflex sympathetic dystrophy of the upper limb
337.22 Reflex sympathetic dystrophy of the lower limb

DEFINITION

Complex regional pain syndrome (CRPS) is a pain syndrome that occurs most often in an extremity in association with abnormal autonomic nervous system activity and trophic changes. The disorder has both nociceptive and neuropathic features and is characterized by persistent pain, allodynia or hyperalgesia, edema, alterations in skin blood flow, and sudomotor dysfunction.[1] In most cases, the syndrome is preceded by an inciting noxious event, trauma, or immobilization.[2]

The classification of CRPS I versus CRPS II depends on the presence or absence of nerve injury, as follows: in CRPS I, there is no known nerve lesion; in CRPS II, there is nerve injury.[3] However, the pain that develops, which is typically severe, deep burning pain, is vastly out of proportion in duration, distribution, and severity to the pain that is expected from the initiating injury.[4] When it is left untreated, permanent hair and nail loss, muscle and skin atrophy, and chronic pain may result. In addition, when it is severe, the disorder may spread to other body areas, including the contralateral limb.[5]

The incidence of CRPS has been estimated at approximately 5.5 per 100,000.[6] The underlying pathophysiologic mechanism of the disease remains incompletely understood at this time. An exaggerated inflammatory response is believed to play a major role, particularly in the early phases of the disease course.[7] Alternatively, autonomic dysregulation with an overly active sympathetic nervous system has been thought to account for the ongoing symptoms. In addition, the site of dysfunction is still unclear, with both central and peripheral mechanisms proposed.[8]

Reflecting this lack of clarity, many terms and definitions have been used to describe the syndrome since its first report by Silas Weir Mitchell, a Civil War surgeon, from his study of gunshot wounds. Previous terms include causalgia, shoulder-hand syndrome, and, most commonly, reflex sympathetic dystrophy. The term *sympathetic* was more recently thought to be inaccurate because of lack of response of a significant number of patients to sympathetic blockade, and the disorder was renamed CRPS by consensus of the International Association for the Study of Pain in 1994.[9] This terminology is meant to emphasize the complexity of the disorder in regard to its pathogenesis and manifestations. The International Association for the Study of Pain established the following four criteria that must be present for a clinical diagnosis of CRPS to be made[9]:

- Preceding noxious event without (CRPS I) or with obvious nerve lesion (CRPS II).
- Spontaneous pain or hyperalgesia-hyperesthesia not limited to a single nerve territory and disproportionate to the inciting event.
- Edema, skin blood flow (temperature) or sudomotor abnormalities, motor symptoms, or trophic changes are present on the affected limb, in particular at distal sites.
- Other diagnoses are excluded.

The disorder has been classically divided into three stages, which are useful descriptively.[10] However, the syndrome may not always follow this stepwise progression. The stages of CRPS are described as follows:

- Stage 1: severe pain; pitting edema; redness; warmth; increased hair and nail growth; hyperhidrosis may begin; osteoporosis may begin.
- Stage 2: continued pain; brawny edema; periarticular thickening; cyanosis or pallor; livedo reticularis;

511

coolness, hyperhidrosis; increased osteoporosis; ridged nails.

- Stage 3: pallor; dry, cool skin; atrophic soft tissue (dystrophy); contracture; extensive osteoporosis.

SYMPTOMS

The hallmarks of CRPS are symptoms, particularly pain, that are disproportionately severe given the underlying trauma that led to their onset and that tend to spread distally from the site of original injury in the affected limb.[4] The hand is the most common site of involvement with spread to the wrist and forearm, followed by the foot and ankle.[11] Further, the symptoms will, by definition, not be confined to a particular nerve territory. Although there is no obvious nerve lesion in CRPS I, the symptoms that develop have neuropathic features. Symptoms include burning spontaneous pain experienced in most of the cases in the deep tissues of the distal part of the affected limb. The majority will have sensory disturbances in a stocking-glove distribution or on the palmar surfaces of the hands or feet. The most common description of the pain will be deep burning, tearing, or stinging that is constant rather than lancinating. Patients with CRPS will typically experience severe stimulus-evoked pains to deep mechanical pressure, application of heat or cold, and sharp stimulation. Pain will commonly be elicited with movement of joints, by wearing of clothes, or with contact of sheets or blankets. Hypoesthesia and hypoalgesia have been found in 50% of patients with CRPS I, occurring on the entire half of the body or in the associated quadrant on the same side as the affected limb. In these patients, quantitative sensory testing has shown that the thresholds to mechanical, cold, warmth, and noxious heat stimuli are higher on the affected side of the body than on the unaffected side, supporting the clinical finding of decreased sensation.[12] In some cases, the symptoms of CRPS can spread beyond the initially affected limb and cause mirror-image pain in the contralateral limb or even spread to affect all four limbs.

Other common symptoms include proximal muscle pain in the affected limb, often associated with myofascial dysfunction. Mood disturbance is common in the chronic stages of the illness. Early in the disease course, patients tend to be euthymic because they expect to get well. From 2 to 6 months of disease progression, patients may begin to become anxious; and by 6 months, all patients will exhibit varying degrees of depression, sleep disturbance, and anxiety. The key point is that although mood disturbance is common in CRPS, it does not predate the disease and in fact can be viewed as an appropriate response to a progressive, unremitting pain disorder.[2]

PHYSICAL EXAMINATION

Although the original International Association for the Study of Pain criteria required only history and subjective symptoms for a diagnosis of CRPS to be made, recent consensus guidelines developed by experts have argued for the inclusion of objective physical findings.[2] Sensory,

motor, and autonomic dysfunction should be thoroughly investigated during the physical examination.

Autonomic disturbances are common; the majority of patients have side-to-side differences in the temperature of the limbs. Skin temperature of the affected limb will depend on the chronicity, with temperature increase in acute stages and temperature decrease in chronic stages. Temperature increase in the acute stages is associated with skin that is white or reddish and with more swelling; temperature decrease in the chronic stage is associated with cyanotic, bluish skin and more atrophy.[13] Other findings include sweating abnormalities and trophic changes, with nail and hair growth in the acute stage and hair loss and nail brittleness in the later stages.

Motor disturbances are often overlooked in CRPS but are a predominant feature. Approximately 70% of patients with CRPS have muscle weakness of the affected limb, exaggerated tendon reflexes or tremor, irregular myoclonic jerks, and dystonic muscle contractions.[14] This muscle dysfunction is frequently associated with significant loss of range of motion of the distal joints. In performing the sensory component of the examination for CRPS, special attention should be focused on the distal extremity. Because of the common finding of regional neuropathic and motor dysfunction, it is still important to broaden the examination both proximally and contralaterally.

For proper assessment of the range of presentations in CRPS, light touch, pinprick, temperature, and vibration sensation should be assessed. Sensory deficits of one modality, such as loss of pinprick sensation, often accompany exaggerated positive responses to another modality, such as pain with light touch. To help distinguish symptom amplification from reliable sensory dysfunction, there should be clear and repeatable findings in the affected area, while the subject is able to respond normally to examination of an unaffected area. In addition to findings of allodynia (pain in response to an innocuous stimulus, such as light touch or brush with a cotton swab) and hyperalgesia (exaggerated pain in response to a painful stimulus, such as pinprick or deep pressure), signs of cutaneous C-fiber dropout should be sought. This can be accomplished by applying hot water in a plastic bag over the skin and comparing the time it takes for the affected limb to be withdrawn with an unaffected area. When loss of C fibers has occurred, the withdrawal latency will be prolonged. Summation can be assessed by repeated application of the same pinprick stimulus with equal force and asking the patient to report any change in pain intensity. The normal nervous system tends to accommodate to repeated painful stimuli, whereas an individual with a facilitated nervous system may report increasing pain.

Findings of autonomic dysfunction, such as abnormal skin temperature, local areas of cutaneous trophedema, and hair loss, should be evaluated. In addition to checking for weakness and difficulty with initiation of motion in the affected limb, regional muscle irritability should be assessed. Specifically, the examination should look for trigger points, spontaneous muscle fasciculations, and cramps in the supporting muscles of the limb. Tendon reflexes may be increased, and presence of a tremor should be noted. Finally, measurement of passive and active range of motion of the joints in the affected limb is important; this information can be used as objective findings to be modified with rehabilitation.

Differential Diagnosis

Cellulitis

Lymphedema

Occult or stress fracture

Acute synovitis

Septic arthritis

Septic tenosynovitis

Upper or lower limb venous thrombosis

Scleroderma

Plexitis, peripheral neuropathy

FUNCTIONAL LIMITATIONS

Chronic pain leads to the well-known syndrome of deconditioning, sleep disturbance, anxiety, and depression. With inadequate treatment, all aspects of the patient's life are affected, often with devastating social, recreational, financial, and vocational consequences. In addition, limb contracture and loss of strength may lead to difficulty in ambulation and basic and advanced activities of daily living.

DIAGNOSTIC STUDIES

CRPS is primarily a clinical diagnosis. However, several diagnostic studies may be helpful in its evaluation and to rule out other pathologic processes. For example, skin temperature can be measured by Doppler flowmeter and infrared thermography; sweat output can be assessed by quantitative sudomotor axon reflex testing; cutaneous blood flow can be measured by vital capillaroscopy; and coexisting nerve injury and muscle fiber loss can be quantified by electromyography and nerve conduction studies.[15] Imaging has historically been used to exclude other diagnoses. Plain films are usually normal except in extreme cases, in which demineralization can occur (Sudeck atrophy). Magnetic resonance imaging may demonstrate marrow edema, soft tissue swelling, and joint effusion. The classic finding on bone scintigraphy is increased periarticular activity in the affected limb.[16] The sensitivity and specificity of three-phase bone scintigraphy are variable.[17,18] Although an abnormal finding on bone scan can confirm the clinical diagnosis of CRPS, the condition cannot be ruled out by a normal study.

A study of brain single-photon emission computed tomography in a small sample of patients with CRPS revealed increased regional cerebral blood flow in the contralateral thalamus in patients with acute CRPS and decreased contralateral thalamic regional cerebral blood flow in patients with chronic CRPS.[19] Further research into the use of nuclear imaging in the evaluation of CRPS is needed.

TREATMENT

Initial

Early in the disease, treatment should focus on aggressive interventional management to control pain and to restore function (see the section on procedures).

Medications play an essential role in the treatment of CRPS, in both the acute and the chronic phases. The following principles should be applied in prescribing drugs for this condition:

- Minimize side effects.
- Minimize medications that could cause dependency.
- Avoid cognitive impairment.
- Avoid organ toxicity.
- Use rational polypharmacy, when appropriate, directed at different components of the pain.

In choosing medications, the findings of the examination together with a basic understanding of the mechanisms of actions of the various drugs can provide some structure to treatment.[20] For example, better medication selection can be made if one can use, within reason, clinical findings and history to distinguish the underlying physiologic mechanism (Table 93-1).

With this approach, a patient with signs and symptoms suggestive of a sensitized peripheral nociceptor may respond better to a topical lidocaine patch, mexiletine, or an anticonvulsant with known sodium channel blocking properties, such as topiramate or lamotrigine, rather than gabapentin. In general, most patients with CRPS will have some combination of symptoms and signs in all four classes; therefore, rational polypharmacy often makes sense. A summary of pharmacologic treatment options available for neuropathic pain is presented in Table 93-2. Many of these medications have not been specifically studied in CRPS.

TABLE 93-1 Physical Findings and Associated Underlying Physiologic Mechanism

Physical Finding	Physiologic Mechanism
Hyperalgesia	Sensitized peripheral nociceptor
Summation of sensory input	Altered central processing of pain (wind-up)
Allodynia, segmental widening of pain, or bilateral findings	Loss of descending pain modulation and loss of inhibitory neurons in the dorsal horn with C-fiber dropout and phenotypic switching of A-B fibers
Trophedema, temperature changes	Altered sympathetic function or responsiveness

TABLE 93-2 Pharmacologic Treatments of Neuropathic Pain (Significant Adverse Events)

Drug	Starting Dose	Dose Range	Usual Dose Schedule	Major Drug Class and Drug-Specific Characteristics and Issues
Antidepressants				
Tricyclic antidepressants				Prolonged QT interval, urinary retention, sedation
Amitriptyline	10 mg	10-150 mg	Once in the evening	More AEs
Nortriptyline	10 mg	10-150 mg	Once in the evening	Moderate AEs
Desipramine	10 mg	10-150 mg	Once in the evening	Fewer AEs
SSNRIs				Sleep disturbance, sexual dysfunction
Venlafaxine	37.5 mg	150-375 mg	Once or twice a day	
Duloxetine	20 mg	40-60 mg	Once or twice a day	
SSRIs				Serotonin syndrome, impotence
Paroxetine	10 mg	20-60 mg	Once a day	
Citalopram	10 mg	20-60 mg	Once a day	
Other				
Bupropion	100 mg	200-400 mg	Once or twice a day	Agitation, tachycardia, seizures All cause some degree of cognitive impairment
Anticonvulsants				
Carbamazepine	200 mg	1000-1200 mg	Twice a day	Highly protein bound, liver metabolism AEs: aplastic anemia, hepatic
Oxcarbazepine	300 mg	1200-2100 mg	Twice a day	Moderately protein bound, liver metabolism AEs: leukopenia, thrombocytopenia
Valproic acid	250 mg	500-1000 mg	Twice a day	AEs: hepatic failure, thrombocytopenia, pancreatitis
Phenytoin	100 mg	300-500 mg	Once a day	AEs: gum hypertrophy, osteomalacia, lymphadenopathy, hepatotoxicity, blood dyscrasias
Gabapentin	100 mg	1800-3600 mg	3 or 4 times a day	<3% protein bound, not metabolized AEs: cognitive
Lamotrigine	25 mg	200-600 mg	Once or twice a day	Moderately protein bound, liver metabolism AEs: Stevens-Johnson syndrome, paresthesias
Topiramate	25 mg	100-800 mg	Once or twice a day	17% protein bound, minimal liver metabolism AEs: cognitive, renal stones, glaucoma
Levetiracetam	250 mg	1000-3000 mg	Once or twice a day	<10% protein bound, minimal liver metabolism AEs: cognitive
Tiagabine	2 mg	4-56 mg	2 to 4 times a day	Highly protein bound, liver metabolism AEs: cognitive; may improve sleep architecture
Clonazepam	0.5 mg	1.5-20 mg	1 to 3 times a day	AEs: cognitive, blood dyscrasias
Pregabalin	50 mg	150-450 mg	3 times a day	AEs: cognitive
Antiarrhythmic				
Mexiletine	150 mg	300-1200 mg	Twice a day	AEs: gastrointestinal, hepatic, arrhythmia Hypotension, sedation
Alpha₂ agonists				
Clonidine	0.1 mg	0.3-2.4 mg	1 to 3 times a day	Hepatic
Tizanidine	2 mg	8-36 mg	1 to 3 times a day	Hepatic
Nonopioid analgesic				
Tramadol	50 mg	150-400 mg	3 or 4 times a day	Risk of serotonin syndrome with use of SSRIs, tricyclic antidepressants
Topical agents				
Lidocaine 5%		Up to 3 patches	12 hours	Potentiates cardiac toxicity from mexiletine
Capsaicin 0.075%			3 times a day	Rash
Doxepin 5%			3 times a day	Potential systemic side effects similar to tricyclic antidepressants

AEs, adverse events; SSNRIs, selective serotonin-norepinephrine reuptake inhibitors; SSRIs, selective serotonin reuptake inhibitors.

The tricyclic antidepressants are traditional choices in neuropathic pain disorders with good evidence to support their use for neuropathic pain.[2] Their sedating side effects are additionally useful in chronic pain conditions in treatment of associated sleep disturbance. The tricyclic antidepressants appear to have some efficacy in treatment of CRPS, although they have not been properly studied in this disorder. A reasonable regimen is to start with amitriptyline at a dose of 10 mg at bedtime with a titration schedule based on patient response up to 75 to 150 mg at bedtime.

Antiepileptic agents are some of the best-studied agents for neuropathic pain, and strong evidence demonstrates their effectiveness. These agents appear to be promising in the treatment of CRPS. Gabapentin has been shown to be effective in large, randomized controlled trials for other neuropathic pain disorders, and a case series suggests its efficacy in CRPS.[21] Dosing is typically started at 300 mg at bedtime with gradual titration to a maximum dose of 1200 mg three times a day (3600 mg daily). Phenytoin and carbamazepine in their usual doses have both been used in the treatment of CRPS with some success. Lamotrigine has been studied in other neuropathic pain conditions and may have some usefulness in the treatment of CRPS, but studies are currently lacking.

Oral corticosteroid agents can be particularly effective early in the disease when significant inflammation is present, and their use is substantially supported by randomized controlled clinical trials.[8] A short course of steroids in the acute stage of the disease may be indicated. A regimen of 30 mg daily tapered during 1 to 2 weeks is reasonable. Longer courses should be avoided because of significant adverse effects, a questionable risk-benefit ratio, and numerous contraindications.

Because of the suspected role of increased sympathetic nervous system activity in CRPS, α-adrenergic antagonists such as phenoxybenzamine and phentolamine have also been used and may be beneficial in cases of sympathetically maintained pain. Phenoxybenzamine may be started at a dose of 10 mg two or three times per day and increased by 10 mg every 2 days to a maximum dose range of 40 to 120 mg daily. The main limiting side effect is postural hypotension that can be treated with abdominal binders and stockings.

The lidocaine patch, a nonwoven patch containing 5% lidocaine, is used topically to deliver medication locally to the affected area. It is approved by the U.S. Food and Drug Administration for the treatment of postherpetic neuralgia and has shown some promise for treatment of CRPS.[22] In particular, it may be useful in diminishing the allodynia frequently associated with this disorder.

Opioids may be useful in the acute stages of CRPS for control of pain. However, their use in chronic pain conditions and conditions with neuropathic features remains controversial. One randomized controlled trial of controlled-release morphine for the treatment of CRPS reported no difference in pain reduction compared with placebo after 8 days of use.[23] However, several studies have suggested the efficacy of opioids for chronic pain.[24] Methadone may be a choice in cases of severe neuropathic pain because of its N-methyl-D-aspartate (NMDA) receptor antagonist activity.[25]

Other pharmacologic treatment options include clonidine, nifedipine, calcitonin, bisphosphonates, nonsteroidal anti-inflammatory drugs, mexiletine, and ketamine, applied topically or as intravenous infusion. The patient with acute CRPS should have close follow-up with treatment aggressively aimed at pain and symptom control so that mobilization becomes possible.

Rehabilitation

The goal of interventional strategies and pharmacologic treatment is to manage pain so that patients may participate in rehabilitation and begin to mobilize the affected limb as early as possible. Stress loading and isometric exercise have shown some benefit in CRPS.[26] Compressive garments are sometimes used to control edema and to desensitize the limb but may not be tolerated because of pain. Densensitization can sometimes be achieved with contrast baths, alternating hot (100°F, 43°C) and cold (65°F, 18°C) water soaks for several minutes. This modality can be taught to patients for home use. Transcutaneous electrical nerve stimulation has been used with mixed results. Paraffin baths or fluidized therapy may be beneficial in the contractures of late-stage CRPS. For chronic CRPS, interdisciplinary pain programs emphasizing functional restoration are often necessary for optimal recovery. The treatment team should consist of medical, psychological, and physical and occupational therapy services.[27] Patients' progress in therapy should be guided by specific functional goals. Inability to progress in therapy because of pain should be addressed with pharmacotherapy, procedures, or other pain control modalities. In the setting of such programs, patients may also require medications to control associated sleep disturbance, anxiety, or depression to progress in an appropriate manner and to regain function.

Procedures

Sympathetic blocks are the traditional and most common early intervention.[28] However, it has become clear that patients can be divided by positive or negative response to selective sympathetic blockade or blockade of the α-adrenergic receptors into those with sympathetically maintained pain and those with sympathetically independent pain.[4] Stellate ganglion blocks for upper limb and lumbar chain blocks for lower limb symptoms can be done by trained anesthesiologists or physiatrists. Intrapleural infusion of local anesthetic can alternatively be used to block the sympathetic chain from T1 to L2. Bier block procedures, involving the intravenous infusion of pharmacologic substances into a limb after gravitational drainage of the venous bed, may also be used. Depending on the substance infused, this can accomplish regional sympathetic blockade with guanethidine, sensorimotor blockade with lidocaine, or a combination of the two.[29] For those patients with sympathetically independent pain, regional sensorimotor blockade with lidocaine should be the early intervention of choice. Such procedures have the possibility of achieving rapid and effective pain relief, allowing more timely progression in rehabilitation.

In addition to the interventional pain control procedures, which should be used aggressively early in the disease course, spinal cord stimulation has been shown to be effective for treatment of both CRPS I and CRPS II for which other less invasive treatment strategies have failed.[30]

Surgery

Surgical sympathectomy has been advocated when chemical block is effective but short lasting. Neurosurgical dorsal root entry zone ablation is another surgical option reserved for chronic severe cases.[31]

POTENTIAL DISEASE COMPLICATIONS

CRPS can lead to severe chronic pain and its typical sequelae. Limb contracture and muscle atrophy can result in loss of extremity function and potentially permanent disability.

POTENTIAL TREATMENT COMPLICATIONS

Adverse effects of pharmacotherapy vary according to the medication selected. Because polypharmacy may be necessary, care should be used in selection of interacting drugs that do not result in untoward side effects. Long courses of corticosteroids can produce significant endocrinologic disturbances and should be avoided. Nonsteroidal anti-inflammatory drugs have well-known adverse effects on the gastric, hepatic, and renal systems. Side effects of opioids may be an issue when high doses are required to control pain, and tolerance can develop with chronic use. Potential complications of stellate ganglion block are inadvertent arterial injection and seizures or recurrent laryngeal nerve injury.[31] Perforation of the aorta, vena cava, or kidney can occur during lumbar sympathetic block. The most common complications of spinal cord stimulation include hardware failure, lead migration, infection, and failure to provide pain relief.[32]

References

1. Ochoa JL, Verdugo RJ. The mythology of reflex sympathetic dystrophy and sympathetically maintained pains. Phys Med Rehabil Clin North Am 1993;4:151-163.
2. Harden N. Pharmacotherapy of complex regional pain syndrome. Am J Phys Med Rehabil 2005;84:S17-S28.
3. Stanton-Hicks M, Janig W, Hassenbusch S, et al. Reflex sympathetic dystrophy: changing concepts and taxonomy. Pain 1995;63:127-133.
4. Janig W, Baron R. Complex regional pain syndrome: mystery explained? Lancet Neurol 2003;2:687-697.
5. Leis S, Weber M, Schmelz M, Birklein F. Facilitated neurogenic inflammation in unaffected limbs of patients with complex regional pain syndrome. Neurosci Lett 2004;359:163-166.
6. Sandroni P, Benrud-Larson LM, McClelland RL, Low PA. Complex regional pain syndrome type I: incidence and prevalence in Olmsted county, a population-based study. Pain 2003;103:199-207.
7. Bonica JJ. Causalgia and other reflex sympathetic dystrophies. In Bonica JJ, ed. Advances in Pain Research and Therapy. New York, Raven Press, 1979:141-166.
8. Cline M, Ochoa JL, Torebjork E. Chronic hyperalgesia and skin warming caused by sensitized C nociceptors. Brain 1989;112:621-647.
9. Birklein F. Complex regional pain syndrome. J Neurol 2005;252:131-138.
10. Schwartzman RJ, McLellan TL. Reflex sympathetic dystrophy: a review. Arch Neurol 1987;44:555-561.
11. Anderson DJ, Falat LM. Complex regional pain syndrome of the lower extremity: a retrospective study of 33 patients. J Foot Ankle Surg 1999;38:381-387.
12. Rommel O, Malin JP, Zenz M, et al. Quantitative sensory testing, neurophysiological and psychological examination in patients with complex regional pain syndrome and hemisensory deficits. Pain 2001;93:279-293.
13. Birklein F, Riedl B, Sieweke N, et al. Neurological findings in complex regional pain syndromes—analysis of 145 cases. Acta Neurol Scand 2000;101:262-269.
14. Van Hilten JJ, Van de Beek WJ, Roep O, et al. Multifocal or generalized tonic dystonia of complex regional pain syndrome: a distinct clinical entity associated with HLA-DR13. Ann Neurol 2000;48:113-116.
15. Law PA, Amadio PC, Wilson PR, et al. Laboratory findings in reflex sympathetic dystrophy: a preliminary report. Clin J Pain 1994;10:235-239.
16. Todorovic-Tirnanic M, Obradovic V, Han R, et al. Diagnostic approach to reflex sympathetic dystrophy after fracture: radiology or bone scintigraphy? Eur J Nucl Med 1999;22:1187-1193.
17. Holder LE, Cole LA, Myerson MS. Reflex sympathetic dystrophy in the foot: clinical and scintigraphic criteria. Radiology 1992;184:531-535.
18. Intenzo C, Kim S, Millin J, et al. Scintigraphic patterns of the reflex sympathetic dystrophy syndrome of the lower extremities. Clin Nucl Med 1989;14:657-661.
19. Intenzo CM, Kim SM, Capuzzi DM. The role of nuclear medicine in the evaluation of complex regional pain syndrome type I. Clin Nucl Med 2005;30:400-407.
20. Dworkin RH, Backonja M, Rowbotham MC, et al. Advances in neuropathic pain: diagnosis, mechanisms, and treatment recommendations. Arch Neurol 2003;60:1524-1534.
21. Mellick GA, Mellick LB. Reflex sympathetic dystrophy treated with gabapentin. Arch Phys Med Rehabil 1997;78:98-105.
22. Devers A, Galer BS. Topical lidocaine patch relieves a variety of neuropathic pain conditions: an open-label study. Clin J Pain 2000;16:205-208.
23. Harke H, Gretenkort P, Ladleif HU, et al. The response of neuropathic pain and pain in complex regional pain syndrome I to carbamazepine and sustained-release morphine in patients pretreated with spinal cord stimulation: a double-blinded randomized study. Anesth Analg 2001;92:488-495.
24. Kalso E, Edwards JE, Moore RA, et al. Opioids in chronic noncancer pain: systematic review of efficacy and safety. Pain 2004;112:372-380.
25. Fishman SM, Wilsey B, Mahajan G, et al. Methadone reincarnated: novel clinical applications with related concerns. Pain Med 2002;3:339-348.
26. Carlson LK, Watson HK. Treatment of reflex sympathetic dystrophy using the stress-loading program. J Hand Ther 1988;5:149-154.
27. Audette JF, Bailey A. Physiatric treatment of pain. In Ballantyne JC, ed. The Massachusetts General Hospital Handbook of Pain Management, 3rd ed. Philadelphia, Lippincott Williams & Wilkins, 2006:236-247.
28. Cepeda MS, Carr DB, Lau J. Local anesthetic sympathetic blockade for complex regional pain syndrome. Cochrane Database Syst Rev 2005;4:CD004598.

29. Paraskevas KI, Michaloglou AA, Briana DD, et al. Treatment of complex regional pain syndrome type I of the hand with a series of intravenous regional sympathetic blocks with guanetheidine and lidocaine. Clin Rheumatol 2005;7:1-7.

30. Taylor RS, Van Buyten JP, Buchser E. Spinal cord stimulation for complex regional pain syndrome: a systematic review of the clinical and cost-effectiveness literature and assessment of prognostic factors. Eur J Pain 2006;10:91-101.

31. Payne R. Neuropathic pain syndromes, with special reference to causalgia and reflex sympathetic dystrophy. Clin J Pain 1986;2:59-73.

32. Stojanovic MP. Neuromodulation techniques for the treatment of pain. In Ballantyne JC, ed. The Massachusetts General Hospital Handbook of Pain Management, 3rd ed. Philadelphia, Lippincott Williams & Wilkins, 2006:193-203.

Headaches 94

Elizabeth Loder, MD, MPH

DEFINITION

The three major primary headache disorders are migraine, cluster, and tension-type headache.[1] Although all three syndromes are characterized by chronic, recurrent, and potentially disabling headaches, specific diagnosis is important because of differing natural history and treatment.

Headache disorders are classified according to criteria outlined in the International Classification of Headache Disorders (ICHD), originally developed by the International Headache Society in 1988 and revised in 2004.[1] Diagnosis of all but a few rare migraine subtypes remains clinical, based on the patient's history and an examination that rules out secondary causes of headache (not covered in this chapter). The ICHD criteria were developed for research purposes and lack sensitivity when they are used in the clinical setting. Both migraine and tension-type headaches are more common in women than in men; cluster headache is generally a male disorder. Peak prevalence of migraine occurs during midlife, when it affects almost a quarter of all women and roughly 10% of men.[2] Recurrent headaches are not rare in children, but accurate diagnosis can be difficult because headache presentation in children varies from that in adults, and children may have difficulty describing the headache characteristics needed for a diagnosis to be made.[3]

Migraine

Migraine is subclassified as migraine without aura (replaces the older term *common migraine;* Table 94-1) and migraine with aura (replaces the older term *classic migraine;* Table 94-2). Twenty percent of patients have aura, usually preceding the headache, which consists of focal neurologic signs or symptoms that begin gradually and fade away within 30 to 60 minutes as the headache begins. The most common type of aura involves visual disturbances, such as field cuts and photopsia. Sensory or motor problems occur far less frequently. Migraine can also be classified as episodic or chronic (more than 15 migraine attacks per month). Three gene mutations have been identified that are associated with a particular subtype of migraine with aura known as familial hemiplegic migraine. These genes influence the stability of neuronal cell membranes.[4,5]

Cluster

Cluster headaches are strictly unilateral headaches that are far more common in men than in women. The pain is sharp and steady, in contrast to the throbbing pain of migraine, and localized to the orbital area. Diagnostic criteria require the presence of at least one autonomic sign or symptom during the headache, including ipsilateral conjunctival injection, lacrimation, rhinorrhea, ptosis, or miosis.

Cluster headache is so called because the headaches occur regularly in most cases, from one to eight times a day, during a period of 2 weeks to 3 months that is referred to as a cluster episode. The headaches then completely remit for months or years. In chronic cluster headache, there are no headache-free periods, or they are less than 2 weeks in duration.[6]

Patients with cluster headache usually describe alcohol intolerance during the cluster episode and generally note intense restlessness during the headache.

Tension Type

Tension-type headaches can vary in length from 30 minutes to 7 days. They are typically bilateral, moderate in intensity, and described as a pressing, squeezing sensation that is not affected by physical activity. Associated symptoms, such as nausea, vomiting, photophobia, and phonophobia, are generally not present or are mild.

Tension-type headache is subclassified as episodic tension-type headache, which occurs less than 15 days per month, and chronic tension-type headache, with attacks occurring 15 or more days per month for at least 6 months.

Patients with tension-type headache typically do not spontaneously report symptoms other than headache. If multiple associated symptoms are reported, a diagnosis of migraine should be reexamined.

SYMPTOMS

In addition to the aforementioned symptoms that are required for diagnosis, many patients with migraine report prodromal symptoms: yawning; neck and shoulder muscle discomfort; excessive salivation; and changes in appetite, mood, sleep, gastrointestinal function, and urination. Postdromal symptoms in migraine include fatigue, exercise intolerance, and neck and shoulder muscle discomfort. If headaches progress untreated, 80% of patients eventually develop allodynia, defined as pain in response to stimuli that normally are nonpainful. Once allodynia develops, treatment may be less successful.[7]

PHYSICAL EXAMINATION

The primary headache disorders are diagnosed by history. With the exception of genetic testing for genes associated with familial hemiplegic migraine, there are currently no laboratory, genetic, or imaging markers that confirm a diagnosis of ordinary migraine with or without aura in individual patients. Biomarkers do exist that can distinguish subgroups of migraineurs from one another or from normal controls.[8] The major purpose of physical and neurologic examination is to rule out the presence of secondary headache disorders. Accordingly, the most important parts of the physical examination are ophthalmoscopic examination to exclude papilledema and neurologic examination to exclude other abnormalities that might suggest a malignant neoplasm, collagen vascular disease, or infectious cause of headaches.

Interictally, the physical and neurologic examination findings will be normal in primary headache disorders, or if another disorder is identified, it must not be causally related to the primary headache. Subtle cerebellar signs, such as dysmetria and balance abnormalities, have been detected in migraineurs compared with normal controls, but these are generally not detectable in a typical examination.[9]

If the patient is examined during a headache attack, the following points should be specifically noted:

- Patients experiencing migraine lie quietly, avoid movement, and may appear pale and diaphoretic. They typically display marked photophobia and phonophobia and may be vomiting.
- Patients experiencing cluster headache are physically restless. Head banging and agitation are common.[10] Autonomic signs should be documented to confirm the diagnosis. Between attacks, persistent ptosis and conjunctival injection may occasionally be seen.
- Patients experiencing tension-type headache may appear uncomfortable but generally are not incapacitated.
- Neck, shoulder, and jaw tightness is common in patients with prolonged episodes of all primary headache types and does not necessarily represent the underlying cause of the headache. In most cases, these complaints will improve with appropriate treatment of the headache and do not need to be treated separately. There is no evidence that patients with tension-type headache as a group have abnormally elevated muscle tension. In fact, electromyographic findings do not have diagnostic or treatment implications in migraine or tension-type headache.[11] Although biofeedback-assisted muscle relaxation is clearly of benefit in migraine and tension-type headache, it may exert its effect through mechanisms other than muscle relaxation.

FUNCTIONAL LIMITATIONS

Quality of life surveys and other data suggest that patients with primary headache disorders are more functionally impaired than is commonly appreciated. Obviously, acute attacks of migraine and cluster headache prohibit function and generally require bed rest if untreated. Visual aura can render driving or other hazardous activities dangerous or even impossible. Tension-type headache does not generally prohibit activities but may inhibit them. Patients commonly report feeling that they are not functioning at "full capacity."

In many cases, severely affected patients report that fear and anxiety about possible attacks lead them to avoid, to cancel, or to decline work, social, and academic opportunities. The depression that can result from poorly controlled headaches also may lead to impaired function. The functional limitations imposed on many patients by nonspecific sedative treatments for migraine or by prophylactic treatments, which can cause fatigue, exercise intolerance, weight gain, and depression, are underappreciated.

DIAGNOSTIC STUDIES

The primary headache disorders are clinical diagnoses, with the exception of the rare hemiplegic migraine syndromes. In general, imaging studies or laboratory tests are done to rule out secondary headache disorders, not to rule in primary disorders.

Differential Diagnosis

Migraine

Seizure disorder

Sinus infection

Early subarachnoid hemorrhage

Collagen vascular disorders

Meningitis

Space-occupying central nervous system lesion

Post-traumatic headache

Cluster

Trigeminal neuralgia

Cavernous sinus thrombosis

Central nervous system or ear, nose, or throat tumor

Orbital cellulitis or fracture

Subarachnoid hemorrhage

Dental abscess

Tension Type

Mild or forme fruste migraine attack

Temporomandibular disorder

Space-occupying central nervous system lesion

TREATMENT

Initial

Headache treatment consists of nonpharmacologic measures, lifestyle changes, and abortive treatment of acute attacks.[12] Prophylactic treatment, in which daily medication is given to decrease the frequency and severity of headache episodes, is reserved for patients who do not obtain acceptable relief from abortive therapy or have more than two headache attacks a week. Although there is some overlap in treatment options among the various headache disorders, there are also important differences. In particular, cluster headache is often erroneously treated for years with migraine medication, to little or no avail.[13]

Migraine

Lifestyle modification includes regular and adequate sleep, avoidance of excess caffeine, avoidance of missed meals, avoidance of alcohol (not a trigger for all migraine patients), and regular aerobic exercise. Although it is commonly advised, there is no scientific evidence that avoidance of chocolate, dairy products, or the myriad other dietary factors anecdotally implicated in migraine is helpful for the majority of patients with migraine. Several studies have exonerated various dietary factors (e.g., chocolate) as a cause of migraine. In the absence of scientific evidence to the contrary, it does not seem wise to promote food anxieties.

Nonpharmacologic treatment encompasses biofeedback-assisted relaxation (thermal or electromyographic) and acupuncture (weak evidence of benefit). Physical therapy has *not* been shown to be useful. One trial compared physical therapy and medication for migraine with medication alone; no benefit was seen with the addition of physical therapy.[14] If physical therapy is used, it should be short term and focus on development of an aerobic or other exercise program rather than on passive modalities.

Abortive therapy consists of nonsteroidal anti-inflammatory drugs, with or without caffeine; isometheptene compounds (Midrin); opioids, with or without aspirin or acetaminophen; barbiturate-containing compounds (e.g., Fiorinal, Fioricet, Esgic, Phrenilin); ergots (e.g., Cafergot, Wigraine, D.H.E. 45); and triptans (sumatriptan, rizatriptan, zolmitriptan, naratriptan, frovatriptan, eletriptan).

Prophylactic therapy consists of nonsteroidal anti-inflammatory drugs; topiramate; β blockers, especially propranolol (except those with sympathomimetic activity); calcium channel antagonists; tricyclic antidepressants, especially amitriptyline; riboflavin (vitamin B_2); sodium valproate; and selective serotonin reuptake inhibitors (weak evidence of benefit).

Cluster

Lifestyle modification includes alcohol avoidance and stress reduction.

Nonpharmacologic therapy employs 100% oxygen; 10 to 12 liters at headache onset by nonrebreather mask for 10 to 15 minutes aborts headache in 80% of patients.

Abortive therapy generally must be parenteral because headaches are short and onset is sudden. Options include oxygen, as previously described; dihydroergotamine, 1 mg subcutaneously; sumatriptan, 6 mg subcutaneously; and parenteral opioids.

Prophylactic therapy includes lithium carbonate; steroids (duration and dose must be limited to avoid side effects; principally used while awaiting results from other prophylactic medications); verapamil (high doses required); sodium valproate (benefit unclear); methysergide (no longer available in the United States but can be obtained from Canada); and topiramate (benefit unclear).

Tension Type

Lifestyle modification includes regular and adequate sleep and aerobic exercise.

Nonpharmacologic therapy includes biofeedback (thermal or electromyographic). Physical therapy focuses on stretching, strengthening, and development of an exercise program rather than on passive modalities.

Acute therapy consists of nonsteroidal anti-inflammatory drugs and isometheptene combinations (Midrin). Potentially sedative or habit-forming opioid or barbiturate-containing compounds should generally be avoided.

Prophylactic therapy consists of nonsteroidal anti-inflammatory drugs, tricyclic antidepressants, and sodium valproate.

Rehabilitation

Patients whose headaches are refractory to currently available treatments suffer significant disability. Secondary depression and medication overuse may develop, along with family dysfunction and poor work performance. The development of chronic pain syndrome (in which patients develop disability out of proportion to the underlying disease, with associated behavioral abnormalities) requires interdisciplinary treatment for best results. The treatment philosophy, which must be accepted by the patient and family, shifts from cure to management. Medication reduction, increased "up" time and regular physical exercise, involvement in hobbies or return to work, and psychological intervention all help return the patient to some semblance of normal living, despite the persistence of headache.[15] Specialized headache treatment programs employing an interdisciplinary approach can be located by contacting the American Council for Headache Education at *www. achenet.org*. Inpatient treatment may be necessary for patients with severe medication overuse, who require special tapering from narcotic or barbiturate drugs, or who have associated medical or psychiatric morbidity that precludes outpatient treatment. Only a handful of such programs exist in the United States.

Procedures

Botulinum toxin injections into the pericranial musculature are currently under investigation for the treatment of chronic daily headaches. Evidence from randomized, controlled clinical trials does not support the use of botulinum toxin for treatment of intermittent migraine or tension-type headache.[16] Headaches associated with significant pericranial muscle spasm or pain may benefit from localized trigger point injections or occipital nerve blocks. Trigger point injections for headache are small-volume injections into one or more tender or painful muscles in the head or neck. The injection may be of a local anesthetic alone, such as 0.5 mL of 2% lidocaine, or in combination with a steroid, such as 1.5 mL of 0.5% bupivacaine and 0.25 mL of methylprednisolone sodium succinate (Solu-Medrol) 20 mg/mL. Trigger point injections may be repeated at 2-month intervals as needed.[17] Greater occipital nerve block is performed by injection of a combination of local anesthetic and steroid 2 cm lateral to the occipital protuberance; a common dose is 2 mL of 2% lidocaine with 5 mg of triamcinolone.[18]

Surgery

Ablative surgical procedures on the fifth cranial nerve (radiofrequency, cryotherapy, and alcohol techniques) are employed in cases of refractory cluster headache. Some women with migraine contemplate oophorectomy, in the belief that elimination of hormonal cycling may eliminate migraine. In fact, abrupt surgical menopause seems to worsen, not improve, migraine, and this procedure should be discouraged. Closure of patent foramen ovale is being investigated as a treatment of migraine with aura.

POTENTIAL DISEASE COMPLICATIONS

Inadequately managed headaches can directly or indirectly lead to depression, suicide, analgesic nephropathy, withdrawal seizures, addiction and dependence syndromes, unemployment, divorce, and poor progress in school and the workplace. Emerging evidence indicates structural brain changes in some patients with long duration, poorly controlled migraine attacks.[19] These include iron deposition in areas of the brainstem, white matter lesions, and reduction in gray matter volume. Migraine is a risk factor for ischemic stroke and may also increase the risk of coronary heart disease. Women with migraine are more likely to develop preeclampsia and to suffer postpartum stroke.[20]

POTENTIAL TREATMENT COMPLICATIONS

Possible complications from injections include an allergic reaction to the medication and infection.

Potential complications from cluster headache surgery include anesthesia dolorosa, dry eye, and facial anesthesia or weakness. Multiple reactions to medications are possible, and the clinician should be aware of the side effect profile for any medications prescribed.

Overuse of symptomatic medications for headache may lead to medication overuse headache syndromes that can be difficult to treat.

References

1. Headache Classification Committee of the International Headache Society. International Classification of Headache Disorders II. Cephalalgia 2004;24(Suppl 1):1-160.
2. Lipton RB, Stewart WF, Diamond S, et al. Prevalence and burden of migraine in the United States: data from the American Migraine Study II. Headache 2001;41:646-657.
3. Laurell K, Larsson B, Mattsson P, Eeg-Olofsson O. A 3-year follow-up of headache diagnoses and symptoms in Swedish schoolchildren. Cephalalgia 2006;26:809-815.
4. Vanmolkot KR, Kors EE, Turk U, et al. Two de novo mutations in the Na,K-ATPase gene ATP1A2 associated with pure familial hemiplegic migraine. Eur J Hum Genet 2006;14:555-560.
5. Kors EE, Melberg A, Vanmolkot KR, et al. Childhood epilepsy, familial hemiplegic migraine, cerebellar ataxia and a new CACNA1A mutation. Neurology 2004;63:1136-1137.
6. Sandrini G, Tassorelli C, Ghiotto N, Nappi G. Uncommon primary headaches. Curr Opin Neurol 2006;19:299-304.
7. Burstein R, Yarnitsky D, Goor-Aryeh I, et al. An association between migraine and cutaneous allodynia. Ann Neurol 2000;47:614-624.
8. Loder E, Harrington MG, Cutrer M, et al. Selected confirmed, probable and exploratory migraine biomarkers. Headache 2006;46:1108-1127.
9. Sándor PS, Mascia A, Seidel L, et al. Subclinical cerebellar impairment in the common types of migraine: a three-dimensional analysis of reaching movements. Ann Neurol 2001;49:668-672.
10. Blau JN. Behavior during a cluster headache. Lancet 1993;342:723-725.
11. Jensen R, Fuglsang-Frederiksen A, Olesen J. Quantitative surface EMG of pericranial muscles in headache. A population study. Electroencephalogr Clin Neurophysiol 1994;93:335-344.
12. Silberstein SD, for the US Headache Consortium. Practice parameter: evidence-based guidelines for migraine headache (an evidence-based review): report of the Quality Standards Subcommittee of the American Academy of Neurology. Neurology 2000;55:754-762.
13. van Vliet JA, Eekers PJ, Haan J, Ferrari MD. Features involved in the diagnostic delay of cluster headache. J Neurol Neurosurg Psychiatry 2003;74:1123-1125.
14. Biondi DM. Physical treatments for headache: a structured review. Headache 2005;45:738-746.
15. McAllister MJ, McKenzie KE, Schultz DM, Epshteyn MG. Effectiveness of a multidisciplinary chronic pain program for treatment of refractory patients with complicated chronic pain syndromes. Pain Physician 2005;8:369-373.
16. Evers S, Olesen J. Botulinum toxin in headache treatment: the end of the road? Cephalalgia 2006;26:769-771.
17. Mellick GA, Mellick LB. Regional head and face pain relief following lower cervical intramuscular anesthetic injection. Headache 2003;43:1109-1111.
18. Ashkenazi A, Young WB. The effects of greater occipital nerve block and trigger point injection on brush allodynia and pain in migraine. Headache 2005;45:350-354.
19. Kruit MC, van Buchem MA, Hofman PAM, et al. Migraine as a risk factor for subclinical brain lesions. JAMA 2004;291:427-434.
20. James AH, Bushnell CD, Jamison MG, Myers ER. Incidence and risk factors for stroke in pregnancy and the puerperium. Obstet Gynecol 2005;106:509-516.

Fibromyalgia 95

Joanne Borg-Stein, MD

Synonym

Fibrositis

ICD-9 Code

729.1   Myalgia and myositis, unspecified

DEFINITION

Fibromyalgia is a syndrome defined by chronic wide-spread pain of at least 6 months' duration. It is a multisystem illness associated with neuropsychological symptoms including fatigue, unrefreshing sleep, cognitive dysfunction, anxiety, and depression. A discrete cause of fibromyalgia has not been identified. Available evidence implicates the central nervous system as key in maintaining pain and other core symptoms of fibromyalgia.[1,2]

According to the 1990 American College of Rheumatology criteria, a patient must have pain in the axial skeleton, pain above and below the waist, and pain to palpation in at least 11 of 18 paired tender points throughout the body. The majority of patients (80%) are women. The prevalence of the condition increases with age and is greater than 7% in women older than 60 years.[2,3]

SYMPTOMS

Fibromyalgia is characterized by widespread and long-lasting pain (>3 months) in the presence of tender points at specific anatomic sites. A series of other symptoms are frequently present. These include marked fatigue, stiffness, sleep disorders, cognitive disturbances, psychological distress, temporomandibular joint syndrome, paresthesias, headache, genitourinary manifestations, irritable bowel syndrome, and orthostatic intolerance.[1,4,5]

PHYSICAL EXAMINATION

The findings of the general medical and neurologic examinations should be normal. Blood pressure recording for orthostatic hypotension is performed. Mood and affect are noted. The 18 paired tender points are palpated with approximately 4 kg/cm² of pressure. This is just enough pressure to blanch the fingernail of the examiner. The patient will experience pain at these locations (Fig. 95-1).

In addition, a comprehensive neurologic and musculoskeletal examination is performed to rule out superimposed pain generators, such as bursitis, tendinitis, radiculopathy, and myofascial trigger points.

FUNCTIONAL LIMITATIONS

Patients are limited in their daily activities and exercise tolerance by both pain and fatigue. Patients also report cognitive dysfunction with difficulty in concentration, organization, and motivation. This has been termed "fibro fog." Approximately 25% of patients with fibromyalgia report themselves disabled and are collecting some form of disability payment. Individuals are more likely to become disabled if they report higher pain scores, work at a job that requires heavy physical labor, have poor coping strategies and feel helpless, or are involved in litigation.[6,7]

DIAGNOSTIC STUDIES

Fibromyalgia is a clinical diagnosis. For other conditions to be excluded, basic laboratory tests may be appropriate, such as complete blood count, erythrocyte sedimentation rate, thyroid-stimulating hormone concentration, and creatine kinase activity. Primary sleep disorders may need to be identified by sleep studies. Radiography or magnetic resonance imaging may be indicated if osteoarthritis, radiculopathy, spinal stenosis, or intrinsic joint disease is suspected.

Electrodiagnostic studies may be useful if an entrapment neuropathy or radiculopathy is suspected.

TREATMENT

Initial

Initial treatment includes education of the patient, pharmacologic treatment, gentle exercise, and relaxation training. Education of the patient includes individual

Differential Diagnosis

Thyroid myopathy

Metabolic myopathy

Mood disturbances

Somatoform pain disorders

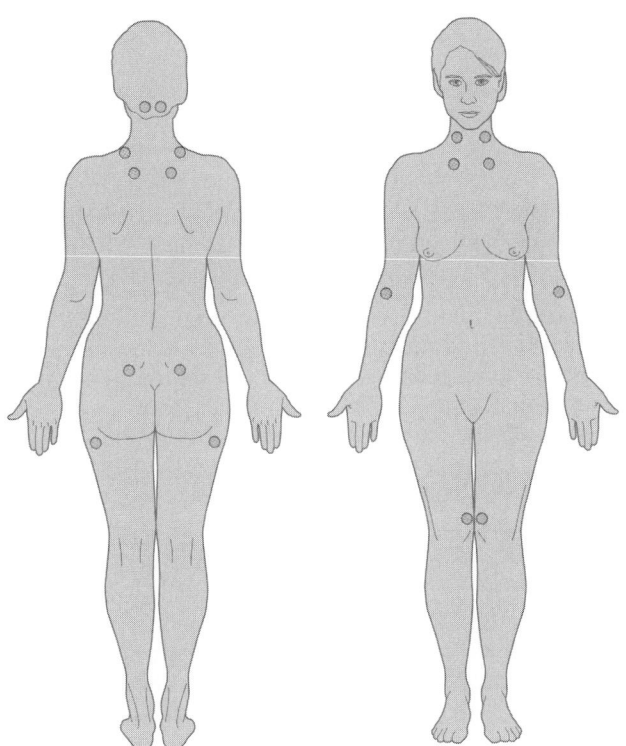

FIGURE 95-1. Locations of tender points.

and group classes that review the symptoms of fibromyalgia; it reassures the patient as to the generally benign course and outlines the treatment path.[8-11]

Pharmacologic management aims to normalize sleep patterns and to diminish pain. Low-dose tricyclic antidepressants at bedtime (e.g., amitriptyline, 10 to 25 mg) with low-dose selective serotonin reuptake inhibitors (e.g., fluoxetine, 20 mg every morning) is an excellent combination. The combination works better than either medication alone. Studies demonstrate that treatments affecting levels of norepinephrine and serotonin have the greatest impact on important symptoms, including pain and sleep.[3,4] The serotonin-norepinephrine reuptake inhibitors venlafaxine and duloxetine demonstrate benefit in patients with fibromyalgia.[11-13]

Pain may be relieved with simple analgesics, such as acetaminophen or a nonsteroidal anti-inflammatory drug. Tramadol is the next-line agent. Pregabalin, a newer anticonvulsant, reduces pain in patients with fibromyalgia at doses of 300 to 450 mg per day, starting with 50 mg three times daily and increasing to 100 mg three times

daily during 7 days. Opioids are rarely necessary. Adjunctive nonpharmacologic pain control methods include acupuncture, massage, and biofeedback.

Rehabilitation

Physical therapy is used to educate the patient in a stretching, gentle strengthening, and cardiovascular fitness program. This can improve fitness and function and decrease pain. Occupational therapy is incorporated to review ergonomics of daily activities, and activities of daily living are reviewed at the work site. Task simplification, pacing, and maximization of function are emphasized.[8,14,15]

Mental health professionals can be helpful in the rehabilitative phase to educate the patients in a mind-body stress reduction program. This provides the patient with positive coping strategies for living with chronic pain.[16] Associated depression and anxiety often need psychopharmacologic treatment as well.

A stepwise approach to fibromyalgia management is recommended. The first step is to confirm the diagnosis, to explain the condition, and to treat any comorbid illness, such as mood or sleep disturbance.

The second step is to try a low-dose tricyclic antidepressant or cyclobenzaprine. The patient should begin a cardiovascular exercise program and be referred for cognitive-behavioral therapy or combine that with exercise.

The third step includes specialty referral (i.e., rheumatology, physiatry, psychiatry, pain management). Trials with selective serotonin reuptake inhibitors, serotonin and norepinephrine reuptake inhibitors, or tramadol should be considered. One may use a combination medication trial or anticonvulsant.[13]

Procedures

Trigger Point Injections

Myofascial trigger points may be injected with 1% lidocaine to decrease local pain. Patients with recalcitrant chronic myofascial pain may respond to injections with botulinum toxin.[17]

If patients have concurrent bursitis, tendinitis, or nerve entrapment, therapeutic injections may be performed to treat these specific diagnoses.

Acupuncture

Acupuncture can be used for treatment of pain and fatigue. Preliminary studies suggest that the benefit may last up to several months.[3] Treatment one or two times per week for at least six visits appears necessary. Improvement lasts at least 1 month but is likely to wane over time (6 months). The optimal number and frequency of acupuncture treatments have not been determined.[3]

Surgery

There is no surgery indicated for fibromyalgia.

POTENTIAL DISEASE COMPLICATIONS

Failure to make the diagnosis early may lead to delay in treatment, deconditioning, and expensive unnecessary medical testing and procedures. Chronic, intractable pain may occur despite treatment.

POTENTIAL TREATMENT COMPLICATIONS

Tricyclic antidepressant medications can be associated with anticholinergic side effects, such as urinary retention, sedation, constipation, and weight gain. Selective serotonin reuptake inhibitor medications may be associated with sexual dysfunction, gastrointestinal intolerance, and anorexia. Overly aggressive exercise programs may transiently increase pain in some patients. Local injections may result in local pain, ecchymosis, intravascular injection, or pneumothorax if they are improperly executed. There is an increased risk of bleeding with use of nonsteroidal anti-inflammatory drugs or selective serotonin reuptake inhibitors. For patients taking high serotonin reuptake antidepressants, consider avoidance or minimal use of nonsteroidal anti-inflammatory drugs.[18] The threshold for seizures is lowered by tramadol. In addition, the risk for seizure is enhanced by the concomitant use of tramadol with selective serotonin reuptake inhibitors.[19]

References

1. Goldenberg DL. Fibromyalgia syndrome a decade later: what have we learned? Arch Intern Med 1999;159:777-785.
2. Bennett R. Fibromyalgia: present to future. Curr Rheumatol Rep 2005;7:371-376.
3. Martin DP, Sletten CD, Williams BA, Berger IH. Improvement in fibromyalgia symptoms with acupuncture: results of a randomized controlled trial. Mayo Clin Proc 2006;81:749-757.
4. Fietta P. Fibromyalgia: state of the art. Minerva Med 2004;95:35-52.
5. Shuer ML. Fibromyalgia: symptom constellation and potential therapeutic options. Endocrine 2003;22:67-75.
6. Goldenberg DL, Mossey CJ, Schmid CH. A model to assess severity and impact of fibromyalgia. J Rheumatol 1995;22:2313-2318.
7. Bennett RM. Fibromyalgia and the disability dilemma. Arthritis Rheum 1996;19:1627-1633.
8. Adams N, Sim J. Rehabilitation approaches in fibromyalgia. Disabil Rehabil 2005;27:711-723.
9. Dadabhoy D, Clauw DJ. Fibromyalgia: progress in diagnosis and treatment. Curr Pain Headache Rep 2005;9:399-404.
10. Borg-Stein J. Treatment of fibromyalgia, myofascial pain and related disorders. Phys Med Rehabil Clin North Am 2006;17:491-510.
11. Crofford L. Pharmaceutical treatment options for fibromyalgia. Curr Rheumatol Rep 2004;6:274-280.
12. Rao SG, Clauw DJ. The management of fibromyalgia. Drugs Today (Barc) 2004;40:539-554.
13. Goldenberg DL, Burckhardt C, Crofford L. Management of fibromyalgia syndrome. JAMA 2004;292:2388-2395.
14. Gowans SE, deHueck A, Voss S, Richardson M. A randomized, controlled trial of exercise and education for individuals with fibromyalgia. Arthritis Care Res 1999;12:120-128.
15. Rosen NB. Physical medicine and rehabilitation approaches to the management of myofascial pain and fibromyalgia syndromes. Baillieres Clin Rheumatol 1994;8:881-916.
16. Kaplan KH, Goldenberg DL, Galvin-Nadeau M. The impact of a meditation-based stress reduction program on fibromyalgia. Gen Hosp Psychiatry 1993;15:284-289.
17. Göbel H, Heinze A, Reichel G, et al. Dysport myofascial pain study group. Efficacy and safety of a single botulinum type A toxin complex treatment for the relief of upper back myofascial pain syndrome: results from a randomized double-blind placebo-controlled multicentre study. Pain 2006;125:82-88.
18. Mansour A, Perace M, Johnson B, et al. Which patients taking SSRIs are at greatest risk of bleeding? J Fam Pract 2006;55:206-208.
19. Gardner JS, Blough D, Drinkard CR, et al. Tramadol and seizures: a surveillance study in a managed care population. Pharmacotherapy 2000;20:1423-1431.

Myofascial Pain Syndrome 96

Martin K. Childers, DO, PhD, Jeffery B. Feldman, PhD,
and H. Michael Guo, MD, PhD

Synonyms

Myogelosis[1,2]
Fibrositis[3-5]
Fibromyalgia[5-10]

ICD-9 Code

729.1   Myofascial pain syndrome

DEFINITION

Myofascial pain syndrome (MPS) is defined as a painful disorder characterized by the presence of myofascial trigger points, distinct sensitive spots in a palpable taut band of skeletal muscle fibers[11,12] that produce local and referred pain. Thus, MPS is characterized by both a motor abnormality (a taut or hard band within the muscle) and a sensory abnormality (tenderness and referred pain).[13] In addition to pain, the disorder is accompanied by referred autonomic phenomena as well as by anxiety and depression.[14] The pathophysiologic process of MPS is not clearly understood, in part because of the scarcity of reliable valid studies.[15] Moreover, concomitant disorders and frequent behavioral and psychosocial contributing factors[16] in patients with MPS contribute to the complexity of human studies. Symptoms of MPS are generally associated with physical activities that are thought to contribute to "muscle overload," either acutely by sudden overload or gradually with prolonged repetitive activity.[17] MPS is reported to be prevalent in regional musculoskeletal pain syndromes; however, the syndrome can be classified as regional or generalized. Some authors broaden the definition of myofascial pain to include a regional pain syndrome of any soft tissue origin. Thus, MPS may be considered either a primary disorder causing local or regional pain syndromes or a secondary disorder that occurs as a consequence of some other condition.[12,13,16,18-20]

The myofascial trigger point is generally considered the hallmark of MPS; therefore, much attention has been given to characteristic features of myofascial trigger points in skeletal muscle. Interestingly, animal studies reported a myofascial trigger spot in taut bands of rabbit skeletal muscle fibers similar to that observed in human myofascial trigger points in several respects.[21] Equine myofascial trigger points have also been identified with features similar to those documented in humans and rabbits, with the exception that referred pain patterns cannot be determined in animals.[22] One such feature of the myofascial trigger point is the so-called twitch response. This local response is considered a characteristic finding of the myofascial trigger point. Mechanical stimulation ("snapping" palpation, pressure, or needle insertion) can elicit a local twitch response that frequently is accompanied by referred pain.[23] The twitch response is accompanied by a burst of electrical activity (end-plate noise) within the muscle band that contains the activated trigger point, whereas no activity is seen at other muscle bands. End-plate noise is significantly more prevalent in myofascial trigger points than in sites that lie outside of a myofascial trigger point but still within the end-plate zone.[24] This observation has been attributed to a spinal reflex,[21,23] as the response is abolished by motor nerve ablation or infusion of local anesthetic. Moreover, spinal cord transection above the neurologic level of the myofascial trigger point fails to permanently alter the characteristic response.

A number of hypotheses[25,26] have been put forward to explain the findings observed in myofascial trigger points. One theory proposes that myofascial trigger points are found only at the muscle spindle in an attempt to explain beneficial effects of α-adrenergic antagonists. However, this idea does not fully explain the electromyographic findings recorded at the myofascial trigger point. Further, there appears to be little evidence that painful muscle areas, such as myofascial trigger points, are associated with any structural changes, such as an alteration in the appearance of the muscle spindle. Another theory is related to excessive release of acetylcholine in abnormal end plates,[21] as the electromyographic activity recorded at trigger points resembles findings described at the end-plate region.[24] This idea has led some clinicians to study effects of botulinum toxin injection into myofascial trigger points in an attempt to reduce release of excessive acetylcholine. To date, results of small cohort studies[27-33] examining effects of botulinum toxin on myofascial trigger points have yielded inconsistent findings.

On the other hand, pain may occur with spasticity, a condition associated with abnormal spindle physiology.[34,35] Although it is not clearly understood or rigorously tested, an association can be made between abnormal spindle physiology and painful muscle conditions or "muscle spasms." It has been our clinical observation that botulinum toxin at doses lower than anticipated for relief of hypertonia are effective for the relief of pain associated with spasticity. One could speculate that these lower doses might be enough to effectively weaken or to "reset" the intrinsic (spindle) fibers and thus indirectly result in pain relief. Therefore, the use of botulinum toxin for some painful muscle conditions stems from the idea that pain relief may result from a decrease in the reflex muscle tone.[36-38]

To test the idea that botulinum toxin might work to relieve regional MPS, a small pilot study[39] was conducted on the use of botulinum toxin type A in a cohort of subjects with regional MPS of the lower limb, in a condition termed piriformis syndrome. Blunt trauma, such as a fall onto the buttocks, has been reported to result in this painful chronic musculoskeletal disorder, thought to involve the piriformis muscle because of its proximity to the sciatic nerve. Piriformis syndrome is associated with buttock, hip, and lower limb pain and occurs predominantly in women. It has been suggested that hip, buttock, and leg pain is a consequence of prolonged or excessive contraction of the piriformis muscle.[40,41] Subsequent to the location of this muscle and its close association with the sciatic nerve, excessive or sustained muscle force might also compress the sciatic nerve and result in lower limb pain. Thus, agents such as botulinum toxin known to locally decrease muscle force[42-44] might bring about pain relief by decreasing muscle tension and also presumably by decreasing tension on nerve axons. Accordingly, it was hypothesized that injection into this muscle with the potent paralytic agent botulinum toxin type A would diminish buttock, hip, and lower limb pain.

Ten women with piriformis syndrome participated in a double-blind crossover pilot to test effects of local intramuscular injection of botulinum toxin type A (100 units) directly into the piriformis muscle. Pain scores and nerve conduction were measured in each participant during several weeks. Results of the main outcome measures (pain scores) suggested clinical benefit, probably as a result of a modest analgesic response from toxin injection. If the benefit was due, at least in part, to local decrease in muscle force and subsequent decrease in motor axon compression, it was anticipated that associated changes would be observed in nerve conduction (H reflex) studies.[45] However, no changes in H reflexes were detected either before or after experimental interventions. Thus, the idea that sciatic nerve compression resulted from local increase in piriformis muscle tension was not supported by the findings. This line of evidence pointed to an alternative mechanism of action[46] of botulinum toxin in pain syndromes and also raised questions about the very nature of MPS.

Fibromyalgia is a chronic, musculoskeletal pain condition that predominantly affects women and is characterized by diffuse muscle pain, fatigue, sleep disturbance, depression, and skin sensitivity.[7,15,47,48] Fibromyalgia may fit the classification of MPS because the diagnosis includes the presence of 11 of 18 tender points.[49-51] Furthermore, treatment of MPS and fibromyalgia is similar; evidence supports the role of exercise, cognitive-behavioral therapy, education, and social support in the management of both fibromyalgia and chronic MPS.[7] However, there is controversy as to whether fibromyalgia and MPS represent specific disease processes or are descriptive terms of clinical conditions.[52] Objective evidence of muscle abnormalities in fibromyalgia has been demonstrated by histologic studies showing disorganization of Z bands and abnormalities in the number and shape of muscle mitochondria. Biochemical studies and magnetic resonance spectroscopy have also shown inconsistent abnormalities of ATP and phosphocreatine levels. It is unclear whether these abnormalities are a result of physical deconditioning or are due to problems in energy metabolism.[49] There are no clear biochemical markers that distinguish patients with fibromyalgia. Thus, although the pathogenesis is still unknown, there has been evidence of increased corticotropin-releasing hormone and substance P in the cerebrospinal fluid of patients with fibromyalgia as well as increased substance P, interleukin-6, and interleukin-8 in their serum.[50] One hypothesis supports the idea that fibromyalgia is an immunoendocrine disorder in which increased release of corticotropin-releasing hormone and substance P from neurons triggers local mast cells to release proinflammatory and neurosensitizing molecules. This hypothesis fits well with recent discoveries of neuropeptides found in the muscles of patients with active myofascial trigger points.[53,54]

SYMPTOMS

The patient generally complains about dull or achy pain, sometimes poorly localized, particularly during repetitive activities or activities requiring sustained postures. Symptoms are exacerbated with digital pressure over tender areas of muscle with reproduction of the patient's usual pain. Symptoms are relieved with rest or cessation of repetitive activities. The presence of sleep disturbances, depressed mood, and fatigue may help distinguish patients with MPS from those with fibromyalgia.

PHYSICAL EXAMINATION

The most important part of the physical examination is generally considered to be the finding and localization of myofascial trigger points to provide an accurate diagnosis of MPS.[12,17,26] *Travell & Simons' Myofascial Pain and Dysfunction: The Trigger Point Manual*[55] is considered the criterion standard reference on location and treatment of myofascial trigger points. Active myofascial trigger points exhibit marked localized tenderness and may refer pain to distant sites, disturb motor function, or produce autonomic changes. Specific clinical training is required to become adept at identification of myofascial trigger points; evidence suggests that "non-trained" clinicians do not reliably detect the taut band and local twitch response.[56] As Simons and Mense pointed out, "The diagnostic skill required depends on considerable innate palpation ability, authoritative training, and extensive clinical experience."[17]

To clinically identify myofascial trigger points, the clinician palpates a localized tender spot in a nodular portion of a taut rope-like band of muscle fibers. Manual pressure over a trigger point should elicit pain at that area and may also elicit pain at a distant site (referred pain) from the point under the fingertip. Myofascial trigger points, when palpated, should also elicit pain that mirrors the patient's experience. Applied pressure often earns the response "That's my pain!" Insertion of a needle, abrupt palpation, or even a brisk tap with the fingertip directly over the trigger point may induce a brief muscle contraction detectable by the examiner. This rapid contraction of muscle fibers of the ropy taut band is termed a local twitch response.[17] In muscles that move a relatively small mass or are large and superficial (like the finger extensors or the gluteus maximus), the response is easily seen and may cause the limb to visibly move when the examiner introduces a needle into the trigger point. Localized abnormal response from the autonomic nervous system may cause piloerection, localized sweating, or even regional temperature changes in the skin attributed to altered blood flow.[25,36,57]

Regional Examination of the Lower Extremity for Piriformis Syndrome

To evaluate individuals for piriformis syndrome,[58,59] their usual buttock, hip, and lower limb pain may be reproduced during the following maneuvers: palpation over a point midway between the sacrum and greater trochanter of the femur, active hip abduction in the lateral recumbent position, and rectal palpation of the ipsilateral side of the involved limb.[39] A number of similar maneuvers have been described. The Freiberg maneuver of forceful internal rotation of the extended thigh elicits buttock pain by stretching the piriformis muscle, and the Pace maneuver elicits pain by having the patient abduct the legs in the seated position, which causes contraction of the piriformis muscle.[60] Beatty[61,62] described a maneuver performed by the patient's lying with the painful side up, the painful leg flexed, and the knee resting on the table. Buttock pain is produced when the patient lifts and holds the knee several inches off the table. Beatty reported that the maneuver he described produced deep buttock pain in three patients with piriformis syndrome. In 100 consecutive patients with surgically documented herniated lumbar discs, the maneuver often produced lumbar and leg pain but not deep buttock pain; and in 27 patients with primary hip abnormalities, pain was often produced in the trochanteric area but not in the buttock. The maneuver described by Beatty presumably relies on contraction of the muscle, rather than stretching, which might reproduce pain from an actively contracting piriformis mus-

cle. A positive finding in at least two of these maneuvers is sufficient to confirm a diagnosis of piriformis syndrome, provided other potential causes have been eliminated from the differential diagnosis (described later). For example, patients with trochanteric bursitis generally present with chronic intermittent aching pain over the lateral aspect of the affected hip. Pain is worsened by sitting in a deep chair or car seat or by climbing stairs. In contrast, patients with regional MPS of the lower limb (piriformis syndrome) complain of pain primarily in the buttocks with occasional radiation into the lateral thigh. Clinical criteria for trochanteric bursitis should include history of lateral aching hip pain, localized tenderness over the greater trochanter, and at least one of the following findings: radiation of pain over the lateral thigh; pain of resisted hip abduction; and pain at extreme ends of rotation, particularly a positive Patrick (FABER) test result.

DIAGNOSTIC STUDIES

No definitive laboratory test or imaging method is diagnostic of MPS. Thus, diagnosis is made primarily by history and physical examination. Whereas no specific laboratory tests confirm (or refute) a diagnosis of MPS,[11,14,63] some tests can be helpful in looking for predisposing conditions, such as hypothyroidism, hypoglycemia, and vitamin deficiencies. Specific tests that may be helpful include complete blood count, chemistry profile, erythrocyte sedimentation rate, and levels of vitamins C, B_1, B_6, and B_{12}, and folic acid. If clinical features of thyroid disease are present, an assay for thyrotropin may be indicated.[64,65] A presumptive diagnosis of piriformis syndrome is based principally on clinical evidence because well-established laboratory or imaging studies to confirm such a diagnosis are not available. Therefore, other sources of buttock, hip, and lower limb pain must be excluded before such a diagnosis can be made. Although laboratory or imaging studies are not diagnostic of this condition, delayed H reflex latencies have been reported in at least one case series,[45] presumably because of sciatic nerve compression by the piriformis muscle.

TREATMENT

A wide variety of therapy is available to patients with MPS. Much of the variation in forms of treatment (and diagnoses) of this disorder probably results from differences in culture, training, and recognition of an often undiagnosed syndrome of pain, dysfunction, and

Differential Diagnosis

Fibromyalgia

Trochanteric bursitis

autonomic dysregulation. This section discusses treatment strategies for patients with MPS, including those individuals in whom chronic pain develops.

Initial

Therapeutic modalities such as biofeedback, ultrasound, lasers, and massage may be useful adjuncts in relieving initial pain to allow participation in an active exercise program. Although therapeutic modalities are commonly used for MPS, most of these modalities have not been rigorously investigated. Appropriate controls, sample sizes, and blinding measures are often lacking. Despite these issues, results from published reports generally indicate therapeutic efficacy.[66] For example, Hou and colleagues[67] investigated the immediate effect of physical therapeutic modalities on myofascial pain in the upper trapezius muscle in 119 subjects with active myofascial trigger points. Their findings suggested that therapeutic combinations such as hot pack plus active range of motion and stretch with spray are effective for pain relief in patients with MPS. To investigate the immediate effectiveness of electrotherapy on myofascial trigger points of the upper trapezius muscle, Hsueh and coworkers[68] studied 60 patients with myofascial trigger points on one side of the upper trapezius muscle. The involved upper trapezius muscles were treated with three different methods according to a random assignment. One group received a placebo treatment, another group was given electrical nerve stimulation therapy, and a third group was given electrical muscle stimulation therapy. The effectiveness of each treatment was assessed by conducting three measurements on each muscle before and immediately after treatment: subjective pain intensity, pressure pain threshold, and range of motion. Results indicated that electrical nerve stimulation is more effective than electrical muscle stimulation for immediate pain relief, whereas muscle stimulation appeared to have a greater benefit on immediate release of muscle tightness compared with nerve stimulation. Together, the results of these and other studies[11,12,16,17,69,70] suggest that addition of therapeutic physical modalities, such as heat and various forms of muscle and nerve stimulation, is beneficial in the initial treatment of MPS.

Rehabilitation

Physical therapy techniques that focus on correction of muscle shortening by targeted stretching, strengthening of affected muscles, and correction of aggravating postural and biomechanical factors are generally considered to be the most effective treatment of MPS.[71-73] This idea is supported by a line of evidence examining the relationship between muscle overload and myofascial trigger points. For example, Itoh and colleagues[74] developed an experimental model of myofascial trigger points in which healthy volunteers underwent repetitive eccentric exercise of the third finger of one hand. Pain thresholds of the skin, fascia, and muscle were measured immediately afterward and for 7 days. After exercise, pressure pain thresholds decreased, then gradually returned to

baseline values. A ropy band was palpated in the exercised forearm muscle, and the electrical pain threshold of the fascia at the palpable band was the lowest among the measured loci and tissues. Needle electromyographic activity accompanied with dull pain sensation was recorded only when the electrode was located on or near the fascia of the palpable band. To explore the effect of exercise for treatment of MPS, a study was conducted in 20 patients with MPS localized to the temporomandibular region.[72] The exercise treatment consisted of jaw movements and correction of body posture. After treatment, six patients had no pain at all and seven patients experienced no impairment. Pain at stress, impairment, and incisal edge clearance also improved. Together, findings from these and other studies suggest a direct relationship between exercise and MPS, although definitive large multicenter trials appear to be lacking.

Cognitive-Behavioral Therapy

The goal for the treatment of MPS is to engage patients in active therapy to prevent the development of chronic pain syndrome or to rehabilitate patients from its disabling interacting symptoms if it has developed. Chronic MPS is not a diagnosis but a descriptive term for individuals who not only report persistent pain but evidence poor coping, self-limitations in functional activities, significant life disruption, and dysfunctional pain behavior.[75] Other common symptoms of chronic pain syndrome related to an accompanying disuse syndrome include the multiple physical systems effects of deconditioning as well as insomnia, fatigue, anxiety, and depression.[76] A central feature of chronic MPS is a disability conviction and resulting avoidance of activity based on the fear that engaging in functional activity will increase pain (fear-avoidance).[76] The critical importance of addressing such a belief is underlined by prior studies that indicated that patients' beliefs about their pain were the best predictors of task performance,[77] medical utilization,[78] and long-term rehabilitation.[79]

Preventing the development of such a disability conviction begins by assisting patients to shift from a biomedical perspective, in which there is an ongoing search for the cause of an illness to be "cured" or "fixed," to a biopsychosocial rehabilitation perspective.[76,79] This perspective views MPS as a multifactorial condition that need not be disabling if it is actively managed by the patient. Cognitive-behavioral therapy is the psychological approach that focuses on changing dysfunctional beliefs or "schemas" by which individuals process, store, and act on information.[80] For individuals with chronic pain syndrome to successfully participate in a functionally oriented rehabilitation approach, they need to understand or to believe the following:

1. The nature of the pain has been thoroughly evaluated, and there is no cure (i.e., surgery or another procedure) for the pain.
2. The rehabilitation approach involving physical activity and conditioning will increase functional capabilities and eventually reduce suffering.
3. The hurt engendered through physical conditioning will not cause harm.

4. Reinjury or worsening of the painful condition is unlikely, and it is in the individual's best interest to become more functional (i.e., the individual will not be fired or laid off if he or she attempts to return to work).

Whereas the first point most often can be addressed by the physician in the office, the critical shift in belief that hurt will not cause harm generally requires the patient to have repeated experiences that contradict prior life experience that if something hurts, you should stop doing it. For a patient with MPS to exercise consistently and sufficiently to contradict the common sense to avoid pain, an interdisciplinary team approach is often required. In such an approach, the physical therapist educates and guides the patient through a progressive physical reconditioning regimen. The physician periodically reevaluates the patient, reassuring and encouraging the patient that there is no problematic change in condition while adjusting medications to facilitate involvement in the program. Concurrently, the psychologist provides training in stress management, pacing, and pain coping strategies. This is often best done in a group setting that normalizes the reactions and experience of the patient and where the social support and encouragement of the patient's peers are of significant benefit. Ultimately, though, it is the patient's repeated mild increases in pain without harm, as functioning improves, that change beliefs about pain and fear-avoidance of activity. It is largely for this reason that multidisciplinary pain programs including a cognitive-behavioral approach have been found to be most effective for individuals with chronic pain on a range of key outcomes.[81] A cognitive-behavioral, functional restoration approach is particularly effective for chronic MPS because unlike with many other chronic pain conditions, one can be fairly certain that the hurt experienced through increased activity will not only not cause harm but will lead to long-term benefit.

Hypnosis

In addition to the cognitive changes noted, patients should be educated on the interacting effects of pain leading to increased sympathetic arousal ("stress response") that leads to increased muscle tension and increased pain. They therefore can reduce pain by reducing their reactivity to pain as well as to other stressors in their life. Techniques for doing so include relaxation training, progressive muscle relaxation, mindfulness meditation, and hypnosis. Hypnosis is increasingly being integrated into multidisciplinary treatment approaches because it enables one to train patients to develop a relaxation response while also interspersing suggestions to encourage the changes in thinking noted earlier.[82-85] It is likely that this is one reason a meta-analytic study found the addition of hypnosis to cognitive-behavioral treatment increased the effectiveness of such treatment for numerous conditions.[86] Furthermore, neuroimaging studies indicated that hypnotic suggestions specifically designed to address the affective dimension of pain reduced activation of the anterior cingulate cortex, found to be most associated with autonomic reactivity to pain.[87-91] In other words, hypnosis is a tool that can be used to assist patients not only to reduce their attention to the sensation of pain but, probably more important, to reduce their affective distress and autonomic reactivity.

Oral Medications

Nonsteroidal anti-inflammatory drugs (NSAIDs) may be a useful adjunct to active exercise-based treatment of MPS, but NSAIDs are generally considered beneficial when they are used in conjunction with an active treatment program. However, no randomized placebo-controlled clinical trials exist to support efficacy of NSAID use in this condition. Interestingly, the NSAID diclofenac, when it is injected into the myofascial trigger point, was shown to be superior to lidocaine in one small clinical trial.[92] Low-dose amitriptyline is widely used in patients with fibromyalgia and is thought to help improve the patient's sleep cycle.[47,50,93,94] Muscle relaxants may provide benefit to patients with MPS. For example, cyclobenzaprine hydrochloride, a commonly prescribed muscle relaxant, is indicated as an adjunct to rest and physical therapy for the relief of muscle spasm associated with acute, painful musculoskeletal conditions. In contrast to low-dose (5 mg three times daily) cyclobenzaprine, a higher dose (10 mg three times daily) is associated with more somnolence and dry mouth. Importantly, there does not appear to be a relationship between somnolence and pain relief. A large, multicenter, community-based trial of patients with acute pain and muscle spasm evaluated low-dose cyclobenzaprine (5 mg three times daily) alone compared with combination therapy with two doses of ibuprofen. It is possible that low-dose cyclobenzaprine or high-dose ibuprofen alone may be sufficient to relieve acute musculoskeletal pain and that no additional benefit is incurred by adding another medication. Future trials comparing various doses of muscle relaxants and NSAIDs alone or in combination will be required to address these questions in the treatment of patients with MPS.

Procedures

When they are combined with other therapies, interventional techniques can be an effective adjunct in the multidisciplinary management of patients with MPS.[95] In treating MPS, other than trigger point injections, interventional procedures (e.g., epidural steroid injections, sacroiliac joint injections, and medial branch blocks) are usually not employed. However, at times, myofascial pain is associated with or caused by other underlying conditions. For instance, lumbar myofascial pain may also have some component of lumbar facet arthropathy. Lumbar medial branch blocks and radiofrequency denervation, alone or in combination with the other therapies (e.g., muscle relaxants), may work together to relieve myofascial pain. Similarly, epidural steroid injection may provide lumbar pain relief in a patient with spondylosis. It has been suggested that epidural steroid injections may be used to treat MPS if conservative treatments fail.[96] Therefore, underlying pathologic changes may respond to more aggressive interventional methods and in turn synergistically provide pain relief to the patient with MPS.

Myofascial trigger point injections should be individualized for both the patient and the clinician. Alcohol, if it is used to clean the skin, should be allowed to dry completely to prevent additional pain. Use of operating rooms or special procedure (sterile) rooms equipped with monitoring devices for the purpose of intramuscular injections with small-caliber needles is not necessary. Most patients can be treated safely in an office setting by experienced clinicians. The diagnostic skill required to find active myofascial trigger points depends on considerable innate palpation ability, authoritative training, and extensive clinical experience.[17] Application of trigger point injection begins, first, with determination of the equipment needs according to the needs of the patient, the clinician's training, and the anatomic target for injection. Typically, a 1.0-mL tuberculin-type syringe with 5/8-inch, 25-gauge needle is adequate for superficial muscles. For small muscles (e.g., facial muscles), a 1-inch, 30-gauge needle is sufficient. For larger muscles, a 1-inch or 1 1/2-inch, 25-gauge needle is adequate. After the patient is placed in a position in which the desired muscle can be relaxed, the myofascial trigger point is located. In the prone position, the myofascial trigger point is ascertained by gentle pressure from the end of a fingertip or a ballpoint pen applied at regular 1-cm intervals. The patient is observed closely during the palpation because pressure on the markedly tender myofascial trigger point usually causes the patient to jump, to wince, or to cry out. Each muscle has a characteristic elicited referred pain pattern that for active myofascial trigger points is familiar to the patient. Thus, the patient will report that this pressure reproduces the usual pain and, when questioned, will describe painful sensations at a site slightly distant to the point under the examiner's finger. Once the myofascial trigger point has been located, the skin is marked, and the site is injected with saline, anesthetic agent, or corticosteroid solution.

Procedures used in the treatment of piriformis muscle syndrome include therapeutic stretch, ultrasound, massage, manipulation, and oral analgesic agents. Caudal epidural steroid injections, local intramuscular steroid injections, and surgical resection of the muscle have also been reported as effective. Childers and colleagues[39] were the first to perform a prospective study to examine the effects of intramuscular botulinum toxin in this condition. Results indicated that compared with placebo, injection with botulinum toxin resulted in significant ($P < .05$) benefit in subjective pain evaluations. Others[97-100] have subsequently reported similar findings. The rationale for use of botulinum toxins in MPS may involve presynaptic blockade of nociceptive peptides in affected muscles, reduction in force of contracting muscles, or some combination of both mechanisms.[37,38,46,101,102]

For injection of the piriformis muscle, the patient is placed in the prone position, the skin over the largest bulk of the buttocks is swabbed with iodine, and sterile drapes are applied. Under pulsed fluoroscopy, the greater trochanter of the femur, the body of the sacrum, and the sciatic notch can easily be identified. The skin is marked corresponding to a location midway between a line that bisects the middle of the sciatic notch and the greater trochanter of the hip. A sterile 5 1/2-inch, 20-gauge dual-purpose injection-electromyographic needle is inserted through the overlying skin marking. The needle should be angled slightly lateral to medial. Once the ileum is encountered, the needle is withdrawn slightly, and the injection site is visualized by fluoroscopy.

To further verify that the needle tip is placed accurately within the piriformis muscle, before injection and subsequent to fluoroscopic localization of needle placement, an electromyograph can be connected to the hub of the needle. A ground and reference electrode is secured to the skin overlying the lateral upper thigh. The patient is instructed to externally rotate the thigh to activate the piriformis muscle. If brisk motor unit action potentials are not observed, the needle should be repositioned slightly, and the procedure repeated; 3 mL of an iodine-based radiotracer dye is subsequently injected. The pattern of radiotracer spread is subsequently examined under pulsed fluoroscopy. If the radiotracer pattern does not correspond with the parallel alignment of piriformis muscle fibers, the needle should be repositioned and the procedure (including electromyography) repeated. If the needle tip is too shallow, radiotracer dye patterns will appear to correlate with those of the gluteus maximus. Similarly, if the needle tip is too proximal or distal, dye patterns will appear to correlate with fibers of the obturator internus or gemelli muscles. After needle tip placement is verified by both fluoroscopic and electromyographic techniques, syringes are changed, and medication is injected.

Surgery

Surgery is not indicated in the treatment of patients with MPS.

POTENTIAL DISEASE COMPLICATIONS

Patients with MPS may go on to develop chronic pain syndrome. Treatment of individuals with chronic MPS is described earlier. Perhaps the biggest complication of untreated and progressive MPS is development of a syndrome of physical inactivity that may lead to cardiovascular disease.[103-106] Evidence of a dose-response relation between physical activity and cardiovascular disease endpoints has been proposed,[104] although the majority of the literature in this area has relied on prospective observational studies, and few randomized trials of physical activity and cardiovascular disease as a clinical outcome have been reported. This notwithstanding, evidence indicates that cardiovascular disease incidence and mortality are causally related to physical activity in an inverse, dose-response fashion. Thus, left untreated, patients with MPS who go on to develop chronic pain and lack physical activity are at high risk for cardiovascular disease and early death.

POTENTIAL TREATMENT COMPLICATIONS

The greatest risk of treatment of the patent with MPS is related to myofascial trigger point injections in the thoracic area. Because of the anatomic location of the apex of the lung to the proximity of the upper trapezius muscle or the scalene muscles, the clinician must be aware of the potential for pneumothorax as a result of myofascial trigger point injection in this area. The use of long (>1 inch) small-gauge needles should be avoided because long, thin needles can easily bend once they are inserted into the muscle, and the tip can inadvertently puncture the pleura. Rather, short (<1 inch) needles should be used for myofascial trigger point injections anywhere near the apex of the lung. In addition, the needle should be directed away from structures at risk for inadvertent puncture. To provide additional proprioceptive feedback during injection, grasping the muscle between the thumb and forefinger will allow the clinician to palpate the thickness of the tissue to be injected. Thin patients or those with reduced lung capacity from underlying diseases are particularly at risk, and thus the clinician should use extra precautions in performing myofascial trigger point injections in these patients.

References

1. Wallraff J. Histology of myogelosis. Munch Med Wochenschr 1951;93:913-916.
2. Windisch A, Reitinger A, Traxler H, et al. Morphology and histochemistry of myogelosis. Clin Anat 1999;12:266-271.
3. Bengtsson A. The muscle in fibromyalgia. Rheumatology (Oxford) 2002;41:721-724.
4. Inanici F, Yunus MB. History of fibromyalgia: past to present. Curr Pain Headache Rep 2004;8:369-378.
5. Schneider MJ. Tender points/fibromyalgia vs. trigger points/myofascial pain syndrome: a need for clarity in terminology and differential diagnosis. J Manipulative Physiol Ther 1995;18:398-406.
6. Buskila D. Fibromyalgia, chronic fatigue syndrome, and myofascial pain syndrome. Curr Opin Rheumatol 2001;13:117-127.
7. Gerwin RD. A review of myofascial pain and fibromyalgia—factors that promote their persistence. Acupunct Med 2005;23:121-134.
8. Goldenberg DL. Fibromyalgia, chronic fatigue syndrome, and myofascial pain syndrome. Curr Opin Rheumatol 1991;3:247-258.
9. Henriksson KG. Is fibromyalgia a distinct clinical entity? Pain mechanisms in fibromyalgia syndrome. A myologist's view. Baillieres Best Pract Res Clin Rheumatol 1999;13:455-461.
10. Pongratz DE, Sievers M. Fibromyalgia—symptom or diagnosis: a definition of the position. Scand J Rheumatol Suppl 2000;113:3-7.
11. Auleciems LM. Myofascial pain syndrome: a multidisciplinary approach. Nurse Pract 1995;20:18, 21-28, passim.
12. Borg-Stein J, Simons DG. Focused review: myofascial pain. Arch Phys Med Rehabil 2002;83(Suppl 1):S40-S49.
13. Gerwin RD. Classification, epidemiology, and natural history of myofascial pain syndrome. Curr Pain Headache Rep 2001;5:412-420.
14. Escobar PL, Ballesteros J. Myofascial pain syndrome. Orthop Rev 1987;16:708-713.
15. Bohr TW. Fibromyalgia syndrome and myofascial pain syndrome. Do they exist? Neurol Clin 1995;13:365-384.
16. Fricton JR. Myofascial pain syndrome. Neurol Clin 1989;7:413-427.
17. Simons DG, Mense S. Diagnosis and therapy of myofascial trigger points [in German]. Schmerz 2003;17:419-424.
18. Aronoff GM. Myofascial pain syndrome and fibromyalgia: a critical assessment and alternate view. Clin J Pain 1998;14:74-85.
19. Buskila D. Fibromyalgia, chronic fatigue syndrome, and myofascial pain syndrome. Curr Opin Rheumatol 1999;11:119-126.
20. Mikhail M, Rosen H. History and etiology of myofascial pain-dysfunction syndrome. J Prosthet Dent 1980;44:438-444.
21. Hong CZ, Simons DG. Pathophysiologic and electrophysiologic mechanisms of myofascial trigger points. Arch Phys Med Rehabil 1998;79:863-872.
22. Macgregor J, Graf von Schweinitz D. Needle electromyographic activity of myofascial trigger points and control sites in equine cleidobrachialis muscle—an observational study. Acupunct Med 2006;24:61-70.
23. Hong CZ. Pathophysiology of myofascial trigger point. J Formos Med Assoc 1996;95:93-104.
24. Simons DG, Hong CZ, Simons LS. Endplate potentials are common to midfiber myofascial trigger points. Am J Phys Med Rehabil 2002;81:212-222.
25. Rivner MH. The neurophysiology of myofascial pain syndrome. Curr Pain Headache Rep 2001;5:432-440.
26. Simons DG. Myofascial pain syndromes: where are we? Where are we going? Arch Phys Med Rehabil 1988;69(pt 1):207-212.
27. Graboski CL, Gray DS, Burnham RS. Botulinum toxin A versus bupivacaine trigger point injections for the treatment of myofascial pain syndrome: a randomised double blind crossover study. Pain 2005;118:170-175.
28. Ho KY, Tan KH. Botulinum toxin A for myofascial trigger point injection: a qualitative systematic review. Eur J Pain 2007;11:519-527.
29. Kamanli A, Kaya A, Ardicoglu O, et al. Comparison of lidocaine injection, botulinum toxin injection, and dry needling to trigger points in myofascial pain syndrome. Rheumatol Int 2005;25:604-611.
30. Kuan TS, Chen JT, Chen SM, et al. Effect of botulinum toxin on endplate noise in myofascial trigger spots of rabbit skeletal muscle. Am J Phys Med Rehabil 2002;81:512-520.
31. Ojala T, Arokoski JP, Partanen J. The effect of small doses of botulinum toxin A on neck-shoulder myofascial pain syndrome: a double-blind, randomized, and controlled crossover trial. Clin J Pain 2006;22:90-96.
32. Qerama E, Fuglsang-Frederiksen A, Kasch H, et al. A double-blind, controlled study of botulinum toxin A in chronic myofascial pain. Neurology 2006;67:241-245.
33. Wheeler AH, Goolkasian P, Gretz SS. A randomized, double-blind, prospective pilot study of botulinum toxin injection for refractory, unilateral, cervicothoracic, paraspinal, myofascial pain syndrome. Spine 1998;23:1662-1666.
34. Bishop B. Spasticity: its physiology and management. Part II. Neurophysiology of spasticity: current concepts. Phys Ther 1977;57:377-384.
35. Schalow G, Zach GA. Reorganization of the human central nervous system. Gen Physiol Biophys 2000;19(Suppl 1):11-240.
36. McPartland JM. Travell trigger points—molecular and osteopathic perspectives. J Am Osteopath Assoc 2004;104:244-249.
37. Mense S. Neurobiological basis for the use of botulinum toxin in pain therapy. J Neurol 2004;251(Suppl 1):I1-I7.
38. Sycha T, Kranz G, Auff E, Schnider P. Botulinum toxin in the treatment of rare head and neck pain syndromes: a systematic review of the literature. J Neurol 2004;251(Suppl 1):I19-I30.
39. Childers MK, Wilson DJ, Gnatz SM, et al. Botulinum toxin type A use in piriformis muscle syndrome: a pilot study. Am J Phys Med Rehabil 2002;81:751-759.
40. Papadopoulos EC, Khan SN. Piriformis syndrome and low back pain: a new classification and review of the literature. Orthop Clin North Am 2004;35:65-71.
41. Parziale JR, Hudgins TH, Fishman LM. The piriformis syndrome. Am J Orthop 1996;25:819-823.
42. Dolly O. Synaptic transmission: inhibition of neurotransmitter release by botulinum toxins. Headache 2003;43(Suppl 1):S16-S24.
43. Dressler D, Saberi FA, Barbosa ER. Botulinum toxin: mechanisms of action. Arq Neuropsiquiatr 2005;63:180-185.

44. Simpson LL. Studies on the mechanism of action of botulinum toxin. Adv Cytopharmacol 1979;3:27-34.

45. Fishman LM, Zybert PA. Electrophysiologic evidence of piriformis syndrome. Arch Phys Med Rehabil 1992;73:359-364.

46. Aoki KR. Review of a proposed mechanism for the antinociceptive action of botulinum toxin type A. Neurotoxicology 2005;26: 785-793.

47. Arnold LM. Biology and therapy of fibromyalgia. New therapies in fibromyalgia. Arthritis Res Ther 2006;8:212.

48. Bennett R. Fibromyalgia, chronic fatigue syndrome, and myofascial pain. Curr Opin Rheumatol 1998;10:95-103.

49. Le Goff P. Is fibromyalgia a muscle disorder? Joint Bone Spine 2006;73:239-242.

50. Lucas HJ, Brauch CM, Settas L, Theoharides TC. Fibromyalgia—new concepts of pathogenesis and treatment. Int J Immunopathol Pharmacol 2006;19:5-10.

51. Meyer HP. Myofascial pain syndrome and its suggested role in the pathogenesis and treatment of fibromyalgia syndrome. Curr Pain Headache Rep 2002;6:274-283.

52. Hayden RJ, Louis DS, Doro C. Fibromyalgia and myofascial pain syndromes and the workers' compensation environment: an update. Clin Occup Environ Med 2006;5:455-469, x-xi.

53. Gerwin RD, Dommerholt J, Shah JP. An expansion of Simons' integrated hypothesis of trigger point formation. Curr Pain Headache Rep 2004;8:468-475.

54. Shah JP, Phillips TM, Danoff JV, Gerber LH. An in vivo microanalytical technique for measuring the local biochemical milieu of human skeletal muscle. J Appl Physiol 2005;99:1977-1984.

55. Simons DG, Travell JG, Simons LS. Travell & Simons' Myofascial Pain and Dysfunction: The Trigger Point Manual, 2nd ed. Baltimore, Williams & Wilkins, 1999:1-940.

56. Hsieh CY, Hong CZ, Adams AH, et al. Interexaminer reliability of the palpation of trigger points in the trunk and lower limb muscles. Arch Phys Med Rehabil 2000;81:258-264.

57. Mense S, Simons DG, Hoheisel U, Quenzer B. Lesions of rat skeletal muscle after local block of acetylcholinesterase and neuromuscular stimulation. J Appl Physiol 2003;94:2494-2501.

58. Burton DJ, Enion D, Shaw DL. Pyomyositis of the piriformis muscle in a juvenile. Ann R Coll Surg Engl 2005;87:W9-12.

59. Jankiewicz JJ, Hennrikus WL, Houkom JA. The appearance of the piriformis muscle syndrome in computed tomography and magnetic resonance imaging. A case report and review of the literature. Clin Orthop Relat Res 1991;262:205-209.

60. Nakamura H, Seki M, Konishi S, et al. Piriformis syndrome diagnosed by cauda equina action potentials: report of two cases. Spine 2003;28:E37-E40.

61. Beatty RA. The piriformis muscle syndrome: a simple diagnostic maneuver. Neurosurgery 1994;34:512-514.

62. Beatty RA. Piriformis syndrome. J Neurosurg Spine 2006;5:101-102.

63. Graff-Radford SB. Myofascial pain: diagnosis and management. Curr Pain Headache Rep 2004;8:463-467.

64. Saravanan P, Dayan CM. Thyroid autoantibodies. Endocrinol Metab Clin North Am 2001;30:315-337, viii.

65. Schussler GC. Diagnostic tests and physiological relationships in thyroid disease. Mod Treat 1969;6:443-464.

66. Harris RE, Clauw DJ. The use of complementary medical therapies in the management of myofascial pain disorders. Curr Pain Headache Rep 2002;6:370-374.

67. Hou CR, Tsai LC, Cheng KF, et al. Immediate effects of various physical therapeutic modalities on cervical myofascial pain and trigger-point sensitivity. Arch Phys Med Rehabil 2002;83: 1406-1414.

68. Hsueh TC, Cheng PT, Kuan TS, Hong CZ. The immediate effectiveness of electrical nerve stimulation and electrical muscle stimulation on myofascial trigger points. Am J Phys Med Rehabil 1997;76:471-476.

69. Graff-Radford SB. Regional myofascial pain syndrome and headache: principles of diagnosis and management. Curr Pain Headache Rep 2001;5:376-381.

70. Wheeler AH. Myofascial pain disorders: theory to therapy. Drugs 2004;64:45-62.

71. McClaflin RR. Myofascial pain syndrome. Primary care strategies for early intervention. Postgrad Med 1994;96:56-59, 69.

72. Nicolakis P, Erdogmus B, Kopf A, et al. Effectiveness of exercise therapy in patients with myofascial pain dysfunction syndrome. J Oral Rehabil 2002;29:362-368.

73. Rosen NB. Physical medicine and rehabilitation approaches to the management of myofascial pain and fibromyalgia syndromes. Baillieres Clin Rheumatol 1994;8:881-916.

74. Itoh K, Okada K, Kawakita K. A proposed experimental model of myofascial trigger points in human muscle after slow eccentric exercise. Acupunct Med 2004;22:2-12.

75. Feldman JB. The neurobiology of pain, affect and hypnosis. Am J Clin Hypn 2004;46:187-200.

76. Aronoff GM, Feldman JB, Campion TS. Management of chronic pain and control of long-term disability. Occup Med 2000;15:755-770, iv.

77. Lackner JM, Carosella AM. The relative influence of perceived pain control, anxiety, and functional self efficacy on spinal function among patients with chronic low back pain. Spine 1999;24:2254-2260.

78. Reitsma B, Meijler WJ. Pain and patienthood. Clin J Pain 1997;13:9-21.

79. Jensen MP, Turner JA, Romano JM. Changes in beliefs, catastrophizing, and coping are associated with improvement in multidisciplinary pain treatment. J Consult Clin Psychol 2001;69:655-662.

80. Butler AC, Chapman JE, Forman EM, Beck AT. The empirical status of cognitive-behavioral therapy: a review of meta-analyses. Clin Psychol Rev 2006;26:17-31.

81. Flor H, Fydrich T, Turk DC. Efficacy of multidisciplinary pain treatment centers: a meta-analytic review. Pain 1992;49:221-230.

82. Malone MD, Strube MJ, Scogin FR. Meta-analysis of non-medical treatments for chronic pain. Pain 1988;34:231-244.

83. Nielson WR, Weir R. Biopsychosocial approaches to the treatment of chronic pain. Clin J Pain 2001;17(Suppl):S114-S127.

84. Osborne TL, Raichle KA, Jensen MP. Psychologic interventions for chronic pain. Phys Med Rehabil Clin North Am 2006;17:415-433.

85. Turner JA, Chapman CR. Psychological interventions for chronic pain: a critical review. II. Operant conditioning, hypnosis, and cognitive-behavioral therapy. Pain 1982;12:23-46.

86. Kirsch I, Montgomery G, Sapirstein G. Hypnosis as an adjunct to cognitive-behavioral psychotherapy: a meta-analysis. J Consult Clin Psychol 1995;63:214-220.

87. Hofbauer RK, Rainville P, Duncan GH, Bushnell MC. Cortical representation of the sensory dimension of pain. J Neurophysiol 2001;86:402-411.

88. Rainville P, Duncan GH, Price DD, et al. Pain affect encoded in human anterior cingulate but not somatosensory cortex. Science 1997;277:968-971.

89. Rainville P, Carrier B, Hofbauer RK, et al. Dissociation of sensory and affective dimensions of pain using hypnotic modulation. Pain 1999;82:159-171.

90. Rainville P, Hofbauer RK, Bushnell MC, et al. Hypnosis modulates activity in brain structures involved in the regulation of consciousness. J Cogn Neurosci 2002;14:887-901.

91. Rainville P, Bao QV, Chretien P. Pain-related emotions modulate experimental pain perception and autonomic responses. Pain 2005;118:306-318.

92. Frost A. Diclofenac versus lidocaine as injection therapy in myofascial pain. Scand J Rheumatol 1986;15:153-156.

93. Borg-Stein J. Treatment of fibromyalgia, myofascial pain, and related disorders. Phys Med Rehabil Clin North Am 2006;17:491-510, viii.

94. Rudin NJ. Evaluation of treatments for myofascial pain syndrome and fibromyalgia. Curr Pain Headache Rep 2003;7:433-442.

95. Criscuolo CM. Interventional approaches to the management of myofascial pain syndrome. Curr Pain Headache Rep 2001;5: 407-411.

96. Murphy DR, Hurwitz EL. A theoretical model for the development of a diagnosis-based clinical decision rule for the management of patients with spinal pain. BMC Musculoskelet Disord 2007;8:75.

97. Fanucci E, Masala S, Sodani G, et al. CT-guided injection of botulinic toxin for percutaneous therapy of piriformis muscle syndrome with preliminary MRI results about denervative process. Eur Radiol 2001;11:2543-2548.

98. Fishman LM, Konnoth C, Rozner B. Botulinum neurotoxin type B and physical therapy in the treatment of piriformis syndrome: a dose-finding study. Am J Phys Med Rehabil 2004;83:42-50.

99. Lang AM. Botulinum toxin type B in piriformis syndrome. Am J Phys Med Rehabil 2004;83:198-202.

100. Monnier G, Tatu L, Michel F. New indications for botulinum toxin in rheumatology. Joint Bone Spine 2006;73:667-671.

101. Raj PP. Botulinum toxin therapy in pain management. Anesthesiol Clin North Am 2003;21:715-731.

102. Reilich P, Fheodoroff K, Kern U, et al. Consensus statement: botulinum toxin in myofascial [corrected] pain. J Neurol 2004;251(Suppl 1):I36-I38.

103. Dubbert PM, Carithers T, Sumner AE, et al. Obesity, physical inactivity, and risk for cardiovascular disease. Am J Med Sci 2002;324:116-126.

104. Kohl HW III. Physical activity and cardiovascular disease: evidence for a dose response. Med Sci Sports Exerc 2001;33(Suppl): S472-S483.

105. Vitale C, Marazzi G, Volterrani M, et al. Metabolic syndrome. Minerva Med 2006;97:219-229.

106. Warburton DE, Nicol CW, Bredin SS. Health benefits of physical activity: the evidence. CMAJ 2006;174:801-809.

Repetitive Strain Injuries 97

Kelly McInnis, DO

Synonyms

Cumulative trauma disorders
Occupational overuse syndromes
Upper extremity musculoskeletal disorders
Nonspecific work-related upper limb disorders
Repetitive overuse disorders

ICD-9 Codes

719.44   Hand pain
729.5   Limb pain

DEFINITION

Repetitive strain injury (RSI) describes nonspecific upper extremity pain that often develops in occupational settings. RSIs are thought to result from the performance of repetitive and forceful hand-intensive tasks. These conditions are also referred to as cumulative trauma disorders, occupational overuse syndromes, and nonspecific work-related upper limb disorders. The varying nomenclature is controversial; it provides little insight into anatomy affected, disease severity, appropriate treatment, or expected prognosis. Classification systems of work-related musculoskeletal disorders often include specific diagnoses, such as carpal tunnel syndrome and de Quervain tenosynovitis, as repetitive strain injuries, but the consensus in recent years has been to consider RSI an entirely separate category of occupational disorder.[1] RSIs have symptom complexes that do not fit neatly into another diagnostic classification, such as specific tendinopathy or nerve entrapment. RSIs typically have few objective physical findings and little in the way of demonstrable pathologic change. There is no standard, data-driven treatment approach.

RSI is a significant medical concern; approximately 65% of reported cases of occupational illness are attributed to repeated trauma annually.[2,3] In fact, occupational musculoskeletal disorders of the hand and wrist are associated with the longest absences from work and have greater lost productivity and wages than those of other anatomic regions.[2] There is evidence that this condition is actually underreported.[4] Important risk factors appear to be repetitive motion of the arm or wrist, movements that require extremes of hand or arm position, prolonged static postures, and vibration. Other risk factors may be poor ergonomic work environment, task invariability, lack of autonomy, and high levels of psychological distress in the workplace. In addition, the female gender appears to be more susceptible to development of RSI.[5] Nonwork exposures also appear to contribute to these disorders. In turn, RSIs can develop outside of the workplace in students and other individuals who participate in hobbies or activities that expose them to repetitive motion and prolonged postures on a consistent basis.

According to the U.S. Department of Labor, Bureau of Labor Statistics, occupations that appear to be at greatest risk for RSIs are those in the service and manufacturing industries, including any job involving computer processing and keyboard use.[2] These occupations have the most demand for upper extremity intensive tasks. Because of limitations in the assessment of risk factors in the epidemiologic research, quantitative levels of exposure that are "acceptable" in each occupation are not available.[6] Clinically, it appears that the onset and perpetuation of RSIs are multifactorial.

There is no proven etiology of RSIs. They are thought to develop from repetitive microtrauma to muscle, tendon, nerve, loose connective tissue, or bone that exceeds the ability of the tissue to heal itself. Despite this postulated mechanism of injury, there is little evidence of pathologic tissue damage. In animal models, when chronic repetitive motion is induced, an acute inflammatory response is stimulated in the tissue. This initial response eventually subsides and is followed by a fibrotic response that may lead to complete tissue repair if loads and repetition are sufficiently low.[7] However, in the presence of high repetition or high force, the acute inflammatory response is followed by tissue degeneration and fibrosis that leads to scarring. It is this tissue reorganization that may lead to a nonspecific pattern of pain in RSI.

Abnormal muscle fatigability may also contribute to pain.[8] Reduction in muscle blood flow and localized tissue hypoxia have been demonstrated in trapezius muscle biopsy specimens taken from assembly-line workers with prolonged, static shoulder postures who developed chronic trapezius myalgia.[9] In addition, diminished local muscle oxygenation and blood flow has been demonstrated in the forearms of individuals with RSI during isometric contraction, compared with controls at similar working intensities. These findings indicate that the underlying vasculature may be impaired in this condition.[10] It is unclear whether these data can be extrapolated to explain the pathophysiologic mechanism of all RSI in the upper extremity.

There may also be a neurogenic origin for RSI. There is evidence of neural reorganization at multiple levels of the central nervous system after the performance of repetitive tasks. The repeated stimulation of nociceptive afferent nerve fibers may cause them to become hypersensitive, to expand their receptive fields, and to increase the excitability of secondary neurons in the spinal cord. These changes may contribute to the hyperalgesia associated with chronic pain in RSIs. Moreover, there may also be an element of central nervous system reorganization at the level of the somatosensory cortex with repetitive tasks. It has been shown that degradation of hand representations occurs with focal hand dystonias that are associated with writer's cramp. The central nervous system basis of dystonia may indeed point to a central nervous system origin of RSI, although this is not currently clear.[2]

Regardless of the factors that contribute to the development of RSI, there is often a complex dynamic in managing patients with work-related musculoskeletal disorders. They are often involved in compensation claims. When the injured patient takes on the additional role of claimant, the perception of both patient and caregiver can change in many aspects of the healing and rehabilitation process. It is paramount for the physician treating RSI to take the medicolegal implications into account. Indeed, the workers' compensation system has a great impact on the reporting and control of work-related disorders.[11]

SYMPTOMS

The predominant symptom in RSI is upper extremity pain. The discomfort often begins as a dull ache in the forearm or hand after the performance of tasks of repetitive motion. Initially, it may be intermittent and alleviated with rest. As the offending activity is repeated with regularity, the pain may increase in intensity and be triggered by minimal exertion in the workplace and even while performing simple activities of daily living, such as dressing or grooming. The symptoms usually begin in one region of the limb in a fairly localized area (e.g., wrist, elbow, or forearm) but may quickly spread to involve the entire arm and at times the contralateral arm. Pain tends to gradually increase during the workday, with peak intensity during the last hours of work. It appears to get better over the weekends and during vacations from work.

Other symptoms may include paresthesias, numbness, and weakness. If these symptoms are present, they may not follow dermatomal or peripheral nerve distributions. Patients may also complain of arm or hand muscle cramping, allodynia, stiffness, and slowing or incoordination of fine motor movements of the hand.

Patients often complain of night pain, resulting in poor sleep. A detailed investigation of sleep habits is important because sleep disruption is common in RSI. Psychological distress and depression may result if pain and sleeplessness persist. In fact, self-reported upper extremity–specific health status measured by the Disabilities of the Arm, Shoulder, and Hand (DASH) questionnaire appears to correlate with depression and pain anxiety in these patients.[12] Some patients may also exhibit maladaptive illness beliefs, such as catastrophizing and fear-avoidance.

In taking a patient's history, the clinician should attain an accurate understanding of the patient's job description and daily workstation. It is important to thoroughly evaluate the biomechanics of body position and posture as well as the physical layout of the work site. Special attention should be given to the details of specific job duties, including the frequency, duration, and conditions under which they are performed. For example, if the patient works a desk job and spends each day on a computer, it is important to inquire about desk and chair setup and placement of the computer monitor and keyboard. The clinician should also take note of the patient's perception and satisfaction with the workplace. This information can give the clinician valuable insight, as dissatisfied workers are notorious for work-related medical claims.

It is important to take into account the patient's past medical history and social history; both can contribute greatly to the current health status. It is critical to elicit any chronic illnesses that the patient might have and to take a detailed medication history. Elements of social history, including family life, child-care issues, and drug or alcohol abuse, can be important factors that influence the patient's complaints on the job.

PHYSICAL EXAMINATION

RSI is a diagnosis of exclusion. Typically, there are no objective physical findings. Hence, the physical examination should be comprehensive and focus on ruling out alternative diagnoses. It should include a thorough musculoskeletal examination with inspection, palpation, and testing of passive and active range of motion of the cervical spine, shoulder, elbow, wrist, and fingers. There is typically no evidence of muscle atrophy or other deformity. There may be pain on active and passive range of motion, but there is generally no restriction of motion when the examiner takes the joint through a full arc. There may be diffuse myofascial pain with palpation over the symptomatic region. In addition, there may be evidence of one or more focal fibromyalgia tender points on the symptomatic as well as on the asymptomatic arm.[13]

Neurologic assessment can rule out localized nerve disease by investigating for dermatomal, myotomal, or peripheral nerve abnormalities. In RSI, deep tendon reflexes are normal and symmetric. Manual muscle strength testing should be performed but is generally inconsistent, depending on the patient's effort and pain level with exertion. Objective and reproducible strength tests can be performed with a hand or pinch dynamometer if level of strength is uncertain with examiner resistance. Computer-driven isokinetic dynamometers can also be used for more reliable measures of strength across uniaxial joints, such as the elbow. Sensory testing should be done by light touch as well as by pinprick. This portion of the neurologic examination is often difficult, as subjective abnormalities are common. The reported impairments in sensation do not typically follow dermatomal distributions.

Provocative tests that reproduce specific pain patterns can help rule out alternative diagnoses. Examples include the Spurling test for cervical radiculopathy, Neer and Hawkins maneuvers for rotator cuff impingement, resisted wrist or finger extension for lateral epicondylitis, Tinel sign at the ulnar groove for ulnar neuritis, and Finkelstein test for de Quervain tenosynovitis. Provocative maneuvers that can rule out carpal tunnel syndrome include Tinel sign at the wrist, Phalen test, reverse Phalen test, and carpal tunnel compression. It is important to keep in mind that percussion over the median nerve at the wrist, the ulnar nerve at the cubital tunnel, or the radial nerve at the elbow may elicit pain or paresthesias in RSI, but this is not necessarily indicative of nerve injury.

FUNCTIONAL LIMITATIONS

RSI can limit upper extremity function to highly variable degrees.[14] Patients may have difficulty in performing activities of daily living at home, such as dressing, grooming, or preparing a meal. The pain impairment may prevent them from participating in recreational activities that they formerly enjoyed. They can also be quite limited in terms of their work-related activity. For example, pain may prevent a patient from being productive at work because he or she finds it difficult to use a keyboard and computer to do different tasks. Employers often advocate functional capacity evaluations to define more objectively the amount of physical labor that the patient can perform safely.

DIAGNOSTIC STUDIES

Diagnostic tests are ordered if the diagnosis is not clear after the history and physical examination, if the results of the testing will change management, or if the testing is needed for medicolegal reasons. The tests are used to exclude other definitive conditions that may remain in the differential diagnosis after examination. Needle electromyography and nerve conduction studies are often necessary to rule out a peripheral nerve lesion, such as median nerve entrapment at the wrist. Electrodiagnostic studies provide the distinct advantage of offering objective data by quantifying the degree of nerve impairment in a manner that is independent of the patient's pain behaviors.[15] This can be very important when injured workers have interest in substantial secondary gain and may not be reliable in their effort or honesty when motor and sensory nerve function is tested on physical examination.

Imaging is likely to be normal in RSI. Plain radiographs of the suspected site of disease will generally not reveal a fracture in the absence of blunt trauma but may reveal underlying degenerative changes that may or may not account for the patient's symptoms. Magnetic resonance imaging of the cervical spine and shoulder is often ordered to rule out disc herniation, neuroforaminal stenosis, and rotator cuff disease. This study may be useful only if there is concern for one of these diagnoses based on physical examination.[16] Magnetic resonance imaging is expensive, and abnormalities such as disc bulging and degenerative spondylosis are often found in asymptomatic individuals and may not explain the current symptom complex.

Laboratory work is seldom necessary at the time of initial evaluation unless an underlying systemic illness is suspected.

Differential Diagnosis

Cervical radiculopathy

Myofascial pain syndrome

Thoracic outlet syndrome

Rotator cuff or biceps tendinitis

Lateral or medial epicondylitis

Compressive neuropathies (e.g., carpal tunnel syndrome)

de Quervain tenosynovitis

Osteoarthritis

Fractures

TREATMENT

Initial

Treatment of RSIs should focus on conservative measures. The first step is to limit exposure to the particular repetitive activities that may have contributed to the development of the RSI and that continue to induce pain. Sick leave should be avoided because it may develop into chronic disability. A substantial proportion of workers experience additional injury-related absences even after their first return to work.[17] Time off work has proved to be a powerful predictor of disability pension; fully following work-related restrictions can ensure that the patient remains a productive employee by going to work.

Unfortunately, there is little evidence for the effectiveness of any specific medical intervention for RSI. Clinical treatment is usually targeted at relief of pain and acute inflammation as well as restoration of range of motion. Inflammatory conditions are often treated with the PRICE regimen: protection (preventing further injury, perhaps by bracing), rest or activity modification (as mentioned before), ice, compression, and elevation to minimize swelling.

Icing of the limb for about 20 minutes three times daily in conjunction with wrist or elbow splinting can decrease symptoms. Other modalities that may be helpful in controlling pain symptoms in the acute phase of treatment include ultrasound, iontophoresis, and transcutaneous electrical nerve stimulation. Manual massage, spray and stretch techniques with a vapocoolant spray, and paraffin baths may also alleviate pain in some patients.

Medications may also be used to control pain and inflammation. Nonsteroidal anti-inflammatory drugs (NSAIDs) are usually the first-line pharmaceuticals for acute inflammation. There are many NSAIDs on the market from which to choose, and some can easily be purchased over-the-counter. It is often useful to try several different types of NSAIDs because patient responses can be idiosyncratic. Anticonvulsant medications, such as gabapentin, pregabalin, and carbamazepine, are also often used for pain. They are generally most effective for neuropathic pain. Local anesthetic patches (e.g., lidocaine) can be helpful if they are placed over a localized area of arm pain. Trigger point injections with local anesthetic or dry needling can also be considered to relieve myofascial pain. Oral narcotics should generally be avoided, given the risk of opioid dependency.

Restoration of sleep can be helpful in reducing pain perception as well as in decreasing the risk for development of depression. The use of low-dose tricyclic antidepressants (e.g., nortriptyline or amitriptyline) can be effective. If signs of depression are present, appropriate antidepressant treatment or referral to a psychiatrist or psychologist is indicated.

Rehabilitation

The rehabilitation of a patient with RSI is best achieved by a multidisciplinary approach with the physician overseeing the treatment plan and following the progress of the patient. A referral to skilled physical and occupational therapy is essential.[18] The therapists may provide several modalities (mentioned before) to decrease pain and to facilitate an active stretching and strengthening program. They not only focus on the affected limb but also work on total body biomechanics and postural control at the workstation and at home. Progressive resistive exercise programs can be used, but worsening of pain symptoms with increasing exertion is often an issue. Progressive resistive exercises can have more benefit if they are introduced with small increments in resistance, allowing the patient to slowly adjust. This approach can improve participation of the patient and thus increase strength gains with treatment. Further physical conditioning with regimented aerobic training, catered to the patient's personal interests, and institution of a home exercise program may reduce pain, improve stress management, and increase work capacity. It is important to encourage physical activity as much as possible. General aerobic conditioning can be effective in encouraging a positive health perception.

Relaxation training may also be helpful for chronic, nonspecific regional arm pain.[19] Continued surveillance and treatment of mental health can be imperative in recovery. Cognitive-behavioral therapy techniques can be used to treat the maladaptive beliefs and misconceptions that may accompany upper extremity dysfunction.[20] Moreover, weight reduction, if needed, and smoking cessation should also be included in any plan to improve overall health.

Other rehabilitative measures for RSI include the fabrication of splints and the introduction of adaptive equipment that may assist in functional activities at home and in the workplace. Some therapists are specially trained to perform work site analysis and to suggest ergonomic modifications. Modifications can range from adjustment in chair height and computer mouse position to the substitution of large-handled tools, depending on the occupation. For computer users, it is generally recommended that chair height be such that the forearms are relatively horizontal to the floor and the wrists are in a neutral position. The volar aspect of the wrist can be supported during typing by a wrist support placed on the desktop or support tray in front of the keyboard. The keyboard should be located in a position directly in front of the typist, minimizing ulnar deviation of either wrist. The mouse should be placed close to midline. Split keyboards and those that provide a trackball can help with forearm and hand positioning. Voice-activated software is also available for those patients whose symptoms are refractory to these modifications.[15] Ergonomically designed computer touch pads, a foot-controlled mouse, and document holders are other tools that can help decrease symptoms in RSI.

There is limited evidence in published literature to confirm the usefulness of ergonomic interventions.[21] However, most clinicians agree that such interventions are a worthwhile component of a comprehensive rehabilitation plan. Ergonomic interventions *may* make the workplace more comfortable, encouraging the patient to return to work and possibly preventing work disability.[22] Education about proper ergonomics should empower patients to make low-cost changes on their own at work and at home.

Many factors can limit the effectiveness of work hardening and work conditioning programs.

Individuals who are having difficulty in returning to their previous level of work activity should be evaluated for alternative jobs. This can involve consideration of a new position with the current employer, if it is mutually agreed on. Job redesign that enriches career development opportunities may be effective. In fact, studies suggest that interventions aimed at altering workers' perceptions of monotonous or tedious work, through better job development opportunities, an increase of latitude over working patterns, and the improvement of communication between employers and employees, may be beneficial and cost-effective to the employer.[23-25] However, in some instances, an entirely different vocation must be pursued. If this is the case, a consultation with a vocational rehabilitation specialist is advised.

Procedures

Procedures are rarely indicated in RSI. In a population of patients with such a nondefinitive diagnosis, treatment failures are frequent. Therefore, trigger point injections, lateral epicondylar injections, carpal tunnel injections, and the like can be attempted to see if symptoms improve. The risk and benefits of each procedure should be explained in detail, including the risk of no relief of pain.

Surgery

Surgery is not indicated for RSI.

POTENTIAL DISEASE COMPLICATIONS

The most feared complication of RSI is increasing functional impairment and disability in all aspects of life. Negative outcomes can occur if the patient feels incapable of using his or her arms and hands. This may result in the inability to participate in home, work, and recreational activities. Depression and social isolation may accompany prolonged periods of absence from work.

POTENTIAL TREATMENT COMPLICATIONS

The risks of treatment complications are rare. Most complications are associated with pain medication side effects. Analgesics and NSAIDs have well-known adverse reactions that most commonly affect the gastric, hepatic, and renal systems. Anticonvulsants can cause fatigue, ataxia, edema, or nausea. Tricyclic antidepressants have a high profile of fatigue, dizziness, dry mouth, and constipation. Patients should be informed of the side effect profile of each medication before administration. The patient's complete medication list should be reviewed to address potential adverse reactions between medications taken concurrently.

References

1. Walker-Bone K, Cooper C. Hard work never hurt anyone—or did it? A review of occupational associations with soft tissue musculoskeletal disorders of the neck and upper limb. Ann Rheum Dis 2005;64:1112-1117.
2. Barr A, Barbe M, Clark B. Work-related musculoskeletal disorders of the hand and wrist: epidemiology, pathophysiology, and sensorimotor changes. J Orthop Sports Phys Ther 2004;34:610-627.
3. Giang GM. Epidemiology of work-related upper extremity disorders: understanding prevalence and outcomes to impact provider performances using a practice management reporting tool. Clin Occup Environ Med 2006;5:267-283.
4. Morse T, Dillon C, Kenta-Bibi E, et al. Trends in work-related musculoskeletal disorder reports by year, type, and industrial sector: a capture-recapture analysis. Am J Ind Med 2005;48:40-49.
5. Lacerda E, Nacul L, Augusto L, et al. Prevalence and associations of symptoms of upper extremities, repetitive strain injuries (RSI) and "RSI-like condition." A cross-sectional study of bank workers in Northeast Brazil. BMC Public Health 2005;5:107-116.
6. Mani L, Gerr F. Work-related upper extremity musculoskeletal disorders. Prim Care 2000;27:845-864.
7. Barr A, Barbe M. Pathophysiological tissue changes associated with repetitive movement: a review of the evidence. Phys Ther 2002;82:173-187.
8. Helliwell P, Taylor W. Repetitive strain injury. Postgrad Med J 2004;80:438-443.
9. Larsson S, Bodegard L, Henriksson K, et al. Chronic trapezius myalgia: morphology and blood flow studied in 17 patients. Acta Orthop Scand 1990;61:394-398.
10. Brunnekreef J, Oosterhof J, Thijssen D, et al. Forearm blood flow and oxygen consumption in patients with bilateral repetitive strain injury measured by near-infrared spectroscopy. Clin Physiol Funct Imaging 2006;26:178-184.
11. Harding W. Worker's compensation litigation of the upper extremity claim. Clin Occup Environ Med 2006;5:483-490.
12. Ring D, Kadzielski J, Fabian L, et al. Self-reported upper extremity health status correlates with depression. J Bone Joint Surg Am 2006;88:1983-1988.
13. Helliwell P, Bennett R, Littlejohn G, et al. Towards epidemiological criteria for soft-tissue disorders of the arm. Occup Med 2003;53:313-319.
14. Ring D, Guss D, Malhotra L, et al. Idiopathic arm pain. J Bone Joint Surg Am 2004;86:1387-1391.
15. Foye P, Cianca J, Prathers H. Cumulative trauma disorders of the upper limb in computer users. Arch Phys Med Rehabil 2002;83:S12-S15.
16. Hassett R. The role of imaging of work-related upper extremity disorders. Clin Occup Environ Med 2006;5:285-298, vii.
17. Baldwin M, Butler R. Upper extremity disorders in the workplace: costs and outcomes beyond the first return to work. J Occup Rehabil 2006;16:303-323.
18. Driver D. Occupational and physical therapy for work-related upper extremity disorders: how we can influence outcomes. Clin Occup Environ Med 2006;5:471-482, xi.
19. Spence S, Sharpe L, Newton-John T, et al. Effect of EMG biofeedback compared to applied relaxation training with chronic, upper extremity cumulative trauma disorders. Pain 1995;63:199-206.
20. Derebery J, Tullis W. Prevention of delayed recovery and disability of work-related upper extremity disorders. Clin Occup Environ Med 2006;5:235-247, vi.
21. Verhagen A, Karels C, Bierma-Zeinstra S, et al. Ergonomic and physiotherapeutic interventions for treating work-related complaints of the arm, neck or shoulder in adults. Cochrane Database Syst Rev 2006;3:CD003471.
22. Pearce B. Ergonomic considerations in work-related upper extremity disorders. Clin Occup Environ Med 2006;5:249-266, vi.
23. Silverstein B, Clark R. Interventions to reduce work-related musculoskeletal disorders. J Electromyogr Kinesiol 2004;14:135-152.
24. Colombini D, Occhipinti E. Preventing upper limb work-related musculoskeletal disorders (UL-WMSDS): new approaches in job (re)design and current trends in standardization. Appl Ergon 2006;37:441-450.
25. Juul-Kristensen B, Jensen C. Self-reported workplace related ergonomic conditions as prognostic factors for musculoskeletal symptoms: the "BIT" follow up study on office workers. Occup Environ Med 2005;62:188-194.

Costosternal Syndromes 98

Marta Imamura, MD, and David A. Cassius, MD

Synonyms

Anterior chest wall syndrome
Costochondritis
Costosternal chondrodynia
Atypical chest pain

ICD-9 Code

733.6   Tietze disease; costochondral junction syndrome and costochondritis

DEFINITION

Costosternal syndrome is a frequent cause of anterior chest wall pain that affects the costosternal[1-6] or the costochondral joints.[2,4-7] The pathogenesis of costosternal syndrome is still unknown.[2,8] Costosternal syndrome is considered an entity distinct from the rarely occurring Tietze syndrome[1-7,9] because it is a frequent cause of benign anterior chest wall pain. Also, as opposed to Tietze syndrome, it is not associated with local swelling of the involved costosternal or costochondral joints,[1-7,9] and it usually occurs at multiple sites. The onset is usually after 40 years of age instead of at a young age as in Tietze syndrome, and it affects more women than men. A traumatic cause has been proposed,[8] and currently it is suspected that repetitive overuse lesions of the costosternal joint and anterior chest[6,10] may be involved in the development of the degenerative changes found at the costosternal joint.[11,12] The costosternal joints may also be inflamed by osteoarthritis, rheumatoid arthritis, ankylosing spondylitis, Reiter syndrome, psoriatic arthritis, and the SAPHO (*s*ynovitis, *a*cne, *p*ustulosis, *h*yperostosis, and *o*steitis) syndrome.[3,7,12] Infections of the costosternal joints are associated with tuberculosis, fungus (mycetoma, pulmonary aspergilloma, candidal costochondritis[13]), and syphilis as well as with viruses. The costosternal joints may also be the site of tumor invasion either from a primary malignant neoplasm, such as a chondrosarcoma or thymoma, or from a metastatic carcinoma, most commonly from the breast, kidney, thyroid, bronchus, lung, or prostate.[12,14] Chondromas and multiple exostoses are the most common benign tumors.

As one can readily see, costosternal syndromes may be a primary condition or secondary to these diseases. The condition occurs more frequently in women (a ratio of 2 to 3:1) and at an older age; two thirds of the patients are older than 40 years.[1-4,7,8] The left side is more often involved. Costosternal joint disease is 1.69 times more frequent in patients who undergo median sternotomy than in normal controls of the same age.[15]

SYMPTOMS

The most common symptom in costosternal syndrome is pain of the anterior chest wall, usually localized at the precordium or at the left parasternal region.[8,16] Pain can radiate superiorly toward the left shoulder and left arm[8,16] and also to the neck, scapula, and anterior chest. Pain mainly develops after postural changes and maneuvers that place stress over the chest wall structures[16] rather than with physical efforts, such as those related to pain of cardiac origin.[16] Cough, deep breathing, and chest and scapular movements usually aggravate pain.[5,11] In contrast to Tietze syndrome, in which only one costal cartilage is involved in the majority of the patients, multiple sites are present in 90% of patients with costosternal syndromes.[1,2,7-9] The second to the fifth costal cartilages are most commonly affected.[1-3,5,8,9] Pain intensity may vary; it usually occurs at rest[12] and lasts for several weeks or months.[8,16]

PHYSICAL EXAMINATION

Inspection of the patient suffering from costosternal syndrome reveals that the patient vigorously attempts to splint the joints by keeping the shoulders stiffly in neutral position.[12] Differing from the Tietze syndrome, the costosternal syndrome has no visible spherical local swelling or any inflammatory signs at the costal cartilages.[1,4,5,7,9] Pain is reproduced by active protraction or retraction of the shoulder, deep inspiration, and elevation of the arm.[12] Palpation of the affected portions of the thoracic cage elicits local tenderness at multiple sites.[9] It may reproduce the patient's spontaneous pain complaint, including its radiation.[9,17,18] Some authors, however, have not found pain reproduction on palpation.[4,5,16-18]

545

Several maneuvers have been found to be helpful in establishing the diagnosis.[8,16] Application of firm steady pressure to the following chest wall structures elicits the patient's pain complaint: the sternum, the left and right parasternal junctions, the intercostal spaces, the ribs, the inframammary area, and the pectoralis major and left upper trapezius muscles.[8,16,17] All of these can precipitate pain similar in quality and location to the spontaneous pain.[16] Another maneuver, called the horizontal flexion test (Fig. 98-1), consists of having the arm flexed across the anterior chest with the application of steady prolonged traction in a horizontal direction while, at the same time, the patient's head is rotated as far as possible toward the ipsilateral shoulder.[2,6,8,10,16,17] Another test, called the crowing rooster maneuver, consists of having the patient extend the neck as much as possible by looking toward the ceiling while the examiner, standing behind the patient, exerts traction on the posteriorly extended arms.[2,8,16,17] Associated myofascial pain syndrome of the intercostal, pectoralis major, pectoralis minor, and sternal muscles is a common feature of the syndrome. These muscles may be tender on palpation. Because this syndrome is usually confused with pain of cardiac,[1,2,11,19,20] abdominal,[2,9,16,21] or pulmonary[19] origin, a comprehensive history and physical examination are essential in all cases,[8,19,20] including athletes.[6,10]

FUNCTIONAL LIMITATIONS

Functional limitations may be due to the severe incapacitating chest pain.[16] Activities such as lifting, bathing, ironing, combing and brushing hair, and other activities of daily living can be very problematic. Patients will need to be at light duty for weeks and to avoid physical efforts of the upper limbs and trunk.[14] Even after a cardiac origin is ruled out for the chest discomfort, many patients do not return to full employment, recreation, or daily activities[22,23] and remain functionally impaired for years.[23] This functional impairment may occur even in patients with chest pain and normal angiographic studies[22,23] without a proven myocardial infarction. Many of these patients may have a costoster-

nal syndrome. However, the continuing regular physician visits, medication consumption, emergency department visits, repeated hospitalizations, and repeated arteriographies may be contributing to the functional impairment.

DIAGNOSTIC STUDIES

The diagnosis of costosternal syndrome is usually a clinical diagnosis based on the detection of chest wall tenderness[11,16] that reproduces the spontaneous pain on physical examination.[8,11,16,17,19,20] Coronary heart disease,[2,4,11,16,19,20] breast conditions,[24] and pulmonary conditions[19,20] may be misdiagnosed with costosternal syndrome because of the anatomic proximity of the involved structures. Costosternal syndrome may also coexist with coronary artery disease[2,4,7,11,16,17] and other types of heart diseases.[16] The differentiation from anginal pain due to coronary heart disease may be judged by the pain characteristics. Typical anginal pain is substernal, provoked by exertion, and relieved by rest or nitroglycerin.[19] Atypical anginal pain has two of these symptoms, and nonanginal chest pain has only one of these symptoms.[19] Swap and Nagurney[20] described a low risk for acute coronary syndrome or acute myocardial infarction, with a likelihood ratio of 0.2 to 0.3, when chest pain is described as stabbing, pleuritic, or positional or is reproducible by palpation. The same authors also described a likelihood ratio of 2.3 to 4.7 for acute coronary syndrome when the chest pain radiates to one or both shoulders or arms or is precipitated by exertion.[20] In most patients with costosternal syndromes, the pain is usually localized in the anterior chest or parasternally at the level of the third or fourth intercostal space. As previously mentioned, it can also radiate superiorly toward the left shoulder and down the left arm. Patients experience pain at rest, and the pain can awaken them from sleep.[8,16] Chest pain characteristics, electrocardiographic abnormalities, or cardiac risk factors should be further evaluated by a cardiologist. Radionuclide cineangiographic testing is a sensitive method to differentiate between costosternal syndromes and cardiac diseases.[16]

Laboratory and imaging procedures are helpful in the diagnosis of the possible secondary causes of the costosternal syndromes and to rule out other causes of anterior chest pain.[11,14]

Plain radiographs are indicated for patients who present with pain possibly emanating from the costosternal joints to rule out occult bone tumors, infections, and congenital defects. If trauma has occurred, costosternal syndrome may coexist with occult rib fractures or fractures of the sternum. These fractures may be missed on plain radiographs and can require radionuclide bone scanning for proper diagnosis. Increased uptake of radioactivity on bone scans is seen in most patients; however, it is not a specific test for making the diagnosis of costosternal syndrome.[25]

Additional testing, including complete blood count, prostate-specific antigen level, sedimentation rate, and antinuclear antibody titer, may be indicated to rule out other diseases that may cause a costosternal syndrome,

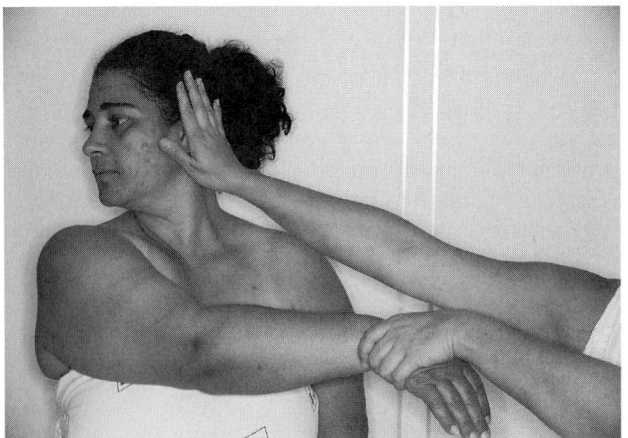

FIGURE 98-1. Horizontal flexion test for the diagnosis of costosternal syndrome.

such as rheumatoid arthritis, ankylosing spondylitis, Reiter syndrome, and psoriatic arthritis. Magnetic resonance imaging of the joints is indicated if joint instability or occult mass is suspected. Diagnostic ultrasonography may also be indicated to investigate the presence of an occult mass.

Neuropathic pain caused by diabetic polyneuropathies and acute herpes zoster involving the chest wall may also be confused or coexist with costosternal syndrome.[12]

A highly reliable test (and an effective differential diagnostic procedure that can confirm the diagnosis of costosternal syndrome) is the complete pain relief noted after an intercostal block at the posterior axillary line.[8] Patients with cardiac disease will have little or no effect on their pain because the nociceptive pathways from the heart are in the sympathetic afferents located in the paravertebral region. This test is both diagnostic and therapeutic.

TREATMENT

Initial

Initial treatment of the pain and functional disability associated with costosternal syndromes should include simple oral analgesics,[2,17] such as acetaminophen and nonsteroidal anti-inflammatory drugs,[12,26] alone or in combination with codeine[8] or tramadol. The use of an elastic rib belt may also provide symptomatic relief and help protect the costosternal joints from additional trauma.[12] Reassurance that the diagnosis is a non–life-threatening musculoskeletal pain syndrome can often by itself reduce the anxiety and fears and lead to symptomatic pain relief.[2,6-9,11,16,26]

In the secondary forms of costosternal syndromes, the underlying conditions should be addressed for good results.[16]

Rehabilitation

Physical modalities, such as local superficial heat for 20 minutes, two or three times a day, or ice for 10 to 15 minutes, three or four times a day, can be performed while symptoms are present.[11,17] Transcutaneous electrical nerve stimulation and electroacupuncture may be applied over the painful area. Gentle, pain-free range of motion exercises should be introduced as soon as tolerated. Vigorous exercises should be avoided because they exacerbate the patient's symptoms. Perpetuating and aggravating factors,[26] such as chronic coughing and bronchospasm, among others, should always be removed.

Procedures

For patients who do not respond to the initial or rehabilitation treatment modalities, a local anesthetic and steroid injection[5,6,9,11,12,24] can be performed as the next symptom control maneuver. Even in patients with coexisting true anginal pain, the relief of local chest pain is evident. Intra-articular injection of the costosternal joint (Fig. 98-2) is performed with the patient in the supine position.[12] The area of maximum tenderness can be infiltrated with a local anesthetic (2% lidocaine[7,24] or 0.25% preservative-free bupivacaine[12]) and methylprednisolone acetate[7,11,12,24] at the dosage of 10 mg per costosternal joint[24] using a 1½-inch, 25-gauge needle with strict aseptic technique.[12] The costosternal joints should be easily palpable as a slight bulging at the point

Differential Diagnosis

Angina pectoris

Acute myocardial infarction

Tietze syndrome

Dislocation and fracture of the ribs, sternum, and clavicle

Congenital sternoclavicular malformations

Myofascial pain syndrome at the anterior chest wall: sternal, pectoralis major, pectoralis minor, scalene, sternocleidomastoid (sternal head), subclavius, and cervical iliocostal muscles

Tumors of the costal cartilages

Costochondral dislocations

Trauma and arthritis of the sternoclavicular joint

Sternoclavicular hyperostosis

Manubriosternal arthritis

Trauma to the sternum

Xiphoidalgia syndrome

Diseases of the lung (pneumonia, lung abscess, atelectasis)

Spontaneous pneumothorax

Mediastinal emphysema

Mediastinitis

T1-12 radiculopathy (herpes zoster, postherpetic neuralgia)

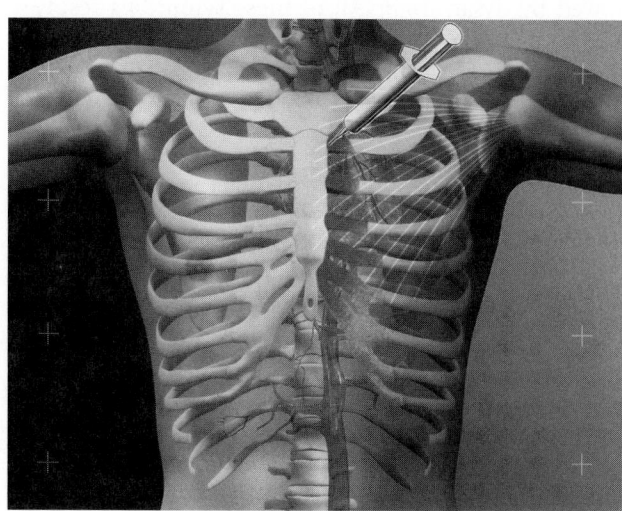

FIGURE 98-2. Schematic representation of the injection site at the second costosternal junction.

where the rib attaches to the sternum.[12] An intercostal block at the posterior axillary line provides complete relief for 6 to 10 hours.[8]

Surgery

Surgical procedures are rarely necessary.[9] Costosternal or sternoclavicular arthrodesis may be performed if conservative measures fail to provide satisfactory results.

POTENTIAL DISEASE COMPLICATIONS

Costosternal syndromes are of benign origin, and complications rarely develop. They are self-limited,[9] and spontaneous recovery usually occurs after 1 year in the majority of the cases.[4] Pain exacerbation due to physical activities and overload is usually followed by spontaneous recovery. However, as mentioned earlier, because of the many pathologic processes that may mimic the pain of costosternal syndrome, the clinician should always be careful to rule out underlying cardiac, lung, breast, and mediastinum diseases.

POTENTIAL TREATMENT COMPLICATIONS

The systemic complications of analgesics such as non-steroidal anti-inflammatory drugs are well known and most commonly affect the gastric, hepatic, and renal systems. Local steroid combined with local anesthetic injections may cause pneumothorax if the needle is placed too laterally or deeply and invades the pleural space.[12] Cardiac tamponade as well as trauma to the contents of the mediastinum, although rare, can occur. This complication can be greatly decreased if the clinician pays close attention to accurate needle placement[12] or performs the injection with ultrasonographic guidance. Transient marked hypophosphatemia has been documented 8 hours after an intra-articular glucocorticoid injection in a patient with chronic costochondritis.[27] In this patient, hypophosphatemia was clinically characterized by limb paresthesia and weakness, followed by dysarthria.[27] All of these symptoms resolved within hours, even before the hypophosphatemia resolved.[27] Iatrogenic infections can also occur if strict aseptic techniques are not followed.[12]

References

1. Carabasi RJ, Christian JJ, Brindley HH. Costosternal chondrodynia: a variant of Tietze's syndrome? Dis Chest 1962;41:559-562.
2. Fam AG, Smythe HA. Musculoskeletal chest wall pain. Can Med Assoc J 1985;133:379-389.
3. Aeschlimann A, Kahn MF. Tietze's syndrome: a critical review. Clin Exp Rheumatol 1990;8:407-412.
4. Disla E, Rhim HR, Reddy A, et al. Costochondritis. A prospective analysis in an emergency department setting. Arch Intern Med 1994;154:2466-2469.
5. Mukerji B, Mukerji V, Alpert MA, et al. The prevalence of rheumatologic disorders in patients with chest pain and angiographically normal coronary arteries. Angiology 1995;46:425-430.
6. Gregory PL, Biswas AC, Batt ME. Musculoskeletal problems of the chest wall in athletes. Sports Med 2002;32:235-250.
7. Freeston J, Karim Z, Lindsay K, et al. Can early diagnosis and management of costochondritis reduce acute chest pain admissions? J Rheumatol 2004;31:2269-2271.
8. Bonica JJ, Sola AF. Chest pain caused by other disorders. In Bonica JJ, ed. The Management of Pain, vol II. Philadelphia, Lea & Febiger, 1990:1114-1145.
9. Calabro JJ, Jeghers H, Miller KA, Gordon RD. Classification of anterior chest wall syndromes. JAMA 1980;243:1420-1421.
10. Rumball JS, Lebrun CM, Di Ciacca SR, et al. Rowing injuries. Sports Med 2005;35:537-555.
11. Wolf E, Stern S. Costosternal syndrome: its frequency and importance in differential diagnosis of coronary heart disease. Arch Intern Med 1976;136:189-191.
12. Waldman SD. Tietze's syndrome. In Waldman SD, ed. Atlas of Common Pain Syndromes. Philadelphia, WB Saunders, 2002:158-160.
13. Yang S-C, Shao P-L, Hsueh P-R, et al. Successful treatment of Candida tropicalis arthritis, osteomyelitis and costochondritis with caspofungin and fluconazole in a recipient of bone marrow transplantation. Acta Paediatr 2006;95:629-630.
14. Wehrmacher WH. The painful anterior chest wall syndromes. Med Clin North Am 1958;38:111-118.
15. Szántó D, Szücs G, Bíró BP, Priska M. Degenerative chondroarthropathy of the sternocostal joint following heart surgery. Orv Hetil 1994;135:2639-2642.
16. Epstein SE, Gerber LH, Borer JS. Chest wall syndrome: a common cause of unexplained cardiac pain. JAMA 1979;241:2793-2797.
17. Levine PR, Mascette AM. Musculoskeletal chest pain in patients with "angina:" a prospective study. South Med J 1989;82:580-591.
18. Wise CM, Semble EL, Dalton CB. Musculoskeletal chest wall syndromes in patients with noncardiac chest pain: a study of 100 patients. Arch Phys Med Rehabil 1992;73:147-149.
19. Cayley WE Jr. Diagnosing the cause of chest pain. Am Fam Physician 2005;72:2012-2021.
20. Swap CJ, Nagurney JT. Value and limitations of chest pain history in the evaluation of patients with suspected acute coronary syndromes. JAMA 2005;294:2623-2629.
21. Scobie BA. Costochondral pain in gastroenterologic practice. N Engl J Med 1976;295:1261.
22. Lavey EB, Winkle RA. Continuing disability of patients with chest pain and normal coronary arteriograms. J Chron Dis 1979;32:191-196.
23. Papanicolau MN, Calif RM, Hlatky MA, et al. Prognostic implications of angiographically normal and insignificant narrowed coronary arteries. Am J Cardiol 1986;58:1181-1187.
24. van Schalkwyk AJ, van Wingerden JJ. A variant of Tietze's syndrome occurring after reconstructive breast surgery. Aesthetic Plast Surg 1998;22:430-432.
25. Mendelson G, Mendelson H, Horowitz SF, et al. Can ^{99m}technetium methylene diphosphonate bone scans objectively document costochondritis? Chest 1997;111:1600-1602.
26. Semble EL, Wise CM. Chest pain: a rheumatologist's perspective. South Med J 1988;81:64-68.
27. Roberts-Thomson KC, Iyngkaran G, Fraser RJ. Intra-articular glucocorticoid injection: an unusual cause of transient hypophosphatemia. Rheumatol Int 2006;27:95-96.

Intercostal Neuralgia 99

Susan J. Dreyer, MD

DEFINITION

Intercostal neuralgia is pain in the chest region emanating from an intercostal nerve. The pain is typically a sharp, shooting, or burning pain radiating around the chest wall. It can be accompanied by altered sensitivity to touch, such as allodynia or an area of hyperalgesia. Intercostal neuralgia occurs commonly after thoracotomy.[1-4] It can also be seen in elderly debilitated patients without a known precipitating event.[5] Other causes include rib trauma, benign periosteal lipoma,[6] and pregnancy.[7]

Intercostal nerves are peripheral nerves that run along with the vascular bundle on the inferior surface of each rib (Fig. 99-1). Intercostal nerves are derived from the ventral rami of the first through twelfth thoracic nerves (Fig. 99-2), with the first, second, third, and twelfth being atypical. Only 17% of intercostal nerves were found in the classic subcostal position in one study.[8] In Hardy's study, a midcostal location was the most prevalent at 73%; an additional 10% were supracostal. The intercostal nerve gives off four main branches as it travels anteriorly: gray rami communicantes, posterior cutaneous branch, lateral cutaneous division, and anterior cutaneous division.

SYMPTOMS

Chest pain is the cardinal symptom. Because intercostal neuralgia involves a peripheral nerve, the pain is neuropathic rather than nociceptive. Neuropathic pain is often unrelenting, shooting, burning, and deep. The International Association for the Study of Pain defines neuropathic pain as "pain initiated or caused by a primary lesion or dysfunction in the nervous system."[9] Neuropathic pain is characterized by three symptoms: dysesthesias, paroxysmal pain, and allodynia.[10] Dysesthetic pain is an abnormal sensation described as unpleasant. Patients commonly use terms such as aching, cramping, pressure, and heat to describe a dysesthetic pain.[11] Paroxysmal pain is pain that comes in waves and is often described as lancinating or electric. Allodynia is the abnormal perception of pain after a normally nonpainful mechanical or thermal stimulus.[11] Patients with allodynia may respond to light touch with an exaggerated pain response or report a sensation of heat when a cold stimulus is applied.

Intercostal neuralgia pain is unilateral. It is common (up to 81%) after thoracotomy for coronary artery bypass grafting to the internal thoracic artery as well as after thoracotomy for tumor excision.[3,4] During thoracotomy (either open or video-assisted thoracoscopic surgery), the intercostal nerve may be directly injured during rib resection, compressed by a retractor, or later entrapped by a healing rib fracture. Intercostal neuralgia may follow other forms of chest trauma. It may mimic the pain of shingles (herpes zoster) but without the rash and can occur without significant trauma in the elderly.

The mechanism of neural injury may be due to ectopic signals from neural "sprouts" after axonal injury. This new nerve growth may become a pain generator, especially if it becomes entrapped in scar tissue, forming a neuroma. Another mechanism may be compression or disruption of the nervi nervorum afferents in the connective tissue covering, producing a peripheral neuropathic pain.

PHYSICAL EXAMINATION

Much of the physical examination in intercostal neuralgia is done to exclude other sources of pain. First, it is important to exclude cardiac and other visceral sources of chest pain (Table 99-1). Although point tenderness is uncommon during myocardial infarction, the presence of point tenderness does not exclude significant cardiac disease. In intercostal neuralgia, there are no constitutional signs, such as fever, dyspnea, diaphoresis, or

549

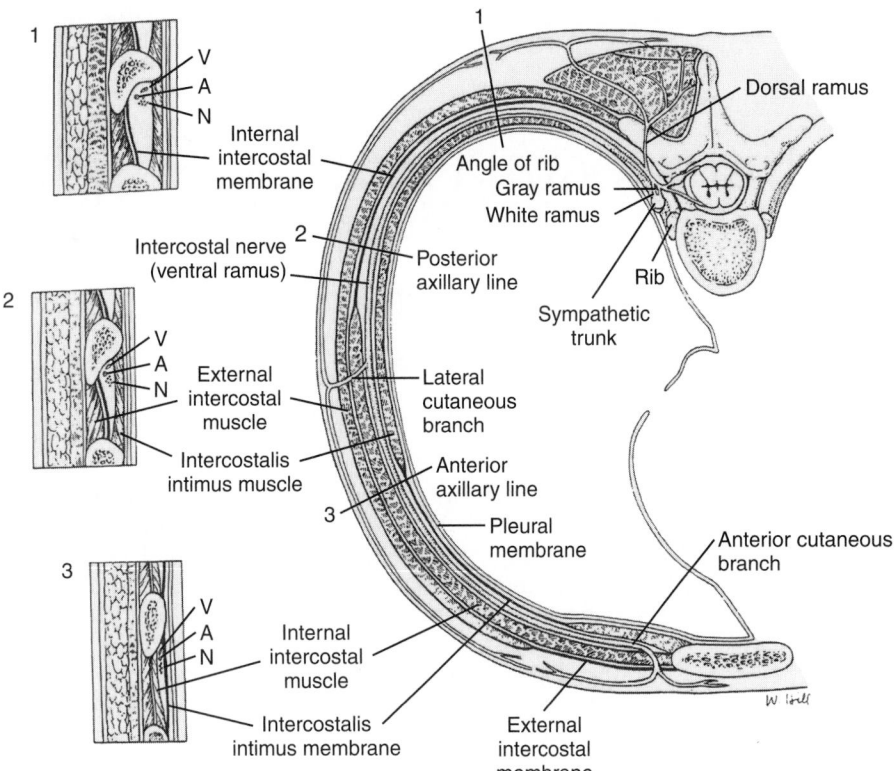

FIGURE 99-1. Intercostal nerve location. The intercostal nerve (N) runs along the inferior rib with the artery (A) and vein (V). (Reprinted with permission from Chung J. Thoracic pain. In Sinatra RS, Hord A, Ginsberg C, Preble L, eds. Acute Pain. St. Louis, Mosby, 1992:230.)

shortness of breath. Cardiopulmonary examination should be normal or stable if prior cardiovascular or pulmonary disease exists.

Intercostal neuralgia is common after thoracotomy.[1-3] Pain that recurs after a pain-free period that follows a thoracotomy for tumor resection is likely (90%) to be

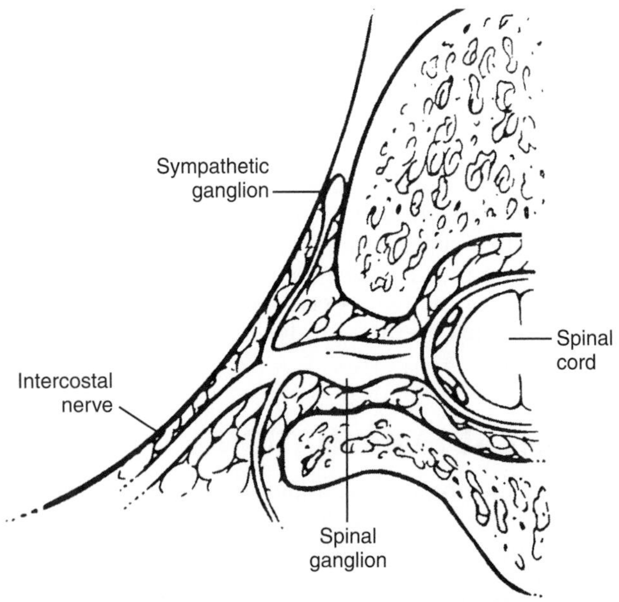

FIGURE 99-2. Intercostal nerves are derived from the ventral rami of the first through twelfth thoracic nerves. (Reprinted with permission from Saberski LR. Cryoneurolysis in clinical practice. In Waldman S, ed. Interventional Pain Management, 2nd ed. Philadelphia, WB Saunders, 2001:226-242.)

due to tumor recurrence. On the other hand, pain that persists for months or years after thoracotomy is most likely (70%) intercostal neuralgia.[12]

Once the chest pain has been determined to be neuromusculoskeletal, the task becomes one of differentiation of intercostal neuralgia from thoracic radiculopathy, herpes zoster, rib fracture, costochondritis, and local contusion. History of trauma, ecchymosis, crepitus, and point tenderness over a rib suggests rib fracture. If the trauma was minor, a contusion or intercostal neuralgia may be the source of discomfort. Contusions typically improve quickly during a period of weeks and are responsive to simple analgesics, such as acetaminophen and nonsteroidal anti-inflammatory medications. Pain from intercostal neuralgia persists and can be quite refractory to acetaminophen, nonsteroidal anti-inflammatory drugs, and even low-dose narcotics.

Careful palpation along the thoracotomy scar or rib may reveal a neuroma with the presence of a Tinel sign. Larger neuromas can often be visualized on magnetic resonance imaging. Sensory examination often reveals a small (1 to 2 cm) band of dermatomal sensory loss.

Examination of the thoracic spine reveals full active range of motion without tenderness. In contrast, thoracic radiculopathy may be accompanied by pain with range of motion and at times thoracic spinal tenderness. Still, pain from thoracic radiculopathy is similar in quality and distribution to intercostal neuralgia. Active denervation potentials in the paraspinal muscles at the affected site confirm a radicular rather than a peripheral (intercostal nerve) source of the pain. Advanced imaging

TABLE 99-1 Other Causes of Chest Pain

Cardiovascular
Myocardial ischemia
Pericarditis
Aortic dissection

Pulmonary
Pneumonia
Pneumothorax
Pleurisy
Pulmonary embolus
Tumor

Gastrointestinal
Esophageal
    Esophagitis
    Reflux
    Perforation
    Spasm
    Cancer
Biliary
    Cholelithiasis
    Cholecystitis
    Cholangitis
    Colic
Pancreatic
    Pancreatitis
    Cancer
Intestinal
    Peptic ulcer
    Gastritis
    Cancer

Musculoskeletal
Vertebral compression fracture
Tietze syndrome
Thoracic radiculopathy
Thoracic disc herniation
Cervical disc herniation
Costochondritis
Rib fracture
Costovertebral pain
Chest contusion
Spondylitis

Infective
Herpes zoster

Psychiatric
Depression
Anxiety
Hyperventilation

Renal
Nephrolithiasis
Pyelonephritis
Tumor

often confirms a thoracic disc herniation or spinal stenosis as the source of the neural compression in thoracic radiculopathy (see Chapter 39).

Intercostal neuralgia is distinct from postherpetic neuralgia (shingles), and no herpes zoster virus can be identified in cases of intercostal neuralgia. Furthermore, in most cases of shingles, the chest pain is followed within a matter of days to weeks by a vesicular, linear eruption. The more debilitating pain of postherpetic neuralgia follows the skin lesions of shingles.

FUNCTIONAL LIMITATIONS

The pain of intercostal neuralgia is commonly mild to moderate but can be debilitating because it may interfere with one's ability to comfortably wear clothes. In one study, nearly 10% of post-thoracotomy patients observed for a mean of 19.5 months had moderate to severe pain that required daily analgesics, nerve blocks, relaxation therapy, acupuncture, or referral to a pain clinic.[4] The pain may also interfere with sleep. Trunk motion may stimulate the intercostal nerve, especially if a neuroma has formed. As a result, patients may begin restricting their activities.

DIAGNOSTIC STUDIES

Final diagnosis of intercostal neuralgia is often one of exclusion. Depending on which intercostal nerve is involved, chest pain from intercostal neuralgia may require an initial workup such as electrocardiography, cardiac enzyme analysis, cardiac computed tomography or magnetic resonance imaging, and other testing to exclude a cardiac source. In the case of pain with a history of chest malignant disease, chest radiography, computed tomography, and bronchoscopy may be necessary to exclude recurrence of tumor. In patients whose history includes chest trauma, rib radiographs and at times bone scans help identify rib fractures.

Thoracic magnetic resonance imaging can exclude a disc herniation in an anatomically related area. Recall that it is not uncommon to identify asymptomatic disc herniations. In cases in which the disc protrusion does not cause clear compression but is abutting a thoracic nerve in the painful distribution, electrodiagnostic testing can exclude thoracic radiculopathy. Lesions of the intercostal nerve do not cause denervation in the thoracic paraspinal muscles.

When a postoperative neuroma is suspected, careful palpation often reveals a Tinel sign. Magnetic resonance imaging of the suspected area may reveal the neuroma. Small neuromas may be missed on magnetic resonance examination only to be identified later at the time of surgical resection.

Historical red flags including history of malignant disease, unexplained weight loss, malaise, and severe night pain raise the index of suspicion for rib metastases rather than intercostal neuralgia as the cause of the patient's chest pain. Appropriate oncologic workup, such as bone scans, laboratory investigation, and at times positron emission tomographic scans, should be performed.

Differential Diagnosis

Thoracic radiculopathy

Malignant neoplasm (primary or metastatic)

Rib fracture

Vertebral compression fracture

Chest wall contusion

Postherpetic neuralgia

Shingles

Referred pain from cardiac, pulmonary, vascular, or gastrointestinal disease

  Angina

  Aortic dissection

  Myocardial infarction

  Esophageal disorders

  Cholecystitis

  Peptic ulcer disease

  Pancreatitis

  Biliary colic

  Pleurisy

  Pulmonary embolism

  Pneumothorax

Costochondritis

Tietze syndrome

Nephrolithiasis

Pyelonephritis

Costovertebral or costochondral arthritis

Spondylitis

TREATMENT

Initial

Thoracic radiculopathy, postherpetic neuralgia, and intercostal neuralgia are all forms of neuropathic pain, and they share many initial conservative treatment options. Principles of treatment of neuropathic pain in general, rather than a specific disease state, are employed.[13,14] Typically, drugs have not been specifically tested on populations of patients with intercostal neuralgia. Instead, physicians are left to extrapolate the data from treatment of other sources of neuropathic pain and to apply those principles in choosing medication to be used for this population. Often, neuropathic pain responds poorly to acetaminophen, nonsteroidal anti-inflammatory drugs, and low-dose narcotics, in contrast to nociceptive pain.[15,16] However, if the pain is mild to moderate, these agents are often tried first. Topical agents may be effective when there is significant allodynia or dysesthesia. The patient may need a family member to help apply the topical agent because it may be difficult to reach the involved area. Capsaicin creams are available both over-the-counter and by prescription. They require frequent application three or four times a day and may initially cause an exacerbation of pain as substance P is depleted. Topical lidocaine applied as a gel, eutectic mixture of local anesthetics (EMLA), or patch (Lidoderm) is another alternative.[17]

Tricyclic antidepressants (e.g., amitriptyline, nortriptyline, desipramine) have been used for neuropathic pain for decades.[18] The dosage for analgesia is typically lower than that required to treat depression. Onset of action may be in days to weeks. The mechanism of action in neuropathic pain is believed to be modulation of descending inhibitory pathways by selective inhibition of norepinephrine or serotonin reuptake. Tricyclic antidepressants all have anticholinergic effects and may cause confusion, increase the risk of falls and injury, and result in urinary retention. For these reasons, it is recommended that amitriptyline be avoided in persons older than 65 years. Despite this, amitriptyline (Elavil) is still a widely prescribed tricyclic antidepressant for neuropathic pain; it is usually started at 10 mg at bedtime and titrated upward as tolerated at 2- to 3-day intervals. Newer antidepressants such as duloxetine (Cymbalta) are approved for treatment of painful diabetic peripheral neuropathy and may be a better choice for elderly or debilitated patients with neuropathic pain.

Anticonvulsants are another mainstay for treatment of neuropathic pain. Anticonvulsants may work in several ways, including suppression of paroxysmal discharges and overall neuronal hyperexcitability.[19] Older agents like carbamazepine and phenytoin have a narrow therapeutic window and risks of serious adverse drug reactions. These agents require careful monitoring if they are used. Bone marrow suppression occurs in up to 1% of patients, and severe dermatologic reactions like Stevens-Johnson syndrome and epidermal necrolysis have also been reported with carbamazepine. Newer anticonvulsants, such as gabapentin (Neurontin) and pregabalin (Lyrica), are often chosen for their more favorable side effect profiles, efficacy, and limited interaction with other drugs. Gabapentin and pregabalin commonly cause sedation and may cause edema; both are indicated for neuropathic pain of diabetic peripheral neuropathy. These agents do not require blood samples for drug levels to be monitored. Dosing typically begins low and at night. For example, many practitioners start with gabapentin 300 mg at bedtime and titrate to 600 to 800 mg two or three times daily. At times, even higher doses are prescribed. Dosages are reduced in patients with renal insufficiency. Gabapentin and other anticonvulsants should be tapered before discontinuance. Like gabapentin and pregabalin, topiramate has also been used off-label for intercostal neuralgia.[20]

Narcotics are often required for intercostal neuralgia. Adequate analgesia is needed to promote continued activity levels and to prevent deconditioning from disuse. Initial treatment should be with short-acting agents. Treatment of intercostal neuralgia can be protracted, and patients are often switched to long-acting agents for maintenance. If the pain is progressive, one should re-evaluate the diagnosis and reconsider the possibility of occult tumor.

In refractory cases of neuropathic pain, clonidine, an adrenergic agonist, and ketamine, an *N*-methyl-D-aspartate (NMDA) receptor antagonist, may be prescribed by pain specialists.[10]

Rehabilitation

Physical and occupational therapy can be instrumental in combating disuse deconditioning. Also, desensitization techniques may be employed. Psychological consultation in patients who exhibit signs of anxiety, depression, or panic disorder may be beneficial to address the negative impact of these psychological stressors on the pain or the patient's behavior in response to the pain. Relaxation therapy and acupuncture have also been employed.[4]

Procedures

Local infiltration of a neuroma with corticosteroids and local anesthetics, intercostal nerve blocks, indwelling epidural catheters, and spinal nerve injections have all been used to control the pain associated with intercostal neuralgia when adequate relief is not achieved with oral and topical medications.

If a focal neuroma is identified, infiltration with several milliliters of local anesthetic with 40 mg of a long-acting corticosteroid, such as methylprednisolone (Depo-Medrol) or triamcinolone (Kenalog), often results in significant analgesia. In addition to its potent anti-inflammatory effect, the corticosteroid may also reduce neural discharges. Care must be taken during the injection to avoid pneumothorax.

Intercostal nerve blocks should be performed with appropriate monitoring. There are several techniques well described in interventional pain management books.[21] One common technique is to position the patient prone and to identify the angle of the rib just lateral to the sacrospinalis muscles (Fig. 99-3). The skin is moved up over the rib, and the needle is introduced down onto the posterior periosteum of the rib and then walked inferior. At the angle of the rib, the rib is typically 8 mm thick. Great care must be taken not to overpenetrate and cause a pneumothorax; 3 to 5 mL of local anesthetic is instilled along with 20 to 40 mg of a long-acting corticosteroid, such as triamcinolone. The needle is then

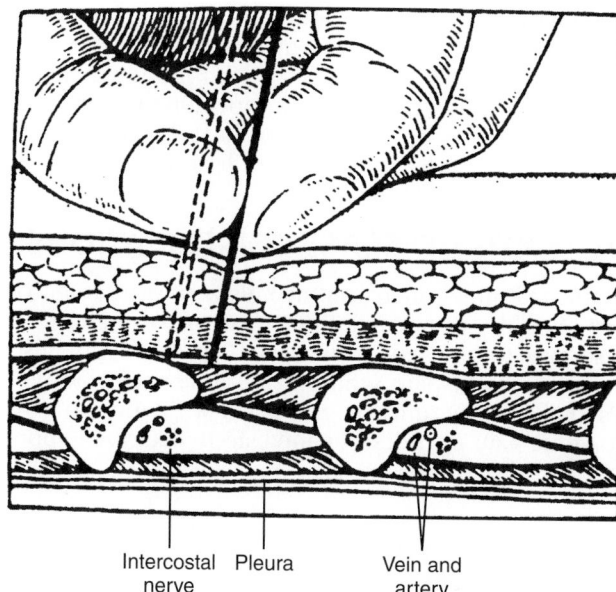

FIGURE 99-3. Intercostal nerve injection technique. The needle is advanced over the rib. Initial contact indicates posterior depth of the nerve. The skin and needle are then moved inferiorly off the rib, with care taken to avoid advancement of the needle too far, causing a pneumothorax. (Reprinted with permission from Chung J. Thoracic pain. In Sinatra RS, Hord A, Ginsberg C, Preble L, eds. Acute Pain. St. Louis, Mosby, 1992:231.)

Labels: Intercostal nerve   Pleura   Vein and artery

withdrawn slightly and moved back over the rib before safe removal. Another approach is midaxillary and may be preferred in postoperative and acutely ill patients who cannot be easily positioned prone.

If symptoms are well controlled with intercostal nerve blocks but recur, neurolytic injection of phenol or alcohol has been used to denervate the peripheral nerve.[21] Indwelling epidural catheters have been used to provide regional anesthesia with minimal drug use. A report of pregnant patients who developed intercostal neuralgias found this technique safe and effective.[7]

Cryotherapy involves another way of interrupting the peripheral nerve's ability to transmit pain by freezing it. Cryotherapy has been used on neuromas and the involved intercostal nerve.[22]

Spinal cord stimulators have been implanted for intercostal neuralgia, but with less success than in neuropathic pain due to diabetic peripheral neuropathy and causalgia.[23] Chronic post-thoracotomy pain and intercostal neuralgia can be difficult to control. In one study, up to 40% of post-thoracotomy patients required pain procedures including trigger point injections, intercostal nerve blocks, epidural steroid injections, and stellate ganglion blocks.[2]

Surgery

Surgical resection of a neuroma can be effective but should be reserved for cases that have failed more conservative care and have demonstrated a temporary response to intercostal blocks. Dorsal root entry zone ablation involves surgical destruction of nociceptive secondary neurons in the spinal cord when pain is not adequately controlled with medical therapy.[24,25] The technique involves laminectomy with intradural exposure of the spinal cord. With an operating microscope, a radiofrequency probe is used to heat the dorsal horn of the affected side with a series of lesions.

POTENTIAL DISEASE COMPLICATIONS

Untreated upper intercostal neuralgia can lead to a frozen shoulder as patients limit their use of the arm in response to the pain. Intercostal neuralgia can also cause a chronic pain syndrome with its comorbidities. Psychosocial dysfunction associated with chronic neuropathic pain includes impaired sleep, decreased appetite, and diminished libido.

POTENTIAL TREATMENT COMPLICATIONS

All medications carry risks. Many of the medications used for neuropathic pain (anticonvulsants, tricyclic antidepressants, narcotics) cause sedation. Injections in the area carry the risk of pneumothorax, bleeding, and infection. Surgical techniques may result in further nerve damage and pain, infection, bleeding, and pneumothorax.

References

1. Landreneau RJ, Mack MJ, Hazelrigg SR, et al. Prevalence of chronic pain after pulmonary resection by thoracotomy or video-assisted thoracic surgery. J Thorac Cardiovasc Surg 1994;107:1079-1085.
2. Keller SM, Carp NZ, Levy MN, et al. Chronic post thoracotomy pain. J Cardiovasc Surg (Torino) 1994;35(Suppl 1):161-164.
3. Mailis A, Umana M, Feindel CM. Anterior intercostal nerve damage after coronary artery bypass graft surgery with the use of internal thoracic artery graft. Ann Thorac Surg 2000;69:1455-1458.
4. Dajczman E, Gordan A, Kreisman H, et al. Long-term postthoracotomy pain. Chest 1991;99:270-274.
5. Jubelt B. Viral infections. In Rowland P, ed. Merritt's Neurology, 11th ed. Philadelphia, JB Lippincott, 2005:Chapter 24.
6. Kim HK. Intercostal neuralgia caused by a periosteal lipoma of the rib. Ann Thorac Surg 2006;85:1901-1903.
7. Samlaska S, Dews TE. Long-term epidural analgesia for pregnancy-induced intercostal neuralgia. Pain 1995;62:295-298.
8. Hardy PAJ. Anatomical variation in the position of the proximal intercostal nerve. Br J Anaesth 1988;61:338-339.
9. International Association for the Study of Pain. IASP pain terminology. Available at: http://www.iasp-pain.org. Accessed February 24, 2007.
10. Milch RA. Neuropathic pain: implications for the surgeon. Surg Clin 2005;85:1-10.
11. Ropper AH, Brown RH. Pain. In Victor M, Ropper AH, eds. Adams and Victor's Principles of Neurology, 8th ed. New York, McGraw-Hill, 2005:Chapter 8.
12. McGarvey ML, Cheung AT, Stecker MM. Neurologic complications of cardiac surgery. UpToDate, April 28, 2006.
13. Woolf CJ. Pain: moving from symptom control toward mechanism-specific pharmacologic management. Ann Intern Med 2004; 140:441-451.
14. Smith HS, Sang CN. The evolving nature of neuropathic pain: individualizing treatment. Eur J Pain 2002;6(Suppl B):13-18.
15. Beydoun A. Neuropathic pain: from mechanisms to treatment strategies. J Pain Symptom Manage 2003;25(5 suppl):S1-3.
16. Portenoy RK, Forbes K, Lussier D. Difficult pain problems: an integrated approach. In Doyle D, Hanks G, MacDonald N. Oxford Textbook of Palliative Medicine, 2nd ed. New York, Oxford University Press, 1998:438-458.
17. Devers A, Galer BS. Topical lidocaine patch relieves a variety of neuropathic pain conditions: an open label study. Clin J Pain 2000;16:205-208.
18. Onghena P, Van Houdenhove B. Antidepressant induced analgesia in chronic non-malignant pain: a meta-analysis of 39 placebo controlled studies. Pain 1992;49:205-219.
19. Tremon-Lukats IW, Megeff C, Backonja MM. Anticonvulsants for neuropathic pain syndromes: mechanisms of action and place in therapy. Drugs 2000;60:1029-1052.
20. Bajwa ZH, Cami N, Warfield CA, et al. Topiramate relieves refractory intercostal neuralgia. Neurology 1999;52:1917-1921.
21. Kopacz DJ, Thompson GE. Intercostal nerve block. In Waldman S, ed. Interventional Pain Management, 2nd ed. Philadelphia, WB Saunders, 2001:401-408.
22. Saberski LR. Cryoneurolysis in clinical practice. In Waldman S, ed. Interventional Pain Management, 2nd ed. Philadelphia, WB Saunders, 2001:226-242.
23. Kumar K, Toth C, Nath RK. Spinal cord stimulation for chronic pain in peripheral neuropathy. Surg Neurol 1996;46:363-369.
24. Brewer R, Bedlack R, Massey E. Diabetic thoracic radiculopathy: an unusual cause of post-thoracotomy pain. Pain 2003;103:221-223.
25. Spaić M, Ivanović S, Slavik E, Antić B. DREZ (dorsal root entry zone) surgery for the treatment of the postherpetic intercostal neuralgia. Acta Chir Iugosl 2004;51:53-57.

Tietze Syndrome 100

Marta Imamura, MD, and Satiko Tomikawa Imamura, MD, PhD

Marta Imamura, MD, and Satiko Tomikawa Imamura, MD, PhD

Synonyms

Parasternal chondrodynia
Costochondral junction syndrome
Thoracochondralgia
Chondropathia tuberosa
Costal chondritis

ICD-9 Code

733.6   Tietze disease; costochondral junction syndrome and costochondritis

DEFINITION

Tietze syndrome is defined as a benign, self-limited, nonsuppurative, localized, painful swelling of the upper costal cartilages that is of unknown etiology.[1-11] It affects the costochondral, costosternal, or sternoclavicular joints.[2,5-7,9] The manubriosternal and xiphisternal joints are less frequently affected.[5,10] First described by a German surgeon in Breslau, Alexander Tietze, in 1921,[12] it is different from costosternal syndrome.[5-11,13,14] Tietze syndrome is a rare cause of benign anterior chest wall pain associated with local swelling of the involved costal cartilages[5,6,14] (Fig. 100-1); on the other hand, costosternal syndrome is a frequent cause of benign anterior chest wall pain without a local swelling of the involved costochondral joints.[5-11,13,14] Tietze syndrome is also typically described in young adults and is a disease of the second and third decades of life.[10,14] Although it is not common, Tietze syndrome may also appear in children, infants,[10,15] and elderly people.[16] It affects both men and women in a 1:1 ratio,[4-6,9,10,17] as opposed to a male-to-female ratio of 2 to 3:1 for costosternal syndrome.[9,10] Lesions are unilateral and single in more than 80% of patients,[4,10] and the second and third costal cartilages are most commonly involved.[1,4,6,9-14] Costosternal syndrome, though, involves multiple costal cartilages in 90% of patients.[5,9,10]

The pathogenesis of Tietze syndrome is unknown.[1-4,6,8-10] Recurrent functional overloading or microtrauma to the costal cartilages from severe coughing, heavy manual work, sporting activities,[11,18] and sudden movement of the rib cage as well as malnutrition, sprain of the intraarticular sternocostal ligament, and respiratory tract infections may influence the development of Tietze syndrome.[2,5,6,8-10,14,17] Costal swelling may be due to focal enlargement,[4,7] ventral angulation or irregular calcification of the affected costal cartilage,[4,19] and thickening of overlying muscle.[19,20] Tietze syndrome may mimic a variety of life-threatening clinical entities[4,6,17,21] and must be considered in the differential diagnosis of any painful mass in the peristernal area. Clinical awareness of this syndrome and of its benign course may minimize performance of invasive diagnostic procedures.[15]

SYMPTOMS

Clinical manifestations include the sudden or gradual onset of pain of variable intensity[3,4,10,17] in the upper anterior chest wall in association with a fusiform and tender swelling of the involved costal cartilage.[4,17] Despite descriptions that pain may radiate to the shoulder, arm, and neck,[3,4,14] its distribution is usually within the segment innervated by the afferent fibers carrying the painful impulse.[2] It is often aggravated by motion of the thoracic wall, sneezing, coughing, deep breathing, bending, exertion,[1-8,17] and lying prone or over the affected side.[10] Some patients report inability to find a comfortable position in bed and have pain on turning over in the bed.[1] Weather change, anxiety, worry, and fatigue may exacerbate the pain.[4] Symptoms are usually unilateral, with no preferential side.[3] There is no reported association with sternotomy.

PHYSICAL EXAMINATION

On physical examination, a slight firm swelling is noted at the involved site.[1-4,17] Systemic manifestations[4,6,10,15,17] and inflammation are usually absent,[1,4,5,7,10,17] but there may be local heat.[17] Pain is reproduced with active protraction or retraction of the shoulder, deep inspiration, and elevation of the arm[14] (Fig. 100-2). A unique visible, spherical, nonsuppurative, tender tumor of elastic-hard and pasty consistency can be palpated, usually over the second and third costochondral joints. Local palpation with firm pressure over the localized tender swelling reproduces the

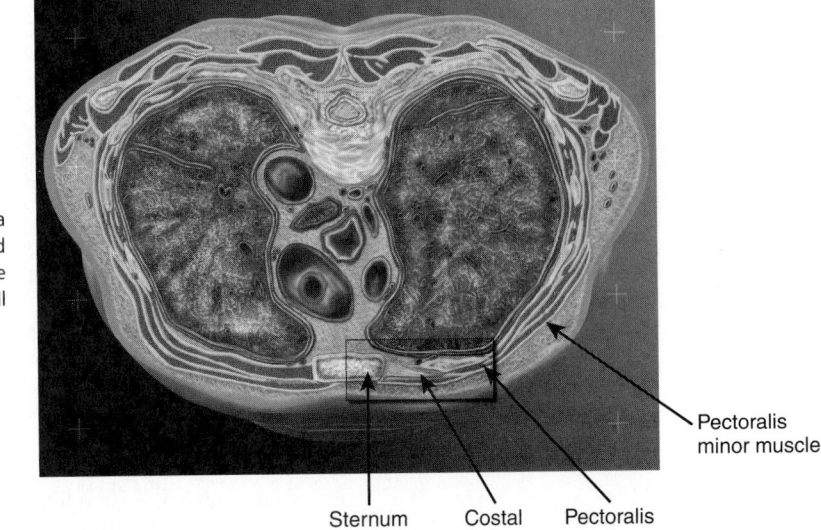

FIGURE 100-1. Schematic representation of the area of Tietze syndrome (costal cartilage, costosternal and costochondral joints) and anatomic relations with the mediastinal structures and other anterior chest wall structures.

Pectoralis minor muscle

Sternum   Costal cartilage   Pectoralis major muscle

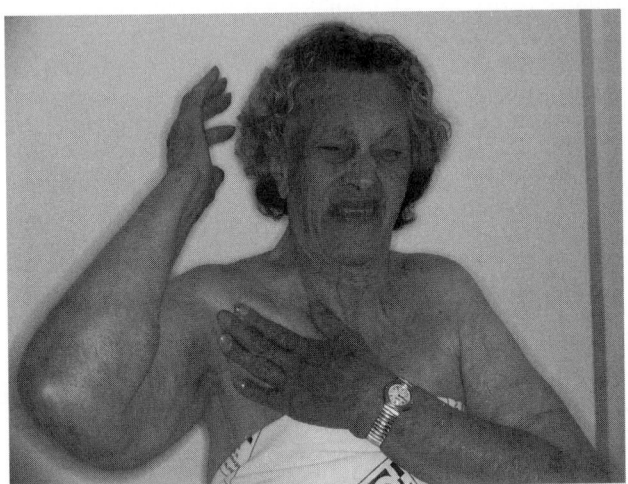

FIGURE 100-2. Reproduction of the spontaneous pain complaint during arm elevation in a patient diagnosed with Tietze syndrome.

spontaneous pain complaint[14] (Fig. 100-3). Physical examination findings of the musculoskeletal and neurologic systems of reported cases from the literature are usually normal except for the local findings.[4-6,15,17,20] Muscle strength and upper limb range of motion may be decreased because of pain. Dermatomal and subcutaneous hyperalgesia (Fig. 100-4) and hyperemia (Fig. 100-5) may be present in the involved thoracic spinal segments. The adjacent intercostal,[14] sternal, and pectoralis major and minor muscles may be tender to palpation.[16]

FUNCTIONAL LIMITATIONS

The disability produced by Tietze syndrome is usually minor, although it can be quite severe with activity restriction involving the trunk and upper limbs. Activities such as lifting, bathing, ironing, combing and brushing hair, and other activities of daily living can be very problematic. Patients who have physically vigorous jobs may need to be assigned light duty for weeks and to avoid physical efforts of the upper limbs and trunk.[1] Functional limitations may also be due to chronic pain[22]; however, even of those patients who continue to have pain after 1 year, most lead a life without disability.

DIAGNOSTIC STUDIES

Diagnosis of Tietze syndrome is essentially made on a clinical basis: anterior chest wall pain confirmed by palpation of a tender swelling at the second or third costochondral junction that reproduces the patient's complaint in the absence of another definite diagnosis.[3-5,7-9,13,17] Results of laboratory analysis, including inflammatory and immunologic parameters, are usually normal.[4-9,17] Some cases may show a slight increase in the erythrocyte sedimentation rate.[7,15,17]

Chest, rib, and sternum plain films and conventional tomograms of the costochondral junction are generally normal.[6,20,23] Plain radiographs may show cartilage enlargement on tangential views, chondral calcification, irregularities at the joint surface, osteosclerosis, and presence of osteophytes at the costal joint. However, these radiographic changes may also be found in physiologic costochondral calcifications.[24] Plain radiographs are therefore mainly indicated to rule out occult bone diseases, including tumors, low-grade infections, tender fat or lipomas, chest wall contusion, and congenital deformity.[4,14,19] Tuberculosis, chondroma, and chondrosarcoma are mostly located at the costochondral junction.[19]

Ultrasonographic findings of the affected costochondral joints are characterized by an increase of the size of the affected costal cartilage compared with the contralateral symmetric joint[25] (Fig. 100-6) and normal age- and gender-matched controls.[26] There is also a nonhomogeneous increase in the echogenicity of the diseased cartilage,[26,27] with a marginal blurring of the costal cartilage

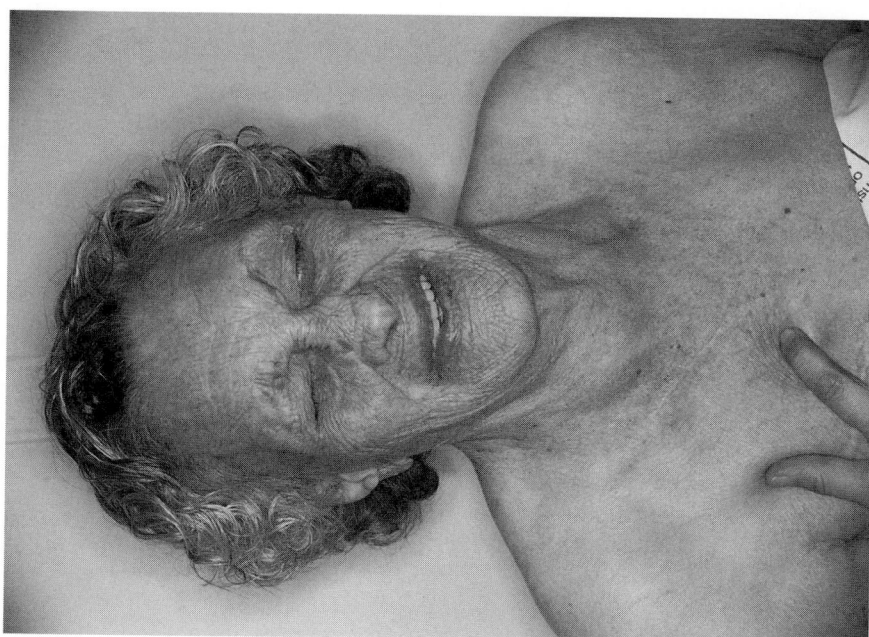

FIGURE 100-3. Local palpation with firm pressure over the localized tender swelling reproduces the spontaneous pain complaint.

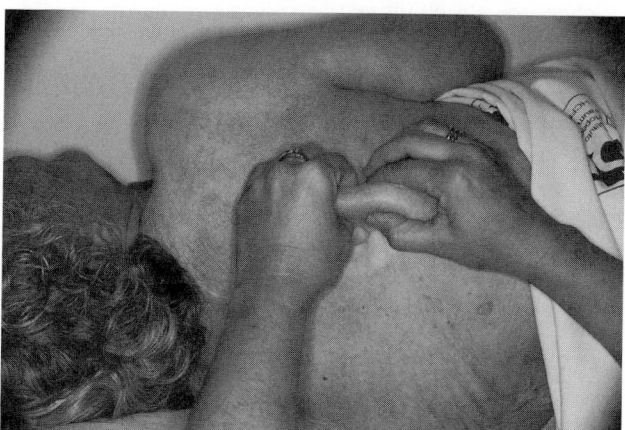

FIGURE 100-4. Subcutaneous hyperalgesia during the pinch and roll maneuver at the thoracic level.

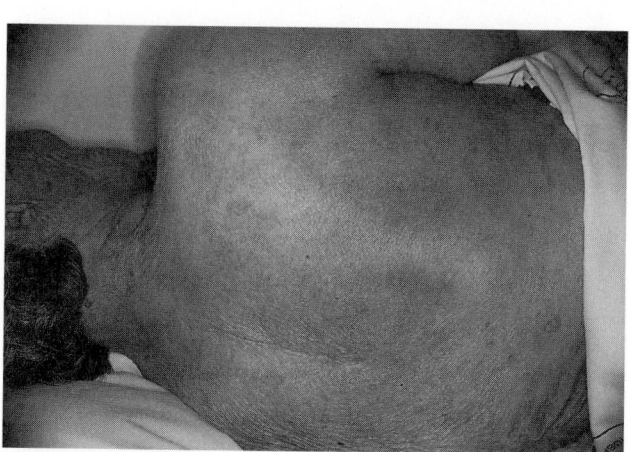

FIGURE 100-5. Hyperemia localized at the involved thoracic spinal segments after the pinch and roll maneuver.

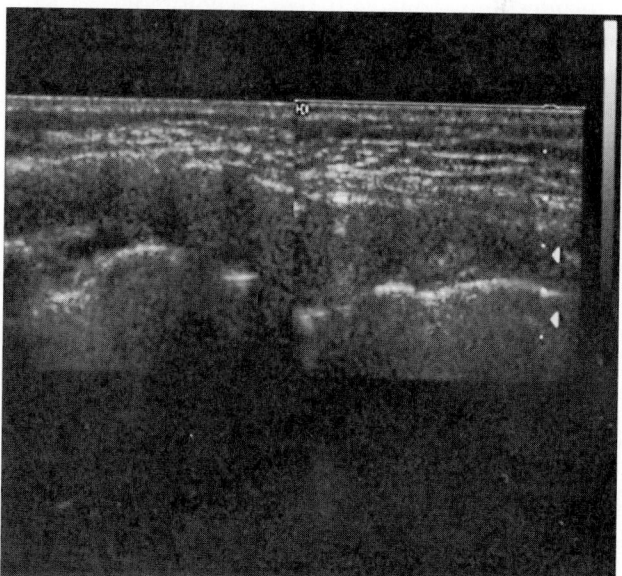

FIGURE 100-6. Comparison of the ultrasonographic findings of the affected costochondral joint (left) and the nonaffected contralateral joint (right) in an 82-year-old woman diagnosed with Tietze syndrome. The affected costochondral joint appears with a discrete increased size and as a nonhomogeneous hyperechoic cartilage with dotty, hyperreflective echoes and broad posterior acoustic shadows. (Courtesy of Marcelo Bordalo Rodrigues.)

at the painful area[27] and dotty, hyperreflective echoes and intense broad posterior acoustic shadow[26] (see Fig. 100-6). The normal ultrasonographic picture of the costal cartilage (Fig. 100-7) appears as a hypoechoic oval area with the absence of posterior acoustic shadows in the longitudinal scans[26]; in the transverse scan, the costal cartilage appears as a ribbon-shaped homogeneous hypoechogenicity with no posterior acoustic shadowing.[26]

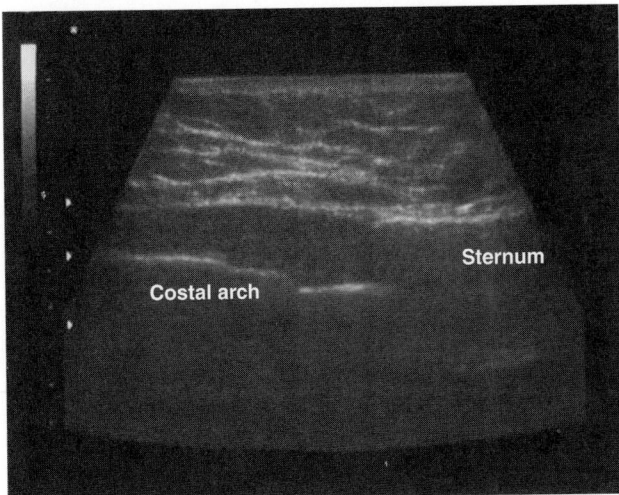

FIGURE 100-7. Normal ultrasonographic appearance of the costal cartilage. The normal costal cartilage appears as the homogeneous hypoechoic oval area between the sternum and the costal arch. (Courtesy of Marcelo Bordalo Rodrigues.)

Computed tomography of the chest is an effective non-invasive means of imaging costal cartilage and adjacent structures in patients with Tietze syndrome.[20,23,26] Costal cartilage is normally symmetric in size and orientation at any level and is normally oriented along the horizontal axis.[20] Cartilage density is uniform and greater than that of the overlying muscle but less than calcium density.[20] Reported computed tomographic abnormalities of patients with Tietze syndrome include focal enlargement of the involved costal cartilage,[6,20,23] ventral angulations,[6,17,20,23] swelling or irregular calcification of the affected costal cartilage,[20,23] perichondral soft tissue swelling, and periarticular bone sclerosis.[5,28] Computed tomographic scan is useful to exclude other possible causes of chest wall or thoracic mass lesions,[6,29,30] such as malignant lymphoma,[20,31] osteosarcoma,[32] mediastinal carcinoma,[33] chest wall metastasis,[29] infection,[30] and costal cartilage fractures.[34] Asymmetric thickening of the pectoralis major muscle simulating a chest wall mass can also be excluded.[20]

Planar bone scanning with technetium Tc 99 usually reveals intense tracer uptake, but the findings are not specific.[4,6,17,24,28] Bone scintigraphy allows the precise localization of the involved joint[6] and delineates the number of involved joints; it should be considered to rule out occult fractures of the ribs and sternum in cases of local trauma.[14]

Pinhole skeletal scintigraphy seems to enhance diagnostic specificity.[24] It is able to show a characteristic appearance of a drumstick-like pattern in acute cases and a C-shaped or inverted C–shaped uptake in the chronically affected costal cartilage.[24]

Magnetic resonance imaging of the joints is indicated if an occult mass is suspected.[9,14]

The histopathologic characteristics of costal cartilage in Tietze syndrome are usually normal[17] or nonspecific.[3,6,7,17] These characteristics include increased vascularity and degenerative changes with patchy loss of ground substance leading to a fibrillar appearance.[6,28,35] Degenerative changes occur with the formation of clefts, which may undergo calcification.[1,28,35]

Differential Diagnosis

Anterior Chest Wall Pain of Local Origin

Costosternal syndrome

Trauma: dislocation and fractures of the ribs, sternum, clavicle, costal cartilage, costochondral or sternoclavicular joint

Arthritis: osteoarthritis, rheumatoid arthritis, ankylosing spondylitis, Reiter syndrome, psoriatic arthritis, SAPHO (*s*ynovitis, *a*cne, *p*ustulosis, *h*yperostosis, and *o*steitis) syndrome, gout

Infection: osteomyelitis, low-grade infection of the costal cartilage (tuberculosis, syphilis, typhoid and paratyphoid infections, blastomycosis, actinomycosis, cryptococcosis, brucellosis)

Tumors of the costochondral cartilages: benign—chondroma, multiple exostoses, lipomas; malignant—Hodgkin and non-Hodgkin lymphoma, metastatic bone diseases (carcinoma of breast, lung, thyroid, kidney, or prostate), multiple myeloma, plasmacytoma, thymoma, chondrosarcoma

Myofascial pain syndrome at the anterior chest wall: sternal, pectoralis major, pectoralis minor, intercostal, scalene, sternocleidomastoid (sternal head), subclavius, and cervical iliocostal muscles

Others: slipping rib syndrome, condensing osteitis of the clavicle, congenital sternoclavicular malformations, xiphoidalgia syndrome, T1-12 radiculopathy, intercostal neuritis (postherpetic neuralgia)

Anterior Chest Pain of Visceral Origin

Cardiac: myocardial infarction, angina pectoris, stenocardia

Pulmonary: pneumonia, pulmonary embolism, pleurisy, lung abscess, atelectasis, spontaneous pneumothorax

Breast: cyclic breast pain, duct ectasia, breast carcinoma

Abdominal: peptic duodenal ulcer, epigastric hernia, gastritis or pancreatitis, acute cholecystitis, diffuse peritonitis

TREATMENT

Initial

Treatment is symptomatic because the pathogenesis of the disease is still unclear.[3,4,6,16,17] The natural history of patients diagnosed with true Tietze syndrome is, in general, good and benign as a result of the self-limited character of the condition. In most cases, pain disappears spontaneously within a few weeks and swelling in a few months[17] without treatment.[9] Symptoms may be exacerbated after manual work and severe cough. During this period, the use of an elastic rib belt may also provide symptomatic relief and help protect the costosternal joints from additional trauma.[9,14] Initial treatment of the pain and functional disability associated with Tietze syndrome should include simple oral analgesics, such as acetaminophen and oral or topical nonsteroidal anti-inflammatory drugs, alone[6,9,13,16] or in combination with codeine[5,8,9,17] or tramadol. Reassurance about the benign nature of the disorder and the diagnosis of a non–life-threatening but real and well-recognized musculoskeletal pain disease can often by itself reduce the anxiety and fears and lead to symptomatic pain relief.[2-5,8-11,13,17,36] Avoidance of iatrogenic worries is usually helpful.[36] Removal of aggravating and perpetuating factors, including physical efforts of the upper limbs and trunk, chronic cough, and bronchospasm, and improved nutrition are also important.[1,5,8-9,16] Human calcitonin at the dosage of 0.25 mg/day was given for a course of 1 month to five women diagnosed with Tietze syndrome who had intense pain not relieved by conventional treatment.[37] Three patients had complete remission of symptoms and imaging findings, and two patients had improved symptoms with disappearance of pain.[37]

Rehabilitation

Physical modalities, including local superficial heat for 20 minutes, two or three times a day, or ice for 10 to 15 minutes, three or four times a day, can be performed until symptoms are improved.[3,14,16] Heat and cold are equally effective, and choice of the modality relies on the patient's preference and tolerance. Transcutaneous electrical nerve stimulation and electroacupuncture may be applied over the painful area.[16] Electroacupuncture is applied by introduction of the acupuncture disposable needle over the skin points of lower electrical skin resistance[16] that are located within the involved spinal segments. Galvanic or faradic low-frequency electrical currents are applied at the inserted needle.[16] Administration of corticosteroids by iontophoresis may provide more prolonged pain relief.[13] Gentle, pain-free range of motion exercises should be introduced as soon as tolerated.[14] Vigorous exercises should be avoided if they exacerbate the patient's symptoms.[14] Proper posture during sitting or working activities should be restored.[5,8,9] Inactivation of associated pectoralis major trigger points followed by relaxation and stretching exercises with relaxation of the involved muscles may also be helpful. Stretching exercises of the pectoralis major muscle can be performed by the standing pushup in the corner for 10 seconds. This exercise can be repeated for 1 or 2 minutes several times a day.[8] Vapocoolant spray applied to the involved areas may also relieve chest wall pain.[8] Patients should be instructed to avoid improper posture or repetitive misuse of chest wall muscles.[8]

Psychological and psychopharmacologic treatment should be considered for patients with continuing symptoms and disability, especially if these are associated with abnormal health beliefs, depressed mood, panic attacks, or other symptoms such as fatigue and palpitations.[36] Both cognitive-behavioral therapy and selective reuptake inhibitors have been shown to be effective.[36] Tricyclic antidepressants are helpful in reducing reports of pain in patients with chest pain and normal coronary arteries.[36]

Procedures

Most patients respond to nonsteroidal anti-inflammatory drugs, heat, and activity modification. For patients who do not respond to the initial and rehabilitation treatment modalities, however, a local anesthetic[2,4,6] and steroid injection can be performed as the next symptom control maneuver.[2,5,6,8,9,11,13,14,17,26] Injection of the costal cartilage is performed by placing the patient in the supine position.[14,26] Proper preparation with antiseptic solution of the skin overlying the affected costal cartilage is carried out with isopropyl alcohol and soluble iodine solution to swab the injection site.[26] The exact position for injection is identified by clinical and ultrasonographic examination.[26] The injection site is the point of maximum tenderness by palpation or the point of maximum cartilaginous hypertrophy by ultrasonographic examination.[26] A refrigerant spray may be used to anesthetize the overlying skin before the needle is inserted.[26] There should be limited resistance to injection.[14] If significant resistance is found, the needle should be withdrawn slightly and repositioned until the injection proceeds with only limited resistance.[14] This procedure is repeated for each affected joint.[14] After the needle is removed, a sterile pressure dressing and ice pack are placed at the injection site.[14]

Local steroid injections associated with local anesthetics have shown good therapeutic results.[26] There is an average of 82% decrease in size of the affected costal cartilage 1 week after the local anesthetic and steroid injection, and the posterior acoustic shadowing is absent.[26] Clinical examination of the injected patients detected complete resolution and substantial improvement of signs and symptoms of pain and swelling. This shows a strong correlation between clinical changes and ultrasonographic findings in patients with Tietze syndrome. An intercostal nerve block performed $1\frac{1}{2}$ to 2 inches proximal to the costochondral joint of the affected level provides even longer lasting pain relief and is indicated if other measures are not effective.[13]

Surgery

Surgical procedures are rarely necessary and indicated only if the symptomatic conservative measures failed to alleviate symptoms.[9] Surgical excision of the localized involved cartilage can be performed in severe and refractory cases.[9] Costosternal or sternoclavicular arthrodesis may be performed if conservative measures fail to provide satisfactory results.

POTENTIAL DISEASE COMPLICATIONS

Tietze syndrome is a benign condition, and complications rarely develop. It is self-limited with spontaneous recovery from the pain after a few weeks or several months[1,3,4,17] to 1 year in the majority of cases. Swelling may persist for months[17] to years.[4] The course of this condition is characterized by periods of recurrence and improvement.[1,3,4,16]

POTENTIAL TREATMENT COMPLICATIONS

The systemic complications of nonsteroidal anti-inflammatory drugs are well known and most commonly affect the gastric, hepatic, and renal systems. The major complication of the local steroid combined with local anesthetic injections is pneumothorax if the needle is placed too laterally or deeply and invades the pleural space.[14] Cardiac tamponade as well as an iatrogenic infection, although rare, can occur if, respectively, the needle is placed in the direction of the heart and strict aseptic techniques are not performed.[14] Trauma to the contents of the mediastinum remains another possibility.[14] This complication can be greatly decreased if the clinician pays close attention to accurate needle placement[14] or performs the injection with ultrasound guidance.[26]

ACKNOWLEDGMENT

The authors are deeply grateful to Marcelo Bordalo Rodrigues, MD, Director of the Radiology Department at the Orthopaedics and Traumatology Institute, Clinics Hospital of the University of São Paulo School of Medicine, for contributing to the radiologic investigation and the ultrasonographic pictures.

References

1. Geddes AK. Tietze's syndrome. Can Med Assoc J 1945;53:571-573.
2. Wehrmacher WH. The painful anterior chest wall syndromes. Med Clin North Am 1958;38:111-118.
3. Kayser HL. Tietze's syndrome: a review of the literature. Am J Med 1956;21:982-989.
4. Levey GS, Calabro JJ. Tietze's syndrome: report of two cases and review of the literature. Arthritis Rheum 1962;5:261-269.
5. Fam AG, Smythe HA. Musculoskeletal chest wall pain. Can Med Assoc J 1985;133:379-389.
6. Boehme MW, Scherbaum WA, Pfeiffer EF. Tietze's syndrome—a chameleon under the thoracic abdominal pain syndromes. Klin Wochenschr 1988;66:1142-1145.
7. Jurik AG, Graudal H. Sternocostal joint swelling—clinical Tietze's syndrome. Report of sixteen cases and review of the literature. Scand J Rheumatol 1988;17:33-42.
8. Semble EL, Wise CM. Chest pain: a rheumatologist's perspective. South Med J 1988;81:64-68.
9. Aeschlimann A, Kahn MF. Tietze's syndrome: a critical review. Clin Exp Rheumatol 1990;8:407-412.
10. Bonica JJ, Sola AF. Chest pain caused by other disorders. In Bonica JJ, ed. The Management of Pain, vol II. Philadelphia, Lea & Febiger, 1990:1114-1145.
11. Gregory PL, Biswas AC, Batt ME. Musculoskeletal problems of the chest wall in athletes. Sports Med 2002;32:235-250.
12. Tietze A. Über eine eigenartige Häufung von Fällen mit Dystrophie der Rippenknorpel. Berl Klin Wochenschr 1921;58:829-831.
13. Jensen S. Musculoskeletal causes of chest pain. Austral Fam Physician 2001;30:834-839.
14. Waldman SD. Tietze's syndrome. In Waldman SD, ed. Atlas of Common Pain Syndromes. Philadelphia, WB Saunders, 2002:158-160.
15. Mukamel M, Kornreich L, Horev G, et al. Tietze's syndrome in children and infants (clinical and laboratory observations). J Pediatr 1997;131:774-775.
16. Imamura ST, Imamura M. Síndrome de Tietze. In Cossermelli W, ed. Terapêutica em Reumatologia. São Paulo, Lemos, 2000:773-777.
17. Hiramuro-Shoji F, Wirth MA, Rockwood CA. Atraumatic conditions of the sternoclavicular joint. J Shoulder Elbow Surg 2003;12:79-88.
18. Rumball JS, Lebrun CM, Di Ciacca SR, et al. Rowing injuries. Sports Med 2005;35:537-555.
19. Jurik AG, Justesen T, Graudal H. Radiographic findings in patients with clinical Tietze syndrome. Skeletal Radiol 1987;16:517-523.
20. Edelstein G, Levitt RG, Slaker DP, et al. Computed tomography of Tietze syndrome. J Comput Assist Tomogr 1984;8:20-23.
21. Von Wichert P. Diagnosis and differential diagnosis in patients with non-coronary related chest pain. Med Klin (Munich) 2006;101:813-822.
22. Mayou RA, Bass C, Hart G, et al. Can clinical assessment of chest pain be made more therapeutic? Q J Med 2000;93:805-811.
23. Edelstein G, Levitt RG, Slaker DP, et al. CT observation of rib anomalies: spectrum of findings. J Comput Assist Tomogr 1985;9:65-72.
24. Yang W, Bahk YW, Chung SK, et al. Pinhole skeletal scintigraphic manifestations of Tietze's disease. Eur J Nucl Med 1994;21:947-952.
25. Martino F, D'Amore M, Angelelli G, et al. Echographic study of Tietze's syndrome. Clin Rheumatol 1991;10:2-4.
26. Choi YW, Im JG, Song CS, et al. Sonography of the costal cartilage: normal anatomy and preliminary clinical application. J Clin Ultrasound 1995;23:243-250.
27. Kamel M, Kotob H. Ultrasonographic assessment of local steroid injection in Tietze's syndrome. Br J Rheumatol 1997;36:547-550.
28. Honda N, Machida K, Mamiya T, et al. Scintigraphic and CT findings of Tietze's syndrome: report of a case and review of the literature. Clin Nucl Med 1989;14:606-609.
29. Seven B, Varoglu E, Cayir K, et al. Chest wall metastasis of ileal carcinoid tumor detected with In-111 octreotide scan. Clin Nucl Med 2006;31:552-553.
30. Mitsuoka S, Kanazawa H. Images in thorax: an unique case of primary pulmonary cryptococcosis with extensive chest wall invasion. Thorax 2005;60:86.
31. Fioravanti A, Tofi C, Volterrani L, et al. Malignant lymphoma mimicking Tietze's syndrome. Arthritis Rheum 2002;47:229-230.
32. Botchu R, Ravikumar KJ, Sudhakar G, et al. Osteosarcoma of rib in a seven-year-old child: a case report. Eur J Orthop Surg Traumatol 2006;16:156-157.
33. Thongngarm T, Lemos LB, Lawhon N, et al. Malignant tumor with chest wall pain mimicking Tietze's syndrome. Clin Rheumatol 2001;20:276-278.
34. Malghem J, Vande Berg B, Lecouvert F, et al. Costal cartilage fractures as revealed on CT and sonography. AJR Am J Roentgenol 2001;176:429-432.
35. Cameron HU, Fornasier VL. Tietze's syndrome. J Clin Pathol 1974;27:960-962.
36. Bass C, Mayou R. ABC of psychological medicine. Chest pain. BMJ 2002;325:588-591.
37. Ricevuti G. Effects of human calcitonin on pain in the treatment of Tietze's syndrome. Clin Ther 1985;7:669-673.

Postherpetic Neuralgia 101

Ariana Vora, MD, and Anita Thompson, PT

Synonyms

Shingles
Herpes zoster

ICD-9 Codes

053.12 Postherpetic trigeminal neuralgia
053.19 Postherpetic neuralgia (intercostal or opthalmic)

DEFINITION

Acute varicella-zoster infection classically results in pruritic, vesicular skin eruptions known as chickenpox. The virus commonly infects children and spreads by aerosol droplets and skin-to-skin exposure to the vesicles, which contain large amounts of virus.

Varicella-zoster is a lipid-enveloped, double-stranded DNA herpesvirus that co-evolved with ancestral primates for more than 70 million years.[1] It expresses its genes sequentially, leading to expression of nonstructural proteins, nonstructural protein enzymes, and late structural proteins.[2] Late structural proteins encapsulate the DNA core, infect host cells, and replicate in host cell nuclei. Two viremic phases are thought to occur in acute zoster infection. Animal studies suggest that the first viremia occurs in regional lymph nodes and viscera, approximately 5 days after exposure.[3] The second viremia, approximately 14 days after exposure, promotes viral spread to the nasopharynx and the skin, causing the hallmark vesicular rash.[4] After acute herpes zoster infection, the virus remains dormant and resides in sensory ganglia, including the dorsal roots and cranial nerves.[5]

Herpes zoster, or shingles, is the reactivation of latent varicella-zoster virus. Reactivation generally results from immunocompromised states such as stress, disease, or advancing age. The virus typically migrates along dermatomes, manifesting as a painful rash. The virus may spread to the spinal sensory nerves, dorsal horn, or cranial nerves. It is a painful condition with a highly age-related incidence, affecting about 50% of individuals who survive to the age of 85 years.[6] It affects men and women equally. Involvement of motor nerves is extremely rare.

Postherpetic neuralgia is defined as pain lasting more than 90 days and occurs in 20% of shingles cases.

SYMPTOMS

Prodromal symptoms include low-grade fever and malaise, which may be combined with hyperesthesia, dysesthesia, paresthesia, or pruritus along the distribution of one to three dermatomes. If there is ophthalmic involvement, photophobia may also be present. The prodromal stage may last up to 1 week.

Fulminant zoster infection is marked by the emergence of erythematous macules accompanied by severe burning, stinging pain in a single sensory or cranial nerve distribution. This is followed by the eruption of fluid-filled papules, clusters, and clear, fluid-filled vesicles. New skin eruptions generally continue to appear for 3 to 5 days. Thoracic dermatomes are most frequently affected. Sensitivity to light touch, intolerance to wearing clothes over the erupted area, and brief jolts of shooting pain are also common. Low-grade fever and malaise may persist, and lymphadenopathy may also be present.

Of the cranial nerves, the ophthalmic branch of the trigeminal nerve is the most often affected and can result in monocular blindness (herpes zoster ophthalmicus); this has an incidence of 1% in the general population.[7] Zoster affecting exposed areas may result in sun or wind sensitivity. In very rare cases, ipsilateral facial paralysis can occur, combined with loss of taste and hearing (Ramsay Hunt syndrome).

In the majority of cases, symptoms tend to resolve shortly after healing of the rash. However, in more than 25% of patients, neuralgia persists for longer than 1 month after resolution of the rash.[8]

PHYSICAL EXAMINATION

Typical skin eruptions follow a dermatomal distribution, appearing as raised, fluid-filled vesicles. Once the vesicles burst (releasing fluid that contains live virus), they crust. Once the vesicles have crusted, the patient is no longer infectious. Lesions are often exquisitely tender to light touch. If deeper dermal involvement is present, scarring and discoloration may be seen.

Ophthalmic zoster is usually accompanied by a rash and is associated with skin lesions in the dermatomal distribution of the nasociliary nerve, along the side of the nose (Hutchinson sign). Periorbital edema, petechial hemorrhages, conjunctivitis, scleritis, and corneal sensitivity are also commonly associated with ophthalmic zoster.[7] Hutchinson sign and an unexplained red eye are indications for ophthalmologic consultation.

FUNCTIONAL LIMITATIONS

If the optic nerve or the ophthalmic branch to the trigeminal nerve is affected, monocular low vision may result in impaired depth perception and decreased field of view. Driving may be affected. Other functional limitations include difficulty with activities involving pressure or heat exposure to the affected area. If the facial divisions of the trigeminal nerve are affected, individuals may not tolerate wearing of protective headgear or facemasks and facial exposure to sun or wind. If the thoracic dermatomes are affected, touching of the back against an office chair may increase pain. Both sex and contact sports may be intolerable. Difficulty sleeping may arise from discomfort from sheets touching the skin. Bathing and toweling often exacerbate pain along the affected dermatome.

DIAGNOSTIC STUDIES

Zoster is usually easy to diagnose on the basis of history and physical examination. In general, laboratory tests for diagnosis of reactivation of herpes zoster virus are not clinically useful.[9] For atypical cases, the Centers for Disease Control and Prevention guidelines suggest direct fluorescent antibody testing for rapid diagnosis.[8] To obtain a specimen, apply a sterile cotton swab to the base of an open lesion or, less preferably, a lesion crust.

Differential Diagnosis

Drug-related allergic infection

Eczema

Contact dermatitis

Other herpetic neuralgias

Nonherpetic viral infection

Complex regional pain disorder

Tertiary syphilis

Radiculitis

TREATMENT

Initial

Oral antiviral medication with any of the following regimens has been found effective for treatment of acute zoster-related pain:

- Acyclovir, 800 mg five times daily for 7 days[10]
- Famciclovir, 750 mg once daily or 500 mg twice daily for 7 days[11]
- Valacyclovir, 1000 mg three times a day for 7 days[12]

For patients with immunocompromise or malabsorption, the intravenous route of antiviral medication delivery is preferred to the oral route. There is limited evidence that a course of intravenous followed by oral antiviral treatment may reduce pain in patients with postherpetic neuralgia of more than 3 months' duration.[13]

When it is given within 72 hours of symptom onset, oral antiviral treatment decreases the incidence of postherpetic neuralgia by 50%.[14] In case series of 18 adults with postherpetic neuralgia, topical lidocaine 5% was found safe and effective in reducing symptoms of postherpetic neuralgia.[15] Studies of corticosteroids, anticonvulsants, opioids, antidepressants, and acupuncture have had small sample sizes; so far, they have not been found to reduce the severity of acute zoster symptoms or the incidence of postherpetic neuralgia.[14]

Rehabilitation

Ultrasound is effective in relieving acute zoster pain. In a clinical trial of acute zoster pain, more than 80% of participants receiving ultrasound were pain free at the end of the treatment, compared with 46% in the placebo group.[16] The treatment parameters used in areas adjacent to the vertebral column were 1 MHz frequency, 25% pulsed cycle, applied for 1 minute per effective radiating area of the transducer at 0.8% W/cm^2 intensity and around the periphery of the vesicles at 0.5 W/cm^2.

Self-administered transcutaneous electrical nerve stimulation (TENS) may be helpful for chronic pain, based on destruction of larger myelinated afferent nerve fibers, leaving a disproportionate number of small delta fibers and nonmyelinated fibers. By driving the remaining large fibers to a higher level of activity, TENS is thought to reduce painful stimuli from the smaller fibers.[17] Electrical stimulation is thought to be more effective for patients with less severe pain because fewer residual myelinated fibers have been destroyed.

TENS should be applied at the maximum setting that is not uncomfortable. If muscle fasciculation can be tolerated, recommended treatment time is 45 to 60 minutes, three times a day.[18] Patients are encouraged to change the voltage, pulse duration, pulse frequency, and pad placements to achieve maximum effectiveness. Large electrode pads are used to reduce painful stimulation.

Desensitizing treatments, such as alternating exposure to heat and cold, vibration, and repeated light tapping of the affected area, may be helpful.

In cases of ophthalmic involvement, occupational therapists can instruct in scanning techniques for low vision and decreased peripheral vision. Occupational therapists can also assist with fall risk reduction, such as by removal of loose rugs, improvement in lighting, and decrease of clutter in the home and work environment.

Other practical measures to improve function include rearrangement of work stations to reduce contact of sensitive areas with seat backs and armrests, use of low-friction fabrics such as silk, use of a hand-held shower-head to direct water flow away from painful dermatomes, and modification of sexual positions.

Procedures

In a randomized, controlled trial of 598 patients receiving standard oral antiviral and analgesic therapy with and without epidural steroid injection, the injection was found to have a modest effect in reducing the pain of postherpetic neuralgia for 1 month and did not prevent long-term postherpetic neuralgia.[19] Paravertebral nerve block, greater occipital nerve block, deep cervical nerve blocks, stellate ganglion blocks, and subcutaneous botulinum toxin A injection have improved symptoms in case reports.[20-22] Although they have not been adequately studied, they may have some efficacy in treatment of recalcitrant postherpetic neuralgia symptoms.

Surgery

Surgery is not indicated for postherpetic neuralgia.

POTENTIAL DISEASE COMPLICATIONS

Chronic postherpetic neuralgia (persistent pain at least 3 months after resolution of rash) is thought to occur in at least 25% of patients who develop zoster symptoms.

Orbital apex syndrome is an inflammation of the oculomotor nerve thought to be related to secondary vasculitis within the orbital apex. It can cause impaired eye motility and often is manifested as dysconjugate gaze and diplopia.

Acute optic neuritis may lead to permanent loss of vision, usually due to virus-induced impairment in retinal perfusion, leading to retinal necrosis. Retinal necrosis generally occurs in severely immunocompromised patients.[23]

POTENTIAL TREATMENT COMPLICATIONS

Gastrointestinal, hepatic, and renal complications may arise from prolonged use of acetaminophen, antiviral medications, or nonsteroidal anti-inflammatory drugs.

References

1. Grose D. Varicella zoster virus: out of Africa and into the research laboratory. Herpes 2006;13:32-35.
2. Cohrs RJ, Hurley MP, Gilden DH. Array analysis of viral gene transcription during lytic infection of cells in tissue culture with varicella-zoster virus. J Virol 2003;77:11718-11732.
3. Dueland AN, Martin JR, Devlin ME, et al. Acute simian varicella infection: clinical, laboratory, pathologic, and virologic features. Lab Invest 1992;66:762-773.
4. Tsolia M, Gershon AA, Steinberg SP, Gelb L. Live attenuated varicella vaccine: evidence that the virus is attenuated and the importance of skin lesions in transmission of varicella-zoster virus. National Institute of Allergy and Infectious Diseases Varicella Vaccine Collaborative Study Group. J Pediatr 1990;116:184-189.
5. Cohrs R, Laguardia J, Gilden D. Distribution of latent herpes simplex virus type-1 and varicella zoster virus DNA in human trigeminal ganglia. Virus Genes 2005;31:223-227.
6. Weiner DK, Schmader K. Postherpetic pain: more than sensory neuralgia? Pain Med 2006;7:243-249.
7. Opstelten W, Zaal MJ. Managing acute herpes zoster in primary care. BMJ 2005;331:147-151.
8. Dubinsky RM, Kabbani H, El-Chami Z, et al. Practice parameter: treatment of postherpetic neuralgia: an evidence-based report of the Quality Standards Subcommittee of the American Academy of Neurology. Neurology 2004;63:959-965.
9. Nicholson B. Differential diagnosis: nociceptive and neuropathic pain. Am J Managed Care 2006;12:S256-S262.
10. Wood MJ, Shukla S, Fiddian AP, Crooks RJ. Treatment of acute herpes zoster: effect on early (<48 h) versus late (48-72 h) therapy with acyclovir and valacyclovir on prolonged pain. J Infect Dis 1998;178(Suppl 1):S81-S84.
11. Tyring S, Barbarash RA, Nahlik JE, et al. Famcyclovir for treatment of acute herpes zoster: effects on acute disease and postherpetic neuralgia. A randomized, double-blind, placebo-controlled trial. Ann Intern Med 1995;123:89-86.
12. Beutner KR, Friedman DJ, Forszpaniak C, et al. Valacyclovir compared with acyclovir for improved therapy for herpes zoster in immunocompetent adults. Antimicrob Agents Chemother 1995;39:1546-1553.
13. Quan K, Hammack B, Kittelson J, Gilden D. Improvement of post-herpetic neuralgia after treatment with intravenous acyclovir followed by oral valacyclovir. Arch Neurol 2006;63:940-942.
14. Alper BS, Lewis PR. Does treatment of acute herpes zoster prevent or shorten postherpetic neuralgia? J Fam Pract 2000;49:255-264.
15. Wasner G, Kleinert A, Binder A, et al. Postherpetic neuralgia: topical lidocaine is effective in nociceptor-deprived skin. J Neurol 2005;252:677-686.
16. Cameron M, ed. Physical Agents in Rehabilitation: From Research to Practice. Philadelphia, WB Saunders, 2003:289.
17. Nathan PW, Hall PD. Treatment of postherpetic neuralgia by prolonged electric stimulation. BMJ 1974;3:645-647.
18. http://www.empi.com/uploadedFiles/Empi_Products/Pain Management_TENS/acute_herpes.pdf. Accessed January 31, 2008.
19. van Wijck AJ, Opstelten W, Moons KG, et al. The PINE study of epidural steroids and local anaesthetics to prevent postherpetic neuralgia: a randomized controlled trial. Lancet 2006;367:219-224.
20. Naja ZM, Maaliki H, Al-Tannir MA, et al. Repetitive paravertebral nerve block using a catheter technique for pain relief in post-herpetic neuralgia. Br J Anaesth 2006;96:381-383.
21. Hardy D. Relief of pain in acute herpes zoster by nerve blocks and possible prevention of post-herpetic neuralgia. Can J Anaesth 2005;52:186-190.
22. Liu HT, Tsai SK, Kao MC, Hu JS. Botulinum toxin A relieved neuropathic pain in a case of post-herpetic neuralgia. Pain Med 2006;7:89-91.
23. Zaal MJ, Völker-Dieben HJ, D'Amaro J. Visual prognosis in immunocompetent patients with herpes zoster ophthalmicus. Acta Ophthalmol Scand 2003;81:216-220.

Arachnoiditis 102

Michael D. Osborne, MD

DEFINITION

Arachnoiditis is the development of chronic inflammation and progressive fibrosis of the arachnoid and pia layers of the meninges. It can occur subsequent to a variety of conditions, although it is most commonly a sequela of spinal surgery or the result of intrathecal injection of radiographic dyes and chemicals with neurotoxic preservatives.[1] Some of the etiologic factors linked to the development of arachnoiditis are listed in Table 102-1.

When microtrauma to the vasculature of the arachnoid membrane and pia mater occurs, it can impair the normal mechanisms for control of excessive meningeal fibrosis.[1] This may result in the deposition of fibrous collagen bands in the arachnoid-pia membranes and cause the nerve roots to adhere to each other as well as to the dural sac. The pathophysiologic mechanism of arachnoiditis involves a progression from root inflammation (radiculitis) to root adherence (fibrosis). In severe cases, the arachnoid fibrosis can cause compressive root ischemia, and progressive neurologic deficits may ensue.[2] When this condition occurs in the meninges of the cervical and thoracic regions, the spinal cord can become enmeshed and constricted as well. Pain is the result of dural adherence with nerve root traction and nerve ischemia. Typically, arachnoiditis develops slowly during the period of months after the initial insult, although it may continue to develop for years, resulting in worsening pain and paresthesias or progressive neurologic injury.[1]

SYMPTOMS

The symptoms associated with arachnoiditis are heterogeneous and often difficult to distinguish from other disease processes, such as radiculopathy, spinal stenosis, cauda equina syndrome, and neuropathies. Also, because arachnoiditis is often acquired iatrogenically during the course of evaluation and treatment of spinal disorders, patients often have concomitant symptoms of mechanical back pain or myofascial pain in addition to the arachnoiditis symptom complex.

Patients with arachnoiditis principally report burning pain or paresthesias; however, these symptoms often do not follow typical radicular patterns. Pain is usually constant but exacerbated by movement. Some patients experience secondary muscle spasms. Weakness and muscle atrophy may also occur, and bowel or bladder sphincter dysfunction is also not uncommon. Onset is insidious, and symptoms may first present years after the inciting event.[3] Symptoms can range from mild (such as slight tingling of the extremities) to severe (such as excruciating pain with progressive neurologic deterioration). The condition may also be asymptomatic and discovered only incidentally on magnetic resonance imaging (MRI).

PHYSICAL EXAMINATION

Neurologic examination typically reveals a patchy distribution of lower motor neuron deficits. Examination findings may include loss of reflexes, muscle weakness, muscle atrophy, anesthesia, gait instability, and reduced rectal tone.[2] Less commonly, arachnoiditis may involve the spinal cord; in these instances, upper motor neuron findings (hyperreflexia, spasticity, presence of Babinski response) can be found on examination.

A complete neurologic examination should be performed at the time of initial diagnosis. In the event that symptoms worsen, this examination may then be used as a benchmark to ascertain whether neurologic deterioration is occurring. In the setting of progressive neurologic decline, it is incumbent on the treating physician to rule out other pathologic processes (such as a new disc herniation) before neurologic deterioration is attributed solely to progressive arachnoid fibrosis.

FUNCTIONAL LIMITATIONS

Patients with arachnoiditis may exhibit a variety of functional limitations, the degree of which corresponds to the extent of the neurologic impairments and the

TABLE 102-1 Some Etiologic Factors Linked to the Development of Arachnoiditis

Agents injected into the subarachnoid space

Contrast media (especially Pantopaque)

Intrathecal chemotherapies (amphotericin B, methotrexate)

Local anesthetics with vasoconstrictors

Corticosteroids with polyethylene glycol or benzyl alcohol preservative

Spinal surgery or trauma

Extradural surgeries, such as laminectomy, discectomy, and fusion

Intradural surgeries

Spinal fractures

Intrathecal blood

Subarachnoid hemorrhage

Bloody spinal tap

Blood patch with inadvertent intrathecal injection

Infection

Discitis, vertebral body osteomyelitis

Spinal tuberculosis

Other

Spinal stenosis

Idiopathic

Adapted from Bourne IH. Lumbo-sacral adhesive arachnoiditis: a review. J R Soc Med 1990;83:262-265.

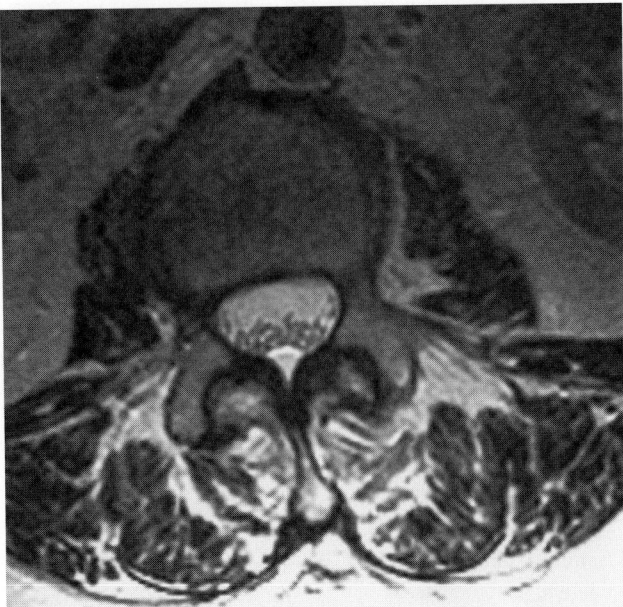

FIGURE 102-1. Normal MRI appearance of lumbar nerve roots on T2-weighted axial sequences.

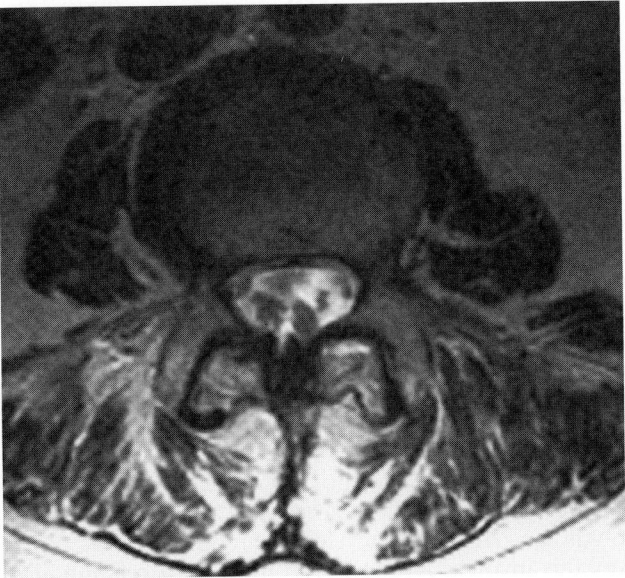

FIGURE 102-2. Lumbar MRI demonstrating the characteristic nerve root clumping indicative of arachnoiditis.

severity of the pain. Gait instability, reduced ambulatory capacity, and impairment in activities of daily living are not uncommon. As time goes by, patients tend to suffer secondary effects of immobilization and deconditioning, causing further functional impairment. The severe pain and impaired mobility tend to isolate patients socially and to limit their ability to work. Because the pain associated with arachnoiditis is usually present even at rest, sedentary work or light duty does not always improve a patient's symptoms enough to facilitate employment despite activity restrictions.

DIAGNOSTIC STUDIES

Presently, the diagnosis of arachnoiditis is most often made through the use of MRI. Historically, myelography was used routinely for diagnosis of arachnoiditis; characteristic findings included the observance of prominent nerve roots as well as various patterns of filling defects. The advent of computed tomography and MRI has made diagnosis easier.

MRI is preferred to computed tomographic myelography because of its noninvasive nature. Typical findings include adherent roots located centrally in the thecal sac (considered mild arachnoiditis), an "empty sac" (where roots are adherent to the wall of the thecal sac), and a

mass of soft tissue replacing the subarachnoid space (severe disease).[4] These findings are well seen on T2-weighted axial images (Figs. 102-1 and 102-2). Although the administration of contrast material with MRI may help rule out other diseases in the differential diagnosis, such as tumors and infection, contrast enhancement is not necessary to visualize the characteristic appearance of arachnoiditis.[5]

The diagnosis can also be made by computed tomographic myelography; even myelography with conventional radiography may be used if spinal instrumentation from prior fusion surgery creates too much artifact on MRI and computed tomography. The water-soluble myelographic contrast media used today (such as io-hexol) are much safer than the prior oil-based media (Pantopaque), and serious adverse reactions involving the central nervous system are extremely rare (<0.1%).[6] There have not been any documented cases of adhesive arachnoiditis with the use of iohexol myelography.[6]

Differential Diagnosis

Spondylosis

Radiculopathy

Cauda equina syndrome

Neuropathy, plexopathy

Neurogenic claudication

Spinal tumors

Spinal infections

Postsurgical epidural fibrosis

Epidural hematoma

Meningitis

TREATMENT

Initial

The treatment of arachnoiditis is palliative, and medications are often used for this purpose. Antidepressant or anticonvulsant analgesics are considered the mainstay of medical management, although other classes of medications may provide benefit as well. Many antidepressants and anticonvulsants have been used for years off-label for the treatment of neuropathic pain with reasonable efficacy; the tricyclic antidepressants (such as amitriptyline) are the most common. The U.S. Food and Drug Administration has more recently approved several newer medications for use in specific neuropathic pain syndromes: duloxetine and pregabalin for diabetic neuropathy, and gabapentin and pregabalin for postherpetic neuralgia. These medications are often tried in patients with arachnoiditis with varying efficacy. Antidepressant and anticonvulsant analgesics are typically started at relatively low doses and titrated upward as tolerated. The precise starting dose and eventual maximal dose usually depend on how well the medication's side effect profile is tolerated. Some examples of dosing regimens are listed in Table 102-2. For most of these medications, it often takes a few weeks at any given dose for optimal analgesic effect to be reached.

Anti-inflammatory medications (nonsteroidal anti-inflammatory drugs) are commonly used as well. This is probably because of the frequent occurrence of back pain in these patients. Often, patients with arachnoiditis have concomitant lumbar disc degeneration or osteoarthritis of the facet joints that may respond in part to anti-inflammatory medications. Likewise, patients with back pain may benefit from trials of muscle relaxants or more potent inhibitors of muscle contractions (antispasticity agents), like baclofen and tizanidine. Baclofen has also been used off-label for treatment of neuropathic pain.

Opiates are often prescribed with varying degrees of success. In general, neuropathic pain seems to be less responsive to opiates. Some advocate the use of methadone because of its N-methyl-D-aspartate (NMDA) receptor antagonist activity, which may make it more effective for neuropathic pain syndromes. One of the chief limitations of opiates is the tendency for development of tolerance, requiring dose escalation.

Rehabilitation

Rehabilitation interventions can be divided into modalities for pain management and therapeutic exercise to improve pain as well as to aid function. Modalities such as heat application (superficial and deep) and ice application are most effective for treatment of the associated mechanical back pain and myofascial pain that often accompany arachnoiditis. Contrast baths can be used for distal extremity pain and can be helpful when the patient exhibits signs of peripheral sympathetic dysfunction. Electrical stimulation is primarily used to treat neuropathic pain, but it may also improve associated musculoskeletal and myofascial pain. Transcutaneous electrical nerve stimulation and percutaneous electrical nerve stimulation can be applied at the paraspinal level or along the course of a peripheral nerve to help attenuate neuropathic pain.

Unfortunately, exercise typically offers the patient very little as a direct means of symptom improvement for severe neuropathic pain, yet exercise is still an important part of treatment. As previously mentioned, patients with arachnoiditis may suffer from other musculoskeletal pain, and therapeutic exercise (such as stretching, strength training, and aerobic exercise) often improves these associated disorders. Patients with intractable pain

TABLE 102-2 Examples of Dosing Regimens for Anticonvulsant and Antidepressant Analgesics

Medication	Starting Dose	Dose Increase and Interval	Maximal Dose
Tricyclic antidepressants	10-25 mg at night	10-25 mg per week	150 mg/day
Duloxetine	20-30 mg/day	20-30 mg per week	60 mg/day
Gabapentin	100-300 mg bid-tid	100-300 mg per week	1800*-3600+ mg/day
Pregabalin	50-75 mg bid-tid	50-75 mg per week	600 mg/day

*denotes the FDA-approved maximal dose.
+ denotes "off-label" dose within standard of care.

often avoid activity because of increased pain or fear of pain provocation. As such, they often become deconditioned and benefit from gentle progressive exercise regimens. Aquatic therapy is generally well tolerated and can be used as a method to improve many of the manifestations of deconditioning and prolonged immobility, such as to improve joint motion, flexibility, aerobic capacity, and muscle strength.

Procedures

There are few data to support the role of neuraxial corticosteroid injections, such as epidural steroids and nerve root blocks, in arachnoiditis treatment. Anecdotally, short-duration improvement may be observed, and any such procedures are usually performed as a "do and see" proposition.

The most promising intervention for the intractable pain associated with arachnoiditis is spinal cord stimulation. Spinal cord stimulation, also known as dorsal column stimulation, involves the placement of a stimulating electrode (either percutaneously or through a laminotomy) over the dorsal aspect of the spinal cord (Figs. 102-3 and 102-4). Exact level and location of electrode placement depend on the location of the patient's pain. Typically, patients undergo a percutaneous trial to test the stimulator's efficacy before permanent implantation. The goal is to stimulate the spinal cord with low levels of electrical impulses that produce a nonpainful paresthesia that modulates (masks) the patient's pain.

The largest studies investigating spinal cord stimulation have included patients with varied diagnoses, the most abundant of which is failed back surgery syndrome. It has been estimated that 11% of patients with failed back surgery syndrome have arachnoiditis. Approximately 50% to 60% of patients with failed back surgery syn-

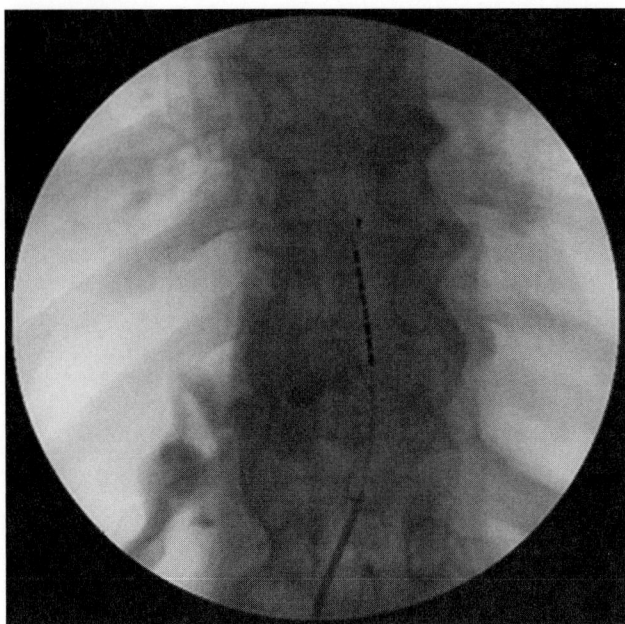

FIGURE 102-4. Fluoroscopic image of a percutaneous spinal cord stimulator lead in the dorsal thoracic spine. (Photograph courtesy of Boston Scientific Neuromodulation, Valencia, CA.)

drome treated with spinal cord stimulation receive more than 50% relief of their symptoms.[7,8] Studies investigating spinal cord stimulation efficacy in patients with a more specific diagnosis of epidural fibrosis or intradural fibrosis (arachnoiditis) have also found improvement in pain (60%), reduction of pain medication requirements (40%), and increased work capacity (25%).[9,10] Spinal cord stimulation seems to be more effective for pain of neuropathic character than for pain of mechanical or musculoskeletal character. In addition, extremity pain is generally more easily treated compared with back pain–predominant symptoms.[10]

Surgery

There is very little role for surgical intervention in the treatment of arachnoiditis. There is no method of surgically untangling the adherent nerve roots. Indications for surgery include rapidly progressive neurologic deterioration, such as myelopathy due to progressive syringomyelia or cauda equina syndrome from arachnoiditis ossificans. In these instances, surgical intervention (shunt placement or removal of the calcific mass) could be contemplated. The emphasis on such interventions is to halt or to retard further neurologic deterioration. The prospect that such procedures will improve pain remains speculative at best.

POTENTIAL DISEASE COMPLICATIONS

In severe cases of arachnoiditis, the fibrous bands that cause adherence of the nerve roots may become so prolific that progressive nerve root injury (radiculopathy, polyradiculopathy) or spinal cord injury (cauda equina syndrome, myelopathy) can ensue. Constriction of the

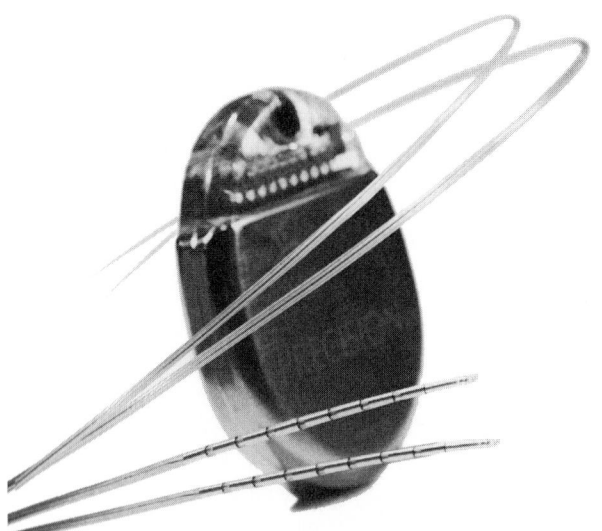

FIGURE 102-3. An example of a spinal cord stimulator with its components: implantable pulse generator and two percutaneous leads. (Photograph courtesy of Boston Scientific Neuromodulation, Valencia, CA.)

spinal cord vasculature causes ischemia and focal areas of spinal cord demyelination. This vascular ischemia and associated alterations of normal cerebrospinal fluid flow have been observed to result in the formation of arachnoid cysts, syringomyelia, and even communicating hydrocephalus.[11,12] Calcification of the fibrotic milieu results in a condition termed arachnoiditis ossificans, which may result in progressive nerve root or spinal cord compression.[13]

POTENTIAL TREATMENT COMPLICATIONS

Medication side effects are common. Anticonvulsant and antidepressant analgesics often produce sedation or alteration of mental status. Opiates, too, can produce sedation as well as severe constipation. Opiate dependence is generally anticipated as a ramification of use of this class of medication long term. Although true psychological addiction to opiates can occur, it is much less common than one might expect. The propensity for nonsteroidal anti-inflammatory drugs to cause gastrointestinal side effects is well known, as is their potential to adversely affect the kidneys and liver as well as to exacerbate hypertension and asthma.

Rehabilitation interventions are generally safe, although patients can suffer thermal injury from inappropriate application of superficial modalities. Transcutaneous electrical nerve stimulation and percutaneous electrical nerve stimulation are generally considered contraindicated in patients with pacemakers. Therapeutic exercise may potentially exacerbate pain symptoms.

Spinal cord stimulation poses some risk; however, complications are usually minor, and the incidence of new neurologic injury from something such as bleeding, infection, or neural trauma is quite small.[8] The most frequent complication usually entails electromechanical failure, such as percutaneous lead migration, when the stimulation no longer covers the symptomatic body region. The majority of electromechanical complications can be remedied with revision of the system.

References

1. Bourne IH. Lumbo-sacral adhesive arachnoiditis: a review. J R Soc Med 1990;83:262-265.
2. Rice I, Wee MY, Thomson K. Obstetric epidurals and chronic adhesive arachnoiditis. Br J Anaesth 2004;92:109-120.
3. Wright MH, Denney LC. A comprehensive review of spinal arachnoiditis. Orthop Nurs 2003;22:215-219.
4. Delamarter RB, Ross JS, Masaryk TJ, et al. Diagnosis of lumbar arachnoiditis by magnetic resonance imaging. Spine 1990;15: 304-310.
5. Johnson CE, Sze G. Benign lumbar arachnoiditis: MR imaging with gadopentetate dimeglumine. AJR Am J Roentgenol 1990;155: 873-880.
6. RxMed, Inc. Comprehensive resource for physicians, drug and illness information: Omnipaque. Available at: http://www.rxmed.com/b.main/b2.pharmaceutical/b2.prescribe.html. Accessed July 25, 2006.
7. Burchiel KJ, Anderson VC, Brown FD, et al. Prospective, multi-center study of spinal cord stimulation for relief of chronic back and extremity pain. Spine 1996;21:2786-2794.
8. Turner JA, Loeser JD, Bell KG. Spinal cord stimulation for chronic low back pain: a systematic literature synthesis. Neurosurgery 1995;37:1088-1096.
9. de la Porte C, Siegfried J. Lumbosacral spinal fibrosis (spinal arachnoiditis). Its diagnosis and treatment by spinal cord stimulation. Spine 1983;8:593-603.
10. Probst C. Spinal cord stimulation in 112 patients with epi-/intradural fibrosis following operation for lumbar disc herniation. Acta Neurochir (Wien) 1990;107:147-151.
11. Tumialan LM, Cawley CM, Barrow DL. Arachnoid cyst with associated arachnoiditis developing after subarachnoid hemorrhage. J Neurosurg 2005;103:1088-1091.
12. Koyanagi I, Iwasaki Y, Hida K, Houkin K. Clinical features and pathomechanisms of syringomyelia associated with spinal arachnoiditis. Surg Neurol 2005;63:350-355.
13. Domenicucci M, Ramieri A, Passacantilli E, et al. Spinal arachnoiditis ossificans: report of three cases. Neurosurgery 2004;55:985-991.

Coccydynia 103

Ariana Vora, MD

DEFINITION

Coccydynia is pain in the vicinity of the coccygeal bone at the base of the spine. Associated symptoms include dyspareunia, dyschezia, and dysmenorrhea. Pain can be insidious or sudden in onset. Symptoms are usually triggered by sitting or rising from a sitting position. The most common inciting factor is trauma to the coccyx or surrounding soft tissue from a vertical blow or difficult vaginal delivery. Pathologic features may range from dislocated sacrococcygeal fracture to ligamentous damage of the caudal coccygeal segments. In most cases, the tip of the coccyx is subluxated or hypermobile[1] (Figs. 103-1 and 103-2).

The fibrous sacrococcygeal joint connects the sacrum to one to four bone segments of the coccyx. This joint is reinforced by sacrococcygeal ligaments, which enclose the final intervertebral foramen through which the S5 roots exit. The S4, S5, and coccygeal roots contribute to the coccygeal plexus, which provides rich somatic and autonomic innervation to the anus, perineum, and genitals.[2] The levator ani (S4 nerve root through perineal branch of pudendal nerve) and coccygeal muscles (S4-5 nerve root branches) attach to and support the coccyx during defecation and childbirth. The gluteus maximus also attaches to the lateral coccyx and can contribute to a sensation of pressure while sitting.

Prevalence of coccydynia is five times higher in women than in men.[3] In addition to obstetric trauma,[4] the increased susceptibility to injury in women is attributed to anatomy, as the female coccyx is more posterior in location and larger than the male coccyx.[5] Coccydynia is three times more frequent in obese women than in nonobese women,[6] and this may be related to decreased pelvic rotation while sitting.

SYMPTOMS

Coccygeal pain is located at the tip or sides of the coccyx. The quality of pain is usually dull and achy at baseline and intermittently sharp during activities that aggravate the symptoms. A sensation of pressure is also commonly described. Symptoms are usually exacerbated by sitting on hard surfaces, prolonged sitting, and moving from the sitting to the standing position. Symptoms are generally relieved by taking weight off the coccyx.

Levator ani syndrome and proctalgia fugax are variants of coccydynia.

Levator ani syndrome is a dull ache or pressure sensation in the rectum, with pain episodes lasting more than 20 minutes at a time. Symptoms tend to be more severe during the day than at night. Symptoms may result from a hypertonic levator ani or puborectalis muscle or from inflammation of the arcus tendon of the levator ani.[7,8] This syndrome is associated with posterior traction of the puborectalis muscle and levator ani muscle tenderness on rectal examination.

Proctalgia fugax is the sudden onset of excruciating anal pain lasting a few seconds or minutes, then disappearing completely. Proctalgia fugax is characterized by spastic muscle contractions of the pelvic floor.[9] Episodes usually occur fewer than five times a year.[10] Symptoms are not related to defecation and are associated with sexual intercourse. Symptoms are usually nocturnal and awaken the patient from sleep. This condition occurs equally in men and women.

PHYSICAL EXAMINATION

Classic findings in coccydynia are exquisite tenderness to direct palpation of the coccyx, sacrococcygeal ligaments, and pubococcygeal ligaments. It is also important to palpate surrounding joints. Pelvic obliquity,

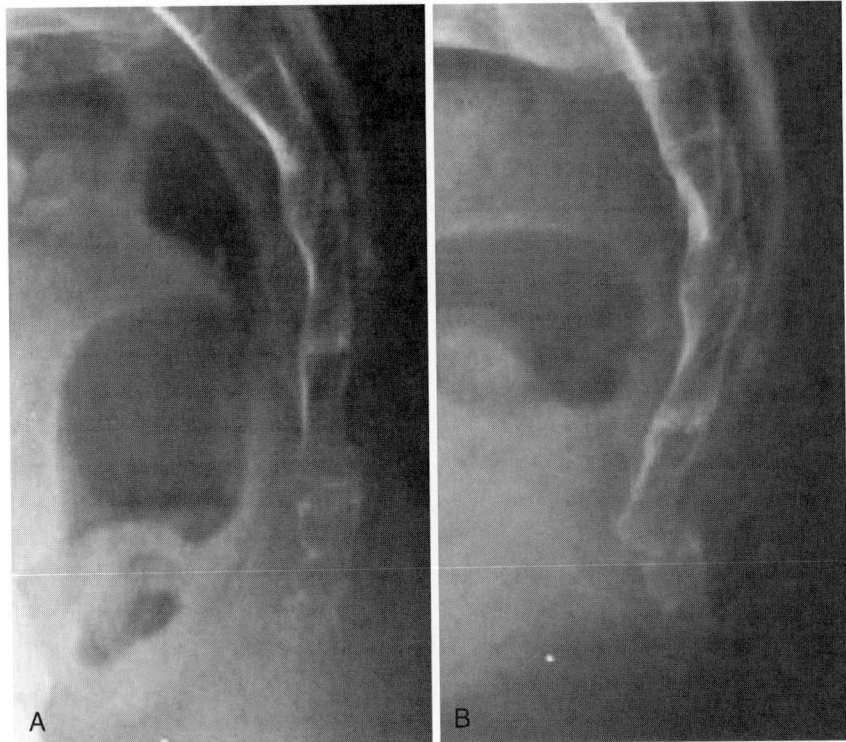

FIGURE 103-1. Lateral radiographs of coccygeal subluxation. (Reprinted with permission from Doursounian L, Maigne JY, Faure F, Chatellier G. Coccygectomy for instability of the coccyx. Int Orthop 2004;28:176-179.)

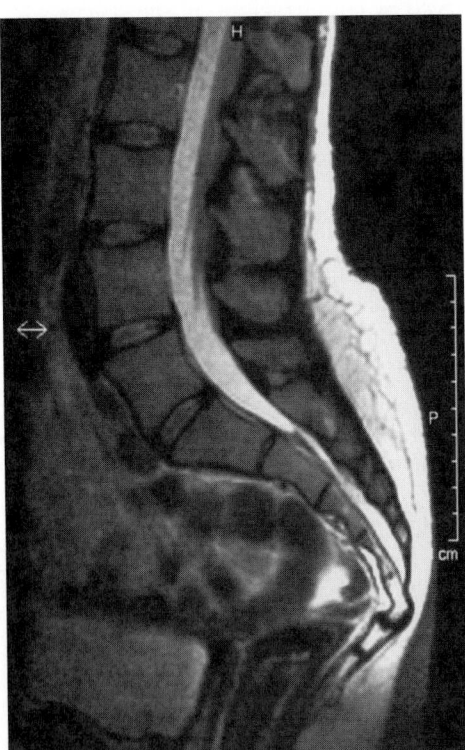

FIGURE 103-2. Sagittal magnetic resonance image of misaligned coccygeal fracture. (Reprinted with permission from Pennicamp PH, Kraft CN, Stuetz A, et al. Coccygectomy for coccygodynia: does pathogenesis matter? J Trauma 2005;59:1414-1419.)

sacroiliac tenderness, and pubic ramus tenderness may be detected if the coccydynia is related to trauma or leg length discrepancy; if so, these underlying problems may be a part of treatment.

Perform a general examination for evidence of lymphadenopathy or pelvic masses to rule out neoplastic or infectious etiology (see the section on differential diagnosis). Assess for point tenderness along the pelvic girdle, including the top of the coccyx. Lower extremity strength, reflexes, and sensation should be assessed for focal neurologic deficits and should be normal in coccydynia. Evaluate leg lengths, pelvic obliquity, sacroiliac motion, and sacroiliac joint tenderness. Examine the anus, surrounding skin, and soft tissue for cysts, fistulas, external hemorrhoids, and fissures. Digital rectal examination should include testing for occult blood, palpation for internal masses, and palpation of the levator ani muscles for tenderness; manipulation of the coccygeal tip, the pubococcygeal ligament, and the sacrococcygeal joint is performed to assess for tenderness and hypermobility.[11]

FUNCTIONAL LIMITATIONS

Because coccydynia is often worsened by sitting, driving can become very painful. It is common to avoid social situations because of pain when sitting or standing. Because of pressure to the coccyx and muscle contractions in the perineum during orgasm, sexual intimacy can worsen symptoms and is often avoided. Equestrian activities and contact sports can be particularly painful. Sedentary work involving prolonged sitting may exacerbate symptoms; frequent breaks may be required.

DIAGNOSTIC STUDIES

Coccydynia is often associated with subluxation or hypermobility of the tip of the coccyx (Fig. 103-3), which is usually seen on dynamic radiographs and may or may not show fusion of the sacrococcygeal joint and superior intercoccygeal joints.[1,12] Dynamic lateral radiographs are done in lateral and oblique views while the patient is sitting and standing. Bone scans and magnetic resonance imaging may show inflammation, fracture, or bone fragments. Because they are static tests, they are no less useful than dynamic radiographs in diagnosis of hypermobility or subluxation.[1] Anal manometry testing has been described in the literature, with conflicting reports on its utility. The basis for manometry testing is the theory that prolonged sphincter contraction or dystonia may contribute to coccygeal pain; abnormal anal manometric pressures support a diagnosis of proctalgia fugax, but the test is unlikely to diagnose proctalgia fugax because episodes are so infrequent.

TREATMENT

Initial

Conservative treatment is viable, as the natural history does not usually lead to deterioration. Sitting on a doughnut-shaped pillow to reduce pressure, acetaminophen, oral nonsteroidal anti-inflammatory drugs, and application of perianal lidocaine jelly may help initially. Although they are relatively safe interventions, the efficacy of muscle relaxants, pelvic floor muscle massage, iontophoresis, biofeedback, electrogalvanic stimulation, and sitz baths has not been established in the literature.

Differential Diagnosis

Coccygeal fracture, ligamentous strain, or dislocation

Bursitis of adventitia at the coccygeal tip

Post-traumatic sacrococcygeal osteoarthritis

Lumbar disc herniation

Internal pudendal nerve entrapment (Alcock canal syndrome)

Lower sacral nerve arachnoiditis

Rectal fissure

Pelvic or perirectal abscess

Pilonidal cyst or sinus

Thrombosed external hemorrhoid

Prostatitis

Pelvic organ prolapse

Tumors of the colorectum, sacrum, prostate, or ovaries

Postsurgical adhesion

Rehabilitation

A trial of a doughnut-shaped pillow is always worthwhile to offload weight on the coccyx while sitting. Physical therapy should include pelvic massage, pelvic relaxation techniques, pelvic floor strengthening exercises, and postural correction. In patients with proctalgia fugax and levator ani symptoms, emphasis is placed on pelvic floor relaxation techniques. Correction of leg length discrepancy can help with referred sacroiliac pain. Psychological support is also crucial.

Procedures

Injection of the sacrococcygeal ligament and coccyx tip with lidocaine 1% can be diagnostic; Depo-Medrol 40 mg can be added to the injection for therapeutic

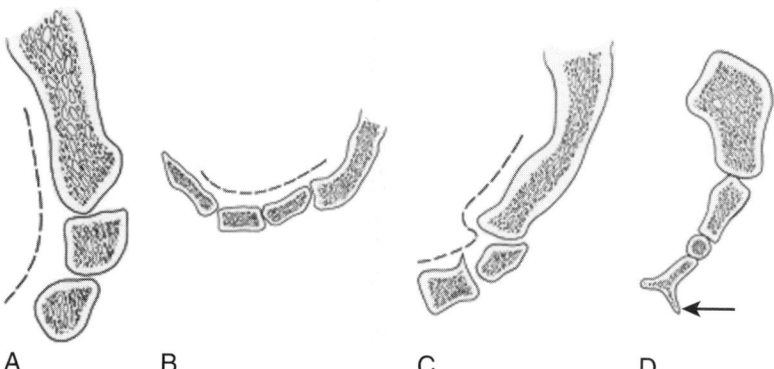

FIGURE 103-3. Schematic drawing of flexion mobility of the coccyx. **A,** Normal standing appearance of the coccyx. **B,** Increased flexion mobility of the coccyx when the patient is seated. **C,** Posterior subluxation of the coccyx when the patient is seated. **D,** Coccygeal spicule *(arrow)* arising from the dorsal surface of coccygeal segment. (Reprinted with permission from Fogel GR, Cunningham PY, Esses SI. Coccygodynia: evaluation and management. J Am Acad Orthop Surg 2004;12:49-54.)

purposes. This procedure can be done blindly by use of landmarks; the utility of fluoroscopic guidance is limited as visualization of ligaments is not possible.

If there is dislocation of the coccyx, manipulation under anesthesia may be helpful, but there are no conclusive data on the efficacy of this approach.

Botulinum toxin injection of the puborectalis and pubococcygeus muscles may relieve pain associated with muscle hypertonicity.[13,14]

Prolotherapy is an injection of proliferant solution that may relieve the pain of enthesopathy and facilitate regeneration of torn or painful sacrococcygeal and pubococcygeal ligaments. Its safety is well established, but there are no clinical trials on its efficacy in coccydynia.

Surgery

Most people recover with conservative treatment alone within weeks to months. A number of uncontrolled studies of patients with refractory coccydynia report pain relief with partial and total coccygectomy.[1,15-19] Successful treatment is usually associated with abnormal coccygeal motion.

POTENTIAL DISEASE COMPLICATIONS

Coccydynia is a symptom and not a disease in itself. The primary complication is functional decline secondary to local pain, generally limiting sitting tolerance, sexual intercourse, and exercise tolerance.

POTENTIAL TREATMENT COMPLICATIONS

Gastrointestinal, hepatic, and renal complications may arise from prolonged use of acetaminophen or non-steroidal anti-inflammatory drugs. Steroid injections may be complicated by skin depigmentation, injection, and transient elevation in blood glucose level. Repeated steroid injections may result in ligamentous breakdown and altered mobility in the sacrococcygeal ligament.

References

1. Fogel GR, Cunningham PY, Esses SI. Coccygodynia: evaluation and management. J Am Acad Orthop Surg 2004;12:49-54.
2. DeAndres J, Chaves S. Coccygodynia: a proposal for an algorithm for treatment. J Pain 2003;4:257-266.
3. Ryder I, Alexander J. Coccydynia: a woman's tail. Midwifery 2000;16:155-160.
4. Kaushal R, Bhanot A, Luthra S, et al. Intrapartum coccygeal fracture, a cause for postpartum coccydynia: a case report. J Surg Orthop Adv 2005;14:136-137.
5. Yamashita K. Radiological study of 1500 coccyces. Nippon Seikeigeka Gakkai Zasshi 1988;62:23-36.
6. Maigne JY, Doursounian L, Chatellier G. Causes and mechanisms of common coccydynia: role of body mass index and coccygeal trauma. Spine 2000;25:3072-3079.
7. Park DH, Yoon SG, Kim KU, et al. Comparison study between local electrogalvanic stimulation and local injection therapy in levator ani syndrome. Int J Colorectal Dis 2005;20:272-276.
8. Mazza L, Formento E, Fronda G. Anorectal and perineal pain: new pathophysiological hypothesis. Tech Coloproctol 2004;8:77-83.
9. Pfenninger JL, Zainea GG. Common anorectal conditions: part I, symptoms and complaints. Am Fam Physician 2001;63:2391-2398.
10. Whitehead WE, Wald A, Diamant NE, et al. Functional disorders of the anus and rectum. Gut 1999;45(Suppl 2):II55-II59.
11. Wald A. Functional anorectal and pelvic pain. Gastroenterol Clin North Am 2001;30:243-251.
12. Hodges SD, Eck JC, Humphreys SC. A treatment and outcomes analysis of patients with coccydynia. Spine J 2002;4:138-140.
13. Jarvis SK, Abbott JA, Lenart MG, et al. Pilot study of botulinum toxin type A in the treatment of chronic pelvic pain associated with spasm of the levator ani muscles. Aust N Z J Obstet Gynaecol 2004;44:46-50.
14. Katsinelos P, Kalomenopoulou M, Christodoulou K, et al. Treatment of proctalgia fugax with botulinum A toxin. Eur J Gastroenterol Hepatol 2001;13:1371-1373.
15. Karalezli K, Iltar S, Irgit K, et al. Coccygectomy in the treatment of coccygodynia. Acta Orthop Belg 2004;70:583-585.
16. Perkins R, Schofferman J, Reynolds J. Coccygectomy for severe refractory sacrococcygeal joint pain. J Spinal Disord Tech 2003;16:100-103.
17. Doursounian L, Maigne JY, Faure F, Chatellier G. Coccygectomy for instability of the coccyx. Int Orthop 2004;28:176-179.
18. Pennicamp PH, Kraft CN, Stuetz A, et al. Coccygectomy for coccygodynia: does pathogenesis matter? J Trauma 2005;59:1414-1419.
19. Wood KB, Mehbod AA. Operative treatment for coccygodynia. J Spinal Disord Tech 2004;17:511-515.

Phantom Limb Pain 104

Moon Suk Bang, MD, PhD, and Se Hee Jung, MD, MS

Synonyms

Painful phantom sensation
Phantom pain
Phantom limb syndrome

ICD-9 Codes

353.6   Phantom limb (syndrome)
729.2   Neuralgia, neuritis, and radiculitis, unspecified
905.9   Late effect of traumatic amputation (injury classifiable to 885-887 and 895-897)
997.60   Stump (surgical) (post-traumatic), abnormal, painful, or with complication (late)

DEFINITION

Phantom pain refers to painful sensation perceived in a body part that is no longer present subsequent to surgical or traumatic removal. It is most common after the amputation of a limb, (i.e., phantom limb pain), but it has also been reported after the surgical removal of other body parts, such as breast, rectum, penis, testicles, eye, tooth, tongue, or lesion of peripheral or central nervous system. Phantom limb pain is distinguished from stump pain, which is pain in the residual limb or stump, and phantom limb sensation, which is nonpainful sensation of the absent part. Peripheral, spinal segmental, central, and psychological mechanisms are considered factors for the development of phantom limb pain.[1-4]

Although phantom limb pain is generally initiated within the first few days after the amputation, it can take several months or years to emerge. The reported prevalence of phantom limb pain differs considerably, ranging from about 40% to 80%.[5-11] However, phantom limb pain is less frequent in congenital amputation and loss of a limb early in childhood. The occurrence of phantom limb pain is independent of gender, age (in adults), level or side of amputation, dominance, and etiology of amputation.[12,13]

In several reports, the incidence and intensity of pain remained constant but both the frequency and duration of pain attacks decreased significantly over time.[14,15] A small percentage of patients experienced a reduction in intensity of pain over time. Phantom limb pain leads to permanent disability in more than 40% of amputees. Phantom limb pain persisting more than 6 months is exceedingly difficult to treat.

Phantom limb pain has been reported to be significantly related to residual limb pain,[16] physical activity,[17] severity and duration of preamputation pain,[14,18] noxious intraoperative inputs (such as pain brought about by cutting of tissues), acute postoperative pain,[19] bilateral amputation, and lower limb amputation.[9]

SYMPTOMS

The pain is most prominent immediately after the operation. Phantom limb pain is not static in nature but changes in quality over the years. Phantom limb pain is usually intermittent, but some patients report constant pain with superimposed exacerbations. The duration of an attack ranges from seconds or minutes to hours or days.[20,21] Phantom limb pain is usually localized in distal parts of the absent limb, usually in the foot or hand.[14]

The pain can be described as tingling, throbbing, aching, pins and needles, squeezing, stabbing, shooting, pinching, or cramping. In some cases, patients report that the amputated limb is positioned in a painful posture, or they sense spasms in the limb. The intensity as well as the quality of the pain varies greatly between patients from mild to severe. Phantom limb pain is triggered or worsened by physical (e.g., rainy weather, low temperature, prosthetic use, urination, defecation, reduced blood flow, and muscle tension), psychosocial (e.g., attention), and emotional (e.g., anxiety and stress) stimuli.[18,22] Phantom limb pain is not relieved with position.

PHYSICAL EXAMINATION

Physical examination is generally unrevealing. However, patients can sometimes identify specific points on the residual limb that trigger phantom limb pain. Therefore, the residual limb should be assessed for any sources of pain or trigger areas. The residual limb is examined for neuromas, cysts, bursae, bone spurs, or sites of excessive pressure. Other precipitating factors should be searched for, such as an ill-fitting prosthesis or mechanical stimulation.

575

Local problems, such as a herniated disc or spinal disease emitting sensations into the phantom limb or neuroma, can cause neuropathic pain. A comprehensive physical evaluation with particular attention to the neurologic examination, including strength, range of motion, muscle stretch reflexes, and muscle tone, should be done to rule out any concomitant central or peripheral neuropathic pain.

FUNCTIONAL LIMITATIONS

Functional complications of phantom limb pain include sleep disorders, interference with prosthesis training and use, reduction in walking ability, inability to return to work, and limitation of participation in social activities. Patients with phantom limb pain experience a greater degree of despair, more symptoms of depression, less satisfaction with social relations, and poorer quality of life than amputees without it.

DIAGNOSTIC STUDIES

The diagnosis of phantom limb pain is generally made clinically on the basis of history and physical examination. Plain radiography and ultrasonography are performed for the diagnosis of underlying conditions, such as neuroma, abscess, bursitis, bone spur or fragment, or nerve entrapment. Magnetic resonance imaging, electrodiagnostic tests, or laboratory tests may be indicated if other diagnoses are suspected.

Nerve block may be attempted as a diagnostic tool to identify candidates for specific procedures. Various pain scales and psychometric questionnaires are used to assess severity, treatment effect, and disability.

Differential Diagnosis

Nonpainful phantom sensation

Stump pain (residual limb pain)

Chronic postsurgical pain

Radicular pain

Neuralgia

Anginal pain

TREATMENT

The treatments commonly used for phantom limb pain are listed in Table 104-1.

Initial

Patients should be taught (if possible, before amputation) that phantom limb pain is not a complication but a normal side effect of some amputations. Education about

TABLE 104-1 Treatments Commonly Used for Phantom Limb Pain

Pharmacologic

Conventional analgesics

Opioids

Anticonvulsants

Antidepressants

NMDA receptor antagonists

Neuroleptics

Ketamine

Barbiturates

β Blockers

Muscle relaxants

Rehabilitation

Physiotherapy

Prosthesis training

Transcutaneous electrical nerve stimulation

Ultrasound

Manipulation

Electromyographic biofeedback

Thermal biofeedback

Sensory discrimination training

Psychological

Cognitive-behavioral pain management

Sensory discrimination training

Relaxation technique

Stress management

Distraction

Hypnosis

Anesthetic

Local anesthesia

Nerve blocks

Sympathetic block

Epidural blockade

Surgical

Stump revision

Neurectomy

Sympathectomy

Dorsal root entry zone ablation

Dorsal rhizotomy

Cordotomy

Thalamotomy

Spinal cord stimulation

Deep brain stimulation

Cortical resection of brain

Other

Acupuncture

phantom limb pain reduces anxiety and distress of patients. The expected course of symptoms after amputation and during the prosthetic fitting process should be carefully reviewed with the patient. Preemptive analgesia, which is attempted to prevent phantom limb pain by epidural or general routes during the preoperative and initial postoperative period, has not been shown to be effective.[1,3,14,23]

Tricyclic antidepressants and anticonvulsants have long been considered to be the drugs of choice. Controlled studies, however, showed conflicting data on the effect of tricyclic antidepressants in phantom limb pain conditions.[24,25] Anticonvulsants such as carbamazepine, gabapentin, topiramate,[26] and lamotrigine are effective in phantom limb pain.

Randomized controlled studies demonstrated that opioids have analgesic efficacy for phantom limb pain and suggested an effect on cortical reorganization.[27-29] Tramadol is an analgesic with both monoaminergic and opioid activity that is effective in long-standing phantom limb pain.[25]

In controlled studies, intravenous calcitonin[30,31] and intravenous ketamine demonstrated reduction of phantom limb pain.[32]

N-Methyl-D-aspartate (NMDA) receptor antagonists, such as dextromethorphan[33,34] and memantine,[35-37] showed efficacy in controlling phantom limb pain in several studies.

Other pharmacologic interventions, such as β blockers, topical capsaicin, nonsteroidal anti-inflammatory drugs, nonopioid analgesics, and botulinum toxin,[38,39] have been suggested, but well-controlled trials have not been published.

Rehabilitation

Transcutaneous electrical nerve stimulation has long been considered an effective treatment modality[40-42]; it can begin early in the postoperative period without significant side effects. Compression stockings or stump shrinkers during the early postoperative period and heat and cold, manipulation, vibration, massage, and acupuncture can all be tried in an attempt to provide relief of phantom limb pain.

Several prior studies have reported positive results of biofeedback, including electromyographic biofeedback, thermal biofeedback, and muscle relaxation procedures.[1,26,42-45] Frequent use of a myoelectric prosthesis that provides sensory, visual, and motor feedback reportedly reduces phantom limb pain.[46]

Sensory discrimination training[47] or tactile stimulation[48] has also been reported to reduce phantom limb pain with a reversal of cortical reorganization. Virtual reality and mirror treatment with use of a "mirror box" or "virtual reality box" to offer visual input on phantom sensations have been suggested as potential treatment.[49-51]

Psychological treatments such as relaxation technique, stress management, distraction, and hypnosis can also provide relief, although very few studies on phantom limb pain were conducted.

Procedures

Regional anesthesia with local anesthetics, including plexus or nerve block, sympathetic block, and epidural block, can be applied to intractable phantom limb pain with pharmacologic measures.

Surgery

Surgery is generally not indicated for phantom limb pain. Stump revision, such as neuroma resection, is indicated in selected patients with stump pain due to neuroma. The purpose of neuroma resection is relief of stump pain, not of phantom limb pain.

Spinal cord stimulation, dorsal root entry zone ablation, neurectomy, sympathectomy, dorsal rhizotomy, cordotomy, thalamotomy, and cortical resection of brain have been used in a few cases of intractable pain.

POTENTIAL DISEASE COMPLICATIONS

Phantom limb pain reportedly causes significant disability. It keeps amputees from their usual activities and causes considerable interference with their daily, social, recreational, and work activities.[8]

The health-related quality of life of amputees with phantom limb pain is poorer than that of amputees without phantom limb pain.[52]

POTENTIAL TREATMENT COMPLICATIONS

Side effects of pharmacologic treatment are well documented. Complications of regional anesthesia are systemic effects of local anesthetics, physiologic effects of the procedure (e.g., hypotension, inadvertent injection or block), and damage to adjacent structures. Spinal cord stimulation has few serious complications. Complications of surgical ablation techniques include Horner syndrome, dysesthesia, sudomotor paralysis, weakness, urinary complications, and respiratory problems. Selection of appropriate patients is important to successful surgical ablation.

References

1. Flor H. Phantom-limb pain: characteristics, causes, and treatment. Lancet Neurol 2002;1:182-189.
2. Ramachandran VS, Hirstein W. The perception of phantom limbs. The D.O. Hebb lecture. Brain 1998;121(pt 9):1603-1630.
3. Hazelgrove JF, Rogers PD. Phantom limb pain—a complication of lower extremity wound management. Int J Low Extrem Wounds 2002;1:112-124.
4. Nikolajsen L, Jensen TS. Phantom limb pain. Br J Anaesth 2001; 87:107-116.
5. Smith DG, Ehde DM, Legro MW, et al. Phantom limb, residual limb, and back pain after lower extremity amputations. Clin Orthop 1999;361:29-38.

6. Wartan SW, Hamann W, Wedley JR, McColl I. Phantom pain and sensation among British veteran amputees. Br J Anaesth 1997;78:652-659.

7. Kooijman CM, Dijkstra PU, Geertzen JH, et al. Phantom pain and phantom sensations in upper limb amputees: an epidemiological study. Pain 2000;87:33-41.

8. Ehde DM, Czerniecki JM, Smith DG, et al. Chronic phantom sensations, phantom pain, residual limb pain, and other regional pain after lower limb amputation. Arch Phys Med Rehabil 2000;81:1039-1044.

9. Dijkstra PU, Geertzen JH, Stewart R, van der Schans CP. Phantom pain and risk factors: a multivariate analysis. J Pain Symptom Manage 2002;24:578-585.

10. Ephraim PL, Wegener ST, MacKenzie EJ, et al. Phantom pain, residual limb pain, and back pain in amputees: results of a national survey. Arch Phys Med Rehabil 2005;86:1910-1919.

11. Hanley MA, Ehde DM, Campbell KM, et al. Self-reported treatments used for lower-limb phantom pain: descriptive findings. Arch Phys Med Rehabil 2006;87:270-277.

12. Sherman RA, Sherman CJ. Prevalence and characteristics of chronic phantom limb pain among American veterans. Results of a trial survey. Am J Phys Med 1983;62:227-238.

13. Jensen TS, Krebs B, Nielsen J, Rasmussen P. Immediate and long-term phantom limb pain in amputees: incidence, clinical characteristics and relationship to pre-amputation limb pain. Pain 1985;21:267-278.

14. Nikolajsen L, Ilkjaer S, Kroner K, et al. The influence of preamputation pain on postamputation stump and phantom pain. Pain 1997;72:393-405.

15. Houghton AD, Nicholls G, Houghton AL, et al. Phantom pain: natural history and association with rehabilitation Ann R Coll Surg Engl 1994;76:22-25.

16. Jensen TS, Krebs B, Nielsen J, Rasmussen P. Phantom limb, phantom pain and stump pain in amputees during the first 6 months following limb amputation. Pain 1983;17:243-256.

17. Geertzen JH, Bosmans JC, van der Schans CP, Dijkstra PU. Claimed walking distance of lower limb amputees. Disabil Rehabil 2005;27:101-104.

18. Katz J, Melzack R. Pain "memories" in phantom limbs: review and clinical observations. Pain 1990;43:319-336.

19. Katz J. Prevention of phantom limb pain by regional anaesthesia. Lancet 1997;349:519-520.

20. Sherman RA, Sherman CJ. Prevalence and characteristics of chronic phantom limb pain among American veterans. Results of a trial survey. Am J Phys Med 1983;62:227-238.

21. Richardson C, Glenn S, Nurmikko T, Horgan M. Incidence of phantom phenomena including phantom limb pain 6 months after major lower limb amputation in patients with peripheral vascular disease. Clin J Pain 2006;22:353-358.

22. Wilkins KL, McGrath PJ, Finley GA, Katz J. Prospective diary study of nonpainful and painful phantom sensations in a preselected sample of child and adolescent amputees reporting phantom limbs. Clin J Pain 2004;20:293-301.

23. Nikolajsen L, Ilkjaer S, Jensen TS. Effect of preoperative extradural bupivacaine and morphine on stump sensation in lower limb amputees. Br J Anaesth 1998;81:348-354.

24. Robinson LR, Czerniecki JM, Ehde DM, et al. Trial of amitriptyline for relief of pain in amputees: results of a randomized controlled study. Arch Phys Med Rehabil 2004;85:1-6.

25. Wilder-Smith CH, Hill LT, Laurent S. Postamputation pain and sensory changes in treatment-naive patients: characteristics and responses to treatment with tramadol, amitriptyline, and placebo. Anesthesiology 2005;103:619-628.

26. Harden RN, Houle TT, Remble TA, et al. Topiramate for phantom limb pain: a time-series analysis. Pain Med 2005;6:375-378.

27. Huse E, Larbig W, Flor H, Birbaumer N. The effect of opioids on phantom limb pain and cortical reorganization. Pain 2001;90:47-55.

28. Wu CL, Tella P, Staats PS, et al. Analgesic effects of intravenous lidocaine and morphine on postamputation pain: a randomized double-blind, active placebo-controlled, crossover trial. Anesthesiology 2002;96:841-848.

29. Bergmans L, Snijdelaar DG, Katz J, Crul BJ. Methadone for phantom limb pain. Clin J Pain 2002;18:203-205.

30. Jaeger H, Maier C. Calcitonin in phantom limb pain: a double blind study. Pain 1992;48:21-27.

31. Wall GC, Heyneman CA. Calcitonin in phantom limb pain. Ann Pharmacother 1999;33:499-501.

32. Nikolajsen L, Hansen CL, Nielsen J, et al. The effect of ketamine on phantom pain: a central neuropathic disorder maintained by peripheral input. Pain 1996;67:69-77.

33. Ben Abraham R, Marouani N, Kollender Y, et al. Dextromethorphan for phantom pain attenuation in cancer amputees: a double-blind crossover trial involving three patients. Clin J Pain 2002;18:282-285.

34. Ben Abraham R, Marouani N, Weinbroum AA. Dextromethorphan mitigates phantom pain in cancer amputees. Ann Surg Oncol 2003;10:268-274.

35. Maier C, Dertwinkel R, Mansourian N, et al. Efficacy of the NMDA-receptor antagonist memantine in patients with chronic phantom limb pain—results of a randomized double-blinded, placebo-controlled trial. Pain 2003;103:277-283.

36. Wiech K, Kiefer RT, Topfner S, et al. A placebo-controlled randomized crossover trial of the N-methyl-D-aspartic acid receptor antagonist, memantine, in patients with chronic phantom limb pain. Anesth Analg 2004;98:408-413.

37. Schley M, Topfner S, Wiech K, et al. Continuous brachial plexus blockade in combination with the NMDA receptor antagonist memantine prevents phantom pain in acute traumatic upper limb amputees. Eur J Pain 2007;11:299-308. Epub 2006 May 22.

38. Kern U, Martin C, Scheicher S, Muller H. Does botulinum toxin A make prosthesis use easier for amputees? J Rehabil Med 2004;36:238-239.

39. Naumann M, Eberhardt B, Laskawi R, et al. Botulinum toxin in rare pain syndromes. J Neurol 2004;251(Suppl 1):I39-I40.

40. Katz J, Melzack R. Auricular transcutaneous electrical nerve stimulation (TENS) reduces phantom limb pain. J Pain Symptom Manage 1991;6:73-83.

41. Wartan SW, Hamann W, Wedley JR, McColl I. Phantom pain and sensation among British veteran amputees. Br J Anaesth 1997;78:652-659.

42. Halbert J, Crotty M, Cameron ID. Evidence for the optimal management of acute and chronic phantom pain: a systematic review. Clin J Pain 2002;18:84-92.

43. Sherman RA, Gall N, Gormly J. Treatment of phantom limb pain with muscular relaxation training to disrupt the pain-anxiety-tension cycle. Pain 1979;6:47-55.

44. Dougherty J. Relief of phantom limb pain after EMG biofeedback-assisted relaxation: a case report. Behav Res Ther 1980;18:355-357.

45. Belleggia G, Birbaumer N. Treatment of phantom limb pain with combined EMG and thermal biofeedback: a case report. Appl Psychophysiol Biofeedback 2001;26:141-146.

46. Lotze M, Grodd W, Birbaumer N, et al. Does use of a myoelectric prosthesis prevent cortical reorganization and phantom limb pain? Nat Neurosci 1999;2:501-502.

47. Flor H, Denke C, Schaefer M, Grusser S. Effect of sensory discrimination training on cortical reorganisation and phantom limb pain. Lancet 2001;357:1763-1764.

48. Huse E, Preissl H, Larbig W, Birbaumer N. Phantom limb pain. Lancet 2001;358:1015.

49. Murray CD, Patchick EL, Caillette F, et al. Can immersive virtual reality reduce phantom limb pain? Stud Health Technol Inform 2006;119:407-412.

50. Ramachandran VS, Rogers-Ramachandran D. Synaesthesia in phantom limbs induced with mirrors. Proc Biol Sci 1996;263:377-386.

51. MacLachlan M, McDonald D, Waloch J. Mirror treatment of lower limb phantom pain: a case study. Disabil Rehabil 2004;26:901-904.

52. van der Schans CP, Geertzen JH, Schoppen T, Dijkstra PU. Phantom pain and health-related quality of life in lower limb amputees. J Pain Symptom Manage 2002;24:429-436.

Cervical Dystonia 105

Moon Suk Bang, MD, PhD, and Shi-Uk Lee, MD, PhD

Moon Suk Bang, MD, PhD, and Shi-Uk Lee, MD, PhD

Synonyms

Spasmodic torticollis
Idiopathic torsion dystonia
Symptomatic torsion dystonia

ICD-9 Codes

333.6   Idiopathic torsion dystonia
333.7   Symptomatic torsion dystonia

DEFINITION

Idiopathic cervical dystonia, the most common form of adult-onset focal dystonia, is defined as involuntary twisting and turning of the neck caused by abnormal involuntary muscle contractures.[1] Cervical dystonia has also been known as spasmodic torticollis, which implies head jerking or neck spasms. However, these features are absent in 25% to 35% of patients with this condition.[2] Furthermore, the term fails to emphasize the dystonic nature of the condition and the frequent association of cervical dystonia with dystonia in adjacent or remote body parts.

The prevalence of cervical dystonia has been estimated at 9 per 100,000, but this low frequency is based on a retrospective chart review.[3] The incidence is sex and age related. Women are affected 1.5 to 1.9 times more often than men are.[2,4] In 70% to 90% of cases, the disease begins between the fourth and sixth decades, with a peak incidence in the fifth decade of life.[5]

The pathogenetic mechanisms are unclear, but increasing evidence suggests that cervical dystonia is influenced by genetic factors. Many patients with cervical dystonia have a family history.[2] Several gene loci, such as DYT1, DYT6, and DYT7, have recently been reported to be associated with cervical dystonia.[6]

Cervical dystonia has also been reported to develop secondary to head, neck, and shoulder trauma.[7] The role of the sensory system is important in pathogenesis (see section on symptoms).[8] Impaired inhibition of sensory Ia afferent fibers, impairment of central sensory pathways, and increased spindle responsiveness secondary to overactive gamma-spindle efferent fibers have been proposed as pathogenic mechanisms.[9] Other mechanisms proposed are vestibular impairment, dysfunction of the subcortical-cortical motor network, and dopaminergic dysfunction.[9]

The natural course of dystonia has been reported.[10] In 68.1% of patients, dystonia had remained focal. Progression of dystonia to sites other than the neck was noted in 31.9% of patients. The only risk factor for progression of dystonia to other body parts was longer duration of disease. The rate of spontaneous remission was 20.8%. In most of the cases (87%), the remission occurred during the first 5 years of illness. The remission was sustained in 60% of the patients. In 40% of the patients who had experienced remission, the disorder relapsed (nonsustained remission). The duration of disease before remission was an important discriminating factor between sustained and nonsustained remission. The patients who experienced nonsustained remission had all done well within the first 2 years of the disorder; whereas in the patients who had sustained remission, the duration of dystonia before remission was more than 2 years.

SYMPTOMS

Symptoms usually begin insidiously with complaints of a "pulling" or "drawing" in the neck or an involuntary twisting or jerking of the head. In a majority of patients, the manifesting symptoms are sensory in nature (described variously as pain, pulling, or stiffness) or a degree of head rotation or deviation, with jerking and tremor of the head being distinctly less common complaints.[2,4,11] In 83% of patients, head deviation was constant rather than jerky (i.e., nonspasmodic) and demonstrated some degree of rotational torticollis (97%). Only a fraction of patients showed head jerks (35%) and neck spasms (37%), which are the cardinal features of "spasmodic" torticollis.[2]

Many patients have signs of dystonia involving other body segments at the time of presentation. Extracervical dystonia is found in 10% to 20% of patients[2,4]; the jaw (oromandibular), eyelids (blepharospasm), arm or hand (writer's cramp,) and trunk (axial) are the most frequently affected parts. A postural or kinetic hand tremor is found in up to 25% of patients.

Several provocative and palliative factors are characteristic of idiopathic dystonia. Most notable is the use of a sensory trick or *geste antagonistique*. Gently touching the chin, back of the head, or top of the head relieves the symptoms. The use of sensory tricks to keep the head in the body midline position was reported by 88.9% of patients in one series.[12] The physiologic mechanism of sensory tricks remains unknown. Other effective maneuvers include leaning against a high-backed chair, placing something in the mouth, and pulling the hair. Early in the illness, these tricks are helpful in most patients, but they tend to lose effectiveness as the disease progresses. Less common palliative factors are relaxation, alcohol, and "morning benefit," when symptoms are improved for a while after waking. Cervical dystonia is commonly exacerbated by activity (e.g., walking), fatigue, or stress.[13]

Pain is a major source of disability in two thirds to three quarters of patients with cervical dystonia.[2,3,14,15] Pain severity was related to the intensity of dystonia and muscle spasms[2] but not to the duration of cervical dystonia and severity of motor dysfunction.[14] Pain was commonly described as tiring, radiating, tugging, aching, and exhausting.[14]

PHYSICAL EXAMINATION

Inspection of the patient's head posture is enough for the diagnosis of cervical dystonia. A wide variety of abnormal head and neck postures can occur. Rotational torticollis is a rotation of the chin around the longitudinal axis toward the shoulder. Laterocollis is a rotation of the head in the coronal plane, moving the ear toward the shoulder. Anterocollis and retrocollis are rotations of the head in the sagittal plane; anterocollis brings the chin toward the chest, and retrocollis elevates the chin and brings the occiput toward the back. By convention, the direction of the rotation is defined by the chin, so right-turning torticollis means that the chin is turning to the right. There may also be sagittal or lateral deviation of the base of the neck from the midline[13]; 66% to 80% of patients present with a combination of these movements.[2,4] The most common component of complex deviations is rotational torticollis, followed by head tilt, retrocollis, and anterocollis. Isolated deviations (e.g., in a single plane) are seen in less than one third of patients. Notably, idiopathic cases of pure anterocollis are extremely uncommon. There is no statistically significant preponderance of right or left deviation.[2,4,5,16] The abnormal posture is present for more than 75% of the time in most patients, but symptoms may change in nature and directional preponderance over time.[2] Although the term *spasmodic torticollis* implies head jerking or neck spasms, this feature is absent in 25.33% of patients. The adjectives spasmodic and spastic are misleading because there is no evidence that

cervical dystonia is a spastic disorder or caused by dysfunction of the pyramidal tracts. Furthermore, the movements are not always spasmodic but may be sustained.

Although abnormal head position is enough for the diagnosis, physical examination in patients with cervical dystonia must be focused on detection of "pseudodystonia" secondary to structural abnormalities.[17] A complete neurologic examination is mandated to exclude secondary dystonia. The presence of corticospinal, sensory, cerebellar, oculomotor, or cortical signs with cervical or extracervical dystonia suggests secondary dystonia.

FUNCTIONAL LIMITATIONS

Functional limitation due to cervical dystonia is found in almost all patients (99% of 220 patients).[16] Severity of disabilities ranged from mild ("subjective feeling of discomfort in social conditions without objective consequences on social life") to severe ("qualitative and quantitative modification of the occupational level with resulting impairment of social life"). One report documented depression in 24% of 67 patients with idiopathic cervical dystonia.[18]

At some point during the illness, 75% of patients complain of pain, and patients usually consider the pain a major source of disability.[2,4,10,15] Pain is associated with constant head turning, greater severity of head turning, and the presence of spasms.[2] Disability is also caused by task-specific limitations (e.g., inability to drive) and avoidance of social interaction due to abnormal posture. Questioning of patients about disability and clarification of the contributing factors are crucial for the optimal care of patients with idiopathic cervical dystonia.

DIAGNOSTIC STUDIES

Screening biochemical studies (blood chemistry screening test, complete blood count, thyroid function) in addition to a ceruloplasmin level should be performed. Because various central nervous system lesions are known to be associated with cervical dystonia, magnetic resonance imaging of the brain and cervical spine should be considered in all patients with a fixed painful neck posture.[19] If there is scoliosis, it may be evaluated with plain radiographs to document the baseline abnormality. In addition, Wilson disease should be excluded in all patients younger than 50 years by measurement of serum ceruloplasmin and a slit-lamp examination.

TREATMENT

Initial

The goals of treatment are to palliate, to improve the quality of life, and to prevent secondary complications. Reassurance is most important. Patients should be reassured that cervical dystonia is not dangerous and be reminded that cervical dystonia does not become

Differential Diagnosis

Atlantoaxial dislocation

Cervical fracture

Degenerative disc

Osteomyelitis

Klippel-Feil syndrome

Congenital torticollis associated with absence or fibrosis of cervical muscles

Postirradiation fibrosis

Acute stiff neck

Pharyngitis

Painful lymphadenopathy, adenitis

Vestibulo-ocular dysfunction (head tilt with fourth nerve paresis or labyrinthine disease)

Posterior fossa tumor

Arnold-Chiari syndrome

Bobble-head doll syndrome (with third ventricle cyst)

Nystagmus

Sandifer syndrome

Spinal cord tumor or syrinx

Extraocular muscle palsies, strabismus

Head thrusts with oculomotor apraxia

Hemianopia

Spasmus nutans

Focal seizures

generalized but may spread locally. However, they should also be told that treatment is symptomatic, not curative. Physicians must understand which aspects of the illness are most limiting because disability in cervical dystonia may be caused by many factors, such as pain, abnormal posture, functional limitation, social embarrassment, and depression. Detection of concomitant depression is crucial because it is a major source of disability, will limit therapeutic benefit, and is itself treatable. Secondary complications, such as radiculopathy, myelopathy, and dysphagia, must be recognized and treated. The evaluation of therapies for cervical dystonia is difficult: the abnormal postures, pain, and disability are not easy to quantitate; there are spontaneous remissions; and most trials are small and not randomized controlled trials.[20] Therefore, no universally accepted treatment protocol exists. However, the treatment of cervical dystonia has been revolutionized by chemodenervation with botulinum toxin. Medications are generally used as adjuncts to botulinum toxin. Adjunctive medications can prevent development of neutralizing antibodies because it is possible to lower dosages and frequency of botulinum toxin injections.

Anticholinergics, benzodiazepines, and baclofen are the most widely used.

Other medications are available, and many patients will require combination therapy. If therapy with botulinum toxin and oral medications fails, surgery may be required.[9]

Rehabilitation

Patients with mild symptoms may be managed with physical measures or pharmacotherapy. Physical measures include the simple *geste antagonistique* (i.e., sensory tricks), biofeedback, mechanical braces, and physiotherapy. Use of the manipulative approach in the treatment of cervical dystonia is not appropriate with the assumption that the condition results from a spinal or orthopedic abnormality. In most patients, it is not possible to physically overcome the brain's disordered central processing commands to displace the head position. Therefore, physiotherapists and chiropractors are advised not to use orthopedic techniques or physical force, as this may result in further discomfort or injury to the patient. However, it is beneficial to assist patients to use their own resources to improve head control by strengthening and enhanced flexibility.

Physical therapy is recommended as an adjunct to botulinum toxin injection. After treatment, there is less opposition from the dystonic musculature. The goal is to facilitate the patient's increased control over head movement and posture once the antagonists are weakened. In a case report, reduction of the effective dose of botulinum toxin was also possible when physiotherapy management was added to a long-term treatment regimen.[21]

Procedures

The prognosis of patients with cervical dystonia has been radically changed after the introduction of chemodenervation with botulinum toxin. Compared with all previous therapies, botulinum toxin benefits the highest percentage of patients in the shortest time, has been proved effective in many double-blind placebo-controlled and open trials,[22] and has fewer side effects than other pharmacologic therapies.[23] For idiopathic cervical dystonia, serotype A is most widely used. The use of serotypes B and F is under investigation in patients who have become immunologically resistant to serotype A.[24]

The identification of the sites of pain and the muscles responsible for the abnormal posture is the most important factor in botulinum toxin administration. The sternocleidomastoid, trapezius, splenius capitis, and levator scapulae are most commonly injected. An electromyographic study of 100 patients found that two or three muscles are most commonly abnormal.[25] The most commonly found abnormal muscles in each head posture are shown in Table 105-1. There is wide variability in the number of muscles injected, the number of injections per muscle, the concentration of botulinum toxin employed, and the use of electromyography-assisted injections among other technical details. Which

TABLE 105-1 Head Postures and the Muscles Most Commonly Responsible for the Posture

Head Posture	Responsible Muscles
Rotational torticollis	Contralateral SCM Ipsilateral SC With or without contralateral SC
Laterocollis	Ipsilateral SCM, SC, TPZ
Retrocollis	Bilateral SC

SCM, sternocleidomastoid; SC, splenius capitis; TPZ, trapezius.
Modified from Deuschl G, Heinen F, Kleedorfer B, et al. Clinical and poly-myographic investigation of spasmodic torticollis. J Neurol 1992;239:9-15.

technique provides optimal results remains to be determined.[26] The average optimal dose for patients with cervical dystonia is 200 units of Botox or 500 units of Dysport. It is important to customize the dosage and the muscles to suit the needs of the individual patients. The optimal dosing in a particular muscle has been assessed only for the sternocleidomastoid muscle by quantitative electromyography. Doses as small as 20 units of Botox reduced dystonic activity in the sternocleidomastoid muscle, whereas doses larger than 20 units offered minimal additional improvement.[27] Similarly, for Dysport, 100 units was sufficient to reduce the sternocleidomastoid muscle activity[27]; doses larger than 100 units were associated with a greater occurrence of dysphagia.[28]

A benefit from botulinum toxin is generally seen within the first week but may rarely be delayed for up to 8 weeks. The benefit lasts for an average of 12 weeks, and most physicians suggest that the injections be repeated every 3 to 4 months. The response to toxin is not affected by the pattern of deviation. Continued toxin injections provide progressive improvement of dystonia.[26]

Patients with cervical dystonia who never benefit from botulinum toxin injection are considered primary nonresponders. This occurs in approximately 15% to 30% of patients.[29] In addition to the occurrence of primary treatment failure (patients never responding to injection), secondary failure may also occur in 10% to 15% of patients. These patients with initial improvement after treatment fail to respond to subsequent injections. Of the secondary failures, 35.7% were found to have antibodies to botulinum toxin by the mouse neutralization assay.[29]

Surgery

Surgical therapy is recommended only for patients whose dystonia is prolonged, unresponsive to adequate trials of medication and botulinum toxin injections, and associated with significant pain or disability. Since the introduction of botulinum toxin, surgery is rarely required. Peripheral denervation procedures designed to denervate dystonic muscles selectively are the most widely practiced surgical procedures. Selective ramisectomy is a procedure that involves the selective section of dorsal rami of the upper cervical spinal nerves.[30] Selective denervation procedures are often combined with selective spinal accessory nerve section, anterior rhizotomy, or myotomy. Deep brain stimulation is becoming the standard of care for medically intractable, disabling dystonias. Advantages of deep brain stimulation include reversibility, adjustability, and continued access to the therapeutic target. Initial reports describing the use of deep brain stimulation in generalized dystonia have been encouraging, and experience in the use of deep brain stimulation to treat various forms of dystonia is continually growing.[31]

POTENTIAL DISEASE COMPLICATIONS

Patients may develop cervical spondylosis with resulting radiculopathy or myelopathy.[32] Extracervical spread of dystonia is a progression of dystonia to a segmental pattern of dystonia. In one third of 72 patients who first had isolated cervical dystonia, the dystonia typically spread to the face, jaw, arms, or trunk.[10]

POTENTIAL TREATMENT COMPLICATIONS

Side effects of botulinum toxin injections have been reported in 20% to 30% of patients per treatment cycle and approximately 50% of patients at some time during therapy. Dysphagia, neck weakness, and local pain at the injection site are the most commonly reported side effects, but dizziness, dry mouth, an influenza-like syndrome, lethargy, dysphonia, and generalized weakness have all been reported. The frequency of side effects varies widely, apparently on the basis of the dosage used.[24]

Failure to spare ventral roots in selective ramisectomy injures the cervical and brachial plexuses and leads to the complications of diaphragmatic paralysis and dysphagia. Other sequelae of the selective denervation procedure include sensory loss in the distribution of the greater occipital nerve, paresthesias, and occasional sudden tic-like pain.

References

1. Fahn S, Marsden CD, Calne DB. Classification and investigation of dystonia. In Marsden CD, Fahn S, eds. Movement Disorders 2. London, Butterworths, 1987:332-358.
2. Chan J, Brin MF, Fahn S. Idiopathic cervical dystonia: clinical characteristics. Mov Disord 1991;6:119-126.
3. Nutt JG, Muenter MD, Aronson A, et al. Epidemiology of focal and generalized dystonia in Rochester, Minnesota. Mov Disord 1988;3:188-194.
4. Jankovic J, Leder S, Warner D, Schwartz K. Cervical dystonia: clinical findings and associated movement disorders. Neurology 1991;41:1088-1091.
5. Duane DD. Spasmodic torticollis. Adv Neurol 1988;49:135-150.
6. Ozelius LJ, Hewett JW, Page CE, et al. The early-onset torsion dystonia gene (DYT1) encodes an ATP-binding protein. Nat Genet 1997;17:40-48.
7. Tarsy D. Comparison of acute- and delayed-onset posttraumatic cervical dystonia. Mov Disord 1998;13:481-485.

8. Tempel LW, Perlmutter JS. Abnormal cortical responses in patients with writer's cramp. Neurology 1993;43:2252-2257.

9. Dauer WT, Burke RE, Greene P, Fahn S. Current concepts on the clinical features, aetiology and management of idiopathic cervical dystonia. Brain 1998;121:547-560.

10. Jahanshahi M, Marion MH, Marsden CD. Natural history of adult-onset idiopathic torticollis. Arch Neurol 1990;47:548-552.

11. Rivest J, Marsden CD. Trunk and head tremor as isolated manifestations of dystonia [see comments]. Mov Disord 1990;5:60-65. Comment in Mov Disord 1990;5:353-354.

12. Jahanshahi M. Factors that ameliorate or aggravate spasmodic torticollis. J Neurol Neurosurg Psychiatry 2000;68:227-229.

13. Consky ES, Lang AE. Clinical assessments of patients with cervical dystonia. In Jankovic J, Hallett M, eds. Therapy with Botulinum Toxin. New York, Marcel Dekker, 1994:211-237.

14. Kutvonen O, Dastidar P, Nurmikko T. Pain in spasmodic torticollis. Pain 1997;69:279-286.

15. Lowenstein DH, Aminoff MJ. The clinical course of spasmodic torticollis. Neurology 1988;38:530-532.

16. Rondot P, Marchand MP, Dellatolas G. Spasmodic torticollis: review of 220 patients. Can J Neurol Sci 1991;18:143-151.

17. Weiner WJ, Lang AE. Idiopathic torsion dystonia. In Weiner WJ, Lang AE, eds. Movement Disorders: A Comprehensive Survey. New York, Futura, 1989:347-418.

18. Jahanshahi M. Psychosocial factors and depression in torticollis. J Psychosom Res 1991;35:493-507.

19. Comella CL, Thompson PD. Treatment of cervical dystonia with botulinum toxins. Eur J Neurol 2006;13(Suppl 1):S16-S20.

20. Lal S. Pathophysiology and pharmacotherapy of spasmodic torticollis: a review. Can J Neurol Sci 1979;6:427-435.

21. Ramdharry G. Case report: physiotherapy cuts the dose of botulinum toxin. Physiother Res Int 2006;11:117-122.

22. Marsden CD, Fahn S. Movement Disorders 3. Oxford, Butterworth-Heinemann, 1994.

23. Brans JW, Lindeboom R, Snoek JW, et al. Botulinum toxin versus trihexyphenidyl in cervical dystonia: a prospective, randomized, double-blind controlled trial. Neurology 1996;46:1066-1072.

24. Jankovic J. Botulinum toxin therapy for cervical dystonia. Neurotox Res 2006;9:145-148.

25. Deuschl G, Heinen F, Kleedorfer B, et al. Clinical and polymyographic investigation of spasmodic torticollis. J Neurol 1992;239:9-15.

26. Jankovic J, Schwartz K, Donovan DT. Botulinum toxin treatment of cranial-cervical dystonia, spasmodic dysphonia, other focal dystonias and hemifacial spasm. J Neurol Neurosurg Psychiatry 1990;53:633-639.

27. Dresler D. Electromyographic evaluation of cervical dystonia for planning of botulinum toxin therapy. Eur J Neurol 2000;7:713-718.

28. Borodic GE, Joseph M, Fay L, et al. Botulinum A toxin for the treatment of spasmodic torticollis: dysphagia and regional toxin spread. Head Neck 1990;12:392-399.

29. Barnes MP, Best D, Kidd L, et al. The use of botulinum toxin type-B in the treatment of patients who have become unresponsive to botulinum toxin type-A—initial experiences. Eur J Neurol 2005;12:947-955.

30. Braun V, Richter HP. Selective peripheral denervation for the treatment of spasmodic torticollis. Neurosurgery 1994;35:58-63.

31. Tagliati M, Shils J, Sun C, Alterman R. Deep brain stimulation for dystonia. Expert Rev Med Devices 2004;1:33-41.

32. Waterston JA, Swash M, Watkins ES. Idiopathic dystonia and cervical spondylotic myelopathy. J Neurol Neurosurg Psychiatry 1989;52:1424-1426.

Post-Thoracotomy Pain Syndrome 106

Justin Riutta, MD

DEFINITION

Post-thoracotomy pain syndrome (PTPS) is defined as pain that recurs or persists at the incision site or in the dermatomal distribution of the intercostal nerves for longer than 2 months after thoracotomy.[1-3] Thoracotomies are used to access intrathoracic contents, such as the lung, esophagus, and heart. The most common indication for a thoracotomy is tumor resection. The classic thoracotomy consists of a posterolateral incision of the thorax, bisection of the latissimus dorsi and serratus anterior, separation of the ribs, disruption of the intercostal nerves, and pleural incision. The thoracotomy is regarded as one of the most painful surgical procedures performed.[1-10] The incidence of PTPS has a wide range (2% to 90%), but on average, approximately 40% of patients will have chronic postoperative pain.[2,4] PTPS is mild to moderate in 92% of cases; 50% of patients will have disruption in capacity to perform daily activities. Sleep disruption occurs in 25% to 30%. Fortunately, severe disabling pain occurs in only 3% to 5% of patients with PTPS.[5,6] Predictive factors for development of PTPS include increased pain 24 hours postoperatively, female gender, preoperative opiate use, and radiation therapy.[4,8]

Intercostal neuralgia is the most commonly implicated cause of chronic PTPS.[1] Other factors contributing to pain are outlined in Table 106-1. Recognizing that local muscle disruption of the serratus anterior and latissimus dorsi results in abnormal scapulohumeral mechanics, shoulder abnormalities are one of the common causes of functional loss after thoracotomy.[7]

SYMPTOMS

PTPS generally presents with symptoms of allodynia, dysesthesias, and lancinating pain typically attributed to intercostal neuralgia.[4] In addition, patients will have symptoms of achiness, pleuritic pain, and focal tenderness over the incision site.[1,4] Shoulder movement, deep breathing, and lying directly on the affected side can aggravate these symptoms.[4] Pain is frequently encountered with shoulder maneuvers and direct contact with the incision site and can present as shoulder dysfunction and sleep disruption.

PHYSICAL EXAMINATION

The examination of the patient with PTPS includes inspection of the incision site and chest wall movement with respiratory excursion. Deep breathing maneuvers to elicit pleuritic pain are another component of the examination. Palpation over the incision site to evaluate for scar adherence, hypersensitivity, or intercostal nerve pain is the next component of the examination. The rib cage is disrupted with surgery and must be assessed for persistent fractures, costochondral avulsions, and costochondritis. Assessment of regional musculature for postoperative disruption, atrophy, and myofascial pain is important. Adhesive capsulitis and shoulder girdle dysfunction are factors in PTPS; therefore, active and passive range of motion of the shoulder and scapulohumeral mechanics should be evaluated. Neurologic examination includes motor testing of the affected extremity compared with the unaffected side, evaluation for scapular winging, and assessment of the dermatomal distribution of the transected intercostal nerves.

FUNCTIONAL LIMITATIONS

PTPS results in daily activity limitations in 50% of those affected.[5] Ochroch and associates[9] identified functional decrement by the 36-item short-form health survey (SF-36) in most patients at 4 to 48 weeks postoperatively. Shoulder restriction secondary to chest wall pain, adhesive capsulitis, and disruption of the serratus anterior and latissimus dorsi has been identified in 15% to 33% of post-thoracotomy patients at 1 year.[7] Shoulder restriction leads to limitations in sleep function, lifting capacity, and full range of motion activities of the shoulder girdle. In addition,

TABLE 106-1 Factors Associated with Post-Thoracotomy Pain[1,4]

Intercostal neuroma
Rib fracture
Adhesive capsulitis
Infection
Pleurisy
Costochondral dislocation
Costochondritis
Local tumor recurrence
Myofascial pain
Vertebral collapse

functional limitations can be attributed to respiratory compromise related to surgery or underlying pulmonary disease.

DIAGNOSTIC STUDIES

The relevant diagnostic studies include baseline radiographs of the rib cage to evaluate for bone disruption. In addition, chest radiographs and computed tomography scans can be used to screen for intrathoracic processes, such as pleura-based dysfunction, pneumonia, and recurrence of primary malignant disease. A diagnostic intercostal nerve block can be performed to identify intercostal neuralgia.

Differential Diagnosis

Rib fracture
Costochondral dislocation
Vertebral collapse
Adhesive capsulitis
Costochondritis
Pleurisy
Myofascial pain
Muscle disruption pain
Tumor recurrence
Thoracic radiculopathy
Intercostal neuroma
Cardiac ischemia
Aortic dissection
Infection of incision, pleura, pleural space, and lung parenchyma

TREATMENT

Initial

The initial aspect of management of PTPS includes early aggressive management of pain. Preemptive analgesia is the concept of diminishing postoperative pain by disrupting pain pathways preoperatively.[1] Aspects of preemptive analgesia include thoracic epidural anesthesia, intercostal nerve blockade, opiates, and nonsteroidal anti-inflammatory drugs (NSAIDs).[1] Thoracic epidural anesthesia has been shown to diminish acute postoperative pain in thoracotomy.[10] Balanced anesthesia with preoperative regional anesthesia, opiates, and NSAIDs diminishes PTPS from 50% to 9.9%.[2,4] The surgical approach does have a bearing on postoperative pain. Smaller surgical incisions and muscle-sparing thoracotomies diminish postoperative pain.[1]

Acute postoperative pain management includes thoracic epidural administration of opiates in combination with regional anesthesia and NSAIDs. Opiates alone decrease PTPS to 23.4%.[11] Opiates plus regional anesthesia decrease PTPS to 14.8%. The opiates, anesthesia, and NSAIDs combine to diminish rates to 9.9%.[11] In addition, early scar management once healing is complete can diminish long-term pain by reduced adherence to chest wall structures and diminishing hypersensitivity. The primary means is gentle massage and repetitive stimulation of the incision site. Transcutaneous electrical nerve stimulation units have also been found to be effective in reducing PTPS.[12]

Pharmacologic management of PTPS includes early postoperative use of opiates and NSAIDs in combination.[2] Delivery of topical anesthetics by patches (Lidoderm) also can be used for pain control.[2] Management of chronic PTPS is usually through use of neuropathic pain medications. The only study specifically for PTPS used gabapentin and found that this was well tolerated and decreased pain in 73% of those studied; 42% of those studied had more than 50% pain relief.[13] Neuropathic pain medications encountered in the literature that have not been studied in PTPS include amitriptyline and nortriptyline. If oral routes of pain control fail, intrathecal administration of opiates is an option.

Rehabilitation

The preoperative management of PTPS begins with nutritional assessment and augmentation. Patients with intrathoracic disease can frequently encounter nutritional issues as a result of their primary disease; it can be beneficial for postoperative recovery to maximize nutritional status. The second factor in preoperative management is to maintain or to obtain normal shoulder range of motion. As mentioned, shoulder dysfunction and muscle dysfunction occur in up to 33% of thoracotomy patients. Maximization of range, function, and strength before surgery can reduce functional loss secondary to postoperative restriction. Pulmonary rehabilitation is important in thoracotomy patients primarily because many have underlying pulmonary disease.

Pulmonary rehabilitation preoperatively includes breathing techniques, energy conservation, medication instruction, secretion management, and aerobic endurance training. The objective is to reduce frequently encountered postoperative complications secondary to decreased depth of breathing, retention of secretions, atelectasis, and pneumonia.[10]

Postoperative rehabilitation includes nutritional assessment as outlined before. Pulmonary rehabilitation begins postoperatively with breathing techniques, secretion management, and assisted coughing with stabilization of the disrupted thorax. Scar mobilization is an important aspect of early pain relief. Scars can increase pain secondary to adherence to chest wall structures, underlying nerve entrapment, and restriction of range of motion of the shoulder. Early scar mobilization consists of gentle massage to maintain mobility of the incision and the soft tissue structures adjacent to the incision. Soft tissue massage techniques are not initiated until adequate wound healing has occurred.

Shoulder dysfunction is a common sequela of PTPS. The shoulder dysfunction has multiple factors including muscle disruption, chest wall pain with shoulder movement, and myofascial pain. Surgical disruption of the latissimus dorsi and serratus anterior can lead directly to shoulder dysfunction. The serratus anterior stabilizes the scapula against the chest wall and aids in protraction. Normal shoulder abduction is limited without serratus anterior function. The latissimus dorsi is a powerful adductor of the arm. Latissimus restriction can lead to lack of forward flexion and abduction at the glenohumeral joint. The disruption of these two muscle groups is less of an issue with muscle-sparing procedures. The rehabilitation process is delayed primarily because of time for muscle continuity to return after disruption. The initial management includes gentle massage of the affected muscle group and pendulum exercises. This is followed by gentle active range of motion exercises that progress to passive range of motion exercises once full muscle continuity has been regained. Strengthening is the next process and can take up to a full year. Weakness in the latissimus muscle group may persist and requires attention and appropriate restrictions. The primary issue with the serratus anterior is obtaining normal scapular mechanics and normalizing scapulohumeral rhythm. This may require dedicated physical therapy by a therapist who understands shoulder mechanics. Shoulder rehabilitation may be delayed by postoperative restrictions. The standard restrictions are active range of motion only and no lifting of more than 10 pounds. These restrictions as standard practice are in place for 6 weeks after surgery. Full lifting as tolerated is typically not recommended until 12 weeks after surgery.

The next step in rehabilitation is regaining and perhaps surpassing of presurgical function with endurance training. Endurance training can include low-impact lower extremity exercise, such as walking and stationary biking once pain allows. The patient can progress to high-load activities (e.g., running, swimming, climbing) after full healing of the chest wall, typically at 12 weeks. The final step is return to work and vocational rehabilitation. It is important to address goals of the rehabilitation process early in management; this helps both physiatrist and patient to set goals that will maximize quality of life.

Procedures

Management of PTPS with interventional procedures consists of perioperative and chronic pain management. The perioperative management involves preemptive analgesia with regional anesthesia preoperatively.[2,4] Thoracic epidural anesthesia is the primary means of early postoperative management, and this typically consists of infusion of an opiate and an anesthetic.[1] Chronic PTPS management usually starts with intercostal nerve blockade.[2] Thoracic nerve root block and radiofrequency ablation of intercostal nerves are other procedures used for PTPS.[2] Long-term maintenance pain management can be accomplished with intrathecal opiate delivery and spinal cord stimulators.[2]

Surgery

There are no surgical treatments for post-thoracotomy pain.

POTENTIAL DISEASE COMPLICATIONS

The potential complications of PTPS include postoperative respiratory dysfunction secondary to decreased depth of breathing, retention of secretions, and atelectasis.[10] In addition, persistent chest wall pain can result in decreased shoulder movement and adhesive capsulitis. Shoulder function also may be affected by the disruption of the serratus anterior and the latissimus dorsi, resulting in scapular dysfunction and glenohumeral dysfunction, respectively. In addition, sleep disruption, depression, loss of employment, and diminished functional and vocational capacities can be seen in PTPS.

POTENTIAL TREATMENT COMPLICATIONS

Complications of PTPS treatment include local complications from interventional procedures, including hematomas, infections, and nerve disruption. In addition, the use of opiates and NSAIDs postoperatively can lead to gastrointestinal dysfunction. The most common side effects identified with the use of gabapentin in this population are sedation (24%) and dizziness (6%).[13]

References
1. Hazelrigg SR, Cetindag IB, Fullerton J. Acute and chronic pain syndromes after thoracic surgery. Surg Clin North Am 2002;82: 849-865.
2. Erdek M, Staats PS. Chronic pain after thoracic surgery. Thorac Surg Clin 2005;15:123-130.
3. Merskey H. Classification of chronic pain: description of chronic pain syndromes and definitions of pain terms. Pain 1986;3: S138-S139.

4. Karmakar M, Ho A. Postthoracotomy pain syndrome. Thorac Surg Clin 2004;14:345-352.

5. Maguire MF, Ravenscroft A, Beggs D, Duffy JP. A questionnaire study investigating the prevalence of the neuropathic component of chronic pain after thoracic surgery. Eur J Cardiothorac Surg 2006;29:800-805. Epub 2006 Apr 3.

6. Perttunen K, Tasmuth T, Kalso E. Chronic pain after thoracic surgery: a follow up study. Acta Anaesthesiol Scand 1999;43:563-567.

7. Li W, Lee T, Yim A. Shoulder function after thoracic surgery. Thorac Surg Clin 2004;14:331-343.

8. Gotoda Y, Kambara N, Sakai T, et al. The morbidity, time course and predictive factors for persistent post-thoracotomy pain. Eur J Pain 2001;5:89-96.

9. Ochroch EA, Gottschalk A, Augostides J, et al. Long-term pain and activity during recovery from major thoracotomy using thoracic epidural analgesia. Anesthesiology 2002;97:1234-1244.

10. Yegin A, Erdogan A, Kayacan N, Karsli B. Early postoperative pain management after thoracic surgery; pre- and postoperative versus postoperative epidural analgesia: a randomised study. Eur J Cardiothoracic Surg 2003;24:420-424.

11. Richardson J, Sabanathan S, Mearns AJ, et al. Post-thoracotomy neuralgia. Pain Clin 1994;7:87-97.

12. Erdogan M, Erdogan A, Erbil N, et al. Prospective, randomized, placebo-controlled study of the effects of TENS on postthoracotomy pain and pulmonary function. World J Surg 2005;29: 1563-1570.

13. Sihoe AD, Lee TW, Wan IY, et al. The use of gabapentin for post-operative and post-traumatic pain in thoracic surgery patients. Eur J Cardiothorac Surg 2006;29:795-799. Epub 2006 Apr 3.

Post-Mastectomy Pain Syndrome

107

Justin Riutta, MD

DEFINITION

Post-mastectomy pain syndrome (PMPS) is defined as a chronic pain condition, typically neuropathic in nature, that can follow surgery to the breast.[1] PMPS can occur with any surgery to the breast, including mastectomy, lumpectomy, reconstruction, and augmentation, although rates seem to be reduced with sentinel lymph node procedures.[2,3] PMPS affects approximately 40% of patients after breast surgery.[3,4] The risk factors for development of PMPS include younger age, more extensive surgery, greater immediate postoperative pain, and anxiety.[2,5]

Classification of PMPS can be divided into three categories: phantom breast pain, intercostobrachial neuralgia, and neuroma pain.[6] Phantom pain is identified in 23% of post-mastectomy patients and consists of painful sensations in the area of the removed breast.[7] The intercostobrachial nerve is the lateral cutaneous nerve of the second thoracic root. It courses along the axillary vein and then provides sensation to the axilla and breast. The intercostobrachial nerve is frequently stretched or sacrificed during axillary lymph node dissections and is a common cause of PMPS.[6,8,9] The scar from breast surgery can be a generator of pain. The pain has been attributed to underlying neuroma formation, axon impingement, and scar retraction.[6,10]

SYMPTOMS

The symptoms associated with PMPS include shooting, stabbing, burning, and pins and needles in the breast, axilla, or medial arm.[1,3,6,11-13] In addition, patients complain of symptoms of tightness and fullness in the axilla. Pain is aggravated by shoulder movement, stretching, straining, and direct contact with clothes.[3,11] The symptoms

of PMPS are usually nonprogressive and have been found to persist in half of patients observed for 9 years.[1,11] PMPS results in functional loss and sleep disruption, and these may be common presenting complaints.[1,10]

PHYSICAL EXAMINATION

The primary aspects of the physical examination include the exclusion of other causes of the identified pain and the classification of PMPS. General inspection is performed to evaluate for muscle wasting, asymmetry, and gross masses. The musculoskeletal examination focuses on shoulder range and function and costovertebral, costochondral, and rib integrity. A careful skin examination is performed to assess for scar adherence, fibrosis, scar tenderness, neuromas, infection, and recurrence of malignant disease. The lymphatic examination is performed to assess for lymphadenopathy in lymphatic distributions not already dissected. The neurologic examination includes motor testing of the shoulder girdle, focusing on motor nerves potentially affected by breast surgery (thoracodorsal, long thoracic, medial and lateral pectoral). Sensory testing includes all affected breast dermatomes T1-5. Particular attention should be paid to the posterior thorax dermatome, as this can be a clue to spinal disease. The sensory examination of the axilla should identify the distribution, severity, and type of sensory abnormality. The complete neurologic examination includes a full assessment of ipsilateral upper extremity motor, reflex, and sensory function.

FUNCTIONAL LIMITATIONS

The major functional limitations with PMPS include loss of shoulder range of motion, lifting restrictions, and sleep disruption. Loss of shoulder range of motion is attributed to maintenance of the more comfortable adducted position, resulting in restricted abduction and external rotation.[11] Limitations with lifting result in diminished capacity to perform household duties (vacuuming, laundry), occupational duties (stocking shelves), and vocational pursuits.[1,10,11] Sleep disruption affects 50% of patients with PMPS and can lead to global daytime dysfunction.[11]

DIAGNOSTIC STUDIES

Diagnostic studies are used primarily to exclude other causes of pain. Recurrent malignant neoplasms can be excluded by mammography, magnetic resonance imaging, or positron emission tomographic scans. Dedicated imaging of the thoracic spine is warranted to exclude another cause of neuropathic pain in the breast dermatomes such as radiculopathy. Electrodiagnosis can be useful to exclude motor nerve abnormalities and plexopathy.

Differential Diagnosis

Tumor recurrence

Rib fracture

Paraneoplastic neuropathy

Intraparenchymal lung disease

Chemotherapy neuropathy

Thoracic nerve root impingement

Radiation plexopathy

Intercostal neuralgia

TREATMENT

Initial

The initial management of PMPS commences perioperatively. This includes minimization of dissection, nerve-sparing procedures, and early control of pain. Early pain control is imperative because severe early postoperative pain is one of the most consistent factors in PMPS.[5] Early postoperative pain control is typically accomplished with judicious use of opiates and nonsteroidal anti-inflammatory drugs. Early desensitization techniques can help limit neuropathic symptoms and can be initiated once the incision is healed. For those with uncontrolled pain that limits sleep and daily function, neuropathic pain medications can be initiated. Pharmaceuticals have not been studied extensively, but capsaicin, amitriptyline, nortriptyline, gabapentin, and Lidoderm patches have been studied and found to be effective.[6,12,14] Long-acting opiates can be used when these agents fail to control symptoms.[12]

Rehabilitation

From a rehabilitation perspective, PMPS management begins immediately postoperatively. The primary factor for rehabilitation management is to identify functional limits, targeting these as goals of both the patient and the caregiver. Clearly, shoulder restriction is a major factor in the functional limitations from PMPS. The initial phase of management includes pain control followed by shoulder range of motion. Shoulder rehabilitation begins with stretching of the pectoralis and latissimus dorsi, followed by glenohumeral range of motion exercises and finally scapulohumeral retraining. Once full shoulder range of motion with normal scapulohumeral mechanics is accomplished, strengthening and task-specific function become the targets of rehabilitation.

Procedures

Procedural management of PMPS is typically limited to regional nerve blocks for pain control.[12] For those with progressive shoulder dysfunction and painful range of motion, local injections in the subacromial space may be beneficial. In addition, myofascial injections with anesthetic preparations or botulinum toxin can be beneficial for myogenic pain.

Surgery

Surgical management for PMPS typically relates to chest wall pain or shoulder dysfunction. Chest wall pain with scar retraction can be managed with scar removal. In addition, soft tissue adherence to chest wall structures may require surgical repair. Adhesive capsulitis as a result of progressive loss of shoulder range of motion may require manipulation under anesthesia for full shoulder range of motion to be obtained.

POTENTIAL DISEASE COMPLICATIONS

The primary potential disease complications of PMPS are loss of shoulder function and diminished carrying capacity of the affected extremity. Resultant to this lack of function, patients can lose employment and vocational and recreational capacity. An insidious and life-altering complication of PMPS is sleep disruption. Sleep disruption can result in global dysfunction and health-related complications.

POTENTIAL TREATMENT COMPLICATIONS

Treatment complications are primarily related to side effects of medications. Capsaicin is known to cause painful skin reactions through its mechanism of action. Tricyclic antidepressants have anticholinergic side effects and must be used with caution in patients with cardiac arrhythmias. The main side effects of gabapentin are sedation, tremors, and dizziness. Topical lidocaine patches can result in skin excoriation. Bleeding, infection, and nerve irritation can complicate interventional procedures.

References

1. Macdonald L, Bruce J, Scott NW, et al. Long-term follow-up of breast cancer survivors with post-mastectomy pain syndrome. Br J Cancer 2005;92:225-230.
2. Schulze T, Mucke J, Markwardt J, et al. Long-term morbidity of patients with early breast cancer after sentinel lymph node biopsy compared to axillary lymph node dissection. J Surg Oncol 2006;93:109-119.

3. Smith WC, Bourne D, Squair J, et al. A retrospective cohort study of post mastectomy pain syndrome. Pain 1999;83:91-95.

4. Tasmuth T, von Smitten K, Hietanen P, et al. Pain and other symptoms after different treatment modalities of breast cancer. Ann Oncol 1995;6:453-459.

5. Katz J, Poleshuck EL, Andrus CH, et al. Risk factors for acute pain and its persistence following breast cancer surgery. Pain 2005;119:16-25.

6. Jung BF, Ahrendt GM, Oaklander AL, Dworkin RH. Neuropathic pain following breast cancer surgery: proposed classification and research update. Pain 2003;104:1-13.

7. Rothemund Y, Grüsser SM, Liebeskind U, et al. Phantom phenomena in mastectomized patients and their relation to chronic and acute pre-mastectomy pain. Pain 2004;107:140-146.

8. Vecht CJ. Arm pain in the patient with breast cancer. J Pain Symptom Manage 1990;5:109-117.

9. Foley KM. Pain syndromes in patients with cancer. Med Clin North Am 1987;71:169-184.

10. Kärki A, Simonen R, Mälkiä E, Selfe J. Impairments, activity limitations and participation restrictions 6 and 12 months after breast cancer operation. J Rehabil Med 2005;37:180-188.

11. Stevens PE, Dibble SL, Miaskowski C. Prevalence, characteristics, and impact of postmastectomy pain syndrome: an investigation of women's experiences. Pain 1995;61:61-68.

12. Kwekkeboom K. Postmastectomy pain syndromes. Cancer Nurs 1996;19:37-43.

13. Wallace MS, Wallace AM, Lee J, Dobke MK. Pain after breast surgery: a survey of 282 women. Pain 1996;66:195-205.

14. Devers A, Galer B. Topical lidocaine patch relieves a variety of neuropathic pain conditions: an open-label study. Clin J Pain 2000;16:205-208.

REHABILITATION

Upper Limb Amputations 108

Timothy R. Dillingham, MD, and Diane W. Braza, MD

Synonyms

Hand amputations
Below-elbow amputations
Above-elbow amputations

ICD-9 Codes

886	Traumatic amputation of other finger(s) (complete) (partial)
886.0	Without mention of complication
886.1	Amputated finger, complicated
887	Traumatic amputation of arm and hand (complete) (partial)
887.0	Unilateral, below elbow, without mention of complication
887.1	Unilateral, below elbow, complicated
887.2	Unilateral, at or above elbow, without mention of complication
887.3	Unilateral, at or above elbow, complicated
887.4	Unilateral, level not specified, without mention of complication
887.5	Unilateral, level not specified, complicated
887.6	Bilateral (any level), without mention of complication
887.7	Bilateral (any level), complicated
905.9	Late effect of traumatic amputation
997.60	Amputation stump complication, unspecified
997.61	Neuroma of amputation stump
997.62	Infection (chronic)
V52	Fitting and adjustment of prosthetic device and implant
V52.0	Artificial arm (complete) (partial)

DEFINITION

Upper limb amputations are devastating occurrences for individuals, with profound functional and vocational consequences. The primary reason for upper limb loss is trauma; cancer is the next most common reason.[1,2] Upper limb amputations from trauma occur at a rate of 3.8 individuals per 100,000; finger amputations are the most common (2.8 per 100,000). Hand amputations from trauma occur at a rate of 0.02 per 100,000.[1] Traumatic transradial amputations occur at a rate of 0.16 per 100,000 persons, and transhumeral limb loss from trauma occurs at a rate of 0.1 per 100,000.[1] The rates for traumatic amputations have declined by 50%

during the period 1988 to 1996,[1] probably because of changing work force patterns and greater concerns for industrial safety.

Limb amputations that result from malignant neoplasms have declined approximately 42% from 1988 to 1996.[1] Their rates of occurrence are lower than for trauma, with an upper limb loss rate in 1996 of 0.09 per 100,000.[1]

These rates of upper limb amputations are lower than the incidence rates for lower limb dysvascular amputations due to diabetes and peripheral arterial diseases, which occur in 45 per 100,000 individuals and disproportionately affect minority individuals.[1,3]

Machinery and power tools are the most common reasons for traumatic upper limb amputations. Men are at far greater risk for traumatic amputation than women are, demonstrating about 6.6 times the female rate for minor amputations of the finger and hand.[2] Traumatic amputations often result in irregularly shaped residual limbs and frequently require skin grafts. Efforts to reduce edema and to promote proper limb shaping should be instituted as soon as possible.[4]

The level of amputation is the single most important determinant of function after amputation. The primary surgical principle is to save as much limb as possible while ensuring removal of devitalized tissues and residual limb wound healing. Saving of the most distal joint possible dramatically improves the amputee's function. The elbow joint, for instance, when it is preserved, allows the arm to function in carrying and supporting activities. For the mangled hand, saving of any fingers or remnants provides reconstructive hand surgeons the possibility of constructing a hand that can perform grasping activities.

Persons sustaining upper limb amputations present complex rehabilitative needs that are ideally best managed by a rehabilitation center with therapists, prosthetists, and physicians possessing specialized knowledge and experience. Proper rehabilitation and a comfortable and functional prosthesis will facilitate functional restoration. Vocational counseling and vocational retraining are vital aspects of any program, as this condition often afflicts young, vocationally productive persons, primarily men.

A continuum of care is vital to successful rehabilitation. Patients must be transitioned effectively from the inpatient postsurgical unit, sometimes to an inpatient rehabilitation unit and always to a long-term outpatient rehabilitation and prosthetic program.

SYMPTOMS

Congenital upper limb amputees may report no specific symptoms except the lack of full upper extremity function. In contrast, traumatic upper limb amputees may describe phantom pain (pain perceived in the missing part of the limb) or phantom sensation (nonpainful perceptions of the missing part of the limb). Discomfort with prosthetic fit or skin breakdown on the residual limb may be reported in prosthetic users.

PHYSICAL EXAMINATION

Upper limb amputees require a thorough musculoskeletal examination that includes muscle strength testing, sensory testing, and examination of the contralateral limb. Examination of the residual limb should assess for areas of skin breakdown, redness, painful neuroma, and volume changes that could affect prosthetic fit. Persons with traumatic amputations of the upper limb can have brachial plexus injuries or rotator cuff tears that weaken the residual upper limb muscles. Insensate skin can predispose a patient to breakdown at the site of contact with a prosthesis. Joint range of motion should be assessed. In particular, the scapulothoracic motion is important, as protraction of the scapulae provides the force for a dual-control cable system for body-powered prostheses. Reduced elbow or shoulder range of motion from heterotopic ossification, joint capsule contracture, or muscle contracture can impede maximum recovery of function or use of a prosthesis.

FUNCTIONAL LIMITATIONS

An upper limb amputee's functional status depends on the level of amputation. Persons with finger loss (not including the thumb) are quite functional without a prosthesis. Persons with thumb amputations lose the ability to grip large objects as well as fine motor skills that require opposition with another finger. Reconstructive surgery by pollicization with another remaining finger dramatically improves hand function.

Transradial and transhumeral amputees lose hand function and have limitations in basic and higher level activities of daily living, such as dressing. They frequently sustain new vocational limitations that can preclude return to their previous work activities. Most persons can adapt to almost all basic daily activities with use of the intact contralateral hand and upper limb. Prosthetic devices may or may not improve

function. Some amputees find upper limb prosthetic devices cumbersome, discarding their use altogether. Datta and colleagues[5] found a 73.2% return to work rate after upper limb amputation, although 66.6% had to change jobs. The overall rejection rate of the prosthesis in this study population of predominantly traumatic upper limb amputees was 33.75%. The vast majority used the prosthesis primarily for cosmesis; 25% of patients reported that the prosthesis was beneficial for driving, and a small proportion used it for employment and recreational activities. Some amputees require a specialized prosthesis to continue their specific work-related activities. Recreational activities such as golf, tennis, and other sports can often be accomplished with the use of adaptive prosthetic devices designed for these specific purposes. Return after amputation to such enjoyable pursuits can be quite therapeutic.

DIAGNOSTIC TESTING

No special diagnostic testing is generally required beyond a careful physical examination. If there is weakness of the limb, electrodiagnostic testing may clarify whether a plexopathy is also present. Radiographs may be necessary to evaluate for osteomyelitis, heterotopic ossification, or a bone spur in the distal limb causing poor prosthetic fit.

TREATMENT

Initial

Perioperative Management

Management of persons with upper limb amputations involves a continuum of care.[1,4,6-9] This begins with provision of preoperative information when the amputation is elective, as in the case of cancer. The overriding concern in planning the amputation is to save all possible length, particularly the elbow joint. This preserves elbow flexion and prevents the need for a dual-control cable system. The early input of a physiatrist, nurse, and therapist with expertise in this area is highly advantageous. Early involvement of the rehabilitation team can provide helpful information about prosthetic options, the rehabilitation continuum, and what can be expected after amputation (such as phantom sensations).

Rehabilitation

Initial Rehabilitation Care

After amputation, the primary goals are wound healing, edema control, and prevention of contractures and deconditioning. Persons sustaining upper limb amputations due to trauma or cancer generally have normal underlying blood supply, and most surgical sites can readily heal. Edema is prevented by use of a shrinker sock, elastic bandage wrapping with a figure-of-eight technique that provides pressure distally without choking the limb, or a rigid dressing system. In sophisticated centers, immediate postoperative prosthesis fitting in the operating room is implemented. The immediate postoperative prosthesis is placed over the limb after padding of the skin with soft dressings. The immediate postoperative prosthesis accommodates surgical drains yet prevents the formation of edema. Prosthetic components can be attached to the immediate postoperative prosthesis and early training implemented.

Postoperative early identification and treatment of adherent scar tissue are important. Scar can form between skin, muscle, and bone. These adherences can cause pain when muscles are contracted or a joint is moved during operation of the prosthesis.[10]

Residual limb pain and phantom pain are two conditions that can affect patients with upper limb amputations.[7] Phantom sensations are common; yet fortunately, disabling phantom pain occurs in only about 5% of amputees.[6] Despite the many interventions used for phantom pain, there are no uniformly effective treatments.[6,8] Medication and physical modalities must be tried in a rational fashion to determine the most effective intervention. Physical modalities include a transcutaneous electrical nerve stimulation unit, physical manipulation, and massage of the residual limb.[6] Fitting of a comfortable prosthesis can often help reduce these painful sensations.

Neuromodulating medications, such as tricyclic antidepressants and antiepileptics (gabapentin), are frequently used with variable results[6,8]; β blockers (propranolol and atenolol) have been found to be somewhat effective in treating phantom pain.[6] If patients require cardiac or hypertension medications, the choice of a β blocker may serve two purposes for these amputees with phantom pain.

Opiates may be effective for these problems when other methods fail to relieve phantom pain.[8] If it is anticipated that the person with phantom pain will need analgesia for a long period, long-acting opiates should be used. Longer acting opiates have less habituation and addiction potential. Most amputees with phantom pain have intermittent severe pain that can be treated with small doses on an as-needed basis of a short-acting opiate, such as oxycodone. For the few patients with severe, unremitting, phantom and residual limb pain, referral to a specialized pain center is suggested.

Rehabilitative and Prosthetic Management

Prevention of contractures in the residual limb and prevention of generalized deconditioning are important goals of early rehabilitation. Any other injuries, as are common in persons sustaining severe trauma, should be identified and rehabilitation efforts directed at their remediation. For body-powered prostheses, scapulothoracic motion provides power through a cable system to operate the prosthesis. Likewise, elbow contractures or shoulder contractures or capsulitis will severely impede

maximal prosthetic use, and these problems should be aggressively addressed. Early training in activity of daily living skills should be pursued as well. Therapies should be directed toward amelioration of weakness through exercises or contractures through active-assisted range of motion exercises and prolonged stretching.

A detailed discussion of prosthetic devices is beyond the scope of this chapter, and consultation with a skilled prosthetist and physiatrist is desirable. In general, there are two types, body-powered and myoelectric devices.[1,9] Body-powered devices are usually less cosmetic yet are less expensive and much more durable. Myoelectric prostheses are controlled by electrical signals generated in muscles from the remaining residual limb or shoulder girdle. Myoelectric prosthetic devices extract signals from remaining muscles under voluntary control to activate and to control drive motors in the prosthesis. These devices are expensive, and special prosthetic skills are required to fabricate and to maintain them, but they are generally more cosmetic in appearance and well suited for selected patients. Prosthetic functional outcomes depend on an individual's goals related to cosmesis, function, and psychological factors.[10] Skin breakdown can occur over bone prominences, where there are skin grafts, or where skin is adherent to underlying bone. Alteration of the prosthetic socket and suspension systems or temporary discontinuation of prosthetic use until the skin has healed may be necessary.

The field of upper extremity prosthetics is changing with the development of implantable neurologic sensing devices and targeted muscle innervation. Targeted motor reinnervation incorporates the transfer of residual peripheral nerves into muscles in or near the residual limb, with subsequent reinnervation of those muscles. By use of these surface electromyographic signals that relate directly to the original function of the limb, control of the externally powered prosthesis occurs.[11] Multidextrous terminal devices may soon be available.[10]

Procedures

Most procedures related to the care of upper extremity amputees focus on pain management techniques, such as injection of local anesthetic around a painful neuroma, nerve blocks, massage, or chiropractic manipulation. Acupuncture, hypnosis, and biofeedback have also been used in the management of phantom limb pain with variable success.[8]

Surgery

Revision surgeries are sometimes necessary to remove bone spurs that interfere with prosthetic fitting. The initial surgery should spare all length possible, particularly the elbow joint. A well-healed surgical site with good distal soft tissue coverage of the bone end is an optimal result that facilitates prosthetic use. In addition, surgical treatment of adherent scar tissue may be necessary to improve function of a prosthesis.

POTENTIAL DISEASE COMPLICATIONS

As a result of the upper limb amputation, residual limb pain, including severe phantom pain, can occur. Joint contractures can develop in the remaining part of the limb, as well as frozen shoulder and adhesive capsulitis. This is a particular concern with coexistent peripheral nerve or brachial plexus injury.

Depression brought on by the difficulties of adjusting to limb loss is reported. Psychological counseling and support groups incorporating peer support are valuable resources.

POTENTIAL TREATMENT COMPLICATIONS

Surgical complications include postoperative wound infections and postoperative failure of the surgical wounds to heal. Neuroma formation can occur after transection of a nerve. Burying the nerve ending under large soft tissue masses may reduce the likelihood of irritation.

Many medications used in the treatment of phantom pain associated with amputations have potential side effects, including dry mouth, constipation, weight gain, mental cloudiness, cardiovascular effects, and addiction. The side effect profiles vary by the medication class and dosage.

Skin breakdown from a poorly fitting prosthesis can occur. This can be aggravated by hyperhidrosis, folliculitis, or poor hygiene.

Overuse injuries in the nonamputated limb reportedly are higher than expected in the normal population.[5]

These include repetitive strain-type injuries due to the individual's performing certain tasks with poor body posture and ergonomics.[12]

References

1. Dillingham TR, Pezzin LE, MacKenzie EJ. Limb amputation and limb deficiency: epidemiology and recent trends in the United States. South Med J 2002;95:875-883.
2. Dillingham TR, Pezzin LE, MacKenzie EJ. Incidence, acute care length of stay, and discharge to rehabilitation of traumatic amputee patients: an epidemiologic study. Arch Phys Med Rehabil 1998;79:279-287.
3. Dillingham TR, Pezzin LE, MacKenzie EJ. Racial differences in the incidence of limb loss secondary to peripheral vascular disease: a population-based study. Arch Phys Med Rehabil 2002;83:1252-1257.
4. Nelson VS, Flood KM, Bryant PR, et al. Limb deficiency and prosthetic management. 1. Decision making in prosthetic prescription and management. Arch Phys Med Rehabil 2006;87:S3-S9.
5. Datta D, Selvarajah K, Davey N. Functional outcome of patients with proximal upper limb deficiency—acquired and congenital. Clin Rehabil 2004;18:172-177.
6. Vaida G, Friedmann LW. Postamputation phantoms: a review. Phys Med Rehabil Clin North Am 1991;2:325-353.
7. Roberts TL, Pasquina PF, Nelson VS, et al. Limb deficiency and prosthetic management. 4. Comorbidities associated with limb loss. Arch Phys Med Rehabil 2006;87:S21-S27.
8. Hanley MA, Ehde DM, Campbell KM, et al. Self-reported treatments used for lower-limb phantom pain: descriptive findings. Arch Phys Med Rehabil 2006;87:270-277.
9. Dillingham TR. Rehabilitation of the upper limb amputee. In Dillingham TR, Belandres P, eds. Rehabilitation of the Injured Combatant. Washington, DC, Office of the Surgeon General, 1998:33-77.
10. Lake C, Dodson R. Progressive upper limb prosthetics. Phys Med Rehabil Clin North Am 2006;17:49-72.
11. Kuiken T. Targeted reinnervation for improved prosthetic function. Phys Med Rehabil Clin North Am 2006;17:1-13.
12. Jones LE, Davidson JH. Save the arm: a study of problems in the remaining arm of unilateral upper limb amputees. Prosthet Orthot Int 1999;23:55-58.

Lower Limb Amputations 109

Michelle Gittler, MD

Synonyms

Below-knee amputation—transtibial amputation
Above-knee amputation—transfemoral amputation
Syme's amputation (foot disarticulation)
Neuropathic pain—dysesthetic pain
Residual limb stump

ICD-9 Codes

353.6	Phantom limb (syndrome)
718.45	Joint contracture (hip), pelvis and thigh
718.46	Joint contracture (knee), lower leg
719.7	Difficulty walking (ankle and foot)
895	Traumatic amputation of toe(s) (complete) (partial)
895.0	Without complication
895.1	Complicated
896	Traumatic amputation of foot (complete) (partial)
896.0	Unilateral, without mention of complication
896.1	Unilateral, complicated
896.2	Bilateral, without mention of complication
896.3	Bilateral, complicated
897	Traumatic amputation of leg(s) (complete) (partial)
897.0	Unilateral, below knee, without mention of complication
897.1	Unilateral, below knee, complicated
897.2	Unilateral, at or above knee, without mention of complication
897.3	Unilateral, at or above knee, complicated
897.4	Unilateral, level not specified, without mention of complication
897.5	Unilateral, level not specified, complicated
897.6	Bilateral (any level), without mention of complication
897.7	Bilateral (any level), complicated
905.9	Late effect of traumatic amputation
997.60	Amputation stump complication, unspecified
997.61	Neuroma of amputation stump
997.62	Infection (chronic)
V52	Fitting and adjustment of prosthetic device and implant
V52.1	Artificial leg (complete) (partial)

DEFINITION

Amputations due to vascular conditions account for most (82%) lower limb loss.[1] More than half of dysvascular amputations (53.6%) are at the transfemoral (25.8%) and transtibial (27.6%) levels; 31% involve the toes.[2] Most of these amputations occur in people aged 60 years and older. In 2001, the rate of lower extremity amputations in the United States was estimated at 6.5 per 1000 people with diabetes. There are approximately 82,000 nontrauma diabetes-related lower extremity amputations each year.[3] Approximately 70% of lower extremity amputations in adults are the result of complications of diabetes and peripheral vascular disease. Trauma is the next most common cause of lower extremity amputation (22%), followed by tumors (5%). However, in children aged 10 to 20 years, tumor is the most common cause of both upper and lower extremity amputations. Male amputees outnumber female amputees 2.1:1 in disease and 7.2:1 in trauma.[3]

SYMPTOMS

The postoperative or post-traumatic sequela of an amputation is that the patient is missing all or part of a limb. In addition, there may be associated symptoms, such as phantom limb sensation, phantom pain, stump pain, and pain from the surgery itself.

Phantom limb sensation is the perception that the extremity is still present and occasionally distorted in position. Phantom limb sensation typically fades away within the first year after amputation, usually in a "telescoping" phenomenon. This includes the perception that the distal aspect of the limb (that is, the foot) is moving closer and closer to the site of amputation.

Phantom limb pain is differentiated as a painful perception within the absent body part. The incidence of phantom limb pain is variable and has been reported from 0.5% to virtually 100% of persons with amputations. This variability is due to differences in study methods and population. The most recent studies suggest that up to 85% of people with amputations will experience phantom pain.[4] Patients may describe the pain in the absent foot or the absent limb as cramping, stabbing, burning, or icy cold.

Pain at the surgical site, including incisional discomfort, is common and should resolve within a few weeks of surgery. Residual limb pain is perceived in the residual limb in the region of the amputation. The incidence of residual limb pain has been reported between 10% and 25%; it may be diffuse or focal and is commonly associated with neuroma, which is palpable around the amputation site.

PHYSICAL EXAMINATION

Wound healing, range of motion, muscle strength, and incisional integrity must be evaluated in the residual limb. Visualization of the contralateral foot is a mandatory component of the examination. Upper extremity strength should be assessed to determine capability for use of assistive devices.

The unaffected foot is assessed for areas of potential breakdown. These include the plantar surface of the foot, web spaces, and areas of bone prominence.

Skin breakdown in the residual limb is typically a result of pressure or shear forces. Skin breakdown can be manifested as abrasions from tape or the unraveling of an elastic wrap or be true partial- or full-thickness (pressure) sores. Pressure sore phenomenon typically occurs at bone prominences. The fibular head, hamstring tendons, patellar tendon, medial and lateral femoral condyles, and anterior distal tibia should routinely be examined for skin breakdown.

Joint contractures are a loss of full range of motion at a joint. They may be conceptualized as functional or mechanical. Functional contractures are the result of (inappropriate) positioning. A transtibial amputee may develop knee or hip flexion contractures merely by sitting with the hip flexed and the knee flexed at 90 degrees (the knee and hip extensors remain intact but are not being used). A mechanical contracture may result from unopposed muscle action. In the transfemoral amputee, the insertion of the hip adductors is sacrificed, leaving the unopposed (and firmly attached) hip abductors. This results in an abduction contracture.

The transtibial and Syme's amputee requires evaluation of range of motion of the knee in flexion and extension. Medial and lateral knee stability must also be assessed. Knee extension muscle strength should be graded higher than 4/5 for successful ambulation with a prosthesis. A knee flexion contracture of 10 to 18 degrees can usually be accommodated in a transtibial prosthesis. A contracture of more than 20 degrees requires that the individual ambulate with a bent socket, weight bearing through the knee.

In the transfemoral (above-knee) amputee, the range of motion evaluation should include hip flexion, hip extension, hip adduction, and hip abduction. A transfemoral prosthesis can functionally accommodate up to a 20-degree hip flexion contracture; a contracture of more than this makes prosthetic fitting and successful ambulation less likely. Strength should also be assessed,

and grades of 4/5 or higher in hip flexion-extension and abduction are required for ambulation.

Stump or residual limb pain is assessed first by inspection. Areas of obvious necrosis indicating poor blood flow may require surgical débridement. Nonhealing incisions are manifestations of ischemia, underlying hematoma, or abscess. The surrounding area should be palpated and assessed for induration and discharge. An attempt should be made to "milk" fluctuance, and drainage is sent for Gram stain and culture. Sutures (if present) may need to be removed to facilitate evacuation of the abscess or hematoma. In some instances, the incision may need to be reopened for drainage and healing to take place.

Stump pain without signs or symptoms of infection should be evaluated for neuroma (palpation of the anatomic course of the sciatic nerve). Stump pain with or without skin breakdown may also be due to poor prosthetic fit, so the fit of the prosthesis ought to be evaluated, preferably with a prosthetist present. Nonblanchable erythema is a pressure sore until proved otherwise, and the prosthesis should not be worn until appropriate adjustments are made. Bruising at the distal aspect of the stump in the prosthetic wearer is indicative of a poor prosthetic fit. That is, the residual limb may be falling too deeply into the socket. Similarly, a choke phenomenon occurs with lack of total contact or inability to get the residual limb all the way into the socket. This can progress to verrucous hyperplasia, which predisposes the individual to fissuring and infection.

Gait evaluation with prosthesis should be performed by use of an appropriate assistive device. Observed gait deviations should be communicated to the prosthetist for prosthesis modifications and to the therapist.

FUNCTIONAL LIMITATIONS

Functional limitations are largely dependent on the premorbid status of the individual. Ambulation with one limb or hopping (with a walker or crutches) requires approximately 60% increased energy over normal human locomotion. The energy cost of ambulation with a prosthesis varies, but for the diabetic or dysvascular amputee, it approaches 38% to 60% increased energy for a below-knee amputee and 52% to 116% higher for an above-knee amputee.[1] An otherwise healthy person who has sustained a traumatic limb amputation or an individual who had been ambulating with crutches or another assistive device before having an amputation (often because of non–weight-bearing status on the affected limb) will probably be discharged from the acute care setting to home with outpatient services, at an "ambulatory" level with the appropriate assistive device; the energy expenditure will be less than that of a dysvascular amputee.

An older individual or person with multiple comorbidities may be at the wheelchair level secondary to deconditioning or inadequate cardiopulmonary reserve to ambulate with an assistive device. This person may have had an acute or subacute rehabilitation hospital stay after the acute care hospitalization.

Functional limitations due to pain are associated with an inability to participate in ongoing activities of daily living. In general, symptoms of phantom sensation tend not to be an issue, whereas phantom pain can be severely limiting, preventing a person from participating in pre-prosthetic and prosthetic rehabilitation. Functional limitations related to stump or residual limb pain include the inability to tolerate stump shrinkage by appropriate modalities and an inability to tolerate gait training with a prosthesis. To accommodate stump pain, the patient may develop gait deviations to decrease pressure under the aspect of the residual limb and may find functional ambulation significantly curtailed.

Individuals with significantly impaired cardiac output may not be able to perform pre-prosthetic training with a walker (or crutches). They may not be prosthetic candidates at all because of the increased energy demands of prosthetic ambulation.

Rates of clinical depression range from 18% to 35% among amputees. Those with amputation-related pain are more prone to depression. Depression should be differentiated from the grief response and postoperative adjustment period.[5]

DIAGNOSTIC STUDIES

The individual with phantom limb pain may benefit from diagnostic as well as therapeutic sympathetic nerve block. On occasion, electrodiagnostic tests (electromyography and nerve conduction studies) are helpful to differentiate symptoms of radiculopathy or other disease in the phantom limb.

In the younger amputee, it is occasionally necessary to obtain plain radiographs of the residual limb to assess the bone overgrowth. This is typically visually evident on inspection; the radiograph confirms the extent of overgrowth.

Differential Diagnosis

Residual Limb

Edema

Neuroma

Incision

  Post surgical

  Infection

Bone Overgrowth

Ischemia

Phantom Pain

Sympathetic Pain

Radiculopathy

Ischemia

TREATMENT

Initial

Initial treatment focuses on edema control and shaping of the residual limb as well as wound healing, prevention of contractures, and pain management. Options for edema control are listed in Table 109-1.[4,6]

Patients with a transtibial amputation have the potential for knee flexion and hip flexion contractures as a result of positioning (usually, sitting in wheelchair or in bed). Therefore, avoidance of pillows under the knee and promotion of lying prone in bed can be helpful.

Persons with a transfemoral amputation may also develop hip flexion contractures as a result of sitting. In addition, there is the tendency for development of hip abduction contractures, so positioning of the hip in relative adduction, avoidance of pillows under the residual limb, and promotion of the prone position are essential.

Phantom sensation is not typically painful, although it can be frightening or disorienting for the patient. The best treatment is to reassure the patient that this is a normal reaction after amputation. Education and reassurance of the patient as well as ongoing tactile input (i.e., massaging the distal residual limb and using the limb) will enhance the treatment of phantom sensation. There are many proposed treatments of phantom pain; however, there is no one definitive treatment that seems to work best. Pharmacologic intervention includes non-narcotic and narcotic analgesics; nonsteroidal anti-inflammatory drugs; anticonvulsants and membrane stabilizers, particularly gabapentin, duloxetine, and pregabalin; and tricyclic antidepressants.[7]

Rehabilitation

Pre-prosthetic training focuses on functional independence in mobility and self-care from the ambulatory (single limb) or wheelchair level, avoidance of hip and knee contractures, and residual limb management. Prosthetic training is initiated once the residual limb is ready, that is, the edema is resolved and the incision has healed; the prosthesis is then fabricated. A description of prostheses is beyond the scope of this chapter; however, the reader is referred to one of several texts on prosthetic components and prescription.[5,6,8] K levels are used by Medicare to determine an individual's functional potential and thus to justify prosthetic components (Table 109-2). When the prosthesis has been fabricated, an outpatient appointment with the ordering physician is scheduled that is attended by the patient and the prosthetist. A basic evaluation of the fit of the prosthesis is conducted, and referral for physical therapy that focuses on prosthetic training is made at that time, or adjustments to the prosthesis are made. The patient must be taught how to put on (don) and take off (doff) the prosthesis as well as when to add socks for a better fit. The patient should also be encouraged to routinely inspect the skin on the residual limb (often done best with a long-handled mirror).

Occupational therapy consists of identifying necessary equipment (e.g., toilet safety frame, tub transfer bench)

TABLE 109-1 Treatment Options for Edema Control

Treatment Options	Advantages	Disadvantages
In a Below-Knee Amputee		
Above-knee cast	Prevents knee flexion contracture Provides protection No patient "skill" or management necessary to remove Very low cost	Bulky, awkward, heavy to move Unable to visualize wound Unable to remove Potential for skin breakdown
"Stump shrinker"	Easy to don and doff Enables visualization of wound Accustoms individual to use of a sock Provides shaping of residual limb	Cost—may need to be replaced after stump has begun to shrink
Rigid removable dressing (Fig. 109-1)	Excellent for preparing residual limb for eventual prosthesis Fosters patient's independence in assessing need for stump socks Good edema management Provides some soft tissue protection Able to view wound	Therapist, physician, and prosthetist must be skilled in fabrication Potential for skin breakdown if applied incorrectly
Elastic bandage (ACE wrap)	Easily available Able to visualize wound Accommodates all shapes and sizes Good edema control	Requires excellent dexterity for patient to don and doff Potential for shear injury if wrap unravels Must be reapplied multiple times a day secondary to potential loosening
In an Above-Knee Amputee		
Stump shrinker, elastic bandage	Same advantages and disadvantages as described for below-knee amputee	

and establishing independence in self-care from the wheelchair or ambulatory level with use of just the unaffected limb (single-limb stance). Occupational therapy should also be ordered when the patient receives the prosthesis to establish independence in self-care, particularly with lower extremity dressing, toileting, and homemaking while the prosthesis is worn.

Return to driving is an important aspect of functional independence. The majority (80.5%) of prosthetic users with major lower extremity amputations are able to return to automobile driving 3.8 months after amputation. People with left-sided amputations have significantly fewer concerns about driving; those with right-sided amputations may need vehicle modifications (40%) or may need to switch to left foot driving style.[9]

Procedures

Treatments of postamputation phantom pain include sympathetic blocks, which are typically performed under fluoroscopic guidance. Neuromas, which typically form 1 to 12 months after amputation, may present as a focal soft tissue mass with reproducible pain on palpation. Local anesthetic injection may provide pain relief. Surgical resection is an option but can result in a new (painful) neuroma.[5]

Surgery

Surgery is indicated when a residual limb requires wound revision or higher level of amputation. Hamstring releases have a limited or no role because they

TABLE 109-2 K Levels

K0 (level 0)	Does not have the ability or potential to ambulate or to transfer safely with or without assistance, and a prosthesis does not enhance the quality of life or mobility
K1 (level 1)	Has the ability or potential to use a prosthesis for transfers or ambulation on level surfaces at fixed cadence—typical of the limited and unlimited household walker
K2 (level 2)	Has the ability or potential for ambulation with the ability to traverse low-level environmental barriers, such as curbs, stairs, or uneven surfaces—typical of the limited community walker
K3 (level 3)	Has the ability or potential for walking with variable cadence—typical of the community walker who is able to traverse most environmental barriers and may have vocational, therapeutic, or exercise activity that demands prosthetic use beyond simple walking
K4 (level 4)	Has the ability or potential for prosthetic use that exceeds basic walking skills, exhibiting high impact, stress, or energy levels—typical of the prosthetic demands of the child, active adult, or athlete

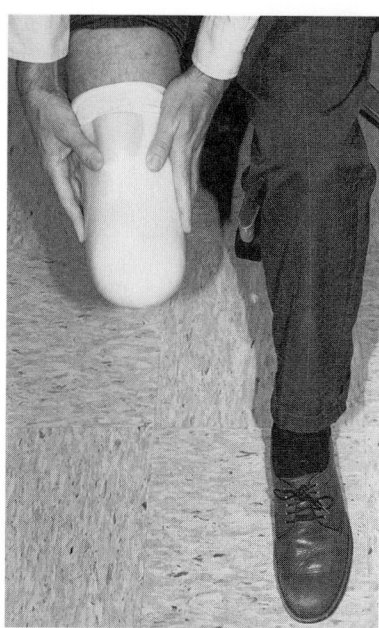

FIGURE 109-1. Application of the removable rigid dressing. (Reprinted with permission from Lennard TA. Pain Procedures in Clinical Practice, 2nd ed. Philadelphia, Hanley & Belfus, 2000:79.)

would inhibit the ability to walk. There does not appear to be any role for surgical stump revision for treatment of phantom pain.

There are few data to promote dorsal root entry zone ablation, dorsal rhizotomy, dorsal column tractotomy, thalamotomy, or cortical resection in the treatment of phantom pain. A small trial to surgically treat phantom pain locally was performed. The sciatic nerve was split proximal to the popliteal fossa, and the two parts were reconnected in a sling fashion. Of 15 patients, 14 reported that the procedure was "very helpful."[10]

Bone overgrowth develops in 10% to 30% of children with congenital amputations, and this must be addressed surgically.[11] This is much less common in the adult with an acquired amputation.

POTENTIAL DISEASE COMPLICATIONS

The most common complications are dehiscence or breakdown of the incision and nonhealing wounds. Infection is the most likely cause of dehiscence or a nonhealing incision. A trial of conservative management including antibiotics (after a culture specimen is obtained) and appropriate local wound care is reasonable. Increasing wound necrosis, foul drainage, and fever or chills warrant reevaluation by the surgeon.

Other potential complications may involve cardiac ischemia as a heretofore inactive (i.e., energy conservative) individual begins using up to 100% more energy for gait training.[12] A reasonable guideline for gait training is assessment of an individual's ability to ambulate with the intact lower extremity with crutches or another assistive device. This consumes approximately 60% more energy than bipedal human locomotion. A person

who is not able to gait train (hop on one foot short distances) with use of an assistive device is probably not a potential prosthetic ambulator. Major limb amputation continues to result in significant morbidity and mortality. One-year survival for dysvascular and diabetic individuals is 50.6% for transfemoral amputees and 74.5% for transtibial amputees. Five-year survival is 22.5% and 37.8% (survival in end-stage renal disease is as low as 14% at 5 years after amputation).[13]

POTENTIAL TREATMENT COMPLICATIONS

Once the prosthesis has been fabricated, skin breakdown is the most common complication. Breakdown commonly occurs at the distal anterior tibia (clapper-in-bell phenomenon, a result of continued forward motion of the distal residual limb in the socket during swing phase), the hamstring tendons (tight brim), and the patellar tendon.

Patients should be instructed to inspect these areas and immediately report to the prosthetist signs of persistent, nonblanchable erythema. The prosthesis should not be worn until modifications are made.

Medication side effects depend on the particular medication being used as well as potential for drug interactions when multiple medications are being used.

References

1. Dillingham TR, Pezzin LE, MacKenzie EJ. Limb amputation and limb deficiency: epidemiology and recent trends in the United States. South Med J 2002;95:875-883.
2. Diabetes and Foot Care. Put Feet First: Prevent Amputations. International Diabetes Federation, Brussels, Belgium, 2005.
3. Leonard EI, McAnelly RD, Lomba M, Faulker VW. Lower limb prosthesis in physical medicine and rehabilitation. In Braddom RL, ed. Physical Medicine and Rehabilitation, 2nd ed. Philadelphia, WB Saunders, 2000:279-310.
4. Ehde DM, Czerniecki JM, Smith DG, et al. Chronic phantom sensations, phantom pain, residual limb pain, and other regional pain after lower limb amputation. Arch Phys Med Rehabil 2000;81:1039-1044.
5. Roberts TL, Pasquina PF, Nelson VS, et al. Limb deficiency and prosthetic management. 4. Comorbidities associated with limb loss. Arch Phys Med Rehabil 2006;87(Suppl 1):S21-S27.
6. Esquenazi A. Gait analysis and the metabolic energy expenditure of amputee ambulation [lecture]. AAPMR, Seattle, 1998.
7. National Limb Loss Information Center. Fact Sheet. Knoxville, Tenn, Amputee Coalition of America, 2004.
8. Aulivola B, Hile CN, Hamdan AD, et al. Major lower extremity amputation: outcome of a modern series. Arch Surg 2004;139:395-399.
9. Prantl L, Schreml S, Heine N, et al. Surgical treatment of chronic phantom limb sensation and limb pain after lower limb amputation. Plast Reconstr Surg 2006;118:1562-1572.
10. Boulias C, Meikle B, Pauley T, Devlin M. Return to driving after lower extremity amputation. Arch Phys Med Rehabil 2006;87:1183-1188.
11. Loesner J. Pain after amputation. In Bonica J, ed. The Management of Pain, 2nd ed. Baltimore, Williams & Wilkins, 1990:244-256.
12. Mueller MS. Comparison of rigid removable dressings and elastic bandages in preprosthetic management of patients with below-knee amputations. Phys Ther 1982;62:1438-1441.
13. Wu Y, Krick H. Rigid removable dressings for below knee amputees. Clin Prosthetics Orthotics 1987;11:33-44.

110
Ankylosing Spondylitis

Steven E. Braverman, MD

DEFINITION

Ankylosing spondylitis is one of a group of rheumatic disorders that affect the spinal column, the sacroiliac joints, and the peripheral joints. It involves inflammation of the entheses (tissues attaching tendons, ligaments, and joint capsules to bone), called enthesitis, and inflammation of the synovium, called synovitis.

It is not associated with the presence of rheumatoid factor or antinuclear antibodies. The onset of symptoms is usually in late adolescence or early adulthood, and it is three times more common in men than in women. There is a genetic association with the HLA-B27 histocompatibility antigen, but this marker is neither specific to the disease nor necessary for the diagnosis to be made.

The most common sites of involvement are sacroiliac, apophyseal, and discovertebral joints of the spine; costochondral and manubriosternal joints; paravertebral ligaments; and attachments of the Achilles tendon and plantar fascia. Peripheral joint involvement is less common but occurs in the more severe forms of the disease.[1]

SYMPTOMS

Ankylosing spondylitis should be considered in any young adult patient who complains of insidious onset of worsening, dull, lumbosacral back pain with progressive morning stiffness. Pain in the area of the sacroiliac joints is common, as is prolonged stiffness after inactivity.

Neurologic symptoms, such as paresthesias and motor weakness, are absent. Tendon and ligament attachment sites may become painful and swollen. One third of patients may develop hip or shoulder pain. Chest pain with deep breathing and eye pain with blurred vision are late symptoms of more severe disease.[2]

PHYSICAL EXAMINATION

The most typical findings involve signs of decreased spine mobility as measured by the modified Schober test, finger to floor distance, occiput to wall distance, and chest expansion. A Gaenslen test result may be positive (Fig. 110-1). The modified Schober test is a test of lumbar spine range of motion.[3] The patient stands erect with normal posture and the examiner marks two lines at the spine, 5 cm above and 5 cm below the posterosuperior iliac spine. The test result is normal if the distance between the two lines is more than 15 cm with full forward flexion at the waist. The inability to touch the occiput to the wall while standing against it and the inability to expand the chest by more than 3 cm in full inhalation are late findings in the disease.

On palpation, the lower paraspinal muscles and sacroiliac joints are tender. Ligamentous and tendinous attachment sites are tender in areas of enthesitis, particularly around the heel and tibial tuberosity.

Peripheral joint swelling and pain with decreased range of motion are found in about one third of patients. A discolored and edematous iris with circumferential corneal congestion occurs in iritis and anterior uveitis.

The neurologic evaluation is typically normal with regard to motor, sensory, and reflex examination findings. Weakness may be noted, but it is usually associated with pain, loss of mobility, or disuse.

FUNCTIONAL LIMITATIONS

The functional limitations of the patient with ankylosing spondylitis are typically related to spine mobility and dysfunction. The three best predictors of decreased function are cervical rotation, modified Schober test,

---

Note: The opinions in this article are those of the author and not necessarily those of the U.S. Army or Department of Defense.

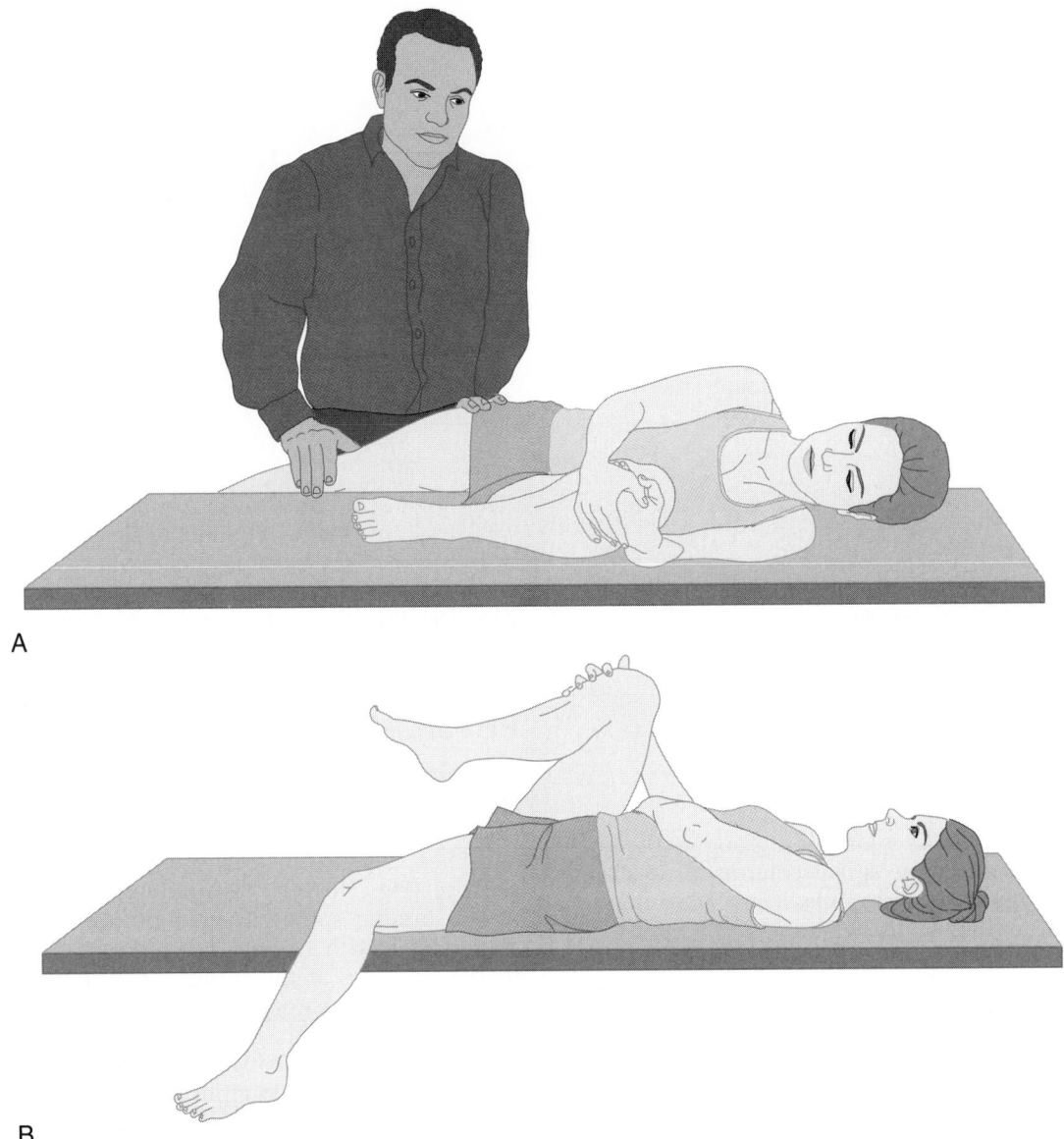

FIGURE 110-1. Gaenslen test. **A,** With the patient in side-lying position, the clinician extends the test leg. **B,** With the patient supine, the test leg is extended over the edge of the table. Pain in the sacroiliac joints indicates a positive test result.

and pain.[4] The Bath Ankylosing Spondylitis Functional Index[5] is a functional assessment measurement index used by clinicians specializing in the care of patients with ankylosing spondylitis.

Early on, decreased spine range of motion is secondary to pain and spasm and improves with treatment. Most dysfunction is mild and self-limited; 90% of patients with ankylosing spondylitis remain employed.

In severe disease, positioning from hip flexion contractures, thoracic kyphosis, and loss of cervical rotation decrease patients' ability to view activities in front of them and side to side. The most commonly reported activity limitations are interrupted sleeping, turning the head while driving, carrying groceries, and having energy for social activities.[6] Limitations in chest wall motion lead to a reliance on diaphragmatic breathing and a secondary drop in aerobic capacity.

DIAGNOSTIC STUDIES

Standard spine and sacroiliac joint radiographs show ossification of spinal ligaments and apophyseal joints with eventual ankylosis, leading to the classic bamboo spine appearance. Sacroiliac joint findings are symmetric; bone erosions, sclerosis, and blurring of the subchondral bone plate eventually progress to complete ankylosis. Bone erosions at entheses are common. Hip radiographs demonstrate symmetric and concentric joint narrowing with subchondral sclerosis. Ankylosis is found in severe disease. Computed tomographic scans and magnetic resonance images are more sensitive in early disease. Early computed tomographic and magnetic resonance imaging findings show pseudowidening of the sacroiliac joints followed by sclerosis, narrowing, and ankylosis. Once initial radiographs are abnormal, further radiographic progression correlates with worsening results of the modified Schober test.[7]

HLA-B27 is present in 90% of patients with ankylosing spondylitis. A negative test result suggests milder disease with a better prognosis. Rheumatoid factor and antinuclear antibodies are absent. Erythrocyte sedimentation rate and C-reactive protein levels correlate with disease activity.

Differential Diagnosis

Rheumatoid arthritis

Other seronegative spondyloarthropathies

Reiter syndrome

Psoriatic arthritis

Enteropathic spondylitis

Behçet syndrome

TREATMENT

Initial

Evidence-based treatment guidelines must be tailored to the disease progression and functional impact on the individual with ankylosing spondylitis. Management must include concurrent medical, rehabilitation, and surgical treatment.[8] The primary medical treatment of ankylosing spondylitis is nonsteroidal anti-inflammatory drugs (NSAIDs). NSAIDs provide symptomatic relief but do not halt progression of the disease. No single NSAID is more effective than any other in ankylosing spondylitis. The choice of NSAID is based on individual therapeutic response, compliance, and side effects.[9] Intermittent NSAID dosing (taking the medication only during periods of exacerbation) is generally as effective as continuous dosing and results in fewer side effects.[10] However, there is some recent evidence that continuous dosing may slow structural damage.[11] Pulsed methylprednisolone at 15 mg/kg for 3 days may be effective for NSAID-resistant flares.[12] However, the use of anti–tumor necrosis factor medications may be more effective in severe disease.[13] Sulfasalazine is ineffective except in cases with a predominance of peripheral disease, inflammatory bowel disease, or psoriasis.[14] Pamidronate, when it is used to treat associated osteoporosis, may also decrease ankylosing spondylitis disease progression.[15]

Rehabilitation

Physical therapy and home exercise programs may improve spine mobility and lead to improvements in flexibility. Exercise programs that include aerobic, stretching, and pulmonary exercises work best.[16,17] The benefit of these programs is lost once the exercise is discontinued. Hip range of motion increases with regular stretching

with use of the contraction-relaxation-stretching technique. Strengthening of back and hip extensors should follow the flexibility exercises. Aerobic activities may maintain chest expansion. However, an exercise stress test should be considered before an aerobic program if aortic insufficiency is suspected. There is no evidence that one type of aerobic exercise is better than another. However, specific exercise programs that target strengthening and flexibility of shortened muscle chains show promise.[18]

In general, splinting and spinal orthoses are not effective, but foot orthotics may help with calcaneal enthesopathies. A firm mattress may help with sleep, along with a small cervical pillow that will help maintain cervical lordosis. Wide mirrors assist drivers with limited cervical mobility.[17]

Procedures

Periarticular corticosteroid injections and fluoroscopically guided sacroiliac joint injections may help during NSAID-resistant flares or when NSAIDs are contraindicated.[19] Local injections for enthesopathies may be effective, but injections in and around the Achilles tendon insertion should be avoided.

Surgery

Hip and knee arthroplasties should be considered before joint ankylosis. Spinal osteotomy is a risky procedure for patients with severe kyphosis.[20]

POTENTIAL DISEASE COMPLICATIONS

Potential complications include iritis or uveitis, inflammatory bowel disease, aortic insufficiency and aortic root dilatation, osteoporosis (best evaluated with bone densitometry of the femur), and spine fracture with spinal cord injury (rare).

POTENTIAL TREATMENT COMPLICATIONS

NSAIDs may produce gastrointestinal and renal toxic effects, and corticosteroids increase risk of osteoporosis. Total hip arthroplasty increases the risk of anterior dislocations. Spinal osteotomy carries the risk of paralysis and a mortality rate of up to 4%.[20]

References

1. Klippel JH. Primer on the Rheumatic Diseases. Atlanta, Arthritis Foundation, 1997:189-193.
2. Ozgul A, Peker F, Taskavnatan MA, et al. Effect of ankylosing spondylitis on health-related quality of life and different aspects of social life in young patients. Clin Rheumatol 2006;25:168-174.
3. Family Practice notebook.com. Schober's test. Available at: http://www.fpnotebook.com/rhe38.htm. Accessed January 11, 2007.
4. Dalyan M, Guner A, Tuncer S, et al. Disability in ankylosing spondylitis. Disabil Rehabil 1999;21:74-79.
5. Calin A, Garrett S, Whitelock H, et al. A new approach to defining functional ability in ankylosing spondylitis: the development of the Bath Ankylosing Spondylitis Functional Index. J Rheumatol 1994;21:2281-2285.

6. Dagfinrud H, Kjeken I, Mowinckel P, et al. Impact of functional impairment in ankylosing spondylitis: impairment, activity limitation, and participation restrictions. J Rheumatol 2005;32:516-523.

7. Wanders A, Landewe R, Dougados M, et al. Association between radiographic damage of the spine and spinal mobility for individual patients with ankylosing spondylitis: can assessment of spinal mobility be a proxy for radiographic evaluation? Ann Rheum Dis 2005;64:988-994.

8. Zochling J, van der Heijde D, Burgos-Varas R, et al. ASAS/EULAR recommendations for the management of ankylosing spondylitis. Ann Rheum Dis 2006;65:432-442.

9. van der Heijde D, Baraf HS, Ramos-Remus C, et al. Evaluation of the efficacy of etoricoxib in ankylosing spondylitis: results of a 52-week randomized controlled study. Arthritis Rheum 2005;52:1205-1215.

10. Koehler L, Kuipers J, Zeidler H. Managing seronegative spondarthritides. Rheumatology (Oxford) 2000;39:360-368.

11. Wanders A, van der Heijde D, Landewe R, et al. Nonsteroidal antiinflammatory drugs reduce radiographic progression in patients with ankylosing spondylitis. Arthritis Rheum 2005;52:1756-1765.

12. Peters ND, Ejstrup L. Intravenous methylprednisolone pulse therapy in ankylosing spondylitis. Scand J Rheumatol 1992;21:134-138.

13. Zochling J, Braun J. Developments and current pharmacotherapeutic recommendations for ankylosing spondylitis. Expert Opin Pharmacother 2006;7:869-883.

14. Clegg DO, Reda DJ, Abdellatif M. Comparison of sulfasalazine and placebo for the treatment of axial and peripheral articular manifestations of the seronegative arthropathies: a Department of Veterans Affairs Comparative Study. Arthritis Rheum 1999;42:2325-2329.

15. Haibel H, Brandt J, Rudwaleit M, et al. Treatment of active ankylosing spondylitis with pamidronate. Rheumatology (Oxford) 2003;42:1018-1020.

16. Ince G, Sarpel T, Drugun B, et al. Effects of a multimodal exercise program for people with ankylosing spondylitis. Phys Ther 2006;86:924-935.

17. Gall V. Exercise in the spondyloarthropathies. Arthritis Care Res 1994;7:215-220.

18. Fernandez-de-Las-Penas C, Alonso-Blanco C, Alguacil-Diego IM, et al. One-year follow-up of two exercise interventions for the management of patients with ankylosing spondylitis: a randomized controlled trial. Am J Phys Med Rehabil 2006;85:559-567.

19. Luukkainen R, Nissila M, Asikainen E, et al. Periarticular corticoid treatment of the sacroiliac joint in patients with seronegative spondyloarthropathy. Clin Exp Rheumatol 1999;17:88-90.

20. Van Royen BJ, de Gast A. Lumbar osteotomy for correction of thoracolumbar deformity in ankylosing spondylitis: a structure review of three methods of treatment. Ann Rheum Dis 1999;58:399-406.

Burns 111

Jeffrey C. Schneider, MD

DEFINITION

There are approximately 1 million injuries, 700,000 emergency department visits, and 45,000 hospitalizations as a result of burns in the United States each year.[1] The incidence of burns has decreased dramatically in the past 50 years as a result of public education and home and work safety efforts. In addition, mortality from burn injury has declined by approximately 50% during the same period.[2] Treatment advances (antimicrobial therapy, early excision, and grafting), advances in the fields of emergency and critical care, and the development of comprehensive burn centers have contributed to this improved survival. Currently, once survival is ensured, treatment is focused on physical healing and, in particular, rehabilitation.

Burn survivors are more likely to be male (75%) and young (mode age, 20 to 40 years). Approximately one third of burn injuries are associated with concomitant alcohol or drug use. The majority of burns result from fire or flame injuries (60%). Other causes that represent the minority of burns are scald, electrical, chemical, tar,

and grease injuries as well as skin diseases. A minority of burn injuries (23%) occur at work.[3]

One of the most common classification systems uses depth of injury to categorize the severity of the burn. Superficial injuries, previously termed first-degree burns, solely affect the epidermal layer. The category of second-degree burns is now divided into superficial and deep partial-thickness burns. The superficial partial-thickness burns interrupt the epidermis and superficial dermis and present with blistering. The deep partial-thickness burns involve the epidermis and deep dermis, including skin appendages, affecting some degree of sensory and apocrine function. Full-thickness burns, formerly third degree, affect the entire epidermal and dermal layers and result in complete loss of skin appendages. Deep injuries may affect muscle, tendon, and bone. Such deep injuries are not part of the newer classification system but were previously classified as fourth-degree burns (Fig. 111-1 and Table 111-1).

SYMPTOMS

The symptoms of burn injury are directly related to the depth of the injury. Deep partial-thickness and full-thickness burns interrupt the function of skin appendages. Damage to the apocrine sweat glands results in dry, friable skin. In larger burns, this may also impair body temperature regulation. Involvement of nerve endings in the dermal layer may result in completely impaired sensation or altered sensations, including neuropathic-like pain and pruritus.

Other symptoms relate to the complications one may experience as a result of the burn injury. Scar tissue commonly develops weeks to months after closure of deep partial-thickness and full-thickness burns, termed hypertrophic scarring. Such scars may be painful and interfere with joint function. Other symptomatic complications include contractures, heterotopic ossification, neuropathy, and amputation. Psychiatric complications include sleep disturbances, depression, anxiety, and post-traumatic stress. Additional complications may result from inhalation injury and prolonged intensive care and hospital stays; these include pulmonary symptoms, possible cognitive effects of anoxia and shock, and generalized deconditioning and malnutrition.

scarring, which initially appears as erythematous, raised, and hardened skin. A complete neurologic examination includes an assessment of motor and sensory function, reflexes, and cognition. The musculoskeletal examination includes assessment of joint range of motion and deformities. A complete cardiac and pulmonary examination is performed with particular attention to signs of respiratory complications and hypermetabolic state. Psychiatric examination should include a thorough screening for signs of sleep disturbance, depression, anxiety, and post-traumatic stress.

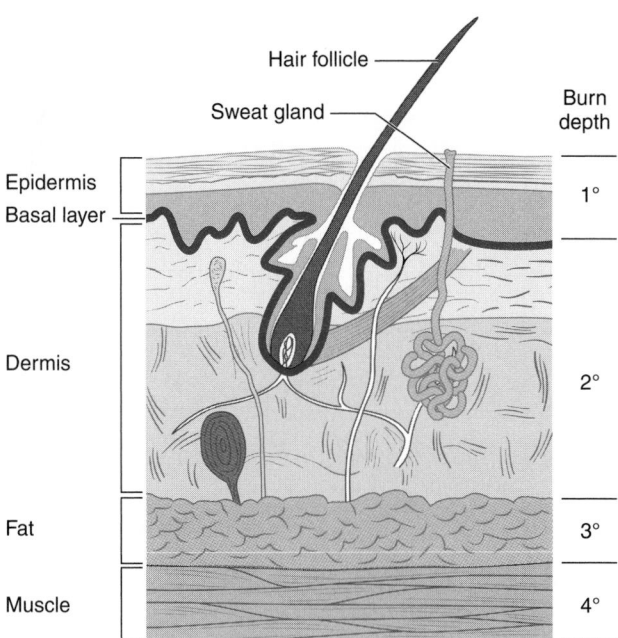

FIGURE 111-1. Diagram of skin anatomy with subdivisions by degree of burn.

FUNCTIONAL LIMITATIONS

Functional limitations are directly related to the location of the burn and complications of the burn injury. Those with burns to the upper extremities may experience impairments in activities of daily living, fine motor tasks, and occupational activities. Burns to the lower extremities may result in impairments in mobility and higher level exercise and sport activities. Another functional effect is impaired psychological function. Reports in the literature vary as to whether hand and face burns are associated with an increased incidence of psychological morbidity.[4,5]

PHYSICAL EXAMINATION

A thorough physical examination is necessary to assess the burn itself as well as the complications of the injury. The skin is examined for burn location, depth, sensation, and signs of infection. Immediately after injury, the sensory examination is primarily by light touch modality. However, after wound closure, the sensory examination thoroughly evaluates for neuropathy of small and large fibers. The motor examination of joints crossed by a deep partial-thickness or full-thickness burn should not be performed until after graft "take" is ensured, usually within a week after skin grafting. After skin grafting and as the skin matures, one should monitor for signs of hypertrophic

DIAGNOSTIC STUDIES

Fiberscopic evaluation of the airway determines the presence of inhalation injury. One may visualize erythema, edema, ulceration, and soot deposition in the tracheobronchial tree in inhalation injury.

Heterotopic ossification is diagnosed as early as 7 days after formation with a triple-phase bone scan. The aberrant ossification is visualized by increased uptake in the third phase of the scan. Plain films may not demonstrate evidence of heterotopic ossification until 3 weeks.[6]

For patients with symptoms of nerve injury, the study of choice is nerve conduction study and electromyography for the diagnosis of neuropathy.

TABLE 111-1 Burn Severity Classifications

Old Classification	New Classification	Appearance and Symptoms	Course and Treatment
First degree (epidermis)	Superficial thickness	Erythematous; dry, mildly swollen; blanches with pressure; painful	Exfoliation; heals spontaneously in 1 week; no scarring
Second degree (dermis)	Superficial partial thickness	Blistering; moist, weeping; blanches with pressure; painful	Reepithelialization in 7-20 days
	Deep partial thickness	No blisters; wet or waxy dry; variable color; less painful; at risk for conversion to full thickness because of marginal blood supply	Reepithelialization in weeks to months; skin grafting may speed recovery; associated with scarring
Third degree (all of dermis and epidermis)	Full thickness	White waxy to leathery gray to charred black; insensate to pain; does not blanch to pressure	Reepithelialization does not occur; requires skin grafting; associated with scarring
Fourth degree (extends to muscle, bone, tendon)	—	Black (eschar); exposed bones, ligaments, tendons	May require amputation or extensive deep débridement

Regular monitoring of the patient's pain with use of standardized measures is recommended. The visual analogue scale, numeric pain rating scale, and other instruments are useful in helping determine the patient's pain and treatment response.

Patients who exhibit symptoms of depression, anxiety, or post-traumatic stress should receive a complete psychiatric evaluation.

TREATMENT

Initial

Management of minor burns includes cooling with room-temperature water, gentle cleansing with mild soap and water, and coverage with a dry sterile dressing. Pain management and tetanus prophylaxis are important. Topical antibiotics should be applied to nonsuperficial burns to prevent infection.

The initial management of the severely burned patient focuses on the ABCs: airway, breathing, and circulation. Aggressive fluid resuscitation to compensate for insensible water loss is a mainstay of the acute management of the burn patient.[7] Other principles of the initial management of the burn patient include relief of ischemic compression (fasciotomy, escharotomy), application of topical antimicrobial agents, and early excision and grafting of open wounds. Sheridan[8] provides a detailed review of the acute management of burn injuries.

Rehabilitation

Contractures

The use of positioning and splinting to prevent development of contracture begins in the intensive care unit on admission. The goal of contracture prevention and treatment is to maximize joint function. The optimal position to minimize contracture development is depicted in Figure 111-2. Positioning should always be paired with passive or active range of motion exercises to prevent the development of contractures. Range of motion exercises can begin immediately if the patient has not undergone skin grafting and usually within 1 week after grafting so as not to interfere with graft take. Particular attention must be given to burns that cross joints and burns that result in exposed tendons. These joints are at high risk for contracture development and should receive empirical splinting and range of motion. Once a contracture develops, rehabilitation interventions such as splinting, positioning, range of motion exercises, and serial casting are employed to prevent worsening of the contracture and to improve the motion of the joint.[9-11]

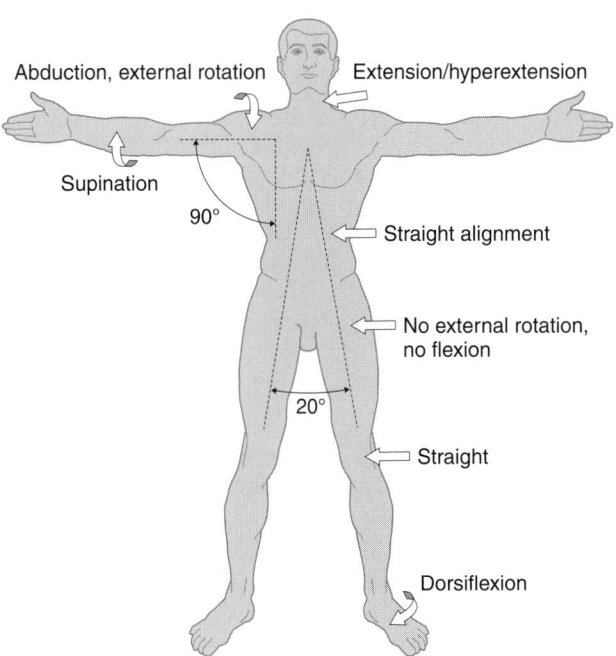

FIGURE 111-2. Optimal positioning to prevent burn contractures.

Exercise

Exercise is an integral component of burn rehabilitation, from the intensive care setting to the outpatient clinic. Passive and active range of motion exercises are used to prevent contracture development. Exercises progress to involve both strength and endurance training. After a severe burn injury, survivors are often severely deconditioned, and long-term exercise training programs are needed for return to the premorbid level of functioning. Aerobic and progressive resistance training programs have been shown to be efficacious in improving strength, peak oxygen consumption, lean body mass, and pulmonary function in burn survivors.[12]

Anabolic Steroids

After severe burns, survivors often experience increased catabolism and loss of lean body mass. Oxandrolone, an anabolic steroid, has been shown in the acute hospital setting in multiple randomized controlled trials to increase muscle protein synthesis and weight gain and to decrease the length of stay. To date, this intervention has not been studied in a rehabilitation setting.[13]

Hypertrophic Scarring

Hypertrophic scarring is commonly treated with compression garments. These garments are recommended to be worn 23 hours per day for up to 1 to 2 years after a burn. Compliance with this schedule is difficult for many patients. Furthermore, the efficacy of this treatment has not been established in the literature[14]; however, it is still considered standard of care.

Pain

Pain management after burn injury is an integral part of the rehabilitation program. Background pain from the injury itself and exacerbations of pain from intermittent débridement dressing changes cause significant discomfort in the burn patient. Long-acting opioid pain medications are commonly used to treat the background pain. Premedication with short-acting opioid analgesics before dressing changes is standard care.[15] Pain is often a multifactorial experience, and therefore clinicians should make extended efforts to treat all possible contributing causes. These additional factors include pruritus, neuropathy, anxiety, sleep disturbance, depression, and post-traumatic stress. Additional adjunctive, nonpharmacologic pain treatments include massage, hypnosis, and distraction techniques.[16]

Pruritus

Pruritus is most commonly treated with antihistaminic agents (diphenhydramine, hydroxyzine) and topical and oral tricyclic antidepressant (doxepin). Additional treatment modalities include massage and transcutaneous electrical nerve stimulation. Patients should also be encouraged to keep their burn wounds moisturized.[17]

Heterotopic Ossification

Conservative treatments include positioning and range of motion exercises. Medications (nonsteroidal anti-inflammatory drugs and bisphosphonates) and radiation therapy have been shown to be efficacious in the prevention of heterotopic ossification in other disease populations (spinal cord injury and hip arthroplasty). Studies have not examined their use in burn injuries.[6]

Psychological

Treatment of depression, post-traumatic stress, and sleep disorders has not been validated in the burn population.[18] However, a large body of evidence documents the efficacy of both pharmacologic and non-pharmacologic treatments of these disorders in other populations.[19-21] Treatment of the burn-injured patient ideally involves the collaboration of a mental health team that can assist in the diagnosis and treatment of these problems.

Procedures

None.

Surgery

In spite of aggressive rehabilitation after a burn injury, significant contractures may develop. Surgical release of the contracted joint is indicated after conservative treatment failure for contractures that result in significant functional impairments.

Surgical resection of heterotopic bone is indicated if it results in significant joint impairment despite a course of conservative treatment or if it results in nerve entrapment.

Scarring, disfigurement, and other cosmetic concerns can be addressed with reconstructive surgical efforts. Severely burned patients may undergo multiple surgeries over the span of years after their burn injury. Planning such reconstruction priorities is a task that should involve multiple members of the burn team, including the patient and his or her family, physiatrist, surgeon, therapists, and mental health professionals.

POTENTIAL DISEASE COMPLICATIONS

Contractures

Contractures are a common and significant complication of burn injury. They result in decreased joint range of motion and may also result in impaired joint function and disability, disfigurement, and cosmetic and psychological impairments. Contractures are most common at the shoulder, elbow, and knee. Length of stay, inhalation injury, and extent of burn are associated with increased incidence and severity of contracture.[22]

Hypertrophic Scars

Hypertrophic scarring is common (32% to 67%) among those severely burned and is more prevalent among darker pigmented individuals.[23] When it crosses a joint, it may result in deformities and contractures and may also have a psychological and cosmetic impact.[6]

Heterotopic Ossification

Heterotopic ossification occurs in approximately 1% of burn injuries and most frequently is located at the elbow. It commonly presents with a decrease in range of motion and may cause impairments in joint function and activities of daily living.

Amputation

Amputations may complicate burn injuries and are most commonly seen after electrical injury. Low-voltage (<1000 V) injuries most commonly result in amputation of the digits. High-voltage injuries frequently result in major amputation (10% to 50%).

Neuropathy

Mononeuropathies, mononeuropathy multiplex, and peripheral neuropathy have all been documented after burn injury. Risk factors for the development of mononeuropathy include electrical injury, days in intensive care, and history of alcohol abuse. Risk factors for the development of a generalized peripheral neuropathy include days in intensive care and the patient's age.[24] It is thought that the neuropathy may result from a combination of compressive phenomenon (including the burn itself, splints, and positioning) and the toxic and metabolic state associated with critical illness.

Thermoregulation

Full-thickness burns damage the sweat glands, present in the dermal layer. After skin grafting, these glands do not regenerate, leading to impaired sweating in involved areas. For those with larger burns, this may affect thermoregulation, particularly with exercise in warm climates.

Psychological Complications

Depression (16% to 53%), post-traumatic stress (11% to 45%), and sleep disturbances (13% to 73%) are common after burn injuries. Routine screening for psychological complications is recommended. Mental health consultation is useful in diagnosis and treatment of these disorders. Furthermore, these issues often require long-term follow-up.

Cognitive impairments may result from anoxia associated with inhalation injury or hypoperfusion associated with shock. A high index of suspicion is needed for diagnosis and treatment of patients with mild cognitive impairments. Brain magnetic resonance imaging and neuropsychological evaluation may assist in diagnosis.

POTENTIAL TREATMENT COMPLICATIONS

Burn injuries crossing major joints that are not aggressively treated with range of motion exercises and splinting may develop clinically significant contractures. Such contractures may result in impaired mobility and activities of daily living. Improper positioning and splinting may lead to compression neuropathies, most commonly seen at the peroneal nerve.

Medications used to treat pruritus and pain may cause sedation.

Psychological complications, such as depression, posttraumatic stress, and anxiety, if they are not recognized and treated, may result in significant functional impairments, additional risk for future injury, and death.

References

1. Burn Incidence and Treatment in the US: 2000 Fact Sheet. Available at http://www.ameriburn.org/pub/burnincidencefactsheet.htm.
2. Ryan CM, Schoenfeld DA, Thorpe WP, et al. Objective estimates of the probability of death from burn injuries. N Engl J Med 1998;338:362-366.
3. National Institute for Disability and Rehabilitation Research. NIDRR Model Systems for Burn Injury Rehabilitation: Adult Facts and Figures. Available at: bms-dcc.uchsc.edu/.
4. Fauerbach JA, Heinberg LJ, Lawrence JS, et al. Coping with body image changes following a disfiguring burn injury. Health Psychol 2002:21:115-121.
5. Lawrence JW, Fauerbach JA, Heinberg L, et al. Visible vs hidden scars and their relation to body esteem. J Burn Care Rehabil 2004;25:25-32.
6. Hunt JL, Arnoldo BD, Kowalske K, et al. Heterotopic ossification revisited: a 21-year surgical experience. J Burn Care Res 2006;27:535-540.
7. Davies J. The fluid therapy given to 1027 patients during the first 24 hours after burning. 1. Total fluid and colloid input. Burns 1975;1/4:319.
8. Sheridan RL. The Trauma Handbook of the Massachusetts General Hospital. Philadelphia, Lippincott Williams & Wilkins, 2004.
9. Richard R, Staley M, Miller S, et al. To splint or not to splint: past philosophy and present practice. Part I. J Burn Care Rehabil 1996;17:444-453.
10. Richard R, Staley M, Miller S, et al. To splint or not to splint: past philosophy and current practice. Part II. J Burn Care Rehabil 1997;18:64-71.
11. Richard R, Staley M, Miller S, et al. To splint or not to splint: past philosophy and present practice. Part III. J Burn Care Rehabil 1997;18:251-255.
12. Cucuzzo NA, Ferrando A, Herndon DN. The effects of exercise programming vs traditional outpatient therapy in the rehabilitation of severely burned children. J Burn Care Rehabil 2001;22:214-220.
13. Wolf SE, Edelman LS, Kemalyan N, et al. Effects of oxandrolone on outcome measures in the severely burned: a multicenter prospective randomized double-blind trial. J Burn Care Res 2006;27:131-139.
14. Kealey GP, Jensen KL, Laubenthal KN, et al. Prospective randomized comparison of two types of pressure therapy garments. J Burn Care Rehabil 1990;11:334-336.
15. Finn J, Wright J, Fong J, et al. A randomised crossover trial of patient controlled intranasal fentanyl and oral morphine for procedural wound care in adult patients with burns. Burns 2004;30:262-268.
16. Frenay MC, Faymonville ME, Devlieger S, et al. Psychological approaches during dressing changes of burned patients: a prospective randomised study comparing hypnosis against stress reducing strategy. Burns 2001;27:793-799.
17. Baker RA, Zeller RA, Klein RL, et al. Burn wound itch control using H1 and H2 antagonists. J Burn Care Rehabil 2001;22:263-268.
18. Esselman PC, Thombs BD, Magyar-Russell G, et al. Burn rehabilitation: state of the science. Am J Phys Med Rehabil 2006;85:383-414.
19. Vieweg WV, Julius DA, Fernandez A, et al. Posttraumatic stress disorder: clinical features, pathophysiology, and treatment. Am J Med 2006;119:383-390.
20. Pagel JF, Parnes BL. Medications for the treatment of sleep disorders: an overview. Prim Care Companion J Clin Psychiatry 2001;3:118-125.
21. Arroll B, Macgillivray S, Ogston S, et al. Efficacy and tolerability of tricyclic antidepressants and SSRIs compared with placebo for treatment of depression in primary care: a meta-analysis. Ann Fam Med 2005;3:449-456.
22. Schneider JC, Holavanahalli R, Goldstein R, et al. A prospective study of contractures in burn injury: defining the problem. J Burn Care Res 2006;27:508-514.
23. Bambaro KM, Egrav LH, Carrougher GJ, et al. What is the prevalence of hypertrophic scarring following burns? Burns 2003;29:299-302.
24. Kowalske K, Holavanahalli R, Helm P. Neuropathy after burn injury. J Burn Care Rehabil 2001;22:353-357.

Cardiac Rehabilitation 112

Alan M. Davis, MD, PhD

Synonyms

None

ICD-9 Codes

410.00–410.92	Acute myocardial infarction
411.0–411.89	Other acute and subacute forms of ischemic heart disease
412	Old myocardial infarction
413.0–413.9	Angina pectoris
414.0–414.9	Other forms of chronic ischemic heart disease
429.2	Cardiovascular disease, unspecified
V42	Cardiac valve replacement status
V42.1	Cardiac transplant status
V45.81	Aortocoronary bypass status

DEFINITION

Cardiac rehabilitation is the integrated treatment of individuals after cardiac events or procedures with the goals of maximizing physical function, promoting emotional adjustment, modifying cardiac risk factors, and addressing return to previous social roles and responsibilities. The American Heart Association estimates that coronary heart disease affects 13,200,000 people in the United States; myocardial infarction affects 7,200,000, and angina pectoris affects 6,500,000.[1] Cardiac diseases, the leading cause of mortality in both men and women, accounted for 29% of all deaths in 2002.[2] Cardiac rehabilitation supports those who survive to change their lifestyle, to maximize their quality of life, and to decrease their risk for future cardiac events. Clinic-based cardiac rehabilitation may benefit individuals after acute coronary syndrome, cardiac surgery (coronary artery bypass, valve replacement, transplantation, ventricular reduction surgery), and compensated congestive heart failure. Those referred to cardiac rehabilitation have improved 3-year survival after myocardial infarction; 95% of participants are alive versus 64% of nonparticipants, with 28% reduction in risk for subsequent myocardial infarction.[3]

SYMPTOMS

The individual with a recent catrdiac event or procedure frequently complains of decreased endurance for walking or climbing stairs, increased dyspnea during physical activity, and fatigue. If arrhythmia is present, the patient may feel palpitations. Chest pain may accompany physical exertion or emotional stress. Pain due to surgical incisions of the extremities or chest wall may also be present. Symptoms of heart failure, such as orthopnea and paroxysmal nocturnal dyspnea, may also be present. The person may feel anxious about any type of physical exercise, resumption of sexual activities, and return to work. In many cases, the patient may complain of depression.

PHYSICAL EXAMINATION

Observation of the patient should look for signs of depression and anxiety. During the examination of the cardiac patient, the clinician should search for signs of complications after the cardiac event or cardiac procedure. Findings of congestive heart failure, such as rales, peripheral edema, and elevated jugular venous distention, should be evaluated. Palpation of decreased or absent pulses in the extremities may suggest the common comorbidity of peripheral vascular disease. Surgical wounds, such as vascular harvest sites, arterial puncture sites, and sternotomy wounds, need evaluation before exercise programs are prescribed. Manual muscle testing of the extremities provides an indication of the degree of skeletal muscle atrophy due to decreased physical activity.

FUNCTIONAL LIMITATIONS

Functional limitations due to cardiac disease alone are related to the workload the myocardium can sustain before signs of cardiac dysfunction result. The workload achieved before symptom onset is generally decreased. Overall endurance is decreased. Most patients with uncomplicated cardiac cases are able to ambulate slowly and to perform self-care on discharge from the hospital.

This alone does not guarantee quality of life for the treated individual. The degree and severity of cardiac impairment may limit a patient's physical progress and ultimate maximum level of function. Decreased endurance for walking, independent living skills, physically demanding labor, and recreational activities is addressed during cardiac rehabilitation. The patient may later return to physically demanding activity, such as heavy labor or competitive singles tennis, after rehabilitation that follows uncomplicated coronary angioplasty or stenting without myocardial infarction. However, for the patient who experienced myocardial infarction complicated by congestive heart failure and arrhythmia, walking to a neighbor's home or performing the household chores may be limited by dyspnea. Further compromise of progress is related to the common comorbidities of cerebrovascular disease, intrinsic lung disease, diabetes mellitus, and peripheral vascular disease. Impairment due to neurologic, rheumatologic, or orthopedic disease may require specific adaptations to allow conditioning and strengthening exercise.

Emotional stress and an individual's response to it may also produce functional limitations when return to social roles and responsibilities is considered. This may range from anxiety about physical exertion to major reactive depression. Dysfunction such as ischemia or arrhythmia may be produced by either physical or emotional demands.[4-6] This is likely to be due to increased sympathetic drive in the autonomic nervous system, which predisposes the individual to more endothelial damage and cardiac arrhythmias mediated by catecholamines. The contribution of psychosocial stress has long been a part of the cardiac literature, but the true magnitude of effect has been shown in a large international study. Depression accounted for approximately the same (35%) risk for myocardial infarction as smoking did.[7] This argues strongly for a clear psychological screening of patients with cardiac events. Patients whose depression was diagnosed and treated by selective serotonin reuptake inhibitors (SSRIs) with their initial myocardial infarction had 43% less new myocardial infarction and cardiac death compared with treatment with non-SSRIs.[8] This is due to an antiplatelet aggregation effect unrelated to aspirin or clopidogrel bisulfate (Plavix).

DIAGNOSTIC STUDIES

The clinician should evaluate the patient's lipid profile to guide pharmacologic and dietary management of hyperlipidemia and hypercholesterolemia. Tight diabetes control may decrease the rate of atheroma formation, and glycosylated hemoglobin (hemoglobin A_{1c}) is used to ascertain the recent success of blood glucose control.

For the individual with dyspnea on exertion and the comorbidity of lung disease, pulmonary function testing will clarify the contribution of obstructive or restrictive lung disease to the symptoms. Treatable conditions, such as reactive airways and hypoxia during exercise,

should be addressed before beginning of cardiac rehabilitation for maximal benefit.

A submaximal exercise test may be administered before or after hospital discharge for risk stratification.[9] *This does not guide the therapeutic exercise prescription.* Submaximal exercise testing is usually limited to 5 metabolic equivalents (METs) for patients older than 40 years or to 7 METs for patients 40 years or younger. A symptom-limited *functional* exercise test administered at 2 to 6 weeks after a cardiac event or procedure provides the best guide to exercise prescription. The specific timing of exercise testing depends on the amount of myocardium damage, the need for return to work, and the practice pattern of the clinician administering the test. Typical functional exercise testing documents work capacity and cardiopulmonary function. Treadmill testing after a modified Naughton, a Naughton-Balke, or a ramp protocol is especially well suited to guide cardiac rehabilitation exercise training because these protocols use smaller increments of workload that more accurately portray functional capacity. Alternatively, bicycle ergometer protocols may also use smaller gradations of workload. These suggested protocols usually start at a lower level than common diagnostic protocols, such as the Bruce protocol, and increase fewer METs per stage. Bicycle ergometry should be considered for individuals with balance deficits, mild neurologic impairment, or orthopedic limitations.

Echocardiographic, pharmacologic, or nuclear medicine stress exercise testing should be considered for patients with marked lower extremity limitations, severe debility, or electrocardiograms that are difficult to interpret. Combined ventilatory gas analysis by use of a metabolic cart and electrocardiographic monitoring may differentiate cardiac versus pulmonary exercise-induced dyspnea, chest pain, or fatigue.

Most patients have had many electrocardiograms during their hospital stay or evaluation. In the outpatient setting, electrocardiograms should be ordered if there is a change in clinical status, such as new symptoms (e.g., the resumption of angina). For the most part, patients are also monitored by telemetry during at least the initial part of their cardiac rehabilitation.

Patients should be screened for psychosocial stressors, such as anxiety and depression. Besides asking the patient about the symptoms of anxiety, anger, persistent sadness, excessive fatigue, and abnormal sleep architecture, commonly used questionnaires that are easy to administer in an office setting are the Beck Depression Inventory the and State-Trait Anxiety Inventory. Both take only a few minutes to complete and can be used to monitor the effectiveness of treatment.

TREATMENT

Initial

Cardiac rehabilitation begins with risk factor reduction. The initial medical management focuses on optimizing the cardiac medication regimen to control or to prevent hypertension, ischemia, arrhythmia, hyperlipidemia, or other complications that follow the patient's cardiac event. Concurrent with medical management, the clinician prescribing cardiac rehabilitation must promote choices for healthy living. Each cardiac patient has choices about smoking, diet, exercise, and stress management.

Smoking cessation has the highest rates of success by combining participation in a smoking cessation support group with pharmacologic management of the craving due to nicotine addiction. Bupropion combined with either a nicotine patch or nicotine gum works well. Have the patient begin taking the bupropion hydrochloride (150 mg every day for the first 3 days, then 150 mg twice daily) 1 to 2 weeks before the chosen date to quit smoking and begin using the nicotine supplement at the time of smoking cessation. This should coincide with the first smoking cessation support group meeting.

Dietary modification has been documented to improve the lipid profile. Ask the patient to keep a food diary for at least 3 days and refer the patient to a registered dietitian for evaluation and education on appropriate dietary choices. The American Heart Association revised cardiac diet recommendations of 2006 are substantially more stringent on the saturated fat intake (Table 112-1).[10] The dietitian may recommend the American Heart Association diet, but other choices could be the Mediterranean diet or the lacto-ovovegetarian diet. None of these three diets has been shown to be superior, and the choice of which diet to recommend is based primarily on the patient's ability to follow the diet.

The individual with cardiac disease often needs to learn tools to decrease the emotional stress of anxiety and depression. Patients with either of these based on the original screening should be treated. SSRIs treat both components fairly well with few side effects. A referral for counseling from a mental health professional can provide patients with an assortment of tools to learn relaxation and provides a forum for the discussion of emotional symptoms surrounding cardiac events in their life. Women have a higher rate of anxiety and psychosomatic complaints than do men beginning cardiac rehabilitation.[11] In the busy clinic, the clinician can also teach the individual a simple stress reduction technique. A relaxation response documented by augmented parasympathetic activity has been noted during the simple exercise of paced breathing. Ask the patient to pace his or her breathing, using a clock, for 5 to 10 minutes twice daily. The patient should time inhalation and exhalation equally for 3 seconds each while avoiding air hunger or hyperventilation. Once he or she performs this exercise with facility, additional relaxation can be achieved from further slowing of the breathing rate or prolonging the period of exhalation.[12]

Return to sexual activity should be frankly discussed with patients and their sexual partners to decrease their anxiety about sexual activity after a cardiac event.[13] Sexual activity between couples with a long-standing relationship requires 3 to 5 METs. A simple test is the two-flight stair test.[14,15] After a few minutes of level walking, the patient rapidly ascends and descends two flights of stairs. If this does not produce cardiac symptoms, sexual relations can be resumed. Extramarital sex causes higher energy demands.

Return to work and recreational activities should be based on patients' clinical status and their previous work. The exercise test performance predicts the level of vocational work capacity. If the patient's work capacity is only 3 to 4 METs or less, return to work may be unrealistic. Even self-care activities are likely to produce symptoms at this low level. With a 5 to 7 MET capacity, the person should be able to perform sedentary work and most domestic roles. If the person can exercise beyond 7 METs, most types of work can be performed without restriction, except those involving heavy physical labor. For recreational activity, the MET level required should be evaluated before return to play is recommended. The following are some common

---

TABLE 112-1 American Heart Association 2006 Diet and Lifestyle Recommendations for Cardiovascular Disease Risk Reduction

Balance calorie intake and physical activity to achieve or maintain a healthy body weight.

Consume a diet rich in vegetables and fruits.

Choose whole-grain, high-fiber foods.

Consume fish, especially oily fish, at least twice a week.

Limit your intake of saturated fat to <7% of energy, *trans* fat to <1% of energy, and cholesterol to <300 mg per day by

　　choosing lean meats and vegetable alternatives;

　　selecting fat-free (skim), 1%-fat, and low-fat dairy products; and

　　minimizing intake of partially hydrogenated fats.

Minimize your intake of beverages and foods with added sugars.

Choose and prepare foods with little or no salt.

If you consume alcohol, do so in moderation.

When you eat food that is prepared outside of the home, follow the American Heart Association Diet and Lifestyle Recommendations.

recreational activities and their MET requirements: tennis, 4 to 7 METs; golf, 2 to 5; skiing, 7 to 18; bowling, 4 to 5; and volleyball, 3 to 4.

Rehabilitation

If the patient is unable to begin a supervised exercise training program on discharge from the hospital because of potential complications (Table 112-2), recommend a self-directed walking program. The patient should walk primarily on level surfaces with the goal of 15 to 30 minutes of walking at least three to five times per week at an intensity that will allow talking. Ask patients to keep a walking journal and review it with them. If no significant cardiac damage has occurred, such as after angioplasty, the period of convalescence may be shortened on the basis of the clinician's judgment and considerations such as the individual's need to return to previous pursuits.

Physical training begins at the end of the convalescence period ideally, based on functional exercise testing described in the preceding discussion of diagnostic testing. Arguments have been made that exercise testing at this stage does not improve the outcome or safety of a supervised cardiac rehabilitation therapy program.[16] Prescription includes type, target intensity, frequency, and duration of exercise. Aerobic exercises, such as walking and bicycling, are the mainstay of most programs. Passive resistive exercises and weight training develop skeletal muscle mass but remain somewhat controversial for patients with congestive heart failure. Prescribe aerobic exercise intensity on the basis of heart rate, workload (METs), or perceived exertion (Table 112-3). The visual

---

TABLE 112-2 Possible Contraindications for Entry into Inpatient or Outpatient Exercise Programs

Unstable angina

Resting systolic blood pressure > 200 mm Hg

Resting diastolic blood pressure > 100 mm Hg

Orthostatic blood pressure drop or drop during exercise training of 20 mm Hg

Moderate to severe aortic stenosis

Acute systemic illness or fever

Uncontrolled atrial or ventricular dysrhythmias

Uncontrolled sinus tachycardia (120 beats per minute)

Uncontrolled congestive heart failure

Third-degree atrioventricular block

Active pericarditis or myocarditis

Recent embolism

Thrombophlebitis

Resting ST displacement (>3 mm)

Uncontrolled diabetes

Orthopedic problems that prohibit exercise

From American College of Sports Medicine. Guidelines for Exercise Testing and Prescription, 4th ed. Philadelphia, Lea & Febiger, 1991.

---

analogue Borg scale rates perceived exertion (Fig. 112-1) that has been shown to correlate linearly with heart rate and oxygen consumption.[17] The frequency of exercise sessions is usually three to five times per week.

Aerobic exercise sessions begin with a warm-up phase of 2 to 5 minutes at a lower intensity of exercise to limber the joints, to open collateral circulation, and to decrease peripheral vascular resistance. The stimulus or conditioning phase may be continuous or discontinuous, with the 3- to 12-month goal of at least 20 to 30 minutes of aerobic exercise. This may be broken down as a discontinuous exercise with rest breaks between periods of conditioning exercise. A cool-down phase at a lower intensity of exercise will prevent hypotension and, later, joint pain. Duration of aerobic exercise sessions depends on the individual's level of fitness. For the poorly debilitated patient, 3 to 5 minutes in the target range will provide benefit initially. The deconditioned individual should be progressed during 4 to 12 weeks to this stimulus duration. Electrocardiographic monitoring during aerobic exercise is recommended for patients with low ejection fraction, abnormal blood pressure response to exercise, ST-segment depression during low-level exercise testing, or serious ventricular arrhythmia.[18]

Strength training or circuit training with resistance exercises adds skeletal muscle strength and facilitates building of local muscle endurance for those with good left ventricular function. This should especially be considered for the cardiac patient who may be returning to a physically demanding job. Patients who use free weights should begin with the lowest weight that produces a perceived exertion of 11 to 13 after 10 to 15 repetitions (see Fig. 112-1). One to three sets will build strength. This should involve enough different exercises to include all major muscle groups of the upper and lower extremities.

The clinic-based supervised exercise program typically lasts 1 to 3 months, with the exercise prescription upgraded monthly. Monthly reevaluation should include consideration of increasing the stimulus-phase intensity or duration of aerobic exercise. After 2 to 3 months of a conditioning exercise program, the individual should have the ability to achieve 7 to 8 METs of sustained exercise. Once the patient has achieved this goal, repeat of the exercise test will show the level of improvement and guide the transition to a self-directed maintenance program. The patient may choose his or her target heart rate or exertion level during exercise.

The benefits of exercise training include increased maximum oxygen uptake, increased endurance for activities of daily living, increased work capacity, decreased heart rate during exercise, decreased rate-pressure product, decreased fatigue, decreased dyspnea, and decreased symptoms of heart failure. Exercise training reduces atherogenic and thrombotic risk factors by managing or preventing excess body weight, increasing high-density lipoprotein cholesterol, decreasing plasma triglycerides, decreasing platelet aggregation, and improving glucose levels. Myocardial perfusion may be improved by increased coronary blood flow. The progress of coronary atherosclerosis may be slowed or possibly reversed.[19-21]

TABLE 112-3 Cardiac Rehabilitation Exercise Prescription

Type	Aerobic	Treadmill Bicycle (circle one)
Include	Strength training?	Yes No (circle one)

Intensity: Based on heart rate

Target heart range

70% to 85% of maximum heart rate if the patient is not taking β-adrenergic blockade

85% maximum completed on treadmill if the patient is taking β-adrenergic blockade

High resting heart rate (HR), by exercise testing results (Karvonen formula):

Target HR = resting HR + [(HRmax − HRrest) × (60 + MTmax/100)]

Intensity: Based on workload

Target 66% MET level completed on treadmill testing

Target 25 watts or 150 kpm less than completed stage on bicycle ergometer testing

Intensity: Based on perceived exertion

Borg scale target 11 to 15

Warm-up phase

Treadmill ambulation at _____ speed _____ grade for _____ minutes.

Bicycle ergometry at _____ kpm/watts for _____ minutes.

Check blood pressure, pulse rate, and perceived exertion.

Advance to stimulus phase.

Stimulus phase

Treadmill ambulation at _____ speed _____ grade _____ minutes with/without rest. Repeat _____ sets.

Bicycle ergometry at _____ kpm/watts for _____ minutes with/without rest. Repeat _____ sets.

Check blood pressure, pulse rate, and perceived exertion.

Advance to cool-down phase.

Cool-down phase

Treadmill ambulation at _____ speed _____ grade for _____ minutes.

Bicycle ergometry at _____ kpm/watts for _____ minutes.

Check blood pressure, pulse rate.

Frequency	3 times per week
Duration	1 hour per visit for 12 weeks

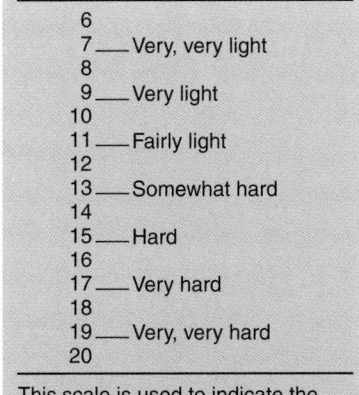

FIGURE 112-1. Borg's scale of perceived exertion. (Reprinted with permission from Borg G. Perceived exertion as an indicator of somatic stress. Scand J Rehabil Med 1970;2-3:92-98.)

Procedures

Medically stabilized cardiac patients need few procedures. Thoracentesis for pulmonary effusion will greatly enhance physical performance. Interventional cardiology procedures may be needed for acutely occluded stents, angioplasty, or grafts. For the patient with significant arrhythmias, pacemaker placement or adjustment may be necessary. The patient with worsening cardiac symptoms may need to repeat coronary angiography or nuclear medicine stress testing if medication adjustment is unsuccessful.

Surgery

Surgical interventions may be needed for failed coronary bypass vascular grafts, infected wounds, or pseudoaneurysms at arterial puncture sites. Permanent pacemaker or implantable defibrillators may be necessary for individuals with arrhythmias not controlled with medications.

POTENTIAL DISEASE COMPLICATIONS

The most common cause of mortality in the United States is cardiac disease. Decreased exercise tolerance and decreased work capacity are the most common functional impairments. Medical complications include congestive heart failure, arrhythmia, repeated infarction, and possible closure of coronary artery grafts and stents or angioplasties. Because coronary artery disease is associated with generalized atherosclerotic vascular disease, one should be aware of possible stroke, peripheral vascular insufficiency, and other end-organ manifestations of compromised vascular supply. Despite referral to cardiac rehabilitation, individuals may still experience loss of social roles, vocational barriers, and difficulty with emotional adjustment despite excellent physical improvement and appropriate psychosocial interventions.

POTENTIAL TREATMENT COMPLICATIONS

There is a slight risk of precipitation of a cardiac event during cardiac rehabilitation. In one study, the risk of a significant cardiac event during exercise training, such as new infarct or death, occurred at a rate of 1/50,000 to 1/120,000 person-hours of exercise.[22] Preventing the enrollment of patients into cardiac rehabilitation who are not medically stabilized can minimize the risk. Exercise testing has relative and absolute contraindications that should be followed; these contraindications have been elucidated in great detail elsewhere.[9] In general, however, do not test patients with unstable angina, malignant cardiac arrhythmia, pericarditis, endocarditis, severe left ventricular dysfunction, severe aortic stenosis, or any other acute noncardiac disease.

References

1. Cardiovascular Disease Statistics. Available at American Heart Association Web site. Accessed January 18, 2007.
2. Anderson RN, Smith BL. Deaths: leading causes for 2002. Natl Vital Stat Rep 2005;53:1-89.
3. Witt BJ, Jacobsen SJ, Weston SA, et al. Cardiac rehabilitation after myocardial infarction in the community. J Am Coll Cardiol 2004;44:988-996.
4. Davis AM, Natelson BH. Brain-heart interactions. The neurocardiology of arrhythmia and sudden cardiac death. Tex Heart Inst J 1993;20:158-169.
5. Thompson DR, Lewin RJ. Coronary disease. Management of the post–myocardial infarction patient: rehabilitation and cardiac neurosis. Heart 2000;84:101-105.
6. Watkins LL, Blumenthal JA, Davidson JR, et al. Phobic anxiety, depression, and risk of ventricular arrhythmias in patients with coronary heart disease. Psychosom Med 2006;68:651-656.
7. Yusuf S, Hawken S, Ounpuu S, et al; INTERHEART Study Investigators. Effect of potentially modifiable risk factors associated with myocardial infarction in 52 countries (the INTERHEART study): case-control study. Lancet 2004;364:937-952.
8. Berkman LF, Blumenthal J, Burg M, et al. Effects of treating depression and low perceived social support on clinical events after myocardial infarction: the Enhancing Recovery in Coronary Heart Disease Patients (ENRICHD) Randomized Trial. JAMA 2003;289:3106-3116.
9. Gibbons RJ, Balady GJ, Bricker JT, et al; American College of Cardiology/American Heart Association Task Force on Practice Guidelines. Committee to Update the 1997 Exercise Testing. ACC/AHA 2002 guideline update for exercise testing: summary article. J Am Coll Cardiol 2002;40:1531-1540.
10. Lichtenstein AH, Appel LJ, Brands M, et al; American Heart Association Nutrition Committee. Diet and lifestyle recommendations revision 2006: a scientific statement from the American Heart Association Nutrition Committee. Circulation 2006;114:82-96.
11. Brezinka V, Kittel F. Psychosocial factors of coronary heart disease in women: a review. Soc Sci Med 1996;42:1351-1365.
12. Davis AM. Respiratory modulation of heart rate variability and parasympathetic influence on the heart [doctoral dissertation]. University of Medicine and Dentistry of New Jersey–New Jersey Medical School, Department of Neurosciences, 1997.
13. Friedman S. Cardiac disease, anxiety, and sexual functioning. Am J Cardiol 2000;86:46F-50F.
14. Larsen JL, McNaughton MW, Kennedy JW, et al. Heart rate and blood pressure response to sexual activity and a stair climbing test. Heart Lung 1980;9:1025-1030.
15. Cheitlin MD. Sexual activity and cardiac risk. Am J Cardiol 2005;96:24M-28M.
16. McConnell TR, Klinger TA, Gardner JK, et al. Cardiac rehabilitation without exercise tests for post–myocardial infarction and post–bypass surgery patients. J Cardiopulm Rehabil 1998;18:458-463.
17. Borg G. Perceived exertion as an indicator of somatic stress. Scand J Rehabil Med 1970;2-3:92-98.
18. American Association of Cardiovascular and Pulmonary Rehabilitation. Guidelines for Cardiac Rehabilitation and Secondary Prevention Programs, 4th ed. Champaign, Ill, Human Kinetics, 2004.
19. Ignaszewski A, Lear SA. Cardiac rehabilitation programs. Can J Cardiol 1999;15(Suppl G):110G-113G.
20. Leon AS. Exercise following myocardial infarction. Current recommendations. Sports Med 2000;29:301-311.
21. Ades PA, Coello CE. Effects of exercise and cardiac rehabilitation on cardiovascular outcomes. Med Clin North Am 2000;84:251-265, x-xi.
22. Franklin BA, Bonzheim K, Gordon S, Timmis GC. Safety of medically supervised outpatient cardiac rehabilitation exercise therapy: a 16-year follow-up. Chest 1998;114:902-906.

Cancer **113**

Andrea Cheville, MD, and Lora Beth Packel, PT, MS

DEFINITION

Cancers vary widely in prognosis, natural history, management, treatment responsiveness, adverse sequelae, and associated physical impairments. As a consequence, cancer rehabilitation is not amenable to reductive therapeutic algorithms. Related impairments depend on the location and stage of cancer as well as on the type of antineoplastic therapy. For example, cancers of the head and neck may require radical neck dissection and subsequent irradiation. Common adverse sequelae include shoulder dysfunction and fibrosis of cervical soft tissue. In contrast, primary breast cancer treatment may cause myofascial pain and upper extremity swelling. The reader is referred to chapters specific to these conditions and anatomic locations (e.g., scapular winging, lymphedema).

A more uniform approach can be applied to the management of cancer-related fatigue, which affects up to 80% of patients.[1] Despite inconsistencies in disease management and clinical course, the majority of cancer patients will have function-limiting fatigue during their illness. For many, fatigue will remain a problem after completion of therapy.[1,2] A robust literature describes how unremitting fatigue undermines patients' function performance and quality of life.[3] A variety of signs and symptoms, including motor weakness, cognitive dysfunction, imbalance, exertional dyspnea, and myalgias, may contribute to patients' complaints of fatigue. Deconditioning is an important contributing factor that may engender and sustain fatigue. Deconditioning also has many potential sources: cancer-related cachexia, inactivity, poor nutrition, chronic steroid exposure, and direct effect of the cancer therapy.[2] Advanced age and extensive medical comorbidity are important additional contributors.

SYMPTOMS

Before formal evaluation is undertaken, it is important to determine the patient's current place on the cancer trajectory, which ranges from active, curative treatment to end-stage palliation. Obviously, all elements of the history and physical examination will be influenced by this knowledge. Three important distinctions must be made:

1. Is the patient receiving active treatment?
2. Does the patient have known cancer?
3. Is the patient deemed curable?

The willingness and capacity of patients to engage in the rehabilitation process will be profoundly affected by the answers to these questions.

A characteristic constellation of symptoms should not be anticipated in patients' reporting of cancer fatigue. As emphasized before, patients' malignant neoplasms, treatment regimens, and disease trajectories are extremely variable. Cancer-related fatigue may therefore present differently, contingent on the unique particulars of each case. Patients' word choices to describe their fatigue may be inconsistent and, at times, puzzling to clinicians. Any of the following subjective complaints should raise concern about possible cancer-related fatigue: weakness (generalized or proximal), dyspnea on exertion, orthostatic hypotension, sedation, hypersomnolence, exertional intolerance, or cognitive compromise (e.g., attention or concentration deficits, short-term memory dysfunction). Patients may report the sensation that their legs are leaden or that they are walking through water. Validated self-report fatigue scales (e.g., Brief Fatigue Inventory, Functional Assessment of Cancer Treatment—Fatigue, Profile of Mood States) can be exceedingly useful to quantify severity and to monitor treatment response.[4] A brief screen for depression or other mood disorders is essential,[5] and validated screening tools are widely available.

Patients' cancer histories should be collected in detail, including prior and ongoing radiation therapy and chemotherapy as well as any surgical procedures. Knowledge of each patient's primary cancer will shift the focus toward particular causes. For example, pancreatic cancer is more likely to produce cachexia, whereas breast and lung cancers are associated with a high incidence of hypercalcemia and neurologic compromise.[3] Attention should be paid to whether radiation fields encompass thyroid, lung, adrenal, or cardiac tissue. If glandular or organ dysfunction is suspected, appropriate serologies and physiologic evaluations may be indicated. Medication use and nutritional status must be carefully reviewed.

Information comparable with that solicited through a good pain history should be elicited for fatigue: acuity of fatigue onset, activity- or treatment-related precipitants, diurnal fluctuation, associated symptoms (e.g., pain, nausea), progressive worsening or improvement, exacerbating and alleviating factors, prior treatments and degree of response, and patients' attributional systems. Questions about sleep patterns, sleep hygiene, and daytime napping are useful. Reports suggest that frequent daytime napping may actually worsen fatigue.[5,6]

The extent to which fatigue limits vocational, avocational, and familial pursuits as well as autonomous mobility and self-care should be comprehensively reviewed. Because fatigue most commonly interferes with activities requiring stamina and exertional tolerance, changes in a patient's comfortable walking distance, duration of physical activity, willingness to climb stairs, and the like will help characterize the impact of fatigue. It is important to determine whether patients have a premorbid history of regular physical activity on which rehabilitation efforts can capitalize.

PHYSICAL EXAMINATION

Special tests are rarely indicated on physical examination. Rather, clinicians should perform a comprehensive evaluation with emphasis on musculoskeletal and neurologic elements. Assessment of range of motion, gait (including tandem), static and dynamic balance, and ability to squat repetitively may identify potential contributing factors amenable to therapy. Examination may reveal evidence of congestive heart failure or pulmonary compromise. Stigmata of hypothyroidism should be sought, particularly in patients with head and neck cancer. For patients without known cancer, the neurologic examination findings should be normal beyond chemotherapy-related peripheral neuropathy. Weakness in proximal hip and shoulder musculature suggests steroid myopathy. Identification of new neurologic deficits should trigger evaluation for malignant progression or emerging treatment toxicity.[4] The mental status examination may reveal evidence of compromised arousal, attention, memory, or concentration, particularly in patients who have received whole-brain radiation therapy or intrathecal chemotherapy.

FUNCTIONAL LIMITATIONS

Although fatigue is rarely so severe that it undermines basic mobility or performance of activities of daily living apart from the palliative context,[7] evaluation of these functional domains is integral to comprehensive evaluation. Severe functional compromise may be a red flag, contingent on the clinical context, that triggers evaluation for significant comorbidity. Ambulation for moderate distances may produce limiting dyspnea in patients with cancer-related cardiac or pulmonary dysfunction. Patients with steroid myopathy or generalized muscle weakness may have difficulty rising from low surfaces, such as a toilet, soft chair, or car seat. These patients may also demonstrate decreased ability to independently complete their activities of daily living in a reasonable time frame. As suggested previously, many patients describe generalized heaviness of the limbs and global decrements in activity level without precise functional limitations.

Dysfunction in social, vocational, psychological, and sexual domains may be present. Patients should be questioned about compromised social interactions, sleep, and intimacy as well as work-related and leisure pursuits. Many patients abandon their avocational activities as a consequence of fatigue, with the potential for isolation and secondary depression. Patients with cognitive deficits related to radiation therapy or chemotherapy may experience difficulty in maintaining their vocational productivity. Financial and domestic management skills may be compromised as well.

DIAGNOSTIC STUDIES

Diagnostic tests vary with the presentation of the patient. Dyspnea should be assessed with pulse oximetry during activity, chest radiography, and electrocardiography. Patients who exhibit severe dyspnea with minimal activity may have pulmonary fibrosis. Definitive diagnosis may be made through computed tomographic scanning.[8] Positron emission tomography may help distinguish fibrosis from cancer involving the lung parenchyma. Patients with cancer are at an elevated risk for venous thrombosis; therefore, a venous duplex study and possibly a ventilation-perfusion scan should be considered for persistent shortness of breath. Patients who have received doxorubicin (Adriamycin) or trastuzumab (Herceptin) should be evaluated with a multigated acquisition scan to rule out possible chemotherapy-related cardiac toxicity. Most patients will have undergone multigated acquisition screening before the administration of chemotherapy. The results of baseline tests can be compared with new evaluations for evidence of deterioration. Pericardial effusions may be a consequence of malignant spread or radiation-induced irritation or occur as a perineoplastic phenomenon. An echocardiogram should be obtained for patients with a suggestive history and physical examination.

Serologic evaluation may include thyroid-stimulating hormone concentration (to screen for thyroid myopathy in patients who have received irradiation to the anterior neck), calcium concentration, electrolyte values (Addison disease may occur with adrenal metastases or irradiation), hemoglobin concentration, and hematocrit. Hypercalcemia or persistent mechanical pain should be evaluated with a bone scan or plain films. *Multiple myeloma and malignant neoplasms producing lytic metastases may fail to generate an abnormal bone scan despite diffuse skeletal involvement.* Blood levels of centrally acting medications (e.g., tricyclic antidepressants, anticonvulsants) should be checked in patients who describe fatigue with a significant cognitive dimension.

For patients with focal neurologic deficits, imaging of those portions of the neural axis implicated on physical examination should be performed. Magnetic resonance images should be obtained with gadolinium. Steroids administered in conjunction with chemotherapy may be of sufficient doses to cause myopathy. Electrodiagnostic studies can rule out alternative, treatable sources of neurologic compromise.

Patients complaining of generalized cognitive dysfunction may benefit from neuropsychological evaluation. Subtle cognitive deficits have been detected after chemotherapy.[9] Multifocal brain metastases may present with a global decrement in mental acuity and capacity to attend. Enhanced computed tomographic scanning of the head may be warranted when there is a high clinical probability of brain metastases (e.g., patients with melanoma and breast or lung cancers).

TREATMENT

Initial

It is important to address any endocrine, hematologic, metabolic, or reversible physical abnormalities before initiation of an exercise program. Uncontrolled pain mandates the initiation or modification of an analgesic regimen. Opioid-based pharmacotherapy has emerged as the cornerstone of cancer pain management.[10] Secondary infections related to cancer therapy–induced neutropenia must be treated before aerobic conditioning can begin. Leukopenia will resolve more rapidly with granulocyte colony-stimulating factor.[11] The discovery of disease progression may warrant initiation or alteration of an antineoplastic regimen or the administration of radiation therapy. Cardiac toxicity may improve after the initiation of digoxin or medications to reduce afterload. Anemia generally responds to therapy with recombinant erythropoietin with associated improvements in the patient's function and quality of life.[12] Patients with pulmonary fibrosis induced by radiation therapy or chemotherapy and those who have undergone lobectomy or pneumonectomy may require supplemental oxygen during rehabilitative efforts. Nutritional evaluation may be needed for cachectic or hypoproteinemic patients.

A psychiatric consultation may be indicated if depression emerges during evaluation. All nonessential centrally acting drugs should be eliminated. Pain medications should be chosen to minimize neuropsychological toxicity. Among the opioids, hydromorphone, fentanyl, and oxycodone have fewer active metabolites than does morphine sulfate.[13] Their use may be associated with a more tolerable side effect profile in the elderly and patients with renal impairment. Pharmacologic approaches for cancer fatigue center predominantly around the administration of psychostimulants.[1] The utility of these agents is supported by studies of methylphenidate and pemoline.[6,7]

Differential Diagnosis

Depression

Nutritional insufficiency

Anemia

Infection

Metabolic or endocrine abnormality (e.g., hypercalcemia, hypothyroidism, adrenal insufficiency)

Steroid myopathy

Medication side effects

Chemotherapy- or radiation therapy–induced cognitive dysfunction

Cachexia

Pulmonary parenchymal disease, bleomycin toxicity, radiation therapy–induced fibrosis

Pleural or pericardial effusion

Doxorubicin- or trastuzumab-related cardiotoxicity

Disturbed sleep-wake cycles

Neural axis compromise (e.g., brain metastasis, epidural metastasis, brachial or lumbosacral plexopathy)

Rehabilitation

A growing body of evidence supports the use of aerobic and resistive exercise to treat cancer-related fatigue. In fact, trials of aerobic conditioning in populations of patients with cancer have been predominantly conducted to characterize effects on fatigue. Breast cancer patients receiving adjuvant chemotherapy constitute the majority of study cohorts, although Dimeo[14-16] has demonstrated the benefits of aerobic conditioning immediately after bone marrow transplantation. Without exception, studies have shown exercise to be well tolerated and free of adverse sequelae irrespective of the cancer population studied.

Trials involving breast cancer patients in active treatment reported amelioration of a range of symptoms: fatigue,[17-23] insomnia,[20] nausea,[24] and emotional distress.[17,20] Benefits are not affected by ongoing anticancer treatment. Exercise interventions have varied in duration, degree of supervision, intensity, and training frequency. Rigorous, tightly structured programs (more than three exercise sessions per week at 60% to 85% of maximal heart rate for 6 weeks or longer) offer a range of benefits including increased relative lean body mass,[25] maximum oxygen consumption,[26] and strength.[27] At an intensity of 50% to 60% maximum oxygen consumption, significant benefits were detected in physical and psychological well-being.[15,28] An exertional threshold, below which physiologic benefits are not appreciable, may exist, yet symptom and mood benefits are still gained with low levels of regular exertion.

Combined aerobic and resistive training programs have generally demonstrated modest improvements in quality of life.[27,29] None specifically measured fatigue. However, because significant improvements in fatigue were achieved with a solely resistance-based program,[30] it is reasonable to assume that a combined aerobic and resistive program will improve fatigue while offering additional fitness benefits. Admittedly, the evidence base is tenuous.

On the basis of the extant literature, clinical recommendations include interval training at 50% to 70% of the heart rate reserve or while working at an exertion of 11 to 14 on the 6 to 20 perceived rate of exertion scale.[8,9] The intensity of the exercise program depends on baseline fitness levels, intensity of cancer treatment, and stage of cancer treatment. While the patient is undergoing treatment, most studies recommend decreasing the intensity to the lower end of the heart rate range. Once active therapy is over, the program should be progressed toward the higher end of the range. The intensity must also take into account daily laboratory values and patterns of fatigue associated with treatment. For example, fatigue peaks within the middle and end of the radiation therapy cycle, and the program should account for this pattern. Finally, duration and frequency should closely match the American College of Sports Medicine guidelines, which recommend that patients exercise for a total of 20 to 30 minutes, three to five times per week.

Exercise precautions for cancer patients are seldom evidence based. They vary significantly between institutions and clinicians. The following limitations are conservative suggestions and should not be interpreted as absolute exercise contraindications.[10] Aerobic and resistive exercise should be carefully reviewed if not discontinued when platelet levels fall below 10,000/μL. Light exercise is allowed when hemoglobin concentration is less than 8 g/dL, with patients closely monitored for symptoms. Contact and high-impact sports should be avoided when platelet levels fall below 50,000/μL or in patients with primary or metastatic bone disease. Exercise should be deferred for febrile patients with temperatures above 101.5°F. Therapeutic activities should be restricted to indoor exercise for patients at nadir with an absolute neutrophil count below 500/μL.

In addition to aerobic conditioning, referral to occupational and physical therapy for training in energy conservation strategies, use of adaptive equipment, and progressive resistive exercise will benefit appropriate patients. Instruction in compensatory strategies for mobility and performance of activities of daily living can optimize autonomy within the constraints imposed by disease. Adaptive equipment, such as canes, crutches, and walkers, may improve mobility; provision with adaptive devices, such as long-handled shoehorns and reachers, may facilitate independent self-care activities. Interventions for mobility and performance of activities of daily living benefit even end-stage cancer patients.[11] For these patients, education and empowerment of caretakers may emerge as the primary therapeutic focus.

Procedures

Patients with pleural or pericardial effusions will benefit from percutaneous drainage of the fluid. Pleurocentesis or pericardiocentesis may be required to prevent the reaccumulation of effusions. Percutaneous stenting procedures have become commonplace when tumor compression narrows the lumen of ureters, bile ducts, bronchi, or blood vessels with adverse physiologic sequelae. When cancer pain cannot be adequately managed with systemic therapy or if side effects become untenable, neuraxial delivery may restore normal arousal, energy, and cognition.[31] Radiation therapy may be used palliatively to treat pain or to reduce tumor bulk that is compressing neurologic structures.

Surgery

Cancer patients with deconditioning and fatigue may benefit from surgical debulking of tumor or resection of isolated lung, liver, bone, or brain metastases. Fatigue, however, is not an independent indication for surgery. If focal sensory or motor deficits result from tumor compression of neural pathways, emergent resection may be required.

POTENTIAL DISEASE COMPLICATIONS

Patients commonly deteriorate functionally because of incremental morbidities as their cancers advance. Consequences of malignant progression may include new or worsening neurologic deficits, dyspnea, cognitive deterioration from intracranial metastases or radiation therapy–induced changes, pathologic fractures, visceral obstruction, and somatic pain syndromes.

POTENTIAL TREATMENT COMPLICATIONS

Potential complications of anticancer modalities are extensive. Radiation therapy can cause fibrosis, neurologic compromise, and worsening of fatigue. Chemotherapy can similarly exacerbate fatigue. Various chemotherapeutic agents have the capacity to impair cognitive, renal, pulmonary, cardiac, and neurologic function. The myriad pharmacologic agents used to manage cancer-associated symptoms and pain can adversely affect neurologic, gastrointestinal, and urinary function as well as exacerbate peripheral edema.

Complications associated with rehabilitative interventions are few when strategies are used appropriately. Patients with bone-avid cancers (e.g., lung, prostate, breast, thyroid, multiple myeloma, and renal) are at risk for pathologic fractures, particularly those with lytic metastases. A recent bone scan or skeletal survey should be reviewed before an exercise program is begun.

Cancer patients should generally be considered more susceptible to common exercise-induced complications. Overly aggressive aerobic conditioning or strengthening programs may worsen fatigue. Uncustomary exertion may aggravate chemotherapeutically induced electrolyte and fluid imbalances. Therapeutic regimens for cancer patients should be adapted and scrutinized accordingly.

References

1. Portenoy RK, Itri LM. Cancer-related fatigue: guidelines for evaluation and management. Oncologist 1999;4:1-10.
2. Morrow GR, Andrews PL, Hickok JT, et al. Fatigue associated with cancer and its treatment. Support Care Cancer 2002;10:389-398.
3. Morrow GR, Shelke AR, Roscoe JA, et al. Management of cancer-related fatigue. Cancer Invest 2005;23:229-239.
4. Schwartz AH. Validity of cancer-related fatigue instruments. Pharmacotherapy 2002;22:1433-1441.
5. Barton-Burke M. Cancer-related fatigue and sleep disturbances. Cancer Nurs 2006;29(Suppl):72-77.
6. Berger AM, Parker KP, Young-McCaughan S, et al. Sleep wake disturbances in people with cancer and their caregivers: state of the science. Oncol Nurs Forum 2005;32:E98-E126.
7. Yennurajalingam S, Bruera E. Palliative management of fatigue at the close of life: "it feels like my body is just worn out." JAMA 2007;297:295-304.
8. Bell J, McGivern D, Bullimore J, et al. Diagnostic imaging of post-irradiation changes in the chest. Clin Radiol 1988;39:109-119.
9. Saykin AJ, Ahles TA, McDonald BC. Mechanisms of chemotherapy-induced cognitive disorders: neuropsychological, pathophysiological, and neuroimaging perspectives. Semin Clin Neuropsychiatry 2003;8:201-216.
10. Foley KM. Treatment of cancer-related pain. J Natl Cancer Inst Monogr 2004;32:103-104.
11. Clark OA, Lyman G, Castro AA, et al. Colony stimulating factors for chemotherapy induced febrile neutropenia. Cochrane Database Syst Rev 2003;3:CD003039.
12. Cortesi E, Gascon P, Henry D, et al. Standard of care for cancer-related anemia: improving hemoglobin levels and quality of life. Oncology 2005;68(Suppl 1):22-32.
13. Mercadante S. The role of morphine glucuronides in cancer pain. Palliat Med 1999;13:95-104.
14. Dimeo FC, Tilmann MH, Bertz H, et al. Aerobic exercise in the rehabilitation of cancer patients after high dose chemotherapy and autologous peripheral stem cell transplantation. Cancer 1997;79:1717-1722.
15. Dimeo FC, Stieglitz RD, Novelli-Fischer U, et al. Effects of physical activity on the fatigue and psychologic status of cancer patients during chemotherapy. Cancer 1999;85:2273-2277.
16. Dimeo F, Schwartz S, Fietz T, et al. Effects of endurance training on the physical performance of patients with hematological malignancies during chemotherapy. Support Care Cancer 2003;11:623-628.
17. Mock V, Pickett M, Ropka ME, et al. Fatigue and quality of life outcomes of exercise during cancer treatment. Cancer Pract 2001;9:119-127.
18. Schwartz AL, Mori M, Gao R, et al. Exercise reduces daily fatigue in women with breast cancer receiving chemotherapy. Med Sci Sports Exerc 2001;33:718-723.
19. Schwartz AL. Exercise and weight gain in breast cancer patients receiving chemotherapy. Cancer Pract 2000;8:231-237.
20. Mock V, Dow KH, Meares CJ, et al. Effects of exercise on fatigue, physical functioning, and emotional distress during radiation therapy for breast cancer. Oncol Nurs Forum 1997;24:991-1000.
21. McNeely ML, Campbell KL, Rowe BH, et al. Effects of exercise on breast cancer patients and survivors: a systematic review and meta-analysis. CMAJ 2006;175:34-41.
22. Kirshbaum MN. A review of the benefits of whole body exercise during and after treatment for breast cancer. J Clin Nurs 2007;16:104-121.
23. Stricker CT, Drake D, Hoyer KA, Mock V. Evidence-based practice for fatigue management in adults with cancer: exercise as an intervention. Oncol Nurs Forum 2004;31:963-976.
24. Winningham ML, MacVicar MG. The effect of aerobic exercise on patient reports of nausea. Oncol Nurs Forum 1988;15:447-450.
25. Winningham ML, MacVicar MG, Bondoc M, et al. Effect of aerobic exercise on body weight and composition in patients with breast cancer on adjuvant chemotherapy. Oncol Nurs Forum 1989;16:683-689.
26. MacVicar MG, Winningham ML, Nickel JL. Effects of aerobic interval training on cancer patients' functional capacity. Nurs Res 1989;38:348-351.
27. Adamsen L, Midtgaard J, Rorth M, et al. Feasibility, physical capacity, and health benefits of a multidimensional exercise program for cancer patients undergoing chemotherapy. Support Care Cancer 2003;11:707-716.
28. Segal R, Evans W, Johnson D, et al. Structured exercise improves physical functioning in women with stages I and II breast cancer: results of a randomized controlled trial. J Clin Oncol 2001;19:657-665.
29. Kolden GG, Strauman TJ, Ward A, et al. A pilot study of group exercise training (GET) for women with primary breast cancer: feasibility and health benefits. Psychooncology 2002;11:447-456.
30. Segal RJ, Reid RD, Courneya KS, et al. Resistance exercise in men receiving androgen deprivation therapy for prostate cancer. J Clin Oncol 2003;21:1653-1659.
31. Portenoy RK. Managing pain in patients with advanced cancer: the role of neuraxial infusion. Oncology (Williston Park) 1999;13(Suppl 2):7-8.

Cerebral Palsy 114

Yong-Tae Lee, MD, and Patrick Brennan, MD

Synonym

Little's disease

ICD-9 Codes

343   Infantile cerebral palsy
343.0   Diplegic
343.1   Hemiplegic; congenital hemiplegia
343.2   Quadriplegic
343.3   Monoplegic
343.4   Infantile hemiplegia; infantile hemiplegia (postnatal) NOS
343.8   Other specified infantile cerebral palsy
343.9   Infantile cerebral palsy, unspecified
V54.8   Orthopedic aftercare: changes, check or removal of casts, splint (external)

DEFINITION

Cerebral palsy is a well-known neurodevelopmental condition that affects children. As medicine has continued to advance, the definition has also been refined over the years. One of the classic and still widely used definitions states that cerebral palsy is a clinical syndrome resulting from a static lesion of an immature brain that primarily affects movement and posture.[1] In 1992, Mutch and colleagues,[2] with further understanding of the development in infants with early brain damage, modified the definition to say that it is "a group of nonprogressive, but often changing, motor impairment syndromes secondary to lesions of the brain arising in the early stages of development."

In 2004, an International Workshop on Definition and Classification of Cerebral Palsy proposed yet another definition that focused on the broader perspective of activity limitation and disability:

> *Cerebral palsy describes a group of disorders of the development of movement and posture, causing activity limitation, that are attributed to non-progressive disturbances that occurred in the developing fetal or infant brain. The motor disorders of cerebral palsy are often accompanied by disturbances of sensation, cognition, communication, perception and/or behavior, and/or by a seizure disorder.[3]*

A commonly accepted criterion for having an immature brain is being younger than 4 years, and therefore a child who sustains a static lesion (e.g., traumatic brain injury, meningitis) before 4 years of age meets the definition of cerebral palsy. Its range of severity is as wide as the list of causes associated with it.

With the improvement of neonatal care, including intensive care, it was noted early on that although there was an increase in cerebral palsy, there was a decreased mortality of very-low-birthweight (<1500 g) preterm babies.[4,5] The Surveillance of Cerebral Palsy in Europe reported a decrease in the frequency of cerebral palsy, finding that the prevalence of cerebral palsy in very-low-birthweight infants and those born before 32 weeks of gestation decreased significantly from 60.6 per 1000 to 39.5 per 1000.[4,6] However with the increasing survival of preterm infants, the stable rate among term infants, and the improved longevity, cerebral palsy overall has increased in prevalence. The reported incidence varies from 2 to 3 per 1000 live births.[7,8]

Neurologic classification divides the syndrome into three types: spastic (pyramidal), dyskinetic (extrapyramidal), and mixed. The spastic group can be further specified by body region involved: monoplegia (one limb), diplegia (both legs affected), triplegia (three limbs affected), quadriplegia (all four limbs affected), and hemiplegia. Spastic cerebral palsy is defined by involuntary contractions of muscles in the extremities, which can lead to a "scissor gait" (simultaneous adduction, knee hyperextension, and plantar flexion of the lower extremities). Dyskinetic types include athetoid cerebral palsy, which is characterized by involuntary writhing movements that can be accompanied by facial grimacing, abnormal tongue movements, or drooling,[9] and ataxic cerebral palsy, in which the primary symptom is a lack of balance and coordination while standing or walking.

Although the neurologic lesion itself is nonprogressive, deterioration of function commonly occurs with aging because of muscle spasticity superimposed on growth, resulting in worsening of contractures and very often chronic joint pain. Ninety-five percent of children with diplegia and 75% of children with quadriplegia survive until the age of 30 years.[10] Lack of basic functional skills (mobility and feeding) was found to be a key predictor of reduced life expectancy, as short as 11 years in the worst functioning groups.[11] One study showed higher than expected mortality from ischemic heart disease, cancer, and stroke in adults with cerebral palsy.[12] A lack of early detection and periodic health care was implicated. Comprehensive care of an adult with cerebral palsy is complex and requires ongoing evaluation by a multidisciplinary team of physicians, therapists, psychologists, and social workers.

Many factors may lead to cerebral palsy. It can occur in the prenatal, perinatal, or postnatal period.[13] In preterm infants, it is most associated with periventricular leukomalacia, with or without severe periventricular hemorrhage or infarction.[14] Other causes are perinatal ischemia, anoxia, perinatal infections (chorioamnionitis), and iatrogenic effects of drugs (steroids) in the postnatal period. It has also been seen with multiple births and maternal or fetal thrombophilia.[4,6,15] Head injuries or other forms of brain damage or infections occurring in the first months or years of life can cause cerebral palsy as well.

SYMPTOMS

Symptoms vary widely, depending on disease severity and chronicity. A cross-sectional survey of 63 adult women aged 20 to 74 years with cerebral palsy living in the community revealed a high incidence of mental retardation (34%), learning disabilities (26%), seizure (40%), pain (84%), hip and back deformities (59%), bowel problems (56%), bladder problems (49%), poor dental health (43%), and gastroesophageal reflux (28%).[16] Symptoms in infants range from muscle weakness or lack of tone to muscle spasticity. There may also be developmental delays. Other symptoms may include drooling, speech impairment, difficulty with bowel and bladder control, seizures, sleep disturbances, and hand tremors.

Musculoskeletal Symptoms and Pain

Pain is a common experience in children with cerebral palsy. It is seen more in children with moderate or severe cerebral palsy and can be associated with educational and social consequences.[17,18] Deterioration in locomotor skills in adults with cerebral palsy is associated with pain, fatigue, and lack of adapted physical activity.[17,19] Chronic musculoskeletal pain is common in cerebral palsy and usually is secondary to spasticity or dystonia.[17,20] It was noted that children with less pain had higher functional walking skills and that pain seemed to interfere with basic activities of daily living and even with getting out of bed.[12,17]

Common manifesting symptoms include neck pain (abnormal tonicity or movements of the neck, especially in athetotic cerebral palsy, can be associated with early cervical spine degeneration and instability[21,22]); low back pain (anecdotally reported as a long-term consequence of hamstring tightness); back deformity (scoliosis is especially common in nonambulatory patients and can progress beyond skeletal maturity[23]); hip pain (hip deformities are common especially in the nonambulatory, are often present in childhood, and can result in disabling osteoarthritis); knee pain (anecdotally reported as a long-term consequence of a crouched [bent-knee] gait pattern, resulting in disabling osteoarthritis at an early age); and loss of range of motion of lower extremity joints due to musculotendinous unit shortening or joint capsule contracture.

Hip subluxation leading to dislocation is a problem seen in spastic cerebral palsy.[24] If it is untreated, it can lead to hip pain, pressure ulcers, lower extremity fractures, coronal decompensation, and sitting problems.[24] Scoliosis can be a significant problem with quadriplegic cerebral palsy; especially at risk are those who are nonambulatory or confined to bed. This can also lead to coronal imbalance and sitting problems and, in severe cases, pulmonary complications, gastrointestinal symptoms, pressure ulcers, pain, and a general decline in function.[24] In one study, there was not a significant relationship between hip dislocation and the rate of scoliosis progression. However, pelvic obliquity was seen much more in patients with persistent hip dislocations. Also, persistent hip dislocations were noted to significantly increase the pelvic obliquity.[24]

Neurologic Symptoms

It is very difficult to base an early diagnosis of cerebral palsy on the neurologic examination findings. A large prospective multicenter study compared the neurologic status in infants from birth to age 7 years and found that only 23% of the children with cerebral palsy at 7 years had abnormal findings on neurologic examination as a newborn.[15,25] Prediction at 4 months was found to be only slightly better; 33% of the children diagnosed with cerebral palsy at age 7 years had abnormal findings on neurologic examination.[15,25,26]

Symptoms can include spasticity, weakness, and deterioration of upper extremity function. Visual problems exist in 25% to 39% of adult patients, hearing deficits in 18%.[27,28] These symptoms commonly worsen with aging.[29] Cognitive deficits may be absent but can range from mild to profound mental retardation. Communication disorders can be severe in athetotic cerebral palsy; these patients are often labeled mentally retarded, although the majority have normal cognition. Thirty percent of individuals with cerebral palsy have a seizure disorder, which is most common in spastic quadriplegia.

Manifesting symptoms of spasticity and underlying weakness (partially attributable to antagonist co-contraction of the muscles)[30] consistent with an upper motor neuron lesion are common. Any worsening of baseline spasticity should prompt an investigation into noxious stimuli, such as impacted bowel or other intra-abdominal processes, urinary tract infection, and musculoskeletal disorders. One thing to note is that increased muscle tone causes an increase in the amount of energy expended by a child and can impede progress.

Functional deterioration of the upper extremity, especially in athetotic cerebral palsy, warrants consideration of cervical myelopathy or radiculopathy. The etiology of visual deficits in adults is likely to be associated with cataracts, optic atrophy, or retinitis known to be present in children.[31]

Sleep

Patients with cerebral palsy are susceptible to sleep disturbances. However, there is a paucity of research to support this observation. Causes such as muscle spasms, pain, and epilepsy as well as other external factors can lead to a disturbance in the sleep architecture.[32] Blindness or severe visual impairment, which can coexist with cerebral palsy, can also affect the maintenance of sleep through an effect on melatonin secretion and light perception.[32,33] Other things, such as gastroesophageal reflux disease and aspiration, can also interrupt sleep. One study found that the principal factor that has been associated with total sleep disturbance is active epilepsy. This was also associated with excessive daytime somnolence.[32] Children with total body involvement (spastic quadriplegia and dystonic-dyskinetic cerebral palsy) were noted to have more sleep disorders.

Cardiopulmonary Symptoms

Symptoms include shortness of breath, irritability, and pallor that may compose a subtle picture of cardiac ischemia. Lower extremity swelling, coolness, and discoloration are common in nonambulatory patients. Chronic gastroesophageal reflux can be associated with symptoms of aspiration pneumonia.

Gastrointestinal and Nutritional Symptoms

Feeding difficulties are common in severely neurologically impaired individuals, and the time required to feed patients can negatively affect the patient's and the caregivers' quality of life. Nutritional problems include malnutrition associated with dysphagia and obesity due to inactivity and overeating. Constipation, diverticula, and hemorrhoids are common, as are dental problems because of difficulties with hygiene, spasticity of oral musculature, and abnormal development.[30] Delayed gastric emptying, gastroesophageal reflux, and constipation are commonly seen.

Some children with cerebral palsy are fed by gastrostomy tube. One study showed that feeding of a commercial formula could lead to excess fat deposition in those children.[34,35] Although the diet can vary per child, it is important to determine the optimal nutritional and calorie intake for these children.

Studies of swallowing have pointed to three problem areas: incomplete lip closure, low suction pressure, and prolonged delay between suction and propelling stage.[36,37] Pathologic drooling (sialorrhea) is drooling in the awake state in a child older than 4 years, particularly in those with moderate or severe developmental disability.[36] These symptoms can be worsened by dental malocclusion, poor head control, diminished intraoral tactile sensitivity, and constant tongue thrusting.[36] This condition can be very hindering, causing aspiration, superficial skin excoriation, infections around the mouth and chin, and dehydration as well as some psychosocial issues.

Urinary Symptoms

Although uncommon in children and not well studied in adults, urinary urgency and frequency with small output are seen, as is a hypotonic enlarged bladder pattern. Urinary tract infections, reflux, and spastic, flaccid, or dyssynergic bladder should also be considered. Daytime urinary incontinence was the most common symptom in one study; the findings of videourodynamic studies were abnormal in about 85% of the participants.[38] One study attempted to determine the age at development of bladder and bowel control and determined that children with cerebral palsy gained bladder and bowel control at an older age compared with healthy children.[39]

Psychosocial Symptoms

With the many symptoms associated with it, cerebral palsy often leads to social isolation and feelings of embarrassment on the part of the parent as well as the child.[36] Depression is often associated with the social isolation that is a consequence of limited independence. Pain can also be a significant contributor to psychological distress, including depression.

PHYSICAL EXAMINATION

The examination of a patient with cerebral palsy can vary, depending on the age of the patient. Important in any examination, especially with children of any age, is observation. Interactions with the environment as well as with people and the caregiver can give important clues to any disabilities or issues that may be present.[40]

General musculoskeletal examination of a patient with cerebral palsy should include range of motion testing, both active and passive. Consider specific tests, such as hip abduction with the knees flexed (to test the flexibility of the adductors) and with the knees extended (gracilis flexibility); Thomas test while the patient is supine with the knee extended (iliopsoas flexibility) and flexed (rectus femoris)[40]; knee extension with hip flexion (popliteal angle, to test the hamstrings); and ankle dorsiflexion with the knees flexed (soleus) and extended (gastrocnemius).

The hips should be examined for symmetry of abduction and external and internal rotation. Common findings may include asymmetry (examination findings mentioned before) and the presence of a Galeazzi sign. With the patient supine, the hips and knees flexed to

90 degrees, and the pelvis neutral, one knee is found to be less prominent than the other, implying hip subluxation on the less prominent side (Fig. 114-1). This asymmetry can lead to bone abnormalities, making the patient more susceptible to subluxation and dislocations. It is also important to examine the spine for scoliosis, which can make the patient more susceptible to other medical problems.

Loss of knee range of motion is common. Inability to fully extend the knee while supine implies posterior joint capsule tightness, especially when the hamstrings are palpably slack. An increased popliteal angle combined with full knee extension when supine indicates hamstring contracture or spasticity.

Examination of the feet is complex, and structural abnormalities are common, including pes planus and pronation with weight bearing. There are also deformities of the hindfoot with exaggerated heel valgus or varus.

Strength testing is important in the evaluation of a patient with cerebral palsy. Observation of the patient doing specific tasks, such as rolling, kicking, crawling, walking, and other activities, can provide valuable information, such as static and dynamic balance along with postural control.[40] Strength testing may reveal weakness that is partly attributable to antagonist muscle co-contraction.

Tone and spasticity should be evaluated to differentiate functional limitations as a result of contracture from motor control issues. Use of the modified Ashworth scale for measurement of spasticity (see Table 150-2) can be helpful in the testing.

Some children will have components of persistent primitive reflexes, such as the asymmetric tonic neck reflex. These can be seen either by passive positioning or by voluntary movement. Some will also have flexion synergy patterns of the upper extremities. Deep tendon reflexes tend to be increased.

Sensation is usually not impaired; however, skin should be inspected for pressure ulcers, especially in the non-ambulatory patient. This may be important for recommendations of rehabilitation and modifications that may be necessary to protect the skin.

When appropriate, gait observation is also part of the examination of a patient with cerebral palsy. Observational gait analysis showing a difference between available (passive) and used range of motion indicates spasticity or weakness and can guide therapeutic alternatives. Common gait abnormalities are initial contact with the forefoot, exaggerated knee extension moment, lack of full knee extension at midstance, narrow base of support with scissoring, and shortened stride length. Formal gait analysis can also provide more information and is mentioned later.

Cognitive testing, when appropriate, is helpful with school- or work-related problems. An initial evaluation by a speech-language pathologist can be helpful with the assessment; however, an evaluation by a neuropsychologist skilled in working with this population is essential.

Given the many impairments and problems that a patient with cerebral palsy may face, it is also important to assess any psychological effects the condition may cause. Five or more positive responses to the SIGECAPS screen (deterioration in *s*leep, *i*nterests; feelings of *g*uilt; decreased *e*nergy, *c*oncentration, *a*ppetite; *p*sychomotor symptoms or *s*uicidal thoughts) are consistent with depression. The presence of anhedonia (lack of pleasure) increases its sensitivity further.

Another consideration in assessing a patient with cerebral palsy is the child's functional ability in daily life. The Gross Motor Function Classification System (GMFCS) was developed to standardize the method for classifying the level of gross motor function in children with cerebral palsy with an emphasis on sitting and walking.[41,42] The motor functions are divided into five levels; level I is the highest level of function and level V, the lowest. Each level provides a description of function for four different age groups. It was found to have a good intraclass correlation coefficient, with excellent agreement between the self-reported and the professional rating. Changes in the level of gross motor function were found to be a matter of choice, given that many participants would go out and used different methods of locomotion, or psychological factors.[42] In one study, the level of GMFCS was found to correlate with at least three impairments present in cerebral palsy, namely, learning disabilities, visual impairments, and epilepsy. The GMFCS can also be used as an indicator of total disability load.

Another classification system for cerebral palsy is the Manual Ability Classification System. It was developed

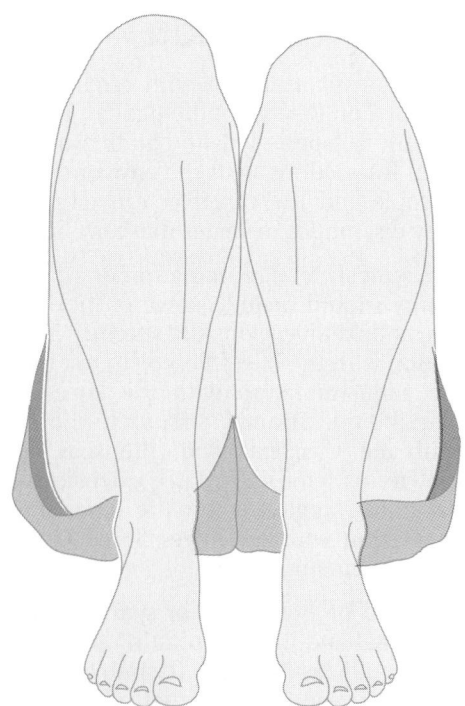

FIGURE 114-1. Galeazzi sign.

to classify how children use their hands to handle objects in daily activities. It was meant to reflect the child's typical manual performance with use of both hands together. This system also takes into account that a child's ability to handle objects can increase with age. Again, it was found to have good validity and reliability as well as a good intraclass correlation coefficient between the parents and the therapist, indicating excellent agreement.[43]

FUNCTIONAL LIMITATIONS

Functional limitations correlate with the degree of severity of cerebral palsy. Investigation into functional status should focus on mobility, self-care, and activities of daily living.

Of adults with cerebral palsy, 40% are nonambulatory, 40% require assistance (e.g., walkers, orthotics, caregivers), and 20% ambulate independently; approximately one third of adults with cerebral palsy live at home.[27] Depending on the degree of impairment, patients may or may not be able to work outside the home. Recreational activities and hobbies may be limited by cognitive and physical impairments. Impairments may affect intimacy and also result in social embarrassment.

One article suggested that the best approach to identify limitations is based on rate of motor development as defined by the motor quotient (motor quotient = motor age/chronologic age; the motor age is determined by the best motor milestone performance).[15] Hence, a motor quotient of less than 0.5 at 8 months of age predicts a delay in walking.[15,44] This had a sensitivity of 87% and a specificity of 89%. However this does not apply to patients who are 6 months of age or younger.

Another objective assessment found to be sensitive and specific was the assessment of a videotape of spontaneous general movements in the first weeks and months of life. It was shown to be predictive of cerebral palsy at a point when neurologic examination was insensitive and a motor quotient was not helpful because of the limited functional motor milestones. It also helped to predict neuromotor functional outcome.[15] In a sample of 84 preterm infants, abnormalities seen with general movements in the first 16 to 20 weeks post term predicted cerebral palsy at age 2 to 3 years with a sensitivity of 100% and a specificity of 92.5% to 100%.[45]

DIAGNOSTIC STUDIES

Musculoskeletal System

Radiographs of the symptomatic joints are indicated to confirm a clinical presentation of osteoarthritis. They can also help with the identification of any bone abnormalities (fractures) as well as help identify children who have certain risks, such as hip subluxation.[46] Magnetic resonance imaging of the cervical spine is indicated when new neurologic symptoms are present, especially in the athetotic patient. Quantitative gait analysis is now a widely accepted tool for both research and teaching. Its use in clinical decision-making remains controversial, partly because of the cost[47] (which can be as much as magnetic resonance imaging). However, gait analysis has helped in clarifying the significance of factors such as skeletal misalignment that compromise muscle function and in determining the treatment of muscles that are too short versus too weak.[47] It has proved useful in guiding surgical and rehabilitative treatments in pediatric patients with cerebral palsy; its use in adults is not widely reported.

Neurologic System

With the ease of access to head computed tomography and magnetic resonance imaging, several types of brain injury underlying cerebral palsy have been described, including brain malformations, hypoxic-ischemic brain injury, focal arterial infarction, and periventricular white matter injury.[48] Brain ultrasonography and magnetic resonance imaging can also detect abnormalities associated with the subsequent diagnosis of cerebral palsy.[15] Cranial ultrasonography has a high correlation with the neuropathologic findings of hemorrhage and cystic periventricular leukomalacia.[15] Infants with very low birth weight should receive an ultrasound examination at term to detect intraventricular hemorrhage, cystic periventricular leukomalacia, and ventricular enlargement.[15] Magnetic resonance imaging can detect abnormalities in the basal ganglia and thalamus in the first 2 to 8 days of life.[15]

Electrodiagnostic testing (e.g., electromyography and nerve conduction studies) is indicated in cases of new focal neurologic deficits. Results of IQ testing that are fine motor dependent should be interpreted with caution because the majority of patients with cerebral palsy have fine motor deficits.

Cardiopulmonary System

Electrocardiography and stress testing are indicated when cardiac dysfunction is suspected.

Gastrointestinal System

Upper gastrointestinal tract imaging and contrast studies, pH probe, and gastric emptying studies may be indicated in patients with symptoms of aspiration pneumonia.

Urinary System

Urodynamic testing can distinguish between upper motor neuron and lower motor neuron patterns of bladder dysfunction and thus help direct treatment.

TREATMENT

Initial

Treatment of musculoskeletal conditions, including osteoarthritis, is based on the specific diagnosis. The goal, however, is to preserve function and to minimize pain as much as possible. Traditional methods of treating

Differential Diagnosis

Many different disorders can mimic cerebral palsy. Each has one or more of the components that can imitate or be manifested like cerebral palsy. Therefore, a thorough workup is important before the diagnosis of cerebral palsy is made. A few are listed here.

Familial spastic paraparesis

Lesch-Nyhan syndrome without self-mutilation[49]

Mental retardation

Kernicterus

Phenylketonuria

Muscular dystrophies

musculoskeletal conditions, such as the use of non-steroidal anti-inflammatory drugs, analgesics, and local icing, are all appropriate interventions in the adult patient with cerebral palsy.

The initial treatment of contracture includes relief of underlying spasticity with oral medications or injections (see Chapters 117 and 144) and application of low-load prolonged stretch with serial casting or dynamic splinting. The use of superficial heat or ultrasound can be an important adjunct to a stretching program. Clear, functional goals should be established before treatment.

Visual and hearing deficits are managed by referral to the appropriate specialists.

Education of patients, family members, and caregivers about the rights of the disabled encourages advocacy. Resources including *Exceptional Parent* magazine and United Cerebral Palsy (*www.ucpa.org*) provide information about employment opportunities, research, and treatment providers specializing in the care of patients with cerebral palsy.

Rehabilitation

For people affected with cerebral palsy, rehabilitation plays an important role in helping them regain function. The different services including physical therapy, occupational therapy, and speech-language pathology all play an important role in the overall rehabilitation of the patient. It is important to have a multidisciplinary approach to the rehabilitation of patients with cerebral palsy.

One important part of physical therapy is strength training, especially in attempting to improve gait. Multiple studies have looked at the effect of strengthening exercise and its effects on spasticity, showing that such exercises do not increase spasticity.[50-52] In fact, these studies showed that not only were there no adverse effects but also there were improvements in walking speed, strength, and motor activity. Another study showed that strength training improved crouched gait as well as the patient's perception of body image in a school-based training program.[53]

Therapy should be adjusted on the basis of the age of the individual. Observation of the patient can also give many important clues as to the needs of the patient.[40] The frequency and duration of physical therapy should be individualized and based on the child's and family's needs. Physical therapy can be obtained both on an outpatient and an inpatient basis. Another avenue is to receive therapy while at school.[40]

Passive stretching is another technique that can be used in patients with cerebral palsy to help with soft tissue tightness. This can be done manually by the therapist or patient or by other external devices, such as splints, casts, or a tilt table.[54] Superficial and deep heating modalities during stretch may relax tone and allow a more permanent elongation of the musculotendinous unit.

Bracing may also be an option for some patients. Lower extremity orthotics are used to address biomechanical limitations and joint alignment to help function.[55] Examples of such orthoses are the ankle-foot orthosis and the dynamic ankle-foot orthosis. In patients with scoliosis, bracing has been shown to slow progression but not to prevent progressive deformity; early referral to an orthopedist is generally indicated.

Occupational therapy can be used to help with activities of daily living, such as dressing, grooming, and holding certain objects (ergonomic spoons).[56] In adults, therapies can focus more on vocational training or basic activities, such as shopping and cooking.

Inquiries into the home environment and a home visit by therapists, when appropriate, can help focus interventions that create the least restrictive and safest environment. Assistive devices provided with input from physical and occupational therapists are essential, and powered mobility should be considered for community access (i.e., walkers and wheelchairs for community mobility and for mobility of longer distances are important).

Speech-language pathologists as well as augmentative equipment providers are essential in assisting patients and their caregivers to maximize communication. Vocational rehabilitation services can help patients access appropriate training and job placement.

When appropriate, other nonconventional adjunctive therapies may be considered, such as hippotherapy (horseback riding therapy). Effects of this therapy seem to improve pelvic movement, co-contraction, joint stability, and weight shift as well as postural and equilibrium responses and dynamic postural stabilization.[57] Some therapists have even used constraint-induced movement therapy, modified to be child friendly, to improve upper extremity functional movement in children with hemiplegic cerebral palsy. There were reported increases in the involved limb use and quality of movement; however, it did not change strength, sensation, or muscle tone.[58]

Procedures

Many procedures may be helpful to manage pain and spasticity and to improve contractures. These are described throughout this text and are based on the specific diagnosis or condition. Joint and soft tissue injections (e.g., trigger point injections) can be helpful in managing pain and improving function. Phenol blocks and botulinum toxin injections may assist in managing spasticity and preventing or improving contractures in combination with low-load prolonged stretch, as provided by serial casting or dynamic splinting. Botulinum toxin has also been seen to be helpful with sialorrhea, especially when it is injected into the parotid and submandibular glands, which can lead to an improvement of quality of life.[36]

Surgery

Children with cerebral palsy should have regular orthopedic consultations, which can help build a relationship between the surgeon and the family if the need for surgery should arise. Physiatrists can help facilitate this by working closely with the therapists and the surgeons. Surgery may be an option for patients with advanced osteoarthritis that limits function or causes pain. Arthroplasty in early or mid adulthood has been shown to be beneficial.[30] Spinal stenosis due to advanced cervical degenerative disease warrants a referral to a neurosurgeon in some cases.

Long-standing contractures may not respond to conservative measures, and referral to an orthopedic surgeon for surgical lengthening or release is often necessary (i.e., hip flexor, hip adductor, hamstring, and Achilles tendon lengthening). These procedures can help conditions such as hip subluxation[59] and spastic ankle equinus deformity.[60] Other surgical procedures include tendon transfers and joint fusions, which can help with function as well as with spasticity.[61,62] A more controversial procedure is selective dorsal rhizotomy for the treatment of spasticity. Whereas many studies did seem to report improvement in spasticity and function, there were concerns about the long-term effects as well as the selection of the root tissue to be transected.[63]

POTENTIAL DISEASE COMPLICATIONS

The spectrum of potential disease complications is vast for individuals with cerebral palsy. As aging occurs, it is important to try to maintain as much function as possible. Progressive weakness, spasticity, and contractures lead to increasing disability. Pain can also limit function. Cognitive changes do not typically occur; but if they are present, a workup is performed to rule out coexisting pathologic processes (e.g., dementia, hydrocephalus).

POTENTIAL TREATMENT COMPLICATIONS

Botulinum toxin injections that are repeated more often than every 4 to 6 months may be associated with antibody production, leading to decreased efficacy. Transient weakness of the injected muscles, malaise, and inflammation at the injection site can occur. Phenol injection of a mixed nerve can result in painful dysesthesias. Overly aggressive stretching can lead to pain, inflammation, and joint damage. Surgical complications are generally well known and depend on the type of surgery performed.

References

1. Bax MC. Terminology and classification of cerebral palsy. Dev Med Child Neurol 1964;11:295-297.
2. Mutch L, Alberman E, Hagberg B, et al. Cerebral palsy epidemiology: where are we now and where are we going? Dev Med Child Neurol 1992;34:547-551.
3. Bax M, Goldstein M, Rosenbaum P, et al. Proposed definition and classification of cerebral palsy, April 2005. Dev Med Child Neurol 2005;47:571-576.
4. Hack M, Costello DW. Decrease in frequency of cerebral palsy in preterm infants. Lancet 2007;369:7-8.
5. Hagberg B, Hagberg G, Olow I, van Wendt L. The changing panorama of cerebral palsy in Sweden. VII. Prevalence and origin in the birth year period 1987-90. Acta Paediatr 1996;85:954-960.
6. Platt MJ, Cans C, Johnson A, et al. Trends in cerebral palsy among infants of very low birthweight (<1500 g) or born prematurely (<32 weeks) in 16 European centres: a database study. Lancet 2007;369:43-50.
7. Keogh JM, Badawi N. The origins of cerebral palsy. Curr Opin Neurol 2006;19:129-134.
8. Paneth N, Kiely J. The frequency of cerebral palsy: a review of population studies in industrialized nations since 1950. In Stanley FJ, Alberman ED, eds. The Epidemiology of the Cerebral Palsies. Oxford, England, Blackwell Scientific, 1984:46-56.
9. Yokochi K, Shimabukuro S, Kodama M, et al. Motor function of infants with athetoid cerebral palsy. Dev Med Child Neurol 1993;35:909-916.
10. Crichton JU, Mackinnon M, White CP. The life-expectancy of persons with cerebral palsy. Dev Med Child Neurol 1995;37:567-576.
11. Strauss D, Shavelle R. Life expectancy of adults with cerebral palsy. Dev Med Child Neurol 1998;40:369-375.
12. Strauss D, Cable W, Shavelle R. Causes of excess mortality in cerebral palsy. Dev Med Child Neurol 1999;41:580-585.
13. Kudrjavcev T, Schoenberg BS, Kurland LT, Groover RV. Cerebral palsy—trends in incidence and changes in concurrent neonatal mortality: Rochester, MN, 1950-1976. Neurology 1983;33:1433-1438.
14. Kuban KC, Leviton A. Cerebral palsy. N Engl J Med 1994;330:188-195.
15. Palmer FB. Strategies for the early diagnosis of cerebral palsy. J Pediatr 2004;145(Suppl):S8-S11.
16. Turk MA, Geremski CA, Rosenbaum PF, Weber RJ. The health status of women with cerebral palsy. Arch Phys Med Rehabil 1997;78(Suppl 5):S10-S17.
17. Tervo RC, Symons F, Stout J, Novacheck T. Parental report of pain and associated limitations in ambulatory children with cerebral palsy. Arch Phys Med Rehabil 2006;87:928-934.
18. Houlihan CM, O'Donnell M, Conaway M, Stevenson RD. Bodily pain and health-related quality of life in children with cerebral palsy. Dev Med Child Neurol 2004;46:305-310.
19. Jahnsen R, Villien L, Egeland T, et al. Locomotion skills in adults with cerebral palsy. Clin Rehabil 2004;18:309-316.
20. Roscigno CI. Addressing spasticity-related pain in children with spastic cerebral palsy. J Neurosci Nurs 2002;34:123-133.
21. Ko HY, Park-Ko I. Spinal cord injury secondary to cervical disc herniation in ambulatory patients with cerebral palsy. Spinal Cord 1998;36:288-292.
22. Nagashima T, Kurimura M, Nishimura M, et al. Late deterioration of functional abilities in adult cerebral palsy [in Japanese]. Rinsho Shinkeigaku 1993;33:939-944.
23. Thometz JG, Simon SR. Progression of scoliosis after skeletal maturity in institutionalized adults who have cerebral palsy. J Bone Joint Surg Am 1988;70:1290-1296.

24. Senaran H, Shah SA, Glutting JJ, et al. The associated effects of untreated unilateral hip dislocation in cerebral palsy scoliosis. J Pediatr Orthop 2006;26:769-772.

25. Nelson KB, Ellenberg JH. Neonatal signs as predictors of cerebral palsy. Pediatrics 1979;64:225-232.

26. Ellenberg JH, Nelson KB. Early recognition of infants at high risk for cerebral palsy: examination at age four months. Dev Med Child Neurol 1981;23:705-716.

27. Granet KM, Balaghi M, Jaeger J. Adults with cerebral palsy. N J Med 1997;94:51-54.

28. Janicki N. Aging, cerebral palsy and older persons with mental retardation. Aust N Z J Dev Disabil 1989;15:311-330.

29. Currie DM, Gershkoff AM, Cifu DX. Geriatric rehabilitation. 3. Mid- and late-life effects of early-life disabilities. Arch Phys Med Rehabil 1993;74(5-S):S413-S416.

30. Brown MC, Bontempo A, Turk MA. Secondary Consequences of Cerebral Palsy: Adults with Cerebral Palsy in New York State. Albany, NY, Developmental Disabilities Planning Council, 1992.

31. Ingram T. Pediatric Aspects of Cerebral Palsy. Edinburgh, E&S Livingstone, 1964.

32. Newman CJ, O'Regan M, Hensey O. Sleep disorders in children with cerebral palsy. Dev Med Child Neurol 2006;48:564-568.

33. Palm L, Blennow G, Wetterberg L. Long-term melatonin treatment in blind children and young adults with circadian sleep-wake disturbances. Dev Med Child Neurol 1997;39:319-325.

34. Gisel E. Gastrostomy feeding in cerebral palsy: too much of a good thing? Dev Med Child Neurol 2006;48:869.

35. Sullivan PB, Juszczak E, Bachlet AM, et al. Gastrostomy tube feeding in children with cerebral palsy: a prospective, longitudinal study. Dev Med Child Neurol 2005;47:77-85.

36. Banerjee KJ, Glasson C, O'Flaherty SJ. Parotid and submandibular botulinum toxin A injections for sialorrhoea in children with cerebral palsy. Dev Med Child Neurol 2006;48:883-887.

37. Lespargot A, Langevin MF, Muller S, Guillemont S. Swallowing disturbances associated with drooling in cerebral-palsied children. Dev Med Child Neurol 1993;35:298-304.

38. Reid CJ, Borzyskowski M. Lower urinary tract dysfunction in cerebral palsy. Arch Dis Child 1993;68:739-742.

39. Ozturk M, Oktem F, Kisioglu N, et al. Bladder and bowel control in children with cerebral palsy: case-control study. Croat Med J 2006;47:264-270.

40. O'Neil ME, Fragala-Pinkham MA, Westcott SL, et al. Physical therapy clinical management recommendations for children with cerebral palsy–spastic diplegia: achieving functional mobility outcomes. Pediatr Phys Ther 2006;18:49-72.

41. Palisano R, Rosenbaum P, Walter S, et al. Development and reliability of a system to classify gross motor function in children with cerebral palsy. Dev Med Child Neurol 1997;39:214-223.

42. Jahnsen R, Aamodt G, Rosenbaum P. Gross motor function classification system used in adults with cerebral palsy: agreement of self-reported versus professional rating. Dev Med Child Neurol 2006;48:734-738.

43. Eliasson AC, Krumlinde-Sundholm L, Rosblad B, et al. The Manual Ability Classification System (MACS) for children with cerebral palsy: scale development and evidence of validity and reliability. Dev Med Child Neurol 2006;48:549-554.

44. Capute AJ, Shapiro BK. The motor quotient. A method for the early detection of motor delay. Am J Dis Child 1985;139:940-942.

45. Ferrari F, Cioni G, Einspieler C, et al. Cramped synchronized general movements in preterm infants as an early marker for cerebral palsy. Arch Pediatr Adolesc Med 2002;156:460-467.

46. Gordon GS, Simkiss DE. A systematic review of the evidence for hip surveillance in children with cerebral palsy. J Bone Joint Surg Br 2006;88:1492-1496.

47. Davids JR. Quantitative gait analysis in the treatment of children with cerebral palsy. J Pediatr Orthop 2006;26:557-559.

48. Wu YW, Croen LA, Shah SJ, et al. Cerebral palsy in a term population: risk factors and neuroimaging findings. Pediatrics 2006;118:690-697.

49. Mitchell G, McInnes RR. Differential diagnosis of cerebral palsy: Lesch-Nyhan syndrome without self-mutilation. Can Med Assoc J 1984;130:1323-1324.

50. Fowler EG, Ho TW, Nwigwe AI, Dorey FJ. The effect of quadriceps femoris muscle strengthening exercises on spasticity in children with cerebral palsy. Phys Ther 2001;81:1215-1223.

51. Dodd KJ, Taylor NF, Damiano DL. A systematic review of the effectiveness of strength-training programs for people with cerebral palsy. Arch Phys Med Rehabil 2002;83:1157-1164.

52. Blundell SW, Shepherd RB, Dean CM, et al. Functional strength training in cerebral palsy: a pilot study of a group circuit training class for children aged 4-8 years. Clin Rehabil 2003;17:48-57.

53. Unger M, Faure M, Frieg A. Strength training in adolescent learners with cerebral palsy: a randomized controlled trial. Clin Rehabil 2006;20:469-477.

54. Pin T, Dyke P, Chan M. The effectiveness of passive stretching in children with cerebral palsy. Dev Med Child Neurol 2006;48:855-862.

55. Bjornson KF, Schmale GA, Adamczyk-Foster A, McLaughlin J. The effect of dynamic ankle foot orthoses on function in children with cerebral palsy. J Pediatr Orthop 2006;26:773-776.

56. van Roon D, Steenbergen B. The use of ergonomic spoons by people with cerebral palsy: effects on food spilling and movement kinematics. Dev Med Child Neurol 2006;48:888-891.

57. Sterba JA. Does horseback riding therapy or therapist-directed hippotherapy rehabilitate children with cerebral palsy? Dev Med Child Neurol 2007;49:68-73.

58. Charles JR, Wolf SL, Schneider JA, Gordon AM. Efficacy of a child-friendly form of constraint-induced movement therapy in hemiplegic cerebral palsy: a randomized control trial. Dev Med Child Neurol 2006;48:635-642.

59. Erken EH, Bischof FM. Iliopsoas transfer in cerebral palsy: the long-term outcome. J Pediatr Orthop 1994;14:295-298.

60. Dietz FR, Albright JC, Dolan L. Medium-term follow-up of Achilles tendon lengthening in the treatment of ankle equinus in cerebral palsy. Iowa Orthop J 2006;26:27-32.

61. Van Heest AE. Surgical management of wrist and finger deformity. Hand Clin 2003;19:657-665.

62. Woo R. Spasticity: orthopedic perspective. J Child Neurol 2001; 16:47-53.

63. McLaughlin J, Bjornson K, Temkin N, et al. Selective dorsal rhizotomy: meta-analysis of three randomized controlled trials. Dev Med Child Neurol 2002;44:17-25.

Chronic Fatigue Syndrome 115

Gerold R. Ebenbichler, MD

Synonyms

Chronic fatigue and immune dysfunction syndrome
Myalgic encephalomyelitis
Neurasthenia
Post-viral fatigue syndrome
Iceland disease
Royal Free disease
Yuppie flu

ICD-9 Code

780.71 Chronic fatigue syndrome

DEFINITION

Chronic fatigue syndrome (CFS) is a debilitating condition of unknown nature and cause, but most medical authorities now accept its existence. CFS is characterized by severe disabling, medically unexplained fatigue of more than 6 months and prominently features subjective impairments in concentration, short-term memory, and sleep as well as musculoskeletal pain.[1] Sufferers experience significant disability and distress, which may be further exacerbated by a lack of understanding from others, including health professionals. CFS affects both adults and children.

Epidemiologic research in Western countries has demonstrated that among adults, between 230 and 500 of every 100,000 persons are affected with CFS.[2-4] Women have CFS more commonly,[5] as do minority groups and people with lower educational status and educational attainment.[2]

The causes of CFS remain uncertain. CFS may start either gradually or suddenly. In the latter case, it is often triggered by an influenza-like viral or similar illness. Some progress in the understanding of the disease has been made when causes were divided into predisposing, triggering or precipitating, and perpetuating factors.[6,7] Personality (neuroticism, introversion) and lifestyle factors, inactivity in childhood and inactivity after infectious mononucleosis, and genetic influence are presumed to influence vulnerability in CFS. Certain infectious illnesses (e.g., Epstein-Barr virus infection, Q fever, and Lyme disease), precipitating somatic events (e.g., serious injuries), and psychological distress (e.g., serious life events) precipitate the disorder. The perceptions, illness attributions, and beliefs of patients may encourage avoidant coping and perpetuate the illness.

Among various pathophysiologic hypotheses tested, some evidence has emerged supporting subtle hypoactivity in the hypothalamic-pituitary-adrenal axis with lower than normal cortisol response to increased corticotropin levels[8] and a hyperserotoninergic state or upregulated serotonin receptors in CFS.[9,10] Whether these alterations are a cause or a consequence of CFS, however, remains unclear. Dysfunction in the immune system in CFS is inconsistently evidenced by findings of abnormal cytokine production, mainly concentrating on proinflammatory ones that are known to be involved in the regulation of the hypothalamic-pituitary-adrenal axis and sympathetic nervous system, such as tumor necrosis factor, interleukin-1, and interleukin-6.[11] On the tissue level, cytokines such as interleukin-6 are involved in the stress response and represent crucial inducers of sickness behavior,[12] which is characterized by avoidance behavior, apathy, sleepiness, impaired memory and concentration, anorexia, mild fever, and increased sensitivity to pain. No convincing evidence exists to support CFS as a continuing viral infection. Perturbed natural killer cells thereby could induce a T_H2-type instead of a T_H1-type antiviral response, resulting in persistent viral activation.[11] Functional magnetic resonance imaging studies in patients with CFS revealed findings indicative of increased neuronal resource allocation[13] or dysfunctional motor planning,[14] which seems to be consistent with cognitive impairment in these patients.

SYMPTOMS

Patients with CFS typically present with a variety of symptoms that may widely overlap with symptoms of functional somatic syndromes, including the irritable bowel syndrome, fibromyalgia, multiple chemical sensitivity, chronic pelvic pain, temporomandibular joint dysfunction, and Gulf War illness.[11]

Patients experience profound, overwhelming exhaustion, both mentally and physically, which is worsened by exertion and is not or not completely relieved by rest.[15] Fatigue is highly subjective, multidimensional, and variable in nature, and it does not necessarily need to be the major and most debilitating symptom in this condition.[1] Patients may express their complaints of fatigue in different ways. Patients' expectations and causal attribution of symptoms to somatic factors, hidden agenda involving insurance issues, and invalidity of benefit claims have been related to an increase in symptoms and may contribute to a diversity of symptoms reported.[7]

In addition to fatigue, patients with CFS usually complain about a wide variety of multisystem symptoms that are nonspecific and variable in both nature and severity over time. These concomitant symptoms may be just as prominent as fatigue and are best summarized in different categories.[15,16]

- Complaints of cognitive dysfunction. CFS patients may experience forgetfulness, confusion, difficulties in thinking, and "mental fatigue" or "brain fog."
- Postexertional malaise. Patients report a period of deep fatigue and exhaustion that lasts for more than 24 hours after physical exertion.
- Complaints of pain. These include headaches of a new type, pattern, or severity; muscle pain; and multijoint pain. Patients may further report pain in bones, eyes, and testicles; abdominal and chest pain; chills; and painful skin sensitivity.
- Unrefreshing sleep and rest is a hallmark of CFS, and insomnia is also common. Patients report more difficulty in falling asleep, more interrupted sleep, and more daytime napping. It is extremely difficult for many patients to maintain a sleep schedule. Patients report that exercise, unlike in healthy persons, worsens the insomnia and unrefreshing sleep symptoms alike.
- Psychological complaints of emotional lability, anxiety, depressive mood, irritability, and sometimes a curious emotional "flattening" most likely due to exhaustion may be reported by CFS patients. CFS patients with preexisting psychiatric symptoms may report that these worsen with the onset of CFS. Treatment of psychiatric symptoms alone does not relieve the physical symptoms of CFS, indicating that the disease is not psychological in nature.
- Other frequently reported complaints refer to general hypersensitivity and poor temperature control; these include low-grade fevers, photophobia, vertigo, nausea, allergies, hot flashes, and rashes.[17,18]

PHYSICAL EXAMINATION

The physical examination is directed toward determination of whether symptoms are caused by any other disease or illness. The findings of the general medical and neurologic examinations should be normal. There may be low-grade fever with temperatures between 37.5°C and 38.5°C orally, nonexudative pharyngitis, and tender cervical or axillary lymph nodes up to 2 cm in diameter. A mild hypotension, elicited mainly with tilt-table testing and reversed by mineralocorticoids, may be observed. In some patients, orthostatic hypotension with wide swings in blood pressure resulting in syncope as well as intermittent hypertension may be found.[19] Complaints of paresthesias usually prove to be odd on sensory testing, particularly numbness in the bones or muscles or fluctuating patches of numbness or paresthesias on the chest, face, or nose. A few patients report blurred or "close to" double vision. In neither case are there physical findings to corroborate the sensory experiences.[19] Unsteadiness on standing with closed eyes may be found.

A thorough mental status examination is performed to rule out any exclusionary psychiatric disorders. The psychological examination may reveal abnormalities in mood, intellectual function, memory, concentration, and personality. Particular attention should be paid to anxiety, self-destructive thoughts, and observable signs such as psychomotor retardation.[1]

The musculoskeletal examination findings should be normal. In CFS patients with arthralgia and myalgia, joint swelling and inflammation and other superimposed pain generators, such as bursitis, tendinitis, and radiculopathy, have to be ruled out. Palpatory examination of muscles may reveal tender muscles, tender points that are not numerous enough to be classified as fibromyalgia, and individual trigger points.

FUNCTIONAL LIMITATIONS

Disablement varies widely among patients with CFS. Whereas some are able to lead a relatively normal life, others are totally bed bound and unable to care for themselves. In a rehabilitative assessment, body functions that represent the patient's core subjective symptoms may reveal the most pronounced impairment; these are energy and drive functions, sensation of pain, sleep functions, attention function, emotional functions, memory functions, and exercise tolerance functions. Both muscle and cardiopulmonary function as demonstrated by cardiopulmonary stress testing may be reduced in these patients. Avoidance behavior as a consequence of patients' experiencing worsening of symptoms after previously well-tolerated levels of exercise and kinesiophobia—a specific kind of fear-avoidance behavior that is defined as an excessive, irrational, and debilitating fear of physical movement and activity resulting from a feeling of vulnerability to painful injury or reinjury—may increase sedentariness in CFS patients. However, kinesiophobia was not correlated with reduced exercise capacity by bicycle ergometer exercise stress testing.[20]

CFS patients may be able to begin but not to complete mental or physical activities that were previously easily accomplished. Thus, tasks that predominantly challenge the cognitive performance, like focusing attention, solving problems, handling stress, making decisions, undertaking multiple tasks, or driving a car, may limit patients in carrying out their daily routine, especially at the workplace. Tasks that require predominantly physical performance, like walking or household tasks, may limit the patient's activities of daily life. Many patients have to modify or give up physical hobbies and exercise and find themselves unable to work full-time or at all.[16] Categories related to intimate relationships, family relationships, communication, and complex interpersonal relationships may be altered in CFS patients, thereby restricting them from participation in social and work life.

Cognitive avoidance coping as a major illness-perpetuating factor was found negatively related to social functioning,[21] and a strong association seems to exist between kinesiophobia and self-reported activity limitations and participation restrictions in CFS patients.[20] In addition to environmental factors related to the immediate family and friends, health professionals may reinforce patients' symptom severity and illness behavior and facilitate further impaired functioning in these patients. Personal beliefs, practices, ideologies, spirituality, laws, and societal norms may also facilitate or hinder functioning in CFS patients. A considerable number of patients with CFS in many countries are receiving disability benefits or private insurance or have made claims and been denied.[22]

DIAGNOSTIC STUDIES

There are no accepted pathognomonic signs of or diagnostic tests for CFS. Diagnosis of CFS is primarily based on the patient's symptoms that fit scientific case definitions of CFS, which aim to effectively distinguish CFS from other types of unexplained fatigue. Among numerous scientific case definitions available, the U.S. Centers for Disease Control and Prevention criteria are the most widely supported.[1] This case definition characterizes CFS by a grouping of nonspecific symptoms and a diagnosis of exclusion (Table 115-1). To receive a diagnosis of CFS, fatigue must have persisted or recurred during 6 or more consecutive months. Concomitant symptoms must have persisted or recurred during 6 or more consecutive months of illness and cannot have predated the fatigue.[15] Clinicians may have difficulties in diagnosis of CFS, especially by not acknowledging the diagnosis of fatigue when its onset is gradual or by the diversity of patients' fatigue reports. Instruments developed to assess fatigue, like the Checklist Individual Strength, the Chalder Fatigue Scale, and the Krupp Fatigue Severity Scale, are widely used in research studies and may assist physicians with objectivation of fatigue and establishment of the medical diagnosis.

Fatigue and similar symptoms can be caused by a wide variety of conditions. Thus, diagnosis of CFS needs to include a diagnostic process that eliminates potential causes of the patient's symptoms (see the section on differential diagnosis). In addition to a thorough history and a meticulous physical examination, diagnostic studies include a mental status examination and a minimum array of laboratory tests.

TABLE 115-1 Case Definition (1994) for Chronic Fatigue Syndrome from U.S. Centers for Disease Control and Prevention

Characterized by persistent or relapsing unexplained chronic fatigue

Fatigue lasts for at least 6 months

Fatigue is of new or definite onset

Fatigue is not the result of an organic disease or of continuing exertion

Fatigue is not alleviated by rest

Fatigue results in a substantial reduction in previous occupational, educational, social, and personal activities

Four or more of the following symptoms, concurrently present for ≥ 6 months: impaired memory or concentration, sore throat, tender cervical or axillary lymph nodes, muscle pain, pain in several joints, new headaches, unrefreshing sleep, or malaise after exertion

Exclusion criteria

Medical condition explaining fatigue

Major depressive disorder (psychotic features) or bipolar disorder

Schizophrenia, dementia, or delusional disorder

Anorexia nervosa, bulimia nervosa

Alcohol or substance abuse

Severe obesity

Modified from Fukuda K, Straus SE, Hickie I, et al; International Chronic Fatigue Syndrome Study Group. The chronic fatigue syndrome: a comprehensive approach to its definition and study. Ann Intern Med 1994;121:953-959; and Prins JB, van der Meer JW, Bleijenberg G. Chronic fatigue syndrome. Lancet 2006;367:346-355.

A structural psychiatric interview is essential to identify permanent psychiatric exclusions (see Table 115-1 and the section on differential diagnosis). Reliable detection instruments may be helpful when physicians perform screening for psychiatric diagnoses. Instruments recommended are the Composite International Diagnostic Interview[23] and the Structured Clinical Interview for DSM-IV Axis I (SCID).[24]

Laboratory examination is intended to detect other disorders, not to find out whether a patient has CFS. Recommendations for laboratory testing have been provided (Table 115-2).

Questionnaires like the Epworth Sleepiness Scale and the Centre for Sleep and Chronobiology Sleep Assessment Questionnaire are useful to screen for and to profile sleep abnormalities.[25] Polysomnography defines sleep architecture, duration and timing of sleep, respiratory obstruction, and abnormal limb movements and may be indicated when primary sleep disorders exclusionary to CFS, such as sleep apnea and narcolepsy, have to be ruled out.

Assessment of a patient's functioning and health according to the International Classification of Functioning, Disability, and Health (ICF)[26] would further complete the diagnostic studies in patients with CFS. The classification might be recommended, but compared with other

TABLE 115-2 Laboratory Tests Recommended for the Exclusion of Diseases That May Cause Chronic Fatigue

Complete blood count with differential cell count

Blood and serum chemistries (serum electrolytes, blood urea nitrogen, glucose, creatinine, calcium)

Erythrocyte sedimentation rate

Urinalysis

Thyroid function studies

Antinuclear antibodies

Serum cortisol

Immunoglobulin levels

Rheumatoid factor

Tuberculin skin test

Human immunodeficiency virus serology

Lyme serology (when endemic)

Magnetic resonance imaging of head (to rule out multiple sclerosis)

Polysomnography (to rule out sleep disorder)

Optional tests to be used when clinically indicated

Quantification of natural killer cells

Quantification of B- and T-cell subsets

Functional elevation of natural killer cells

T-cell response to mitogenic stimulation

Measurements of delayed hypersensitivity

Production of and response to cytokines

Enzyme-linked immunosorbent assay/activated cell test

Serologic tests for *Candida albicans*

RNase L enzymatic activity assay or RNase L protein quantification

Spinal tap for oligoclonal bands

Tilt table

Catecholamine testing

Nerve conduction studies including electromyography

Anti–acetylcholine receptor antibodies

Vitamin B_{12} deficiency

Circulating immune complexes including CD3 and CD4

Viral serologies

Modified from Craig T, Kakumanu S. Chronic fatigue syndrome: evaluation and treatment. Am Fam Physician 2002;65:1083-1090; and Wikipedia 2007/results from an NIH consensus conference.

Differential Diagnosis

Patients may present with apparently unexplained fatigue with these medical conditions, which are exclusionary or differential diagnoses for CFS.[31,32]

Blood
- Anemia
- Hemochromatosis

Infections
- Chronic Epstein-Barr virus infection
- Influenza
- Hepatitis
- Human immunodeficiency virus infection
- Lyme disease
- Occult abscess
- Poliomyelitis, post-poliomyelitis syndrome
- Tuberculosis
- Bacterial endocarditis
- Chronic brucellosis

Parasitic infections

Fungal infections

Autoimmune disease
- Behçet syndrome
- Dermatomyositis
- Lupus erythematosus
- Polyarteritis
- Polymyositis
- Reiter syndrome
- Rheumatoid arthritis
- Sjögren syndrome
- Vasculitis

Liver disease

Chronic heart disease

Chronic lung disease

Metabolic and toxic conditions

Endocrine disease
- Diabetes mellitus
- Hyperthyroidism and hypothyroidism
- Addison disease
- Cushing syndrome
- Panhypopituitarism

Ovarian failure

Malignant neoplasms

Neuromuscular disorders
- Fibromyalgia
- Multiple sclerosis
- Parkinson disease
- Myasthenia gravis
- Head injuries

Sleep disorders
- Obstructive sleep syndromes (sleep apnea, narcolepsy)

Psychiatric
- Bipolar affective disorders
- Schizophrenia of any subtype
- Delusional disorders of any subtype
- Dementias of any subtype
- Organic brain disorders and alcohol or substance abuse within 2 years before onset of the fatiguing illness

chronic conditions like osteoarthritis and back pain, ICF core sets that best describe the prototypical spectrum of disability have not yet been developed for CFS.[27,28] Furthermore, ICF core sets have to be psychometrically validated after they have been developed. This can be best accomplished by item response theory–based computerized adaptive testing, a method selecting only those items out of the item pool that are most relevant for the individual patient.[29,30] For the time being, instruments that have been recommended in a consensus conference may be used to measure the symptom-specific disablement and quality of life of patients with CFS.[15]

Other
    Pharmacologic side effects
    Alcohol and substance abuse
    Body weight fluctuation (severe obesity or
    marked weight loss)

TREATMENT

Initial

Treatment of CFS is symptom based and aims to improve fatigue and comorbid conditions, such as sleep disturbances, depression, and painful symptoms.

Treatment of CFS with pharmacologic therapies has had disappointing results in most cases. So far, no pharmacologic treatments have been proved effective in the treatment of fatigue. The subtle changes found in the hypothalamic-pituitary-adrenal axis have led to a few randomized controlled trials that overall did not establish steroids as a treatment of choice.[33] For immunologic therapies like immunoglobulin G, staphylococcus toxoid, ribonucleic acid, and others, there is insufficient evidence about the effectiveness of these therapies in CFS.[33]

Anecdotal evidence suggests that low doses of antidepressant medication (e.g., 10 to 30 mg of nortriptyline) administered at bedtime improve sleep and diminish pain, although the benefit of these medications has not been demonstrated in CFS.[33,34] In addition, the use of acetaminophen, nonsteroidal antiinflammatory drugs, and opioids may be worthwhile in patients with prominent musculoskeletal complaints or headaches.

Complementary medicine has gained increasing popularity among patients with chronic diseases. These treatments include homeopathy, herbal remedies, supplements, megavitamins, special diets, and energy healing. Although individual studies revealed beneficial effects for homeopathy and supplements in the treatment of CFS, there is insufficient evidence for the effectiveness of these interventions.[33]

Rehabilitation

Management based on a rehabilitation model is now recommended for patients with CFS. The individual rehabilitative assessment is necessary to identify those treatment targets that are most likely to reach the rehabilitation aims of the patient with CFS. These rehabilitation programs may involve different professions and therapies, and increasing evidence for the effectiveness of individual rehabilitation interventions has emerged.[33-36]

Cognitive-behavioral therapy for CFS addresses changing of condition-related cognitions and behaviors and incorporates two elements: (1) a cognitive element focusing on the modification of thoughts and beliefs thought relevant for the disease process and (2) a behavioral element consisting of a graded increase of activity. Several systematic reviews suggest that cognitive-behavioral therapy for adults with CFS is an effective treatment in improving both physical functioning and symptoms such as fatigue, anxiety, and mood compared with either routine care or relaxation therapy.[33-35] Furthermore, one study provided evidence supporting the effectiveness of cognitive-behavioral therapy in children and adolescents.[37] In this study, cognitive-behavioral therapy was associated with a significant positive effect on fatigue, symptoms, physical functioning, and school attendance.

Graded exercise addresses deconditioning and is designed to overcome deconditioning and to increase strength and cardiovascular health. Cycle ergometer training, swimming, or walking may be varied according to the patients' preferences. Graded exercise has no intentions of explicitly treating cognitions but should incorporate considerable education wherein the sufferer learns to start at an appropriate level of activity (based on intensity and duration) that is incrementally increased, at a rate that does not substantially increase symptoms. If severe fatigue follows exercise, lasting more than 24 hours, the exercise prescription is adjusted so it is less demanding; there are no specific and firm guidelines because of the wide spectrum found in this syndrome. Overall results from systematic reviews suggest that graded aerobic exercise therapy, at intensities between 40% and 70% maximum oxygen consumption performed three to five times per week for 30 minutes, is a promising intervention with positive effects on CFS patients' symptoms and quality of life.[33,36] A few patients may find health benefits and pain relief from other than aerobic exercises, like gentle stretching and gentle strengthening including yoga or Tai Chi.

Education of the individual as to what is known and not known about CFS, its impact on function at work and home, and its prognosis should be included in the rehabilitation programs. Patients' education in self-management strategies that consider when, how, and why people change their behavior over time (transtheoretical model)[38] is of utmost importance in modern rehabilitation. The transtheoretical model describes a "meta" model and critically incorporates aspects of other models into its theoretical framework. These are self-initiated and professionally facilitated changes in health beliefs, behavioral intentions, decision-making processes, self-efficacy, and coping to overcome the temptations component of the transtheoretical model.

Patients are better prepared for coping on a daily basis, have more realistic expectations, and think that the physician is not ignoring their concerns. In addition, when appropriate, the individual should be informed that periodic reassessment for a possible treatable underlying process may ensue. This may help relieve anxiety about abandonment. Avoidance of heavy meals, alcohol, caffeine, and total rest can help, as can minimizing intake of substances that alter sleep patterns or alter one's self-image.[39]

Procedures

Treatment is symptomatic; therefore, procedures may be chosen to help with trigger points, dizziness, headache, or other symptoms as they occur. If trigger points are noted, appropriate therapy may be initiated. Spray and stretch techniques, dry needling, and trigger point injection with a local anesthetic or small amount of steroid have all met with some success.[40]

Acupuncture is an important constituent of traditional Chinese medicine. It is believed in traditional Chinese medicine that acupuncture can strengthen the vital essence of the human body and remove the blockage in channels. The application of acupuncture for CFS is mainly empirically based; a few Chinese clinical trials that included a control group have reported beneficial effects with success rates ranging from 88% to 94%.[41]

Surgery

No specific surgery is performed for CFS.

POTENTIAL DISEASE COMPLICATIONS

Recovery without treatment is rare, with a median recovery rate of 5% and improvement rate of 39.5%.[5] Recovery episodes seem more likely in patients with less severe fatigue and if patients do not attribute the illness to physical causes.[5] The primary complication of the disease is continued fatigue and loss of function, which commonly occur despite treatment. Predictors of poor treatment outcome were membership in a self-help group, receipt of a sickness benefit, claiming of a disability-related benefit, low sense of control, strong focus on symptoms, and pervasively passive activity pattern.[7]

Both reduced functioning and sedentariness may increase the progress or severity of chronic diseases of the cardiovascular and metabolic system, thereby further increasing the disablement of patients with CFS.

POTENTIAL TREATMENT COMPLICATIONS

Physicians who convey understanding and compassion to patients, despite the lack of a known "cure," can alter a patient's quality of life; fear, or the perception of being abandoned, can markedly accentuate frustration and accelerate a decline in function. Medication side effects should be reviewed on an intermittent basis to be certain that the nonspecific symptoms found in CFS are not being accentuated. Care should be taken to avoid too strenuous an exercise program because the fatigue that may ensue can be both physically and mentally debilitating. Despite optimal care, depression, fatigue, and a loss of function may still occur. Physicians and patients should both be aware that symptoms found in CFS may persist for months or years but that remittance or recovery is still possible.

ACKNOWLEDGMENT

I am indebted to Dr. Thomas Brockow, FBK German Institute for Health Care Research, for his valuable comments on the manuscript.

References

1. Fukuda K, Straus SE, Hickie I, et al; International Chronic Fatigue Syndrome Study Group. The chronic fatigue syndrome: a comprehensive approach to its definition and study. Ann Intern Med 1994;121:953-959.
2. Reyes M, Nisenbaum R, Hoaglin DC, et al. Prevalence and incidence of chronic fatigue syndrome in Wichita, Kansas. Arch Intern Med 2003;163:1530-1536.
3. Jason LA, Richman JA, Rademaker AW, et al. A community-based study of chronic fatigue syndrome. Arch Intern Med 1999;159:2129-2137.
4. Wessely S. The epidemiology of chronic fatigue syndrome. Epidemiol Psichiatr Soc 1998;7:10-24.
5. Cairns R, Hotopf M. A systematic review describing the prognosis of chronic fatigue syndrome. Occup Med (Lond) 2005;55:20-31.
6. White PD. What causes chronic fatigue syndrome? BMJ 2004;329:928-929.
7. Prins JB, van der Meer JW, Bleijenberg G. Chronic fatigue syndrome. Lancet 2006;367:346-355.
8. Cleare AJ. The neuroendocrinology of chronic fatigue syndrome. Endocr Rev 2003;24:236-252.
9. Cleare AJ, Messa C, Rabiner EA, Grasby PM. Brain 5-HT$_{1A}$ receptor binding in chronic fatigue syndrome measured using positron emission tomography and [^{11}C]WAY-100635. Biol Psychiatry 2005;57:239-246.
10. Yamamoto S, Ouchi Y, Onoe H, et al. Reduction of serotonin transporters of patients with chronic fatigue syndrome. Neuroreport 2004;15:2571-2574.
11. Cho HJ, Skowera A, Cleary A, Wessely S. Chronic fatigue syndrome: an update focusing on phenomenology and pathophysiology. Curr Opin Psychiatry 2006;19:67-73.
12. Konsman JP, Parnet P, Dantzer R. Cytokine-induced sickness behaviour: mechanisms and implications. Trends Neurosci 2002;25:154-159.
13. Lange G, Steffener J, Cook DB, et al. Objective evidence of cognitive complaints in chronic fatigue syndrome: a BOLD fMRI study of verbal working memory. Neuroimage 2005;26:513-524.
14. de Lange FP, Kalkman JS, Bleijenberg G, et al. Neural correlates of the chronic fatigue syndrome—an fMRI study. Brain 2004;127(pt 9):1948-1957.
15. Reeves WC, Lloyd A, Vernon SD, et al. Identification of ambiguities in the 1994 chronic fatigue syndrome research case definition and recommendations for resolution. BMC Health Serv Res 2003;3:25.
16. Afari N, Buchwald D. Chronic fatigue syndrome: a review. Am J Psychiatry 2003;160:221-236.
17. CFIDS Association of America Web site. Available at http://www.cfids.org/. Accessed 11/1/07.
18. Levine PH. Chronic fatigue syndrome comes of age. Am J Med 1998;105:2s-4s.
19. Ropper AH, Brown RH. Fatigue, asthenia, anxiety, and depressive reactions. In Ropper AH, Brown RH, eds. Adams and Victor's Principles of Neurology, 8th ed. New York, McGraw-Hill, 2005:433-447.
20. Nijs J, de Meirleir K, Duquet W. Kinesiophobia in chronic fatigue syndrome: assessment and associations with disability. Arch Phys Med Rehabil 2004;85:1586-1592.
21. Heijmans MJ. Coping and adaptive outcome in chronic fatigue syndrome: importance of illness cognitions. J Psychosom Res 1998;45(Spec No):39-51.
22. Ross SD, Estok RP, Frame D, et al. Disability and chronic fatigue syndrome: a focus on function. Arch Intern Med 2004;164:1098-1107.
23. Andrews G, Peters L. The psychometric properties of the Composite International Diagnostic Interview. Soc Psychiatry Psychiatr Epidemiol 1998;33:80-88.

24. Taylor RR, Friedberg F, Jason LA. A Clinician's Guide to Controversial Illnesses: Chronic Fatigue Syndrome, Fibromyalgia, and Multiple Chemical Sensitivities. Sarasota, Fla, Professional Resource Press, 2001.

25. Unger ER, Nisenbaum R, Moldofsky H, et al. Sleep assessment in a population based study of chronic fatigue syndrome. BMC Neurol 2004,4:6.

26. World Health Organization. International Classification of Functioning, Disability and Health (ICF). Geneva, World Health Organization, 2001.

27. Cieza A, Stucki G, Weigl M, et al. ICF Core Sets for low back pain. J Rehabil Med 2004;44(Suppl):69-74.

28. Dreinhöfer K, Stucki G, Ewert T, et al. ICF Core Sets for osteoarthritis. J Rehabil Med 2004;44(Suppl):75-80.

29. Weiss DJ. Adaptive testing by computer. J Consult Clin Psychol 1985;53:774-789.

30. Ware JE Jr, Bjorner JB, Kosinski M. Practical implications of item response theory and computerized adaptive testing: a brief summary of ongoing studies of widely used headache impact scales. Med Care 2000;38(Suppl):II73-II82.

31. Royal College of Paediatrics and Child Health. Evidence Based Guidelines for the Management of CFS/ME (Chronic Fatigue Syndrome/Myalgic Encephalopathy) in Children and Young People. London, RCPCH, Dec. 2004, 1-22. Available at www.rcpch.ac.uk/recent_publications.html.

32. Craig T, Kakumanu S. Chronic fatigue syndrome: evaluation and treatment. Am Fam Physician 2002;65:1083-1090.

33. Chambers D, Bagnall A, Hempel S, Forbes C. Interventions for the treatment, management and rehabilitation of patients with chronic fatigue syndrome/myalgic encephalomyelitis: an updated systematic review. J R Soc Med 2006;99:506-520.

34. Whiting P, Bagnall A, Sowden A, et al. Interventions for the treatment and management of chronic fatigue syndrome: a systematic review. JAMA 2001;286:1360-1368.

35. Price JR, Couper J. Cognitive behaviour therapy for adults with chronic fatigue syndrome. Cochrane Database Syst Rev 2000;2: CD001027.

36. Edmonds M, McGuire H, Price J. Exercise therapy for chronic fatigue syndrome. Cochrane Database Syst Rev 2004;3: CD003200.

37. Stulemeijer M, de Jong LW, Fiselier TJ, et al. Cognitive behaviour therapy for adolescents with chronic fatigue syndrome: randomised controlled trial. BMJ 2005;330:14-17.

38. Prochaska J, DiClemente CC, Norcross JC. In search of how people change. Am Psychol 1992;47:1102-1114.

39. Manningham R. The Symptoms, Nature and Causes, and Cure of the Febricula, or Little Fever. London, J. Robinson, 1750.

40. Robinson J, Arendt Nielsen L. Muscle pain syndromes. In Braddom RL. Physical Medicine and Rehabilitation. Philadelphia, WB Saunders, 2006:989-1020.

41. Zhang W, Liu ZS, Wu T, Peng WN. Acupuncture for chronic fatigue syndrome. Cochrane Database Syst Rev 2006;2:CD006010.

Chronic Kidney Disease 116

Ajay K. Singh, MD

Synonyms

Chronic kidney disease
Chronic kidney failure
Pre-ESRD

ICD-9 Codes

585   Chronic kidney disease
585.1 Chronic kidney disease, stage I
585.2 Chronic kidney disease, stage II (mild)
585.3 Chronic kidney disease, stage III (moderate)
585.4 Chronic kidney disease, stage IV (severe)
585.5 Chronic kidney disease, stage V
585.6 End-stage renal disease
586   Chronic kidney disease (unspecified)
593.9 Unspecified disorder of kidney and ureter

DEFINITION

Chronic kidney disease (CKD) is defined as a clinical syndrome characterized by a progressive decline in kidney function such that the kidney's ability to adequately excrete waste products and to contribute to the constancy of the body's homeostatic functions becomes progressively impaired. CKD at its mildest stage is asymptomatic; at its most severe stage, it is characterized by uremia. End-stage kidney failure denotes CKD that necessitates kidney replacement therapy (dialysis or transplantation). The National Kidney Foundation has developed a consensus definition of CKD that has been widely accepted. CKD is defined as an absolute reduction in glomerular filtration rate (GFR) to below 60 mL/min/1.73 m² for 3 months or more, with or without other evidence of kidney damage; or the presence of kidney damage for 3 months or more, as evidenced by structural or functional abnormalities of the kidney, with or without reduction in GFR. Kidney damage can be manifested by pathologic changes on kidney biopsy specimens, abnormalities in the composition of the blood or urine (such as proteinuria or changes in the urine sediment examination), or abnormalities in imaging tests. This definition of CKD does leave unaddressed the significance of a reduced GFR below 60 mL/min/1.73 m² in certain subgroups, such as the elderly, the undernourished, and those of specific ethnic groups. For example, elderly individuals with reduced GFR may never develop end-stage renal disease. However, the classification serves as a useful starting point in evaluation of a patient with depressed GFR and provides an impetus either to refer the patient to a nephrologist for further workup or to identify a patient at higher risk for development of kidney disease.

CKD is classified into five stages, depicted in Table 116-1. Each stage has a corresponding level of GFR. Patients with stage V CKD have advanced kidney disease; this includes patients receiving dialysis and those with a kidney transplant. Approximately 98% of patients beginning dialysis for CKD in the United States have an estimated GFR of less than 15 mL · min⁻¹ per 1.73 m². Nevertheless, this definition is not synonymous with end-stage kidney failure defined earlier. In essence, end-stage renal disease (ESRD) is an administrative term in the United States signifying eligibility for coverage by Medicare for payment for dialysis and transplantation.

The incidence of kidney failure in the United States is approximately 268 cases per 1 million population per year.[1] However, the incidence of CKD is greater among black Americans (829 per million population per year, compared with 199 per million population per year among white Americans). The major causes of CKD in the United States are diabetes mellitus (40%), hypertension (30%), glomerular disease (15%), polycystic kidney disease, and obstructive uropathy (Table 116-2).[1] Elsewhere in the world, where the incidence of diabetes mellitus has not reached epidemic proportions (e.g., in Europe and parts of the developing world), chronic glomerulonephritis (20%) and chronic reflux nephropathy (25%) are the most common causes of CKD. The progressive decline in kidney function in individuals with CKD is variable and depends on both the cause of the underlying insult and patient-specific factors. Furthermore, evidence also points to the importance of several factors in modulation of kidney disease progression. These include proteinuria, the presence of systemic hypertension, age, gender, genetic factors, and smoking.[2]

At an early stage, insidious effects on target organs may be manifested. For example, patients may have mild to

TABLE 116-1 National Kidney Foundation Classification of Chronic Kidney Disease

Stage I	Kidney damage with normal or supranormal GFR	GFR ≥ 90
Stage II	Kidney damage with mild reduction in GFR	GFR 60-89
Stage III	Moderate reduction in GFR	GFR 30-59
Stage IV	Severe reduction in GFR	GFR 15-29
Stage V	Kidney failure or on dialysis	GFR < 15

moderate hypertension, mild anemia, left ventricular hypertrophy, and subtle changes in bone structure due to kidney osteodystrophy. It is imperative to investigate the abnormal kidney function and to refer the patient to a nephrologist. As kidney function gradually declines further, with the GFR reaching 10 to 30 mL/min, hypertension is usually present and subtle biochemical and hematologic abnormalities may become evident, such as mild hyperkalemia, mild hypobicarbonatemia (from uremic acidosis), and anemia of chronic disease.[3]

As kidney dysfunction becomes severe (GFR in the range of 10 to 15 mL/min), the syndrome of uremia is invariably present. Uremia reflects the accumulation of metabolic toxins, some characterized and others unknown, that influences the functioning of a variety of organ systems. In this late stage, the need for kidney

TABLE 116-2 Causes of Chronic Kidney Disease

Prekidney

Cardiogenic
    Severe cardiac failure
Vascular
    Kidney artery stenosis

Kidney

Immunologic
    Glomerulonephritis (primary or secondary)
Neoplastic
    Multiple myeloma
Toxic
    Gold, pennicillamine, cyclosporine
Tubulointerstitial
    Infection or reflux
Cystic diseases
    Polycystic kidney disease

Postkidney

Stones
Pelviureteric obstruction
Retroperitoneal fibrosis
Prostatic hypertrophy
Urethral stricture

replacement therapy is imminent, and dialysis or transplantation is required to sustain life. The indications for initiation of kidney replacement therapy include severe refractory abnormalities in biochemistry (severe hyperkalemia and acidosis), severe pulmonary edema, bleeding, metabolic encephalopathy, and pericarditis.[4] More subtle but no less important indications include malnutrition and severe disability (marked tiredness and lethargy).

SYMPTOMS

CKD may be asymptomatic when kidney function is only mildly impaired; when the GFR is markedly reduced, the patient is usually symptomatic and may be severely disabled. Early in kidney disease, individuals may present simply with elevated serum creatinine and blood urea nitrogen levels but no symptoms. These individuals are usually unaware that they have any abnormalities in kidney function and usually fail to register on the "radar screen" of their clinicians. Edema may also be observed for the first time, reflecting the kidney's inability to excrete salt and water. With a further decline in kidney function, there is often a concomitant decline in cognitive and physical functioning. This is usually due to anemia, kidney osteodystrophy, and onset of the uremic syndrome. In addition, appetite declines, and there is often a significant loss of lean body mass.

PHYSICAL EXAMINATION

One or more of a spectrum of abnormalities that reflect the multisystem nature of the uremic syndrome may be manifested on physical examination of patients with CKD. Patients may appear generally ill, gaunt, and pale. Mucous membranes may be pale from anemia, and poor platelet function may result in easy bleeding of the gums. The cardiovascular system may exhibit no abnormality, or there may be evidence of hypertension, extracellular fluid overload (elevated jugular venous pressure, pulmonary venous congestion manifested by rales, and pitting edema), and acute pericarditis. The presence of a pericardial rub on physical examination is usually highly suggestive of uremic pericarditis. The pulmonary system may demonstrate rales from fluid overload on physical examination. Gastrointestinal abnormalities include stomatitis, cheilosis, and halitosis. Patients may also experience epigastric tenderness compatible with gastritis secondary to uremia. Abnormalities in the musculoskeletal system may include generalized weakness on physical examination. Proximal weakness may be an early sign of kidney osteodystrophy. Patients with dialysis-associated amyloidosis may experience bone tenderness, carpal tunnel syndrome, and amyloid accumulations or tumors in various parts of the body, such as the skin. Hematologic abnormalities evident on physical examination may include bruising from platelet function abnormalities. Findings of the neurologic examination may, quite commonly, be abnormal in patients with uremia. Patients may have mild abnormalities, such as intermittent confusion, or more severe manifestations, such as delirium, seizure activity, and psychosis. In extreme cases, the patient may become co-matose. Common abnormalities on physical examination include evidence of confusion, a flapping tremor (as-terixis), and fasciculations. A peripheral neuropathy is quite rare because most patients have started dialysis treatment before a neuropathy has time to develop.

It is unclear why some patients demonstrate the "full-blown" physical abnormalities of the uremic syndrome, whereas others exhibit relatively mild findings on physical examination. The physical examination is important in the diagnosis of uremia. In particular, abnormalities such as encephalopathy, acute pericarditis, and pulmonary edema are indications for initiation of kidney replacement therapy.

FUNCTIONAL LIMITATIONS

Functional limitations in individuals with CKD depend on the degree of lethargy, fatigue, and neuropsychological symptoms that are present. Individuals may go from being mobile to nonmobile because of weakness. Elderly individuals with underlying comorbidities may be the most affected. Endurance and the ability to perform activities of daily living may be reduced, and modifications in lifestyle may become necessary, including a change from full-time to part-time work, reduction in travel, and discontinuation of driving.[5-7] In diabetic patients, the onset of symptomatic CKD in the setting of other underlying complications of diabetes mellitus, including impaired visual acuity and peripheral neuropathy, presents challenging functional limitations.

DIAGNOSTIC STUDIES

Diagnostic testing in individuals with CKD essentially focuses on two areas: monitoring of the progression of CKD and assessment of the complications of CKD. Monitoring of kidney disease progression involves regular measurement of serum creatinine, blood urea nitrogen, electrolyte, calcium, phosphorus, albumin, and magnesium concentrations. A complete blood count is also necessary.

Creatinine and urea have several major limitations in estimation of kidney function accurately.[8] Muscle mass is perhaps the single most important factor for the limited accuracy of creatinine as a measure of kidney function. This is because creatinine is a byproduct of creatine metabolism, which is a product of muscle breakdown. Thus, individuals with large muscle mass generate greater amounts of endogenous creatine and therefore have a higher steady-state serum creatinine level, even though their kidney function as measured by GFR is in the normal range.[9] On the other hand, individuals with smaller muscle mass, such as elderly patients, will have a serum creatinine concentration within the normal range but will have lower than normal kidney function as measured by the GFR.[9] Urea levels reflect the metabolic state of the body. In highly anabolic individuals, a "normal" level may even suggest significant abnormal-

ity in kidney function (e.g., pregnant women will have blood urea levels that are markedly depressed). In contrast, a very high urea level may be observed in highly catabolic patients, such as those who are critically ill or receiving large doses of corticosteroids. Therefore, interpretation of a very high blood urea nitrogen level should be done in concert with the serum creatinine measurement.

Kidney function can be measured more accurately by calculation of the creatinine clearance and urea clearance with 24-hour collection of urine. These methods also have limitations because they are dependent on the compulsiveness of the patient in collection procedures; however, they are very useful in practice—often more so than a serum creatinine measurement. A creatinine clearance measurement is reasonably accurate until kidney function is severely impaired. This is because creatinine is both filtered freely by glomeruli and secreted by the proximal tubule. Thus, as kidney function declines, the proportion of creatinine that is secreted over that which is filtered increases. Hence, as kidney function declines, the creatinine clearance tends to underestimate the impairment of GFR. In contrast, urea clearance is an overestimation of GFR; despite the fact that urea is freely filtered by the glomerulus and not secreted by the proximal tubule, it undergoes a variable degree of reabsorption in the distal nephron—its reabsorption being crucial for the maintenance of a hyperosmolar medullary interstitium. In low-flow states, such as dehydration, urea is reabsorbed in the collecting duct of the distal nephron. Consequently, urea clearance values overestimate impairment in GFR.

More accurate measurement of kidney function is feasible through the measurement of inulin clearance and iothalamate or ethylenediaminetetraacetic acid clearance. These methods are not widely available, are expensive, and may be inconvenient for the patient to have performed. Most recently, the use of cimetidine-blocked creatinine clearance and of estimating equations, such as the Modification of Diet in Renal Disease (MDRD) formula, have become popular.[10,11]

The National Kidney Foundation recommends the use of either the full (MDRD 1) or abbreviated MDRD formula because among patients with CKD, it most closely approximates actual kidney function (Table 116-3). The MDRD equation to predict GFR was developed in 1999. The equation is based on 1628 nondiabetic subjects, aged 18 to 70 years, with renal insufficiency. The formula uses urea, creatinine, and albumin as well as demographics of age, gender, and race (black or white). If race is unavailable and white race is assumed, the GFR will be underestimated by 18% if the patient is black. The equation has been validated in both diabetic and nondiabetic patients and in kidney transplant recipients. It works well in estimating kidney function in whites and in blacks. However, it has not been adequately validated in Latinos, Chinese and other Asians, and individuals with extremes of body mass. It is important to know that the MDRD equation underestimates kidney function among

TABLE 116-3 MDRD Equations*

MDRD 1

$$GFR = 170 \times [S_{Cr}]^{-0.999} \times [age]^{-0.176} \times [0.762 \text{ if patient is female}] \times [1.18 \text{ if patient is black}] \times [BUN]^{-0.170} \times [Alb]^{0.318}$$

MDRD abbreviated

$$GFR = 186 \times [S_{Cr}]^{-1.154} \times [age]^{-0.203} \times [0.742 \text{ if patient is female}] \times [1.212 \text{ if patient is black}]$$

*MDRD 1 is the complete equation; MDRD abbreviated is the shortened version and is most widely used clinically.
Alb, albumin; BUN, blood urea nitrogen; GFR, glomerular filtration rate; S_{Cr}, serum creatinine concentration.

individuals with normal or nearly normal kidney function. In 2000, a simplified MDRD equation (MDRD 2) was made available. It is based on serum creatinine as the only laboratory value—in the absence of urea or albumin. The MDRD formula yields an estimated GFR (eGFR) normalized to 1.73 m² body surface area. Adjustment for body surface area is necessary in comparing a patient's eGFR with normal values or in determining the stage of CKD. However, an uncorrected eGFR may be preferred for clinical use in some situations, such as drug dosing.

Measurement of iron stores (serum iron, ferritin, and total iron-binding capacity) and parathyroid hormone is recommended approximately every 3 months or more frequently if the patient is unstable or there is active treatment modification. In patients with early to moderate kidney dysfunction, measurement of proteinuria—either by a spot urine specimen to determine protein to creatinine ratio or by a 24-hour urine collection for protein excretion—is necessary, given the important role that proteinuria plays as a risk factor in kidney disease progression.

Screening for complications of CKD is important to reduce morbidity and mortality. In assessing for cardiovascular complications, annual echocardiography is increasingly being recommended to assess for early left ventricular hypertrophy.[12] An electrocardiographic study may also be used for this purpose, but its sensitivity is limited, particularly for early detection. Measurement of serum total cholesterol, low-density lipoprotein, high-density lipoprotein, triglycerides, and homocysteine levels is recommended because nearly 50% of individuals with end-stage kidney disease die of cardiovascular causes—commonly coronary artery disease. To screen for malnutrition, regular assessment by a dietitian is also recommended. Individuals with CKD spontaneously eat less than healthy age-matched controls do. Furthermore, the majority of patients who reach end-stage kidney failure in the United States have hypoalbuminemia, despite good evidence that suggests the importance of albumin as a marker for a poor outcome among patients receiving dialysis. Although anemia is a common complication in individuals with CKD, as a result of erythropoietin deficiency, it is important to rule out other causes of anemia, particularly if the patient has erythropoietin resistance. Screening for fecal occult blood and measurement of iron stores and serum folate are recommended.

Differential Diagnosis

Acute kidney failure

TREATMENT

Initial

The timely referral of the patient with CKD to a nephrologist is of great importance.[13] Studies demonstrate that early referral is associated with optimal management of the complications of CKD.[14,15] As well, there is time for elective construction of an arteriovenous fistula, rather than resorting to either a temporary catheter or a synthetic graft. In addition, early referral saves money and reduces the days of hospitalization.

The focus of treatment before dialysis becomes necessary is treatment of complications (such as anemia and bone disease), slowing of the progression of CKD, and management of complications. The treatment of complications rests on consensus and widely adopted guidelines from the National Kidney Foundation called the KDOQI guidelines.[16-18] The main thrusts of antiprogression therapy are the use of an angiotensin-converting enzyme (ACE) inhibitor (or, if the patient cannot tolerate an ACE inhibitor, an angiotensin receptor blocker); the optimal management of hypertension, targeting a mean arterial blood pressure of 92 mm Hg (120/80 mm Hg), particularly in patients who have CKD associated with significant (more than 1 g/24 hour) proteinuria; the implementation of strategies to reduce proteinuria; and the judicious use of a low-protein, high-calorie diet. In addition, the use of a hypolipidemic agent and early treatment of anemia with epoetin are important. A protocol to comprehensively manage the protean manifestations of CKD is highly recommended. One such protocol focuses on the 10 A's of CKD: anemia, atherosclerosis (cardiovascular disease), antiangiotensin therapy, albumin (nutrition), anions and cations (acidosis, hyperkalemia, hypermagnesemia), arterial blood pressure, arterial calcification (calcium × phosphorus product), access (vascular access), avoidance of nephrotoxic drugs, and allograft (timely referral for a kidney transplant evaluation).

Rehabilitation

Rehabilitation ensures that the patient remains intact both physically and psychologically as major changes in health and life status occur. In this regard, rehabilitation strategies have emerged as adjuncts in management of patients with CKD, especially those nearing the initiation of dialysis.[19-27] These strategies focus on two issues: an assessment of function and then a prescriptive component targeted at muscle strengthening and restoration of function. This is accomplished in some dialysis programs with exercise machines.

Referral to a physical or occupational therapist as an outpatient is an important part of the overall management. Initially, a physical medicine consultation is sought to assess the degree of physical and functional impairment. Evaluation of the patient in the home setting is particularly valuable and is usually orchestrated by the social worker in concert with the physical therapist, the occupational therapist, and a visiting nurse. Adaptations in the home may be necessary, particularly for elderly patients. These could range from obtaining new housing for patients who need ground floor accommodation or more space to facilitate equipment such as a dialysis machine to adaptations in the bathroom (e.g., raised toilet seat, railings to steady the patient, and shower adaptations). Modifications such as a bed with railings, safety adaptations to the kitchen, and a chair lift may also become necessary.

Education of patients with CKD is of crucial importance.[26,27] In addition to having an improved understanding of the treatment protocol, an informed patient is likely to make better choices about dialytic options and about whether he or she wishes to be considered for kidney transplantation. Many options for education are now available, but the most focused program is the "People Like Us" program of the National Kidney Foundation.[27]

Procedures

Temporary line insertion procedures are a much less desirable method to obtain vascular access for dialysis and should be contemplated only in patients who cannot undergo construction of an AV fistula or placement of an AV graft. On occasion, because patients present late or in cases in which CKD ensues after a devastating acute kidney insult, insertion of a tunneled internal jugular double-lumen dialysis catheter is necessary. It is important to insert the catheter into the jugular vein and not a subclavian vein because studies demonstrate that the subclavian vein has a substantially higher risk of stenosis in the setting of an indwelling line.

Surgery

The most common surgical procedure in patients with CKD is dialysis access. An early assessment of the patient's vascular access options by a vascular surgeon is very important. Patients are asked to save their nondominant veins during blood draws to facilitate future construction of vascular access. In the United States, an arteriovenous (AV) graft is the most common form of vascular access for dialysis, outnumbering AV fistulas in some centers by three to one. In contrast, in Europe, Canada, and even some American centers, AV grafts are in the minority. The reasons behind this variation include a higher rate of patients with diabetes with CKD in the United States, a higher rate of small-vessel disease (because of the higher prevalence of diabetes mellitus coupled with an older population), and a higher level of time and skill required to construct an AV fistula compared with an AV graft.

Although transplantation is the preferred option once the patient reaches end-stage kidney disease, this may not be feasible. Individuals may have comorbidities that preclude transplantation (e.g., there may be no readily available living related or unrelated donor, and the patient may have to wait 3 or 4 years for a cadaver kidney). Alternatively, the patient may prefer dialysis to transplantation as a lifestyle option. Because the failure and complication rates of an AV fistula are much lower than those of an AV synthetic graft (approximately 80% of AV grafts have failed 3 years after placement, whereas the reverse is true for AV fistulas), an AV fistula is highly recommended. Surgery is usually performed when the GFR has reached 25 to 30 mL/min and can be done on an outpatient basis. An AV fistula takes approximately 6 months to mature before it can be used, and therefore surgery should be planned at least 6 to 9 months before the anticipated initiation of dialysis treatment.

If the patient is to start hemodialysis, the dialysis access is either an AV fistula or an AV graft. In a minority of patients in whom dialysis is required emergently or in whom surgical construction or insertion of a dialysis access is not feasible, the use of a tunneled double-lumen catheter is the treatment of choice. On the other hand, in patients targeted to start peritoneal dialysis, surgical insertion of a tunneled peritoneal dialysis catheter (Tenckhoff catheter) into the anterior abdominal wall is necessary.

Vascular access for hemodialysis requires early planning, rigorous counseling of the patient about the choices available for dialysis access, and a good vascular surgeon. Access through an AV fistula is preferred in all patients receiving hemodialysis because of its advantage of long-term patency (more than 80% are patent at 3 years after construction) and a low complication rate. An AV fistula is the native anastomosis of an arm vein with an arm artery (e.g., the cephalic vein in the arm with the radial artery). In contrast, AV grafts have a low patency rate (nearly 80% fail by 3 years after surgery) and a higher complication rate. An AV graft is the surgical connection of a native vein and a native artery (e.g., an AV graft connects the cephalic vein with the radial artery).

If the patient is a viable candidate for kidney transplantation, this procedure is the treatment of choice from medical, quality of life, and cost perspectives. Potential contraindications include cardiopulmonary disease that places the patient at risk from the surgery; an underlying malignant disease; active infection, including positive human immunodeficiency virus (HIV) status; and active intravenous drug abuse. Age is not considered an absolute contraindication, although few elderly patients undergo transplantation. The inability to comply with medications and psychiatric disability are also relative contraindications. The workup for a kidney transplant recipient consists of a thorough physical examination, screening for infections (including HIV infection), and screening for underlying malignant disease. In patients with diabetes mellitus, formal cardiac testing, such as an exercise tolerance stress test and echocardiography, is recommended. Many centers also perform pulmonary function testing.

POTENTIAL DISEASE COMPLICATIONS

CKD may be associated with protean disease complications. However, complications in the cardiovascular system, bone and mineral metabolism, and hematologic system are of the greatest significance.

Life expectancy for a 49-year-old patient with CKD is approximately 7 years—lower than in colon and prostate cancer and one quarter that of the general population.[28] This staggering reduction in life expectancy is largely attributable to cardiovascular complications.[28,29] Nearly 50% of all deaths in patients with end-stage kidney failure are due to cardiovascular causes.[29] The risk is 17 times that of the general population. Remarkably, this gap is largest in young patients with end-stage kidney disease.[29] The risk factors for cardiovascular disease in individuals with CKD include but are not limited to the magnitude of the calcium-phosphorus product with its attendant risk of coronary calcification and the presence of dyslipidemia, hypertension, hyperhomocysteinemia, and left ventricular hypertrophy.[28,29] The clinical manifestations of cardiovascular disease in patients with CKD include left ventricular hypertrophy, left ventricular dilatation, diastolic dysfunction, macrovascular and microvascular disease, and abnormalities in autonomic function including increased sympathetic discharge and increased circulating catecholamine levels.[30] Indeed, there is now an extensive literature that addresses the role of traditional and nontraditional risk factors for cardiovascular disease in patients with CKD.[31] Traditional risk factors are those factors that have been used to estimate the risk for development of symptomatic ischemic heart disease in the Framingham study. Traditional Framingham cardiovascular disease risk factors (older age, diabetes mellitus, systolic hypertension, left ventricular hypertrophy) are highly prevalent in patients with CKD, and their relationship to cardiovascular disease is the same regardless of CKD status. On the other hand, there appears to be what has been termed a reverse epidemiology for other factors, such as hypertension and low-density lipoprotein cholesterol, among dialysis patients. The increased risk at lower levels of blood pressure and cholesterol may reflect confounding from cardiomyopathy and malnutrition, respectively, although this has not been proved. The role of nontraditional risk factors in influencing cardiovascular disease

risk in CKD is more controversial. Observational studies strongly suggest that factors such as proteinuria, hemoglobin level, inflammation, and calcium-phosphorus abnormalities are important; however, definitive evidence remains lacking. Some of these nontraditional risk factors are specific to kidney disease and worsen with progressive impairment of kidney function. It is likely that the increase in cardiovascular risk in patients with CKD is a multifactorial composite of both traditional cardiovascular risk factors and nontraditional kidney-specific risk factors. Many of these traditional factors and the nontraditional risk factors are modifiable and therefore need to be studied to assess whether treatment of these factors improves outcome.

Abnormalities in bone and mineral metabolism are common in individuals with CKD.[32,33] Patients may have both biochemical and skeletal abnormalities. Hypocalcemia, hyperphosphatemia, hypermagnesemia, and hyperparathyroidism are usually observed in some combination. In addition, bone effects may range from an abnormally high to an abnormally low bone turnover.[32] Kidney osteodystrophy is characterized by increased osteoclast and osteoblast activity coupled with peritrabecular fibrosis. Bone pain is the single most common manifestation of kidney osteodystrophy; it occurs mostly in the hips, lumbosacral spine, and legs and is usually nonspecific in nature. Acute periarthritis from metastatic calcification may also occur. Muscle weakness is also common. Other clinical manifestations of kidney osteodystrophy include pruritus, metastatic calcification, and calciphylaxis. All of these clinical manifestations progressively impair the patient's strength and functionality.

Anemia is an early and easily recognized complication of CKD.[34] Erythropoietin is produced predominantly by kidney interstitial cells and to a lesser degree by the liver. Erythropoietin production is markedly decreased in individuals with CKD, and as a consequence, anemia ensues. Other causes of anemia in CKD include direct marrow suppression by uremic toxins, shortened red cell survival, increased blood loss, and iron deficiency. The benefits of treating anemia with epoetin have been well established in the literature and include a better sense of well-being, enhanced cognitive function, regression of left ventricular hypertrophy, improved sleep pattern, and reduced hospitalizations. Current recommendations center on a target hemoglobin level of 11 to 13 g/dL and a hematocrit level of 33% to 39%.[17]

POTENTIAL TREATMENT COMPLICATIONS

Strategies to slow progression are now the centerpiece of management of CKD. Nevertheless, treatment complications may occur. Because ACE inhibitor therapy is a central component of antiprogression therapy (i.e., all patients with chronic kidney insufficiency and CKD should be targeted for ACE inhibitor therapy), complications include, most commonly, hyperkalemia, a dry cough, and a feeling of lassitude. In patients who have not reached the stage of advanced CKD, the use of the resin polystyrene in conjunction with a low-potassium diet allows continued use of an ACE inhibitor. Often, the patient's potassium level may stabilize on the high side of the normal range when polystyrene is taken every other day. Patients who experience a dry cough (about 15% of the ACE inhibitor–treated population) can instead be sufficiently treated with an angiotensin receptor blocker. ACE inhibitors may result in hemodynamically associated acute kidney failure in patients with bilateral kidney artery stenosis.

The use of low-protein diets in patients who are borderline malnourished may precipitate even worse malnutrition. Withdrawal of the low-protein diet in these circumstances is important. In addition, it is important to ensure that the patient is consuming sufficient calories. Referral to a dietitian is an important adjunct to management that specifically addresses these issues.

Complications of AV grafts (and, to a lesser extent, of AV fistulas) include, most commonly, thrombosis and infection. Thrombosis of an AV graft is probably the most common reason for a patient with end-stage kidney disease to be admitted to the hospital.

Kidney transplantation is very successful. One-year kidney survival rates are more than 95% for transplants from living related and unrelated donors, whereas the 1-year rate is 90% to 95% for cadaver kidney transplantation. Longer term survival is in the 80% range at 5 years. The most common complications are early nonfunction, acute rejection, mechanical issues (such as obstruction of the allograft), and chronic allograft rejection. As well, depending on the underlying kidney disease, recurrent disease in the allograft may be manifested as a complication. Immunosuppressive treatment includes a calcineurin inhibitor (cyclosporine or FK506), mycophenolate mofetil (CellCept), and prednisone. Treatment of rejection involves pulsing with methylprednisolone acutely and a "rescue" strategy with either muromonab-CD3 (OKT3) or antithymocyte globulin.

References

1. Incidence and prevalence of ESRD. United States Renal Data System. Am J Kidney Dis 1998;32:S38-S49.
2. El Nahas M. Progression of CKD. In Johnson RJ, Freehally J, eds. Comprehensive Clinical Nephrology. London, Mosby, 2000: 67.1-67.10.
3. Winearls CG. In Johnson RJ, Freehally J, eds. Comprehensive Clinical Nephrology. London, Mosby, 2000:68.1-68.14.
4. Hakim RM, Lazarus JM. Initiation of dialysis. J Am Soc Nephrol 1995;6:1319-1328.
5. Furr LA. Psycho-social aspects of serious kidney disease and dialysis: a review of the literature. Soc Work Health Care 1998; 27:97-118.
6. Iborra MC, Pico VL, Montiel CA, Clemente R. Quality of life and exercise in kidney disease. EDTNA ERCA J 2000;26:38-40.
7. Fitts SS, Guthrie MR, Blagg CR. Exercise coaching and rehabilitation counseling improve quality of life for predialysis and dialysis patients. Nephron 1999;82:115-121.
8. Levey AS. Measurement of kidney function in chronic kidney disease. Kidney Int 1990;38:167-184.
9. Perrone RD, Madias NE, Levey AS. Serum creatinine as an index of kidney function: new insights into old concepts. Clin Chem 1992;38:1933-1953.
10. Walser M. Assessing kidney function from creatinine measurements in adults with CKD. Am J Kidney Dis 1998;32:23-31.
11. Levey AS, Bosch JP, Lewis JB, et al. A more accurate method to estimate glomerular filtration rate from serum creatinine: a new prediction equation. Modification of Diet in Renal Disease Study Group. Ann Intern Med 1999;130:461-470.
12. Murphy SW, Parfrey PS. Screening for cardiovascular disease in dialysis patients. Curr Opin Nephrol Hypertens 1996;5:532-540.
13. Pereira BJ. Optimization of pre-ESRD care: the key to improved dialysis outcomes. Kidney Int 2000;57:351-365.
14. Obrador GT, Ruthazer R, Arora P, et al. Prevalence of and factors associated with suboptimal care before initiation of dialysis in the United States. J Am Soc Nephrol 1999;10:1793-1800.
15. Arora P, Obrador GT, Ruthazer R, et al. Prevalence, predictors, and consequences of late nephrology referral at a tertiary care center. J Am Soc Nephrol 1999;10:1281-1286.
16. National Kidney Foundation. K/DOQI clinical practice guidelines for bone metabolism and disease in chronic kidney disease. Am J Kidney Dis 2003;42(Suppl 3):S1-S201.
17. Kidney Disease Outcomes Quality Initiative (KDOQI) Group; National Kidney Foundation. KDOQI clinical practice guidelines and clinical practice recommendations for anemia in chronic kidney disease. Am J Kidney Dis 2006;47(Suppl 3):S11-S145.
18. Kidney Disease Outcomes Quality Initiative (K/DOQI) Group. K/DOQI clinical practice guidelines for management of dyslipidemias in patients with kidney disease. Am J Kidney Dis 2003;41(Suppl 3):I-IV, S1-S91.
19. Tawney KW, Tawney PJ, Hladik G, et al. The life readiness program: a physical rehabilitation program for patients on hemodialysis. Am J Kidney Dis 2000;36:581-591.
20. Thornton TA, Hakim RM. Meaningful rehabilitation of the end-stage kidney disease patient [review]. Semin Nephrol 1997;17:246-252.
21. Cowen TD, Huang CT, Lebow J, et al. Functional outcomes after inpatient rehabilitation of patients with end-stage kidney disease. Arch Phys Med Rehabil 1995;76:355-359.
22. Oberley ET, Sadler JH, Alt PS. Kidney rehabilitation: obstacles, progress, and prospects for the future. Am J Kidney Dis 2000;35(Suppl 1):S141-S147.
23. Kutner NG, Cardenas DD, Bower JD. Rehabilitation, aging and chronic kidney disease. Am J Phys Med Rehabil 1992;71:97-101.
24. Callahan MB, LeSage L, Johnstone S. A model for patient participation in quality of life measurement to improve rehabilitation outcomes. Nephrol News Issues 1999;13:33-37.
25. Orr ML. Pre-dialysis patient education. J Nephrol Nurs 1985; 2:22-24.
26. Gorrie S. Patient education: a commitment. ANNA J 1992;19: 504, 506.
27. King K. People like us, live: an interactive patient education program. EDTNA ERCA J 1997;23:34-35, 50.
28. Port FK. Morbidity and mortality in dialysis patients. Kidney Int 1994;46:1728-1737.
29. Sarnak MJ, Levey AS, Schoolwerth AC, Coresh J. Kidney disease as a risk factor for development of cardiovascular disease: a statement from the American Heart Association Councils on Kidney in Cardiovascular Disease, High Blood Pressure Research, Clinical Cardiology, and Epidemiology and Prevention. Circulation 2003;108:2154-2169.
30. Foley RN, Parfrey PS, Sarnak MJ. Clinical epidemiology of cardiovascular disease in chronic kidney disease. Am J Kidney Dis 1998;32(Suppl 3):S112-S119.
31. Shlipak MG, Fried LF, Cushman M, et al. Cardiovascular mortality risk in chronic kidney disease: comparison of traditional and novel risk factors. JAMA 2005;293:1737.
32. Llach F, Yudd M. Pathogenic, clinical, and therapeutic aspects of secondary hyperparathyroidism in CKD. Am J Kidney Dis 1998;32(Suppl 2):S3-S12.
33. Sherrard DJ, Hercz G, Pei Y, et al. The spectrum of bone disease in end-stage kidney failure—an evolving disorder. Kidney Int 1993;43:436-442.
34. Pendse S, Singh AK. Complications of chronic kidney disease: anemia, mineral metabolism, and cardiovascular disease. Med Clin North Am 2005;89:549-561.

Joint Contractures 117

Nancy Dudek, MD, MEd, and Guy Trudel, MD

Synonyms

Arthrofibrosis
Capsulitis
Ankylosis

ICD-9 Codes

M24.5 Contracture of joint
M24.6 Ankylosis of joint

DEFINITION

A joint contracture is a limitation in the passive range of motion of a joint. Changes in articular structures (bone, cartilage, capsule), muscles, tendons, or skin can prevent a joint from moving passively through its full range. A classification according to the tissue limiting the range of motion is proposed in Table 117-1.

By this definition, regardless of the nature of the tissue alteration, if it results in joint motion limitation, the joint condition is called a joint contracture. For example, a muscle with adaptive shortening or fibrosis restricting joint motion is classified as "joint contracture—myogenic type." It should not be referred to as a muscle contracture.

As such, joint motion limited by pain or spasticity qualifies as a joint contracture only if the limitation is demonstrated after the pain or the influence of the hyperactive upper motor neuron (increased tone, spasticity, co-contraction) has been removed. For example, when a person with a spinal cord injury is treated for spasticity, the tone in the lower extremities will be reduced and an apparent chronic ankle plantar flexion contracture may disappear.

Conventionally, a joint contracture is named according to the joint involved and the direction *opposite* the lack of range. Some examples: a knee flexion contracture lacks full extension; an elbow extension contracture lacks full flexion; and an ankle plantar flexion contracture lacks dorsiflexion.

A contracture is the final common path of numerous conditions preventing movement of a joint through its full range of motion. Pain, trauma, immobility, weakness, and edema commonly contribute to reduced joint range of motion. The body's natural reaction to a painful joint is to "splint" or immobilize it. This results in the joint's not moving through its full range and places it at risk for development of a contracture. Joints traumatized by fracture or reconstructive surgery, such as anterior cruciate ligament repair or arthroplasty, are susceptible to contractures.[1] Joint contractures can happen as a consequence of the disease (prolonged immobility in bed in intensive care units; Fig. 117-1) or as part of the treatment (casting after fracture or prolonged use of a brace). Any joint can be affected.

Neurologic conditions that increase muscle tone or cause weakness contribute to contractures because of unequal strength in opposing muscle groups. In upper motor neuron conditions, such as after a stroke or traumatic brain injury, spasticity and excessive muscle tone prevent a joint from accessing portions of its normal range.[2] Similarly, in lower motor neuron injuries, such as a plexopathy or peripheral nerve injury, the unopposed muscle pull will limit joint motion toward the paralyzed muscle. The range of motion not accessed will eventually be lost, resulting in a joint contracture.

A number of other local conditions, such as arthritis, joint infections, and burns, will cause contractures.[3] In addition, systemic conditions, such as muscular dystrophy, diabetes, Parkinson disease, and Alzheimer disease, can limit mobility or initiation and put the patient at risk for contractures.

Data on incidence and prevalence of joint contractures are limited and often describe one specific joint.[4] Nevertheless, these studies indicate a common problem. At least one joint contracture was noted in 7% to 51% of persons after a spinal cord injury.[5-7] Between 16% and 81% of persons with an acquired brain injury developed a joint contracture,[2,8,9] and 51% of children who had an obstetric brachial plexus injury were found to have a shoulder contracture.[10] In institutionalized elderly, one research reported that 71% of those who were immobile had a joint contracture, whereas none of the mobile patients had a joint contracture.[11]

TABLE 117-1   Classification of Contractures According to the Tissue Causing Restriction in the Range of Motion of the Joint

Type	Example*
Arthrogenic	
Bone	Intra-articular fracture
Cartilage	Osteochondritis dissecans
Synovium	Pigmented villonodular synovitis, synovial chondromatosis
Capsular	Secondary to immobility, adhesive capsulitis, arthrofibrosis
Other	Meniscal tear, labrum tear
Myogenic	
Muscle	Muscle fibrosis, myositis ossificans, muscle adaptation to altered neurologic supply (spasticity, flaccidity)
Fascia	Eosinophilic fasciitis
Tendinous	Tendon transposition, shortening
Cutaneous	Burn, scleroderma
Mixed (any combination of the above types)	Burn and adhesive capsulitis

*One or more clinical conditions illustrate each type of joint contracture.

SYMPTOMS

Joint contractures develop insidiously and progress asymptomatically. They are painful only with attempts to move the joint through its full range beyond the restriction. Many daily activities do not require a joint to move through its entire range. Therefore, a contracture may develop unnoticed for extended periods until the joint restriction interferes with functional activity. In the outpatient setting, patients with hand and finger joint contractures might present with complaints of a weak or ineffective grasp. A patient with a knee flexion contracture may present with complaints of a limp[3] or of hip or low back pain.

PHYSICAL EXAMINATION

The patient must be relaxed, properly positioned, and in no pain. The clinician inspects the patient for abnormalities of limb shape, size, symmetry, and position. Edema or deformity of the joints is noted. Skin is also assessed for any areas of breakdown or thickening complicating a contracture. Palpation of joints for swelling and tenderness must be completed.

Passive range of motion is particularly important when weakness prevents normal active movement. The most precise tool for joint measurement is a universal goniometer (Fig. 117-2). Comparison is made with the contralateral side or with normative values.[12]

It is important to complete a neuromuscular examination. Particular attention must be paid to strength and specifically to the presence of any muscle imbalance. Reflexes and tone are assessed, and in the presence of spasticity, the clinician should optimize medication and then apply prolonged passive stretch (sometimes by use of therapeutic heating modalities) to determine whether a full range of motion can be achieved by overcoming the increased muscle tone. Finally, a sensory examination is completed because abnormal sensation will influence the choice of treatment modalities.

FUNCTIONAL LIMITATIONS

Joint contractures affect the performance of activities of daily living. Functional limitations depend on the underlying medical condition and the joints affected.

Upper extremity contractures of the elbow, wrist, and fingers impair the performance of all basic activities of daily living, such as dressing and grooming, as well as advanced skills requiring fine motor coordination, like writing. In continuing care, half as many residents with an upper limb contracture fed themselves compared with those without a contracture.[13]

Lower extremity contractures interfere with mobility. Multiple joint contractures exacerbate disability. The

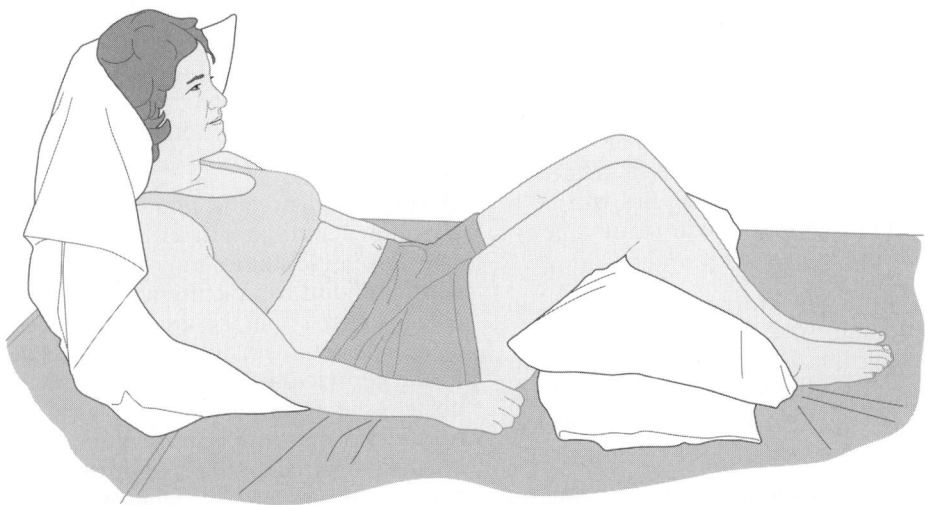

FIGURE 117-1. Prolonged bed rest is a risk factor for contractures in multiple joints.

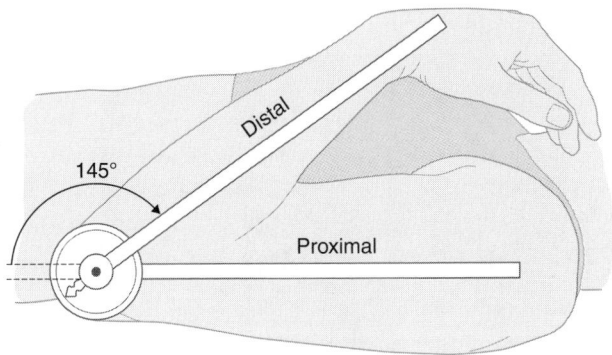

FIGURE 117-2. Example of how to measure a joint with a universal goniometer. (Modified from Norkin CC, White DJ. Measurement of Joint Motion: A Guide to Goniometry, 3rd ed. Philadelphia, FA Davis, 2003.)

mobility of continuing care residents with a lower limb contracture is significantly reduced.[13] Hip and knee flexion contractures alter gait pattern, energy expenditure, wheelchair mobility, and car transfers. Patients with transtibial amputations are at risk for development of a knee flexion contracture after their amputation (Fig. 117-3A). This may result in an inability to fit that patient with the most functional below-knee prosthesis. Instead, a bent-knee prosthesis, offering the patient less function and increased energy cost, must be used (Fig. 117-3B).

DIAGNOSTIC STUDIES

The diagnosis of a joint contracture is clinical. Radiographic evaluation can identify contributing conditions, such as osteophytes and heterotopic ossification. If a systemic cause is suspected, specific investigations are indicated.

Differential Diagnosis

Spasticity

Heterotopic ossification

Degenerative joint disease

Fracture

Dislocation

Loose body in a joint

Meniscal tears

Psychogenic

These conditions could present as a joint contracture, but the apparent contracture would resolve with treatment. However, these conditions can also be present alongside a true contracture, so a stepwise assessment may be needed to arrive at the correct diagnosis.

TREATMENT

Initial

The initial "treatment" of contractures is prevention. Moving joints actively or passively through their full range on a daily basis prevents contractures. Continuous passive motion devices, such as those used after total knee joint arthroplasty, can achieve this in postoperative situations.[14]

Pain control is essential to the prevention and treatment of contractures, particularly after a surgical procedure.[15] Appropriate use of analgesics will promote the patient's comfort and compliance with stretching sessions.

Therapeutic positioning and splinting prevent contractures in immobilized patients.[15] These measures maintain the correct length of connective tissue and rotate between different positions of the joint. An example of therapeutic positioning is lying prone to stretch the hip joint in extension. External rotation and abduction of the shoulders with an arm support attached to the bed of patients in the intensive care unit will maintain shoulder range. Standing upright will help stretch the ankle joints. Hand and finger as well as ankle static orthoses are useful for preventing finger and ankle contractures.

Rehabilitation

Once contractures have developed, rehabilitation includes sustained stretching and range of motion exercises. Again, analgesia and control of spasticity should be optimized to benefit the stretching sessions.

Therapeutic modalities are commonly used to potentiate the effect of stretching sessions. The combination of modalities that heat soft tissues with stretching is an effective treatment. Ultrasound, for example, heats soft tissues around large joints to a therapeutic temperature range of 40°C to 43°C, improving their elasticity.[15] Small joints can be heated by the use of paraffin bath dips or hydrotherapy (e.g., for hand and finger contractures in scleroderma or nerve injury).

Dynamic bracing can achieve prolonged, continuous stretching of joint contractures. Serial casting or serial splinting is also used with the same intent. After maximal stretching, a cast or orthosis is applied. The cast or orthosis is removed every 2 or 3 days, stretching is repeated, and the cast or orthosis is reapplied at an enhanced angle (Fig. 117-4). Serial casting or splinting should be carefully monitored on limbs with circulatory or sensory compromise.

Provision of assistive devices to lessen specific disability and of gait aids to try to normalize gait completes the rehabilitation process.

Procedures

If spasticity is thought to maintain contractures, despite optimized oral medication, treatments such as motor point blocks with phenol, botulinum toxin injections, or intrathecal baclofen are considered. These procedures

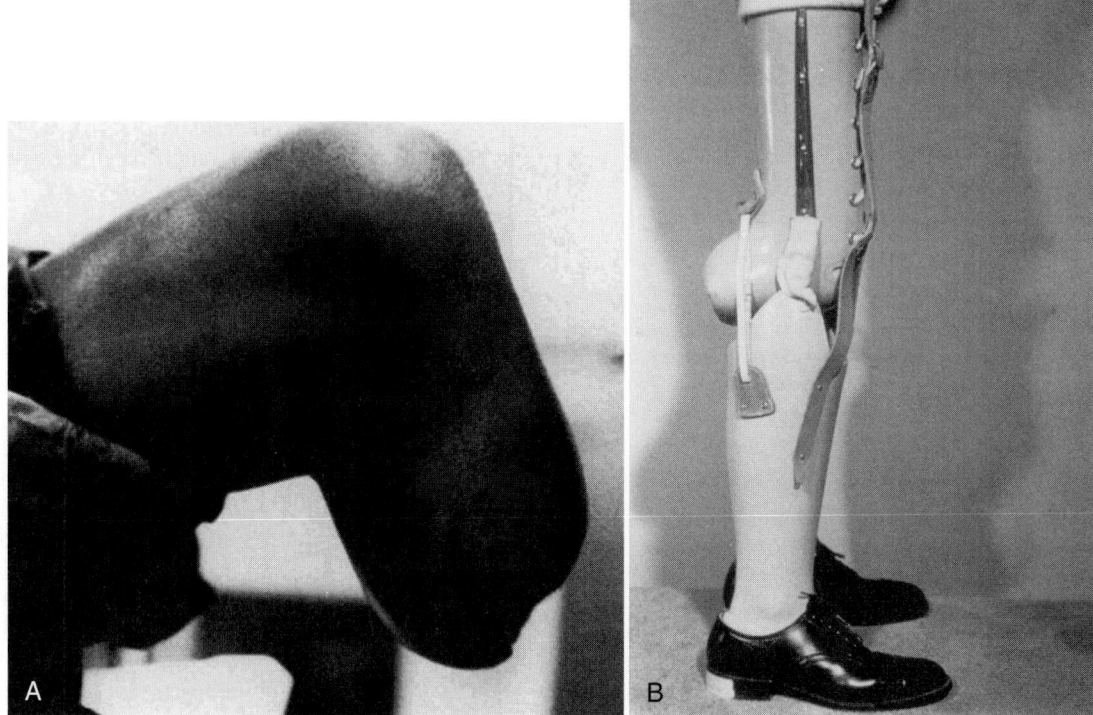

FIGURE 117-3. **A,** Knee flexion contracture in a below-knee (transtibial) amputee. **B,** Example of a bent-knee prosthesis.

can be diagnostic as well as therapeutic because they can differentiate a joint contracture from spasticity. The injection can constitute an adjunct to dynamic bracing and serial casting or splinting.

Surgery

In fixed contractures, surgical treatments include tenotomy, tendon lengthening, joint capsule release, and joint reconstruction. These procedures are reserved for patients in whom less aggressive methods of treatment have failed and the fixed contractures significantly affect function.[15]

POTENTIAL DISEASE COMPLICATIONS

Joint contracture can lead to ankylosis of a joint with corresponding loss of function. Upper limb contractures, especially if they are affecting multiple joints, can lead to dependency for all aspects of care. Mobility can be decreased to a bedridden state. Pressure sores can develop because of the limited options for mobility and weight-bearing areas. Infection by bacteria and fungal agents can occur in the skin folds if contractures prevent adequate access for hygiene.

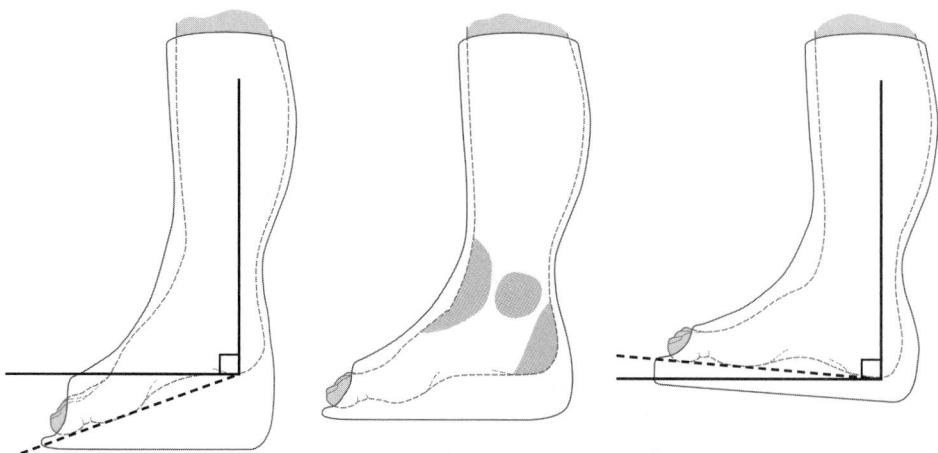

FIGURE 117-4. Serial short leg casts depicting a reduction of plantar flexion contracture of 20 degrees to a final holding cast at 5 degrees of dorsiflexion. Several intermediate casts between the initial and final holding casts may be required to achieve gradual dorsiflexion range.

POTENTIAL TREATMENT COMPLICATIONS

Aggressive stretching can inadvertently result in pain; tears in muscle, ligament, or capsule; and joint subluxation. These complications can lead to bleeding, especially in patients with thrombocytopenia or receiving anticoagulation.

Splinting and casting can result in skin ulceration or limb ischemia if patients are inappropriately selected or not closely monitored. This risk is increased if the patient lacks protective sensation because of the underlying disease.

References

1. Scuderi GR. The stiff total knee arthroplasty—causality and solution. J Arthroplasty 2005;20:23-26.
2. Singer BJ, Jegasothy GM, Singer KP, et al. Incidence of ankle contracture after moderate to severe acquired brain injury. Arch Phys Med Rehabil 2004;85:1465-1469.
3. Buschbacher RM, Porter CD. Deconditioning, conditioning, and the benefits of exercise. In Braddom RL, ed. Physical Medicine and Rehabilitation, 2nd ed. Philadelphia, WB Saunders, 2000:706-708.
4 Fergusson D, Hutton B, Drodge A. The epidemiology of major joint contractures: a systematic review of the literature. Clin Orthop and Related Res 2007;456:22-29.
5. Krause JS. Aging after spinal cord injury: an exploratory study. Spinal Cord 2000;38:77-83.
6. Vogel LC, Krajci KA, Anderson CJ. Adults with pediatric-onset spinal cord injury: part 2: musculoskeletal and neurological complications. J Spinal Cord Med 2002;25:117-123.
7. Bryden AM, Kilgore KL, Lind BB, Yu DT. Triceps denervation as a predictor of elbow flexion contractures in C5 and C6 tetraplegia. Arch Phys Med Rehabil 2004;85:1880-1885.
8. Pohl M, Mehrholz J. A new shoulder range of motion screening measurement: its reliability and application in the assessment of the prevalence of shoulder contractures in patients with impaired consciousness caused by severe brain damage. Arch Phys Med Rehabil 2005;86:98-104.
9. Yarkony GM, Sahgal V. Contractures. A major complication of craniocerebral trauma. Clin Orthop Relat Res 1987;219:93-96.
10. Hoeksma A, Ter Steeg AM, Dijkstra P, et al. Shoulder contracture and osseous deformity in obstetrical brachial plexus injuries. J Bone Joint Surg Am 2003;85:316-322.
11. Selikson S, Damus K, Hamerman D. Risk factors associated with immobility. J Am Geriatr Soc 1988;36:707-712.
12. Norkin CC, White DJ: Measurement of Joint Motion: A Guide to Goniometry, 3rd ed. Philadelphia, FA Davis, 2003.
13. Yip B, Stewart DA, Roberts MA. The prevalence of joint contractures in residents in NHS continuing care. Health Bull (Edinb) 1996;54:338-343.
14. Salter RB. Continuous Passive Motion (CPM). A Biological Concept. For the Healing and Regeneration of Articular Cartilage, Ligaments, and Tendons. From Origination to Research to Clinical Applications. Baltimore, Williams & Wilkins, 1993.
15. Halar EM, Bell KR. Immobility and inactivity: physiological and functional changes, prevention, and treatment. In DeLisa JA, ed. Physical Medicine and Rehabilitation: Principles and Practice, 4th ed. Philadelphia, Lippincott Williams & Wilkins, 2004:1452-1463.

Deep Venous Thrombosis 118

Jonas Sokolof, DO, and Ricardo Knight, MD, PT

Synonyms

Venous thromboembolism
Blood clot
Thrombophlebitis
Phlebothrombosis

ICD-9 Code

451.1   Phlebitis and thrombophlebitis, of deep vessels of lower extremities

DEFINITION

Deep venous thrombosis (DVT) occurs when a fibrin clot abnormally occludes a vein in the deep venous system. The circumstances that are necessary for DVTs to develop are classically described by Virchow's triad, which includes venous stasis, intimal injury, and hypercoagulopathy. The risk for development of DVT varies according to specific characteristics of the patient, the surgical procedure, or the medical condition (Table 118-1).

Surgical patients can be placed in categories according to their risk for development of venous thromboembolism (VTE),[1] with orthopedic surgery patients carrying the highest risk[2] (Table 118-2). It is believed that orthopedic procedures carry such a high risk for VTE because the mechanical destruction of bone marrow during most orthopedic procedures causes intravasation of marrow cells and cell fragments and elevations of plasma tissue factor.[3] Tissue factor is a potent trigger of blood clotting[4] and is found in high concentration in bone marrow and the adventitia surrounding the major blood vessels and the brain, putting neurosurgical patients at great risk for development of VTE. After neurosurgery, the incidence of VTE has been reported to be as high as 50%.[5] Risk factors that increase the rates of VTE in neurosurgery patients include intracranial surgery, malignant tumors, duration of the surgery, and presence of paresis or paralysis of the lower limbs.[6] Patients can remain in this postsurgical hypercoagulable state for weeks after surgery.[7]

In addition to surgical patients, victims of orthopedic and neurologic trauma are at great risk for development of DVT, especially if long bone fracture or paralysis is involved. Patients who suffer spinal cord injury are in high jeopardy of VTE because of stasis and hypercoagulability. Other conditions that may predispose one to VTE are malignant disease, morbid obesity, previous history of VTE, stroke, irritable bowel syndrome, and congestive heart failure.

Pregnancy, prolonged immobility, advanced age, and certain hereditary conditions also predispose to development of VTE. Hereditary conditions include deficiencies in protein C and protein S and familial thrombophilia. Acquired deficiencies of the natural anticoagulant system include antibodies directed against antiphospholipid. The frequency of thromboembolism increases with age; this may be related to a heterozygous factor V Leiden mutation.[8]

SYMPTOMS

Venous thrombosis often occurs asymptomatically. If this is not the case, a pulmonary embolus is typically the first symptom. Other symptoms of VTE may include lower extremity edema, fever, extremity warmth, and pain. Symptoms can serve only as a trigger for further diagnostic inquiry; they cannot, by themselves, rule VTE in or out.

PHYSICAL EXAMINATION

The classic signs of DVT are tenderness, swelling, and warmth; a palpable cord can sometimes be felt. In the past, emphasis was placed on the presence of Homans sign and calf tenderness in making a clinical diagnosis of DVT; however, these physical examination findings have been found to be nonspecific with poor positive predictive values.[9] Significant asymmetric calf edema is an important sign and can be determined by taking the circumferential measurement of the calf 10 cm below the tibial tuberosity. A 3-cm difference in calf girth is considered a significant clinical difference. Like symptoms, physical examination findings are not sensitive or

TABLE 118-1 Risk Factors for Deep Venous Thrombosis

Patient Factors	Diseases	Procedures
Age > 40 years	Thrombophilia	Pelvic surgery
Obesity	Antithrombin III,	Lower limb
Varicose veins	protein C, protein	orthopedic
Immobility	S deficiency	surgery
Pregnancy	Antiphospholipid	Neurosurgery
High-dose	antibody, lupus	
estrogen therapy	anticoagulant	
Previous DVT	Malignant disease	
	Major medical illness	
	Trauma	
	Spinal cord injury	
	Paralysis	

specific; in more than 50% of the instances in which there was verified DVT, there was a normal physical examination.

FUNCTIONAL LIMITATIONS

DVT rarely causes functional compromise, except calf pain during walking. Absolute bed rest is generally not indicated, but patients should suspend their lower extremity exercise program until they are fully anticoagulated.

Pretest Probability

The Wells prediction rules (Table 118-3) are a group of clinical characteristics that are useful in estimating the pretest probability of DVT. High-quality evidence exists to support the validity of these rules, and their use is recommended as a practice guideline by the American Academy of Family Physicians and the American College of Physicians.[10] They are easily implemented before more definitive testing is performed on patients.[11]

DIAGNOSTIC STUDIES

Venography is the reference or "gold standard" for the diagnosis of DVT and is the only test that can reliably detect DVT isolated to the calf veins, the iliac veins, and the inferior vena cava (Figs. 118-1 and 118-2). The drawbacks to venography are its technical complexity, the requirement for the use of contrast dye, and the risk of allergic reaction.

Real-time, B-mode venous ultrasonography is the procedure of choice for the investigation of patients with suspected DVT. Venous ultrasonography allows direct visualization of the vein lumen; inability to compress that lumen is the main criterion for a positive test result. Other adjunctive findings include vein distention, absence of flow, echogenic signals within the vessel lumen, and visualization of filling defects by color Doppler study. Systematic reviews have demonstrated high sensitivities and specificities for the diagnosis of DVT in the proximal lower extremity by ultrasonography. However, sensitivities were poor for determination of the presence of calf vein thrombosis.

Visualization of calf veins by ultrasonography is technically more difficult and less reliable than diagnosis of venous thrombus in the area between the trifurcation of the popliteal vein and the femoral vein in the groin. Other noninvasive diagnostic methods include Doppler ultrasonography, impedance plethysmography, and ^{125}I-fibrinogen scanning for the presence or absence of fibrin accretion.

TABLE 118-2 Risk Categories of Venous Thromboembolism in Surgical Patients without Prophylaxis

Risk Category	Calf DVT	Proximal DVT	Fatal PE
High	40%-80%	10%-30%	1%-5%
Major orthopedic surgery of the lower limb			
Major general surgery in patients >40 years with cancer or recent DVT or PE			
Multiple trauma			
Thrombophilia			
Moderate	10%-40%	2%-10%	0.1%-0.8%
General surgery in patients >40 years that lasts 30 minutes or more without additional risk factors			
General surgery in patients <40 years receiving estrogen or with a history of DVT or PE			
Emergency cesarean section in women >35 years			
Low	<10%	<1%	<0.01%
Minor surgery (i.e., <30 minutes in patients >40 years without additional risk factors)			
Uncomplicated surgery in patients <40 years without additional risk factors			

DVT, deep venous thrombosis; PE, pulmonary embolism.
Modified from Bounameaux H. Integrating pharmacologic and mechanical prophylaxis of venous thromboembolism. Thromb Haemost 1999;82:931-939.

TABLE 118-3 Wells Prediction Rules: Clinical Evaluation Table for Predicting Pretest Probability of Deep Venous Thrombosis

Clinical Characteristic	Score
Active cancer (treatment ongoing, within previous 6 months, or palliative)	1
Paralysis, paresis, or recent plaster immobilization of the lower extremities	1
Recently bedridden > 3 days or major surgery within 12 weeks requiring general or regional anesthesia	1
Localized tenderness along the distribution of the deep venous system	1
Entire leg swollen	1
Calf swelling 3 cm larger than asymptomatic side (measured 10 cm below tibial tuberosity)	1
Pitting edema confined to the symptomatic leg	1
Collateral superficial veins (nonvaricose)	1
Alternative diagnosis at least as likely as deep venous thrombosis	−2

Clinical probability: low ≤ 0; intermediate 1-2; high ≥ 3. In patients with symptoms in both legs, the more symptomatic is used.
From Wells PS, Anderson DR, Bormanis J, et al. Value of assessment of pretest probability of deep-vein thrombosis in clinical management. Lancet 1997;350:1795-1798. Copyright 2002, Elsevier.

D-dimer assay has emerged as a method to help predict the presence of VTE. D-dimer is a degradation product of the cross-linked fibrin blood clot and as such is typically elevated in patients with VTE. D-dimer levels may also be elevated in a variety of nonthrombotic disorders, including recent major surgery, hemorrhage, trauma, malignant disease, and sepsis. Because of the high sensitivity (but low specificity) of the D-dimer assay, it is a good tool for exclusion of VTE if the test result is negative.

The first step in the diagnostic approach is the determination of risk. Patients can be separated by clinical criteria into high-, moderate-, and low-risk categories. A nine-point clinical criteria scoring system has been developed to determine a patient's pretest probability for DVT, and it can be a useful adjunct to noninvasive testing (see Table 118-3).[12,13] All symptomatic patients thought to have DVT should, at the very least, undergo venous ultrasound imaging of the proximal venous system. Patients at moderate or high risk should have the ultrasound study repeated in 1 week, or DVT may be ruled out on the basis of a negative result of the D-dimer assay. If the D-dimer assay result is positive, a follow-up ultrasound study in 1 week is indicated.

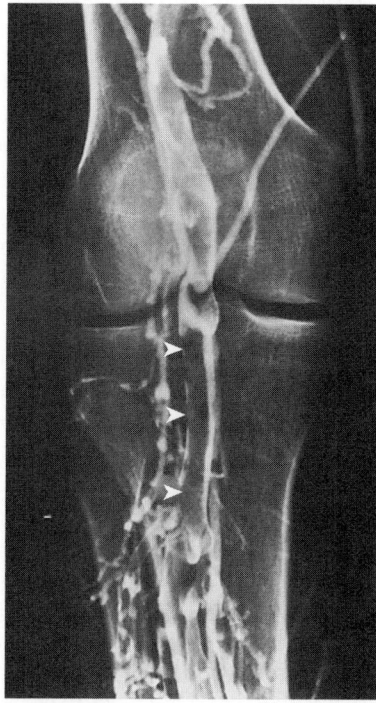

FIGURE 118-1. Acute deep venous thrombosis of popliteal vein. Note the intraluminal filling defect *(arrowheads)* and "tram-tracking" of contrast material around the thrombus.

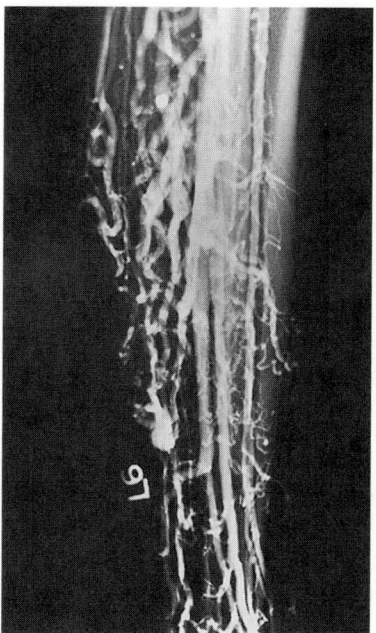

FIGURE 118-2. Chronic lower extremity deep venous thrombosis with abundant collaterals. (Reprinted with permission from Katz DS, Math KR, Groskin SA. Radiology Secrets. Philadelphia, Hanley & Belfus, 1998:527.)

Differential Diagnosis

Claudication

Ruptured Baker's cysts

Cellulitis

Hematoma

Lymphedema

TREATMENT

Initial

Nowhere in medicine is the aphorism "an ounce of prevention is worth a pound of cure" more appropriate than when the prevention of DVT is considered. The choice of the most appropriate prophylactic method depends on the clinical scenario and the risk-benefit profile for the particular patient. Unfractionated low-dose subcutaneous heparin (5000 units every 8 to 12 hours), although appropriate for most medical patients, has been slowly replaced by low-molecular-weight heparin (LMWH) as the agent of choice in many clinical situations. Large meta-analyses comparing LMWH with unfractionated heparin in general and orthopedic surgery[14] have shown LMWH as safe and more efficacious than unfractionated heparin. Antiplatelet agents such as aspirin also reduce the risk of VTE in some patients; however, the evidence is not overwhelming for use with more than low-risk patients. Low-dose warfarin is better than aspirin or placebo in patients with hip fractures but may not be satisfactory in preventing VTE after elective hip and knee surgery.

Mechanical VTE prophylaxis can be achieved with intermittent pneumatic leg compression, intermittent pneumatic foot compression, or graduated compression stockings. Intermittent pneumatic leg compression provides increase in peak flow velocity and flow in the common femoral vein and is better than placebo in preventing DVT. Intermittent pneumatic foot compression is a high-pressure system that exerts a compression limited to the foot. These devices are best for patients who undergo lower extremity orthopedic surgery and cannot be fitted with the intermittent pneumatic leg compression devices. The intermittent pneumatic foot compression devices offer no advantage over LMWH in the prevention of DVTs, except for a lower rate of bleeding complications. Graded compression elastic stockings work by increasing venous blood flow velocity. Knee-length stockings are sized to fit, and they deliver graduated pressure of 40 mm Hg at the ankle, 36 mm Hg at the lower calf, and 21 mm Hg at the upper calf.

The optimal duration of pharmacologic prophylaxis also varies with individual risk and clinical situation. Current standard of care is to stop prophylaxis 7 to 10 days after a surgical procedure or, in medical patients, when the patient is ambulating freely. After major orthopedic surgery, prolongation of prophylaxis to 4 to 6 weeks is most advantageous. In patients with spinal cord injuries, prophylaxis is best maintained for 6 to 10 weeks.

The goal of treatment is to prevent local extension of thrombosis, embolization, and recurrent thrombosis. The cornerstone of medical treatment of DVT is anticoagulation therapy. Evidence for its efficacy comes from a study that showed death in 26% of patients who had clinically suspected pulmonary embolism and did not receive anticoagulation, compared with no deaths in the treatment group.[15]

An analysis of 16 systematic reviews of clinical trials revealed that there is high-quality evidence to support the use of LMWH over unfractionated heparin in the treatment of established DVT.[16] Furthermore, the risk of major bleeding during initial therapy appears to be reduced with these agents.[16] When unfractionated heparin is used, the early establishment of an activated prothrombin time in the therapeutic range is essential. Many medical centers have adopted some kind of weight-adjusted nomogram to increase the likelihood of obtaining a therapeutic anticoagulation effect early. The nomogram that has been found to achieve the most rapid acquisition of the target activated prothrombin time is one in which the initial bolus of 80 units/kg is followed by an infusion rate of 18 units/kg per hour. Activated prothrombin time should be checked every 4 to 6 hours until a therapeutic range of 1.5 is achieved.

The duration of heparin treatment ranges between 4 and 10 days. Patients with large iliofemoral vein thrombosis or major pulmonary embolism require a 7- to 10-day course of heparin, with a delay in the initiation of warfarin until the activated prothrombin time is in the therapeutic range. Studies demonstrate that a 4- to 5-day course of heparin with warfarin administered within 24 hours of heparin initiation in patients without major pulmonary embolism of large proximal clots was as effective as 9 to 10 days of heparin.

LMWHs are fragments of unfractionated heparin produced by either chemical or enzymatic depolymerization. LMWHs display improved bioavailability, dose-independent clearance, and more predictable dose response compared with unfractionated heparin. These agents can therefore usually be given once or twice daily subcutaneously in weight-adjusted doses without laboratory monitoring.

The U.S. Food and Drug Administration has approved two LMWHs, dalteparin (Fragmin) and enoxaparin (Lovenox), for perioperative VTE prophylaxis (Table 118-4). There are two other LMWHs available for use in DVT treatment, tinzaparin (Innohep) and nadroparin. Enoxaparin and tinzaparin are approved for DVT treatment in the United States and Canada. Dalteparin and nadroparin are approved for this use only in Canada. Ardeparin (Normiflo) is another LMWH previously used for DVT treatment, but it was later withdrawn from the market. Enoxaparin can be used for the inpatient with DVT with

TABLE 118-4 U.S. Food and Drug Administration–Approved Uses of Low-Molecular-Weight Heparins

Name	FDA-Approved Indications	Dosage
Dalteparin (Fragmin)	DVT prophylaxis	5000 units SC daily
Enoxaparin (Lovenox)	DVT prophylaxis after knee surgery	30 mg SC q12h
	DVT prophylaxis after hip surgery	30 mg SC q12h or 40 mg SC daily
	DVT prophylaxis after abdominal surgery	40 mg SC daily
	Inpatient treatment of acute DVT with or without PE	1 mg/kg SC q12h or 1.5 mg/kg SC daily
	Outpatient treatment of acute DVT without PE	1 mg/kg SC q12h

DVT, deep venous thrombosis; PE, pulmonary embolism.

or without pulmonary embolism and for outpatient treatment of DVT without pulmonary embolism.

Unmonitored outpatient therapy with LMWH is thought to be as safe and effective as in-hospital intravenous unfractionated heparin in patients with proximal DVT.[17] Like patients receiving unfractionated heparin, those treated with LMWH should begin taking warfarin within 24 to 48 hours. LMWH can be discontinued after a minimum of 5 days, provided the international normalized ratio (INR) has been therapeutic for 2 consecutive days.

Thrombolytic therapy has a limited role in the treatment of DVT. It has been suggested that pharmacologic lysis of DVT could prevent post-thrombotic syndrome if complete lysis can be achieved before valve destruction occurs. However, thrombolysis, whether it is given systemically or by catheter, is expensive; the risk of bleeding complications is higher, and the evidence of additional benefit is not convincing. Thrombolysis should be reserved for patients with massive iliofemoral thrombosis or unstable cardiac or pulmonary disease with no contraindications to thrombolytic therapy.

After initial treatment with LMWH, long-term anticoagulation therapy to prevent recurrent DVT is needed. An INR goal of 2 to 3 is generally considered effective in preventing recurrent DVT, and risk of bleeding is lower than with higher INR levels. Treatment duration ranges between 3 and 6 months; the short duration is reserved for those who had some risk factor (e.g., immobility before surgery). Patients who wear compression stockings for 1 year after initial DVT have a lower incidence of post-thrombotic syndrome.

The risk of recurrent DVT is serious on the cessation of anticoagulation treatment. There is some evidence to suggest that post-treatment residual thrombus increases the risk of recurrent DVT and mortality.[18] The monitoring of serial D-dimer levels has been shown to be useful in determining the likelihood of DVT recurrence.[19] Treatment is indicated for more than 12 months in patients with recurrent DVT or for individuals with continuous risk factors for thromboembolic disease, such as malignant disease.[17]

Untreated calf vein thrombosis does not commonly result in clinically important pulmonary embolism unless the thrombus extends into the proximal venous segments, which occurs in about one quarter of the cases. It is safe to monitor calf thrombi with serial venous ultrasound examinations or impedance plethysmography and to initiate therapy only if the thrombus extends into the popliteal or more proximal veins. Treatment of superficial venous thrombosis is usually not indicated.

Pregnant women with DVT are classically treated with unfractionated heparin for 5 days, followed by adjusted-dose subcutaneous heparin every 12 hours until delivery. Warfarin is contraindicated during pregnancy but is safe for the mother and nursing child after delivery.

Rehabilitation

There is no strict contraindication to therapeutic exercises and ambulatory activities after DVT, but it is recommended that these activities be suspended until the patient is in the therapeutic range for heparin or has been receiving LMWH for 24 hours.

On the other hand, physical and occupational therapy ordered immediately after high-risk surgical procedures can greatly improve a patient's postoperative mobility and lessen the chance for development of DVT.

Procedures

Vena cava filters are indicated in patients with DVT who have a high risk of bleeding or who suffered a pulmonary embolism or recurrent pulmonary embolism despite adequate anticoagulation. Caval interruption has been found to be effective in preventing subsequent pulmonary embolism; however, this is counterbalanced by the increased incidence of recurrent DVT. Patients who have significant but temporary contraindications to the use of anticoagulants who receive caval interruption devices should begin taking anticoagulation medication as soon as possible.

Surgery

Surgical removal of acute DVT by thrombectomy or embolectomy is rarely used. It should be considered only in patients with massive thrombosis and compromised arterial circulation who do not respond to or who have an absolute contraindication to thrombolytic therapy.

POTENTIAL DISEASE COMPLICATIONS

If untreated, proximal DVT is linked with a 10% immediate risk of fatal pulmonary embolism and approximately 20% higher risk of development of a severe post-thrombotic syndrome 5 to 10 years later[20] (Fig. 118-3). There are two predominant patterns of DVT: an ascending pattern, with DVT arising in the calf veins; and a descending pattern, with DVT occurring initially in the iliac or common femoral vein. The descending pattern more commonly results in pulmonary embolus. Post-thrombotic syndrome is a condition characterized by chronic edema and debilitating pain and can lead to ulceration, infection, or in rare cases amputation. Heparin use and the wearing of graduated compression stockings have been associated with a lower risk for development of post-thrombotic syndrome.

POTENTIAL TREATMENT COMPLICATIONS

All pharmacologic anticoagulation agents alter the hemostatic mechanisms to some extent by decreasing blood coagulation or platelet function, and all carry a risk of bleeding. Both unfractionated heparin and LMWH are associated with similar increased risk of bleeding complications. Heparin-induced thrombocytopenia is a potential complication of heparin use and is seen slightly less commonly with LMWH than with unfractionated heparin because of the lower affinity of LMWH for platelet binding. A diagnosis of heparin-induced thrombocytopenia is made when there is a 50% reduction in platelet count or with the presence of antiplatelet antibodies. Once the diagnosis is made, all heparins are contraindicated. Skin necrosis is a rare complication of warfarin use, and it can be prevented if high-dose warfarin is delayed until the activated prothrombin time is therapeutic with heparin.

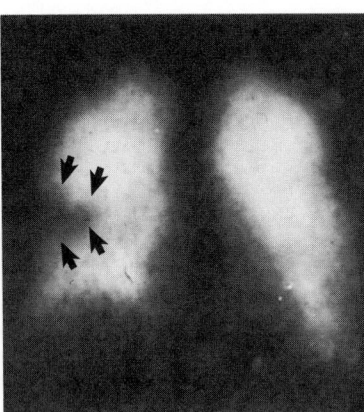

FIGURE 118-3. Frontal image from subsequent perfusion lung scan shows a corresponding peripheral, pleura-based area of absent perfusion in the right midlung. The ventilation study showed diminished ventilation in this area, consistent with pulmonary embolus with infarction, and multiple unmatched perfusion defects were seen in the left lung, indicating that the probability of pulmonary embolism is high. (Reprinted with permission from Katz DS, Math KR, Groskin SA. Radiology Secrets. Philadelphia, Hanley & Belfus, 1998:55.)

Complications from caval interruption include problems related to the deployment of the device; these are hemorrhage, hematomas, femoral artery injury, femoral nerve injury, infections, and site pain. Other potential complications are pulmonary embolism from embolization of the device itself or from failure of the device to capture an embolus. A clot-laden caval interruption device can impede venous flow and lead to lower extremity venous stasis and edema.

Osteoporosis and risk of bone fracture are associated with long-term use of unfractionated heparin[21]; the risk may be less with LMWH.[22]

Contraindications to the use of warfarin include advanced liver disease, alcoholism, poor compliance with follow-up, poorly controlled hypertension, major bleeding, and pregnancy.[23]

References

1. Clagett GP, Anderson FA Jr, Geerts W, et al. Prevention of venous thromboembolism. Chest 1998;114:531s-560s.
2. Pineo GF, Hull RD. Prophylaxis of venous thromboembolism following orthopedic surgery: mechanical and pharmacological approaches and the need for extended prophylaxis. Thromb Haemost 1999;82:918-924.
3. Giercksky KE, Bjorklid E, Prydz H, Renck H. Circulating tissue thromboplastin during hip surgery. Eur Surg Res 1979;11:296-300.
4. Camerer E, Kolsto AB, Prydz H. Cell biology of tissue factor, the principal initiator of blood coagulation. Thromb Res 1996; 81:1-14.
5. Joffe SN. Incidence of postoperative deep vein thrombosis in neurosurgical patients. J Neurosurg 1975;42:201-203.
6. Flinn W, Sandager G, Silva M. Prospective surveillance for perioperative venous thrombosis: experience in 2643 patients. Arch Surg 1996;131:472-480.
7. Dahl OE, Aspelin T, Arnesen H, et al. Increased activation of coagulation and formation of late deep venous thrombosis following discontinuation of thromboprophylaxis after hip replacement surgery. Thromb Res 1995;80:299-306.
8. Ridker PM, Glynn RJ, Miletich JP, et al. Age-specific incidence rates of venous thromboembolism among heterozygous carriers of factor V Leiden mutation. Ann Intern Med 1997;126:528-531.
9. Handler J, Hedderman M, Davodi D, et al. Implementing a diagnostic algorithm for deep venous thrombosis. Permanente J 2003;7:54-60.
10. Qaseem A, Snow V, Barry P, et al; Joint American Academy of Family Physicians/American College of Physicians Panel on Deep Venous Thrombosis/Pulmonary Embolism. Current diagnosis of venous thromboembolism in primary care: a clinical practice guideline from the American Academy of Family Physicians and the American College of Physicians. Ann Fam Med 2007;5:57-62.
11. Segal JB, Eng J, Tamariz LJ, Bass EB. Review of the evidence on diagnosis of deep venous thrombosis and pulmonary embolism. Ann Fam Med 2007;5:63-73.
12. Anderson DR, Wells PS. Improvements in the diagnostic approach for patients with suspected deep vein thrombosis or pulmonary embolism. Thromb Haemost 1999;82:878-886.
13. Wells PS, Hirsh J, Anderson DR, et al. A simple clinical model for the diagnosis of deep-vein thrombosis combined with impedance plethysmography: potential for an improvement in the diagnostic process. J Intern Med 1998;243:15-23.
14. Nurmohamed MT, Rosendaal FR, Buller HR, et al. Low-molecular-weight heparin versus standard heparin in general and orthopaedic surgery: a meta-analysis. Lancet 1992;340:152-156.
15. Barritt DW, Johnson SC. Anticoagulation drugs in the treatment of pulmonary embolism trial. Lancet 1960;1:1309-1312.
16. Snow V, Qaseem A, Barry P, et al. Management of venous thromboembolism: a clinical practice guideline from the American College

of Physicians and the American Academy of Family Physicians. Ann Fam Med 2007;5:74-78.

17. Siragusa S, Cosmi B, Piovella F, et al. Low-molecular-weight heparins and unfractionated heparin in the treatment of patients with acute venous thromboembolism: results of a meta-analysis. Am J Med 1996;100:269-277.

18. Young L, Ockelford P, Milne D, et al. Post-treatment residual thrombus increases the risk of recurrent deep vein thrombosis and mortality. J Thromb Haemost 2006;4:1919-1924.

19. Shrivastava S, Ridker PM, Glynn RJ, et al. D-dimer, factor VIII coagulant activity, low intensity warfarin and the risk of recurrent venous thromboembolism. J Thromb Haemost 2006;4:1208-1214.

20. Bounameaux H, Ehringer H, Gast A, et al. Differential inhibition of thrombin activity and thrombin generation by a synthetic direct thrombin inhibitor (napsagatran, Ro 46-6240) and unfractionated heparin in patients with deep vein thrombosis. ADVENT Investigators. Thromb Haemost 1999;81:498-501.

21. Dahlman T. Osteoporotic fractures and the recurrence during pregnancy and puerperium in 94 women undergoing thromboprophylaxis with heparin. Am J Obstet Gynecol 1983;168:1265-1270.

22. Monreal M, Lafoz E, Olive A, et al. Comparison of subcutaneous unfractionated heparin with a low molecular weight heparin (Fragmin) in patients with thromboembolism and contraindications to coumadin. Thromb Haemost 1994;71:7-11.

23. Hoppenfeld S. Physical Examination of the Spine and Extremities. Norwalk, Conn, Appleton & Lange, 1976.

Dementia 119

Jatin Dave, MD, MPH, and Melvyn Hecht, MD

Synonyms

Senile dementia
Alzheimer dementia
Multi-infarct dementia

ICD-9 Codes

042	Human immunodeficiency virus (HIV) disease
046.1	Jakob-Creutzfeldt disease
046.2	Subacute sclerosing panencephalitis
046.3	Progressive multifocal leukoencephalopathy
290.0	Senile dementia, uncomplicated
290.1	Presenile dementia
290.2	Senile dementia with delusional or depressive features
290.3	Senile dementia with delirium or confusion
290.4	Arteriosclerotic dementia
291.1	Alcohol amnestic syndrome
291.2	Other alcoholic dementia
292.82	Drug-induced dementia
292.83	Drug-induced persisting amnestic disorder
293.0	Acute delirium (use for acute metabolic encephalopathy)
293.1	Subacute delirium (use for subacute metabolic encephalopathy)
294.0	Amnestic syndrome
294.1	Dementia in conditions classified elsewhere
294.8	Other specified organic brain syndromes (chronic)
294.9	Unspecified organic brain syndrome (chronic)
310.0	Specified nonpsychotic mental disorders due to organic brain damage
311	Depressive disorder, not elsewhere specified
331.0	Alzheimer disease
331.11	Pick disease
331.19	Other frontotemporal dementia
331.2	Senile degeneration of the brain
331.3	Communicating hydrocephalus
331.4	Obstructive hydrocephalus
331.82	Dementia with Lewy bodies
	Dementia with parkinsonism
331.89	Other cerebral degenerations
331.9	Cerebral degeneration, unspecified
332.0	Parkinson disease
348.1	Anoxic brain damage
348.30	Encephalopathy, unspecified

434.91	Ischemic stroke
434.11	Embolic stroke
434.01	Thrombotic stroke
437.0	Cerebral atherosclerosis
437.7	Transient global amnesia
780.93	Memory loss of unknown cause
784.69	Agraphia, apraxia, acalculia, agnosia

DEFINITION

Dementia is a syndrome of acquired deterioration in cognitive abilities severe enough to interfere with social or occupational functioning. More than 55 illnesses causing dementia can be categorized by localization (cortical, frontal, or subcortical) or by etiology (Table 119-1).[19] Cortical dementias like Alzheimer disease predominantly affect the cerebral cortex; subcortical forms like Parkinson disease and vascular dementia primarily affect the basal ganglia, thalamus, and deep white matter. Subcortical dementias are characterized by a slowness and rigidity of thinking rather than by prominent memory loss, language problems, and impairment of visual-spatial functioning. Some disorders, like dementia with Lewy bodies, display signs of both cortical and subcortical dysfunction. Although its prevalence increases steadily with age, nearly doubling every 5 years after the age of 60 years, dementia is never a normal part of aging even in the oldest old.[20]

According to the *Diagnostic and Statistical Manual of Mental Disorders*, dementia is characterized by memory impairment and one (or more) of the following cognitive disturbances: aphasia (language disturbance), apraxia (impaired ability to carry out motor activities despite intact motor function), agnosia (failure to recognize or to identify objects despite intact sensory function), and disturbance in executive functioning (i.e., planning, organizing, sequencing, abstracting). Cognitive impairment causes significant impairment in social or occupational functioning, and these disturbances are not due to delirium or depression. Prevalence, clinical presentation, risk factors, and other characteristics of common subtypes of dementia are summarized in Table 119-1.

TABLE 119-1 Characteristics of Common Types of Dementia*

	Alzheimer Disease	Vascular Dementia[1]	Dementia with Lewy bodies[2,3]	Mixed Dementia[4]
Prevalence[5]	50%	15%	15%	15%
Clinical presentation	Insidious onset and slow progression with profound memory loss	Relatively abrupt onset, fluctuating stepwise progression; often history of stroke, focal neurologic signs, gait abnormalities Left hemisphere: language problems Right hemisphere: visual-spatial/ simultaneous processing	Visual hallucinations, fluctuating cognition, parkinsonism with rapid progression	Usually combination of AD + VaD
Diagnostic criteria	NINDS	Hachinski Ischemic Scale or NINDS-AIREN[6-9]	McKeith 1996 and 2006[10-15]	Hachinski Ischemic Scale ADDTC NINDS-AIREN DSM-IV-TR
Neuropathology hallmark	Extracellular amyloid plaques and intracellular neurofibrillary tangles	Cerebral infarctions, often multiple lacunar infarctions and periventricular leukoencephalopathy (white matter changes)	Lewy body, a spherical intraneuronal cytoplasmic inclusion	Features of both AD and VaD
Risk factors	Age, family history, sex, apolipoprotein E	History of stroke, age, smoking, obesity, hypertension, and diabetes		Both AD and VaD
Imaging	Hippocampal atrophy	Lacunes, infarctions on imaging[16,17]	—	Mixed features of AD and VaD
Estimated natural course	5-7 years[18]	5-7 years	3-4 years	5-7 years
Treatment	ChE-I	ChE-I; therapy for vascular risk factors	Avoid neuroleptics, ChE-I	ChE-I; therapy for vascular risk factors

*Other causes of dementia, which contribute less than 5% in aggregate, are frontotemporal dementia (including Pick disease), Parkinson disease–associated dementia, Huntington disease, progressive supranuclear palsy, and Wilson disease.
AD, Alzheimer disease; VaD, vascular dementia; NINDS, National Institute of Neurological Disorders and Stroke; AIREN, Association Internationale pour la Recherché et l'Enseignement en Neurosciences; ADDTC, Alzheimer Disease Diagnostic and Treatment Centers; DSM-IV-TR, Diagnostic and Statistical Manual of Mental Disorders, 4th edition, text revision; ChE-I, cholinesterase inhibitors.

Alzheimer disease is the most common cause of dementia, accounting for up to two thirds of cases and affecting 4.5 million people in the United States. It is also the eighth leading cause of death, and its prevalence is predicted to rise even more, to 13.5 million by 2050, without advances in therapy.[21] Of those affected by Alzheimer disease, 7% are 65 to 74 years old, 53% are 75 to 84 years old, and 40% are older than 85 years; thus, it is predominantly a disease of older adults.[22] The exact etiology of Alzheimer disease is not known; many hypotheses based on amyloid, tangle-tau protein, cholinergic pathway, and inflammation have been proposed. Neuronal loss with decreased acetylcholine is the hallmark of Alzheimer disease. Intracellular clumps of tau proteins–neurofibrillary tangles and extracellular ß-amyloid plaques contribute to neuronal loss. Whether neuronal loss is mediated through inflammation remains controversial. ß-Amyloid plaques develop when amyloid precursor protein is cleaved at a ß- or γ-secretase site instead of an α-secretase site. Common risk factors for Alzheimer disease are age, female sex, genetic factors (apolipoprotein E e4 allele), history of head injury, and Down syndrome.[23-27] The current diagnostic approach is a diagnosis of inclusion based on defined criteria rather than the previously recommended diagnosis of exclusion.

Although vascular dementia was traditionally thought to be associated with a stroke, studies support cognitive impairment in patients with small-vessel disease with white matter changes. Dementia with Lewy bodies is a dementia sharing clinical and pathologic characteristics with both Parkinson disease and Alzheimer disease. To differentiate this from Parkinson disease–associated dementia, current diagnostic criteria restrict a diagnosis of dementia with Lewy bodies to patients with parkinsonism who develop dementia within 12 months of the onset of motor symptoms. Considering that many patients with dementia have pathologic findings consistent with more than one type of dementia, mixed dementia is likely to be the second most common type of dementia. The most common type of mixed dementia is a combination of Alzheimer disease and vascular dementia. Recent research supports a common pathway based on vascular disease leading to Alzheimer disease.[28]

Although the distinction between normal and pathologic cognitive changes still remains controversial, studies suggest that many of the changes attributed to aging in the past in fact reflect the effect of unrecognized mild cognitive disorder. Considering the insidious nature of the symptoms of dementia, many early warning signs are often dismissed as "normal aging." The continuum between normal aging, mild cognitive impairment, and dementia is described in Table 119-2. Although the exact distinction between these entities across the continuum is not clear, recent data support the contention that a decrease in episodic memory (learning and retention, but no impairment in retrieval) and preserved implicit memory (ability to perform a learned skill) could be associated with normal aging. Mild cognitive impairment is a transitional state between normal aging and dementia in which cognitive deficits are present but have not yet affected function.[29-36]

SYMPTOMS

A careful history of the presentation with special attention to symptom duration and course, impact on work and family life, and issues of driving and home safety is essential to narrow the differential and to assess the severity. This often requires a detailed clinical history involving the individual with cognitive deficit and a reliable primary informant, with a focus on a previous baseline of education and evidence of changes in occupational role and functionality. Interview of the patient and caregiver separately not only enables the cooperation and language skills to be assessed without being masked by interruptions or assistance from the caregiver but provides information on poor insight. Symptoms associated with dementia can be grouped into cognitive, functional, and behavioral disturbances.

Common cognitive changes include memory loss (forgetting names of loved ones, missing multiple appointments, inability to remember recent important family gatherings, and inability to manage medications), language disturbances (word-finding difficulties, paraphasic errors), and loss of writing or reading abilities often noticed by family members of patients. Recent classification of memory based on type of information is preferred to traditional distinction of short-term or long-term memory loss. Useful classification includes declarative (explicit) and nondeclarative (implicit) memory. Declarative memory is further classified into episodic (events, context related: What did you eat this morning?), semantic (factual: Who is the president?), and working memory. Nondeclarative memory includes procedural memory (such as driving). Improved understanding of the types of memory may aid clinicians in diagnosis and treatment. Patients with Alzheimer disease commonly progress from anterograde episodic memory loss (e.g., forgetting recent personal and family events, repetitive questioning) and delayed recall during earlier stages to semantic memory loss (e.g., loss of verbal fluency and previously known facts).[37]

Impaired function often resulting in social withdrawal includes difficulty in driving, shopping, cooking, housekeeping, dressing, and feeding.

Common behavioral disturbances are apathy, poor insight into symptoms, agitation with verbal abuse, sundowning, wandering, crying spells, poor impulse control, poor safety awareness or judgment, and change in sleep habits.

In addition to focusing on clues to confirm and to differentiate the diagnosis of dementia, it is important to look for potentially reversible causes of cognitive impairment (e.g., depression, medications) and other contributing factors (e.g., stroke).

PHYSICAL EXAMINATION

Physical examination in patients thought to have dementia focuses on assessment of cognition, neurologic and other relevant systems, and functional limitations to establish the diagnosis of dementia, to look for clues of specific subtypes, and to assess the severity of dementia.

Cognition

Cognitive assessment is a two-step process: detection of high-risk patients through screening and confirmation of cognitive impairment through detailed cognitive assessment, history, physical examination, and caregiver interview. The use of cognitive screening and assessment in real life remains limited despite availability of more than 25 instruments from which to choose.[38,39] Clinicians often do not screen for cognitive problems even in high-risk older adults unless they receive complaints from either the patient or the caregivers. This is unfortunate because the majority of patients with dementia do not complain about it to their health care

TABLE 119-2 Normal Aging, Mild Cognitive Impairment, and Dementia

	Normal Aging	Mild Cognitive Impairment	Dementia
Cognition	Decline in ability to learn new information, working memory, simultaneous processing, and perceptual speed	Memory loss only	Memory loss and at least one of the following: aphasia, apraxia, agnosia, executive dysfunction
Social and occupational functioning	Preserved	Preserved	Impaired
IADL, ADL	Can be preserved	Can be impaired/preserved	Impaired/usually impaired

IADL, instrumental activities of daily living; ADL, activities of daily living.

providers. Barriers to assessment of patients cognitively include lack of time, potential for causing the patient discomfort, and inadequacies of available tests and effective treatment.[40] Nonetheless, we recommend a brief screening test in all older adults (arbitrarily defined as older than 65 years) and targeted detailed cognitive assessment in patients with abnormal screening test results. For clinicians who are not comfortable in assessing cognition in detail, a referral to a neuropsychologist may be considered. Newer computer-based cognitive testing can also be used. Neuropsychological assessment includes assessment of executive function (letter and category frequency), orientation (to time and place), attention (naming of days or months), memory (three-item recall, address recall), language (naming, writing, comprehension), visual-spatial function (clock drawing, overlapping pentagons), problem solving, and personality.

Neurologic and Other Relevant Systems

A thorough neurologic examination focusing on any focal signs, involuntary movements, fasciculations, and gait disturbances and an ocular examination are important. Examination of other systems is useful in looking for a multisystem disease. This includes signs suggestive of immune (lymphadenopathy), infective (rash, organomegaly), malignant (hepatomegaly), nutritional (cachexia), or vascular (abnormal pulses) disorders.

DIAGNOSTIC STUDIES

Commonly recommended diagnostic studies include full blood count, electrolyte determinations, liver function, thyroid function, and serum vitamin B_{12} concentration.[41,42] Specialized tests are indicated only when historical features or clinical circumstances suggest infections, inflammatory diseases, or exposure to toxins. Unless the patient has some specific risk factor or evidence of prior syphilitic infection or resides in one of the few areas in the United States with high numbers of syphilis cases, screening for the disorder in patients with dementia is not justified.

A non–contrast-enhanced computed tomographic scan or magnetic resonance imaging examination to exclude rare but potentially correctable causes of dementia (e.g., subdural hematoma, hydrocephalus) is recommended. The role of functional and quantitative neuroimaging is currently being defined and awaits further studies. Cerebral biopsy is rarely indicated in patients thought to have a treatable cause (cerebral vasculitis) and in the absence of an alternative diagnosis.

Differential Diagnosis

Reversible dementia (also called pseudodementia)

Mild cognitive impairment

Age-associated cognitive impairment (see Table 119-2).

Other Causes of Potentially Reversible Cognitive Impairment

Delirium (commonly due to medications, infections, electrolyte abnormalities, and renal failure)

Depression

Anemia

Thyroid disorder

Intracranial pathologic processes (subdural hematoma, brain tumors).[43]

Earlier studies suggested that reversible dementia accounts for up to one fifth of all dementia cases. However, studies have shown that although 10% of cases appear to have a potentially reversible cause, dementia is actually reversed in less than 1% of cases.[44-47] Thus, many cases of reversible dementia are associated with comorbid conditions. The course of dementia is usually progressive, and many so-called reversible dementias may not be cured, but the disease course may be modified through treatment of the potentially reversible cause. Differential diagnosis of dementia from delirium is characterized in Table 119-3.

In addition, it is important to differentiate various subtypes of dementia. For example, in patients with Alzheimer disease, the progression is usually steady decline, whereas the decline in patients with vascular dementia tends to be stepwise.

TABLE 119-3 Differentiation of Dementia from Delirium and Depression

	Dementia	Depression	Delirium
Onset	Insidious (years)	Subacute (weeks to months)	Abrupt (days)
Consciousness	Clear	Clear	Altered
Primary defect	Memory	Mood	Attention
Hallmark	Progression	Response to treatment	Fluctuation
Patient may report	"I do not have memory problems." (reflecting lack of insight)	"I have very serious memory problems." (reflecting hopelessness)	"Why do we care about memory?" (reflecting disorganized thinking)

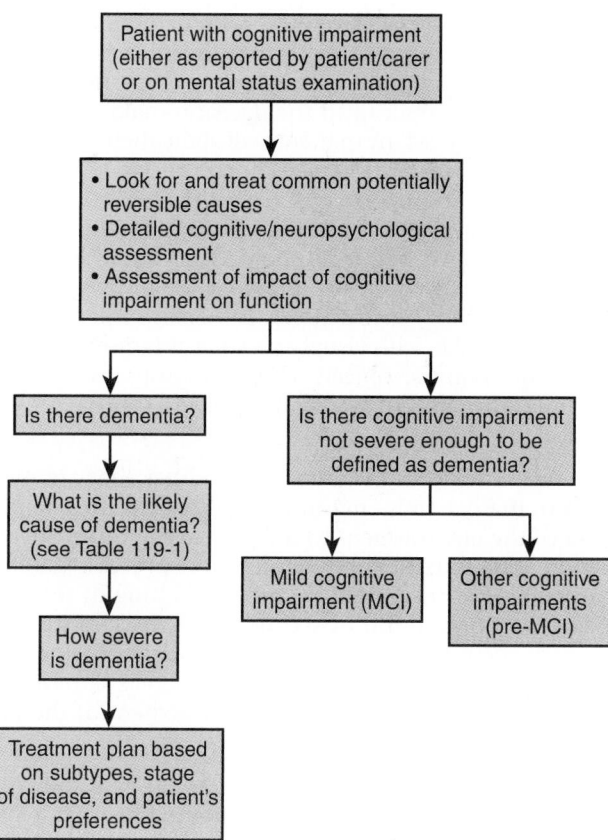

FIGURE 119-1. An approach to a patient with cognitive impairment.

TREATMENT

Initial

An approach to patients with persistent cognitive impairment is illustrated in Figure 119-1.

The treatment of dementia halts the progression of disease, minimizes disability, and reduces caregiver stress (Table 119-4).[48] The focus of management shifts from reducing the rate of progression, vascular risk reduction, and family and patient education in earlier stages to palliative care or hospice, discussion of artificial feeding, and management of behavioral symptoms during later stages.

Goals for halting the progression of dementia are to stop neuronal death and to replace dead neurons. No drugs have been definitively shown to alter the histopathologic progression of dementia. As a result of the awareness of a common vascular pathway, aggressive treatment of vascular risk factors (hypertension, hypercholesterolemia, and diabetes) may help mitigate the progressive course.[49]

Although studies question the efficacy of cholinesterase inhibitors and suggest a minimal benefit on a rating scale, we recommend a trial of cholinesterase inhibitors after discussion of risks and benefits in patients with mild to moderate Alzheimer disease. Our recommendation is based on current guidelines and individual studies. Current evidence does not support superiority of one agent over others despite frequent claims by individual studies. Three commonly used cholinesterase inhibitors are donepezil (starting dose: 5-mg tablet daily; the dose can be increased to 10 mg in 4 to 6 weeks), rivastigmine (starting dose: 1.5-mg capsule daily; the dose can be increased in 2 weeks to 1.5 mg twice daily to a target dose of 6 to 12 mg during the next 4 to 6 weeks; also available in liquids), and galantamine (starting dose: 4-mg tablet twice daily; the dose can be increased in 4 weeks to 8 mg twice daily). Memantine is an N-methyl-D-aspartate receptor antagonist approved for moderate to severe Alzheimer disease. Studies support the beneficial effect of memantine on neuropsychiatric symptoms.

These drugs will not cure Alzheimer disease but only slow its progression. Another challenge in use of cholinesterase inhibitors is the difficulty in accurately measuring the patient's response, given the progressive nature of the disease. Currently, this requires measurement of the slope of decline, which is not practical for most clinical settings. Data on non–Alzheimer disease dementia are limited; however, the current literature supports use of cholinesterase inhibitors in vascular dementia, dementia with Lewy bodies, and mixed dementia.

TABLE 119-4 Overview of Management of Patients with Dementia

	Halting the Progression	Noncognitive Symptoms	Caregiver Support
Early	Cholinesterase inhibitors Vascular risk factor management and management of comorbid condition	Treatment of depression if appropriate Reorientation therapy	Education on manifestation and natural history as well as tips on communicating with patients with dementia Advanced care planning Support groups
Moderate	Cholinesterase inhibitors plus memantine	Cautious and time-limited trial of antipsychotics Memantine	Introduce palliative care
Late	Role unclear at this stage	Sedatives Round-the-clock low-risk analgesics like acetaminophen if pain suspected	Hospice

Other pharmacologic interventions, including the use of antioxidants, anti-inflammatory agents, and hormone replacement therapy, are not recommended. Studies have shown an increase in risk of dementia with hormone replacement therapy[50] and an increase in all-cause mortality with high-dose vitamin E ($\geq$400 IU/day).[51] A trial of anti-inflammatory drugs in Alzheimer disease was suspended because of safety concerns.[52]

Abnormal behaviors not controlled by nonpharmacologic measures can be managed with cautious use of low-dose antipsychotics, anxiolytics, and antidepressants. Depression is especially common, and consideration of the use of antidepressants early in the disease is important. The management of behavior needs to be balanced with the high side effect profile of these drugs. A trial of collaborative care for the treatment of Alzheimer disease resulted in significant improvement in the quality of care and in behavioral and psychological symptoms of dementia among primary care patients and their caregivers.[53]

After a relationship has been established with the clinician, but early in the treatment, the patient and family should be counseled about a living will, health care proxy, and guardianship. An excellent resource for this information is the local chapter of the Alzheimer's Association.

Caregiver Support

Caring for patients with dementia can be difficult and challenging. Education about common symptoms, strategies to deal with those symptoms, and available resources including caregiver support groups offered through local Alzheimer disease associations may help in preventing caregiver burnout.

Rehabilitation

The importance of dementia for rehabilitation is twofold. The first focuses on the importance of dementia in the rehabilitation of general patients, the second on cognitive rehabilitation of patients with dementia.

The rehabilitation of patients with dementia is complicated by their cognitive status. Dementia is one of the key contributors to the development of functional dependence and decline.[54] It is also likely to be associated with less favorable outcome of rehabilitation after hip fracture.[55-57] Whereas there is no specific literature on the interventions for recovery of patients with dementia, several factors aid in their rehabilitation. These factors include motivation and socialization, limited reality orientation (when possible, but it is not always practical, especially in advanced stages), and cognitive training. For motivation training, the team often looks for early success, such as recognition of the patient's room. In reality orientation, opportunities are taken as often as possible to orient the patient to time and place. In cognitive training, patients are given techniques to aid memory (e.g., use of cue cards to recite the names of objects).

The rehabilitation of the patient with dementia calls for a coordinated approach with the clinical therapist and family. Obviously, the patient should participate as much as he or she can in the decision-making process and treatment. Many patients, despite their cognitive dysfunction, are able to make choices and to rationalize their choices appropriately and are therefore competent to make clinical decisions. Therapists and family members who are working with the patients should be well versed in the use of diversionary tactics and visual, tactile, and auditory instructions. The environment needs to be home-like, with visual aids such as family portraits and other familiar objects. Use of appropriate lighting to prevent reversal of day-night cycle and sundowning is critical.

Repeated measures of functional abilities that are relevant to the patient's environment as well as the adaptation of the environment to the patient's abilities are essential elements of the rehabilitation process. Careful assessment of the patient's function, setting of realistic goals, and prevention of secondary disabilities such as urinary incontinence, depression, and weight loss, as well as complications of immobility such as skin breakdown, are all key to successful management of the patients with dementia.

Physical therapy intervention focuses on gait and mobility. As dementia progresses, impairment in gait becomes a problem. This impairment can be complicated by degenerative joint changes and orthopedic injuries. The physical therapist needs to provide a good deal of repetition with respect to the exercise program. Technique should be individualized to the level of cognition and abnormal behaviors.

Occupational therapy is especially important in the rehabilitation of the patient with dementia. The primary focus in this area is on dressing, toileting, and cognition. The occupational therapist is a key member of the treatment team, responsible for structuring activities such as reminiscence, reality orientation, and group-based therapies. The speech and language pathologist evaluates and guides decisions in regard to feeding and swallowing.

Most data on the effectiveness of rehabilitation come from studies of geriatric assessment units, and results to date have been both positive and negative.[58] In addition to functional goals, focus on improvement of medical conditions and reduction of polypharmacy is vital. Certainly, rehabilitation of the patient with dementia needs further research focus to improve techniques.

Cognitive rehabilitation in patients with dementia includes both pharmacologic and nonpharmacologic interventions. In recent years, nonpharmacologic intervention has gained more attention because of limited efficacy of drug treatments. Two key interventions are multistrategy approaches (reality orientation, reminiscence therapy, and validation therapy) and cognitive methods.[59] A Cochrane review concluded that there is no evidence for the effectiveness of cognitive training and insufficient evidence to evaluate individualized cognitive rehabilitation.[60]

Assessment of functional limitations, especially in driving, is often an important yet challenging issue because of the potential change in lifestyle that the loss of driving privileges would entail. Patients with mild dementia (defined as dementia rating score of 0.5) should be referred for independent driving assessment; those with more advanced dementia (defined as dementia rating score of 1) should not be allowed to drive.[61]

Procedures

The only procedural intervention currently performed is shunting for normal pressure hydrocephalus. Results are mixed but can be dramatic in patients diagnosed early with this disorder.

Surgery

In a rare form of dementia caused by normal pressure hydrocephalus, ventriculoperitoneal shunt is indicated.

POTENTIAL DISEASE COMPLICATIONS

Complications from dementia become more devastating with progression of the disease. Three of the most significant complications are depression, loss of cognitive function, and loss of motor function.

Depression can be a significant issue, especially early during the disease process, when patients recognize their deficits. Untreated and undiagnosed depression can produce worsening cognitive function, increased confusion, and social isolation. Loss of cognitive function brings the loss of independence. Driving should be assessed as discussed earlier. Patients may benefit from alert devices like Lifeline and may require 24-hour supervision. Swallowing difficulties and decrease in oral intake are common with advanced disease. The role of artificial nutrition is often limited and has not been shown to be of any benefit in almost all studies. However, this should be discussed early in the course to incorporate the patient's preferences.

Loss of motor function often results in falls, fractures, aspiration pneumonia, and contractures, eventually causing skin breakdown. The most common cause of death remains infection.

POTENTIAL TREATMENT COMPLICATIONS

Common side effects of cholinesterase inhibitors are gastrointestinal (diarrhea, nausea, anorexia) and neuropsychiatric (agitation, nightmares). If the patient or family requests artificial feeding, the patient commonly removes the tube because of limited cognitive abilities. Postsurgical patients with dementia often have worsening of their cognitive abilities, requiring, on average, 6 weeks to return to baseline functioning.

References

1. Vermeer SE, Prins ND, den Heijer T, et al. Silent brain infarcts and the risk of dementia and cognitive decline. N Engl J Med 2003;348:1215-1222.
2. McKeith IG, Galasko D, Kosaka K, et al. Consensus guidelines for the clinical and pathologic diagnosis of dementia with Lewy bodies (DLB): report of the Consortium on DLB International Workshop. Neurology 1996;47:1113-1124.
3. McKeith IG. Consensus guidelines for the clinical and pathologic diagnosis of dementia with Lewy bodies (DLB): report of the Consortium on DLB International Workshop. J Alzheimer's Dis 2006;9:417-423.
4. Langa KM, Foster NL, Larson EB. Mixed dementia: emerging concepts and therapeutic implications. JAMA 2004;292:2901-2908.
5. Ebly EM, Parhad IM, Hogan DB, Fung TS. Prevalence and types of dementia in the very old: results from the Canadian Study of Health and Aging. Neurology 1994;44:1593-1600.
6. Chui HC, Mack W, Jackson JE, et al. Clinical criteria for the diagnosis of vascular dementia: a multicenter study of comparability and interrater reliability. Arch Neurol 2000;57:191-196.
7. Dichgans M, Mayer M, Uttner I, et al. The phenotypic spectrum of CADASIL: clinical findings in 102 cases. Ann Neurol 1998;44:731-739.
8. Schneider JA, Wilson RS, Cochran EJ, et al. Relation of cerebral infarctions to dementia and cognitive function in older persons. Neurology 2003;60:1082-1088.
9. Knopman DS, Parisi JE, Boeve BF, et al. Vascular dementia in a population-based autopsy study. Arch Neurol 2003;60:569-575.
10. Hohl U, Tiraboschi P, Hansen LA, et al. Diagnostic accuracy of dementia with Lewy bodies. Arch Neurol 2000;57:347-351.
11. Ballard C, O'Brien J, Gray A, et al. Attention and fluctuating attention in patients with dementia with Lewy bodies and Alzheimer disease. Arch Neurol 2001;58:977-982.
12. McKeith IG, Fairbairn AF, Bothwell RA, et al. An evaluation of the predictive validity and inter-rater reliability of clinical diagnostic criteria for senile dementia of Lewy body type. Neurology 1994;44:872-877.
13. Mega MS, Masterman DL, Benson DF, et al. Dementia with Lewy bodies: reliability and validity of clinical and pathologic criteria. Neurology 1996;47:1403-1409.
14. Stern Y, Jacobs D, Goldman J, et al. An investigation of clinical correlates of Lewy bodies in autopsy-proven Alzheimer disease. Arch Neurol 2001;58:460-465.
15. Minoshima S, Foster NL, Sima AA, et al. Alzheimer's disease versus dementia with Lewy bodies: cerebral metabolic distinction with autopsy confirmation. Ann Neurol 2001;50:358-365.
16. Gorelick PB. Risk factors for vascular dementia and Alzheimer disease. Stroke 2004;35:2620-2622.
17. Gorelick PB. Status of risk factors for dementia associated with stroke. Stroke 1997;28:459-463.
18. Brookmeyer R, Corrada MM, Curriero FC, Kawas C. Survival following a diagnosis of Alzheimer disease. Arch Neurol 2002;59:1764-1767.
19. Kukull WA, Bowen JD. Dementia epidemiology. Med Clin North Am 2002;86:573-590.
20. Ritchie K, Kildea D, Robine J-M. The relationship between age and the prevalence of senile dementia: a meta-analysis of recent data. Int J Epidemiol 1992;21:763-769.
21. Hebert LE, Beckett LA, Scherr PA, Evans DA. Annual incidence of Alzheimer disease in the United States projected to the years 2000 through 2050. Alzheimer Dis Assoc Disord 2001;15:169-173.
22. Hebert LE, Scherr PA, Bienias JL, et al. Alzheimer disease in the US population: prevalence estimates using the 2000 census. Arch Neurol 2003;60:1119-1122.
23. Bretsky P, Guralnik JM, Launer L, et al. The role of APOE-ϵ 4 in longitudinal cognitive decline: MacArthur Studies of Successful Aging. Neurology 2003;60:1077-1081.
24. Truelsen T, Thudium D, Gronbaek M. Amount and type of alcohol and risk of dementia: the Copenhagen City Heart Study. Neurology 2002;59:1313-1319.

25. Daly E, Zaitchik D, Copeland M, et al. Predicting conversion to Alzheimer disease using standardized clinical information. Arch Neurol 2000;57:675-680.

26. Green RC, Cupples LA, Go R, et al. Risk of dementia among white and African American relatives of patients with Alzheimer disease. JAMA 2002;287:329-336.

27. Mayeux R, Saunders AM, Shea S, et al. Utility of the apolipoprotein E genotype in the diagnosis of Alzheimer's disease. Alzheimer's Disease Centers Consortium on Apolipoprotein E and Alzheimer's Disease. N Engl J Med 1998;338:506-511.

28. Iadecola C, Gorelick PB. Converging pathogenic mechanisms in vascular and neurodegenerative dementia. Stroke 2003;34:335-337.

29. Morris JC, Storandt M, Miller JP, et al. Mild cognitive impairment represents early-stage Alzheimer disease. Arch Neurol 2001;58:397-405.

30. Bennett DA, Wilson RS, Schneider JA, et al. Natural history of mild cognitive impairment in older persons. Neurology 2002;59:198-205.

31. Bowen J, Teri L, Kukull W, et al. Progression to dementia in patients with isolated memory loss. Lancet 1997;349:763-765.

32. Collie A, Maruff P, Shafiq-Antonacci R, et al. Memory decline in healthy older people: implications for identifying mild cognitive impairment. Neurology 2001;56:1533-1538.

33. Petersen RC, Doody R, Kurz A, et al. Current concepts in mild cognitive impairment. Arch Neurol 2001;58:1985-1992.

34. Storandt M, Grant EA, Miller JP, Morris JC. Rates of progression in mild cognitive impairment and early Alzheimer's disease. Neurology 2002;59:1034-1041.

35. Tabert MH, Albert SM, Borukhova-Milov L, et al. Functional deficits in patients with mild cognitive impairment: prediction of AD. Neurology 2002;58:758-764.

36. Tuokko H, Frerichs R, Graham J, et al. Five-year follow-up of cognitive impairment with no dementia. Arch Neurol 2003;60:577-582.

37. Milner B, Squire LR, Kandel ER. Cognitive neuroscience and the study of memory. Neuron 1998;20:445-468.

38. Siu AL. Screening for dementia and investigating its causes. Ann Intern Med 1991;115:122-132.

39. Tangalos EG, Smith GE, Ivnik RJ, et al. The Mini-Mental State Examination in general medical practice: clinical utility and acceptance. Mayo Clin Proc 1996;71:829-837.

40. Bush C, Kozak J, Elmslie T. Screening for cognitive impairment in the elderly. Can Fam Physician 1997;43:1763-1768.

41. Knopman DS, DeKosky ST, Cummings JL, et al. Practice parameter: diagnosis of dementia (an evidence-based review). Report of the Quality Standards Subcommittee of the American Academy of Neurology. Neurology 2001;56:1143-1153.

42. Clarke R, Smith AD, Jobst KA, et al. Folate, vitamin B_{12}, and serum total homocysteine levels in confirmed Alzheimer disease. Arch Neurol 1998;55:1449-1455.

43. Kaye JA. Diagnostic challenges in dementia. Neurology 1998;51:S45-S52; discussion S65-S67.

44. Hejl A, Hogh P, Waldemar G. Potentially reversible conditions in 1000 consecutive memory clinic patients. J Neurol Neurosurg Psychiatry 2002;73:390-394.

45. Piccini C, Bracco L, Amaducci L. Treatable and reversible dementias: an update. J Neurol Sci 1998;153:172-181.

46. Clarfield AM. The decreasing prevalence of reversible dementias: an updated meta-analysis. Arch Intern Med 2003;163:2219-2229.

47. Clarfield AM. Reversible dementia—the implications of a fall in prevalence. Age Ageing 2005;34:544-545.

48. Doody RS, Stevens JC, Beck C, et al. Practice parameter: management of dementia (an evidence-based review). Report of the Quality Standards Subcommittee of the American Academy of Neurology. Neurology 2001;56:1154-1166.

49. Simons M, Schwarzler F, Lutjohann D, et al. Treatment with simvastatin in normocholesterolemic patients with Alzheimer's disease: a 26-week randomized, placebo-controlled, double-blind trial. Ann Neurol 2002;52:346-350.

50. Shumaker SA, Legault C, Rapp SR, et al. Estrogen plus progestin and the incidence of dementia and mild cognitive impairment in postmenopausal women: the Women's Health Initiative Memory Study: a randomized controlled trial. JAMA 2003;289:2651-2662.

51. Miller ER 3rd, Pastor-Barriuso R, Dalal D, et al. Meta-analysis: high-dosage vitamin E supplementation may increase all-cause mortality. Ann Intern Med 2005;142:37-46.

52. Alzheimer's Disease Anti-Inflammatory Prevention Trial (ADAPT). Available at: http://www.alz.org/news_and_events_alzheimer_news_01-06-2005.asp.

53. Callahan CM, Boustani MA, Unverzagt FW, et al. Effectiveness of collaborative care for older adults with Alzheimer disease in primary care: a randomized controlled trial. JAMA 2006;295:2148-2157.

54. Aguero-Torres H, Fratiglioni L, Guo Z, et al. Dementia is the major cause of functional dependence in the elderly: 3-year follow-up data from a population-based study. Am J Public Health 1998;88:1452-1456.

55. Kyo T, Takaoka K, Ono K. Femoral neck fracture. Factors related to ambulation and prognosis. Clin Orthop Relat Res 1993;292:215-222.

56. Parker MJ, Palmer CR. Prediction of rehabilitation after hip fracture. Age Ageing 1995;24:96-98.

57. Heruti RJ, Lusky A, Barell V, et al. Cognitive status at admission: does it affect the rehabilitation outcome of elderly patients with hip fracture? Arch Phys Med Rehabil 1999;80:432-436.

58. Wieland D, Hirth V. Comprehensive geriatric assessment. Cancer Control 2003;10:454-462.

59. Cotelli M, Calabria M, Zanetti O. Cognitive rehabilitation in Alzheimer's disease. Aging Clin Exp Res 2006;18:141-143.

60. Clare L, Woods RT. Cognitive rehabilitation and cognitive training for early-stage Alzheimer's disease and vascular dementia. Available at: http://www.cochrane.org/reviews/en/ab003260.html. Accessed September 9, 2006.

61. Dubinsky RM, Stein AC, Lyons K. Practice parameter: risk of driving and Alzheimer's disease (an evidence-based review): report of the Quality Standards Subcommittee of the American Academy of Neurology. Neurology 2000;54:2205-2211.

Management of the Patient with a Foot at Risk: Peripheral Arterial Disease and Diabetes 120

Timothy R. Dillingham, MD, and Diane W. Braza, MD

DEFINITION

The incidence of lower limb amputations due to vascular disease has increased in the United States by approximately 20% during the last decade, disproportionately in minorities.[1] Persons with diabetes mellitus and peripheral vascular disease should be identified and prophylactic foot education and preventive care instituted to reduce the risk of limb loss.[2]

Atherosclerosis is a vascular disease that can involve the peripheral arterial system. The American Heart Association estimates that 8 to 12 million Americans have peripheral arterial disease and that nearly 75% of them are asymptomatic. Annually, approximately 1 million Americans develop symptomatic peripheral arterial disease.[3] Despite its association with other cardiovascular risks including stroke and heart disease, only 25% of Americans with peripheral arterial disease are undergoing active treatment.[4] Major risk factors associated with the development of peripheral arterial disease or that accelerate its progression are high plasma cholesterol and lipoprotein levels, cigarette smoking, hypertension, diabetes, hyperhomocysteinemia, older age, and positive family history.[5,6] African American ethnicity is a strong and independent risk factor for peripheral arterial disease.[7] Given that men have more risk factors for peripheral arterial disease, they are more commonly affected than women.

Diabetes mellitus, a multisystem disease, causes two conditions that place the foot at high risk for amputation: polyneuropathy and peripheral arterial disease.

Diabetes affects about 20.8 million Americans.[8] Diabetes is also on the rise in the United States, particularly in African American and Hispanic populations.[9] Risk factors for diabetic ulcers include male sex, hyperglycemia, and diabetes duration. Foot ulcers often result from severe macrovascular disease, and diabetic neuropathy exacerbates the risk.[10] More than 60% of nontraumatic lower limb amputations occur in people with diabetes, underscoring the need to prevent foot ulcers and subsequent limb loss.[7] Multidisciplinary clinics that identify and manage patients with at-risk feet have demonstrated impressive reductions of 44% to 85% in the incidence of foot ulcers and lower limb amputations.[11] Minor foot trauma in a person with poor underlying circulation and reduced sensation can lead to skin ulceration. Skin ulcers can fail to heal and progress such that an amputation becomes necessary. This sequence of events can often be prevented before it starts.

Numerous studies have further shown that attention to lifestyle modification can dramatically reduce progression to type 2 diabetes.[12] The importance of identifying and treating a core set of risk factors (pre-diabetes, hypertension, dyslipidemia, and obesity) cannot be overstated.[13]

SYMPTOMS

The patient with a diabetic foot may demonstrate no symptoms because peripheral neuropathy can result in a lack of sensation. Peripheral neuropathy can mask painful ulcers and ischemic skin. Foot collapse due to Charcot joints can progress asymptomatically. Alternatively, diabetic patients can have pain sensations in the feet from sensory polyneuropathy, including burning, tingling, and painful numbness. Because of impaired sensation, patients may report imbalance and falls.

Persons with peripheral arterial disease have claudication pain with walking because of insufficient arterial blood supply to meet the demand of exercising muscles. Pain with vascular claudication is typically in the calf and worsened with ambulation. Patients with neurogenic claudication due to spinal stenosis can have similar leg or calf pain with walking but must bend at the waist or sit to relieve the symptoms. Persons may present with gangrene, ischemic ulcers on the distal foot, or, when peripheral arterial disease is severe, pain at rest.

PHYSICAL EXAMINATION

In addition to a standard physical examination, special neurovascular areas must be highlighted.[14]

Inspect the skin for ulcerations, cracks, callus, or trophic changes (thin, shiny skin; distal hair loss).

Evaluate for any foot deformities that predispose it to abnormal stress distribution. These include hammer toes, collapsed foot arches due to Charcot joints, high arched feet due to intrinsic muscle atrophy from polyneuropathy, and changes in stress distribution from previous toe or ray amputations.

Assess distal pulses, particularly dorsalis pedis and posterior tibial. If they are absent or weak, it suggests the need for further testing for vascular integrity.

Assess sensation because persons with loss of protective sensation are at risk for skin ulceration. The instrument most frequently used for detection of neuropathy is the nylon Semmes-Weinstein monofilament. Inability to perceive the 10-g force applied by a 5.07 monofilament is associated with clinically significant large-fiber neuropathy.[15]

Evaluate gait and balance. Peripheral neuropathy predisposes to falls and skin trauma.

Probe any ulcers with sterile cotton-tipped applicators or surgical instruments. If bone is reached, this identifies persons with osteomyelitis, and other special bone imaging is unnecessary.[16]

Assess shoes for uneven wear patterns, areas of breakdown, and width of the toe box. Assess skin for redness and pressure points.

FUNCTIONAL LIMITATIONS

Persons with diabetes can develop peripheral polyneuropathy with loss of position sense and weakness. These can lead to gait instability and falls. Persons with peripheral arterial disease are often limited in community ambulation and vocational activities because of pain from claudication.

DIAGNOSTIC STUDIES

There are many noninvasive and invasive tests for peripheral arterial disease that are beyond the scope of this discussion. Angiography can identify surgically remediable lesions.

In the outpatient setting, the ankle-brachial index, a ratio of Doppler-recorded systolic pressures in the lower and upper extremities, is a convenient, accurate, noninvasive test that provides objective assessment of lower limb vascular status for screening and diagnosis of peripheral arterial disease.[17] An index of 0.9 or higher is normal; 0.7 to 0.9 indicates mild disease, 0.4 to 0.6 reflects moderate to severe disease, and less than 0.4 indicates severe disease.[11] Measurement of systolic pressure in the foot also provides a measure of arterial integrity.

Transcutaneous oximetry is the best method for assessment of cutaneous ischemia.[11] Transcutaneous oximetry pressures of more than 40 mm Hg are normal; pressures of 20 to 40 mm Hg indicate moderate disease, and potential for healing of a skin ulcer is less likely. With pressures below 20 mm Hg, severe skin ischemia is present, and skin healing is poor.

Systolic blood pressures in the foot are also helpful in quantifying the severity of ischemia. Persons with ischemic ulcers and ankle systolic pressures of less than 40 to 60 mm Hg are considered to have severe ischemia. Persons with persistently recurring ischemic rest pain and ankle systolic pressures of 50 mm Hg or less are severely involved. Frank ulceration and gangrene of the foot or toes with an ankle pressure of less than 50 mm Hg reflects severe limb ischemia.[11]

If a person complains of numbness in the legs or feet or has low back pain, electrodiagnostic testing should be conducted to identify whether peripheral polyneuropathy is present or whether lumbosacral radiculopathy is responsible for these symptoms. Nerve conduction study findings may include reduced sensory and motor amplitude, latencies, and slowed conduction velocity. Electromyographic findings in radiculopathy include increased insertional activity, abnormal spontaneous activity, and changes in motor unit morphology; when these electromyographic findings are seen in a myotomal pattern, this suggests radiculopathy.

Differential Diagnosis[5]

Nonvascular

Neurogenic claudication from lumbar spinal stenosis

Calf pain due to S1 radiculopathy

Foot pain due to plantar fasciitis

Pain in legs and feet due to polyneuropathy

Arthritis of the hips

Restless legs syndrome

Vascular

Arterial embolus

Deep venous thrombosis

Thromboangiitis obliterans (Buerger disease)

TREATMENT

Initial

Risk Factor Modification

Cigarette smoking is the most important risk factor for development of peripheral arterial disease.[18] Smoking cessation reduces the disease progression, lowering rates of amputation and the incidence of rest ischemia.[19]

For diabetes control, minimize hyperglycemia. For hypertension control, management of blood pressure is required.

Elevated total and low-density lipoprotein cholesterol levels, reduced high-density lipoprotein level, and hypertriglyceridemia are associated with lower extremity peripheral arterial disease.[20] Several clinical trials have demonstrated the benefits of lipid-lowering therapy in patients with peripheral arterial disease and coexistent coronary and cerebral arterial disease.[5]

High serum homocysteine levels are associated with a twofold to threefold increased risk for peripheral arterial disease.[21] Dietary supplementation with B vitamins and folate may lower homocysteine levels, but no controlled trials to date demonstrate this clinical benefit in peripheral arterial disease.[5]

Given the role of aerobic exercise in modifying lipid profiles, weight, blood pressure, and glycemic control, it plays a strong role in primary prevention of peripheral arterial disease.

Cilostazol, a phosphodiesterase type 3 inhibitor, has vasodilator and platelet inhibitory effects. Cilostazol, 100 mg orally twice daily, is indicated as an effective therapy to improve symptoms and to increase walking distance in patients with lower extremity peripheral arterial disease and intermittent claudication.[18] It is contraindicated in heart failure. Other antiplatelet drugs, including aspirin, clopidogrel, and dipyridamole, are frequently prescribed for patients with peripheral arterial disease.

Rehabilitation

Exercise

A program of supervised exercise is recommended for patients with intermittent claudication. A meta-analysis of training programs performed up until the mid-1990s suggested that an optimal exercise program aimed at improvement of walking performance should use walking as the mode of exercise.[22] A study comparing the efficacy of cycle training versus treadmill exercise in the treatment of intermittent claudication concluded that cycle exercise is not effective in improving walking performance in all claudication patients. A cross-transfer effect between training modes was noted for patients reporting common limiting symptoms at baseline for both cycling and walking. Therefore, the current recommendation for exercise in intermittent claudication is walking.[23] Exercise should be performed for a minimum of 30 to 45 minutes, at least three times per week. Supervised exercise can induce increases in maximal walking ability that exceed those attained with drug therapies alone and translate into improved functional ability.[18] Exercise is contraindicated in the presence of an ischemic ulcer or rest pain.

Foot Care

Meticulous attention to the feet by both patient and physician and detailed education of the patient are the mainstays of preventive foot care.

Deformities should prompt the clinician to consider custom shoe inserts to distribute pressures evenly over the foot. Extra-depth shoes may be necessary to accommodate hammer toes. Tennis shoes are an inexpensive alternative for persons without foot deformities. However, if there are any aberrations in foot bone architecture, custom footwear with molded sole inserts is desirable.

Skin Ulcers

Early treatment of skin infections with antibiotics is warranted along with minimization or elimination of weight bearing during healing. Achievement of a therapeutic antibiotic concentration at the site of infection is key. Intravenous antibiotics may therefore be necessary for patients with severe infection or systemic illness and for treatment of pathogens that are not susceptible to oral agents.[24]

For more involved wounds, débridement with dressing changes or whirlpool is sometimes necessary. Deep infections into bone or infections that extend along fascial planes require débridement. If osteomyelitis is suspected, at least a 6-week course of parenteral or oral antibiotic therapy guided by culture samples obtained during débridement is an effective clinical approach.[20] Other wound care measures, such as total contact casting, can assist with resolution of plantar surface ulcers.

Hyperbaric oxygen therapy may improve wound healing and reduce the rate of amputation.[25] However, given its expense and limited resource, it is mostly limited to deep infections unresponsive to standard therapy.

Edema hinders wound healing. Measures to control edema, such as leg elevation, compression stockings, and pneumatic compression devices, are often used.[26]

Procedures

An acute painful, pale, pulseless limb should be evaluated emergently as this indicates acute arterial compromise. Likewise, gangrene or an ulcer extending to bone should prompt surgical consultation. Sharp débridement for a necrotic wound is often necessary to remove devitalized tissue and to promote healing of ulcers.

Percutaneous endovascular interventions to treat peripheral arterial occlusion include transluminal angioplasty with balloon dilatation, stents, atherectomy, laser, cutting balloons, thermal angioplasty, and fibrinolysis or fibrinectomy. This intervention may be necessary to provide enough oxygenated arterial blood to a limb to heal open sores, to improve symptoms of claudication, or to save an extremity at risk for amputation.[21]

Endovascular procedures are indicated for individuals with severe vocational or lifestyle-limiting disability due to intermittent claudication for whom exercise and pharmacologic therapy have failed. Clinical features must suggest a reasonable likelihood of symptomatic improvement with endovascular intervention with a favorable risk-benefit ratio.[21]

Outcomes of percutaneous transluminal angioplasty and stents depend on anatomic and clinical factors. Durability of patency after percutaneous transluminal angioplasty is greatest for lesions in the common iliac artery and decreases distally. Durability decreases with increasing length of the stenosis, multiple and diffuse lesions, poor-quality runoff, diabetes, renal failure, and smoking. Hormone replacement in women has been shown to decrease patency of iliac stents.[21]

Surgery

Surgical treatment of intermittent claudication is indicated in individuals who do not derive adequate functional benefit from nonsurgical therapies, who have limb arterial anatomy favorable to a durable clinical result, and in whom the risk of cardiovascular complications is low.

The exact surgical procedure (aortobifemoral bypass, aortoiliac bypass, iliofemoral bypass, axillofemoral-femoral bypass) is determined by the site and severity of the occlusive lesion, prior revascularization attempts, general medical condition, and desired outcome.[21]

Similar considerations are given in the management of limb-threatening ischemia. Surgical lower limb amputation may be necessary if revascularization attempts are unsuccessful in the management of limb-threatening ischemia or gangrene.

POTENTIAL DISEASE COMPLICATIONS

As a result of peripheral arterial disease, patients may develop ischemic pain from arterial insufficiency defined as claudication (pain with ambulation) or rest pain. Other potential complications include nonhealing or slow to heal foot ulcers, cellulitis, and deeper wound infections in the foot. If those complications cannot be treated medically, amputation of a portion of the lower limb may be necessary to save the remaining viable limb and to prevent disseminated infection. Charcot joints and bone fractures in the foot due to diabetic polyneuropathy can be seen, potentially leading to skin ulcer and breakdown.

POTENTIAL TREATMENT COMPLICATIONS

Potential treatment complications depend on the intervention implemented. For example, in surgical revascularization, infection of arterial bypass grafts, ischemic cardiac disease, and worsening of renal azotemia are potential complications. Patients undergoing wound débridement should be closely observed for possible infection of foot ulcers after débridement.

For peripheral arterial disease patients initiating an exercise program, potential complications include cardiac ischemic events, given the strong correlation of arterial disease and cardiovascular disease. Therefore, in such patients, supervised exercise instruction after cardiac stress testing is initially recommended to stratify patients at potential risk.[21]

References

1. Dillingham T, Pezzin L, MacKenzie E. Limb amputation and limb deficiency: epidemiology and recent trends in the United States. South Med J 2002;95:875-883.
2. Sanders L. Diabetes mellitus: prevention of amputation. J Am Podiatr Med Assoc 1994;84:322-328.
3. American Heart Association. Peripheral Arterial Disease—Statistics. Available at: http://www.americanheart.org/presenter.jhtml?identifier=3020262. Accessed April 20, 2006.
4. Becker GJ, McClenny TE, Kovacs ME, et al. The importance of increasing public and physician awareness of peripheral arterial disease. J Vasc Interv Radiol 2002;13:7-11.
5. Gey DC, Lesho EP, Manngold J. Management of peripheral arterial disease. Available at: http://www.aafp.org/afp/20040201/525.html. Accessed April 20, 2006.
6. Meijer WT, Grobbee DE, Hunink MG, et al. Determinants of peripheral arterial disease in the elderly: the Rotterdam study. Arch Intern Med 2000;160:2934-2938.
7. Criqui MH, Vargas V, Denenberg JO, et al. Ethnicity and peripheral arterial disease: the San Diego Population Study. Circulation 2005;112:2703-2707.
8. National Diabetes Fact Sheet, 2005. Available at: http://www.diabetes.org/uedocuments/NationalDiabetesFactSheetRev.pdf. Accessed April 20, 2006.
9. Harris MI. Diabetes in America: epidemiology and scope of the problem. Diabetes Care 1998;21(Suppl 3):C11-C14.
10. Beckman JA, Creager MA, Libby P. Diabetes and atherosclerosis: epidemiology, pathophysiology, and management. JAMA 2002;287:2570-2581.
11. Pandian G, Hamid F, Hammond MC. Rehabilitation of the patient with PVD and diabetic foot problems. In DeLisa J, Gans BM, eds. Rehabilitation Medicine: Principles and Practice. Philadelphia, Lippincott-Raven, 1998:1517-1544.
12. Tuomilehto J, Lindstrom J, Eriksson JG, et al; the Finnish Diabetes Prevention Study Group. Prevention of type 2 diabetes mellitus by changes in lifestyle among subjects with impaired glucose tolerance. N Engl J Med 2001;344:1343-1350.
13. Eckel RH, Kahn R, Robertson RM, Rizza RA. Preventing cardiovascular disease and diabetes mellitus: a call to action from the ADA and AHA. Circulation 2006;113:2943-2946.
14. Standards of Medical Care in Diabetes—2006. Diabetes Care 2006;29:S4-S42.
15. Singh N, Armstrong DG, Lipsky BA. Preventing foot ulcers in patients with diabetes. JAMA 2005;293:217-228.
16. Grayson M, Gibbons G, Balough K, et al. Probing to bone in infected pedal ulcers: a clinical sign of underlying osteomyelitis in diabetic patients. JAMA 1995;273:721-723.
17. U.S. Preventive Services Task Force Recommendation Statement. Screening for peripheral arterial disease. Am Fam Physician 2006;73:1-8.
18. Regensteiner JG, Hiatt WR. Current medical therapies for patients with peripheral arterial disease: a critical review. Am J Med 2002;112:49-57.
19. Girolami B, Bernardi E, Prins MH, et al. Treatment of intermittent claudication with physical training, smoking cessation, pentoxifylline, or nafronyl: a meta-analysis. Arch Intern Med 1999;159:337-345.

20. Hirsch AT, Haskal ZJ, Hertzer NR, et al. ACC/AHA guidelines for the management of patients with peripheral arterial disease: a collaborative report. Available at: http://www.acc.org/clinical/guidelines/pad/index.pdf. Accessed April 20, 2006.

21. Graham IM, Daly LE, Refsum HM, et al. Plasma homocysteine as a risk factor for vascular disease. JAMA 1997;277:1775-1781.

22. Gardner AW, Poehlman ET. Exercise rehabilitation programs for the treatment of claudication pain. JAMA 1995;274:975-980.

23. Sanderson B, Askew C, Stewart I, et al. Short-term effects of cycle and treadmill training of exercise tolerance in peripheral arterial disease. J Vasc Surg 2006;44:119-127.

24. Lipsky BA. Medical treatment of diabetic foot infections. Clin Infect Dis 2004;39:S104-S114.

25. Wunderlich RP, Peters EJD, Lavery L. Systemic hyperbaric oxygen therapy: lower-extremity wound healing and the diabetic foot. Diabetes Care 2000;23:1551-1555.

26. Armstrong DG, Nguyen HC. Improvement in healing with aggressive edema reduction after débridement of foot infection in persons with diabetes. Arch Surg 2000;135:1405-1409.

Dysphagia 121

Jeffrey B. Palmer, MD, and Koichiro Matsuo, DDS, PhD

Synonyms

Swallowing disorder
Swallowing impairment
Deglutition disorder

ICD-9 Codes

438.82 Other late effects of cerebrovascular disease, dysphagia
787.2 Dysphagia, difficulty in swallowing

DEFINITION

Dysphagia generally refers to any difficulty with swallowing, including occult or asymptomatic impairments. It is a common problem, affecting one third to one half of all stroke patients[1] and about one sixth of elderly individuals.[2] It is frequent in head and neck cancer, traumatic brain injury, degenerative disorders of the nervous system, gastroesophageal reflux disease, and inflammatory muscle disease (Table 121-1). Dysphagia is classified according to the location of the problem as oropharyngeal (localized to the oral cavity or pharynx, not just the oropharynx) or esophageal. It may also be classified as mechanical (due to a structural lesion of the foodway) or functional (caused by a physiologic abnormality of foodway function).[3]

Sudden onset is suggestive of stroke. Concomitant limb weakness suggests a neurologic or neuromuscular disorder. Medication-induced dysphagia is commonly overlooked. Medications that impair level of consciousness (such as sedatives and tranquilizers), have anticholinergic effects (tricyclics, propantheline), or can damage mucous membranes (nonsteroidal anti-inflammatory drugs, aspirin, quinidine) may also cause dysphagia.[4]

SYMPTOMS

The most common symptoms of dysphagia are coughing or choking during eating[5] and the sensation of food sticking in the throat or chest.[3] Some of the many symptoms and signs of dysphagia are listed in Table 121-2. A history of drooling, significant weight loss, or recurrent pneumonia suggests that the dysphagia is severe. The history is most useful for identification of esophageal dysphagia; the complaint of food sticking in the chest is usually associated with an esophageal disorder. In contrast, the complaint of food sticking in the throat has little localizing value and is often caused by an esophageal disorder. Coughing and choking during swallowing suggest an oropharyngeal origin and may be elicited by aspiration (penetration of material through the vocal folds and into the trachea). However, some patients have impaired cough reflexes, resulting in silent aspiration (without cough).[5,6] Silent aspiration occurs in 28% to 94%, depending on the population of patients.[6-8] Patients with neurologic disorder have a higher incidence of silent aspiration. Pain on swallowing (odynophagia) may occur transiently in pharyngitis, but persistent pain is unusual and is suggestive of neoplasia. Heartburn is a nonspecific complaint that is usually not associated with swallowing but occurs after meals. Heartburn may occur in gastroesophageal reflux disease, but a more specific symptom of gastroesophageal reflux disease is regurgitation of sour or bitter-tasting material into the throat after eating.

PHYSICAL EXAMINATION

An examination of the oral cavity and neck may identify structural abnormalities, weakness, or sensory deficits. The finding of dysarthria (abnormal articulation of speech) or dysphonia (abnormal voice quality) is often associated with oropharyngeal dysphagia. However, the examination is primarily useful for finding evidence of underlying neurologic, neuromuscular, or connective tissue disease. The examination should always include trial swallows of water.[9-11] During the swallow, there should be prompt elevation of the hyoid bone and larynx. Changes in voice quality or spontaneous coughing after swallowing suggest pharyngeal dysfunction. The history and physical examination are limited in their ability to detect and to characterize dysphagia, so instrumental studies are usually necessary.[12]

Neurologic examination is important in the evaluation of dysphagic individuals because neurologic disorders commonly cause dysphagia. Disorders of either upper or lower motor neuron may produce dysphagia. The

TABLE 121-1 Selected Causes of Oral and Pharyngeal Dysphagia

Neurologic Disorders and Stroke	Structural Lesions	Connective Tissue Diseases
Cerebral infarction	Thyromegaly	Polymyositis
Brainstem infarction	Cervical hyperostosis	Muscular dystrophy
Intracranial hemorrhage	Congenital web	Psychiatric disorders
Parkinson disease	Zenker diverticulum	Psychogenic dysphagia
Multiple sclerosis	Caustic ingestion	
Amyotrophic lateral sclerosis	Neoplasm	
Poliomyelitis	Post–ablative surgery	
Myasthenia gravis	Radiation fibrosis	
Dementias		

TABLE 121-2 Symptoms and Signs of Dysphagia

Oral or pharyngeal dysphagia

Coughing or choking with swallowing

Difficulty with initiation of swallowing

Food sticking in the throat

Drooling

Unexplained weight loss

Change in dietary habits

Recurrent pneumonia

Change in voice or speech

Nasal regurgitation

Dehydration

Esophageal dysphagia

Sensation of food sticking in the chest or throat

Oral or pharyngeal regurgitation

Drooling

Unexplained weight loss

Change in dietary habits

Recurrent pneumonia

Dehydration

findings of atrophy or fasciculations of the tongue or palate suggest lower motor neuron dysfunction of the brainstem motor nuclei. In contrast to the prevailing wisdom, the gag reflex is not strongly predictive of the ability to swallow. It may be absent in normal individuals and normal in individuals with severe dysphagia and aspiration.[13]

FUNCTIONAL LIMITATIONS

These depend on the nature and severity of the dysphagia. Many individuals modify their diets to eliminate foods that are difficult to swallow. Some require inordinate amounts of time to consume a meal. In severe cases, tube feeding is necessary. These alterations in the ability to eat a meal may have a profound effect on psychological and social function.[14] Interaction with family and friends often centers on mealtime—family dinners, "going out" for a drink or for dinner, "coming over" for a snack or for dessert. Difficulty in eating a meal may disrupt relationships and result in social isolation. Some patients may require supervision during meals or feel unsafe when they eat alone, causing further disruption of social and vocational function.

DIAGNOSTIC TESTING

Because the mechanics of swallowing are largely invisible to the naked eye, diagnostic studies are commonly needed. The sine qua non for diagnosis of oropharyngeal swallowing disorders is the videofluorographic swallowing study (VFSS).[15] In this test, the patient eats and drinks a variety of solids and liquids combined with barium while images are recorded with videofluorography (radiographic videotaping). The VFSS is usually performed jointly by a physician (physiatrist or radiologist) and a speech-language pathologist. A unique benefit of the VFSS is that therapeutic techniques (such as modification of food consistency, body position, or respiration) can be tested and their effects on swallowing observed during the study. A routine barium swallow study is frequently sufficient if the problem is clearly esophageal.

If a VFSS cannot be performed because of the physical limitation of the patient, the fiberoptic endoscopic evaluation of swallowing is useful to visualize the anatomy of the pharynx and larynx and vocal fold function during eating with no x-ray exposure.[16] It is also highly sensitive for detection of aspiration[8]; but it does not visualize essential aspects of swallowing, such as the oral and esophageal stages of swallowing, or critical events of pharyngeal swallowing including opening of the upper esophageal sphincter, elevation of the larynx, and contraction of the pharynx.

In cases of esophageal dysphagia, esophagoscopy is frequently necessary to detect mucosal lesions or masses. Biopsy is indicated when mucosal abnormalities are detected. Manometry is useful for detection and characterization of motor disorders of the esophagus. Electromyography is indicated when neuromuscular disease is suspected and is useful for detection of lower motor neuron dysfunction of the larynx and pharynx.

TREATMENT

Initial

The treatment of dysphagia depends on its causes and mechanism. Common treatments are listed in Table 121-3. Whenever possible, initial treatment should be

Differential Diagnosis

Myocardial ischemia

Globus sensation

Heartburn due to gastroesophageal reflux disease

Indirect aspiration (aspiration of refluxed gastric contents)

TABLE 121-3 Principal Treatments of Selected Disorders Affecting Swallowing

Problems	Principal Treatments
Amyotrophic lateral sclerosis	Dietary modification
	Compensatory maneuvers
	Counseling and advance directives
Carcinoma of esophagus	Esophagectomy
Gastroesophageal reflux disease	Dietary modification
	No eating at bedtime
	Pharmacologic therapy
	Smoking cessation
Parkinson disease, polymyositis, myasthenia gravis	Pharmacologic treatment of underlying disease (dietary modification, compensatory maneuvers, and dysphagia therapy only if necessary)
Esophageal stricture or web	Dilatation
Stroke, multiple sclerosis	Dietary modification
	Compensatory maneuvers
	Dysphagia therapy

directed at the underlying disease process; for example, levodopa for Parkinson disease, or steroids for polymyositis. Esophageal dysphagia necessitates evaluation and treatment by a gastroenterologist. When no therapy exists for the underlying disease or the therapy is ineffective or contraindicated, rehabilitative strategies are appropriate. Patients and their family members are encouraged to learn the Heimlich maneuver; this is important because airway obstruction is potentially fatal.

Rehabilitation

Many patients benefit from a structured swallowing therapy provided by a speech-language pathologist, including instruction and supervision about diet, compensatory maneuvers, and exercise.[17] The goals of therapy are to reduce aspiration, to improve the ability to eat and drink, and to optimize nutritional status. Ther-

apy is individualized according to the patient's specific anatomic and structural abnormalities and the initial responses to treatment trials observed at the bedside or during the VFSS.[18] A fundamental principle of rehabilitation is that the best therapy for any activity is the activity itself; swallowing is generally the best therapy for swallowing disorders, so the rehabilitation evaluation is directed at identification of circumstances for safe and effective swallowing for each individual patient.

Diet modification is a common treatment of dysphagia.[19,20] Patients vary in ability to swallow thin and thick liquids, and that determination is usually best made by VFSS. A patient can usually receive adequate oral hydration with either thin (e.g., water or apple juice) or thick liquids (e.g., apricot nectar, tomato juice). Rarely, a patient may be limited to pudding consistency if thin and thick liquids are freely aspirated. Most patients with significant dysphagia are unable to safely eat meats or similarly tough foods and require a mechanical soft diet. A pureed diet is recommended for patients who exhibit oral preparatory phase difficulties, pocket food in the buccal recesses (between the teeth and the cheek), or have significant pharyngeal retention with chewed solid foods. Maintenance of oral feeding often requires compensatory techniques to reduce aspiration or to improve pharyngeal clearance. A variety of behavioral techniques are used, including modifications of posture, head position (Fig. 121-1),[21,22] and respiration,[23] as well as specific swallow maneuvers.[24-26]

Exercise therapy for dysphagia is indicated when the problem is related to weakness of the muscles of swallowing.[27] The choice of exercises must be individualized according to the physiologic assessment. The full range of exercises is beyond the scope of this chapter, but several examples illustrate the principles.

- Tongue weakness can be treated with lingual resistance exercise.[28]
- Strengthening of the anterior suprahyoid muscles is useful when the upper esophageal sphincter opens poorly. Flexing the neck against gravity while lying supine can strengthen these muscles (Fig. 121-2).[29,30]
- Vocal fold adduction exercises may be useful in cases of aspiration due to weakness of these muscles. These exercises are done on a daily basis whenever possible.

Procedures

VFSS functions as both a diagnostic and a therapeutic procedure for dysphagia, especially oropharyngeal dysphagia, because it can be used to test the effectiveness of modifying food consistency and other compensatory techniques.[31] Endoscopy with dilatation of the esophagus is often indicated in cases of partial esophageal obstruction due to stricture or web. Dilatation is also appropriate in stenosis of the upper esophageal sphincter. Endoscopy can also be used for biofeedback, especially to demonstrate movements of the larynx during swallowing maneuvers. Electromyography is also used for biofeedback. Activities of the infrahyoid

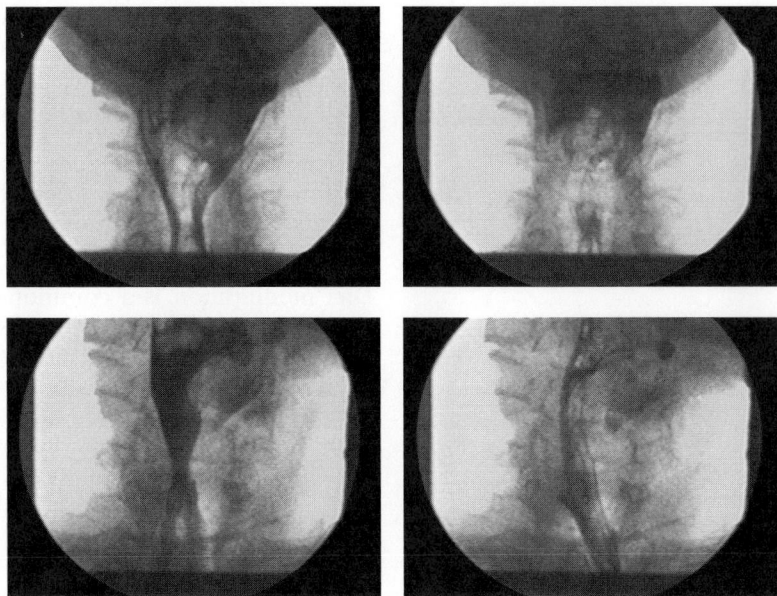

FIGURE 121-1. Turning the head toward the weak side improves pharyngeal emptying in some individuals with dysphagia due to lateral medullary infarction. This series of videoprints is taken from a videofluorographic swallowing study of an individual with severe dysphagia due to lateral medullary infarction. The top images show an anteroposterior projection of swallowing with the head in anatomic position. The top left image was obtained in mid-swallow. There is stasis of barium in the left piriform recess, with only minimal flow of barium through the upper esophageal sphincter. The top right image shows the large amount of residual barium in the pharynx after swallowing. The bottom images show swallowing with the head turned toward the weak left side. The lower left figure, in mid-swallow, shows enhanced flow of barium. The lower right figure shows dramatically reduced retention of barium after the swallow.

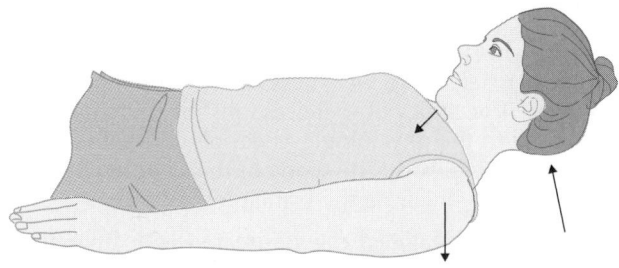

FIGURE 121-2. Shaker exercise to augment upper esophageal sphincter opening by strengthening of the anterior suprahyoid muscles. The neck is actively flexed, raising the head so the patient can see the toes, touching the chin to the chest, without lifting the shoulders.

and suprahyoid muscles are recorded with surface electrodes during swallowing therapy. Biofeedback itself is not a dysphagia therapy but can be a useful adjunct to therapy. Surface electrical stimulation on the submental or anterior cervical muscles is a controversial new treatment of dysphagia. There is little evidence for its safety and efficacy.[32-34]

Surgery

Surgery is rarely indicated in the care of patients with oral or pharyngeal dysphagia. The most common procedure for pharyngeal dysphagia is cricopharyngeal myotomy, during which the upper esophageal sphincter is disrupted to reduce the resistance of the pharyngeal outflow tract. However, the effectiveness of myotomy is highly controversial.[35] Esophagectomy may be necessary in case of esophageal cancer or obstructive stric-

tures. Feeding gastrostomy (usually percutaneous endoscopic gastrostomy) is indicated when the severity of the dysphagia makes it impossible for adequate alimentation or hydration to be obtained orally, although intravenous hydration or nasogastric tube feedings may be sufficient on a time-limited basis.[36] Orogastric tube feedings have been used successfully by patients who have absent gag reflexes and can tolerate intermittent oral catheterization.

POTENTIAL DISEASE COMPLICATIONS

Severe dysphagia may result in aspiration pneumonia,[1] airway obstruction, bronchiectasis, dehydration, or starvation[37] and is potentially fatal. Severe dysphagia often causes social isolation because of the inability to consume a meal in the usual manner. This may lead to depression, sometimes severe. Suicide has been reported.

POTENTIAL TREATMENT COMPLICATIONS

The VFSS is safe and well tolerated. Prescription of a modified diet often means the substitution of thick for thin liquids. Some patients find these unpalatable and reduce fluid intake to the point of dehydration and malnutrition. Failure to reevaluate patients in a timely manner may lead to unnecessary prolongation of dietary restrictions, increasing the risk of malnutrition and adverse psychological effects of dysphagia. Dilatation of the esophagus or sphincters may result in perforation, but this complication is uncommon.

Percutaneous endoscopic gastrostomy may have direct or indirect sequelae. Direct sequelae, such as pain, infection, and obstruction of the feeding tube, are common. Percutaneous endoscopic gastrostomy tube feeding may promote aspiration pneumonia in individuals with severe gastroesophageal reflux disease.

References

1. Martino R, Foley N, Bhogal S, et al. Dysphagia after stroke: incidence, diagnosis, and pulmonary complications. Stroke 2005;36:2756-2763.
2. Achem SR, Devault KR. Dysphagia in aging. J Clin Gastroenterol 2005;39:357-371.
3. Palmer JB, Drennan JC, Baba M. Evaluation and treatment of swallowing impairments. Am Fam Physician 2000;61:2453-2462.
4. Buchholz DW. Oropharyngeal dysphagia due to iatrogenic neurological dysfunction. Dysphagia 1995;10:248-254.
5. Smith Hammond CA, Goldstein LB. Cough and aspiration of food and liquids due to oral-pharyngeal dysphagia: ACCP evidence-based clinical practice guidelines. Chest 2006;129:154S-168S.
6. Smith CH, Logemann JA, Colangelo LA, et al. Incidence and patient characteristics associated with silent aspiration in the acute care setting [see comments]. Dysphagia 1999;14:1-7.
7. Arvedson J, Rogers B, Buck G, et al. Silent aspiration prominent in children with dysphagia. Int J Pediatr Otorhinolaryngol 1994;28:173-181.
8. Leder SB, Sasaki CT, Burrell MI. Fiberoptic endoscopic evaluation of dysphagia to identify silent aspiration. Dysphagia 1998;13:19-21.
9. DePippo KL, Holas MA, Reding MJ. Validation of the 3-oz water swallow test for aspiration following stroke [see comments]. Arch Neurol 1992;49:1259-1261.
10. Tohara H, Saitoh E, Mays KA, et al. Three tests for predicting aspiration without videofluorography. Dysphagia 2003;18:126-134.
11. Wu MC, Chang YC, Wang TG, et al. Evaluating swallowing dysfunction using a 100-ml water swallowing test. Dysphagia 2004;19:43-47.
12. Palmer JB. Evaluation of swallowing disorders. In Grabois M, ed. Physical Medicine and Rehabilitation: The Complete Approach. Malden, Mass, Blackwell Science, 1999:277-290.
13. Leder SB. Gag reflex and dysphagia. Head Neck 1996;18:138-141.
14. Kumlien S, Axelsson K. Stroke patients in nursing homes: eating, feeding, nutrition and related care. J Clin Nurs 2002;11:498-509.
15. Palmer JB, Kuhlemeier KV, Tippett DC, et al. A protocol for the videofluorographic swallowing study. Dysphagia 1993;8:209-214.
16. Langmore SE. Endoscopic Evaluation and Treatment of Swallowing Disorders. New York, Thieme, 2001.
17. Carnaby G, Hankey GJ, Pizzi J. Behavioural intervention for dysphagia in acute stroke: a randomised controlled trial. Lancet Neurol 2006;5:31-37.
18. Ott DJ, Hodge RG, Pikna LA, et al. Modified barium swallow: clinical and radiographic correlation and relation to feeding recommendations. Dysphagia 1996;11:187-190.
19. Bisch EM, Logemann JA, Rademaker AW, et al. Pharyngeal effects of bolus volume, viscosity, and temperature in patients with dysphagia resulting from neurologic impairment and in normal subjects. J Speech Hear Res 1994;37:1041-1059.
20. McCallum SL. The National Dysphagia Diet: implementation at a regional rehabilitation center and hospital system. J Am Diet Assoc 2003;103:381-384.
21. Welch MV, Logemann JA, Rademaker AW, et al. Changes in pharyngeal dimensions effected by chin tuck. Arch Phys Med Rehabil 1993;74:178-181.
22. Ohmae Y, Ogura M, Kitahara S, et al. Effects of head rotation on pharyngeal function during normal swallow. Ann Otol Rhinol Laryngol 1998;107:344-348.
23. Bulow M, Olsson R, Ekberg O. Videomanometric analysis of supraglottic swallow, effortful swallow, and chin tuck in patients with pharyngeal dysfunction. Dysphagia 2001;16:190-195.
24. Hind JA, Nicosia MA, Roecker EB, et al. Comparison of effortful and noneffortful swallows in healthy middle-aged and older adults. Arch Phys Med Rehabil 2001;82:1661-1665.
25. Ding R, Larson CR, Logemann JA, et al. Surface electromyographic and electroglottographic studies in normal subjects under two swallow conditions: normal and during the Mendelsohn maneuver. Dysphagia 2002;17:1-12.
26. Logemann JA. Behavioral management for oropharyngeal dysphagia. Folia Phoniatr Logop 1999;51:199-212.
27. Logemann JA. The role of exercise programs for dysphagia patients. Dysphagia 2005;20:139-140.
28. Robbins J, Gangnon RE, Theis SM, et al. The effects of lingual exercise on swallowing in older adults. J Am Geriatr Soc 2005;53:1483-1489.
29. Shaker R, Kern M, Bardan E, et al. Augmentation of deglutitive upper esophageal sphincter opening in the elderly by exercise. Am J Physiol 1997;272:G1518-1522.
30. Shaker R, Easterling C, Kern M, et al. Rehabilitation of swallowing by exercise in tube-fed patients with pharyngeal dysphagia secondary to abnormal UES opening. Gastroenterology 2002;122:1314-1321.
31. Palmer JB, Carden EA. The role of radiology in rehabilitation of swallowing. In Jones B, ed. Normal and Abnormal Swallowing: Imaging in Diagnosis and Therapy, 2nd ed. New York, Springer-Verlag, 2003:261-273.
32. Freed ML, Freed L, Chatburn RL, et al. Electrical stimulation for swallowing disorders caused by stroke. Respir Care 2001;46:466-474.
33. Ludlow CL, Humbert I, Saxon K, et al. Effects of surface electrical stimulation both at rest and during swallowing in chronic pharyngeal dysphagia. Dysphagia 2006;21:1-10.
34. Suiter DM, Leder SB, Ruark JL. Effects of neuromuscular electrical stimulation on submental muscle activity. Dysphagia 2006;21:56-60.
35. Jacobs JR, Logemann J, Pajak TF, et al. Failure of cricopharyngeal myotomy to improve dysphagia following head and neck cancer surgery. Arch Otolaryngol Head Neck Surg 1999;125:942-946.
36. Dennis MS, Lewis SC, Warlow C. Effect of timing and method of enteral tube feeding for dysphagic stroke patients (FOOD): a multicentre randomised controlled trial. Lancet 2005;365:764-772.
37. Finestone HM, Greene-Finestone LS, Wilson ES, et al. Malnutrition in stroke patients on the rehabilitation service and at follow-up: prevalence and predictors. Arch Phys Med Rehabil 1995;76:310-316.

Enteropathic Arthritides 122

Karen Atkinson, MD, MPH

DEFINITION

The term *enteropathic arthritis* describes arthritis that is associated with disease of the bowel. This category includes the arthritis associated with infection (Reiter syndrome), inflammatory bowel disease, Whipple disease, intestinal bypass surgery, and celiac disease (gluten-sensitive enteropathy).[1]

Reiter syndrome (reactive arthritis) usually occurs in young to middle-aged adults after genitourinary (*Chlamydia*) or gastrointestinal (typically, *Salmonella, Shigella, Campylobacter,* or *Yersinia*) infection. Men are affected more often in cases that occur after genitourinary infection, but the sex distribution is equal in cases occurring after gastrointestinal infection. The term originally described patients with the classic triad of nongonococcal urethritis, arthritis, and conjunctivitis. Peripheral joint arthritis occurs in 90% of patients with Reiter syndrome, whereas axial involvement (spondylitis or sacroiliitis) affects less than 50% of patients.[1,2]

Arthritis associated with inflammatory bowel disease also typically affects young to middle-aged adults. The sex distribution is equal. Peripheral arthritis occurs in 10% to 20% of patients and axial disease in 10% of patients.[1,2]

Whipple disease, intestinal bypass, and celiac disease can have associated arthritis. Typically, the joint involvement occurs in a symmetric peripheral polyarticular pattern that resembles rheumatoid arthritis. Whipple disease can have axial involvement (spondylitis or sacroiliitis) in 8% to 20% of cases.[3]

SYMPTOMS

Constitutional symptoms are common to all forms of enteropathic arthritis. Patients can experience fever, malaise, weight loss, and fatigue. Morning stiffness of more than 30 to 60 minutes indicates inflammatory disease. The stiffness may be located in the hands or other peripheral joints or in the back of patients with axial involvement. Other symptoms vary according to the type of enteropathic arthritis.[2-7]

Inflammatory Bowel Disease–Associated (Crohn Disease and Ulcerative Colitis) Arthritis

Patients experience pain and swelling in joints that can be transient or migratory but recurrent. Lower extremity joints are affected more frequently than are those of the upper extremity. Patients with dactylitis complain of diffusely swollen digits. Active bowel inflammation leads to diarrhea or bloody stools. Peripheral arthritis flares with the bowel; axial involvement does not correlate with active bowel disease and can be asymptomatic. Heel or foot pain occurs secondary to enthesitis, which is inflammation at the site of tendon or ligament insertion onto bone. Patients with spondylitis or sacroiliitis describe back or buttock pain. Painful oral ulcer may be described. Red or violet bumps (erythema nodosum) can develop; they are painful and most commonly located over the shins. Ulcerating lesions (pyoderma gangrenosum) are less common. Red eyes indicate conjunctivitis or iritis. In iritis (anterior uveitis), the patient experiences pain and decreased vision.

Reiter Syndrome

Patients experience painful, swollen joints. The minority of patients report preceding diarrhea, even on direct questioning. Arthritis involves lower extremity joints more often than upper extremity joints. Heel or foot pain occurs secondary to enthesitis. As in inflammatory bowel disease, back or buttock pain occurs with spondylitis and sacroiliitis. Some form of skin involvement occurs in almost 50% of patients. Lesions include rash over the palms and soles (keratoderma blennorrhagicum), penile lesions (circinate balanitis), and nail changes (onycholysis but not nail pitting). About 15% of patients develop oral ulcers. Urogenital symptoms include penile or vaginal discharge and ulcers. As in inflammatory bowel disease–associated arthritis, eye symptoms include redness, pain, and decreased vision. Symptoms of left-sided heart failure or heart block (syncope) can result from aortic root or valve inflammation.

Whipple Disease

Whipple disease is characterized by fever, diarrhea, foul-smelling or floating stools (steatorrhea), and profound weight loss. Patients with Whipple disease complain of migratory arthralgias or transient episodes of swollen joints. Swollen glands may be a feature. If pleural effusions are present, patients may experience chest pain or shortness of breath. Complaints of double vision (ocular palsies) or mental status changes accompany nervous system involvement.

Intestinal Bypass

Patients complain of painful, swollen joints. Cutaneous vasculitis causes rash in some patients.

Celiac Disease

Joint aches or swelling, usually affecting the large joints, can develop in patients with gluten-sensitive enteropathy. Only 50% of patients have diarrhea. Patients with associated dermatitis herpetiformis complain of burning and itching of the skin.

PHYSICAL EXAMINATION

Physical examination findings vary with the cause of enteropathic arthritis.[2-7]

Inflammatory Bowel Disease–Associated Arthritis

Patients with inflammatory bowel disease usually have monarticular (one joint) or oligoarticular (two to four joints) asymmetric arthritis involving the peripheral joints. The knees, ankles, and feet are most commonly affected. Large effusions occur, especially in the knee. Limited lumbar mobility secondary to spondylitis is documented with an abnormal Schober maneuver (Fig. 122-1). To perform this maneuver, the clinician makes a mark at the level of the posterior superior iliac spines (dimples of the pelvis) and another mark 10 cm above the first mark with the patient standing. The patient is then asked to bend forward, attempting to touch the toes. The distance between the two marks is

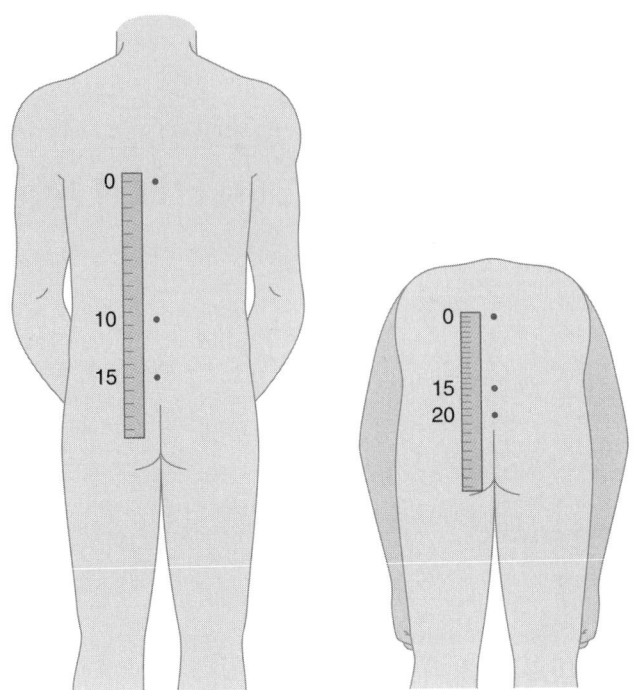

FIGURE 122-1. Schober maneuver.

measured again. With normal lumbar motion, the distance between the two points increases by at least 5 cm. Maneuvers such as pelvic distraction or compression to elicit pain associated with sacroiliitis lack specificity. Thickening of the Achilles tendon or pain at the insertion site of the Achilles or plantar fascia on the calcaneus is found in patients with enthesitis. Examination of the skin may reveal red or violet subcutaneous nodules (erythema nodosum) or painful ulcers with irregular borders (pyoderma gangrenosum). Conjunctivitis causes a red or injected eye. Pericorneal injection, corneal clouding, and miosis suggest anterior uveitis (usually iritis with sparing of the ciliary body). Slit-lamp examination reveals cells in the anterior chamber.

Reiter Syndrome

Like inflammatory bowel disease, Reiter syndrome causes monarticular or oligoarticular asymmetric peripheral arthritis that usually affects the lower limbs. Enthesitis, dactylitis, conjunctivitis, and uveitis also occur, and evaluation of these is as previously described. Urogenital evaluation may reveal a mucoid discharge secondary to inflammation (urethritis or cervicitis). Some skin manifestation will occur in 50% of patients. Keratoderma blennorrhagicum and circinate balanitis each occur in about 25% of patients with Reiter syndrome. Keratoderma blennorrhagicum is a papulosquamous lesion that appears identical to psoriasis but is usually limited to the palms and soles. Circinate balanitis occurs on the shaft or glans; the appearance in men who are circumcised (dry, plaque-like lesions resembling keratoderma) is different from that in uncircumcised men (shallow, serpiginous penile ulcers surrounding the meatus). Nail changes include onycholysis and hyperkeratosis. Lack of pitting may distinguish this from psoriatic changes. Pyoderma gangrenosum can occur. Oral or genital ulcers can be found and are often painless. Aortitis and valve insufficiency can cause a murmur.

Whipple Disease

The arthritis of Whipple disease is typically a symmetrical peripheral polyarthritis (more than four joints). Lymphadenopathy may be noted. Pleural effusions can occur and are detected during pulmonary examination. Neurologic examination may demonstrate ocular palsies or encephalopathy.

Intestinal Bypass

Patients who have undergone intestinal bypass can develop a symmetric peripheral nondeforming polyarthritis. Lesions that can be found on the skin include vesiculopustular lesions, erythema nodosum, urticaria, and ecchymosis.

Celiac Disease

Joint examination reveals a symmetrical peripheral polyarthritis. Dermatitis herpetiformis can be associated with this disorder; it appears as urticarial wheals, vesicles, bullae, and erythema that occur symmetrically on limbs or the trunk.

FUNCTIONAL LIMITATIONS

Functional limitations depend on the location and severity of joint involvement. The criteria for the assessment of functional status that have been established for rheumatoid arthritis (see Chapter 142) are also applied to patients with psoriatic arthritis. These criteria are based on activities of daily living, including self-care (dressing, feeding, bathing, grooming, and toileting), vocational (work, school, and homemaking), and avocational activities (recreational and leisure).[8] Visual impairment can result from inflammatory eye disease.

DIAGNOSTIC STUDIES

Laboratory testing in all of these diseases may reveal anemia and an elevated sedimentation rate. Rheumatoid factor and antinuclear antibodies are usually absent. Synovial fluid is inflammatory (more than 2000 white blood cells) with negative cultures and no crystals when it is examined under polarized microscopy. HLA-B27 is highly associated with Reiter syndrome, occurring in 81% of patients. There is no increased frequency of HLA-B27 in patients with inflammatory bowel disease alone, but 50% of patients with inflammatory bowel disease with spondylitis are B27 positive.[1]

Radiographic evaluation of the axial skeleton may confirm spondylitis or sacroiliitis. In inflammatory bowel disease, sacroiliitis is usually symmetrical, and syndesmophytes usually insert marginally on the vertebral body—findings that are indistinguishable from ankylosing spondylitis (Fig. 122-2). Asymmetric sacroiliitis is found in Reiter syndrome. Peripheral joints in both inflammatory bowel disease and Reiter syndrome may show erosion, but adjacent bone proliferation may distinguish these changes from rheumatoid arthritis. In patients with a history suggestive of enthesitis, calcaneal films will often show proliferative bone formation at the tendon or ligament insertion site.[4] There are usually no radiographic changes in patients with Whipple disease, intestinal bypass, or celiac disease.

Other tests are directed toward the underlying illness or symptom. In patients without confirmed inflammatory bowel disease, evaluation of the bowel with endoscopy or colonoscopy and biopsy is indicated. Skin biopsy may be helpful when clinical findings are not typical or are in question. Patients with ocular symptoms are referred for ophthalmologic (slit-lamp) examination.

In patients with suspected Reiter syndrome, cervical or urethral smears should be performed to rule out gonorrhea and to evaluate for *Chlamydia*. Stool samples from patients who report preceding or concurrent diarrhea should also be sent. If aortitis and aortic insufficiency are suspected, electrocardiography and echocardiography are indicated.

The diagnosis of Whipple disease may be confirmed with characteristic periodic acid–Schiff staining of deposits on small bowel biopsy specimen or lymph node or synovial biopsy specimen. Diagnosis is also now possible by polymerase chain reaction analysis for *Tropheryma whipplei* on blood or tissue samples.

Celiac disease can be diagnosed by small bowel biopsy. Antibody tests are now available, including antigliadin and endomysial antibodies. A presumptive diagnosis can be made if symptoms resolve on a gluten-free diet.

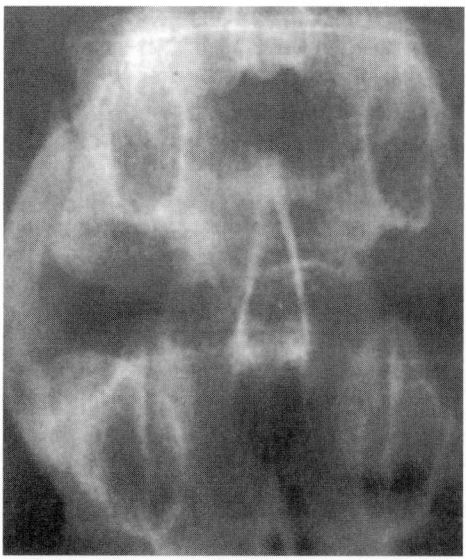

FIGURE 122-2. Radiograph of spine showing a large "jug-handle" syndesmophyte. (Reprinted with permission from West SG. Rheumatology Secrets. Philadelphia, Hanley & Belfus, 1997.)

TREATMENT

Initial

The treatment of inflammatory bowel disease–associated arthritis and the arthritis of Reiter syndrome is generally the same as that of other spondyloarthropathies.[5,9] Nonsteroidal anti-inflammatory drugs are effective in many patients. Cyclooxygenase 2–specific anti-inflammatories may reduce the incidence of gastrointestinal symptoms in patients who have a history of bleeding or who are intolerant of traditional nonsteroidal anti-inflammatory drugs.

For patients with inadequate response or progressive, erosive disease, disease-modifying antirheumatic drugs should be initiated. Antimalarials, intramuscular gold, sulfasalazine, azathioprine, methotrexate, and cyclosporine have all been shown to be effective. As for other inflammatory arthritides, combination therapy can be effective, although controlled data supporting this approach are unavailable. Corticosteroids can be very useful and can be administered systemically as a bridge to therapy with disease-modifying antirheumatic drugs or intra-articularly for monarticular or oligoarticular involvement. Antibiotic treatment targeting the precipitating infection does not improve Reiter syndrome but should be administered if a microbe is isolated to prevent spread of infection.

Patients with Whipple disease can achieve remission with long-term (≥1 year) antibiotic treatment with tetracyclines.[5]

The arthritis associated with intestinal bypass is sometimes controlled with nonsteroidal anti-inflammatory drugs or glucocorticoids. Resolution of the arthritis can be achieved with normalization of gut anatomy.[5]

In patients with celiac disease, the arthritis responds to a gluten-free diet.[4]

Rehabilitation

Approaches to rehabilitation are identical to those in rheumatoid and other inflammatory arthritis. The role of occupational and physical therapy in early or established disease may be different from that in end-stage disease. In early disease, occupational therapy is directed toward education of the patient about how to use the joints to minimize joint stress in performing activities of daily living. Splints may be used to provide joint rest and to reduce inflammation. Splints may also allow functional use of joints that would otherwise be limited by pain; however, not all clinicians advocate this use. Paraffin baths can provide relief of pain and stiffness in the small joints of the hands. In end-stage disease, the occupational therapist plays an important role, providing aids and adaptive devices such as raised toilet seats, special chairs and beds, special grips, and other devices that can assist in self-care.

Physical therapy can help reduce joint inflammation and pain. The therapist may employ a variety of techniques, including the application of heat or cold, transcutaneous nerve stimulation, and iontophoresis. Water exercise (hydrotherapy) is used to increase muscle strength without joint overuse. In patients with foot involvement, such as dactylitis, a high toe box or extra-depth shoe may provide decreased pain and a more normal gait. Shoe inserts are often used in Achilles tendinitis and plantar fasciitis. For patients with axial involvement, the goal of therapy is to maintain a normal upright posture through stretching of paravertebral musculature and correction of the tendency toward kyphotic posture. In end-stage disease, the goals of therapy are to reduce joint inflammation, to loosen fixed position of joints, to improve the function of damaged joints, and to improve strength and general condition. Local immobilization may be used to reduce inflammation and pain. Nonfixed contractures may be prevented or improved with periods of splinting combined with goal-oriented exercise. Muscle strength and overall conditioning may be improved by static, range of motion, and relaxation exercises. In recent years, aerobic exercises and weight training have been used without detrimental effect on the joints. These dynamic exercises are more effective in increasing muscle strength, range of motion, and physical capacity. The motivation and encouragement provided by the therapist should not be underestimated.

Procedures

For monarticular or oligoarticular involvement, local steroid injection may be used when oral medications fail to control joint inflammation.

Surgery

Joint replacement, tendon repair, or synovectomy may be required. Reversal of intestinal bypass is curative in patients with this disorder.

POTENTIAL DISEASE COMPLICATIONS

For patients with inflammatory bowel disease–associated arthritis and Reiter syndrome, progressive damage to joints, including ankylosis, results in loss of function. Tendons can rupture secondary to chronic enthesitis. Visual loss may occur secondary to chronic or poorly controlled inflammatory eye disease. Patients with inflammatory bowel disease, especially Crohn disease, may develop secondary amyloidosis.

POTENTIAL TREATMENT COMPLICATIONS

Side effects vary according to the drug used (Table 122-1).[10]

TABLE 122-1 Toxic Effects of Medications Used in the Treatment of Enteropathic Arthritis

Medication	Side Effects
Nonsteroidal anti-inflammatory drugs	Dyspepsia, ulcer, or bleeding Renal insufficiency Hepatotoxicity Rash Inhibited platelet function
Cyclooxygenase 2 inhibitors	Same as traditional nonsteroidal anti-inflammatory drugs, but gastrointestinal side effects occur less often No platelet effect
Glucocorticoids	Increased appetite, weight gain, cushingoid habitus Acne Fluid retention Hypertension Diabetes Glaucoma, cataracts Atherosclerosis Avascular necrosis Osteoporosis Impaired wound healing Increased susceptibility to infection
Antimalarials	Dyspepsia Macular damage Abnormal skin pigmentation Neuromyopathy Rash
Gold	Myelosuppression Proteinuria or hematuria Oral ulcers Rash Pruritus
Sulfasalazine	Myelosuppression Hemolysis (glucose-6-phosphate dehydrogenase–deficient patients) Hepatotoxicity Photosensitivity, rash Dyspepsia, diarrhea Headaches Oligospermia
Azathioprine	Myelosuppression Hepatotoxicity Pancreatitis (rarely) Lymphoproliferative disorders (long-term risk)
Methotrexate	Hepatic fibrosis, cirrhosis Pneumonitis Myelosuppression Mucositis Dyspepsia Alopecia
Cyclosporine	Renal insufficiency Hypertension Anemia

References

1. Taurog JD. Seronegative spondyloarthropathies: epidemiology, pathology and pathogenesis. In Klippel JH, ed. Primer on the Rheumatic Diseases, 11th ed. Atlanta, Ga, Arthritis Foundation, 1997:180-183.
2. Gladman DD. Clinical aspects of the spondyloarthropathies. Am J Med Sci 1998;316:234-238.
3. Dobbins WO. Whipple's disease: an historical perspective. Q J Med 1985;56:523-531.
4. Veys EM, Hielants H. Enteropathic arthropathies. In Klippel JH, Dieppe PA, eds. Rheumatology, 2nd ed. London, Mosby, 1998:24.1-24.8.
5. Wollheim FA. Enteropathic arthritis. In Kelley WN, Ruddy S, Harris ED Jr, Sledge CB, eds. Textbook of Rheumatology, 5th ed. Philadelphia, WB Saunders, 1997:1006-1014.
6. Arnett FC. Reactive arthritis (Reiter's syndrome) and enteropathic arthritis. In Klippel JH, ed. Primer on the Rheumatic Diseases, 11th ed. Atlanta, Ga, Arthritis Foundation, 1997:184-188.
7. Leirisalo-Repo M, Repo H. Gut and spondyloarthropathies. Rheum Dis Clin North Am 1992;18:23-35.
8. Hochberg MC, Chang RW, Dwosh I, et al. The American College of Rheumatology 1991 Revised Criteria for the classification of global functional status in rheumatoid arthritis. Arthritis Rheum 1992;35:493-502.
9. Haslock I. Ankylosing spondylitis: management. In Klippel JH, Dieppe PA, eds. Rheumatology, 2nd ed. London, Mosby, 1998:19.1-19.10.
10. Cash JM, Klippel JH. Drug therapy: second-line drug therapy for rheumatoid arthritis. N Engl J Med 1994;330:1368-1375.

Heterotopic Ossification 123

Amanda L. Harrington, MD, Philip J. Blount, MD,
and William L. Bockenek, MD

Synonyms

Myositis ossificans
Ossifying fibromyopathy
Neurogenic heterotopic ossification
Periarticular ossification
Heterotopic ossification in paraplegia
Neurogenic ossifying fibromyositis
Neurogenic osteoma
Paraosteoarthropathy

ICD-9 Codes

728.1   Muscular calcification and ossification
728.10   Calcification and ossification, unspecified
         Massive calcification (paraplegic)
728.11   Progressive myositis ossificans
728.12   Traumatic myositis ossificans
         Myositis ossificans (circumscripta)
728.13   Postoperative heterotopic calcification
733.99   Other and unspecified disorders of bone and cartilage
         Hypertrophy of bone

DEFINITION

Heterotopic ossification is the formation of mature, lamellar bone in nonskeletal tissue, usually in soft tissue surrounding joints.[1,2] Its exact etiology is unknown. Heterotopic ossification is commonly seen in patients with traumatic brain injury, spinal cord injury, cerebrovascular accident, burns, fractures, trauma, or muscle injuries and after total joint arthroplasty. More recently, heterotopic ossification has been described in patients after prolonged sedation, ventilation, critical illness, and immobilization.[3,4] Riedel first described heterotopic ossification after trauma to the spinal cord in 1883.[5] The term *neurogenic heterotopic ossification* has been commonly used for heterotopic ossification in patients with traumatic brain injury, spinal cord injury, and cerebrovascular accident.[2,6] The bone formation in heterotopic ossification differs from that in other disorders of calcium deposition in that heterotopic ossification results in encapsulated bone between muscle planes, which is not intra-articular or connected to periosteum.[7]

The incidence rate reported in the literature varies from 11% to 75% in patients with severe traumatic brain injury and spinal cord injury. Lower rates have been reported in patients with cerebrovascular accident. In the populations of patients with traumatic brain injury and spinal cord injury diagnosed with heterotopic ossification, studies have shown a 33% rate of loss of joint range of motion; 10% to 16% progress to complete joint ankylosis.[2,8] The incidence of heterotopic bone formation after total hip arthroplasty and acetabular fracture is estimated at 16% to 53% and 18% to 90%, respectively.[9]

Heterotopic ossification is both more common and more extensive in patients with severe spasticity. Increased spasticity and lower level of limb function not only increase the risk for development of heterotopic ossification but also increase the rate of recurrence after surgical resection.[6] When ectopic bone is discovered in paraplegic patients, it is never found above the level of injury. Heterotopic ossification is rarely seen in flaccid limbs.[6] Interestingly, heterotopic ossification is infrequently reported in cerebral palsy or in children with anoxic brain injury.[2]

The pathogenic mechanisms of heterotopic ossification are still being investigated. Whether genetic factors or local phenomena (trauma, tissue hypoxia, venous insufficiency, edema) are triggering factors, the final common pathway is inflammation and increased blood flow in the tissues.[1,6,10] Undifferentiated mesenchymal cells in connective tissue surrounding muscle or vasculature are transformed by bone morphogenic proteins into osteoblasts, which lay down new bone matrix.[4,9-12] The temporal relationship between injury and initiation of ossification is not clear; however, clinical signs, symptoms, and positive diagnostic test results may appear as early as 2 weeks after injury.[9] Mineralization and true bone formation are usually completed by 6 to 18 months.[6] The extent of bone formation has been described in Brooker's classification[2,12-14] for heterotopic ossification of the hip:

- Class I: islands of bone within soft tissue
- Class II: bone spurs from the pelvis or proximal femur, leaving at least 1 cm between bone surfaces

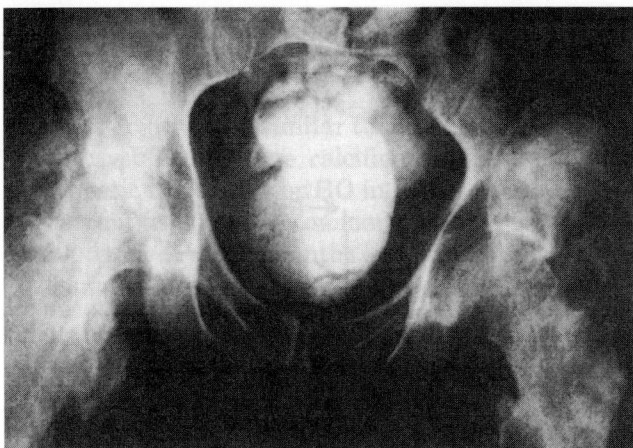

FIGURE 123-1. Radiograph of Brooker class IV heterotopic ossification of the right hip.

- Class III: bone spurs from the pelvis or proximal femur, reducing the space between opposing surfaces to less than 1 cm
- Class IV: apparent bone ankylosis of the hip (Fig. 123-1)

Only class III and class IV are clinically significant. Although modifications to the Brooker classification have been suggested, most clinicians continue to use the Brooker system to describe the extent of heterotopic bone formation.

SYMPTOMS

Individuals demonstrate great variability in initial manifestation of symptoms and degree of heterotopic bone involvement. Patients are often asymptomatic.[1,15] In neurogenic heterotopic ossification, the most common symptom is pain (although this is often absent in spinal cord injury because of sensory deficits). Limitation to joint range of motion is a common finding.[6,9] Symptoms range in onset from 2 weeks to 12 months after the inciting event and include warmth, erythema, swelling, low-grade fever, pain, and tenderness.[2,13,16,17] Heterotopic ossification may trigger autonomic dysreflexia in patients with spinal cord injury at or above the T6 level.[18]

PHYSICAL EXAMINATION

Time at onset, location, and degree of heterotopic bone formation vary between individuals. Therefore, joints should be examined frequently to assess range of motion and to assist in early diagnosis. The clinician should also inspect each joint for erythema and palpate the joints for point tenderness or masses. The most common physical finding is decreased range of motion of the joint.

Distal joints of the hands and feet are almost never involved. Heterotopic ossification is typically limited to hips, knees, shoulders, and elbows.[6] In neurogenic het-

erotopic ossification secondary to traumatic brain injury or spinal cord injury, the hip is the most common joint affected.[10] Ossification is usually found inferomedial to the joint and is typically associated with adductor spasticity.[2]

FUNCTIONAL LIMITATIONS

The loss of range of motion secondary to heterotopic ossification inhibits optimal rehabilitative efforts and interferes with hygiene, transfers, and daily activities; it can ultimately cause catastrophic complications, such as nerve entrapment, joint ankylosis, and spinal cord compression.[17] Pain from heterotopic ossification can be a significant cause of functional limitation.

DIAGNOSTIC STUDIES

The three-phase bone scan is the current "gold standard" for early detection of heterotopic ossification. It is possible to discover increased metabolic activity as early as 2 to 4 weeks after injury. This procedure involves intravenous injection of technetium Tc 99m–labeled polyphosphate, which is known to accumulate in areas of active bone growth. The three phases are as follows[6,17] (Fig. 123-2):

- Phase 1: Dynamic blood flow occurs immediately after injection.
- Phase 2: Immediate static scan detects areas of blood flow after injection.
- Phase 3: Static phase involves a repeated bone scan after several hours.

A disadvantage of the three-phase bone scan is its lack of specificity. It therefore may be difficult to differentiate bone tumor, metastasis, or osteomyelitis from heterotopic ossification.[6]

Radiographs are readily available and economical but may not show calcification until after clinical signs and symptoms have developed (see Fig. 123-1). Heterotopic ossification may not be evident on radiographs until 4 to 6 weeks after an abnormality is detected on the bone

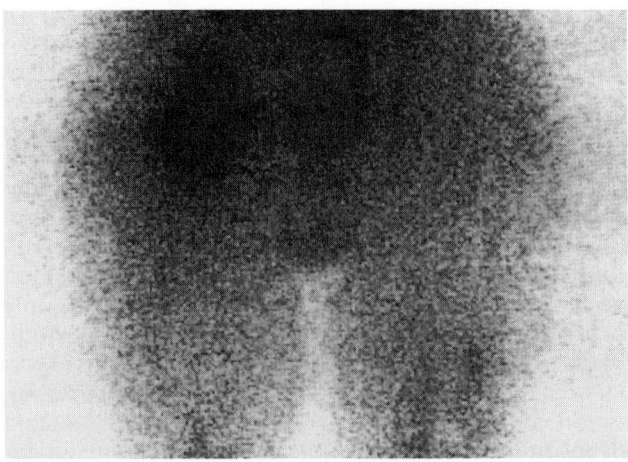

FIGURE 123-2. Three-phase bone scan showing increased activity at the right hip juxta-articular ossification site.

scan.[9] Heterotopic ossification has been described in three radiologic stages with variable time frames[2,19]:

1. early: increased activity on bone scan, no radiologic evidence;
2. intermediate: radiographically appearing immature bone; and
3. mature: well-developed, mature-appearing bone

Both mature and immature bone can coexist. It is not uncommon for mature ossification to radiographically obscure immature bone.[2] Therefore, radiographic determination of the maturity of heterotopic bone is often unreliable.[2,6]

Computed tomographic scanning is rarely used in detection of heterotopic ossification. However, both computed tomography and magnetic resonance imaging have proved especially helpful in preoperative planning for resection to establish relationships of bone to muscle and neurovascular bundles.[6,9]

Ultrasonography and angiography are not often used for the diagnosis of heterotopic ossification. Cases have been reported in which ultrasound examination has been used to help differentiate heterotopic ossification from primary bone tumor, hematoma, or abscess. Similarly, angiography has been used to differentiate traumatic myositis ossificans from tumor and to define anatomy before surgical resection.[6,9]

Many laboratory tests have been investigated for use in the diagnosis of heterotopic ossification. No one test has been found to be completely reliable with high sensitivity and specificity for heterotopic ossification. Although it is nonspecific, a widely used laboratory test for monitoring of heterotopic bone formation is the alkaline phosphatase (ALP) level. ALP has been shown to be elevated during the active bone formation of heterotopic ossification (normal range is 38 to 126 U/L). ALP levels rise as early as 2 weeks after injury, reaching a peak around 10 weeks.[6] ALP is helpful for diagnosis because it may be elevated up to 7 weeks before development of clinical symptoms.[4] Because the specificity of ALP elevation is low, it is recommended that three-phase bone scan be used to confirm suspected cases of heterotopic ossification.[20]

Serum and urinary calcium concentrations, frequently nonspecific responses to trauma, do not provide any information about the ongoing ossification process and are therefore not used for diagnosis and monitoring of heterotopic ossification.[10] Other urinary markers, including hydroxyproline, deoxypyridinoline, and prostaglandin E_2, have been suggested for use in detection of heterotopic ossification.[3,4,6,9] Serum intact osteocalcin, C-reactive protein, erythrocyte sedimentation rate, and creatine kinase have been used as markers for heterotopic bone formation in studies. In the population of spinal cord–injured patients, the inflammatory phase of heterotopic bone formation can be monitored by C-reactive protein levels, and creatine kinase can be used to estimate the severity of heterotopic ossification.[3,11] Both C-reactive protein and creatine kinase levels may be used to assist in therapeutic and treatment decisions.

Differential Diagnosis

Deep venous thrombosis

Cellulitis or infection

Acute arthritis

Superficial thrombophlebitis

Contracture

Complex regional pain syndrome

Spasticity

Tumoral calcinosis

Secondary hyperparathyroidism

Hypervitaminosis D

Fracture

Gout

Pseudogout

Para-articular chondroma

Calcinosis circumscripta

Hematoma or hemorrhage

TREATMENT

Initial

Nonsurgical strategies for treatment of heterotopic ossification include mobilization of the joint, medications to decrease inflammation or to decrease bone formation, and prophylactic low-dose radiation therapy. Therapies and preventive strategies may be combined to improve outcome.[2,15] Spasticity and pain can be barriers to providing proper range of motion. Both should be managed appropriately to ensure that mobilization occurs. Nonsteroidal anti-inflammatory drugs (NSAIDs) can be used not only for analgesia of the patient but also to reduce bone formation by the inhibition of prostaglandin synthetase. NSAIDs inhibit arachidonic acid metabolism, thereby inhibiting prostaglandin production, reducing inflammation, and slowing bone metabolism.

Studies have shown that indomethacin, ibuprofen, and other NSAIDs have been effective for prevention of heterotopic ossification in total hip arthroplasty and in high-risk spinal cord–injured patients.[2,6,9,11,16,21] Indomethacin has been the most widely used NSAID in prophylaxis for heterotopic ossification and is commonly used after surgical resection to prevent recurrence. Traditionally, indomethacin is started on postoperative day 1 at a dose of 25 mg three times a day for 3 weeks and is continued for up to 2 months.[2,6,12] More recently, shorter treatment durations have been found effective for prophylaxis.[22]

Etidronate disodium (EHDP), a bisphosphonate, is structurally similar to inorganic pyrophosphate and is shown to delay the aggregation of apatite crystals into large, calcified clusters in patients with traumatic brain injury and spinal cord injury.[2,6,8] Although EHDP does not eradicate bone that has already formed, it reduces further progression of surrounding cells.[11] EHDP is not routinely used for prophylaxis, but some clinicians advocate prophylactic use in high-risk spinal cord–injured patients. The current treatment recommendation for established heterotopic ossification in spinal cord injury is 300 mg intravenously daily for 3 days followed by 20 mg/kg daily orally for 6 months.[23] Intravenous EHDP is no longer available, and the use of alternate bisphosphonates in intravenous form has not yet been investigated for the treatment of heterotopic ossification. For patients with traumatic brain injury, it has been suggested that treatment be initiated at 20 mg/kg per day orally for 3 months, then reduced to 10 mg/kg per day for 3 months.[8]

Rehabilitation

Comprehensive physical and occupational therapy can be considered preventive and a first-line treatment modality. Several studies have shown that early range of motion exercises are beneficial in the prevention and treatment of heterotopic ossification.[7] Controversy exists that joint manipulation may increase the inflammatory response, thereby increasing production of heterotopic bone. There has been no objective evidence to show this to be true.[2] Joint manipulation may not alter bone formation, but it can prevent soft tissue contractures and maintain functional range of motion. Because physical therapy is often difficult secondary to pain or spasticity, forceful manipulation under anesthesia has been tried but is not a standard treatment modality. Range of motion is still considered the mainstay for prevention of heterotopic ossification.[2,16] Continuous passive motion machines are beneficial in increasing range of motion after surgical resection of heterotopic bone.[4,9]

Procedures

Radiation therapy has been shown to help prevent heterotopic ossification after total hip arthroplasty and after resection of mature heterotopic bone.[1,20] It is the only therapy for heterotopic ossification that acts locally.[6] Although opinions differ as to the most effective treatment method, single doses of 5 to 8 Gy are more frequently used than fractionated doses, and similar results are found when preoperative and postoperative treatments are compared.[1] Radiation therapy has been used successfully after heterotopic bone resection in patients with traumatic brain injury and spinal cord injury to help prevent recurrence; more recently, it has been used for local treatment of heterotopic ossification in spinal cord injury.[2,11,12,24]

Surgery

Although recurrence is common, surgical resection is the only definitive treatment for mature heterotopic bone. Surgical indications include joint immobility causing difficulty in activities of daily living, ankylosed joints leading to pressure sores or skin breakdown, and conditions in which heterotopic ossification contributes to peripheral neuropathy.[2] Preoperative planning often requires three-dimensional computed tomography and magnetic resonance imaging to assess the relationship between heterotopic bone and neurovascular structures at risk. Careful dissection with isolation of neurovascular bundles reduces risk of morbidity associated with hemorrhage, sepsis, or repeated ankylosis.[2] Functional range of motion can typically be reached with a wedge resection of the ectopic bone.[2]

Controversy exists as to the timing of the procedure because bone maturity is difficult to assess. It has been shown that immature heterotopic bone has a greater incidence of recurrence.[11,20] Traditionally, three-phase bone scan and ALP levels have been used to monitor bone maturity. However, because both may remain abnormal indefinitely, many clinicians no longer wait for normalization of bone scans and ALP levels to proceed with resection.[11] Still, it is not uncommon for surgery to be delayed for up to 2 years in patients with traumatic brain injury or spinal cord injury. After heterotopic bone resection, radiation therapy and NSAIDs are often used to prevent recurrence.[2,6]

POTENTIAL DISEASE COMPLICATIONS

Heterotopic bone deposition impairs normal joint range of motion and causes secondary soft tissue contractures, which involve surrounding skin, muscles, ligaments, and neurovascular bundles.[2] The resulting restrictive position predisposes the patient to the development of pressure sores and subsequent infections. Direct pressure or chronic spasticity can cause nerve ischemia and compression, resulting in peripheral neuropathy.[2] Vascular compression, deep venous thrombosis, and lymphedema may also result. Decreased range of motion predisposes to osteoporosis and subsequent pathologic fracture during transfer or lifting of the patient.[2]

POTENTIAL TREATMENT COMPLICATIONS

NSAIDs have well-known side effects that most commonly affect the gastric, hepatic, and renal systems. There is also a risk of defective bone-prosthesis union and poor bone healing in orthopedic populations while NSAIDs are used for the prevention of heterotopic ossification.[6,22]

EHDP is generally a safe method for treatment of heterotopic ossification. The most common side effects are nausea and diarrhea. Twice-daily divided dosing of EHDP helps alleviate these symptoms. EHDP also carries a potential risk of bone fracture secondary to osteomalacia; if it is withdrawn after a short treatment duration, a rebound ossification secondary to prolonged osteoclast inhibition may result.[8,23]

Radiation therapy is rarely associated with malignant neoplasia and does not disrupt wound healing, provided wounds are not in the field of irradiation.[6,25] In orthopedic populations after total hip arthroplasty, increased rates of trochanteric nonunion have been described with both high-dose fractionated and single-dose protocols.[22,25]

Surgical complications, which carry a high morbidity and are not uncommon, include hemorrhage, sepsis, wound infection, repeated ankylosis, and heterotopic bone recurrence.[6,20] Chronic pain and recurrent contracture may also result. The distorted anatomy in heterotopic ossification makes dissection visibility difficult, endangering neurovascular structures.[2] Postoperative blood loss requiring transfusion is not uncommon despite good surgical hemostasis.[2]

References

1. Balboni TA, Gobezie R, Mamon HJ. Heterotopic ossification: pathophysiology, clinical features, and the role of radiotherapy for prophylaxis. Int J Radiat Oncol Biol Phys 2006;65:1289-1299.
2. Botte MJ, Keenan ME, Abrams RA, et al. Heterotopic ossification in neuromuscular disorders. Orthopedics 1997;20:335-341.
3. Sugita A, Hashimoto J, Maeda A, et al. Heterotopic ossification in bilateral knee and hip joints after long-term sedation. J Bone Miner Metab 2005;23:329-332.
4. Pape HC, Marsh S, Morley JR, et al. Current concepts in the development of heterotopic ossification. J Bone Joint Surg Br 2004;86:783-787.
5. Riedel B. Demonstration eine durch achttägiges Umhergehen total destruirten Kniegelenkes von einem Patienten mit Stichverletzung des Rückens. Verh Dtsch Ges Chir 1883;12:93.
6. Buschbacher R. Heterotopic ossification: a review. Crit Rev Phys Med Rehabil 1992;4:199-213.
7. Venier LH, Ditunno JF. Heterotopic ossification in the paraplegic patient. Arch Phys Med Rehabil 1971;52:475-479.
8. Spielman G, Gennarelli TA, Rogers CR. Disodium etidronate: its role in preventing heterotopic ossification in severe head injury. Arch Phys Med Rehabil 1983;64:539-542.
9. Bossche LV, Vanderstraeten G. Heterotopic ossification: a review. J Rehabil Med 2005;37:129-136.
10. McCarthy EF, Sundaram M. Heterotopic ossification: a review. Skeletal Radiol 2005;34:609-619.
11. Banovac K, Sherman AL, Estores IM, et al. Advanced clinical solutions: prevention and treatment of heterotopic ossification after spinal cord injury. J Spinal Cord Med 2004;27:376-382.
12. Puzas JE, Miller MD, Rosier RN. Pathologic bone formation. Clin Orthop Relat Res 1989;245:269-281.
13. Garland DE. Clinical observations on fractures and heterotopic ossification in the spinal cord and traumatic brain injured populations. Clin Orthop Relat Res 1988;233:86-101.
14. Brooker AF, Bowerman JW, Robinson RA, et al. Ectopic ossification following total hip replacement. Incidence and a method of classification. J Bone Joint Surg Am 1973;55:1629-1632.
15. Pakos EE, Pitouli EJ, Tsekeris PG, et al. Prevention of heterotopic ossification in high-risk patients with total hip arthroplasty: the experience of a combined therapeutic protocol. Int Orthop 2006;30:79-83.
16. Stover SL, Hataway CJ, Zeiger HE. Heterotopic ossification in spinal cord–injured patients. Arch Phys Med Rehabil 1975;56:199-204.
17. Johns JS, Cifu DX, Keyser-Marcus L, et al. Impact of clinically significant heterotopic ossification on functional outcome after traumatic brain injury. J Head Trauma Rehabil 1999;14:269-276.
18. Blackmer J. Rehabilitation medicine: 1. Autonomic dysreflexia. CMAJ 2003;169:931-935.
19. Haider T, Winter W, Eckholl D, et al. Primary calcification as a mechanism of heterotopic ossification. Orthop Trans 1990;14:309-310.
20. Garland DE. A clinical perspective on common forms of acquired heterotopic ossification. Clin Orthop Relat Res 1991;263:13-29.
21. Moore KD, Goss K, Anglen JO. Indomethacin versus radiation therapy for prophylaxis against heterotopic ossification in acetabular fractures: a randomized, prospective study. J Bone Joint Surg Br 1998;80:259-263.
22. Dahners LE, Mullis BH. Effects of nonsteroidal anti-inflammatory drugs on bone formation and soft-tissue healing. J Am Acad Orthop Surg 2004;12:139-143.
23. Banovac K. The effect of etidronate on late development of heterotopic ossification after spinal cord injury. J Spinal Cord Med 2000;23:40-44.
24. Sautter-Bihl ML, Hultenschmidt B, Liebermeister E, et al. Fractionated and single-dose radiotherapy for heterotopic bone formation in patients with spinal cord injury. Strahlenther Onkol 2001;177:200-205.
25. Coventry MB, Scanlon PW. The use of radiation to discourage ectopic bone. A nine-year study in surgery about the hip. J Bone Joint Surg Am 1981;63:201-208.

Lymphedema 124

Mabel E. Caban, MD, Sandra S. Hatch, MD, and Atul Patel, MD

Synonyms

Primary lymphedema
Secondary lymphedema
Postmastectomy lymphedema
Noone-Milroy-Meige syndrome
Familial lymphedema

ICD-9 Codes

457.0   Postmastectomy lymphedema syndrome
457.1   Lymphedema
     Acquired
     Praecox
     Secondary
757.0   Hereditary edema of legs
     Chronic hereditary
     Congenital
997.99 Surgical

DEFINITION

Lymphedema is chronic edema of the arm, leg, trunk, or face secondary to accumulation of lymph fluid.[1,2] A normal lymphatic system can handle modest increases in protein and water loads without formation of edema. Lymphedema, however, represents an imbalance in the lymphatic load and lymphatic transport capabilities.[3,4] Figures 124-1 and 124-2 demonstrate the anatomy of the lymphatic system. Imbalance can be due to either high-output lymph failure or low-output lymph failure. High-output lymph failure refers to factors that increase blood capillary filtration; low-output lymph failure occurs with impaired lymphatic drainage. Either contingency alters the equilibrium between lymph formation and lymph absorption, resulting in frank edema.[3,5] One example of high-output lymph failure is ascites secondary to portal hypertension associated with cirrhosis of the liver. An example of low-output lymph failure is post-mastectomy edema from the resection of lymph nodes.

Lymphedema is typically progressive[6] and exists when there is impaired return of the lymph into the circulatory system. Long-standing lymphedema is associated with chronic inflammatory cells and subsequent fibrosis of the soft tissue.[7]

Four major physiologic mechanisms cause lymphedema: increased blood capillary hydrostatic pressure, decreased plasma protein concentration, increased blood permeability, and blockage of lymph return.[8]

Lymphedema is classified into primary (congenital) and secondary. Primary lymphedema is associated with aplasia, hypoplasia, or obstruction of the lymphatic vessels. The three major categories are congenital (noted early in infancy), lymphedema praecox (onset at puberty), and lymphedema tarda (manifested around the age of 35 years). Secondary lymphedema is associated with damage or obstruction of the lymphatic vessels by infectious etiology (filariasis, bacteria), lymph node dissection, radiotherapy, and other causes[9] (Fig. 124-3).

The most common cause of secondary lymphedema in the world is filariasis.[9] More than 120 million people have been infected and about 40 million people are subjected to serious disfigurement and disability. In the United States and other industrialized countries, lymphedema is most commonly secondary to cancer therapies (lymph node dissection and radiation therapy). Petrek and Heelan[10] estimated the incidence of lymphedema after breast cancer treatment from 6% to 30% in five Western countries; but in a cohort of breast cancer survivors examined 20 years after diagnosis, 49% presented the sensation of lymphedema and 13% had severe lymphedema.[11] Erickson and colleagues[12] estimated a 41% incidence of lymphedema after breast cancer therapy (range, 21% to 51%) but a lower incidence of 17% in women who did not receive axillary irradiation. The effect of sentinel node biopsy on the incidence of lymphedema is still unknown.

The combination of cancer treatments increases the likelihood of lymphedema. Resection of lymph nodes remains the highest risk for surgery-related lymphedema, but the risk is greatly enhanced when patients receive adjuvant radiation treatment to the operative nodal basin. Adjuvant chemotherapeutic agents such as paclitaxel (Taxol) and docetaxel (Taxotere) may also elevate the incidence of secondary lymphedema. Lymphedema from cancer treatment may develop months to years after therapeutic intervention. Events associated with late onset of lymphedema include infection, injury, and post–cancer treatment weight gain.[11] Research is needed to determine the association of air travel, venipuncture, and blood pressure monitoring as events provocative of lymphedema.

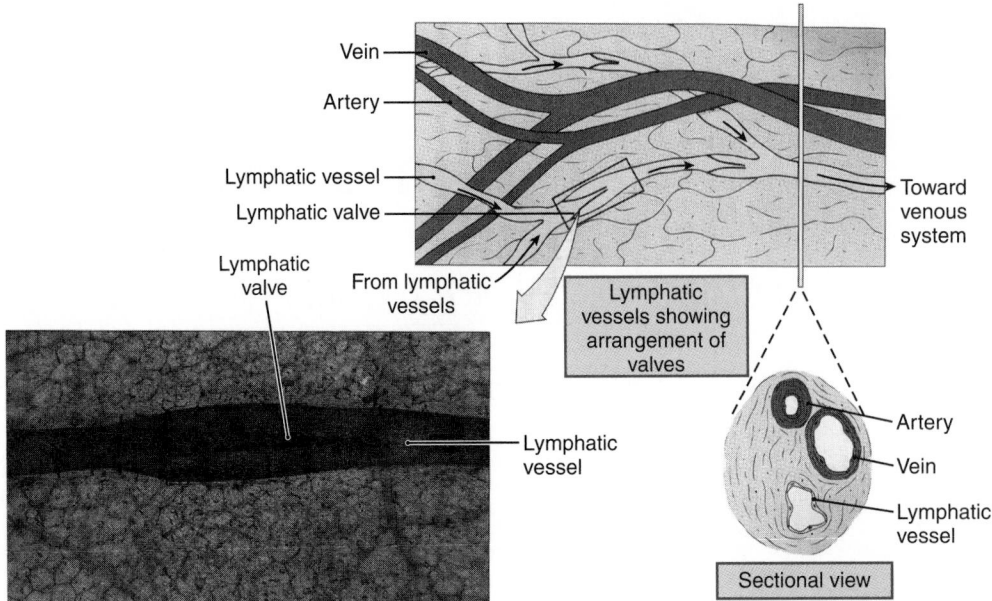

FIGURE 124-1. Association of lymphatic collectors with the arteries and veins. The lymphatic collectors have smooth muscle in their walls and are able to move the lymph unidirectionally until final evacuation in the thoracic duct. (Reproduced with permission of Pearson Education, Inc., Glenview, Ill.)

FIGURE 124-2. Blind lymphatic vessels and their relationship with capillaries. The lack of a primitive basal membrane of the superficial lymphatics allows the transport of proteins and particles. The lymphatic system regulates the absorption of interstitial fluid and the response to infection. (Reproduced with permission of Pearson Education, Inc., Glenview, Ill.)

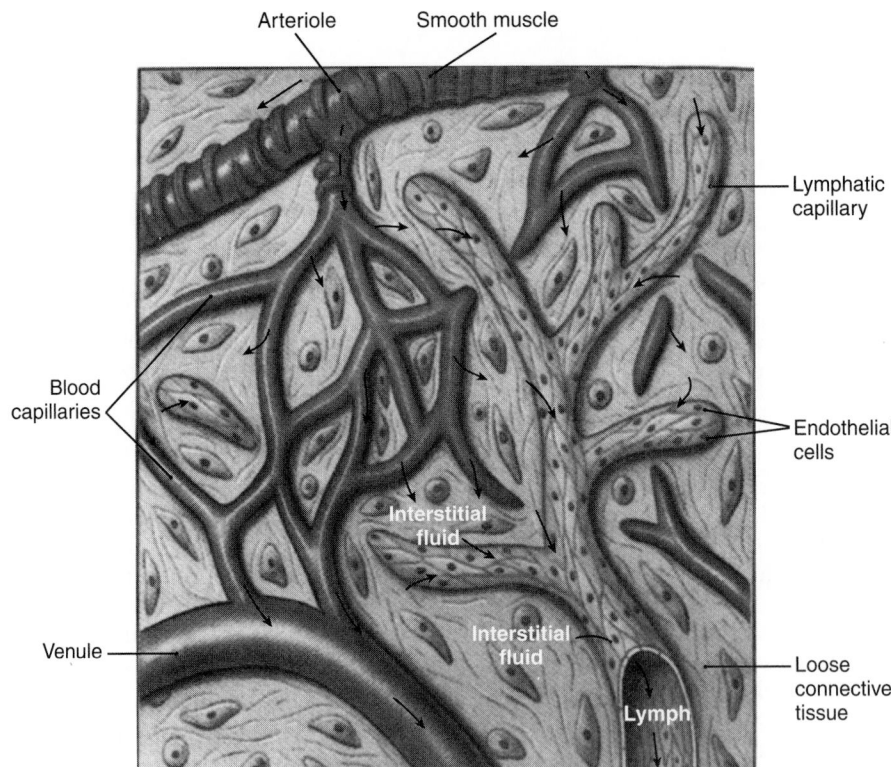

SYMPTOMS

Early symptoms are described as heaviness, tightness, hardness, numbness, stiffness, pain, or weakness from stagnant protein-rich fluid in a limb. Pain-free swelling develops after a latent phase that may be manifested with limitation of motion of the fingers on the involved extremity. Postoperative swelling after cancer surgery is usually transitory, although there is a group of patients who progress to long-standing swelling of the limb from lymphedema.

PHYSICAL EXAMINATION

Emphasis is placed on the description and possibly the measurement of the subjective symptoms of lymphedema. These components provide feedback to the initial therapy on repeated measures over time. Table 124-1

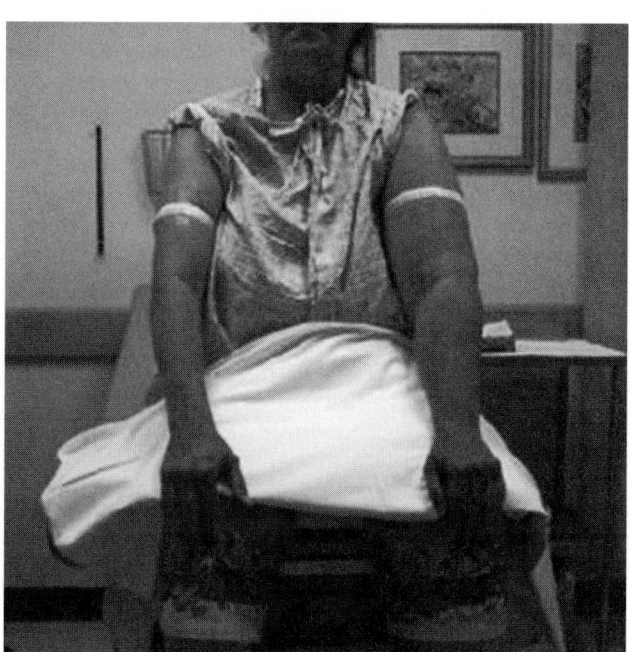

FIGURE 124-3. Post-mastectomy patient with secondary lymphedema due to cancer therapy.

TABLE 124-2	Grading of Lymphedema by the International Society of Lymphedema Criteria
Staging	**Description**
Stage 0	Latent or subclinical Swelling is not evident despite lymph transport.
Stage I	Early accumulation of edema This stage responds to elevation of the arm and may exhibit pitting.
Stage II	Tissue fibrosis This stage shows no pitting and no response to arm elevation.
Stage III	Elephantiasis This stage has no pitting and manifests trophic skin changes (acanthosis, warty overgrowth, and fat deposits).

TABLE 124-1 Physical Examination of the Swollen Limb

Measurable circumference of the swollen limb

Number of skin folds from side to side

Skin color (erythema, brownish pigmentation)

Skin texture (soft, hard, shiny, taut)

Asymmetric increase in subcutaneous adipose tissue

Pitting edema 0-4

Arterial pulses of the extremities

Range of motion

Neurologic deficits

Measurement of limb volume

Venous collaterals or congestion

Modified with permission from Caban ME. Trends in the evaluation of lymphedema. Lymphology 2002;35:28-38.

shows the physical examination for the evaluation of a swollen limb. The International Society of Lymphology has established criteria to grade lymphedema on the basis of circumference measures[13] (Table 124-2). The International Society of Lymphology Consensus Document added a stage 0 to recognize the latent or subclinical phase in which swelling is not overt in spite of impaired lymph transport capabilities. Criteria for grading of lymphedema in clinical trials were summarized by Cheville and associates,[14] including the criteria established by the Lymphedema Working Group. These criteria account for the clinical manifestations of lymphedema, graded 1 to 3, after cancer treatment. Grade 1 represents mild swelling and grade 3 represents the most severe and disabling. These criteria need to be tested for validity and reliability.

Failure to control the swelling may lead to repeated infections, progressive skin changes (elephantiasis), and sometimes a deformed limb. Although it is rare, a lethal angiosarcoma, also known as Stewart-Treves syndrome, is sometimes associated with chronic lymphedema. For this reason, it is important to inspect the skin for changes. After 1 to 30 years of lymphedema, a purplish patch develops into a plaque or nodule in the area of chronic edema. The manifestation of Stewart-Treves syndrome can vary from a subcutaneous nodule or a poorly healing eschar with recurrent bleeding and oozing to small satellite lesions that become confluent and enlarged. The dismal prognosis for this condition will most likely include amputation.[15]

FUNCTIONAL LIMITATIONS

About 40 million live disabled and seriously disfigured by lymphedema, whether or not it is associated with filariasis.[16,17] Severe limitations are most often related to extreme or advanced disease, such as in elephantiasis, a rare manifestation of lymphedema. Functional limitations are associated with swelling and heaviness with or without discomfort of the upper extremities. For patients in treatment, the bandaging or wearing of a sleeve chronically is a constant reminder of the cancer experience. Limitations of the lower extremity are due to inability to fit into appropriate clothing, even closed-toe shoes. Patients with lower extremity lymphedema can have difficulty in walking and climbing stairs or limited participation in physical activities. Both upper and lower extremity lymphedema can progress, resulting in disfigurement.

Premorbid maladaptive behaviors are usually predictive of the need for psychological intervention after the diagnosis of lymphedema.[18] Psychological therapy is recommended in those with lymphatic filariasis and the additional physical disfigurement.[19] In particular, elephantiasis of the penis or scrotum affects sexuality and potency, and it is often severe enough to be accompanied by mental anguish and limitations in physical function.

Most of the time, the functional limitation is massive swelling of the arm or leg from complications associated with lymphedema. For instance, infections like erysipelas, lymphangitis, and cellulitis will be associated with temporary disability until resolution with antibiotic therapy.

DIAGNOSTIC STUDIES

Lymphedema is a clinical diagnosis that follows a thorough history and physical examination. In new-onset lymphedema, it is helpful to rule out deep venous thrombosis as the cause of the swelling. This can be excluded through the use of noninvasive Doppler studies. Such studies have high clinical value and have also proved practical in documenting the dance of worms in scrotal lymphatic filariasis.

In some instances, the diagnosis can be confounded by other conditions like obesity, venous insufficiency, occult trauma, and repeated infections.

Lymphoscintigraphy or lymphangioscintigraphy is the study of choice to visualize the lymphatic system. Although it has not been standardized, it offers tremendous insight into the lymphatic dysfunction.

Other diagnostic tools, less often used, are magnetic resonance imaging, computed tomography, ultrasonography, indirect lymphangiography (water soluble), and fluorescent microlymphangiography. The utility of these tools is described elsewhere.[20]

Genetic testing is another area that has advanced the understanding of a number of specific hereditary syndromes with discrete gene mutations. Lymphedema distichiasis (*FOXC2*) and other forms of Milroy disease (*VEGFR3*) are two examples.

Differential Diagnosis

The differential diagnosis includes causes of unilateral edema of the limb, trunk, or face; the most common conditions are deep venous thrombosis and cellulitis. Confounding comorbidities are chronic venous insufficiency, renal failure, stroke, obesity, injury, underlying fractures, and diabetes mellitus.[13]

TREATMENT

The best treatment of lymphedema is prevention. Other treatment strategies include meticulous skin care, exercises, and compression.

Initial

Prevention of lymphedema after cancer therapies is crucial.

It is unlikely that lymphedema can be completely prevented, although the patient may undertake measures to lessen the impact or to delay its onset. Unfortunately, no randomized controlled trials establish the role of preventive measures. In general, the patient should be instructed to avoid constriction of the affected limb, weight gain, repetitive strenuous activity to the point of fatigue, heavy lifting, extreme heat, and rapid altitude changes. The patient must undertake measures to prevent injury and infection. In practice, preventive measures have focused on minimizing the extent of surgical resection by moving from a full lymphadenectomy to a more targeted resection, such as sentinel node dissection, and additionally minimizing the use of adjuvant radiation therapy directed to the nodal resection bed.

Comorbidities that require attention for control of the edema include congestive heart failure, hypertension, and stroke.[13]

The presence of cellulitis, erysipelas, and lymphangitis requires antibiotic treatment before initiation of manual massage and therapy.

Drug use in the treatment of lymphedema is controversial. Diuretics are useful only in the presence of effusion, like ascites and hydrothorax, or in cases of malignant lymphedema for a short course of the diuretic treatment. Long-term diuretic therapy is not recommended as it may cause electrolytic disturbances.

Benzopyrones hydrolyze the tissue proteins to facilitate their absorption and to stimulate the collectors; their exact role, however, is not understood, and some of them, like coumarin, are associated with liver toxicity.[21,22] Selenium, a free radical scavenger, is reported to reduce lymphedema after radiation therapy. It has a low side effect profile, making it attractive for treatment.[23,24]

Rehabilitation

Decongestive lymphatic therapy is the mainstay of treatment and consists of skin care and hygiene, light manual massage or manual lymph drainage, range of motion exercises, and compression by multiple layers of low-stretch bandage. Two phases are described. Phase 1 contains these modalities. Phase 2 occurs promptly after phase 1; a low-stretch stocking or sleeve is provided to the patient with remedial exercises and massage as needed to drain the affected area into the lymphatic system.[25-28] Relative contraindications to the use of manual lymphatic drainage are acute cellulitis, uncontrolled infections of the affected part, deep venous thrombosis of the affected limb, and renal dysfunction. Poor response to decongestive lymphatic therapy may be related to underlying peripheral vascular disease[29] or malignant lymphedema.[4]

Pneumatic devices facilitate the initial reduction of swelling by sequential and multi-pressure gradient pumps.

However, use of these devices is not meant to replace decongestive lymphatic therapy, and their use is mostly limited by cost, size, and complexity of the treatment. Moreover, research on their efficacy is limited. The development of a sclerotic ring at the proximal end of the limb or edema of the genitalia needs to be avoided.[13,28]

It is essential to make measurements at baseline, at follow-up, and at the end of the treatment. Circumferential measurements can be transformed to volume measures, particularly for clinical trials. Also, if it is available, more expensive equipment to determine volume is helpful. For example, the Perometer takes multiple measures of vertical and horizontal diameter as the frame moves along the leg.[30] Bioelectrical impedance will measure the fluid resistance but does not assess the skin texture.[31] Even magnetic resonance imaging has been used to calculate volume, but it is expensive and slow.

Repeated measures of the visual analogue scale for the patient's symptoms (heaviness, tightness, hardness, numbness, stiffness, pain, or weakness) are also appropriate to quantify the patient's progress.[20]

Exercise for patients with lymphedema has been an area of controversy. The movement exercises, including passive and active movements plus tension (isometric) of the surrounding muscles of the limb after manual lymphatic drainage, are well accepted.[32] Clinical trials using progressive resistive exercises after cancer treatments are showing benefits and no increased risk for aggravation of lymphedema.[33,34] For those with lymphedema, exercises are recommended with the affected limb bandaged or with a compression elastic sleeve.

Surgery

Debulking Surgery

Debulking is the removal of excess skin on a severely edematous limb. The major disadvantage is the removal of superficial lymphatics and collaterals and further obliteration of the lymphatic system. Debulking is useful in cases of elephantiasis with advanced fibrosclerotic lymphedema[23] (Fig. 124-4).

Microsurgery

This is a surgical technique that uses a lymphatic collector or vein segment to restore lymphatic continuity. It appears to be beneficial if it is performed in early lymphedema.[5,35-37]

Liposuction

In some cases, nonpitting lymphedema is caused by excess fat deposition that does not respond to nonoperative treatment; these have, reportedly, been improved with liposuction. Still, patients will need to wear a low-stretch elastic garment long term.[38]

Lymph Node Dissection

Whereas the number of lymph nodes dissected is a major risk factor for the development of lymphedema after cancer treatment, the advent of sentinel node

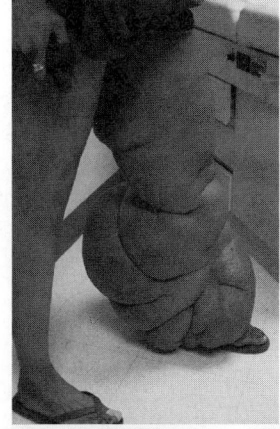
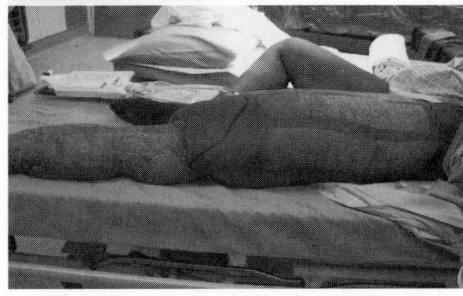

FIGURE 124-4. Patient with elephantiasis before and after debulking surgery and graft. (Courtesy of Dr. Lori Pounds, University of Texas Medical Branch, Galveston, Tex.)

biopsy has also helped reduce the dreadful complication of lymphedema.[39] Sentinel node biopsy reduces the number of lymph nodes resected by the injection of a subcutaneous blue dye or a radioactive tracer on the affected breast that will travel to the first lymph node (sentinel node). A Geiger counter then traces the injected dye. The sentinel node is sampled, and the biopsy specimen is sent for pathologic examination. No further excision is necessary if no cancer cells are found in that node.

POTENTIAL DISEASE COMPLICATIONS

Cellulitis can be a risk factor for development of lymphedema or a complication of lymphedema. Other infections that can occur are erysipelas and lymphangitis (Fig. 124-5). These cases require immediate therapy with antibiotics.

Malignant lymphedema is a condition in which cancer cells invade the lymph nodes or the tumor bulk directly compresses the lymph nodes. This condition necessitates treatment of the underlying disease, and although patients can receive physical therapy, the response is poor.[4]

POTENTIAL TREATMENT COMPLICATIONS

Potential treatment complications that usually arise from underlying conditions are congestive heart failure and malignant effusions, which might tilt the balance

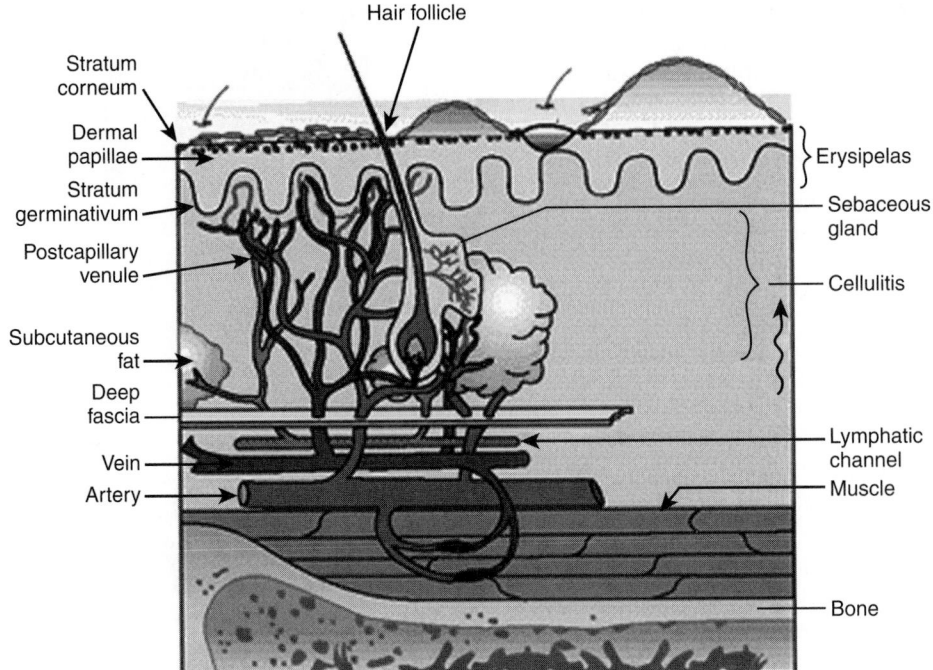

FIGURE 124-5. Layers of the skin affected by various infections. Erysipelas originates at the dermal papillae. Cellulitis is subcutaneous, and lymphangitis originates at the lymphatic vessels. (Modified with permission of The McGraw-Hill Companies.)

to a high-output failure because of massive fluid or venous return. Medical management is crucial to successful volume reduction.

In malignant lymphedema, manual lymphatic drainage raises concerns about spreading of cancer cells throughout the body by mobilization of tumor thrombi that have already spread to the lymph collectors. The prognosis in this population is already poor, and therefore any reduction in swelling is perceived as palliative and capable of improving quality of life.[13,25]

References

1. Stanton AW, Levick JR, Mortimer PS. Current puzzles presented by postmastectomy oedema (breast cancer related lymphoedema). Vasc Med 1996;1:213-225.
2. Stanton AW, Levick JR, Mortimer PS. Cutaneous vascular control in the arms of women with postmastectomy oedema. Exp Physiol 1996;81:447-464.
3. Mortimer PS. The pathophysiology of lymphedema. Cancer 1998;83:2798-2802.
4. Földi E, Földi M, Clodius L. The lymphedema chaos: a lancet. Ann Plast Surg 1989;22:505-515.
5. Campisi C, Boccardo F. Frontiers in lymphatic microsurgery. Microsurgery 1998;18:462-471.
6. Casley-Smith JR. Alterations of untreated lymphedema and its grades over time. Lymphology 1995;28:174-185.
7. Olszewski WL. Clinical picture of lymphedema. In Olszewski WL, ed. Lymph Stasis: Pathophysiology, Diagnosis and Treatment. Boca Raton, Fla, CRC Press, 1991:347.
8. Brennan MJ, DePompolo RW, Garden FH. Focused review: postmastectomy lymphedema. Arch Phys Med Rehabil 1996;77:S74-S80.
9. Creager MA, Dzau VJ. Vascular diseases of the extremities. In Kasper DL, Braunwald E, Fauci AS, et al, eds. Harrison's Principles of Internal Medicine. New York, McGraw-Hill, 2005:1491-1492.
10. Petrek JA, Heelan MC. Incidence of breast carcinoma–related lymphedema. Cancer 1998;83:2776-2781.
11. Petrek JA, Senie RT, Peters M, Rosen PP. Lymphedema in a cohort of breast carcinoma survivors 20 years after diagnosis. Cancer 2001;92:1368-1377.
12. Erickson VS, Pearson ML, Ganz PA, et al. Arm edema in breast cancer patients. J Natl Cancer Inst 2001;93:96-111.
13. International Society of Lymphology Executive Committee. The diagnosis and treatment of peripheral lymphedema. Consensus document of the International Society of Lymphology. Lymphology 2003;36:84-91.
14. Cheville AL, McGarvey CL, Petrek JA, et al. Semin Radiat Oncol 2003;13:214-225.
15. Roy P, Clark MA, Thomas JM. Stewart-Treves syndrome—treatment and outcome in six patients from a single centre. Eur J Surg Oncol 2004;30:982-986.
16. Lymphatic filariasis. World Health Organization Web site. Available at: http://www.who.int/topics/filariasis/en. Accessed May 16, 2006.
17. Schellekens SM, Ananthakrishnan S, Stolk WA, et al. Physicians' management of filarial lymphoedema and hydrocele in Pondicherry, India. Trans R Soc Trop Med Hyg 2005;99:75-77.
18. Passik SD, McDonald MV. Psychosocial aspect of upper extremity lymphedema in women treated for breast carcinoma. Cancer 1998;83(12 Suppl American):2817-2820.
19. Krishna Kumari A, Harichandrakumar KT, Das LK, Krishnamoorthy K. Physical and psychosocial burden due to lymphatic filariasis as perceived by patients and medical experts. Trop Med Int Health 2005;10:567-573.
20. Caban ME. Trends in the evaluation of lymphedema. Lymphology 2002;35:28-38.
21. Casley-Smith JR. Benzo-pyrones in the treatment of lymphoedema. Int Angiol 1999;18:31-41.
22. Loprinzi CL, Kugler JW, Sloan JA, et al. Lack of effect of coumarin in women with lymphedema after treatment for breast cancer. N Engl J Med 1999;340:346-350.
23. Bruns F, Micke O, Bremer M. Current status of selenium and other treatments for secondary lymphedema. J Support Oncol 2003;1:121-130.

24. Micke O, Bruns F, Mucke R, et al. Selenium in the treatment of radiation-associated secondary lymphedema. Int J Radiat Oncol Biol Phys 2003;56:40-49.
25. Földi E. The treatment of lymphedema. Cancer 1998;83:2833-2834.
26. Kasseroller RG. The Vodder School: the Vodder method. Cancer 1998;83:2840-2842.
27. Badger CM, Peacock JL, Mortimer PS. A randomized, controlled, parallel-group clinical trial comparing multilayer bandaging followed by hosiery versus hosiery alone in the treatment of patients with lymphedema of the limb. Cancer 2000;88:2832-2837.
28. Cheville AL, McGarvey CL, Petrek JA, et al. Lymphedema management. Semin Radiat Oncol 2003;13:290-301.
29. Gironet N, Baulieu F, Giraudeau B, et al. Lymphedema of the limb: predictors of efficacy of combined physical therapy [in French]. Ann Dermatol Venereol 2004;131:775-779.
30. Stanton AW, Northfield JW, Holroyd B, et al. Validation of an optoelectronic limb volumeter (Perometer). Lymphology 1997;30:77-97.
31. Mikes DM, Cha BA, Dym CL, et al. Bioelectrical impedance analysis revisited. Lymphology 1999;32:157-165.
32. Kurz I. Textbook of Dr. Vodder's Manual Lymph Drainage, 3rd ed. Treatment Manual, vol 3. Brussels, Haug, 1996.
33. McKenzie DC, Kalda AL. Effect of upper extremity exercise on secondary lymphedema in breast cancer patients: a pilot study. J Clin Oncol 2003;3:463-466.
34. Ahmed RL, Thomas W, Yee D, Schmitz KH. Randomized controlled trial of weight training and lymphedema in breast cancer survivors. J Clin Oncol 2006;24:2765-2772.
35. Campisi C, Boccardo F, Zilli A, et al. Peripheral lymphedema: new advances in microsurgical treatment and long-term outcome. Microsurgery 2003;23:522-525.
36. Campisi C, Davini D, Bellini C, et al. Lymphatic microsurgery for the treatment of lymphedema. Microsurgery 2006;26:65-69.
37. Campisi C, Davini D, Bellini C, et al. Is there a role for microsurgery in the prevention of arm lymphedema secondary to breast cancer treatment? Microsurgery 2006;26:70-72.
38. Brorson H. Liposuction in arm lymphedema treatment. Scand J Surg 2003;92:287-295.
39. Mendez JE, Fey JV, Cody H, et al. Can sentinel lymph node biopsy be omitted in patients with favorable breast cancer histology? Ann Surg Oncol 2005;12:24-28.

Motor Neuron Disease 125

Lisa S. Krivickas, MD

Synonyms

Amyotrophic lateral sclerosis (Lou Gehrig's disease)
Progressive muscular atrophy
Primary lateral sclerosis
Progressive bulbar palsy
Adult spinal muscular atrophy
Spinobulbar muscular atrophy (Kennedy disease)

ICD-9 Codes

335.1	Spinal muscular atrophy
335.2	Motor neuron disease
335.10	Spinal muscular atrophy, unspecified
335.11	Kugelberg-Welander disease
	Spinal muscular atrophy: familial, juvenile
335.19	Other
	Adult spinal muscular atrophy
335.20	Amyotrophic lateral sclerosis
	Motor neuron disease (bulbar) (mixed type)
335.21	Progressive muscular atrophy
	Duchenne-Aran muscular atrophy
	Progressive muscular atrophy (pure)
335.22	Progressive bulbar palsy
335.23	Pseudobulbar palsy
335.24	Primary lateral sclerosis
335.29	Other

DEFINITION

The term *motor neuron disease* refers to a progressive neuro-muscular disorder in which upper or lower motor neurons degenerate. The most common form of motor neuron disease is amyotrophic lateral sclerosis (ALS), which is the primary focus of this chapter. Management principles for other forms of motor neuron disease are similar. To meet diagnostic criteria for ALS, an individual must have both upper and lower motor neuron dysfunction. If only lower motor neuron dysfunction is present, the disease is called progressive muscular atrophy; if only upper motor neuron dysfunction is present, it is called primary lateral sclerosis. If only bulbar dysfunction is present, the disease is called progressive bulbar palsy. Most patients initially diagnosed as having progressive muscular atrophy, primary lateral sclerosis, or progressive bulbar palsy eventually have full-blown ALS. Those who do not convert to ALS have a slower rate of disease progression.

Most cases of ALS are idiopathic. However, 5% to 10% of patients have a familial form, usually transmitted in an autosomal dominant fashion. In approximately 20% of these familial cases, mutations in *SOD1* (superoxide dismutase) can be identified. Other rare forms of inherited adult motor neuron disease are Kennedy disease (X-linked recessive) and adult spinal muscular atrophy (autosomal recessive), which both have only lower motor neuron dysfunction.

ALS rapidly produces skeletal muscle weakness, eventually leading to the requirement for ventilatory support or death from respiratory failure. The onset of weakness may be in any limb, the bulbar muscles, or the respiratory muscles. The extraocular muscles and bowel and bladder function are generally spared. Mean survival, without tracheostomy, is 3 years from symptom onset, but the range may be less than 1 year to more than 20 years. One explanation for the extreme variability in rate of disease progression is that ALS is probably a heterogeneous group of diseases rather than a single disease.[1] The mean age at onset is in the mid-50s, but ALS may develop in adults of any age. The cause of the disease is unknown, but leading theories concerning pathogenesis implicate glutamate excitotoxicity, oxidative stress, neuroinflammation, microglial cell activation, apoptosis, and mitochondrial dysfunction.

SYMPTOMS

Patients with upper motor neuron syndrome may present with spasticity, loss of dexterity, stiffness, weakness due to spasticity, and loss of voluntary motor control.

Patients with lower motor neuron syndrome may present with weakness, fasciculations, muscle atrophy, and muscle cramps.

Bulbar symptoms include dysarthria, dysphagia, sialorrhea (drooling), aspiration, and pseudobulbar affect (laughter or crying discordant with mood).

Respiratory failure and constitutional symptoms of weight loss and generalized fatigue may be present.

Cognitive symptoms include behavioral or executive dysfunction and frontotemporal dementia in a minority of patients.

PHYSICAL EXAMINATION

The emphasis of the physical examination of a patient with suspected or diagnosed motor neuron disease is on the neurologic, musculoskeletal, and cardiorespiratory systems. On neurologic examination, one is looking for evidence of upper and lower motor neuron dysfunction. The mental status, non-motor cranial nerve function, sensory examination, and cerebellar examination findings are usually normal. The "gold standard" for the diagnosis of upper motor neuron disease is the presence of pathologic reflexes—the Babinski sign, Hoffmann sign, and brisk jaw jerk. Patients with ALS may be hyperreflexic or hyporeflexic, depending on the stage at which they are in the disease process and whether they have a predominance of upper or lower motor neuron disease. Evidence of lower motor neuron disease includes muscle weakness, atrophy, hypotonia, hyporeflexia, and fasciculations. Atrophy often appears first in the hand intrinsic muscles. Although fasciculations are not a necessary criterion for the diagnosis of ALS, one should question the diagnosis when none are observed. The tongue is examined for fasciculations and atrophy, and tongue strength and range of motion are assessed. The musculoskeletal examination focuses on assessment of range of motion and evaluation of painful joints or soft tissue structures. Because progressive respiratory failure develops, the cardiorespiratory system should be assessed at each visit. Forced vital capacity (FVC) can be measured with a hand-held spirometer in the office setting.

FUNCTIONAL LIMITATIONS

The majority of the functional limitations that develop in patients with ALS are the direct or indirect result of muscle weakness. As the disease progresses, patients have impaired mobility and difficulties with performance of even the most basic activities of daily living, such as feeding themselves. Bulbar muscle weakness produces dysarthria (difficulty speaking) and dysphagia (difficulty swallowing); eventually, some patients become anarthric and unable to swallow even their own saliva. Reactive depression, generalized fatigue, and musculoskeletal pain may further limit function.

DIAGNOSTIC STUDIES

The diagnosis of ALS is based on appropriate physical examination and electrodiagnostic findings and the use of neuroimaging and clinical laboratory studies to exclude other conditions that may mimic ALS. All patients should undergo electrodiagnostic testing. The revised El Escorial criteria are currently used to diagnose ALS.[2] They classify the certainty level of the diagnosis into one of five categories: definite, probable, probable with laboratory support, possible, and suspected (Fig. 125-1).

SCHEMA

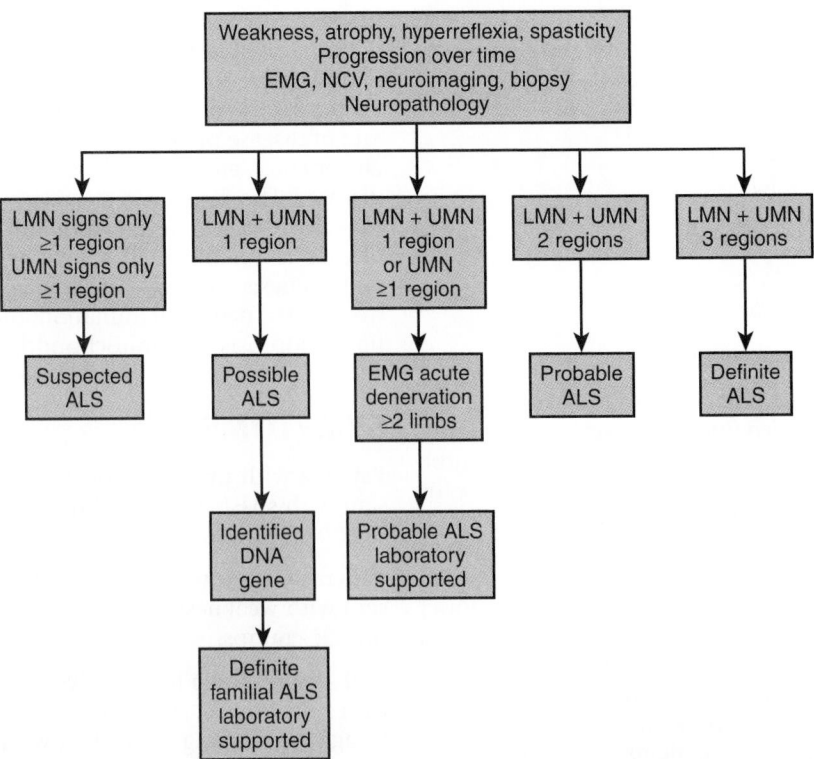

FIGURE 125-1. El Escorial criteria for the diagnosis of ALS. EMG, electromyography; NCV, nerve conduction velocity; LMN, lower motor neuron; UMN, upper motor neuron.

The motor system is divided into four regions: bulbar, cervical, thoracic, and lumbosacral. Clinical evidence of upper and lower motor neuron disease is sought in each region. The certainty level of diagnosis depends on how many regions reveal upper motor neuron or lower motor neuron disease. Electrophysiologic findings can be used both to confirm lower motor neuron dysfunction in clinically affected regions and to detect lower motor neuron dysfunction in clinically uninvolved regions.

Imaging studies are used to exclude possibilities other than motor neuron disease from the differential diagnosis. Magnetic resonance imaging is the primary imaging modality in the evaluation of patients with suspected ALS. Almost all patients should have magnetic resonance imaging of the cervical spine to exclude cord compression, syrinx, or other spinal cord disease. The location of symptoms will dictate whether other regions of the spinal cord should be imaged. In those presenting with bulbar symptoms, brain magnetic resonance imaging should be performed to exclude stroke, tumor, syringobulbia, and other pathologic processes.

In most neuromuscular clinics, a routine panel of laboratory tests is performed for all patients thought to have ALS. A suggested set of such tests is provided in Table 125-1. The rationale behind the performance of this extensive battery of tests is to assess the general health of the patient and to exclude treatable conditions. The differential diagnosis, developed after the history and physical examination, may suggest that more specialized testing be performed. Table 125-2 suggests additional tests that may be warranted when the presentation is with the progressive muscular atrophy, primary lateral sclerosis, or progressive bulbar palsy phenotype. When there is a family history of motor neuron disease, *SOD1* testing may be considered.

TREATMENT

Initial

Pharmacologic

Although there is not yet a cure for ALS, significant research advances are being made in an attempt to identify drugs that will slow disease progression. Offering patients pharmacologic treatment of their disease has psychological benefits that may outweigh the actual slowing of disease progression that currently can be achieved. Riluzole (Rilutek) is the only drug approved by the Food and Drug Administration (FDA) specifically for treatment of ALS. However, many neuromuscular experts recommend that their patients also take a combination of antioxidant vitamins and supplements.

Riluzole, an antiglutamate agent, was approved by the FDA for treatment of ALS in 1995 after two clinical trials showed that the drug slowed disease progression.[3,4] A Cochrane review reporting a meta-analysis of riluzole clinical trials showed a survival benefit of approximately 2 months.[5] Unfortunately, no functional benefit was derived as strength declined at a similar rate in those

TABLE 125-1 Suggested Laboratory Studies

Hematology
Complete blood count
Sedimentation rate

Chemistry
Electrolytes, blood urea nitrogen, creatinine
Glucose
Hemoglobin A_{1c}
Calcium
Phosphorus
Magnesium
Creatine kinase
Liver function tests
Serum lead level
Urine heavy metal screen
Vitamin B_{12}
Folate

Endocrine
Thyroxine
Thyroid-stimulating hormone

Immunology
Serum immunoelectrophoresis
Urine assay for Bence Jones proteins
Antinuclear antibody
Rheumatoid factor

Microbiology
Lyme titer
VDRL test

Optional
Human immunodeficiency virus test (if risk factors are present)
Anti-Hu antibody (if malignant disease is suspected)
DNA test for *SOD1* mutation (with family history)

taking riluzole and placebo. The recommended dose of riluzole is 50 mg twice daily. The most common adverse side effects are fatigue, nausea, and elevation of hepatic enzymes. Riluzole is contraindicated in those with hepatic enzyme activity of more than five times the upper limit of normal.

Because oxidative stress due to excessive free radical production in motor neurons is one of the proposed pathogenic factors in ALS, many physicians recommend a variety of antioxidants; vitamin E, vitamin C, and coenzyme Q10 are the most frequently used. No double-blind, placebo-controlled trials have proved the efficacy of these treatments. Safe recommended daily doses are 1000 to 3000 mg of vitamin C, 400 IU of vitamin E, and up to 1200 mg of coenzyme Q10.

TABLE 125-2 Specialized Laboratory Testing

Phenotype	Test	Diagnosis Excluded
Progressive muscular atrophy	DNA test: CAG repeat on X chromosome	Kennedy disease
	DNA test: *SMN* gene mutation	Spinal muscular atrophy
	Hexosaminidase A	Hexosaminidase A deficiency (heterozygous Tay-Sachs disease)
	Voltage-gated calcium channel antibody test	Lambert-Eaton myasthenic syndrome
	Cerebrospinal fluid examination	Polyradiculopathy, infectious or neoplastic
	GM$_1$ antibody panel	Multifocal motor neuropathy
Primary lateral sclerosis	Very long chain fatty acids	Adrenoleukodystrophy
	Human T-lymphotropic virus 1 (HTLV-1) antibodies	HTLV-1 myelopathy (tropical spastic paraparesis)
	Parathyroid hormone	Hyperparathyroid myelopathy
	Cerebrospinal fluid examination	Multiple sclerosis
Progressive bulbar palsy	Acetylcholine receptor antibodies	Myasthenia gravis
	DNA test: CAG repeat on X chromosome	Kennedy disease
	Cerebrospinal fluid examination	Multiple sclerosis

Differential Diagnosis

The differential diagnosis depends on whether the presentation is primarily lower motor neuron, upper motor neuron, bulbar, or mixed lower and upper motor neuron.

Lower Motor Neuron Only

Progressive muscular atrophy

Spinal muscular atrophy

Kennedy disease

Poliomyelitis, post-poliomyelitis syndrome

Benign monomelic amyotrophy

Hexosaminidase A deficiency

Polyradiculopathy

Multifocal motor neuropathy with conduction block

Chronic inflammatory demyelinating polyneuropathy

Motor neuropathy or neuronopathy

Lambert-Eaton syndrome

Plexopathy

Benign fasciculations

Upper Motor Neuron Only

Primary lateral sclerosis

Multiple sclerosis

Adrenoleukodystrophy

Subacute combined systems degeneration

Hereditary spastic paraparesis

Myelopathy

Syringomyelia

Bulbar

Progressive bulbar palsy

Myasthenia gravis

Multiple sclerosis

Foramen magnum tumor

Brainstem glioma

Stroke

Syringobulbia

Head and neck cancers

Polymyositis

Oculopharyngeal muscular dystrophy

Kennedy disease

Upper and Lower Motor Neurons

ALS

Cervical myelopathy with radiculopathy

Syringomyelia

Spinal cord tumor or arteriovenous malformation

Lyme disease

Recent negative ALS clinical trials have tested a number of growth factors, creatine, glutamate antagonists, anti-inflammatory agents (celecoxib), calcium channel blockers, and amino acids.[6] At present, trials of neurotrophic factors, antioxidants, glutamate antagonists, coenzyme Q10, and tamoxifen are ongoing. In the future, a cocktail approach to slowing of disease progression may be the ideal treatment strategy.[7]

A number of drugs are useful for treatment of spasticity, sialorrhea, pseudobulbar affect, depression, and anxiety.

Spasticity requires treatment only if it interferes with function. Nonpharmacologic management involves teaching patients stretching exercises and positioning techniques that decrease muscle tone. Baclofen (Lioresal) is the most effective pharmacologic agent, followed by tizanidine (Zanaflex). Diazepam (Valium) should be avoided because it may suppress respiration, and dantrolene (Dantrium) is not recommended because it causes excessive muscle weakness. In general, pharmacologic management of spasticity is less successful in ALS than in multiple sclerosis or spinal cord injury because the lower motor neuron component of ALS makes patients extremely susceptible to the development of excessive weakness.

Patients with bulbar dysfunction experience sialorrhea because they have difficulty swallowing and managing the oral secretions they normally produce. A variety of anticholinergic drugs may be used to dry the mouth. Tricyclic antidepressants are often tried first but may not be tolerated because of adverse side effects (dry mouth, somnolence, urinary retention). One benefit of the tricyclic antidepressants is that they may treat other ALS-related symptoms, such as pseudobulbar affect (see next paragraph for definition), insomnia, and pain. Tricyclic antidepressants are contraindicated in patients with cardiac arrhythmia or conduction disorder. When tricyclic antidepressants are not tolerated, a scopolamine patch (Transderm Scop) or glycopyrrolate (Robinul) may be helpful. If these treatments are inadequate, patients may benefit from injection of botulinum toxin into the salivary glands.[8]

Pseudobulbar affect, also sometimes called emotional incontinence, refers to the patient's inability to accurately portray emotions being experienced. Patients laugh or cry when they are experiencing sadness or happiness, respectively. They also may have an exaggerated response to situationally appropriate feelings. Amitriptyline (Elavil), a combination of dextromethorphan (Robitussin, Drixoral) and quinidine, or fluvoxamine (Luvox) may help blunt the intensity of these inappropriate or exaggerated reactions. A combination preparation of dextromethorphan and quinidine was found to be effective in a large randomized clinical trial,[9] but this combination has not yet been approved by the FDA.

Reactive depression and anxiety are both normal responses to a diagnosis of ALS.[10] Patients and their families may benefit from individual counseling and participation in ALS support groups. Anxiety may be treated with benzodiazepines as long as the patient does not have significant reduction of vital capacity. Undetected hypoventilation may produce or contribute to preexisting feelings of anxiety. Depression should be treated pharmacologically because not treating it may have a significant negative impact on the quality of life remaining.[11,12] Selective serotonin reuptake inhibitors are good first choices because of their minimal side effects. However, the tricyclic antidepressants may be preferred if they are also needed to treat other symptoms, such as sialorrhea or pseudobulbar affect.

Rehabilitation

Skeletal muscle weakness is the primary impairment in ALS and causes the majority of the clinical problems. In the early stages of ALS, patients often inquire about the role of exercise in preventing or forestalling the development of weakness. Later in the disease, rehabilitation strategies must be used to maintain function and to compensate for muscle weakness.

Three forms of exercise training are relevant to patients with ALS: flexibility, strengthening, and aerobic exercise. Flexibility training helps prevent the development of painful contractures, nonpharmacologically decreases spasticity, and aborts painful muscle spasms. Traditionally, physicians have been reluctant to recommend strengthening exercises because they fear that overuse weakness will accelerate disability. This philosophy promotes the development of disuse weakness and muscle deconditioning, which may compound the weakness produced by ALS itself. The literature supporting the development of overwork weakness in neuromuscular patients is anecdotal, and overuse weakness has not been demonstrated in any controlled prospective studies. A single study of strength training has been published in ALS. It demonstrates a slowing of decline in physical function and no adverse effects.[13] Studies of patients with more slowly progressive neuromuscular diseases and post-poliomyelitis syndrome suggest that muscles only mildly affected by the disease process can be strengthened by a moderate resistance strengthening program.[14-16] High-resistance eccentric exercise should be avoided because it may damage muscle.

I recommend that interested ALS patients begin or continue with a strengthening program to maximize the strength of unaffected or mildly affected muscles in an attempt to delay the time at which function becomes impaired. Weight training should be performed with a weight that can be lifted 20 times, and the individual should be instructed to perform submaximal sets of 10 to 15 repetitions; this ensures that the training is performed at a low to moderate level of resistance. If an exercise regimen consistently produces muscle soreness or fatigue lasting longer than half an hour after exercise, it is too strenuous.

Aerobic exercise helps maintain cardiorespiratory fitness. A study of moderate aerobic activity in patients with ALS demonstrated a short-term positive effect on disability; patients who exercised remained in a milder disease state longer.[17] In addition, studies in a transgenic mouse model of ALS have shown that aerobic exercise prolongs survival.[18-20] Given the lack of any apparent contraindication, aerobic exercise training is recommended for patients with ALS as long as it can be performed safely without a risk of falling or injury. In addition to the physical benefits, strengthening and aerobic exercise may have a beneficial effect on mood, psychological well-being, appetite, and sleep.

As ALS progresses, the rehabilitation focus shifts from exercise to maintenance of independent mobility and function for as long as possible. Interventions include assistive devices, such as canes, walkers, braces, hand splints, wheelchairs, and scooters; home equipment, such as dressing aids, adapted utensils, grab bars, raised toilet seats, shower benches, and lifts; home modifications (ramps, wide doorways); and automobile adaptations such as hand controls, environmental control units, and voice-activated software. These rehabilitation interventions are best provided by a multidisciplinary team that includes physiatrists, physical therapists, occupational therapists, and orthotists.

Patients frequently develop musculoskeletal pain syndromes, such as adhesive capsulitis (frozen shoulder) and low back pain and neck pain due to muscle weakness and inability to change positions. Measures to prevent adhesive capsulitis include range of motion exercises and support of the arm as much as possible rather than allowing it to dangle at the side. Low back pain can be triggered by an uncomfortable seating system. Preventive measures include a lumbar support for the wheelchair, a good cushion on a solid seat, encouragement of frequent weight shifts, and a reclining back or tilt-in-space wheelchair. Neck pain associated with head drop is one of the most difficult musculoskeletal pain issues to remedy. A variety of cervical collars may be tried. A head support on the wheelchair or a reclining lounge chair may be more comfortable than a collar. Acetaminophen, nonsteroidal anti-inflammatory drugs, Lidoderm patches, and, if necessary, opioids should be used to alleviate musculoskeletal pain. Transcutaneous electrical nerve stimulation can also be used. The major concerns with opiate use are respiratory depression and constipation. The respiratory depression may be acceptable in the late stages of the disease; in fact, morphine is a good way to relieve air hunger in the terminal stage.

Adequate swallowing function is necessary to maintain the nutritional status of the patient with ALS (unless a feeding tube is in place). If nutritional status is not properly maintained, patients tend to use muscle as fuel and thus lose muscle mass and strength earlier than they would otherwise.[21] Swallowing dysfunction may also precipitate aspiration pneumonia or respiratory failure. Early signs and symptoms of dysphagia are drooling, a wet voice, coughing during or after drinking thin liquids, nasal regurgitation, and requiring an excessive amount of time to complete meals. Patients should be referred to a speech pathologist when the first signs of dysphagia develop. Those with mild swallowing difficulties can be taught compensatory techniques to reduce the risk of aspiration and choking.[22] Recommendations may be given concerning modification of food consistencies. The development of aspiration pneumonia, loss of more than 10% of body weight, and requiring an excessive amount of time to eat such that quality of life is impaired are indications for feeding tube placement.

Early or mild dysarthria may be managed by having a speech therapist teach patients adaptive strategies, such as overarticulation and slowing of the speaking rate. In patients with hypernasal speech caused by palatal weakness and primarily lower motor neuron dysfunction, a palatal lift or augmentation prosthesis often improves speech clarity.[23] As dysarthria worsens, patients will require alternative forms of communication. Writing is a good alternative while hand function is intact. For those unable to write, low-technology interventions include letter and word boards. Higher technology solutions are augmentative communication devices that may have a voice synthesizer. As long as one muscle somewhere in the body can be voluntarily activated (including the extraocular muscles), the patient should be able to operate a communication device. High-technology solutions to communication problems are not suitable for all patients. Systems must be flexible so that the method of access can be modified as weakness progresses.

Respiratory failure is the primary cause of death in ALS. In the absence of underlying intrinsic pulmonary disease, the respiratory failure in ALS is purely mechanical. Because of muscle weakness, the lungs do not inflate fully on inspiration. Most patients with ALS remain asymptomatic until the FVC is less than 50% of predicted. Pulmonary function tests, particularly the FVC, should be monitored every few months, depending on rate of disease progression. The earliest symptoms of respiratory failure are caused by nocturnal hypoventilation and include poor sleep with frequent awakening, nightmares, early morning headaches, and excessive daytime fatigue and sleepiness. Another early sign of respiratory muscle weakness is a weak cough and difficulty in clearing secretions.

The management of respiratory failure in ALS involves prevention of infection when possible and provision of mechanical ventilatory assistance. All patients with ALS should receive a pneumococcal vaccination and a yearly influenza vaccination. If the expiratory muscles are too weak to generate an adequate cough, patients can be helped by either manually assisted coughing or the Cough Assist (J.H. Emerson Co., Cambridge, Mass).[24,25] Providing patients with supplemental oxygen can relieve symptoms of air hunger and dyspnea but also may suppress respiratory drive, exacerbate alveolar hypoventilation, and ultimately lead to carbon dioxide retention and respiratory arrest.[26] Supplemental oxygen is recommended only for patients with concomitant pulmonary disease or as a comfort measure for those who decline assisted ventilation. Discussion concerning the possibility of respiratory failure should be initiated soon after the diagnosis of ALS so that patients and their families can learn about their choices and, ideally, make a decision about ventilator use in a noncrisis situation. Noninvasive respiratory muscle aids are not a permanent solution to respiratory failure but do provide many patients with additional time to make a decision concerning tracheostomy. Ultimately, less than 5% of ALS patients choose long-term ventilatory support by tracheostomy.[27,28]

Noninvasive positive-pressure ventilation (NIPPV) can be delivered through a variety of oral or nasal masks and interfaces by use of bilevel positive airway pressure (BiPAP) machines or portable volume-cycled ventilators. BiPAP is the most commonly used form of NIPPV. Several studies suggest that use of NIPPV may prolong survival and slow the decline of FVC.[29,30] The American Academy of Neurology's practice parameter on ALS recommends that NIPPV be introduced when the FVC falls to 50% of predicted, or earlier if the patient is symptomatic.[31] However, others have suggested that earlier introduction of NIPPV may improve survival and quality of life.[32,33] Initially, NIPPV is used only at night. As FVC continues to decline, ventilator use extends into the day for varying periods and eventually becomes continuous.

Procedures

Management of Sialorrhea

Transtympanic neurectomy, salivary duct ligation, and parotid gland irradiation have been used to decrease saliva production but are associated with high failure and complication rates.[34] Botulinum toxin injection into the salivary glands is a preferred method of management for patients who do not respond to pharmacologic therapy.[8]

Gastrostomy Tube

Either a percutaneous endoscopic gastrostomy (PEG) tube or a radiologically inserted gastrostomy tube is recommended when a feeding tube is needed. The American Academy of Neurology's practice parameter on ALS states that the morbidity and mortality of PEG tube placement increase when the FVC is below 50% of predicted[31] and recommends placement before that time. However, later studies have shown that PEG tubes can be safely placed with BiPAP assistance in patients with lower FVCs.[35,36] In addition, radiologically inserted gastrostomy tubes may be preferable in patients with low FVCs; less sedation is required, incidence of aspiration is lower, and tube placement is more often successful.[37] Two studies have suggested longer survival in patients choosing PEG tube placement[38,39] when they are compared with comparable patients refusing PEG.

Surgery

Tracheostomy

This is best performed on a planned basis when patients choose long-term ventilatory support. However, it is more frequently performed in a crisis situation. A cuff-

less tracheostomy tube or a tube with a deflated cuff is preferred.

POTENTIAL DISEASE COMPLICATIONS

The potential disease complications are progressive weakness, joint contractures, musculoskeletal pain syndromes, dysphagia, aspiration, dysarthria, depression, progressive respiratory failure, and death.

POTENTIAL TREATMENT COMPLICATIONS

The potential treatment complications include drug reactions (e.g., to riluzole, tricyclic antidepressants) and malfunction or infection of the PEG tube or radiologically inserted gastrostomy tube.

Complications of long-term ventilation by tracheostomy are tracheomalacia, loss of extraocular movements, totally locked-in state, and dementia.

References

1. Rosenfeld J, Swash M. What's in a name? Lumping or splitting ALS, PLS, PMA and other motor neuron diseases. Neurology 2006;66:624-625.
2. Brooks BR, Miller RG, Swash M, Munsat TL; World Federation of Neurology Research Group on Motor Neuron Diseases. El Escorial revisited: revised criteria for the diagnosis of amyotrophic lateral sclerosis. ALS Other Motor Neuron Disord 2000;1:293-299.
3. Bensimon G, Lacomblez L, Meininger V, et al. A controlled trial of riluzole in amyotrophic lateral sclerosis. N Engl J Med 1994;330:585-591.
4. Lacomblez L, Bensimon G, Leigh PN, et al. Dose-ranging study of riluzole in amyotrophic lateral sclerosis. Lancet 1996;347:1425-1431.
5. Miller R, Mitchell J, Lyon M, Moore D. Riluzole for amyotrophic lateral sclerosis (ALS)/motor neuron disease (MND). Cochrane Database Syst Rev 2002;2:CD001447.
6. de Carvalho M, Costa J, Swash M. Clinical trials in ALS: a review of the role of clinical and neurophysiological measurements. ALS Other Motor Neuron Disord 2005;6:202-212.
7. Rosenfeld J. ALS combination treatment. Drug cocktails. ALS Other Motor Neuron Disord 2004;5:115-117.
8. Tan E. Botulinum toxin treatment of sialorrhea: comparing different therapeutic preparations. Eur J Neurol 2006;13:60-64.
9. Brooks B, Thisted R, Appel S, et al. Treatment of pseudobulbar affect in ALS with dextromethorphan/quinidine: a randomized trial. Neurology 2004;63:1364-1370.
10. Ganzini L, Johnston WS, Hoffman WF. Correlates of suffering in amyotrophic lateral sclerosis. Neurology 1999;52:1434-1440.
11. Lou J, Reeves A, Benice T, Sexton G. Fatigue and depression are associated with poor quality of life in ALS. Neurology 2003;60:122-123.
12. Kubler A, Winter S, Ludolph A, et al. Severity of depressive symptoms and quality of life in patients with amyotrophic lateral sclerosis. Neurorehabil Neural Repair 2005;19:182-193.
13. Dal Bello-Haas V, Florence JM, Kloos AD, et al. A randomized controlled trial of resistance exercise in individuals with ALS. Neurology 2007;68:2003-2007.
14. Lindeman E, Leffers P, Spaans F, et al. Strength training in patients with myotonic dystrophy and hereditary motor and sensory neuropathy: a randomized clinical trial. Arch Phys Med Rehabil 1995;76:612-620.
15. Aitkens SG, McCrory MA, Kilmer DD, Bernauer EM. Moderate resistance exercise program: its effect in slowly progressive neuromuscular disease. Arch Phys Med Rehabil 1993;74:711-715.

16. Agre JC, Rodriquez AA, Franke TM. Strength, endurance, and work capacity after muscle strengthening exercise in postpolio subjects. Arch Phys Med Rehabil 1997;78:681-686.

17. Drory V, Goltsman E, Reznik J, et al. The value of muscle exercise in patients with amyotrophic lateral sclerosis. J Neurol Sci 2002;191:133-137.

18. Kirkenezos I, Hernandez D, Bradley W, Moraes C. Regular exercise is beneficial to a mouse model of amyotrophic lateral sclerosis. Ann Neurol 2003;53:804-807.

19. Veldink J, Bar P, Joosten E, et al. Sexual differences in onset of disease and response to exercise in a transgenic model of ALS. Neuromuscul Disord 2003;13:737-743.

20. Kaspar B, Frost L, Christian L, et al. Synergy of insulin-like growth factor-1 and exercise in amyotrophic lateral sclerosis. Ann Neurol 2005;57:649-655.

21. Heffernan C, Jenkinson C, Holmes T, et al. Nutritional management in MND/ALS patients: an evidence based review. ALS Other Motor Neuron Disord 2004;5:72-83.

22. Strand EA, Miller RM, Yorkston KM, Hillel AD. Management of oral-pharyngeal dysphagia symptoms in amyotrophic lateral sclerosis. Dysphagia 1996;11:129-139.

23. Esposito S, Mitsumoto H, Shanks M. Use of palatal lift and palatal augmentation prostheses to improve dysarthria in patients with amyotrophic lateral sclerosis: a case series. J Prosthet Dent 2000;83:90-98.

24. Bach J. Respiratory muscle aids for the prevention of morbidity and mortality. Semin Neurol 1995;15:72-83.

25. Winck J, Gonclaves M, Lourenco C, et al. Effects of mechanical insufflation-exsufflation on respiratory parameters for patients with chronic airway secretion encumbrance. Chest 2004;126:774-780.

26. Gay P, Edmonds L. Severe hypercapnia after low flow oxygen therapy in patients with neuromuscular disease and diaphragmatic dysfunction. Mayo Clin Proc 1995;70:327-330.

27. Moss A, Casey P, Stocking C, et al. Home ventilation for amyotrophic lateral sclerosis patients: outcomes, costs, and patient, family, and physician attitudes. Neurology 1993;43:438-443.

28. Lechtzin N, Weiner C, Clawson L, et al. Use of noninvasive ventilation in patients with amyotrophic lateral sclerosis. ALS Other Motor Neuron Disord 2004;5:9-15.

29. Kleopa KA, Sherman M, Neal B, et al. BiPAP improves survival and rate of pulmonary function decline in patients with ALS. J Neurol Sci 1999;164:82-88.

30. Aboussouan L, Khan S, Banerjee M, et al. Objective measures of the efficacy of noninvasive positive-pressure ventilation in amyotrophic lateral sclerosis. Muscle Nerve 2001;24:403-409.

31. Miller R, Rosenberg J, Gelinas D, et al. Practice parameter: the care of the patient with amyotrophic lateral sclerosis (an evidence based review). Neurology 1999;52:1311-1323.

32. Jackson C, Rosenfeld J, Moore D, et al. A preliminary evaluation of a prospective study of pulmonary function studies and symptoms of hypoventilation in ALS/MND patients. J Neurol Sci 2001;191:75-78.

33. Bourke S, Tomlinson M, Williams T, et al. Effects of non-invasive ventilation on survival and quality of life in patients with amyotrophic lateral sclerosis: a randomised controlled trial. Lancet Neurol 2006;5:140-147.

34. Yorkston KM, Miller RM, Strand EA. Management of Speech and Swallowing in Degenerative Diseases. Tucson, Communication Skill Builders, 1995:253.

35. Gregory S, Siderowf A, Golaszewski A, et al. Gastrostomy insertion in ALS patients with low vital capacity: respiratory support and survival. Neurology 2002;58:485-487.

36. Boitano L, Jordan T, Benditt J. Noninvasive ventilation allows gastrostomy tube placement in patients with advanced ALS. Neurology 2001;56:413-414.

37. Thornton F, Fotheringham T, Alexander M, et al. Amyotrophic lateral sclerosis: enteral nutrition provision—endoscopic or radiologic gastrostomy? Radiology 2002;224:713-717.

38. Mathus-Vliegen L, Louwerse L, Merkus M, et al. Percutaneous endoscopic gastrostomy in patients with amyotrophic lateral sclerosis and impaired pulmonary function. Gastrointest Endosc 1994;40:463-469.

39. Mazzini L, Corra T, Zaccala M, et al. Percutaneous endoscopic gastrostomy and enteral nutrition in amyotrophic lateral sclerosis. J Neurol 1995;242:695-698.

Movement Disorders 126

Kenneth H. Silver, MD

Synonyms

Extrapyramidal disease
Hypokinesias
Hyperkinesias
Dyskinesias

ICD-9 Codes

307.2	Tics
307.20	Tic disorder, unspecified
307.22	Chronic motor tic disorder
307.23	Gilles de la Tourette disorder
332	Parkinson disease
332.0	Parkinsonism or Parkinson disease: primary, idiopathic
332.1	Secondary parkinsonism
	Parkinsonism due to drugs
333.0	Other degenerative diseases of the basal ganglia
	Progressive supranuclear ophthalmoplegia
	Shy-Drager syndrome
333.1	Essential and other specified forms of tremor
333.2	Myoclonus
333.4	Huntington chorea
333.5	Other choreas
333.6	Idiopathic torsion dystonia
333.84	Organic writers' cramp
781.0	Abnormal involuntary movements: abnormal head movements, spasms, fasciculation, tremor

DEFINITION

Involuntary movement disorders can be characterized by either too little (hypokinetic) or too much (hyperkinetic) movement. Hypokinetic problems include Parkinson disease and Parkinson-like conditions, such as progressive supranuclear palsy, vascular or trauma-induced parkinsonism, and multisystem atrophy (which encompasses the related disorders of Shy-Drager syndrome, striatonigral degeneration, and olivopontocerebellar degeneration). Hyperkinetic disorders include parkinsonian and non-parkinsonian tremor, tics, Gilles de la Tourette syndrome, dystonia, dyskinesias (including tardive dyskinesias), hemifacial spasm, athetosis, chorea (including Huntington disease), hemiballismus, myoclonus, and asterixis.

Depending on which diagnostic criteria are used, essential tremor has a prevalence ranging from 0.1% to 22%, roughly 20 times more common than Parkinson disease. Idiopathic Parkinson disease constitutes approximately 85% of all the Parkinson-like conditions; neuroleptic-induced Parkinson disease (7% to 9%), vascular parkinsonism (3%), multisystem atrophy (2.5%), and progressive supranuclear palsy (1.5%) represent much smaller fractions. Relatively rare, Huntington disease occurs with a frequency in the population as low as 0.004% by some estimates.

SYMPTOMS

Parkinsonian patients commonly show a resting tremor, slowness of movement or bradykinesia, and a form of increased muscle tone called rigidity (see Chapter 132 for more details). Other common features are reduction in movements of facial expression resulting in "masked facies," stooped posture, and reduction of the amplitude of movements (hypometria). Also seen are changes in speech to a soft monotone (hypophonia) and small, less legible handwriting (micrographia). Walking becomes slower, stride length is reduced, and pivoting is replaced with a series of small steps (turning "en bloc").[1-4] The following syndromes typically present with the listed features in addition to the characteristic symptoms of Parkinson disease (tremor and rigidity)[5]:

- Shy-Drager syndrome: autonomic failure with prominent postural hypotension
- Progressive supranuclear palsy: reduction in vertical gaze and slowing of eye movements
- Vascular parkinsonism: early dementia with brisk tendon reflexes
- Multiple head trauma, "parkinsonism pugilistica": early dementia with brisk tendon reflexes
- Olivopontocerebellar degeneration: prominent intention tremor, imbalance, and ataxia

Tremors, the most common form of involuntary movement disorders, are characterized by rhythmic oscillations of a body part. Tremors can be classified as to the situation in which they are most prominent. Is the tremor most pronounced at rest or with movement? Tremors with movement are subdivided into those occurring with maintained posture (postural or static tremor, tested by holding the arms out in front), with movement from point to point (kinetic or intentional tremor, tested by finger to nose pointing), or only with a specific type of movement (task-specific tremor). Tremors that are at their worst at rest are exclusively associated with Parkinson disease or other parkinsonian states (such as those produced by neuroleptics).[6-10]

Tics are sustained nonrhythmic muscle contractions that are rapid and stereotyped, often occurring in the same extremity or body part during times of stress. The muscles of the face and neck are usually involved, with movement of a rotational sort away from the body's midline. They are commonly familial and often seen in otherwise normal children between the ages of 5 and 10 years and usually disappear by the end of adolescence. Tourette syndrome is characterized by motor and vocal tics lasting for more than 1 year and may involve involuntary use of obscenities and obscene gestures, although such behavior may be mild and transient and occurs only in a minority of afflicted persons.[11,12]

Dystonias are slow, sustained contractions of muscles that frequently cause twisting movements or abnormal postures. The disorder resembles athetosis but shows a more sustained static contraction. When rapid movements are involved, they are usually repetitive and continuous. Dystonia often increases with emotional or physical stress, anxiety, pain, or fatigue and disappears with sleep. The dystonias are further classified as focal, segmental, or multifocal on the basis of the distribution of muscles affected. Symptoms of hemifacial spasm usually begin in the orbicularis oculi and later involve other muscles innervated by cranial nerve VII.[2,10,13,14]

Tardive dyskinesia is a condition characterized by involuntary, choreiform movements of the face and tongue associated with chronic neuroleptic medication use. Common movements include chewing, sucking, mouthing, licking, "fly-catching movements," puckering, and smacking (buccal-lingual-masticatory syndrome). Choreiform movements of the trunk and extremities can also occur along with dystonic movements of the neck and trunk.[8]

Athetosis is characterized by involuntary, slow, writhing, and repetitious movements. They are slower than choreiform movements and less sustained than dystonia. Athetosis may be seen alone or in combination with other movement disorders and itself leads to bizarre but characteristic postures. Any part of the body can be affected, but it is usually the face and distal upper extremities that are involved. Chorea presents as nonsteretyped, unpredictable, and jerky movements that interfere with purposeful motion. The movements are rapid, erratic, and complex and can be seen in any or all body parts but usually involve the oral structures, causing abnormal speech and respiratory patterns. Hemiballismus is an uncommon disorder consisting of extremely violent flinging of the arms and legs on one side of the body.[8,15]

Myoclonus is one of the most common involuntary movement disorders of central nervous system origin. It is characterized by sudden, jerky, irregular contractions of a muscle or groups of muscles. It can be subdivided into stimulus-sensitive myoclonus (reflex myoclonus), appearing with volitional movement, muscle stretch, or superficial stimuli such as touch, and nonstimulus-sensitive myoclonus, which occurs at rest (spontaneous myoclonus). Myoclonic movements can be either irregular or periodic.[16,17]

PHYSICAL EXAMINATION

A complete general history and physical examination are key to ruling out treatable causes of the presenting movement disorder, such as infectious (encephalitis), medication side effect (tardive dyskinesia), genetic (Tourette syndrome), or endocrinologic (tremor-associated thyrotoxicosis).

A good neurologic examination of patients thought to have a movement disorder helps identify an underlying causative condition, such as stroke (e.g., cerebrovascular-based Parkinson disease, hemiballismus, or ataxia), tumor, brain trauma, or even peripheral nerve injury–associated focal dystonias. Other aspects of physical examination focus on characterization of the type of abnormal movements by detailing of their body distribution (limb, trunk, head, face, or widespread), their quality (tremor, writhing, explosive, rigidity), their frequency (rapid and repetitive or slow and sustained), and their general quantity or lack thereof (hyperactive or hypoactive).

For instance, essential tremor (senile tremor) is usually rapid and fine and occurs when the patient is asked to hold the arms outstretched, whereas parkinsonian tremor decreases with voluntary movement. Intention (cerebellar) tremor is slow and broad, occurring at the end of a purposeful motion, as when the patient executes a finger to nose task. In addition to tests of cerebellar function, tests for upper motor neuron syndrome (hyperreflexia, spasticity, presence of Babinski sign) may assist the examiner in distinguishing movement disorders more commonly associated with stroke or brain injury.

FUNCTIONAL LIMITATIONS

Functional limitations depend on the severity of the movement disorder. Some tremors and tics may be more a cosmetic and psychological concern, whereas severe postural disturbance in Parkinson disease or stroke-induced ataxia can clearly impair ambulation or upper extremity control. In Parkinson disease, postural changes, such as stooping with the development of permanent kyphosis, can occur after years of disease. Depression and social isolation are commonly seen in patients with Parkinson disease. Many physical activities require additional effort to be performed. This has a negative impact on quality of life, leading to declining efficiency at work and, in many cases, abandonment of many leisure activities. Manual dexterity is invariably impaired as Parkinson disease worsens, affecting many daily activities, such as dressing, cutting food, writing, and handling small objects such as coins.[3,18,19]

In cervical dystonia (torticollis), social stigmatization is a major concern, as are functional impairments, which can include driving, reading, and activities that involve looking down and using the hands. In another focal dystonia, writer's or occupational cramp, the symptoms present in a certain posture or position; for instance, a patient may be able to write at a blackboard but not seated at a desk. With lingual involvement in oromandibular dystonia, the tongue has abnormal movements during speaking or deglutition. The result of such dystonias is impairment of speech and eating.[14] In Huntington chorea, along with the choreiform movement, progressive dementia and emotional and behavioral abnormalities are seen. As the disease progresses, the presentation becomes less choreiform and more parkinsonian and dystonic (i.e., restricted motions, immobility, and unsteadiness of gait). Intellectual impairment and psychosis invariably occur and progress rapidly to become the most disabling features.[15]

DIAGNOSTIC STUDIES

In most cases of movement disorders, such as Parkinson disease, tardive dyskinesia, essential tremor, and dystonia, the diagnosis is made on the grounds of clinical examination and history; no one specific test is pathognomonic for the disease.[4,5] However, underlying causes of many of the movement disorders, such as stroke, traumatic brain injury, tumor, infection, and metabolic or endocrinologic disease, should be evaluated with appropriate tests, including head and spinal magnetic resonance imaging and computed tomography, cerebrospinal fluid analysis, and blood serum analysis. Electrodiagnostic tests (electromyography and nerve conduction studies) may be useful in some cases, such as focal dystonias, to rule out coexisting or causative peripheral nerve entrapment. Electroencephalography is often helpful in distinguishing focal seizures from myoclonus or other repetitive movement presentations.[16] More tests may be necessary to confirm or to exclude other diagnoses, such as human immunodeficiency virus–related diseases, central nervous system infection, toxic exposures, and psychiatric illnesses.

Differential Diagnosis

Seizures

Psychiatric illness

Spasticity, spasms

TREATMENT
Initial

Treatment is highly dependent on which specific category of movement disorder is present. Typically, pharmacologic treatment is initiated when the symptoms become severe enough to cause discomfort or disability.

Antiparkinson medications either replace dopamine (levodopa), acting as a postsynaptic (dopamine) agonist, or reestablish the dopamine-acetylcholine balance in the striatum (anticholinergics). In addition, The catechol O-methyltransferase inhibitors and monoamine oxidase B inhibitors increase the availability of levodopa or dopamine by preventing their metabolism. Levodopa in combination with carbidopa (Sinemet) is the most effective medication for the relief of Parkinson disease, but it is usually not the first medication given to a newly diagnosed patient. Loss of levodopa efficacy usually develops within 3 to 5 years after the medication is begun, so an effort is made to manage early Parkinson disease with other medications. A guiding principle is to start levodopa treatment in patients with symptoms that interfere with the performance of daily life functions despite other treatment. Anticholinergic drugs such as trihexyphenidyl (Artane) are widely used to treat patients with early Parkinson disease, with tremor as their primary symptom. Amantadine (Symmetrel) is another useful medication in early Parkinson disease. Although its usefulness in early Parkinson disease is controversial, the monoamine oxidase inhibitor deprenyl or selegiline (Eldepryl) is widely given to newly diagnosed patients. Within 1 to 2 years, most patients will have sufficient difficulty with movement and daily activities to require levodopa. Gradually over the years, the patient's frequency of dosing will increase and the total dose needed will increase, along with the need for other supplemental medications. The two most useful are bromocriptine (Parlodel) and pergolide (Permax).[3,4,20,21]

Propranolol is the most useful medication in treating essential tremor (the most common symptomatic tremor), task-specific tremor, and action tremor. Other β blockers have fewer side effects but are less effective. The anticonvulsant primidone and the benzodiazepine clonazepam are also effective antitremor drugs. Gabapentin and botulinum toxin injections have also been demonstrated to be effective in tremor management.[7,9,22,23] Tics can be managed with neuroleptics; pimozide and haloperidol are generally effective, but sedation limits their use. Newer atypical neuroleptics may have fewer or different side effects, including risperidone, quetiapine, olanzapine, and clozapine. Other medications shown to be of use include benzodiazepines, clonazepam, clonidine, calcium channel blockers, and antidepressant agents.[11,12] Anticholinergic medications, such as trihexyphenidyl and benztropine, are the most effective oral agents for both generalized and focal dystonias. Baclofen, carbamazepine, and the benzodiazepines, such as diazepam and clonazepam, are sometimes helpful. Dopamine-blocking or dopamine-depleting agents may be used to treat some patients with dystonia. Focal dystonias are now commonly treated with botulinum toxin injections.[14,24] (See the section on procedures.)

Replacement of the neuroleptic drug with substitute drugs may help some patients with tardive dyskinesia. The atypical neuroleptics clozapine and risperidone are useful to control psychosis in patients with tardive dyskinesia without worsening of symptoms. Other drugs, such as benzodiazepines, adrenergic antagonists, and dopamine agonists, may also be beneficial for suppression of the movements. The most important step in the treatment of tardive dyskinesia is prevention by limiting the use of neuroleptic medications.[25] The response to drug therapy has been poor in patients with ataxia; many agents have been touted as useful (propranolol, isoniazid, carbamazepine, clonazepam, tryptophan, buspirone, thyroid-stimulating hormone), but none has demonstrated efficacy.[26] A number of drugs have been used to treat myoclonus and can be effective in some situations. These include diazepam, clonazepam, valproate, and levetiracetam (Keppra) as well as botulinum toxin injections.[27]

Rehabilitation

In general, the patient with Parkinson disease needs to be counseled to maintain a reasonable level of activity at all costs as physical exertion becomes more difficult and the risk of deconditioning increases. Exercises focus on proper body alignment (upright posture) and postural reflexes (response to dynamic balance challenges) as well as limb range of motion and strengthening of proximal musculature to assist in stair climbing and coming to a stand. Exercises are also aimed at the restoration of diminished reciprocal limb motions and an increase in step length and can include treadmill training. The tendency to freeze can be reduced with visual targets, such as markers on the floor, counting, or marching rhythmically. The difficulty in rising from sitting surfaces can be addressed with elevated sitting surfaces (chair, toilet) and strategically placed grab rails or bars (bed, bathtub). Although wheeled walkers are useful in assisting ambulation, particularly by preventing backward instability, patients with significant postural deficits may prefer more stable devices, such as a supermarket shopping cart or walking behind a wheelchair. Adaptive equipment is provided when deficits in upper extremity control limit efficient and safe function.[28-31] Speech therapy is useful in patients with Parkinson disease to improve articulation and loudness as well as to diagnose and to manage dysphagia.[32]

In tremor, measures to reduce or to alleviate anxiety (e.g., biofeedback, relaxation exercises) are useful, as are strategies to control oscillation excursion with weights or other mechanical compensations.[8] Lifestyle changes may include restriction of caffeine intake or other stimulants that may temporarily augment symptoms. In addition, alcohol consumption may lead to transient improvement for many with essential tremor.[9]

Stretching exercises may be important for maintenance or recovery of range of motion for affected joints in a dystonic limb. Certain types of occupation-based focal limb dystonias (e.g., writer's or musician's cramp) may be treated with muscle reeducation techniques, including biofeedback. A regular program of stretching exercises may assist affected individuals in regaining full range of motion after a botulinum toxin injection has weakened a dystonic muscle. Some patients use so-called sensory tricks to temporarily relieve their symptoms. These commonly involve touching or stroking a particular spot on the skin. In addition, in some patients, certain types of braces may provide the same stimulation and be equally effective.[8,14]

Ataxic patients may benefit from rehabilitation to help them learn compensatory techniques for performance of basic self-care and occupational activities and to assess the benefits of weighted bracelets or similar devices to damp the oscillations. Gait training and education in the use of assistive devices for walking can prevent falls and enhance mobility in the ataxic individual.[8] In disorders involving athetosis, ballismus, or Huntington disease, careful weighting of the extremities can help at times. Rehabilitation techniques involving improvement of coactivation and trunk stability, rhythmic stabilization, and traditional relaxation techniques including biofeedback have been mentioned as reasonable strategies. Some have suggested value in oral desensitization when hyperreactivity to sensory stimuli exists for reducing excessive facial movements in tardive dyskinesia, but other rehabilitation strategies are not of proven utility.[8]

Procedures

Botulinum toxin injections are beneficial in numerous hyperkinetic movement disorders including focal dystonias, tremor, and myoclonus. Trigger point injections may provide relief in painful muscles associated with focal dystonias (e.g., cervical torticollis).

The muscles selected for botulinum toxin injection are based on understanding of the primary clinical patterns of spasticity or dystonia.

Direct injection by palpation technique may be appropriate for superficial muscles; electromyography or electrical stimulation guidance is commonly used to identify deeper muscles. Each muscle is injected in one or more sites, the number being a function of the size of the muscle. Dosage is variable but typically does not exceed 400 units total body dose for a 3-month period. Botulinum toxin A is reconstituted in the vial with preservative-free normal saline, at varying dilutions depending on the muscle size: very small muscles need 20 units per 0.1 mL; average size muscle, 10 units per 0.1 mL; and large muscles, 5 units or less per 0.1 mL.

The skin is cleaned with an alcohol or iodine swab and allowed to dry. When electromyography or electrical stimulation guidance is used, a specialized needle with an exposed tip connected by wire to the recording or stimulating device is needed. Needles are typically 37 mm in length and 27-gauge; larger or smaller needles are often needed, depending on muscle size and depth. In adults, preanesthetization of the skin is usually unnecessary; in children, local anesthetic creams are helpful. When botulinum toxin is injected, aspiration of the syringe to prevent injection into a blood vessel is standard technique. Before the injection, informed consent is obtained.

Surgery

Deep brain stimulation, thalamotomy, and pallidotomy have been used with success in some patients with Parkinson disease as well as other movement disorders (e.g. dystonia and tremor). In addition, peripheral destructive procedures such as myectomy, rhizotomy, and peripheral nerve denervation are occasionally performed on individuals with dystonic limbs who have proved refractory to more conventional management. Cell transplants and gene therapies continue as experimental tools under investigation.[33,34]

POTENTIAL DISEASE COMPLICATIONS

Many of the movement disorders, particularly Parkinson disease, are progressive and can result in muscle weakness and immobility, severe limb contractures, aspiration of food and respiratory compromise, social isolation and depression, and intellectual impairment and dementia.

POTENTIAL TREATMENT COMPLICATIONS

Antiparkinson medications may have numerous side effects including nausea and other gastrointestinal symptoms, drowsiness, confusion, hallucinations, psychosis, and motor dyskinesia.[4,20] Similar adverse medication effects are described with other agents used to suppress unwanted movements. Botulinum toxin is generally well tolerated but can cause transient unwanted weakness in target or adjacent muscles, including dysphagia. Risks associated with surgical approaches to central nervous system structures are considerable and need to be properly weighed before these options are selected.[20]

References

1. Weiner W, Lang A. Movement Disorders. New York, Futura, 1989.
2. Pentland B. Parkinsonism and dystonia. In Greenwood R, Barnes M, McMillan T, Ward C, eds. Neurological Rehabilitation. London, Churchill Livingstone, 1997:475-484.
3. Olanow C, Watts R, Koller W, eds. An algorithm for the management of Parkinson's disease. Treatment guidelines. Neurology 2001;56(Suppl 5):S1-S88.
4. Nutt J, Wooten G. Diagnosis and initial management of Parkinson's disease. N Engl J Med 2005;353:1021-1027.
5. Weiner WJ. A differential diagnosis of parkinsonism. Rev Neurol Dis 2005;2:124-131.
6. Elbe R, Koller W. Tremor. Baltimore, Johns Hopkins Press, 1990.
7. Hallett M. Classification and treatment of tremor. JAMA 1991; 266:1115.
8. Francisco G, Kothari S, Schiess M, Kaldis T. Rehabilitation of persons with Parkinson's disease and other movement disorders. In DeLisa JA, Gans BM, Walsh NE, eds. Physical Medicine and Rehabilitation: Principles and Practice, 4th ed. Philadelphia, Lippincott Williams & Wilkins, 2005:809-828.
9. Evidente VG. Understanding essential tremor. Differential diagnosis and options for treatment. Postgrad Med 2000;108:138-149.
10. Chen JJ, Lee KC. Nonparkinsonism movement disorders in the elderly. Consult Pharm 2006;21:58-71.
11. Evidente VG. Is it tic or Tourette's? Clues for differentiating simple from more complex tic disorders. Postgrad Med 2000;108: 175-176, 179-182.
12. Scahill L, Sukhodolsky DG, Williams SK, Leckman JF. Public health significance of tic disorders in children and adolescents. Adv Neurol 2005;96:240-248.
13. Berardelli A, Rothwell J, Hallett M, et al. The pathophysiology of primary dystonia. Brain 1998;121:1195-1212.
14. Tarsy D, Simon DK. Dystonia. N Engl J Med 2006;355:818-829.
15. Ranen N, Peyser C, Folstein S. A Physician's Guide to the Management of Huntington's Disease. New York, Huntington's Disease Society of America, 1993.
16. Vercueil L, Krieger J. Myoclonus in the adult: diagnostic approach. Neurophysiol Clin 2001;31:3-17.
17. Rivest J. Myoclonus. Can J Neurol Sci 2003;30(Suppl 1):S53-S58.
18. Duvaisin R. Parkinson's Disease: A Guide for Patients and Families. New York, Raven Press, 1991.
19. Chapuis S, Ouchchane L, Metz O, et al. Impact of the motor complications of Parkinson's disease on quality of life. Mov Disord 2005;20:224-230.
20. Pahwa R, Factor D, Lyons K, et al. Practice Parameter: treatment of Parkinson disease with motor fluctuations and dyskinesia (an evidence-based review). Report of the Quality Standards Subcommittee of the American Academy of Neurology. Neurology 2006;66:983-995.
21. Fahn S, Oakes D, Shoulson I, et al. Levodopa and the progression of Parkinson's disease. N Engl J Med 2004;351:2498-2508.
22. Wasielewski P, Burns J, Koller W. Pharmacologic treatment of tremor. Mov Disord 1998;13(Suppl 3):90-100.
23. Gironell A, Kulisevsky J, Barbanoj M, et al. A randomized placebo-controlled comparative trial of gabapentin and propranolol in essential tremor. Arch Neurol 1999;56:475-480.
24. Jankovic J, Hallett M. Therapy with Botulinum Toxin. New York, Marcel Dekker, 1994.
25. Margolese HC, Chouinard G, Kolivakis TT, et al. Tardive dyskinesia in the era of typical and atypical antipsychotics. Part 2: incidence and management strategies in patients with schizophrenia. Can J Psychiatry 2005;50:703-714.
26. Ogawa M. Pharmacological treatments of cerebellar ataxia. Cerebellum 2004;3:107-111.
27. Frucht SJ, Louis ED, Chuang C, Fahn S. A pilot tolerability and efficacy study of levetiracetam in patients with chronic myoclonus. Neurology 2001;57:1112-1114.
28. Turnbull G, ed. Physical Therapy Management of Parkinson's Disease. New York, Churchill Livingstone, 1992.
29. De Goede C, Keus S, Kwakkel G, Wagenaar R. The effect of physical therapy in Parkinson's disease: a research synthesis. Arch Phys Med Rehabil 2001;82:509-515.
30. Deane K, Jones D, Playford E, et al. Physiotherapy for patients with Parkinson's disease: a comparison of techniques. Cochrane Database Syst Rev 2001;3:CD002817.
31. Suchowersky O, Gronseth G, Perlmutter J, et al. Practice Parameter: neuroprotective strategies and alternative therapies for Parkinson disease (an evidence-based review). Report of the Quality Standards Subcommittee of the American Academy of Neurology. Neurology 2006;66:976-982.
32. Ramig L, Sapir S, Fox C, Countryman S. Changes in vocal loudness following intensive voice treatment (LSVT) in individuals with Parkinson's disease: a comparison with untreated patients and normal age-matched controls. Mov Disord 2001;16:79-83.
33. Lyons K, Pahwa R. Deep brain stimulation in Parkinson's disease. Curr Neurol Neurosci Rep 2004;4:290-295.
34. Anderson W, Lenz F. Surgery insight: deep brain stimulation for movement disorders. Nat Clin Pract Neurol 2006;2:310-320.

Multiple Sclerosis 127

Ann-Marie Thomas, MD, PT

Synonyms

Disseminated sclerosis
Focal sclerosis
Insular sclerosis

ICD-9 Code

340   Disseminated or multiple sclerosis
         Brain stem
         Cord
         Generalized

DEFINITION

Multiple sclerosis (MS) can be defined as an inflammatory disorder that results in damage primarily to myelin sheaths and oligodendrocytes and less so to axons and nerve cells in the central nervous system.[1,2]

The prevalence of MS has been estimated at 300,000 to 400,000 in the United States and 2 million worldwide.[3] The estimated cost in the United States is $10 billion.[4-6] The disease usually becomes clinically apparent between the ages of 20 and 40 years, with a peak incidence at 24 to 30 years and onset as late as the seventh decade.[3,7] The disease appears twice as likely to develop in women as in men, and whites are more frequently diagnosed than are other races.[3,7] Although African Americans may experience greater MS-related disability than white individuals do, the disease progresses similarly for both races.[8,9]

There are four common clinical courses in MS:

- Relapsing-remitting MS: Patients experience episodes of acute worsening of neurologic function followed by periods of remission. Patients may exhibit residual deficits after the episode of exacerbation. Most patients start with this course.
- Secondary progressive MS: Patients initially experience a relapsing-remitting course followed by progression of the disease with or without additional episodes of exacerbation and improvement. Most patients eventually transition to this disease course.

- Primary progressive MS: Patients experience a relentless progression of symptoms from the onset.
- Progressive relapsing MS: Patients experience a baseline progressive course with episodes of acute relapses followed by a return to the baseline progressive course.

MS can be diagnosed if there is evidence of two attacks separated by at least 1 month with clinical, laboratory, or imaging evidence of at least two lesions in the brain or spinal cord.[2,3,10] Evidence may be obtained from clinical findings, magnetic resonance imaging, cerebrospinal fluid analysis, or visual evoked potentials.[2,3] The most recent guidelines do not recommend the use of "clinically definite MS" or "probable MS"; the outcome of a diagnostic evaluation is MS, "possible MS," or "not MS" (Table 127-1).[2]

SYMPTOMS

Symptoms of MS may involve multiple systems[11] (Table 127-2). Motor symptoms typically include weakness and spasticity.[12] Up to 85% of patients with MS may experience spasticity, and as many as a third may be affected by spasticity that is severe enough to diminish their quality of life.[13] Patients with MS may report paroxysmal spasms or nocturnal spasms, and MS may be responsible for the rapid development of a progressive paraparesis in association with sphincter dysfunction.

MS may be the cause of decreased or even absent sensation in various body parts, including sensory levels that most often affect the trunk. Paresthesia (uncomfortable abnormal sensation that may be described by the patient as pain, pins and needles, or tingling) can occur in up to 50% of patients with MS and most commonly is neuropathic.[14,15] Lhermitte sign is an electric shock–like sensation that radiates down the spine to the legs when the neck is flexed.[16] It may occur in up to 40% of patients with MS.[17] Multiple pain syndromes may occur in patients with MS[18] (Table 127-3). Visual symptoms may include optic neuritis that results from inflammation of the optic nerves and typically is manifested as retro-orbital pain or painful eye movements. Visual deficits

719

TABLE 127-1 Diagnostic Criteria for Multiple Sclerosis

Clinical Presentation	Additional Data Needed for MS Diagnosis
Two or more attacks Objective clinical evidence of 2 or more lesions	None
Two or more attacks Objective clinical evidence of 1 lesion	Dissemination in space, demonstrated by MRI *or* Two or more MRI-detected lesions consistent with MS plus positive CSF *or* Await further clinical attack implicating a different site
One attack Objective clinical evidence of 2 or more lesions	Dissemination in time, demonstrated by MRI *or* Second clinical attack
One attack Objective clinical evidence of 1 lesion (monosymptomatic presentation; clinically isolated syndrome)	Dissemination in space, demonstrated by MRI *or* Two or more MRI-detected lesions consistent with MS plus positive CSF *and* Dissemination in time, demonstrated by MRI *or* Second clinical attack
Insidious neurologic progression suggestive of MS	Positive CSF *and* Dissemination in space, demonstrated by (1) 9 or more T2 lesions in brain, or (2) 2 or more lesions in spinal cord, or (3) 4-8 brain lesions plus 1 spinal cord lesion *or* Abnormal VEPs associated with 4-8 brain lesions, or with fewer than 4 brain lesions plus 1 spinal cord lesion demonstrated by MRI *and* Dissemination in time, demonstrated by MRI *or* Continued progression for 1 year

If criteria indicated are fulfilled, the diagnosis is multiple sclerosis (MS); if the criteria are not completely met, the diagnosis is "possible MS"; if the criteria are fully explored and not met, the diagnosis is "not MS."
CSF, cerebrospinal fluid; MRI, magnetic resonance imaging; VEPs, visual evoked potentials.
Reprinted with permission from McDonald WI, Compston A, Edan G, et al. Recommended diagnostic criteria for multiple sclerosis: guidelines from the International Panel on the diagnosis of multiple sclerosis. Ann Neurol 2001;50:124.

TABLE 127-2 Common Symptoms in Multiple Sclerosis

Bladder symptoms	Urgency, frequency, hesitancy, retention, incontinence
Bowel symptoms	Constipation, urgency, incontinence
Cerebellar symptoms	Incoordination, imbalance, tremor
Cognition	Concentration, memory, executive dysfunction
Fatigue	Lassitude, reduced endurance
Mood disorders	Depression, anxiety, emotional lability
Motor	Weakness, spasticity
Sensory symptoms	Loss of sensation, positive sensations
Sexual dysfunction	Decreased libido, erectile dysfunction
Vision	Visual loss and double vision

Reprinted with permission from Goldman MD, Cohen JA, Fox RJ, Bethoux FA. Multiple sclerosis: treating symptoms, and other general medical issues. Cleve Clin J Med 2006;73:178.

can range from mild distortions to complete visual loss.[19] Scotoma may be present as an area in the visual field with absent or impaired vision and dyschromatopsia as imperfect color vision.[19] Ocular motor deficits usually include internuclear ophthalmoplegia and nystagmus and are manifested as diplopia, blurry vision, and reading fatigue.[19]

Cerebellar symptoms may include tremor, which can range from mildly annoying to disabling, be gross or fine, and occur at rest or with purposeful actions. Various parts of the body may be involved, including the head, the upper or lower limbs, and the trunk.

Constipation and bowel incontinence may occur in up to 54% of patients with MS.[16] Factors contributing to bowel dysfunction include slowed colonic transit, decreased pelvic muscle function, sensory deficits, and adverse effects of medications.[20,21] More than 80% of patients with MS may suffer from bladder dysfunction.[21-23] MS lesions in the spinal cord can result in a small spastic bladder due to detrusor overactivity. This

TABLE 127-3 Multiple Sclerosis Pain Syndromes and Their Treatment

Pain Syndrome	Acute or Chronic	Clinical Example	Treatment Approaches
Neuralgia	Both	Trigeminal neuralgia	Gabapentin, 100-900 mg three or four times daily Carbamazepine, 200-400 mg three times daily (extended-release form also available) Dilantin, 300-600 mg daily Oxcarbazepine, 150-900 mg daily Amitriptyline, 10-100 mg daily at bedtime Other tricyclic antidepressants Baclofen (oral or intrathecal) as adjuvant therapy
Meningeal irritation	Acute	Optic neuritis	Intravenous corticosteroids directed at underlying inflammation
Sensory pain	Both	Paresthesias	Same as for neuralgia
Skeletal muscle pain	Chronic	With spasticity or limited mobility	Rehabilitation (physical and occupational therapy) Assistive devices Nonsteroidal anti-inflammatory drugs

Reprinted with permission from Goldman MD, Cohen JA, Fox RJ, Bethoux FA. Multiple sclerosis: treating symptoms, and other general medical issues. Cleve Clin J Med 2006;73:182.

usually is manifested as urinary urgency, frequency, voiding of small amounts of urine, and eventually incontinence.[21,22] Bladder underactivity can result in retention and overflow incontinence. Bladder dysfunction is often associated with urinary tract infections that can worsen MS symptoms. Sexual dysfunction commonly includes erectile and ejaculatory dysfunction in men, vaginal dryness in women, and increased time to arousal, decreased genital sensation, and decreased libido in men and women.[24] Factors contributing to sexual dysfunction include disease progression, antidepressants, fatigue, and depression.[16,21,24]

Involvement of cranial nerves VII, IX, X, and XII may result in dysphagia or swallowing difficulties. These are manifested as coughing, frequent throat clearing, complaints of food "sticking" in the throat, weight loss, weak voice, choking, or even aspiration pneumonia.[25]

Fatigue has been reported to occur in more than 90% of MS patients and is regarded as the most disabling symptom in as many as 40% of these patients.[26] MS-related fatigue has been described as "an overwhelming feeling of tiredness in those who have done little and are not depressed."[15]

As many as 50% of patients with MS may have cognitive deficits that are manifested as problems with memory, planning, concentration, judgment, problem solving, and processing speed.[15,27,28] MS patients frequently report heat intolerance with an exacerbation of symptoms in warm or humid environments.

PHYSICAL EXAMINATION

Inflammation of the optic nerve may result in optic or retrobulbar neuritis manifesting as acute vision loss. Even after treatment, vision deficits may persist in the form of poor vision, especially in dim light, or blind spots in the visual field known as scotomas. Demyelination in the medial longitudinal fasciculus may result in varying degrees of horizontal nystagmus; involvement of the third cranial nerve may be manifested as a persistently enlarged pupil. Patients with MS may also complain of double vision attributable to weakened strength and coordination in the eye muscles. Cataracts may develop at an earlier age in the MS population because of the use of steroids. Visual problems may worsen with stress, increased temperature, and infection.[29]

Speech dysfunction may include dysarthria with diminished fluency, slurring, decreased speed, and eventually incomprehensibility.

Sensory testing may reveal deficits in pinprick, temperature, proprioception, or vibration. A sensory level may be evident.

Manual muscle testing can show varying degrees of muscle weakness. The patient may exhibit poor control of a limb or insufficient clearance of the foot during gait. Spastic gait may be another motor finding. Cerebellar involvement may be manifested as dysmetria with past pointing on finger to nose testing and uncoordinated heel to shin movements. The Ashworth scale (or modified Ashworth scale)[30] is commonly used to measure the amount of spasticity, and the 88-item Multiple Sclerosis Spasticity Scale is a reliable and valid measure of the impact of spasticity in patients with MS.[31]

Early in the course, deep tendon reflexes tend to be hyperactive. Decreased or absent reflexes can represent segmental levels of deficit. Corticospinal tract involvement may be evident with an asymmetric plantar response or loss of the abdominal reflex. Deep tendon reflexes can also be asymmetric; testing them in more than one position can determine the consistency of the findings.

Cognitive testing may reveal multiple deficits. These include deficits in memory, problem solving, judgment, and concentration.

FUNCTIONAL LIMITATIONS

The combinations of deficits in MS lead to difficulties with activities of daily living and mobility. Weakness, incoordination, spasticity, or sensory deficits may each or in combination contribute to falls. In addition to possible injuries, these falls may lead to decreased mobility due to fear of repeated falls. Decreased mobility itself leads to further weakness, decreased endurance, and less independence. Weakness or spasticity can also lead to difficulties with feeding and self-care, resulting in the need for personal care attendants. The MS Functional Composite[32] is a relatively new clinical measure developed by a task force of the National MS Society. It measures ambulation, arm and hand function, and cognition and has been found to have greater reliability, sensitivity, and validity than the Kurtzke Expanded Disability Status Scale.[3]

Bowel and bladder dysfunction can contribute to many embarrassing moments in the community, causing patients with MS to fear leaving home or to become distracted by seeking out the locations of bathrooms in areas they plan to visit. Many resort to wearing diapers or catheters. Fear of bladder incontinence may also lead a patient to decrease fluid intake, resulting in dehydration.

Depression, insomnia, and fatigue can all contribute to activity intolerance.

Visual deficits may limit activities such as driving and reading, thus limiting participation in work and recreation.

DIAGNOSTIC STUDIES

Magnetic resonance imaging is the most important test in the diagnosis and management of MS.[2,33] The use of gadolinium allows enhancement of active inflammatory lesions that represent areas with blood-brain barrier breakdown. These hyperintense lesions on T2-weighted images are more specific for MS if they are located in the cerebral white matter, especially the corpus callosum, periventricular area, and brainstem.[2,3]

Cerebrospinal fluid studies, visual evoked potentials, and brainstem auditory evoked potentials can assist in the diagnosis of MS when magnetic resonance imaging findings but not clinical findings support a diagnosis of MS.[2,3]

TREATMENT

Initial

Treatment of patients with MS requires a multidisciplinary approach that should involve careful identification of the symptoms with consideration given to the consequences of these symptoms. Symptoms then need to be prioritized and a treatment plan formulated with use, where appropriate, of nonpharmacologic interventions first.[11]

Differential Diagnosis

Acute disseminated encephalomyelitis

Cerebrovascular disease

Primary cerebral vasculitis

Systemic lupus erythematosus

Polyarteritis nodosa

Familial cavernous hemangiomas

Eales disease with neurologic involvement

Sjögren syndrome

Inflammatory central nervous system disease

Migratory sensory neuritis

Behçet disease

Lyme disease

Chronic fatigue syndrome

Neurobrucellosis

Neurosarcoidosis

Metastatic and remote effects of cancer

Multiple metastases

Paraneoplastic syndromes

Vitamin B_{12} deficiency

Myasthenia gravis

Human T-lymphotropic virus 1–associated myelopathy

Acquired immunodeficiency syndrome myelopathy

Other human immunodeficiency virus syndromes

Adult-onset leukodystrophy

Herpes zoster myelitis

Arachnoiditis

Education of the patient and family should be included in any initial treatment plan involving patients with MS. This provides information about a balanced diet,[34] including adequate fluid intake, weight control, and appropriate exercise.[35] The patient is encouraged to continue working and participating in recreational activities for as long as possible. Modifications may be necessary to allow these activities to continue. The health care providers, the family, and the patient should closely monitor emotional stability, especially mood, because such conditions as depression can contribute to disability. Disabled parking placards can make the task of driving and parking more convenient for the disabled patient with MS.

High-dose methylprednisolone for 3 to 5 days has been established as effective treatment of acute relapses.[36-39] This can be given in a home or hospital setting with similar efficacy.[40] Tapering doses of oral prednisone that follow the intravenous administration of corticosteroids may be helpful, but more definitive evidence is needed to support the need for this. The medications approved by the Food and Drug Administration that are available as first-line treatment to decrease the relapse rate in relapsing-remitting MS include interferon beta-1a (Avonex, Rebif), interferon beta-1b (Betaseron), and glatiramer acetate (Copaxone).[41-45] These therapies were shown to decrease the relapse rate by about 30% during a 2-year period. Early use of interferon beta-1a has been shown to delay the onset of definite MS after the first demyelinating event of MS,[43] and treatment with interferon beta-1b may delay the conversion to MS in patients with clinically isolated syndromes.[46] The every-other-day administration of interferon beta-1b was shown to be more effective than once-weekly interferon beta-1a in reducing ongoing inflammation and demyelination in MS.[47]

Spasticity management can be complex. Some patients use their spasticity to assist with transfers or gait; therefore, spasticity should be treated only if it interferes with mobility or activities of daily living. The first step is seeking and treatment of noxious stimuli, such as pain or infection, especially urinary tract infections, because such stimuli can exacerbate spasticity. Multiple treatment options include physical therapy (see the section on rehabilitation), oral or intrathecal medications, and nerve or muscle blocks.

Oral baclofen is the usual first-line treatment, starting with 5 mg two or three times per day and titrating up to a maximum of 80 mg per day in divided doses. Patients with severe spasticity may require and have been shown to tolerate higher doses (up to 160 mg/day).[48] Weakness is a potential side effect of baclofen, especially at the higher doses. Tizanidine, an α-adrenergic receptor antagonist, has been shown to be effective in reducing muscle tone in patients with MS.[49,50] Dosing should be started at 2 mg and slowly increased to the effective dose of 24 to 36 mg/day in three divided doses.[51] Side effects can include sedation, dry mouth, and weakness. Tizanidine may cause less weakness but more severe dry mouth compared with baclofen.[49] Overall side effects were found to be minimal and temporary, with linear correlations between the dose, concentration, and antispasticity effect of tizanidine.[52]

The newer antiepileptic gabapentin (Neurontin) has antispasticity properties[53,54] and can be used as monotherapy or in addition to baclofen or tizanidine. It is usually started at 100 mg three times a day and can be titrated up to 3600 mg/day. Sedation is the most common side effect. An initial nighttime dose of 300 mg may be given for primarily nocturnal spasms, especially if they are accompanied by insomnia. Levetiracetam (Keppra), another newer anticonvulsant, showed promise for treatment of phasic spasticity.[55] It may be added to a regimen when sedation limits the increase of other antispasticity medications.

Benzodiazepines such as diazepam (Valium) at 5 to 7.5 mg and clonazepam (Klonopin) at 0.5 to 1.5 mg can be sedating and so are best used at bedtime for nocturnal spasms. They have addiction potential.

A third-line oral antispasticity option is dantrolene sodium, a direct-acting muscle relaxant. It may be best for the nonambulatory patient with MS with severe spasticity who may be unaffected by the resultant weakness.[11] Patients receiving dantrolene need to be monitored for toxic hepatitis, which can be fatal. Additional research is needed to fully determine the comparative efficacy and tolerability as well as dosing guidelines for antispasticity medications.[50]

Paroxysmal spasms, which can be quite severe, may be managed with the antiseizure medications carbamazepine (Tegretol, Carbatrol), topiramate (Topamax), gabapentin (Neurontin), and oxcarbazepine (Trileptal).[15] Back spasms in patients with MS may respond to cyclobenzaprine (Flexeril). Intractable spasticity may be managed with muscle or nerve blocks or intrathecal administration of baclofen (see the section on procedures).

Bladder dysfunction can be assessed with a urodynamic study, which can help determine the presence (or absence) of detrusor hyperreflexia, detrusor-sphincter dyssynergia, or detrusor areflexia. Nonpharmacologic interventions for bladder dysfunction include timed voiding, minimizing the intake of bladder irritants such as caffeine, and regulation of fluid intake. Detrusor hyperactivity may respond to anticholinergic medications,[21,22,56,57] such as oxybutynin (Ditropan), 2.5 to 5 mg three times a day, or tolterodine (Detrol), 2 mg twice per day. Tolterodine may have fewer anticholinergic side effects.[58] Transdermal oxybutynin may offer even fewer side effects.[59] Solifenacin succinate (VESIcare) is a newer anticholinergic shown to be effective for overactive bladder.[60] Detrusor underactivity may respond to cholinergic agents such as bethanechol (Urecholine), 10 to 50 mg titrated up to four times a day. An α blocker used in combination with bethanechol was shown to be more effective than monotherapy in the treatment of voiding dysfunction in patients with an underactive detrusor.[61] Detrusor-sphincter dyssynergia may respond to botulinum toxin type A injections in the urethral sphincter.[62] It is not infrequent for patients with bladder dysfunction eventually to need an intermittent catheterization program or continuous drainage by a suprapubic catheter. Urology consultation may be necessary for further workup and treatment in complicated cases that are not responding well to medications or for those patients requiring suprapubic catheterization. Surgical procedures may be necessary (see the section on surgery). Sexual dysfunction can be treated with oral medications such as sildenafil, vardenafil, and tadalafil if the problem is erectile dysfunction.[63] Intraurethral or penile injections of papaverine or alprostadil,[64,65] mechanical vibrators, and vacuum devices can enhance arousal and orgasm.[11] Treatment of sexual dysfunction should include counseling.[66]

Bowel dysfunction manifesting as constipation is best managed by establishment of a bowel program. This consists of adequate fluid intake, incorporation of fiber, adherence to a bowel elimination schedule, and judicious use of medications. Fluid intake should be at least 8 cups each day. Fiber can be found in such foods as raw fruits and vegetables, whole grains, nuts, and seeds.[15] Bowel elimination is most likely to occur shortly after a meal when the gastrocolic reflex results in an increase in the movement of intestinal contents; allow up to 30 minutes of uninterrupted time. Depending on the cause of the constipation, bulk formers, stool softeners, laxatives, suppositories, or occasional use of enemas may be necessary. Diarrhea may be managed by bulk formers taken once per day without the extra fluid as in treatment of constipation.[29] Medications such as loperamide, to slow bowel activity, may be necessary in extreme cases. Workup should seek to eliminate other causes of diarrhea, such as *Clostridium difficile* infection or lactose intolerance.

Factors contributing to or mimicking fatigue should be ruled out or identified and addressed. Common factors are thyroid dysfunction, anemia, sleep disturbance, and sedating medications.[11] Treatment should include nonpharmacologic[16] (Table 127-4) and, if necessary, pharmacologic interventions. First-line medications include amantadine[26] (Symmetrel), started at 100 mg in the morning and early afternoon, or modafinil[67] (Provigil), 100 to 400 mg in the morning. Pemoline (Cylert) and methylphenidate (Ritalin) are third-line medications.[11,15] Aspirin has been shown to improve fatigue in patients with MS.[68]

The multiple pain syndromes in patients with MS are amenable to nonpharmacologic and pharmacologic interventions (see Table 127-3).[11] Lhermitte sign may respond to lidocaine or mexiletine.[69]

Cognitive impairment can be detected during daily interactions with family, colleagues, and friends or during interactions with speech-language pathologists, physical therapists, and occupational therapists. Formal neuropsychological testing can determine the presence and severity of even subtle cognitive impairments. Speech-language pathologists can teach compensatory techniques, such as repetition and maintaining a memory book. Antidepressant medication and counseling can help improve the patient's quality of life.[15]

Acute visual deficits attributable to inflammation may improve more rapidly after high-dose intravenous administration of methylprednisolone. Prism lenses may help compensate for double vision. Regular patching should be avoided because this may prevent the brain from learning to compensate for double vision; patching can be limited to specific activities, such as watching television or reading.[29]

Rehabilitation

Physical therapy interventions to decrease spasticity include range of motion exercises, stretching, positioning, aerobic exercise, and relaxation techniques.[15]

The physical therapist may also improve mobility by training the patient to use various assistive devices to compensate for weakness and fatigue. The physical therapist may also use transcutaneous electrical nerve stimulation to assist with pain management. Physical therapists can teach aerobic exercises to prevent deconditioning, to improve endurance, and thus to delay or to minimize the effects of fatigue.[70,71] Weakness due to the "short circuiting" in demyelinated nerves, as can occur in MS, may be made worse if the patient exercises to the point of fatigue. Exercise programs should be individualized and updated as the patient's condition changes. Occupational therapists can help mitigate the effects of fatigue by teaching energy conservation and work simplification through the use of various devices and techniques.

Ataxia and tremor can be difficult symptoms to manage. Weighted utensils and weights on the distal limbs or assistive devices may lessen the effect of the tremor on a patient's function. Compensatory techniques taught by occupational therapy may improve activities of daily living. Medications for tremor may include β blockers, buspirone, and clonazepam.[15]

A speech-language pathologist can teach the patient techniques to improve speech intelligibility. Various oromotor exercises can help maintain oral muscle coordination.[29] Swallowing dysfunction should be evaluated with a videofluoroscopy study. The speech-language pathologist can also help determine the safest food texture for a patient with dysphagia. Severe dysphagia may require placement of a gastrostomy tube for nutrition to be maintained.

A vocational rehabilitation counselor can play an important role in integrating the disabled MS patient back into the workforce.

Procedures

Muscle or nerve blocks should be reserved for patients with focal spasticity or generalized spasticity with a focal target, such as hip adductor spasticity that interferes with toileting. The most commonly used agents are botulinum toxin and phenol.[72,73] Intramuscular injection of

TABLE 127-4 Nonpharmacologic Interventions for Management of Fatigue in Patients with Multiple Sclerosis

Intervention	Method
Treat underlying factors that exacerbate fatigue	Correction of sleep disturbances Treatment of depression Reversal of thyroid abnormalities Management of medication adverse effects
Improve physical fitness	Aerobic exercise
Improve mobility	Physical and occupational therapy Instruction in proper use of mobility aids and techniques
Teach energy conservation	Timed rest periods Work simplification techniques
Teach cooling techniques	Avoidance of heat Use of cooling vests or other garments

Reprinted with permission from Crayton HJ, Rossman HS. Managing the symptoms of multiple sclerosis: a multimodal approach. Clin Ther 2006;28:449.

botulinum toxin to specific muscles usually takes effect within a week, peaks in 2 to 3 weeks, and lasts 3 to 4 months. Side effects may include muscle weakness, atrophy, and diffusion to other muscles. The maximum recommended dose of botulinum toxin is 400 units at a minimum interval of 3 months.[74,75] Resistance may develop in 10% of patients by antibodies to the toxin.[75] The neurolytic effect from phenol usually lasts 3 to 12 months. Side effects of the procedure include local soreness, edema, and fibrosis.

Surgery

Intrathecal administration of baclofen from a pump implanted in the abdomen is a reasonable option when oral antispasticity medications or muscle and nerve blocks are not tolerated or effective. In rare cases, severe spasticity may need to be treated with rhizotomy, cordectomy, or myelotomy[76] and refractory tremors with deep brain stimulation,[77] dorsal column stimulation,[78] or thalamotomy.[79,80] Augmentation cystoplasty may be an option in patients with detrusor hyperreflexia that is refractory to conservative treatments.[81]

POTENTIAL DISEASE COMPLICATIONS

MS has the potential to progress in such a way as to render the patient severely disabled both physically and cognitively. Dysphagia may lead to aspiration pneumonia that can cause death. Cervical myelopathy or severe demyelination in the brainstem may lead to respiratory failure. Complications related to the relative immobility include pneumonia, deep venous thrombosis, pulmonary embolism, and decubitus ulcers. Neurogenic bladder may contribute to urinary tract infections and even urosepsis. Half the deaths are due to pneumonia, pulmonary embolism, aspiration, urosepsis, and decubitus ulcers; respiratory complications account for most of the deaths.[82] The other deaths are similar to those in the general population. There may be a higher incidence of suicide in patients with MS.[83] If suicides are excluded, the life expectancy of patients with MS may be 6 to 7 years less than that of the general population.[84]

POTENTIAL TREATMENT COMPLICATIONS

Corticosteroids may cause myriad adverse effects, including osteoporosis, immunosuppression, edema, cataracts, glaucoma, avascular necrosis, and myopathy. Interferon beta-1b and beta-1a may result in influenza-like symptoms and injection site reactions. Continued use of interferons may lead to the development of antibodies, rendering them less effective.[85] Baclofen and other antispasticity medications can lead to weakness. If oral or intrathecal baclofen is abruptly withdrawn, hallucinations or seizures may occur. Medications such as opiates for severe pain and benzodiazepines for tremor and spasticity have abuse potential. Dantrolene for spasticity may result in toxic hepatitis. Antidepressants may contribute to sexual dysfunction.

References

1. Polman CH, Reingold SC, Edan G, et al. Diagnostic criteria for multiple sclerosis: 2005 revisions to the "McDonald Criteria." Ann Neurol 2005;58:840-846.
2. McDonald WI, Compston A, Edan G, et al. Recommended diagnostic criteria for multiple sclerosis: guidelines from the International Panel on the diagnosis of multiple sclerosis. Ann Neurol 2001;50:121-127.
3. Fox RJ, Bethoux F, Goldman MD, Cohen JA. Multiple sclerosis: advances in understanding, diagnosing, and treating the underlying disease. Cleve Clin J Med 2006;73:91-102.
4. Sloan FA, Viscusi WK, Chesson HW, et al. Alternative approaches to valuing intangible health losses: the evidence for multiple sclerosis. J Health Econ 1998;17:475-497.
5. Whetten-Goldstein K, Sloan FA, Goldstein LB, Kulas ED. A comprehensive assessment of the cost of multiple sclerosis in the United States. Mult Scler 1998;4:419-425.
6. O'Brien JA, Ward AJ, Patrick AR, Caro J. Cost of managing an episode of relapse in multiple sclerosis in the United States. BMC Health Serv Res 2003;3:17.
7. Victor AA. Neurology 2001.
8. Kaufman MD, Johnson SK, Moyer D, et al. Multiple sclerosis: severity and progression rate in African Americans compared with whites. Am J Phys Med Rehabil 2003;82:582-590.
9. Marrie RA, Cutter G, Tyry T, et al. Does multiple sclerosis-associated disability differ between races? Neurology 2006;66:1235-1240.
10. Polman CH, Wolinsky JS, Reingold SC. Multiple sclerosis diagnostic criteria: three years later. Mult Scler 2005;11:5-12.
11. Goldman MD, Cohen JA, Fox RJ, Bethoux FA. Multiple sclerosis: treating symptoms, and other general medical issues. Cleve Clin J Med 2006;73:177-186.
12. Lance JW. What is spasticity? Lancet 1990;335:606.
13. Rizzo MA, Hadjimichael OC, Preiningerova J, Vollmer TL. Prevalence and treatment of spasticity reported by multiple sclerosis patients. Mult Scler 2004;10:589-595.
14. Beiske AG, Pedersen ED, Czujko B, Myhr KM. Pain and sensory complaints in multiple sclerosis. Eur J Neurol 2004;11:479-482.
15. Schapiro RT. Managing symptoms of multiple sclerosis. Neurol Clin 2005;23:177-187, vii.
16. Crayton HJ, Rossman HS. Managing the symptoms of multiple sclerosis: a multimodal approach. Clin Ther 2006;28:445-460.
17. Al-Araji AH, Oger J. Reappraisal of Lhermitte's sign in multiple sclerosis. Mult Scler 2005;11:398-402.
18. Solaro C, Brichetto G, Amato MP, et al. The prevalence of pain in multiple sclerosis: a multicenter cross-sectional study. Neurology 2004;63:919-921.
19. Chen L, Gordon LK. Ocular manifestations of multiple sclerosis. Curr Opin Ophthalmol 2005;16:315-320.
20. Munteis E, Andreu M, Tellez MJ, et al. Anorectal dysfunction in multiple sclerosis. Mult Scler 2006;12:215-218.
21. DasGupta R, Fowler CJ. Bladder, bowel and sexual dysfunction in multiple sclerosis: management strategies. Drugs 2003;63:153-166.
22. Kalsi V, Fowler CJ. Therapy insight: bladder dysfunction associated with multiple sclerosis. Nat Clin Pract Urol 2005;2:492-501.
23. Carr LK. Lower urinary tract dysfunction due to multiple sclerosis. Can J Urol 2006;13(Suppl 1):2-4.
24. Demirkiran M, Sarica Y, Uguz S, et al. Multiple sclerosis patients with and without sexual dysfunction: are there any differences? Mult Scler 2006;12:209-214.
25. Calcagno P, Ruoppolo G, Grasso MG, et al. Dysphagia in multiple sclerosis—prevalence and prognostic factors. Acta Neurol Scand 2002;105:40-43.
26. Bakshi R. Fatigue associated with multiple sclerosis: diagnosis, impact and management. Mult Scler 2003;9:219-227.
27. Achiron A, Polliack M, Rao SM, et al. Cognitive patterns and progression in multiple sclerosis: construction and validation of percentile curves. J Neurol Neurosurg Psychiatry 2005;76:744-749.
28. Bobholz JA, Rao SM. Cognitive dysfunction in multiple sclerosis: a review of recent developments. Curr Opin Neurol 2003;16:283-288.

29. Schapiro RT. Managing the Symptoms of Multiple Sclerosis, 4th ed. New York, Demos, 2003:94-95.

30. Platz T, Eickhof C, Nuyens G, Vuadens P. Clinical scales for the assessment of spasticity, associated phenomena, and function: a systematic review of the literature. Disabil Rehabil 2005;27:7-18.

31. Hobart JC, Riazi A, Thompson AJ, et al. Getting the measure of spasticity in multiple sclerosis: the Multiple Sclerosis Spasticity Scale (MSSS-88). Brain 2006;129(pt 1):224-234.

32. Rudick R, Antel J, Confavreux C, et al. Recommendations from the National Multiple Sclerosis Society Clinical Outcomes Assessment Task Force. Ann Neurol 1997;42:379-382.

33. Bakshi R. Magnetic resonance imaging advances in multiple sclerosis. J Neuroimaging 2005;15(Suppl):5S-9S.

34. Schapiro RT. Diet and nutrition. In Schapiro RT. Managing the Symptoms of Multiple Sclerosis. 4th ed. New York, Demos, 2003: 111-124.

35. Schapiro RT. Exercise. In Schapiro RT. Managing the Symptoms of Multiple Sclerosis. 4th ed. New York, Demos, 2003:125-128.

36. Moreira MA, Tilbery CP, Monteiro LP, et al. Effect of the treatment with methylprednisolone on the cerebrospinal fluid and serum levels of CCL2 and CXCL10 chemokines in patients with active multiple sclerosis. Acta Neurol Scand 2006;114:109-113.

37. Chapman C, Tubridy N, Cook MJ, et al. Short-term effects of methylprednisolone on cerebral volume in multiple sclerosis relapses. J Clin Neurosci 2006;13:636-638.

38. Sellebjerg F, Barnes D, Filippini G, et al. EFNS guideline on treatment of multiple sclerosis relapses: report of an EFNS task force on treatment of multiple sclerosis relapses. Eur J Neurol 2005;12:939-946.

39. Mirowska-Guzel DM, Kurowska K, Skierski J, et al. High dose of intravenously given glucocorticosteroids decrease IL-8 production by monocytes in multiple sclerosis patients treated during relapse. J Neuroimmunol 2006;176:134-140.

40. Chataway J, Porter B, Riazi A, et al. Home versus outpatient administration of intravenous steroids for multiple-sclerosis relapses: a randomised controlled trial. Lancet Neurol 2006;5:565-571.

41. Patti F, Pappalardo A, Florio C, et al. Effects of interferon beta-1a and -1b over time: 6-year results of an observational head-to-head study. Acta Neurol Scand 2006;113:241-247.

42. Koch-Henriksen N, Sorensen PS, Christensen T, et al. A randomized study of two interferon-beta treatments in relapsing-remitting multiple sclerosis. Neurology 2006;66:1056-1060.

43. Kinkel RP, Kollman C, O'Connor P, et al. IM interferon beta-1a delays definite multiple sclerosis 5 years after a first demyelinating event. Neurology 2006;66:678-684.

44. Gottesman MH, Friedman-Urevich S. Interferon beta-1b (betaseron/betaferon) is well tolerated at a dose of 500 microg: interferon dose escalation assessment of safety (IDEAS). Mult Scler 2006;12: 271-280.

45. Etemadifar M, Janghorbani M, Shaygannejad V. Comparison of Betaferon, Avonex, and Rebif in treatment of relapsing-remitting multiple sclerosis. Acta Neurol Scand 2006;113:283-287.

46. Kappos L, Polman CH, Freedman MS, et al. Treatment with interferon beta-1b delays conversion to clinically definite and McDonald MS in patients with clinically isolated syndromes. Neurology 2006;67:1242-1249.

47. Barbero P, Bergui M, Versino E, et al. Every-other-day interferon beta-1b versus once-weekly interferon beta-1a for multiple sclerosis (INCOMIN Trial) II: analysis of MRI responses to treatment and correlation with Nab. Mult Scler 2006;12:72-76.

48. Smith CR, LaRocca NG, Giesser BS, Scheinberg LC. High-dose oral baclofen: experience in patients with multiple sclerosis. Neurology 1991;41:1829-1831.

49. Chou R, Peterson K, Helfand M. Comparative efficacy and safety of skeletal muscle relaxants for spasticity and musculoskeletal conditions: a systematic review. J Pain Symptom Manage 2004;28:94-95.

50. Shakespeare DT, Boggild M, Young C. Anti-spasticity agents for multiple sclerosis. Cochrane Database Syst Rev 2003;4: CD001332.

51. A double-blind, placebo-controlled trial of tizanidine in the treatment of spasticity caused by multiple sclerosis. United Kingdom Tizanidine Trial Group. Neurology 1994;44(Suppl 9):S70-S78.

52. Emre M, Leslie GC, Muir C, et al. Correlations between dose, plasma concentrations, and antispastic action of tizanidine (Sirdalud). J Neurol Neurosurg Psychiatry 1994;57:1355-1359.

53. Paisley S, Beard S, Hunn A, Wight J. Clinical effectiveness of oral treatments for spasticity in multiple sclerosis: a systematic review. Mult Scler 2002;8:319-329.

54. Cutter NC, Scott DD, Johnson JC, Whiteneck G. Gabapentin effect on spasticity in multiple sclerosis: a placebo-controlled, randomized trial. Arch Phys Med Rehabil 2000;81:164-169.

55. Hawker K, Frohman E, Racke M. Levetiracetam for phasic spasticity in multiple sclerosis. Arch Neurol 2003;60:1772-1774.

56. Chancellor MB, Anderson RU, Boone TB. Pharmacotherapy for neurogenic detrusor overactivity. Am J Phys Med Rehabil 2006;85:536-545.

57. De Ridder D, Ost D, Van der Aa F, et al. Conservative bladder management in advanced multiple sclerosis. Mult Scler 2005;11: 694-699.

58. Abrams P, Freeman R, Anderstrom C, Mattiasson A. Tolterodine, a new antimuscarinic agent: as effective but better tolerated than oxybutynin in patients with an overactive bladder. Br J Urol 1998;81: 801-810.

59. Davila GW, Starkman JS, Dmochowski RR. Transdermal oxybutynin for overactive bladder. Urol Clin North Am 2006;33: 455-463, viii.

60. Garely AD, Kaufman JM, Sand PK, et al. Symptom bother and health-related quality of life outcomes following solifenacin treatment for overactive bladder: the VESIcare Open-Label Trial (VOLT). Clin Ther 2006;28:1935-1946.

61. Yamanishi T, Yasuda K, Kamai T, et al. Combination of a cholinergic drug and an alpha-blocker is more effective than monotherapy for the treatment of voiding difficulty in patients with underactive detrusor. Int J Urol 2004;11:88-96.

62. Karsenty G, Baazeem A, Elzayat E, Corcos J. Injection of botulinum toxin type A in the urethral sphincter to treat lower urinary tract dysfunction: a review of indications, techniques and results. Can J Urol 2006;13:3027-3033.

63. Fowler CJ, Miller JR, Sharief MK, et al. A double blind, randomised study of sildenafil citrate for erectile dysfunction in men with multiple sclerosis. J Neurol Neurosurg Psychiatry 2005;76: 700-705.

64. Betts CD, Jones SJ, Fowler CG, Fowler CJ. Erectile dysfunction in multiple sclerosis. Associated neurological and neurophysiological deficits, and treatment of the condition. Brain 1994;117 (pt 6):1303-1310.

65. Landtblom AM. Treatment of erectile dysfunction in multiple sclerosis. Expert Rev Neurother 2006;6:931-935.

66. Bitzer J, Platano G, Tschudin S, Alder J. Sexual counseling for women in the context of physical diseases—a teaching model for physicians. J Sex Med 2007;4:29-37.

67. Stankoff B, Waubant E, Confavreux C, et al. Modafinil for fatigue in MS: a randomized placebo-controlled double-blind study. Neurology 2005;64:1139-1143.

68. Wingerchuk DM, Benarroch EE, O'Brien PC, et al. A randomized controlled crossover trial of aspirin for fatigue in multiple sclerosis. Neurology 2005;64:1267-1269.

69. Sakurai M, Kanazawa I. Positive symptoms in multiple sclerosis: their treatment with sodium channel blockers, lidocaine and mexiletine. J Neurol Sci 1999;162:162-168.

70. Newman MA, Dawes H, van den Berg M, et al. Can aerobic treadmill training reduce the effort of walking and fatigue in people with multiple sclerosis? a pilot study. Mult Scler 2007;13: 113-119.

71. Rampello A, Franceschini M, Piepoli M, et al. Effect of aerobic training on walking capacity and maximal exercise tolerance in patients with multiple sclerosis: a randomized crossover controlled study. Phys Ther 2007;87:545-555.

72. Borg-Stein J, Pine ZM, Miller JR, Brin MF. Botulinum toxin for the treatment of spasticity in multiple sclerosis. New observations. Am J Phys Med Rehabil 1993;72:364-368.

73. Sheean G. Botulinum toxin treatment of adult spasticity: a benefit-risk assessment. Drug Saf 2006;29:31-48.

74. Francisco GE. Botulinum toxin: dosing and dilution. Am J Phys Med Rehabil 2004;83(Suppl):S30-S37.

75. O'Brien CF. Treatment of spasticity with botulinum toxin. Clin J Pain 2002;18(Suppl):S182-S190.

76. Smyth MD, Peacock WJ. The surgical treatment of spasticity. Muscle Nerve 2000;23:153-163.

77. Nandi D, Aziz TZ. Deep brain stimulation in the management of neuropathic pain and multiple sclerosis tremor. J Clin Neurophysiol 2004;21:31-39.

78. Siegfried J. Treatment of spasticity by dorsal cord stimulation. Int Rehabil Med 1980;2:31-34.

79. Niranjan A, Kondziolka D, Baser S, et al. Functional outcomes after gamma knife thalamotomy for essential tremor and MS-related tremor. Neurology 2000;55:443-446.

80. Schuurman PR, Bosch DA, Bossuyt PM, et al. A comparison of continuous thalamic stimulation and thalamotomy for suppression of severe tremor. N Engl J Med 2000;342:461-468.

81. Zachoval R, Pitha J, Medova E, et al. Augmentation cystoplasty in patients with multiple sclerosis. Urol Int 2003;70:21-26; discussion 26.

82. Cottrell DA, Kremenchutzky M, Rice GP, et al. The natural history of multiple sclerosis: a geographically based study. 5. The clinical features and natural history of primary progressive multiple sclerosis. Brain 1999;122(pt 4):625-639.

83. Sadovnick AD, Eisen K, Ebers GC, Paty DW. Cause of death in patients attending multiple sclerosis clinics. Neurology 1991;41:1193-1196.

84. Sadovnick AD, Ebers GC, Wilson RW, Paty DW. Life expectancy in patients attending multiple sclerosis clinics. Neurology 1992;42:991-994.

85. Rosenblum D, Saffir M. Therapeutic and symptomatic treatment of multiple sclerosis. Phys Med Rehabil Clin North Am 1998;9: 587-601, vi-vii.

Myopathies 128

Kristian Borg, MD, PhD, and Erik Ensrud, MD

DEFINITION

Myopathy is the common name for diseases derived from the muscle. Myopathies have different causes and different courses, that is, they may have acute, subacute, or chronic presentations (Table 128-1). Myopathies affect proximal or distal muscle groups; some of them also affect heart muscle, leading to cardiomyopathy.[1] Many myopathies are inherited disorders. An updated gene table is published online by *Neuromuscular Disorders*.[2]

Muscular Dystrophies

Muscular dystrophies are inherited disorders of muscle due to abnormal structural muscle proteins. They are characterized by progressive course and early onset (Table 128-2).

Congenital Myopathies

Congenital myopathies are a clinically heterogeneous group characterized by findings on muscle biopsy. They are slowly progressive or nonprogressive and usually present in the neonatal period.

Metabolic Myopathies Including Mitochondrial Myopathies

Metabolic myopathies are a clinically heterogeneous group of muscle disorders resulting from inherited defects in intracellular energy production. They may be manifested as cramps and myoglobinuria. Patients with cramps and myoglobinuria often have disorders in the glycogen or lipid metabolism pathways. They may be asymptomatic at rest but develop symptoms after exercise. Mitochondrial myopathies may be a part of a neurologic syndrome often involving the central nervous system.

Inflammatory Myopathies

Inflammatory myopathies are characterized by inflammatory changes in the muscle and are associated with infections or an immunologic process.[3] They are divided into polymyositis, dermatomyositis, and inclusion body myositis.[4] The course is acute or subacute and is almost always associated with an elevated serum creatine kinase (CK) level.

Drug-Induced and Endocrine Myopathies

Drug-induced myopathies are caused by different drugs, for example, colchicine, azidothymidine (AZT), chloroquine, hydroxychloroquine, and corticosteroids. Myopathy due to intake of statins, the cholesterol-lowering agents, has been reported.[5] Endocrine myopathies include both hyperthyroid and hypothyroid myopathies as well as myopathy due to hyperparathyroidism.

Myotonic Syndromes

A number of disorders are associated with clinical or electrical myotonia. The myotonic disorders are divided into myotonic dystrophies and "pure" myotonia.[6] The myotonias are inherited disorders due to alterations in ion channels in the muscle and seldom give rise to persistent muscle weakness. Myotonic dystrophy or Steinert disease exists in a congenital and an adult form. Individuals with myotonic dystrophy may

TABLE 128-1 Myopathic Disorders

Muscular dystrophies

X-linked (dystrophinopathy)

Limb-girdle

Congenital

Facioscapuloperoneal

Scapuloperoneal

Distal myopathy

Congenital myopathies

Central core disease

Nemaline myopathy

Myotubular myopathy

Centronuclear myopathy

Desmin-related myopathy

Other

Metabolic myopathies

Glycogenosis

Lipid storage myopathies

Mitochondrial myopathies

Periodic paralysis

Inflammatory myopathies

Polymyositis

Dermatomyositis

Inclusion body myositis

Other (e.g., viral)

Endocrine myopathies

Thyroid

Parathyroid

Adrenal, steroid

Pituitary

Drug induced/toxic
Myotonic syndromes

Myotonic dystrophy (DM type 1)

Proximal myotonic myopathy (PROMM; DM type 2)

Chloride channel myotonia (myotonia congenita Thomsen)

Sodium channel myotonia (paramyotonia congenita Eulenburg, hyperkalemic periodic paralysis)

Schwartz-Jampel

Drug induced

TABLE 128-2 Muscular Dystrophies

Disorder	Inheritance[*]
Duchenne muscular dystrophy	X-linked recessive
Becker muscular dystrophy	X-linked recessive
Facioscapulohumeral dystrophy	Autosomal dominant
Scapuloperoneal dystrophy	Autosomal dominant
Limb-girdle dystrophy	Autosomal recessive/dominant
Oculopharyngeal dystrophy	Autosomal dominant
Distal myopathy/muscular dystrophy	Autosomal dominant/recessive
Congenital muscular dystrophy	Autosomal recessive/sporadic
Myotonic dystrophy	Autosomal dominant

[*]Major forms of inheritance are noted, although several variations are also possible.

Reprinted with permission from Dumitru D. Electrodiagnostic Medicine. Philadelphia, Hanley & Belfus, 1995:1067.

to myotonic dystrophy is an expansion of a CTG repeat in chromosome 19 (*DMPK* gene). The gene encodes a protein kinase that occurs in different tissues, leading, for example, to cardiomyopathy. The clinical affection is correlated to the number of repeats, and the number of repeats increases between generations, leading to a clinical anticipation.

SYMPTOMS

Muscle weakness, most often affecting proximal muscles, is the cardinal symptom. Nearly all myopathies affect the proximal muscles to the greatest extent. Another prominent symptom is muscle fatigue. The earliest symptoms are often related to weakness of the hip and proximal leg muscles; patients experience difficulty in rising from a chair and often require support of their arms. Compensation for leg extensor weakness by bracing of the legs with the hands and climbing with the hands on the legs in rising to a standing position is known as the Gower maneuver. Walking up and down stairs may be difficult because of quadriceps and hip extensor weakness, respectively. Weakness of proximal muscles in the upper extremities can be manifested as fatigue or inability with overhead tasks, such as hair brushing, brushing teeth, and lifting objects to elevated shelves.

In hereditary distal myopathies[8] and inclusion body myopathy, the distal muscle weakness leads to footdrop and ankle instability as well as difficulty with manual tasks, such as turning doorknobs and opening jars.

Pain is not a common symptom in myopathies. However, inflammatory and metabolic myopathies are associated with pain. Exercise-induced pain suggests a metabolic myopathy; an exercise-induced weakness suggests a neuromuscular junction disorder. The pain has an aching, dull, and crampy quality and is usually poorly localized.

not notice any problems until adolescence or early adult life.[7] The first symptom may be difficulty in releasing an object due to myotonia. Progressive weakness with onset in distal muscles follows. A newly recognized form has proximal muscle weakness (proximal myotonic myopathy, PROMM). The genetic background

Symptoms of hypoventilation and cardiac failure should be considered.

PHYSICAL EXAMINATION

A general examination is performed to assess for signs of cardiac failure and rashes. Muscle atrophy assessment and testing of muscle strength are central and should involve examination of proximal and distal muscles in all extremities as well as facial muscles and neck flexors and extensors. Hip girdle muscles are best isolated for strength testing while the patient is in the supine and prone positions. The tasks of walking, rising from a chair (or floor in pediatric patients), and stepping onto a low chair are often helpful in evaluating leg weakness. Examination of the shoulder may reveal winging of the scapula, a characteristic finding in facioscapulohumeral muscular dystrophy. Facial weakness and temporalis muscle wasting are also present in facioscapulohumeral muscular dystrophy and in myotonic dystrophy.

Range of motion at joints should be examined because contractures may have marked functional effects. Reflexes should be normal or decreased proportional to muscle weakness in myopathies. Abnormalities on sensory testing should suggest involvement of sensory nerves (i.e., a neuromuscular disorder).

FUNCTIONAL LIMITATIONS

The most common functional limitations are related to the prominent symptom of proximal weakness, which can have a marked effect on transfers, ascending and descending stairs, and ambulation. In severe myopathies, patients may be restricted to wheelchair mobility. Proximal upper extremity weakness can interfere with activities of daily living, such as dressing, grooming, and cooking. Fatigue is common secondary to the increased effort required with weakened muscles. Cardiac failure and respiratory insufficiency requiring ventilation can result in difficulty with daily activities and increased fatigue. The dysphagia involved in some myopathies may make eating time-consuming and difficult.

DIAGNOSTIC STUDIES

The serum CK concentration is the most important test in myopathies. Patients with Duchenne muscular dystrophy may have very high CK values. Serum CK concentration is usually elevated in inflammatory myopathies and metabolic myopathies. It is often normal or nearly normal in congenital myopathies.

Exercise, especially if it is strenuous or performed in a sedentary individual, can cause marked CK elevation. Thus, patients should be advised to abstain from strenuous exercise for 5 days before serum CK testing. CK concentration may also be elevated in neuromuscular disorders, such as motor neuron disease.

Nerve conduction studies are important in cases of suspected myopathy. The findings of the sensory and motor nerve conduction studies are usually normal. However, distal compound muscle action potentials may be reduced. Exceptions include patients with inclusion body myositis (30% have a sensory or sensorimotor polyneuropathy).[4] In cases with abnormal nerve conduction velocities, coexisting neuropathies such as diabetic polyneuropathy should be considered.

The electromyographic examination is helpful in the evaluation of myopathies. Primarily, the size of motor units is decreased by the dysfunction or loss of individual muscle fibers, leading to motor unit action potentials that characteristically have decreased duration, decreased amplitude, and increased phases in contrast with the neuropathic motor unit action potential findings. In addition, denervating potentials (fibrillations and positive sharp waves) occur in many myopathic disorders.

Muscle biopsy is often useful in the diagnosis of myopathy. The selection of muscle for biopsy is important because a muscle that is end stage is likely to show only fibrotic replacement of muscle tissue, and an unaffected muscle may be normal. In an acute myopathy, it is best to select a muscle for biopsy that is clinically weak; in a chronic myopathy, it is best to select a muscle that is only mildly weak. The muscle selected should not have been sampled by needle electromyography, which may result in temporary inflammation. The pathologist, to investigate possible causes, performs specific histochemical stains and occasionally electron microscopy on the specimen.

Magnetic resonance imaging may be an additional diagnostic tool in clinical practice. The pattern of muscle involvement is specific for the different entities.[9]

Genetic testing has become routine in the evaluation of many of the muscular dystrophies and is also useful in the evaluation of other chronic myopathies. A helpful resource is the journal *Neuromuscular Disorders*, which each month publishes a list of all known genetic neuromuscular disorders on the Web.[2]

Differential Diagnosis

Motor neuron disease
- Amyotrophic lateral sclerosis
- Late-onset spinal muscular atrophy

Neuromuscular junction disorders
- Myasthenia gravis
- Lambert-Eaton myasthenic syndrome

Motor neuropathies
- Demyelinating motor neuropathies, such as multifocal motor neuropathy and diabetic amyotrophy

Spinal stenosis or myelopathy

Parkinson disease

Poliomyelitis, post-poliomyelitis syndrome

TREATMENT

Initial

Of great importance is an initial detailed explanation to the patient and the people in the near surrounding (e.g., relatives). Patients are informed that they must not exert themselves to the point of exhaustion. Referral to the Muscular Dystrophy Association is helpful for education and support of the patient.

Steroids are often effective in the treatment of inflammatory myopathies (as are other immunosuppressants) and have been shown to slow progression in some muscular dystrophies. Carnitine is used in lipid storage myopathies. Otherwise, the only therapeutic option is symptomatic treatment (e.g., pain treatment with different analgesics).

Rehabilitation

Physical therapy and occupational therapy are often necessary for gait training and stretching. Assistive devices, such as canes, walkers, and wheelchairs, as indicated in a particular patient, can minimize disability. Assistive devices should be used, preferably after training with a physical therapist. Bracing may be helpful for footdrop.

Adaptive equipment may be prescribed to assist a patient with daily activities. Home adaptations, such as tub bars and entrance ramps, may be of great assistance to patients with proximal muscle weakness.

Exercise can help maintain joint range of motion. There has been debate about whether patients with muscle disorders benefit from muscle training. An increasing knowledge based on the results from studies has led to new recommendations.[10] High-resistance training at submaximal level seems to be beneficial in slowly progressive disorders in the short perspective. In rapidly progressive disorders, such as Duchenne muscular dystrophy, high-resistance training is questionable. On the basis of this, moderate exercise not to the point of exhaustion is preferable. Of importance is to start muscle training early in the course of the disease so that there are still trainable muscle fibers left.

The common opinion on muscle training in inflammatory myopathies has changed during recent years. Patients with inflammatory myopathies have been strongly advised to avoid exercise. However, a result from training studies has shown that muscle training has beneficial effects on muscle function.[11]

Procedures

Assisted ventilation, including negative-pressure ventilation, noninvasive positive-pressure ventilation, and invasive positive-pressure ventilation (i.e., endotracheal tube or tracheostomy), may be indicated for patients with insufficient ventilation.[12] Feeding tubes may be necessary for patients with dysphagia due to severe bulbar myopathy.

Surgery

Patients with muscular dystrophies may require contracture release and spine stabilization surgeries.

POTENTIAL DISEASE COMPLICATIONS

Severe myopathies, including muscular dystrophies, can cause restrictive pulmonary disease by chest wall muscle weakness and scoliosis. Assisted ventilation, including negative-pressure ventilation, noninvasive positive-pressure ventilation, and invasive positive-pressure ventilation (endotracheal tube or tracheostomy), may be indicated. Decreased mobility can result from proximal lower and upper extremity weakness. Contractures can be caused by disuse and fibrosis as well as by scoliosis due to paraspinal muscle weakness. Cardiac involvement is present in some forms of muscle disorders.[1] Gastrointestinal symptoms due to smooth muscle involvement are common in patients with muscular dystrophies.

POTENTIAL TREATMENT COMPLICATIONS

Immunosuppression may have associated side effects. Steroid use and decreased mobility may lead to osteoporosis and the subsequent risk of pathologic fractures, and analgesics have well known side effects. Special attention should be paid to patients undergoing general anesthesia.

References

1. Goodwin FC, Muntoni F. Cardiac involvement in muscular dystrophies: molecular mechanisms. Muscle Nerve 2005;32: 577-588.
2. GeneTable of Neuromuscular Disorders. Available at: http://www.musclegenetable.org.
3. Briani C, Doria A, Sarzi-Puttini P, Dalakas MC. Update on idiopathic inflammatory myopathies. Autoimmunity 2006;39: 161-170.
4. Oldfors A, Lindberg C. Diagnosis, pathogenesis and treatment of inclusion body myositis. Curr Opin Neurol 2005;18:497-503.
5. Miller JAL. Statins—challenges and provocations. Curr Opin Neurol 2005;18:494-496.
6. Davies NP, Hanna MG. The skeletal muscle channelopathies: distinct entities and overlapping syndromes. Curr Opin Neurol 2003;16:559-568.
7. Schara U, Schoser BG. Myotonic dystrophies type 1 and 2: summary on current aspects. Semin Pediatr Neurol 2006;13:71-79.
8. Mastaglia FL, Lamont PJ, Laing NL. Distal myopathies. Curr Opin Neurol 2005;18:504-510.
9. Mercuri E, Jungbluth H, Muntoni F. Muscle imaging in clinical practice: diagnostic value of muscle magnetic resonance imaging in inherited neuromuscular disorders. Curr Opin Neurol 2005;18:526-537.
10. Ansved T. Muscle training in muscular dystrophies. Acta Physiol Scand 2001;171:359-366.
11. Alexandersson H, Lundberg IE. The role of exercise in the rehabilitation of idiopathic inflammatory myopathies. Curr Opin Rheumatol 2005;17:164-171.
12. Mellies U, Dohna-Schwake C, Voit T. Respiratory function assessment and intervention in neuromuscular disorders. Curr Opin Neurol 2005;18:543-547.

Neurogenic Bladder 129

Ayal M. Kaynan, MD, and Inder Perkash, MD

ICD-9 Codes

344.61	Cauda equina syndrome with neurogenic bladder
596.4	Atony of bladder
596.51	Hypertonicity of bladder
596.52	Low bladder compliance
596.53	Paralysis of bladder
596.54	Neurogenic bladder NOS
596.55	Detrusor-sphincter dyssynergia
596.59	Other functional disorder of bladder
596.9	Unspecified disorder of bladder

DEFINITION

The term *neurogenic bladder* describes a process of dysfunctional voiding as the result of neurologic injury. In one way or another, this type of injury can interfere with urine storage at low bladder pressures or with voluntary coordinated voiding. Approximately 2,138,408 patients are discharged from hospital care annually in the United States for neurologic disorders.[1] Neurologic control of bladder function is at multiple levels throughout the central nervous system and subject to multiple pathophysiologic processes. Voiding dysfunction occurs in most of these patients.

SYMPTOMS

The symptoms of neurogenic bladder have a wide spectrum of presentation and include urinary incontinence, urinary retention, suprapubic or pelvic pain, incomplete voiding, paroxysmal hypertension with diaphoresis (autonomic dysreflexia), urinary tract infection, and occult deterioration in renal function. The symptoms vary according to the pathophysiologic process and are detailed later. To understand the pathophysiologic processes, the clinician must have a thorough understanding of the relevant anatomy.

The micturition reflex center has been localized to the pontine mesencephalic reticular formation in the brainstem.[2,3] Efferent axons from the pontine micturition center travel down the spinal cord in the reticulospinal tract to the detrusor motor nuclei located in the S2, S3, and S4 segments in the sacral gray matter (vertebral levels T12 to L2).[4]

Parasympathetic nerves take their origin from nuclei at the intermediolateral gray column of the spinal cord at S2, S3, and S4 and travel by the pelvic nerve and pelvic plexus to ganglia in the bladder wall. The predominant parasympathetic nerve root supplying the bladder is usually S3. Acetylcholine is released from the postganglionic nerves, which in turn excites muscarinic receptors.[5]

Preganglionic sympathetic neurons originate in the intermediolateral gray column of the spinal cord from spinal segments T10 to L2. These nerves course to the sympathetic chain ganglion and ultimately through the pelvic plexus to the bladder neck, which constitutes the internal (smooth muscle, involuntary) urethral sphincter, as well as to the fundus of the bladder. Receptors at the bladder neck are primarily α-adrenergic,[6] stimulation of which results in closure of the internal sphincter during urinary storage and, in men, during ejaculation as well. In contrast to the bladder neck, the fundus of the bladder is populated with β-adrenergic receptors, which contribute to bladder relaxation (and therefore urinary storage) during sympathetic activation.

The external urethral sphincter (striated muscle, voluntary) surrounds the membranous urethra and extends up and around the distal part of the prostatic urethra. The pudendal nerves, which innervate the external sphincter, take their origin from the somatic motor nuclei in the anterior gray matter of the sacral cord (conus, S2 to S4); however, it is the S2 spinal segment that provides the principal motor contribution. Toe plantar flexors also have S1 and S2 innervation. Thus, the preservation of toe plantar flexors after spinal cord injury suggests that the external urethral sphincter is intact.

The central control of the bladder is a complex, multilevel process. Advances in functional brain imaging have allowed research into this control in humans. The regions of the brain that have been implicated in the central control of continence include the pons (pontine micturition center), periaqueductal gray, thalamus, insula, anterior cingulate gyrus, and prefrontal cortices. The pontine micturition center and the periaqueductal gray are thought to be crucial in the supraspinal control of continence and micturition. Higher centers, such as the insula, anterior cingulate gyrus, and prefrontal regions, are probably involved in the modulation of this control and cognition of bladder sensations and, in the case of the insula and anterior cingulate, modulation of autonomic function. Further work should aim to examine how the regions interact to achieve urinary continence.[7]

Abnormalities in the midbrain (e.g., Parkinson disease) lead to detrusor hyperreflexia due to loss of dopamine. Lesions in segmental areas of the spinal cord lead to detrusor-sphincter dyssynergia. Cortical lesions (lesions above the pontine micturition center) usually result in loss of voluntary inhibition of the micturition reflex. Lesions in the forebrain, such as cerebrovascular accidents with change in blood flow to the cingulate gyrus, can lead to hyperreflexic bladder because of reduced dopamine D_1 with increased glutamate activity. Thus, the cingulate gyrus plays an important role in urine storage. Patients with Parkinson disease have less severe urinary dysfunction with little evidence of internal or external sphincter denervation. By contrast, in multiple system atrophy, patients have more symptoms and wide-open bladder neck. The result is a hyperreflexic bladder with coordinated (synergic) sphincter function.[8] In the absence of outflow obstruction (e.g., urethral stricture, benign prostatic hyperplasia, large uterine leiomyoma, fecal impaction), complete bladder evacuation with some incontinence is the outcome. The findings of postmicturition residuals of more than 100 mL, detrusor–external sphincter dyssynergia, and open bladder neck at the start of bladder filling, with significant postural hypotension and neurogenic sphincter motor unit potentials, are highly suggestive of multiple system atrophy.[9] The patient can have unstable blood pressure, which is aggravated with a postural change, indicating some degree of autonomic failure. Similarly, after a severe head injury, an autonomic failure can result in unstable postural hypotension and wide-open bladder neck.

All lesions from the pons to spinal cord level S2 result in a loss of cortical inhibition and loss of coordinated sphincter activity during reflex voiding. Micturition reflex is without an inhibitory or coordinated control from higher centers. This results in a hyperreflexic bladder with dyssynergic sphincter function (detrusor-sphincter dyssynergia), which often results in incomplete voiding and high bladder pressures; it can lead to ureteral reflux.[10] Urinary retention from functional obstruction occurs, and overflow incontinence may occur with an overdistended bladder.

Spinal cord lesions above T5-6 result in autonomic dysreflexia, in which the bladder is allowed to fill to excess. This is virtually always seen in conjunction with detrusor-sphincter dyssynergia.[11] This is due to loss of cortical and medullary inhibitory reflexes modulating sympa-

thetic activity of the splanchnic bed (T5-8). Accentuated visceral activity (e.g., full bladder, fecal impaction), which causes sympathetically mediated vasoconstriction, is normally inhibited by secondary output from the medulla and is countered by vasodilation in the splanchnic bed through the greater splanchnic nerve. Without the proper inhibitory reflexes or control of the splanchnic bed to redistribute circulating blood volume, blood pressure rises sharply. With the carotid bodies and vagal nerves intact, bradycardia results. The full syndrome is characterized by paroxysmal and extreme elevation in blood pressure, facial flushing, perspiration, goose pimples, headache, and some degree of bradycardia.

Spinal cord lesions in the conus at S2 or below result in lower motor neuron injury to the bladder and external sphincter. The effect on the bladder is predictable: areflexia. Because the parasympathetic ganglia reside in or near the bladder wall, bladder tone is generally maintained. Bladder compliance therefore tends to decrease with time as a result of neural decentralization (or infection-related fibrosis).[12] The result on the bladder neck and external sphincter is not as intuitive. Although an atonic synergic sphincter system might be expected, the external sphincter usually retains some fixed tone, although not under voluntary control, and the bladder neck is often competent because of an intact sympathetic innervation (α-adrenergic activity) but nonrelaxing. Even though bladder pressures are generally low during filling and storage, obstructive physiology is often the case during voiding.[13] Overflow incontinence is possible.

In the acute phase of injury, most central nervous system lesions result in a temporarily areflexic bladder.[14,15] This phase, termed central nervous system shock, is variable and can last several weeks. Reappearance of knee jerks heralds recovery from the shock phase.

The specific patterns of voiding dysfunction with the most common neurologic abnormalities in the chronic phase are detailed in Table 129-1 and Figure 129-1.

Confounding medical problems, such as diabetes and many cardiovascular drugs (Table 129-2), will profoundly affect bladder function. Patients who catheterize themselves intermittently should be asked about the size of catheter used and whether there is any resistance or trauma during catheterization—clues to the presence of a urethral stricture. Patterns of voiding should be elicited, and changes in voiding habits should be scrutinized. Patients with suprasacral spinal cord injury, for example, often give a history of intermittent stream coinciding with spasticity of their lower extremities, a strong clue to detrusor-sphincter dyssynergia. Spinal cord–injured patients with incomplete lesions can void with excessive Valsalva maneuver and can produce very high intra-abdominal pressures. This can lead to vesicoureteral reflux, upper tract changes, repeated pyelonephritis, and even stone disease. They therefore need to be monitored frequently with urodynamics and managed appropriately to achieve low-pressure voiding. Approximately 50% of men ultimately have benign

TABLE 129-1 Patterns of Voiding Dysfunction in Chronic Neurologic Disease

Neurologic Disorder	Detrusor Activity	Striated Sphincter	Comments
Suprapontine	**Hyperreflexic**	**Synergic**	
Brain tumor, cerebral palsy			Detrusor-sphincter dyssynergia may occur in those with spinal cord damage; voluntary control may be impaired
Cerebrovascular accident			Voluntary control may be impaired
Delayed central nervous system maturation			Persistence of uninhibited bladder beyond age 2-3 years; enuresis later
Dementia			Voluntary control is impaired
Parkinson disease			Detrusor contractility and voluntary control may be impaired
Pernicious anemia			Bladder compliance may be decreased
Shy-Drager syndrome			Bladder neck remains open; bladder compliance may be decreased; autonomic instability (low blood pressure)
Pons-S1	**Hyperreflexic**	**Dyssynergic**	
Anterior spinal cord ischemia			Bladder compliance may be decreased
Multiple sclerosis			Varies with lesions
Myelodysplasia, trauma			Variable
Below S1	**Areflexic**	**Fixed tone**	
Acute transverse myelitis			Bladder neck may be closed but nonrelaxing
Diabetes, Guillain-Barré syndrome, herniated intervertebral disc			Usually overdistended bladder
Myelodysplasia, poliomyelitis			Decreased bladder compliance may develop; bladder neck may be open (sympathetic denervation)
Radical pelvic surgery			Bladder neck is open
Tabes dorsalis, trauma			Bladder neck may be closed but nonrelaxing

prostatic hyperplasia. Thus, even in the case of stable neurologic disease, these men may develop difficulty in voiding from progressive outflow obstruction. Typical symptoms include nocturia, decreased force of stream, hesitancy, and postvoid dribbling. However, patients with outflow obstruction frequently have irritative voiding symptoms as well. It is important to make sure that these symptoms are not due to symptomatic infection: back pain, suprapubic pain, fever, dysuria, urgency, frequency, or hematuria. These symptoms are not specific and can reflect many of the processes discussed. Their presence must therefore be interpreted according to context.

PHYSICAL EXAMINATION

General considerations include the level of disability and the capability to use upper and lower extremities. The neurologic examination focuses on the strength and dexterity of the upper extremities and the tone and reflexes of the lower extremities. Neurourologic examination includes perianal sensation for evidence of sacral sparing, anal sphincter voluntary contraction, and bulbocavernosus reflex.

The genitalia are examined for the condition of the penis: whether it is circumcised, its size, and adequacy of the meatus; attention is paid to the presence of meatal erosion. In women, it is important to note the appearance of the urethral meatus; this structure erodes quite readily with long-standing catheterization. Pelvic examination will identify confounding factors to voiding dysfunction, such as uterine prolapse or leiomyoma. Rectal examination yields information on anal tone, size of prostate, and presence of fecal impaction. Voluntary contraction of the anal sphincter indicates control over the perineal muscles; in the presence of quadriplegia, it indicates an incomplete central cord–type lesion. To determine voluntary contraction, the clinician places a finger in the patient's anal canal. The bulbocavernosus reflex should be tested. Because deep tendon reflexes at the patella reflect status of the spinal cord at L3-4, hyperreflexia at the knee almost certainly indicates increased tone at the pelvic diaphragm and thus detrusor-sphincter dyssynergia. Absence of the toe plantar flexors reflects either damage to S2 or a supraconal lesion, and it therefore predicts damage to the external urinary sphincter (detrusor-sphincter dyssynergia) and possible involvement of the bladder. For patients with spinal cord injury,

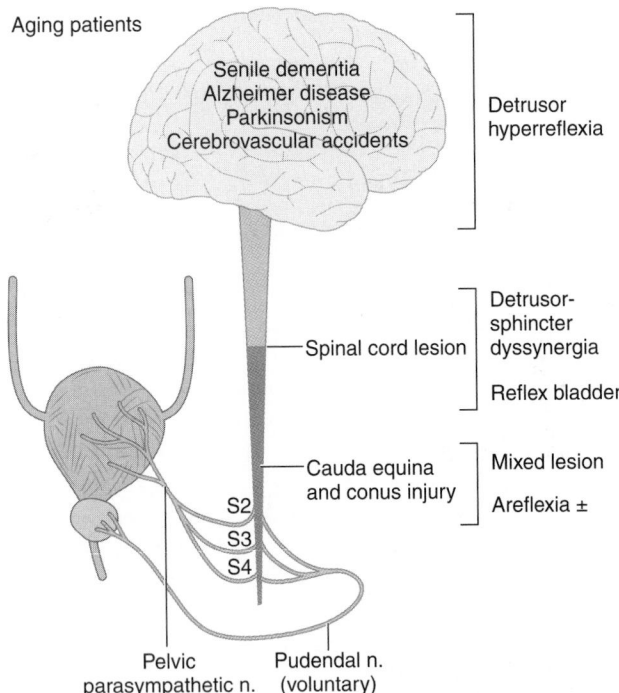

Aging patients

Senile dementia
Alzheimer disease
Parkinsonism
Cerebrovascular accidents

Detrusor
hyperreflexia

Spinal cord lesion

Detrusor-
sphincter
dyssynergia

Reflex bladder

Cauda equina
and conus injury

Mixed lesion

Areflexia ±

S2
S3
S4

Pelvic
parasympathetic n.

Pudendal n.
(voluntary)

FIGURE 129-1. Diagrammatic illustration of central nervous system disorders leading to different neurologic manifestations. (Reprinted with permission from Perkash I. Incontinence in patients with spinal cord injuries. In O'Donnell P, ed. Geriatric Urology. Boston, Little, Brown, 1994:321-325.)

the return of deep reflexes below the level of injury heralds the conclusion of spinal cord shock. Acute-phase physiology then switches to chronic physiology.

The first and most important determination with regard to bladder function is the establishment of good bladder evacuation. The abdomen must therefore be examined for bladder palpability after a trial of voiding. Either a bladder ultrasound scan or urinary catheterization should be performed to determine the postvoid residual.

FUNCTIONAL LIMITATIONS

Functional limitations are typically due to incontinence and include social rejection and isolation. Incontinence may also affect a patient's ability to work, to participate in recreational activities, and to sustain interpersonal relationships.

DIAGNOSTIC STUDIES

All patients with neural injury should have blood chemistries at baseline and periodically during follow-up for blood urea nitrogen and creatinine concentrations. Renal and bladder ultrasound examination should be performed to assess the status of the urinary tract: size, shape, and echogenicity of the kidneys; presence of hydronephrosis or hydroureter; presence of renal or bladder stones; change in hydronephrosis during and after voiding; and completeness of the void. If vesicoureteral reflux or urethral strictures are suspected, voiding cystourethrography may be performed.

If renal stones are suspected, non–contrast-enhanced computed tomography (renal stone protocol) is an excellent tool for identification of the size and location of the stones. In dealing with renal stones, it is sometimes important to assess calyceal or ureteral anatomy or differential renal function, in which case intravenous urography may be performed. Finer qualitative assessment of differential renal function may be performed by technetium Tc 99m mertiatide (^{99m}Tc-MAG3) nuclear renal scan. When compromise of renal function is suspected, this test may be useful.

Transrectal linear array ultrasonography may be performed to assess prostate size, prominent median prostatic lobe, ledge at the bladder neck,[16] or proximal urethra–bladder neck strictures. Voiding videofluoroscopy or ultrasonography can show abrupt cessation of urine flow.

Cystoscopy is an excellent tool for studying bladder and urethral anatomy; it quickly identifies the presence of a urethral stricture (although it may not determine its length or depth), provides an assessment of internal prostatic size, provides indirect evidence of high intravesical pressures (bladder trabeculation), and readily demonstrates bladder stones. Cytoscopy is essential in the assessment of hematuria (more than five red blood cells per high-power field on two or more urine specimens). Whereas hematuria in neurally injured patients is commonly related to infection or traumatic catheterization, the use of indwelling catheters for a long time places these patients at a significantly higher risk for bladder cancer.[17] It has been suggested, therefore, that these patients undergo surveillance cystoscopy annually, particularly if they have other risk factors for bladder cancer, such as smoking or a family history with bladder cancer. After bladder irrigation with normal saline, a urine specimen for malignant cell cytology may be helpful as a screening test. No test is as sensitive for the detection of bladder tumors as the cystoscopic examination and biopsy of a suspicious area.

Note that cystoscopy does not provide functional information. The best single test for bladder function is urodynamic testing.

Formal urodynamic testing, including cystometrography and electromyography, is crucial to the proper documentation of bladder and outlet function. The test is subject to inherent errors in technique, interpretation, and cooperation of the patient; however, the astute clinician must interpret the results in light of the entire clinical scenario. Properly performed, it will elucidate and quantify postvoid residual of urine, bladder capacity, bladder compliance, bladder pressures during filling and voiding, and external sphincteric coordination. In conjunction with videofluoroscopic monitoring, ureteral reflux, bladder position, and internal and external sphincteric function may be visualized. Urodynamics should be performed at baseline for all patients with neurologic disease. Because of central nervous system shock in the acute phase of injury, it is best to perform urodynamics after the shock resolves—on return of distal reflexes. Figure 129-2 illustrates a normal voiding pattern. Figure 129-3 illustrates the urodynamic findings of an areflexic bladder. Figure 129-4A shows detrusor-sphinc-

TABLE 129-2 Pharmacologic Action on the Bladder

Drug	Indication	Mechanism	Side Effects and Cautions
Cholinergics Bethanechol	Areflexic bladder	Muscarinic receptor agonists Bladder has M_2 and M_3 receptors; M_3 receptors are responsible for normal detrusor contraction	Bronchospasm, miosis

Anticholinergics
  Hyoscyamine
  Oxybutynin
  Tolte rodine
  Trospium chloride
    (quaternary amine)
  Darifenacin
  Solifenacin
	Hyperreflexic bladder	Muscarinic receptor antagonists	Constipation, dry mouth, tachycardia

Sympathomimetics
  Norepinephrine
  Pseudoephedrine
	Open bladder neck	α-Receptor antagonists	Arrhythmia, hypertension, coronary vasospasm, excitability, tremors

Antiadrenergics
  (α blockers)
  Phenoxybenzamine
  Phentolamine
  Terazosin
  Doxazosin
  Tamsulosin
  Alfuzosin
	Smooth sphincter dyssynergia (competent, nonrelaxing bladder neck)	α-Receptor agonists	Orthostatic hypotension, dizziness, rhinitis, retrograde ejaculation

Tricyclic antidepressants
  Amitriptyline
  Imipramine
	Hyperreflexic bladder with stress incontinence	Anticholinergic and sympathomimetic properties	Myocardial infarction, tachycardia, stroke, seizures, blood dyscrasias, dry mouth, drowsiness, constipation, blurred vision

Benzodiazepines Chlordiazepoxide	Extremity spasticity with detrusor-sphincter dyssynergia	GABA channel activator, centrally acting muscle relaxant	Dizziness, drowsiness, extrapyramidal effects, ataxia, agranulocytosis
Baclofen	Extremity spasticity with detrusor-sphincter dyssynergia	GABA-B channel activator (?); exact mechanism unknown; centrally acting muscle relaxant	Central nervous system depression, cardiovascular collapse, respiratory failure, seizures, dizziness, weakness, hypotonia, constipation, blurred vision*
Dantrolene	Extremity spasticity with detrusor-sphincter dyssynergia	Direct muscle relaxant by calcium sequestration in the sarcoplasmic reticulum	Hepatic dysfunction, seizures, pleural effusion, incoordination, dizziness, nausea, vomiting, abdominal pain
Botulinum toxin	Detrusor-sphincter dyssynergia	Inhibits release of acetylcholine	Repeated injections necessary

*Note that baclofen is also administered intrathecally by an implanted pump in these patients, and adverse effects are primarily limited to the central nervous system. Bladder contractility may also be reduced. No significant change occurs in detrusor-sphincter dyssynergia.

ter dyssynergia. The sonographic correlate of detrusor-sphincter dyssynergia is shown in Figure 129-4B (nonrelaxation of the external urethral sphincter is demonstrated).

TREATMENT

Initial

The priorities of bladder management relate first to preservation of renal function and abolition of infection and second to social concerns. Overflow incontinence, ureteral reflux, or high bladder pressures in the presence of renal insufficiency or active infection must be managed aggressively by ensuring proper egress for urine. A source for persistent infection, such as urinary lithiasis, must be sought and, if found, eliminated. High bladder pressure, particularly if it is sustained (>40 cm

Differential Diagnosis

The diseases listed in Table 129-1 are the most common causes of neurogenic bladder.

H_2O), ultimately results in deterioration of renal function and should therefore be addressed actively, even if renal function is normal.[18]

Patients at risk for degenerative neurogenic bladders, particularly those with (or at risk for) sensory neuropathies (e.g., diabetic patients, phenytoin users), should

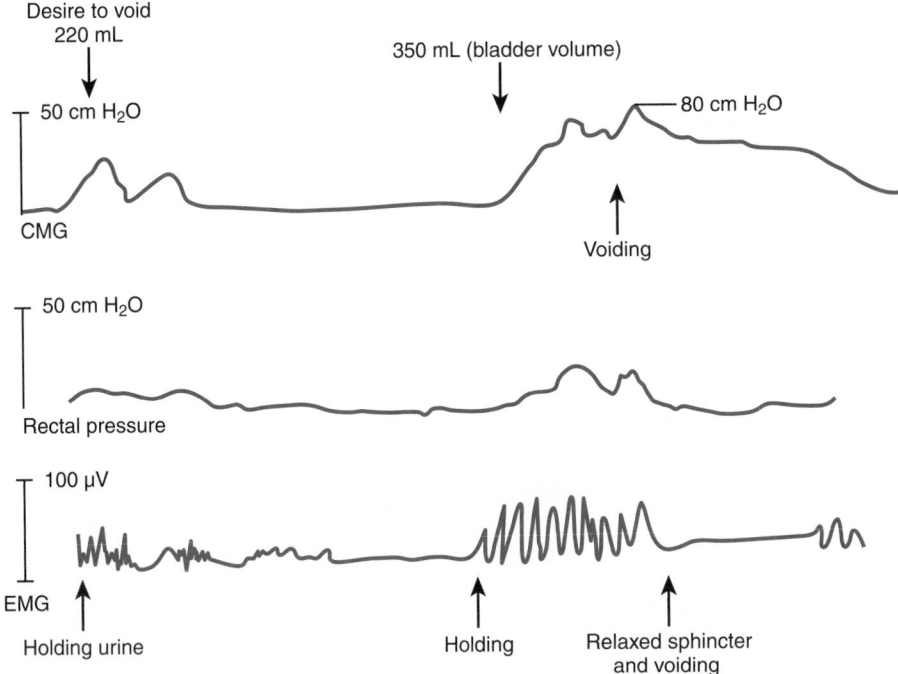

FIGURE 129-2. Urodynamic study consisting of simultaneous cystometrography (CMG), rectal pressure, and electromyography (EMG) of the external urethral sphincter. During bladder filling, the desire to void is usually expressed between 300 and 400 mL. When the normal person is asked to hold urine, the external urethral sphincter contracts and the bladder relaxes. When asked, this person voided voluntarily at a filling volume of approximately 350 mL; the external urethral sphincter relaxed just before voiding, indicating a normal study.

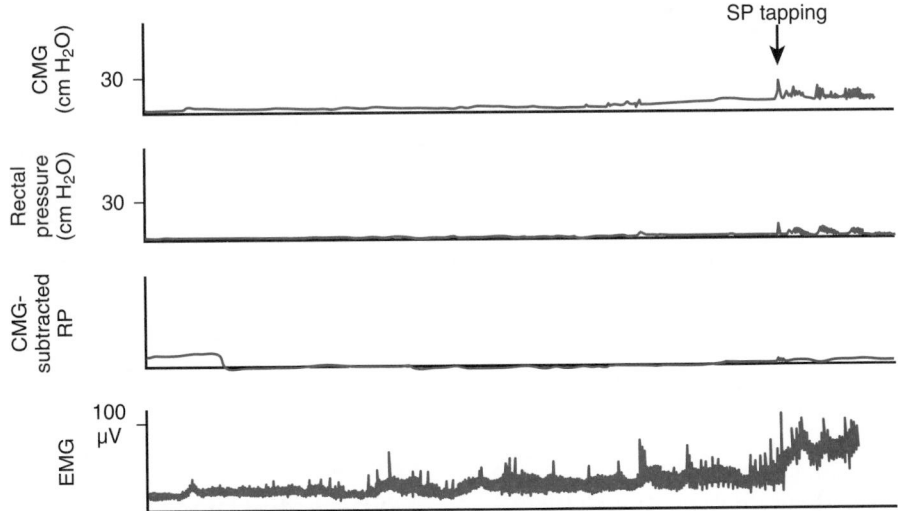

FIGURE 129-3. Urodynamic study demonstrating an areflexic bladder in a patient with spinal cord injury. There is minimal increase in electromyographic (EMG) activity during filling of the bladder. There is no bladder contraction, even after suprapubic (SP) tapping, indicating overdistention areflexia or a lower motor neuron lesion. CMG, cystometrography; RP, rectal pressure.

have a timed voiding schedule to prevent overdistention and progression to bladder areflexia. A 24-hour voiding diary, including fluid intake, time and quantity voided, and postvoid residual (by catheterization or ultrasound evaluation), should be recorded periodically. These patients should void every 6 hours, void again immediately after the first void, and adjust their fluid intake and voiding frequency according to the voiding diary. Patients with diabetes should be careful to maintain good

glycemic control, not only for global prevention of related degenerative disease but also to prevent osmotic diuresis.

Most neurogenic injuries to the bladder are associated with impaired bowel function. Fecal impaction and obstipation not only place the patient at risk for colon perforation, they may also cause mechanical obstruction to the passage of urine. Further, many of the

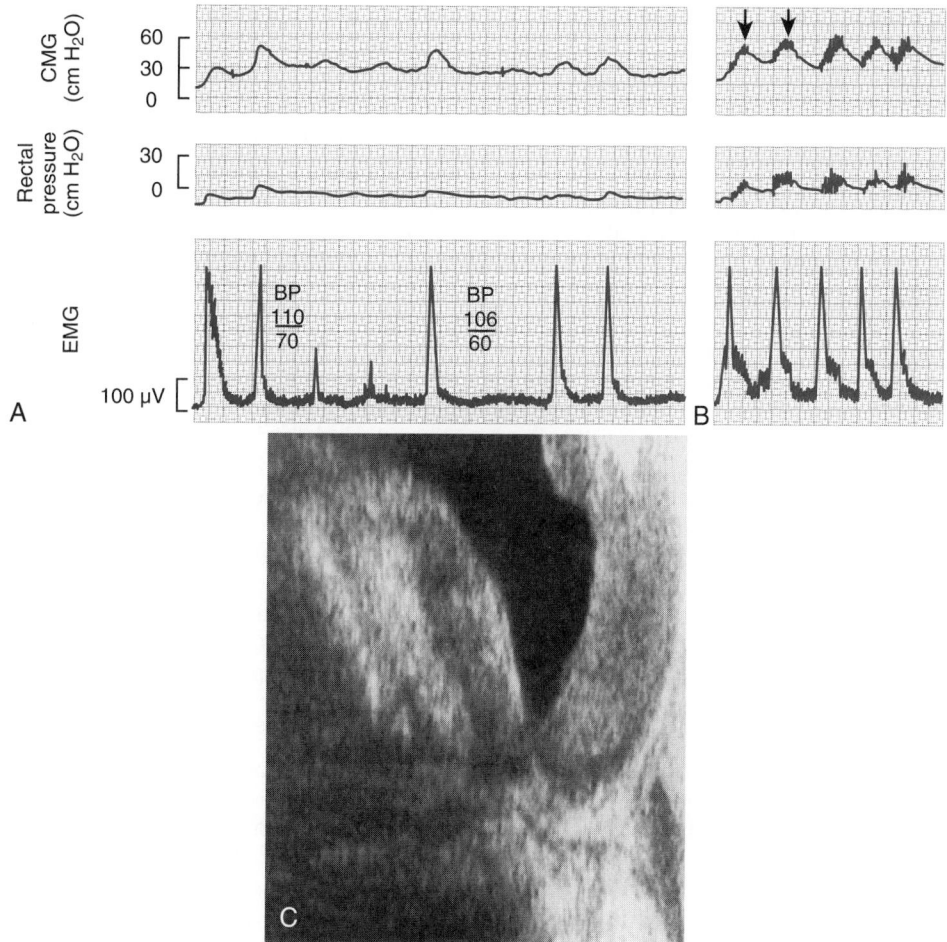

FIGURE 129-4. **A** and **B,** Detrusor-sphincter dyssynergia in a patient with spinal cord injury; each bladder contraction on the cystometrogram (CMG) is accompanied by a marked increase in electromyographic (EMG) activity of the external urethral sphincter. BP, blood pressure. **C,** Ultrasound cystourethrogram during an attempted void in a patient with spinal cord injury with detrusor-sphincter dyssynergia. The passage of urine is abruptly stopped by closure of the external urethral sphincter, and the posterior urethra is dilated.

medications used to reduce bladder contractility, particularly the anticholinergics, exacerbate bowel motile dysfunction. It is therefore important that these patients be routinely prescribed high-fiber diets, stool softeners (e.g., docusate, 100 mg orally, three times daily), laxatives (e.g., psyllium, 1 packet orally every day), and suppositories (e.g., bisacodyl, 10 mg per rectum every day) and undergo digital stimulation either daily or every other day. Digital stimulation is best performed after either a meal or coffee or tea to take advantage of the gastrocolic reflex.

The Credé method (suprapubic pressure) alone can lead to high intravesical pressures and even vesicoureteral reflux. Such pressure, or persistent tapping of the suprapubic region for 2 minutes at a time, should be performed only when methods to relieve bladder outlet obstruction have been ensured. This should not be performed in patients with active detrusor-sphincter dyssynergia because it will only exacerbate already high bladder pressures, and urine will not be completely evacuated.

Acute Phase and Central Nervous System Shock

This phase usually lasts days to weeks but sometimes persists for months. The bladder is areflexic during this period, and adequate bladder drainage should be secured to prevent the areflexic bladder from developing overdistention and myogenic failure. Indwelling continuous Foley catheterization (14 Fr) is the easiest way to ensure bladder drainage. Alternatively, intermittent catheterization may be performed (after the initial phase of diuresis) and, when it is used from the onset, reduces the incidence of infection and stone disease.[19]

Catheterization is performed every 4 to 6 hours and fluid is restricted to 2 liters per day, if possible. The frequency of catheterization should be adjusted so that residuals are no more than 300 to 400 mL. For patients with a hyperreflexic bladder, long-term intermittent catheterization requires mitigation of the detrusor reflex with anticholinergic medication (see Table 129-2) to reduce bladder pressures to safe levels (below 40 cm H_2O) and to achieve continence between catheterizations.

Anticholinergic Drugs (Drugs to Increase Bladder Capacity)

In the human being, bladder (detrusor muscle) has muscarinic receptors (M_2 and M_3 receptors). M_3 compared with M_2 are small in number but are mainly responsible for bladder contraction. The antimuscarinic drugs oxybutynin, tolterodine, darifenacin, solifenacin, and trospium are the five major drugs (Table 129-3) currently available to modulate detrusor hyperreflexia, to increase bladder capacity, and to reduce bladder voiding pressures. Comparative clinical studies have shown that oxybutynin and solifenacin may be marginally more effective than tolterodine, although tolterodine seems to be better tolerated. Dry mouth and constipation are still major problems for compliance of patients with all of them because of the widespread existence of M_3 receptors, particularly in the salivary glands. Except for trospium chloride, most others shown in Table 129-3 are tertiary amines and cross the blood-brain barrier, enhancing anticholinergic factor. There is evidence that they may lead to some loss of memory.[20]

Autonomic Dysreflexia

The control of widespread sympathetic activity below the spinal lesion is the key factor in the management of autonomic dysreflexia, and prevention is the first concern. Noxious stimuli, such as overdistention of the bladder, should be reversed immediately by catheter drainage. Local instillation of 25 to 50 mL of 0.3% tetracaine through the Foley catheter or suprapubic tube may provide topical anesthesia of the vesical mucosa and reduce triggering impulses to the spinal cord. Consideration of procedures for patients at risk (spinal lesions above T6) should include spinal anesthesia, use of ganglion blockers, and use of adrenergic blockers.

In the acute episode, if reversal of the noxious stimulus fails to control symptoms, administration of nifedipine (30 mg orally)[21] or nitropaste (about 1 inch applied on the body surface) is usually adequate to reduce blood pressure. Note that normal blood pressure for a patient with spinal cord injury is less than 100 mm Hg systolic. If nifedipine fails, hydralazine (10 to 20 mg intravenously or 10 to 50 mg intramuscularly) may be administered. Use lower doses initially and repeat every 20 to 30 minutes as necessary to maintain a low blood pressure. Other useful drugs include α blockers (such as prazosin, terazosin, guanethidine, and clonidine) and anticholinergics (such as oxybutynin and tolterodine). For long-term management of subacute autonomic dysreflexia, clonidine (0.1 to 0.3 mg orally twice daily) is useful. Note that the chronic form of this syndrome is often related to active detrusor-sphincter dyssynergia, and methods aimed at control of this phenomenon, such as transurethral sphincterotomy, may alleviate the patient of autonomic dysreflexia.[22]

Urinary Tract Infections

For those who have had indwelling Foley catheters for an extended period (more than several days) and require catheter removal or exchange, antibiotics should be administered prophylactically before, during, and after removal of the existing catheter. Gentamicin (80 mg intramuscularly once just before removal of the

TABLE 129-3 Summary of Anticholinergic Agents

Anticholinergic*	$T_{1/2}$(h)	Typical Side Effects	Comments
Oxybutynin Ditropan	2-3	Dry mouth, constipation, blurry vision, headaches Elderly: cognitive impairment, hallucinations	Typical dose is 5 mg orally tid
Ditropan XL	13	Same as oral oxybutynin	Slower absorption with more stable blood concentration Typical dose is 10 mg orally daily, but doses up to 40 mg daily are generally safe
Oxytrol (oxybutynin patch)	2-5	Same as oral oxybutynin, plus local skin irritation	Bypasses first pass of the liver, which reduces the concentrations of active metabolites that are thought to contribute to side effects Dosed at 3.9 mg/day, 1 patch 2 times/week, alternating skin sites
Tolterodine Detrol	2-10	Same as oral oxybutynin	Possibly more selective to urinary M receptors, resulting in fewer side effects Typical dose is 2 mg orally bid
Detrol LA	2-10	Same as oral oxybutynin	Slower absorption with more stable blood concentration Typical dose is 4 mg orally daily
Darifenacin (Enablex)	13-19	Same as oral oxybutynin	Typical dose is 7.5 mg or 15 mg orally daily
Trospium	20	Same as oral oxybutynin	Quaternary amine does not cross the blood-brain barrier well, resulting in minimal central nervous system anticholinergic effect, and it may limit cognitive side effects (particularly in the elderly) Typical dose is 20 mg orally bid
Sanctura XR	36	Same as oral oxybutynin	More stable blood concentration Typical dose is 60 mg orally daily
Solifenacin (VESIcare)	45-68	Same as oral oxybutynin	Typical dose is 5 mg or 10 mg orally daily

*Unless patients with urinary retention are managed with a catheter, anticholinergic therapy is contraindicated for them. Anticholinergics are also contraindicated in patients with gastric retention and patients with uncontrolled narrow-angle glaucoma.
$T_{1/2}$(h), pharmacokinetic half-life (hours).

catheter) is appropriate for most patients with stable renal function, even if function is impaired, and has both gram-positive and gram-negative coverage. Those with prosthetics, aortic stenosis, or other risk factors for seeding should have coadministration of ampicillin (1 g intravenously) for enterococcus coverage. Alternatively, amoxicillin–clavulanic acid (750 mg) or ciprofloxacin (500 mg) may be given orally twice daily around catheter removal. In addition, the bladder should be irrigated gently through the catheter with 50 mL of normal saline (at body temperature) containing 120 µg/mL Neosporin and 60 µg/mL polymyxin B. Irrigation is continued while the catheter is being pulled through the urethra. This method has been shown to significantly reduce urinary tract infection related to catheter changes.[23,24]

Attention to hygiene is paramount in the prevention of urinary tract infections in the spinal cord–injured population. Those who wear condom catheters should change the catheter once a day. Leg bags should be routinely disinfected with 6% Clorox solution or bleach (most cost-efficient) and then washed well with running water. Wheelchair seat cushions should be changed and cleaned, and the patient should take a shower daily to reduce colony counts at the perineum. Suppressive treatment should be considered for patients who demonstrate recurrent infections. Nitrofurantoin, 100 mg orally daily, is sufficient. Methenamine hippurate (1 g orally twice a day) and ascorbic acid (500 mg orally daily) acidify the urine and are good for prophylaxis of urinary tract infection.[25]

Rehabilitation

Supervised physical or occupational therapy is not typically indicated in neurogenic bladder except when patients need training or assistance in self-catheterization. Rehabilitation nurses may also be involved in this educational process.

Procedures

Another alternative to long-term management of bladder drainage is placement of a suprapubic catheter. This is preferable to chronic transurethral catheterization because it eliminates the risk of urethral or meatal erosion and is less often the cause of epididymitis or orchitis. Urinary tract infections, however, are just as likely, and these catheters require changing once a month. They are best placed either in the operating room under cystoscopic guidance or, better, through suprapubic incision to ascertain that the catheter ultimately resides as superiorly as possible, far from the bladder neck. This helps prevent irritation at the bladder neck, which often causes reflex bladder contractions, particularly if the catheter balloon (also in an indwelling Foley catheter) drops down into the posterior urethra (Fig. 129-5).

For patients with hyperreflexic bladders, electrical stimulation through peripheral patch electrodes or implantation of a sacral nerve root stimulator may be of some benefit. The treatment is dependent on an intact sacral reflex and works by inhibition of the pudendal–pelvic nerve reflex. Patients must be able to empty their bladders voluntarily (or by Valsalva maneuver) when the device is turned off or be capable of performing intermittent self-catheterization. Its effectiveness varies; the majority of users reported no benefit, and approximately one third have a 30% decrease in urinary frequency.[26] The studies reported are primarily in able-bodied populations with idiopathic detrusor hyperreflexia.[27]

Surgery

Transurethral sphincterotomy has been used in suprasacral lesions in the past and has fallen into disfavor because of intraoperative and delayed bleeding potential. Use of a laser[28] causes virtually no intraoperative bleeding. This procedure results in global incontinence

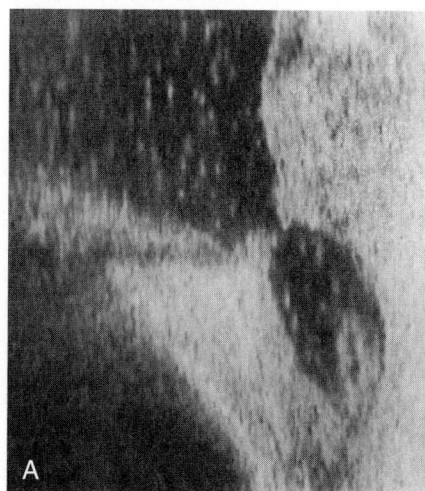
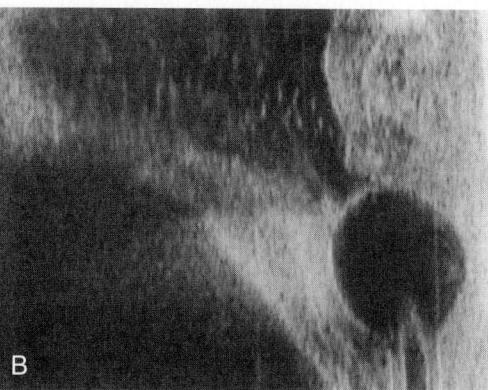

FIGURE 129-5. A, Linear array ultrasound–voiding cystourethrogram shows a contracted bladder neck and dilated prostatic urethra. **B,** The balloon of the urethral Foley catheter is lodged in the prostatic urethra. This occurs uncommonly; however, it may lead to inadequate bladder drainage and, in patients with lesions above T6, autonomic dysreflexia.

postoperatively and requires the use of an external condom catheter.

There are rare circumstances in which bladder management has aggravated renal function, evidenced by recurrent ascending urinary tract infections or a bladder that is too contracted to store sufficient volumes. Some patients find it socially unacceptable to be incontinent and are willing to perform intermittent self-catheterization, but the body habitus precludes them from this. In such cases, there are certain reconstructive options that should be considered. Cystectomy and either incontinent diversion (ureteroileal conduit) or continent diversion (ureteroileocecal conduit) may be performed. Patients must have reasonably good renal function to qualify for continent diversion, lest they suffer from electrolyte and metabolic disturbances.[29]

The most common reconstructive alternative is an ileovesical conduit. The bladder is augmented by a segment of ileum that acts as a conduit to the skin, where a stoma is fashioned. The ureters remain in their native locations. Bladder pressure is reduced because the system is opened, and pelvic urinary continence is dependent on a hyperactive sphincter.

For bladders that have low pressures and good compliance but leak through fixed sphincters, the Mitrofanoff and bladder neck closure may be an excellent option. Spina bifida patients with conus lesions might be good candidates for this procedure. Egress through the bladder neck is eliminated, and the appendix is interposed between the bladder and the umbilicus where it is opened. In the common event that the bladder has poor compliance, an ileal bladder augmentation will raise bladder volume and lower bladder pressure. Patients would then catheterize their augmented bladders through the umbilicus.

POTENTIAL DISEASE COMPLICATIONS

Urinary tract infections, kidney stones, and autonomic dysreflexia are common disease complications associated with neurogenic bladder. Social isolation due to incontinence may lead to depression.

Patients with spinal cord injury who have a urinary tract infection commonly may not present with symptoms.[4] Fevers, chills, back pain, suprapubic pain, dysuria, frequency, and testicular swelling in the setting of positive urine cultures should be regarded as a urinary tract infection. Patients without overt symptoms of pyelonephritis, prostatitis, epididymitis-orchitis, or cystitis are more difficult to diagnose, particularly if they have an indwelling catheter or are being managed by intermittent catheterization. Those using catheters are virtually always colonized with bacteria,[30] and the injudicious use of antibiotics will only select out resistant strains. Factors indicating a need for treatment include urinary lithiasis, as this is most often related to infection (struvite, magnesium ammonium phosphate), and pyuria (8 to 10 white blood cells per high-power field, or 100 white blood cells per milliliter) in the setting of bacteri-

uria (more than 10,000 colony-forming units per milliliter).[4] Urine pH should be checked periodically; pH above 7 is invariably associated with infection from urea-splitting organisms, which may lead to struvite stone formation.

Patients with detrusor-sphincter dyssynergia or urinary retention of any kind should have the bladder drained expeditiously with a fresh Foley catheter during the course of their treatment to ascertain good egress of infected urine. If prostatitis is suspected, transurethral insertion of a Foley catheter is relatively contraindicated, and drainage should be ensured suprapubically. Fluoroquinolones are an excellent first choice for most urinary tract infections; therapy may then be tailored to culture and sensitivity results. Three to five days is sufficient for cystitis. Pyelonephritis requires 2 weeks of therapy. Epididymitis requires at least 3 weeks of therapy, and prostatitis often requires 6 weeks.

POTENTIAL TREATMENT COMPLICATIONS

Stoma care is a source of great consternation for many who have it because of frequent appliance leaks and skin irritation. Also, the stoma must be situated properly on the abdomen according to the patient's habitus and positioning in the wheelchair. Bladder augmentations of any kind are susceptible to perforations and life-threatening infections (as much as 10%). These patients have a 3% chance of small bowel obstruction from adhesions during their lifetime.[31] Chronic indwelling Foley catheters carry the potential for urinary infection, meatal erosion, epididymitis-orchitis, stone disease, and urethral fistula. In women, the urethra becomes patulous in time and incontinence ensues with or without a catheter. Finally, with time and repeated infections, indwelling catheters put patients at risk for development of squamous cell cancer of the bladder. Although the incidence is low, gross hematuria should be evaluated with great suspicion in these patients because this disease is often advanced at the time of discovery and is often fatal.[32]

References

1. H-CUPnet 2004 National Statistics, Department of Health and Human Services, Agency for Healthcare Research and Quality. Available at: http://hcup.ahrq.gov/HCUPnet.asp.
2. Bradley WE, Timm GW, Scott FB. Innervation of the detrusor muscle and urethra. Urol Clin North Am 1974;1:3-27.
3. Denny-Brown D, Robertson EG. On the physiology of micturition. Brain 1933;56:149.
4. Perkash I. Long-term urologic management of the patient with spinal cord injury. Urol Clin North Am 1993;3:423-434.
5. Igawa Y. Discussion: functional role of M_1, M_2, and M_3 muscarinic receptors in overactive bladder. Urology 2000;55(Suppl 5A):47-49.
6. Gosling JA, Dixon JS. The structure and innervation of smooth muscle in the wall of the bladder neck and proximal urethra. Br J Urol 1975;47:549-558.
7. Kavia RB, Dasgupta R, Fowler CJ. Functional imaging and the central control of the bladder [review]. J Comp Neurol 2005;493:27-32.

8. Khan A, Hertanu J, Yang WC, et al. Predictive correlation of urodynamic dysfunction and brain injury after cerebrovascular accident. J Urol 1981;126:86-88.

9. Sakakibara R, Hattori T, Uchiyama T, Yamanishi TJ. Videourodynamic and sphincter motor unit potential analyses in Parkinson's disease and multiple system atrophy. J Neurol Neurosurg Psychiatry 2001;71:600-606.

10. deGroat WC, Steers WD. Autonomic regulation of the urinary bladder and sexual organs. In Loewy AD, Spyer KM, eds. Central Regulation of Autonomic Functions. Oxford, Oxford University Press, 1990:313-314.

11. Perkash I. Pressor response during cystomanometry in spinal injury patients complicated with detrusor-sphincter dyssynergia. J Urol 1979;121:778-782.

12. Fam B, Yalla SV. Vesicourethral dysfunction in spinal cord injury and its management. Semin Neurol 1988;8:150-155.

13. Wein AJ. Neuromuscular dysfunction of the lower urinary tract and its treatment. In Walsh PC, Retik AB, Vaughan ED, et al, eds. Campbell's Urology, 7th ed. Philadelphia, WB Saunders, 1998:961.

14. Burney TL, Senapti M, Desai S, et al. Acute cerebrovascular accident and lower urinary tract dysfunction: a prospective correlation of the site of brain injury with urodynamic findings. J Urol 1996;156:1748-1750.

15. Borrie MJ, Campbell A, Caradoc-Davies TH, et al. Urinary incontinence after stroke: a prospective study. Age Ageing 1986;15:177-181.

16. Perkash I, Friedland GW. Posterior ledge at the bladder neck: crucial diagnostic role of ultrasonography. Urol Radiol 1986;8:175-183.

17. West DA, Cummings JM, Longo WE. Role of chronic catheterization in the development of bladder cancer in patients with spinal cord injury. Urology 1999;53:292-297.

18. Flood HD, Ritchey ML, Bloom DA, et al. Outcome of reflux in children with myelodysplasia managed by bladder pressure monitoring. J Urol 1994;152:1574-1577.

19. Guttman L, Frankel H. The value of intermittent catheterization in early management of traumatic paraplegia and teraplegia. Paraplegia 1966;4:63-84.

20. Katz IR, Prouty Sands L, Bilker W, et al. Identification of medications that cause cognitive impairment in older people: the case of oxybutynin chloride. J Am Geriatr Soc 1988;46:8-13.

21. Messerli FH, Grossman E. The use of sublingual nifedipine: a continuing concern. Arch Intern Med 1999;159:2259-2260.

22. Gasparini ME, Schmidt RA, Tanagho EA. Selective sacral rhizotomy in the management of the reflex neuropathic bladder: a report on 17 patients with long-term followup. J Urol 1992;148:1207-1210.

23. Rhame FS, Perkash I. Urinary tract infections occurring in recent spinal cord injury patients on intermittent catheterization. J Urol 1979;122:669-673.

24. Pearman JW. Prevention of urinary tract infections following spinal cord injury. Paraplegia 1971;9:95-104.

25. Banovac K, Wade N, Gonzalez F, et al. Decreased incidence of urinary tract infections in patients with spinal cord injury: effect of methenamine. J Am Paraplegia Soc 1991;14:52-54.

26. Ohlsson BL, Fall M, Frankenberg-Sommars D. Effects of external and direct pudendal nerve maximal electrical stimulation in the treatment of the uninhibited overactive bladder. Br J Urol 1989;64:374-380.

27. Jonas U, Fowler CJ, Chancellor MB, et al. Efficacy of sacral nerve stimulation for urinary retention: results 18 months after implantation. J Urol 2001;165:15-19.

28. Perkash I. Contact laser sphincterotomy: further experience and longer follow-up. Spinal Cord 1996;34:227-233.

29. McDougal WS. Use of intestinal segments and urinary diversion. In Walsh PC, Retik AB, Vaughan ED, et al, eds. Campbell's Urology, 7th ed. Philadelphia, WB Saunders, 1998:3146.

30. Brisset L, Vernet-Garnier V, Carquin J, et al. In vivo and in vitro analysis of the ability of urinary catheter to microbial colonization [in French]. Pathol Biol (Paris) 1996;44:397-404.

31. Rink RC, Adams MCL. Augmentation cystoplasty. In Walsh PC, Retik AB, Vaughan ED, et al, eds. Campbell's Urology, 7th ed. Philadelphia, WB Saunders, 1998:3167-3189.

32. Serretta V, Pomara G, Piazza F, Gange E. Pure squamous cell carcinoma of the bladder in western countries. Report on 19 consecutive cases. Eur Urol 2000,37:85-89.

Osteoarthritis 130

Allen N. Wilkins, MD, and Edward M. Phillips, MD

DEFINITION

Osteoarthritis represents a family of disorders characterized by a relentless process in which all components of cartilage are destroyed.[1] Osteoarthritis is steadily becoming the most common cause of disability for the middle-aged and has become the most common cause of disability for those older than 65 years.[2] It has been estimated that the total cost for arthritis, including osteoarthritis, is more than 2% of the United States gross domestic product.[3]

Osteoarthritis involves all structures in the joint. Subchondral bone, synovial fluid, and the synovial membrane are major sites of change in the course of the disease process. In addition to degradation and loss of articular cartilage, osteoarthritis is characterized by hypertrophic bone changes with osteophyte formation, subchondral bone remodeling, and, in many cases, chronic inflammation of the synovial membrane.[1]

Joint involvement is usually asymmetrical, with a predilection for weight-bearing joints. Common sites of involvement are the hip, knee, distal and proximal interphalangeal joints, and facet joints of the spine. Less common sites of involvement are the ankle, wrist, and shoulder. Inflammation and joint effusion are present in some cases.

Osteoarthritis is classified into two groups, primary and secondary. Primary osteoarthritis can be localized or generalized; primary generalized osteoarthritis is more commonly found in postmenopausal women, with development of Heberden nodes. Secondary osteoarthritis has an underlying cause (Table 130-1).

Risk factors for osteoarthritis include advanced age, obesity, bone density, and genetics (Table 130-2). Epidemiologic data suggest increased risk of osteoarthritis in persons with low levels of vitamins D and C and estrogen deficiency.[8]

The pathophysiologic mechanism of osteoarthritis involves a combination of mechanical, cellular, and biochemical processes. The interaction of these processes leads to changes in the composition and mechanical properties of the articular cartilage. The normal remodeling process is disrupted in osteoarthritis, leading to increased degenerative changes and an abnormal repair response.[9]

The mechanisms of cartilage degeneration, pain, and functional loss in osteoarthritis are not completely understood (Fig. 130-1).

SYMPTOMS

Patients usually complain of pain, stiffness, reduced movement, and swelling in the affected joints that is exacerbated with activity and relieved by rest. Pain at rest or at night suggests severe disease or another diagnosis. Early morning stiffness, if it is present, is typically less than 30 minutes. Joint tenderness and crepitus on movement may also be present. Swelling may be due to bone deformity, such as osteophyte formation, or an effusion caused by synovial fluid accumulation. Systemic symptoms are absent.[10]

In early disease, pain is usually gradual in onset and mild in intensity. Pain is typically self-limited or intermittent. Patients with advanced disease may describe a sense of grinding or locking with joint motion and buckling or instability of joints during demanding tasks. Spasm of periarticular muscles may be prominent and painful. Patients may complain of fatigue if biomechanical

TABLE 130-1 Causes of Secondary Osteoarthritis

Calcium deposition

Congenital or developmental disorders

Endocrine disorders

Genetic defects

Infectious diseases

Metabolic disorders

Neuropathic disorders

Trauma

Inflammatory arthritis

Obesity

Paget disease

TABLE 130-2 Risk Factors for Osteoarthritis

Risk Factor	Related Studies
Age	Of people older than 65 years, 80% have some radiographic evidence of osteoarthritis, but that incidence and prevalence of symptomatic osteoarthritis leveled off or declined in men and women at around 80 years of age.[4]
Obesity	Increased risk for development of progressive osteoarthritis seems to be apparent in overweight people with localized disease.[5]
Bone density	There is an inverse relationship between bone density and osteoarthritis.[6]
Genetics	There is increased concordance for osteoarthritis in monozygotic twins compared with dizygotic twins, indicating that there is a genetic susceptibility to the disease. The defective genes are often coding for structural proteins of the extracellular matrix of the joint and collagen proteins. Children of parents with early-onset osteoarthritis are at higher risk.[7]
Gender	Before the age of 50 years, men have a higher prevalence and incidence than women do. However, once older than 50 years, women have a higher overall prevalence and incidence than men do.[5]

changes lead to increased energy requirements for activities of daily living. Overuse of alternative muscle groups can lead to development of pain syndromes in other parts of the musculoskeletal system.

PHYSICAL EXAMINATION

Joint Examination

Diagnosis of osteoarthritis involves assessment of the affected joint's range of clinical features. Table 130-3 outlines the pertinent features of an osteoarthritic joint. These features include tenderness, bone enlargement,

and malalignment. In many cases, the patient presents with a warm, swollen joint. Osteophytes, joint surface irregularity, periarticular muscle spasm, or chronic disuse may also result in decreased range of motion, pain, and crepitus. Locking during range of motion suggests loose bodies or floating cartilage fragments in the joint. Joint contracture can result from holding a joint in slight flexion, which is less painful for inflamed or swollen joints. There may be secondary abnormalities in joints above or below the primarily involved joint.

Neuromuscular Examination

Periarticular muscle atrophy and weakness may also be present in chronic osteoarthritis. It is notable that manual muscle testing is typically unreliable in the lower extremities because of the high baseline strength of these muscle groups. A careful neurologic examination should be performed to ensure that pain is not a result of nerve impingement or neuropathic process.

In addition, gait should be observed. There may be antalgia (a limp secondary to pain) and a slow gait pattern because of pain in a specific joint. If the patient uses a cane, appropriate use of the cane should be assessed during gait.

Flexibility in both the affected and unaffected joints should also be evaluated. Messier and colleagues[11] suggested that patients with symptomatic osteoarthritis of the knee have poorer flexibility in both the affected and unaffected legs and demonstrate significantly less knee angular velocity and knee range of motion during gait. They have an increased loading rate in the unaffected leg after heel strike, exert less peak vertical force during push-off, and are significantly weaker in both the dominant and nondominant legs compared with adults with no lower extremity disease.

Because obesity has been identified as a risk factor for osteoarthritis, assessment of the patient's body mass index may also be useful.

FUNCTIONAL LIMITATIONS

Functional limitations depend on the joints involved. Patients with disease in the hips and knees can suffer from reduced walking speed and efficiency, difficulty in climbing stairs, trouble with transfers (in and out of cars, chairs, or toilet facilities), and problems with lower body dressing and grooming. Degeneration in the shoulders or hands can limit vocational and recreational activities, grooming, eating, and other activities of daily living. Spinal degeneration can result in limitations with all mobility.

DIAGNOSTIC STUDIES

Plain radiographs are important in confirming the diagnosis of osteoarthritis. The classic findings include asymmetric joint space narrowing, osteophytes at joint margins, cortical sclerosis, and subchondral cyst

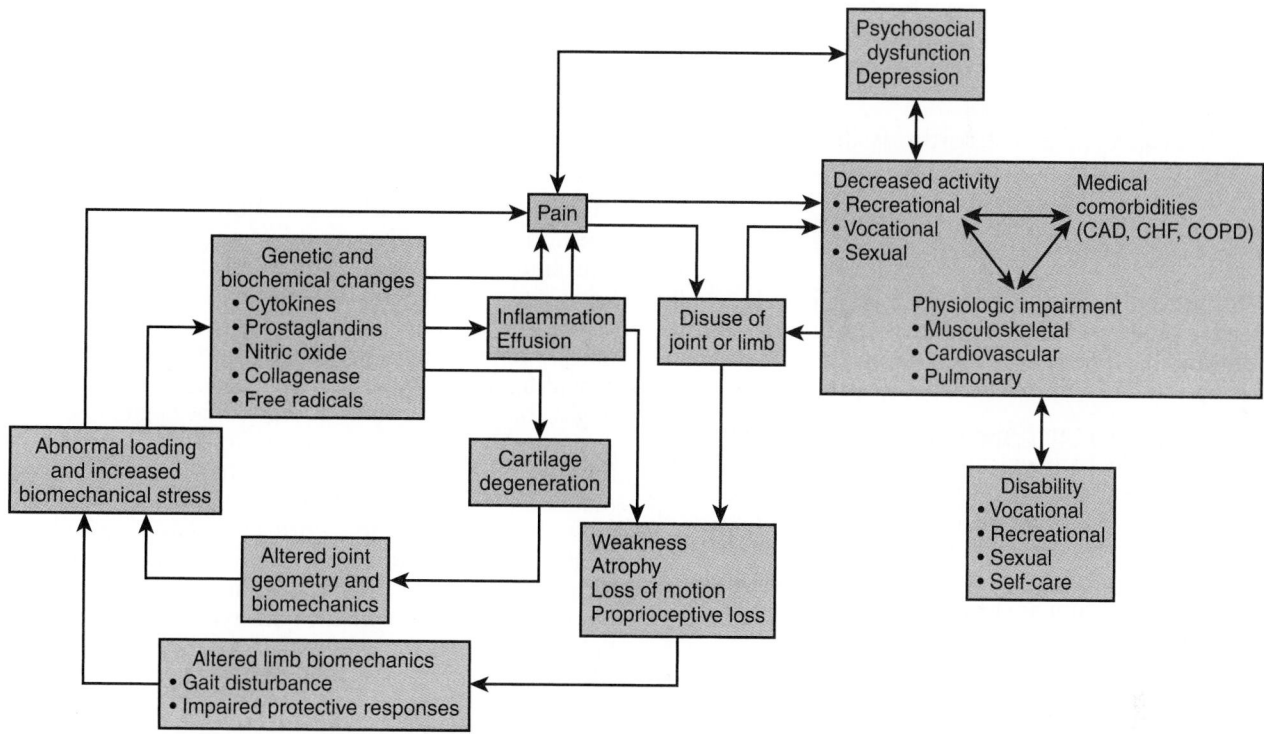

FIGURE 130-1. Model of multifactorial process of degeneration, pain, psychosocial and physiologic dysfunction, and disability that may occur in osteoarthritis. CAD, coronary artery disease; CHF, congestive heart failure; COPD, chronic obstructive pulmonary disease.

formation. There is a well-demonstrated discordance between radiographic findings and symptoms in osteoarthritis. Asymptomatic individuals may have significant radiographic disease, and severe pain and dysfunction can occur in the setting of limited radiologic changes. Magnetic resonance imaging is typically not needed for diagnosis of osteoarthritis but can be helpful in ruling out early osteonecrosis if osteoarthritis is not evident on plain radiographs of painful joints.

Because osteoarthritis is a noninflammatory arthritis, routine laboratory test results are usually normal. Because of the high prevalence of laboratory abnormalities in elderly people, such as a raised erythrocyte sedimentation rate and anemia, however, these will commonly be detected and may prompt an unnecessary investigation.

Joint fluid analysis can be helpful in ruling out crystal deposition disease (gout, pseudogout), inflammatory

arthritis, or infectious arthritis and should be pursued in patients with significant joint inflammation. In osteoarthritis, synovial fluid leukocyte counts are typically less than 2000 cells/mm^3.

Differential Diagnosis

Neoplasm

Deep venous thrombosis

Osteomyelitis

Occult fracture

Aseptic necrosis

Chondromalacia

Soft tissue infection

Bursitis

Tendinitis

Ligamentous injury

Overuse injury

Radiculopathy

Neuropathy

Polymyalgia rheumatica

Inflammatory arthritis

Crystal arthritis (gout, pseudogout)

TABLE 130-3 Clinical Features of an Osteoarthritic Joint

Tenderness to palpation

Bone enlargement

Malalignment

Warmth

Joint effusion or swelling

Crepitus

Periarticular muscle spasm, atrophy, or weakness

Decreased, painful range of motion

TREATMENT

Initial

The management of osteoarthritis involves attention to four important principles: avoid drug toxicity, limit physical disability, relieve pain and other symptoms, and maximize physical function and psychosocial adjustment.

No intervention has been shown conclusively to alter disease progression in osteoarthritis. A number of interventions have been demonstrated to reduce pain and stiffness and to improve functional status.

Acetaminophen and nonsteroidal anti-inflammatory drugs (NSAIDs) are typically first-line agents and useful in reducing pain. Head-to-head randomized trials showed that NSAIDs are more efficacious than acetaminophen.[12,13] However, the superiority of NSAIDs over acetaminophen (at doses of 4 g/day) is modest.[12] The literature is not as clear about the role of NSAIDs in both acute and chronic soft tissue injury.[14]

A quantitative systematic review of 86 trials evaluating the efficacy of topical NSAIDs in osteoarthritis and tendinitis found them significantly more effective than placebo.[15] However, no one topical NSAID seems to be better than the others.[16] Topical capsaicin cream has also been shown to reduce pain in joints affected by osteoarthritis. This derivative of cayenne pepper causes exuberant release and depletion of substance P, which is involved in pain transmission. Limited data from controlled trials have shown improvements in pain with capsaicin.[17] It is worthwhile to caution patients that they may experience increased pain while beginning therapy with capsaicin.

Topical capsaicin or NSAIDs may also help reduce the use of systemic NSAIDs.

The American Pain Society guidelines recommend a tramadol-acetaminophen combination for treatment of osteoarthritis pain when NSAIDs alone cannot provide adequate relief. It is considered to be safe and effective in a subset of elderly patients.[18] Oxycodone has been shown to be useful in the treatment of osteoarthritis pain. Patients with moderate to severe pain from osteoarthritis can achieve effective pain relief when opioids are included as part of a comprehensive pain management program. Studies have also indicated that relief with low-dose opioids can be achieved without deterioration in function.[19]

Recent attention has focused on the use of chondroitin or glucosamine. Chondroitin and glucosamine are naturally occurring substrates for the synthesis of articular cartilage. To date, there have been no large-scale randomized controlled trials of these compounds in humans with osteoarthritis. Small controlled studies have shown that glucosamine affords pain relief that is similar in magnitude to that of NSAIDs.[20] Meta-analyses of both chondroitin and glucosamine found moderate to large reduction in symptoms of pain and immobility.[21] Studies that have evaluated the time course of improvement have shown a delay of up to 1 month in onset of pain relief after treatment begins. The benefit has persisted for several weeks or months after glucosamine is discontinued. Patients considering the use of glucosamine or chondroitin should be cautioned that no long-term trials have evaluated their safety and that these products are not subject to regulation of purity or accuracy of labeling.

Patients with osteoarthritis should be screened for depression and treated appropriately with nonpharmacologic and pharmacologic interventions. Nonpharmacologic interventions are also important and effective in promoting wellness and reducing disability. Multifactorial self-management programs improve self-efficacy by providing experiential skills in disease management, physiologic self-regulation, emotional hygiene, and interpersonal communication. Studies have demonstrated reduced pain, improvements in health behavior, and reduction in use of health care resources in patients with chronic pain and arthritis.[22-25] Group-based self-management programs are often available through a local chapter of the Arthritis Foundation and may overlap significantly in content with typical hospital-based behavioral medicine programs.

Rehabilitation

A comprehensive rehabilitative approach addresses prevention and treatment of pain and disability through counseling, education and encouragement of weight loss, exercise, adaptive equipment, and superficial modalities such as heat and cold.

A physical therapist can guide and encourage a stretching program that can ease the stiffness associated with sleep or prolonged immobility and prevent or reduce impairment in range of motion. Patients should be educated in appropriate positioning during extended inactivity or sleep. Appropriate use of heat before stretching can help loosen tight periarticular muscles, and application of ice packs after exercise can reduce the need for analgesic medications. Treatment time with the therapist should focus on education in the use of these interventions, rather than passive treatment. Gait and transfer training can improve functional mobility in patients with limitations in range of motion or strength. Finally, a program of aerobic and resistance exercise can safely decrease pain, prevent disability, and promote general conditioning.

Occupational therapy can provide training in energy conservation techniques to reduce fatigue in patients with reduced activity tolerance. In the setting of significant functional impairments, the therapist can provide assistive devices that help with feeding, grooming, dressing, and other activities of daily living.

As there is currently no cure for osteoarthritis, most research continues to evaluate the use of exercise as a treatment to alleviate symptoms of the disease and to enhance functional capacity. Two meta-analyses published in 2004 focus specifically on the efficacy of strengthening[26] and aerobic exercise[27] for osteoarthritis.

With muscle strengthening, improvements in strength, pain, function, and quality of life were noted. However, there was no evidence that the type of strengthening exercise influences outcome. Static or dynamic strengthening exercises can maintain or improve periarticular muscle strength, thereby reversing or preventing biomechanical abnormalities and their contribution to joint dysfunction and degeneration.

In regard to aerobic exercise, results indicated that aerobic exercise alleviates pain and joint tenderness and promotes functional status and respiratory capacity. Aerobic exercise improves activity tolerance, increases pain threshold, and can have positive effects on mood and motivation for participation in other activities.

Whereas strengthening appears to be superior to aerobic exercise in the short term for specific impairment-related outcomes (e.g., pain), aerobic exercise appears more effective for functional outcomes during the longer term.[28] There is also evidence that exercise can improve proprioception,[29] thus improving biomechanics and protective responses.

Clinical trials have demonstrated the effectiveness of structured exercise programs in reducing pain and disability due to osteoarthritis.[30,31] Compared with patients who received health education, patients assigned to aerobic and resistance exercise programs had fewer self-reported disabilities, less pain, and greater strength. The greatest effect was seen after the initial 3 months of supervised exercise.[32]

Adaptive equipment, such as a cane or walker, can reduce joint loading, thereby reducing pain. It may also prevent falls in patients with impaired balance. Orthotic devices, bracing, or taping can also mitigate abnormal joint loading and localized stress concentration. However, reliable clinical trials have not been performed to demonstrate whether bracing or orthoses actually decrease pain and increase function.

There are no consistent data from clinical trials supporting the use of therapeutic cold, heat, or ultrasound in patients with osteoarthritis. Clinical experience suggests that cold and heat can be helpful in decreasing pain and increasing mobility.

The use of transcutaneous electrical nerve stimulation is supported by a few small, short-term trials. For most patients, pain relief was experienced only during periods of active use of the device, although the beneficial effect was sustained for several hours in a few.[33]

Acupuncture, a technique in existence for thousands of years, has gained renewed interest for treatment of osteoarthritis. A multicenter, 26-week National Institutes of Health–funded randomized controlled trial found acupuncture to be effective as adjunctive therapy for reducing pain and improving function in patients with knee osteoarthritis.[31]

Procedures

In randomized trials, intra-articular injection of corticosteroids provided slightly improved pain relief compared with placebo injection of saline, although the effects typically last for only 1 to 3 weeks.[34] The intra-articular injection of corticosteroid cannot prevent the pain derived from weight-bearing forces across the joint. The literature has shown that intra-articular corticosteroid injections for the treatment of osteoarthritis can be variable. Jones and Doherty,[35] in a double-blind, placebo-controlled study of 59 patients, reported a significant reduction in pain scores 3 weeks after an intra-articular injection of corticosteroid. Another comparison of intra-articular triamcinolone and placebo showed greater pain relief with a steroid injection at 1 week but similar results at later intervals.[36] Intra-articular corticosteroid injections are commonly used for rheumatoid arthritis and show excellent long-term pain relief. Therefore, it is thought that the primary effect of the corticosteroid is on the synovium.

The intra-articular injection of hyaluronic acid is supported by theoretical considerations and limited data from controlled studies.[37] Intra-articular injection of hyaluronic acid is also referred to as viscosupplementation. Clinical trials of hyaluronic acid injections have focused on patients with knee osteoarthritis. The data on efficacy are inconsistent. Side effects included local inflammation and increased pain at the injection site. There is no evidence that hyaluronic acid injection in humans alters biologic processes or progression of cartilage damage. No clear dose-response trial has been published to determine ideal number of injections or dosage.[38]

Surgery

In patients for whom pain and loss of mobility are disabling despite conservative management, orthopedic consultation should be obtained to assess risks and benefits of surgery.

Arthroscopic lavage and removal of loose bodies or osteophytes may be helpful in some patients for whom conservative therapy has failed. Osteotomy has been used with some success to correct biomechanics and to unload areas of high stress. Fusion may be helpful when joint replacement is not appropriate.

In the past few decades, joint replacement surgery has provided tremendous improvements in quality of life for people with severe osteoarthritis (see Chapters 53 and 71). In older patients who experience functional limitations due to osteoarthritis, hip replacement surgery has been shown to be cost-effective. A systematic review of hip replacement surgery trials concluded that in 70% of subjects, pain and function scores were rated good or excellent at 10 years postoperatively.[39] Observational studies have suggested that better outcomes are associated with the following patient characteristics: age 45 to 75 years, weight less than 70 kg, good social support, higher educational level, and less preoperative morbidity.[40] A small percentage of patients require revision because of persistent or recurrent pain, which is most often a result of aseptic loosening of the prosthetic joint. Similar results have been achieved in total knee replacement. In older patients with medical comorbidities, early inpatient rehabilitation after hip or knee arthroplasty has been shown to reduce hospital stays and cost of care.[41]

POTENTIAL DISEASE COMPLICATIONS

Potential complications include pain; immobility; loss of capacity to perform occupational, recreational, and social roles; and loss of self-care skills.

POTENTIAL TREATMENT COMPLICATIONS

Analgesics and NSAIDs have well-known side effects that most commonly affect the gastric, hepatic, and renal systems. It is notable that gastrointestinal bleeding from NSAID-induced ulcers commonly occurs without pain or abdominal discomfort as a warning sign. Risk for gastrointestinal toxicity is dose dependent and increases with prolonged use, concurrent medical illness, and advanced age. Unfortunately, osteoarthritis is a chronic disease that requires long-term treatment and is most common in older patients, who are at risk for gastrointestinal complications.

However, the combination of NSAIDs and misoprostol or proton pump inhibitors has been shown in randomized trials to reduce the number of endoscopically confirmed ulcers associated with NSAIDs.[42] Potential benefit of NSAIDs in individual patients must be weighed against the increased risk of gastrointestinal toxicity.

Acetaminophen carries the risk of hepatic toxicity, and topical NSAIDs or capsaicin may produce local irritation. The possible side effects of glucosamine and chondroitin are gastrointestinal discomfort. Some basic science, nonhuman studies suggest the possibility that glucosamine raises blood glucose concentration.[43]

Intra-articular injection of steroids or hyaluronic acid can result in infection and local irritation and pain.

The risk factors of joint replacement surgery are bleeding, prosthetic failure, infection, pain, venous thrombosis, pulmonary embolism, and complications of general anesthesia.

References

1. Pearl AD, Warren RF, Rodeo SA. Basic science of articular cartilage and osteoarthritis. Clin Sports Med 2005;24:1-12.
2. Brashaw RT, Tingstad EM. Rehabilitation of the osteoarthritic patient: focus on the knee. Clin Sports Med 2005;24:101-131.
3. Felson DT, Lawrence RC, Dieppe PA, et al. Osteoarthritis: new insights. Part 1: the disease and its risk factors. Ann Intern Med 2000;133:635-646.
4. Saxon L, Finch C, Bass S. Sports participation, sports injuries and osteoarthritis: implications for prevention. Sports Med 1999;28:123-135.
5. Felson DT, Zhang Y. An update on the epidemiology of knee and hip osteoarthritis with a view to prevention. Arthritis Rheum 1998;41:1343-1355.
6. Hunter DJ, March L, Sambrook PN. Knee osteoarthritis: the influence of environmental factors. Clin Exp Rheumatol 2002;20:93-100.
7. Loughlin J. Genome studies and linkage in primary osteoarthritis. Rheum Dis Clin North Am 2002;28:95-109.
8. Felson DT. Preventing hip and knee osteoarthritis. Bull Rheum Dis 1998;47:1-4.
9. Hinton R, Moody RL, Davis AW, et al. Osteoarthritis: diagnosis and therapeutic considerations. Am Fam Physician 2002;65:841.
10. Haq I, Murphy E, Dacre J. Osteoarthritis. Postgrad Med J 2003;79:377-383.
11. Messier SP, Loeser RF, Hoover JL, et al. Osteoarthritis of the knee: effects on gait, strength, and flexibility. Arch Phys Med Rehabil 1992;73:252.
12. Pincus T, Koch GG, Sokka T, et al. A randomized, double-blind, crossover clinical trial of diclofenac plus misoprostol versus acetaminophen in patients with osteoarthritis of the hip or knee. Arthritis Rheum 2001;44:1587-1598.
13. Felson DT. The verdict favors nonsteroidal antiinflammatory drugs for treatment of osteoarthritis and a plea for more evidence on other treatments. Arthritis Rheum 2001;44:1477-1480.
14. Gorsline RT, Kaeding CC. The use of NSAIDs and nutritional supplements in athletes with osteoarthritis: prevalence, benefits, and consequences. Clin Sports Med 2005;24:71-82.
15. Moore RA, Tramer MR, Carroll D, et al. Quantitative systematic review of topically applied non-steroidal anti-inflammatory drugs. BMJ 1998;316:333-338.
16. Dickson DJ. A double-blind evaluation of topical piroxicam gel with oral ibuprofen in osteoarthritis of the knee. Curr Ther Res Clin Exp 1991;49:199-207.
17. Zhang WY, Po ALW. The effectiveness of topically applied capsaicin: a meta-analysis. Eur J Clin Pharmacol 1994;46:517-522.
18. Rosenthal NR, Silverfield JC, Wu SC, et al; the CAPSS-105 Study Group. Tramadol/acetaminophen combination tablets for the treatment of pain associated with osteoarthritis flare in an elderly patient population. J Am Geriatr Soc 2004:52:374-380.
19. Apgar B. Controlled-release oxycodone for osteoarthritis-related pain. Am Fam Physician 2000;62:1405-1406.
20. Delafuente JC. Glucosamine in the treatment of osteoarthritis. Rheum Dis Clin North Am 2000;26:1-11.
21. McAlindon TE, LaValley MP, Gulin JP, Felson DT. Glucosamine and chondroitin for treatment of osteoarthritis: a systematic quality assessment and meta-analysis. JAMA 2000;283:1469-1475.
22. Caudill M, Schnable R, Zuttermeister P, et al. Decreased clinic use by chronic pain patients: response to behavioral medicine intervention. Clin J Pain 1991;7:305-310.
23. Lorig K, Mazonson PD, Holman HR. Evidence suggesting that health education for self-management in patient with chronic arthritis has sustained health benefits while reducing health care costs. Arthritis Rheum 1993;36:439-446.
24. Lorig KR, Sobel DS, Stewart AL, et al. Evidence suggesting that a chronic disease self-management program can improve health status while reducing hospitalization: a randomized trial. Med Care 1999;37:5-14.
25. Sobel D. Rethinking medicine: improving health outcomes with cost-effective psychological interventions. Psychosom Med 1995;57:234-244.
26. Pelland L, Brosseau L, Wells G, et al. Efficacy of strengthening exercises for osteoarthritis. Part I: a meta-analysis. Phys Ther Rev 2004;9:77-108.
27. Brosseau L, Pelland L, Wells G, et al. Efficacy of aerobic exercises for osteoarthritis. Part II: a meta-analysis. Phys Ther Rev 2004;9:125-145.
28. Bennell K, Hinman R. Exercise as a treatment for osteoarthritis. Curr Opin Rheumatol 2005;17:634-640.
29. Hurley MV. The role of muscle weakness in the pathogenesis of osteoarthritis. Rheum Dis Clin North Am 1999;25:283-298.
30. Taylor P, Hallett M, Flatherty L. Treatment of osteoarthritis of the knee with transcutaneous electrical nerve stimulation. Pain 1981;11:233-240.
31. Hochberg M, Lixing L, Bausell B, et al. Traditional Chinese acupuncture is effective as adjunctive therapy in patients with osteoarthritis of the knee [abstract]. Arthritis Rheum 2004;50:S644.
32. Ettinger WH Jr, Burns R, Messier SP, et al. A randomized trial comparing aerobic exercise and resistance exercise with a health

education program in older adults with knee osteoarthritis: the Fitness Arthritis and Seniors Trial (FAST). JAMA 1997;277:25-31.

33. Puett DW, Griffin MR. Published trials of nonmedicinal and noninvasive therapies for hip and knee osteoarthritis. Ann Intern Med 1994;121:133-140.

34. Creamer P. Intra-articular corticosteroid treatment in osteoarthritis. Curr Opin Rheumatol 1999;11:417-421.

35. Jones A, Doherty M. Intra-articular corticosteroids are effective in osteoarthritis but there are no clinical predictors of response. Ann Rheum Dis 1996;55:829-832.

36. Freidman DM, Moore MF. The efficacy of intraarticular steroids in osteoarthritis: a double blind study. J Rheumatol 1980;7:850-856.

37. Lo GH, LaValley M, McAlindon T, et al. Intra-articular hyaluronic acid in treatment of knee osteoarthritis: a metaanalysis. JAMA 2003;290:3115-3121.

38. Simon LS. Viscosupplementation therapy with intra-articular hyaluronic acid: fact or fantasy. Rheum Dis Clin North Am 1999;25:345-357.

39. Faulkner A, Kennedy LG, Baxter K, et al. Effectiveness of hip prostheses in primary total hip replacement: a critical review of evidence and an economic model. Health Technol Assess 1998;2:1-33.

40. Young NL, Cheah D, Waddell JP, et al. Patient characteristics that affect the outcome of total hip arthroplasty: a review. Can J Surg 1998;41:188-195.

41. Munin MC, Rudy TE, Glynn NW, et al. Early inpatient rehabilitation after elective hip and knee arthroplasty. JAMA 1998;279:847-852.

42. Wolfe MM, Lichtenstein DR, Singh G. Gastrointestinal toxicity of nonsteroidal anti-inflammatory drugs. N Engl J Med 1999;340:1888-1899.

43. Morelli V, Naquix CR, Weaver V. Alternative therapies for traditional disease states: osteoarthritis. Am Fam Physician 2003;67:339-344.

Osteoporosis 131

David M. Slovik, MD, and Jonas Sokolof, DO

DEFINITION

Osteoporosis is a skeletal disorder characterized by compromised bone strength predisposing a person to an increased risk for fracture. Bone strength primarily reflects the integration of bone density and bone quality. Bone quality refers to architecture, turnover, damage accumulation (e.g., microfractures), and mineralization.[1] Bone has a normal ratio of mineral to matrix.

Osteoporosis can also be defined according to World Health Organization criteria on the basis of bone mineral density (BMD) and bone mineral content (BMC) measurements:

- Normal: A value for BMD or BMC that is not more than 1 SD below the young adult mean value.
- Low bone mass (osteopenia): A value for BMD or BMC that lies between 1 and 2.5 SDs below the young adult mean value.
- Osteoporosis: A value for BMD or BMC that is more than 2.5 SDs below the young adult mean value.
- Severe osteoporosis (or established osteoporosis): A value for BMD or BMC more than 2.5 SDs below the young adult mean value in the presence of one or more fragility fractures.

A fragility fracture is one that occurs without any trauma, after a fall from a height of less than 12 inches, or after abrupt deceleration from a speed slower than a run.

Osteoporosis is the most common metabolic bone disease. The National Osteoporosis Foundation estimates that at least 10 million Americans have osteoporosis and another 18 million have decreased bone mass, putting them at increased risk for osteoporosis and fractures. Of the 10 million, 8 million are women and 2 million are men. Annually in the United States, more than 1.5 million fractures attributable to osteoporosis occur, including approximately 700,000 vertebral, 300,000 hip, and 250,000 wrist fractures. The annual cost of caring for osteoporosis-related fractures in the United States is in excess of $16 billion. In addition, there is a 10% to 20% excess mortality within the first year after a hip fracture.

Osteomalacia refers to a group of disorders characterized by an abnormality in bone mineralization. The ratio of mineral to matrix is diminished as a result of an excess of unmineralized osteoid.

SYMPTOMS

Osteoporosis is a silent disease until a fracture occurs. Pain and deformity are usually present at the site of fracture. Vertebral fractures often occur with little trauma, such as coughing, lifting, or bending over. Acute back pain may be related to a vertebral compression fracture with pain localized to the fracture site or in a radicular distribution. New back pain or chronic back pain in a patient with osteoporosis and prior vertebral fractures may be related to new fractures, muscle spasm, or other causes.

With vertebral fractures, there may be a gradual loss of height and the development of a kyphosis. Breathing may be difficult, and bloating—a sensation of fullness and dyspepsia—may develop because of less room in the abdominal cavity.

PHYSICAL EXAMINATION

In evaluating patients with osteoporosis, it is important to diagnose treatable and reversible causes and to assess the risk factors for development of osteoporosis and osteoporotic fractures. Table 131-1 lists common causes of osteoporosis. Table 131-2 lists risk factors for osteoporosis.

The physical examination focuses on findings suggestive of secondary causes of osteoporosis (e.g., hyperthyroidism and Cushing syndrome). One should also examine

TABLE 131-1 Common Causes of Osteoporosis

Age related
Postmenopausal
Senile

Endocrine related
Hypogonadism
Hyperthyroidism
Hyperparathyroidism
Adrenal-cortical hormone excess
Diabetes mellitus, type 2

Genetics
Osteogenesis imperfecta
Ehlers-Danlos syndrome
Homocystinuria

Immobilization
Hematologic disorders
Multiple myeloma
Systemic mastocytosis
Thalassemia

Drug related
Glucocorticoids
Thyroid hormone excess
Cyclosporine
Anticonvulsant drugs
Aromatase inhibitors
Androgen deprivation therapy (men)

Miscellaneous
Rheumatoid arthritis

TABLE 131-2 Risk Factors for Osteoporosis

Advanced age
Female
Small-boned, thin women
White and Asian women
Estrogen deficiency
Personal history of fracture as adult
Fracture in first-degree family members
Inactivity
Low calcium intake
Cigarette smoking
Alcoholism
Medications such as glucocorticoids, excessive thyroid hormone, cyclosporine, antiseizure drugs, aromatase inhibitors; androgen deprivation therapy in men

areas previously involved with fractures (e.g., back, hip, and wrist) to assess for deformity and limitation of function. A baseline measurement of height should be obtained and reevaluated at subsequent visits.

FUNCTIONAL LIMITATIONS

Functional limitations are related to the type of fracture and its long-term consequences and disabilities. With vertebral fractures, the functional limitation may initially be related to the acute pain and inability to move. The chronic limitations may be related to loss of height, chronic back pain, difficulty in moving, abdominal distention, and difficulty in breathing.

The functional limitations after a hip fracture are related to the decreased functional mobility, often the need for long-term use of assistive devices, the lack of independence, and the long-term need for assistive care. An assistive device will be needed permanently for ambulation by 50% of people with a hip fracture, and two thirds will lose some of their ability to perform ordinary daily activities.

Wrist fractures usually heal completely, but some people have chronic pain, deformity, and functional limitations.

DIAGNOSTIC STUDIES

Bone density measurements are the standard for assessment of risk, diagnosis, and observation of patients with osteoporosis. Available techniques include single-photon absorptiometry, dual-energy x-ray absorptiometry, quantitative computed tomography, and quantitative ultrasonography. Dual-energy x-ray absorptiometry, although it is not as sensitive as quantitative computed tomography for detection of early trabecular bone loss, is now the method of choice for measurement of bone mineral density because of its good precision, low radiation dose, and fast examination time.

Bone mineral density testing should be performed only if the results will influence a treatment decision. The National Osteoporosis Foundation suggests bone mineral density testing in the following circumstances: all postmenopausal women younger than 65 years who have one or more additional risk factors for osteoporosis (besides menopause); all women 65 years and older, regardless of additional risk factors; postmenopausal women who present with fractures; women who are considering therapy for osteoporosis, if bone mineral density testing would facilitate the decision; and women who have been receiving hormone replacement therapy for prolonged periods.[2] Bone mineral density should also be obtained in patients receiving chronic glucocorticoid therapy, in those with primary hyperparathyroidism, and in those with conditions placing them at high risk for osteoporosis (e.g., aromatase inhibitors to treat breast cancer and androgen deprivation therapy to treat prostate cancer). Bone mineral density testing is also performed to assess the response to treatment programs.

TABLE 131-3 Bone Mineral Density Reporting

T score	Standard deviations (SDs) above or below peak bone mass in young, normal, sex-matched adults
Z score	Standard deviations (SDs) above or below age- and sex-matched adults

Bone mineral density is reported by T and Z scores (Table 131-3). The T score is the best measurement for risk assessment and can help confirm a diagnosis of osteoporosis. A value that is more than 2.5 SDs below the young adult mean indicates osteoporosis. The lower the T score, the higher the risk for subsequent fractures. However, the score will not predict who will fracture because other factors come into play (e.g., fall velocity, type of fall, direction of fall, and protective padding).

Quantitative ultrasonography has shown promise for predicting the occurrence of fractures in patients with osteoporosis.[3] The most common sites for ultrasound measurement are the patella and calcaneus. Advantages of ultrasound measurement include cost-effectiveness, absence of radiation exposure, and portability.

Specific laboratory tests are obtained to help in the differential diagnosis of osteoporosis and to rule out osteomalacia. The general laboratory tests include a complete blood count, chemistry profile including liver and kidney tests, serum and urine protein electrophoresis, and thyroid-stimulating hormone concentration. A 24-hour collection of urine for calcium and creatinine measurement is also helpful. Because of the high prevalence of vitamin D deficiency in the adult population, especially elderly individuals, a serum 25-hydroxyvitamin D level should be obtained. A parathyroid hormone level should be determined in suspected cases of primary or secondary hyperparathyroidism. Blood and urine test results are usually normal in uncomplicated cases of osteoporosis. After a fracture, the alkaline phosphatase activity may be elevated. Biochemical markers of bone turnover, including urine N-telopeptide, may be helpful in selective patients to assess for bone turnover and whether someone is responding to treatment.

Differential Diagnosis

Common causes of osteoporosis are listed in Table 131-1.

TREATMENT

Initial

The initial approach to the prevention and treatment of osteoporosis involves nonpharmacologic intervention and, in appropriate patients, the use of various pharmacologic agents (Table 131-4). Prevention and treatment guidelines are presented in Tables 131-5 and 131-6.

Calcium

Epidemiologic studies suggest that long-standing dietary calcium deficiency can result in lower bone mass. The average dietary calcium intake in postmenopausal women is less than 500 mg/day. Several studies have shown that calcium supplementation, especially in the

TABLE 131-4 Treatment Options

Nonpharmacologic intervention

Calcium

Vitamin D

Exercise

Smoking cessation

Fall prevention

Pharmacologic agents

Hormone replacement therapy

Selective estrogen receptor modulators

   Raloxifene (Evista)

Bisphosphonates

   Alendronate (Fosamax)

   Risedronate (Actonel)

   Ibandronate (Boniva)

   Zoledronic acid (Reclast)

Calcitonin (Miacalcin nasal spray)

Teriparatide (Fortéo)

TABLE 131-5 Osteoporosis Prevention Guidelines

Hormone replacement therapy for menopausal symptoms

Raloxifene, 60 mg/day

Alendronate, 5 mg/day or 35 mg once weekly by mouth (prevention dose)

Risedronate, 5 mg/day or 35 mg weekly by mouth

Ibandronate, 2.5 mg daily or 150 mg monthly by mouth

TABLE 131-6 Osteoporosis Treatment Guidelines

Alendronate, 10 mg/day or 70 mg once weekly (treatment dose)

Risedronate, 5 mg/day or 35 mg weekly by mouth

Ibandronate, 2.5 mg/day or 150 mg monthly orally; 3 mg intravenously every 3 months

   Zoledronic acid, 5 mg intravenously yearly

Raloxifene, 60 mg/day

Calcitonin (nasal spray) once daily

Teriparatide 20 μg subcutaneously daily for 2 years

elderly, may slow bone loss and reduce vertebral and nonvertebral fracture rates.[4] A total calcium intake of 1200 to 1500 mg/day is recommended for postmenopausal women. This can be achieved by consumption of foods that have a high calcium content, such as milk and dairy products, especially yogurt. Calcium supplementation is often required, especially in elderly individuals.

Vitamin D

Vitamin D deficiency is common in postmenopausal women, especially in those who have sustained a hip fracture and those who are chronically ill, housebound, institutionalized, and poorly nourished.[5] A dose of 800 to 1000 IU per day (from multivitamins and other sources) should be administered to prevent vitamin D deficiency. Many calcium supplements now contain vitamin D. A serum 25-hydroxyvitamin D level of more than 30 ng/mL (70 nmol/L) should be maintained.

Exercise

There is increasing evidence that exercise is beneficial to bone in helping achieve peak bone mass and preserving bone later in life.[6] Bone adapts to physical and mechanical loads placed on it by altering its mass and strength. This occurs either by the direct impact from the weight-bearing activity or by the action of muscle attached to bone. Exercising can also help strengthen back muscles, improve balance, lessen the likelihood of falling, and give one a sense of well-being.[7] Back extension exercises and abdominal strengthening exercises are helpful. However, acute stresses to the back must be avoided to lessen the likelihood of fracture. A proper exercise program should be established. Older postmenopausal women and even the frail elderly can tolerate and potentially show improvements in muscle strength and bone mineral density in response to strength training and resistive exercise programs.

Smoking Cessation

A link between smoking and bone mineral loss has been reported. In one particular study, a 5% to 10% reduction in bone density was demonstrated in women who smoked one pack per day in adulthood.[8] Therefore, it is recommended that physicians aggressively pursue smoking cessation in their treatment plans.

Fall Prevention

Many factors can lead to falls, including poor vision, frailty, medication (especially hypotensive agents and psychotropic agents), and balance disturbances.[9] Each area needs to be assessed appropriately.

Prevention measures include keeping rooms free from clutter and having good lighting. Advise patients to wear supportive shoes, to be aware of thresholds, and to avoid slippery floors; rugs should be tacked down. Grab bars are useful in the bathroom. A portable telephone and a personal alarm activator are helpful, and someone should check on the individual regularly.

Hormone Replacement Therapy

Hormone replacement therapy can be used in the short-term management of postmenopausal women with symptoms of estrogen deficiency, including hot flashes, memory deficits, urinary frequency, and vaginal dryness. Long-term hormone replacement therapy can slow bone loss and lower the incidence of fractures. In the Women's Health Initiative with estrogen and progestin, there was a 34% reduction in vertebral and hip fractures. However, there was an increase in breast cancer, coronary heart disease, stroke, and thromboembolic disease.[10] The mean age of patients in the Women's Health Initiative was 63 years. A recent reanalysis from the Women's Health Initiative showed no increase in coronary heart disease risk in women when hormone replacement therapy was started within 10 years of the onset of menopause.[11] Hormone replacement therapy is indicated to treat menopausal symptoms. The lowest dose of estrogen and progesterone should be used to effectively relieve these symptoms. Women who have had a hysterectomy should be given estrogen alone. A progestin should be added to the estrogen regimen if the uterus is still present.

Selective Estrogen Receptor Modulators

Selective estrogen receptor modulators are synthetic compounds that have both estrogen-antagonistic and estrogen-agonistic properties. Raloxifene (Evista) is approved by the Food and Drug Administration (FDA) for the prevention and treatment of osteoporosis at an oral dose of 60 mg daily. Raloxifene is also approved for the reduction in risk of invasive breast cancer in postmenopausal women with osteoporosis and in postmenopausal women at high risk of invasive breast cancer. Raloxifene reduces new vertebral fractures by 40% to 50% but not the risk of nonspine fractures.[12] Raloxifene acts as an antiestrogen on breast tissue, and in the STAR (Study of Tamoxifen and Raloxifene) trial involving almost 20,000 postmenopausal women, raloxifene reduced the risk of invasive breast cancer similar to the reduction by tamoxifen.[13] Raloxifene does not produce uterine hypertrophy. In another report, the RUTH (Raloxifene Use for The Heart) trial involving more than 10,000 postmenopausal women who had either coronary heart disease or multiple risk factors for coronary heart disease, raloxifene did not significantly affect the risk of coronary heart disease.[14] Raloxifene has no beneficial effects on menopausal symptoms and may increase hot flashes and the risk of deep venous thrombosis.

Bisphosphonates

The bisphosphonates are a group of compounds related chemically to pyrophosphate. They are characterized by a P-C-P structure. Changes in the side chains affect the binding and potency of the bisphosphonates. They are potent inhibitors of osteoclastic bone resorption. Alendronate (Fosamax) was the first approved by the FDA in 1995 for the prevention and treatment of postmenopausal osteoporosis. Alendronate is also approved for the treatment of glucocorticoid-induced osteoporosis[15] and osteoporosis in men.[16] In postmenopausal women, the dose for prevention is 5 mg/day or 35 mg once weekly; the dose for treatment is 10 mg/day or 70 mg once weekly. Alendronate significantly increases bone mineral density at various sites. In addition, there is a significant decrease in the incidence of vertebral, hip, and wrist fractures as well as painful vertebral fractures, hospitalization days, and other measurements of functional impairment.[17]

Risedronate (Actonel) is approved by the FDA for the prevention and treatment of postmenopausal osteoporosis with an oral dose of 5 mg daily or 35 mg weekly. Studies have shown an increase in bone mineral density at various sites along with a decrease in vertebral and nonvertebral fractures.[18] Risedronate is also approved for the prevention and treatment of glucocorticoid-induced osteoporosis and osteoporosis in men.

Ibandronate (Boniva) is approved by the FDA for the prevention and treatment of postmenopausal osteoporosis. The oral dose is either 2.5 mg daily or 150 mg monthly. An intravenous preparation is also available for the treatment of postmenopausal osteoporosis in a dose of 3 mg intravenously every 3 months. Studies have shown an increase in bone density and a reduction in vertebral fractures.[19]

The bisphosphonates are poorly absorbed and must be given on an empty stomach to maximize their absorption. Alendronate and risedronate must be taken at least 30 minutes (ibandronate, 60 minutes) before the first food, beverage, or medication with a full glass of plain water, and patients should not lie down for at least 30 minutes (ibandronate, 60 minutes) to avoid the potential side effect of esophagitis. Patients with a history of reflux should not be given these medications.

Zoledronic acid was recently approved by the Food and Drug Administration for the treatment of postmenopausal osteoporosis. It is administered as a once-yearly injection of 5 mg. In a study of 7765 postmenopausal women with osteoporosis, at the end of 3 years, there was a 70% reduction in morphometric vertebral fractures, 41% reduction in hip fractures, and 25% reduction in nonvertebral fractures. Bone density improved. However, serious atrial fibrillation occurred significantly more frequently in the zoledronic acid group.[23]

Calcitonin

For more than 15 years, synthetic salmon calcitonin given parenterally by injection has been approved for the treatment of postmenopausal osteoporosis. In 1995, the nasal spray of calcitonin was approved in a dose of 200 units (one spray) daily. A reduction in new vertebral fractures has been reported but no effect on nonvertebral fractures.[20] Occasional nasal irritation or headache may be seen with the nasal spray.

Parathyroid Hormone

As long ago as the late 1920s, there was evidence that parathyroid extract, administered in an intermittent once-a-day injection, stimulated osteoblast activity in animal models. This is in contrast to bone loss seen with chronic elevations in parathyroid hormone in primary hyperparathyroidism. After human parathyroid hormone was sequenced in the early 1970s, clinical studies with use of the 1-34 amino-terminal fragment started. Early results in osteoporosis trials showed increases in bone accretion, calcium balance, and trabecular bone volume with normal skeletal architecture.[21] In the multicenter trial of recombinant human parathyroid hormone 1-34 fragment (teriparatide), 20 µg administered subcutaneously daily produced an increase in vertebral and hip bone density and a 55% reduction in vertebral fracture risk.[22] Teriparatide (Fortéo) is generally well tolerated and is self-administered for up to 2 years by use of a 31-gauge needle and a prefilled syringe with a 28-day supply of medication. It is the only anabolic agent available (in contrast to the antiresorptive agents) and is approved for the treatment of postmenopausal women with osteoporosis who are at high risk for fracture. It is also approved for osteoporosis in men. In rats given teriparatide in doses up to 60 times the exposure in humans, there was an increase in osteosarcoma, which was dose and duration dependent. Thus, teriparatide should not be administered to patients who have an increased baseline risk for osteosarcoma, including patients with Paget disease of bone, those with unexplained elevated alkaline phosphatase, and those who have received prior external beam or implant radiation therapy involving the skeleton.

Future Therapies

Many new therapies have potential in the treatment of osteoporosis. A few are given as examples.

Strontium ranelate has shown increases in bone mineral density and decreased vertebral fracture incidence.[24]

Denosumab is a monoclonal antibody directed against RANKL, a cytokine mediator responsible for accelerating osteoclast formation. In one clinical trial, osteoporotic patients treated with denosumab showed clinically significant increases in lumbar spine and hip bone mineral density of 3.0 to 6.7 and 1.9 to 3.6, respectively.[25]

Rehabilitation

Rehabilitation efforts in osteoporosis should commence long before a fracture. Either a physical or occupational therapist can be involved in assessing the patient's home to make sure it is safe and to decrease the risk of falls. Specialized equipment, such as grab bars for the bathroom and hand-held reachers for high cupboards, can be very helpful. It is important to educate patients about keeping the floors clear of clutter and throw rugs. Small pets also can be a hazard underfoot.

Therapists can assess whether the patient would be safer ambulating with an assistive device (e.g., cane or walker) in the home and community. It is important for all assistive devices to be appropriately prescribed and fitted for the patient.

Finally, therapists can instruct patients about how to exercise to improve strength, flexibility, and balance. All of these activities can help prevent falls, and weight-bearing strengthening exercises may also improve bone density.

In patients with a hip fracture or other disabling fracture, a multidisciplinary coordinated team approach involving the physician, therapists, and other rehabilitation specialists (e.g., nurse, social worker) is necessary for the patient to regain maximal function and to lead a productive life. The initial rehabilitation program also involves pain control, bowel and bladder care, and maintenance of skin integrity. The therapists, in addition to working on a program involving bed mobility, transfers, gait activities, safety precautions, and activities of daily living, must be cognizant of the medical problems in each patient. After an acute rehabilitation stay, some patients may need an additional stay in a transitional setting on their way to eventually going home or else require long-term placement. For those able to go home, the team needs to teach the patient a home exercise program, to order appropriate equipment, and to arrange for continued therapy, either at home or in an outpatient setting.

Procedures

Other than surgery for fracture repair, procedures are generally not needed in the management of osteoporosis. Two procedures—vertebroplasty and kyphoplasty—are available to stabilize vertebral fractures and to alleviate pain.

Surgery

Surgical repair and stabilization is the preferred treatment for hip fracture and some other fractures.

POTENTIAL DISEASE COMPLICATIONS

As bone density decreases, the risk for sustaining a fracture increases. Osteoporosis is asymptomatic until a fracture occurs. Thereafter, all complications are related to the problems from these fractures, to the surgery (if it is required), and to the recuperative period.

After vertebral fractures, acute pain may limit mobility. Bed rest and narcotic analgesics may be necessary. Severe constipation and urinary retention may ensue. Chronically, patients may suffer from severe back pain and have respiratory problems, abdominal distention, bloating, and constipation. Many patients who wear a back brace complain about the discomfort and difficulty in using it.

POTENTIAL TREATMENT COMPLICATIONS

The complications of treatment can be related either to the surgical repair of the fracture and the recuperative phase or to medications used to prevent or to treat osteoporosis.

Most osteoporotic fractures occur in older patients and result in loss of function and loss of independence and the need for long-term care. Because surgery is required to repair a hip fracture, complications from surgery, anesthesia, bed rest, and pain medications (often narcotics) are common. Pneumonia, phlebitis, urinary tract infection, constipation, and respiratory problems also are frequent.

Complications from drug therapy for osteoporosis include the following: potential increase in breast cancer, heart disease, thromboembolic problems, and endometrial cancer (in those using only estrogen) with hormone replacement therapy; hot flashes and increase in clotting from raloxifene; upper gastrointestinal symptoms and esophagitis from oral alendronate, risedronate, and ibandronate; influenza-like symptoms from intravenous ibandronate and zoledronic acid; running nose and headache from calcitonin; and transient mild hypercalcemia with teriparatide.

References

1. NIH Consensus Development Panel on Osteoporosis Prevention, Diagnosis, and Therapy. Osteoporosis prevention, diagnosis, and therapy. JAMA 2001;285:785-795.
2. National Osteoporosis Foundation in collaboration with American Academy of Orthopaedic Surgeons. Physician's Guide to Prevention and Treatment of Osteoporosis. Washington, DC, National Osteoporosis Foundation, 1998.
3. Marin F, Gonzalez-Macias J, Dies-Perez A, et al. Relationship between bone quantitative ultrasound and fractures: a meta-analysis. J Bone Miner Res 2006;21:1126-1135.
4. Dawson-Hughes B, Harris SS, Krall EA, Dallal GE. Effect of calcium and vitamin D supplementation on bone density in men and women 65 years of age or older. N Engl J Med 1997;337:670-676.
5. Leboff MS, Kohlmeier L, Hurwitz S, et al. Occult vitamin D deficiency in postmenopausal US women with acute hip fracture. JAMA 1999;281:1505-1511.
6. Slovik DM. Osteoporosis. In Frontera WF, Slovik DM, Dawson DM, eds. Exercise in Rehabilitation Medicine, 2nd ed. Champaign, Ill, Human Kinetics, 2006:221-248.
7. Nelson ME, Wernick S. Strong Women, Strong Bones. New York, Putnam, 2000.
8. Hopper JL, Seeman E. The bone density of female twins discordant for tobacco use. N Engl J Med 1994;330:387-392.
9. Greenspan SL, Myers ER, Kiel DP, et al. Fall direction, bone mineral density, and function: risk factors for hip fracture in frail nursing home elderly. Am J Med 1998;104:539-545.
10. Writing Group for the Women's Health Initiative Investigation. Risks and benefits of estrogen plus progestin in healthy postmenopausal women: principal results from the Women's Health Initiative randomized controlled trial. JAMA 2002;288:321-333.
11. Rossouw JE, Prentice RL, Manson JE, et al. Postmenopausal hormone therapy and risk of cardiovascular disease by age and years since menopause. JAMA 2007;297:1465-1477.
12. Ettinger B, Black DM, Mitlak BH, et al; Multiple Outcomes of Raloxifene Evaluation (MORE) Investigators. Reduction of vertebral fracture risk in postmenopausal women with osteoporosis treated with raloxifene: results from a 3-year randomized clinical trial. JAMA 1999;282:637-645.
13. Vogel VG, Costantino JP, Wickerham DL, et al; National Surgical Adjuvant Breast and Bowel Project (NSABP). Effects of tamoxifen vs raloxifene on the risk of developing invasive breast cancer and other disease outcomes: the NSABP Study of Tamoxifen and Raloxifene (STAR) P-2 Trial. JAMA 2006;295:2727-2741.
14. Barrett-Connor E, Mosca L, Collins P, et al; Raloxifene Use for The Heart (RUTH) Trial Investigators. Effects of raloxifene on cardiovascular events and breast cancer in postmenopausal women. N Engl J Med 2006;355:125-137.
15. Saag KG, Emkey R, Schnitzer TJ, et al; Glucocorticoid-Induced Osteoporosis Intervention Study Group. Alendronate for the prevention and treatment of glucocorticoid-induced osteoporosis. N Engl J Med 1998;339:292-299.

16. Orwoll E, Ettinger M, Weiss S, et al. Alendronate for the treatment of osteoporosis in men. N Engl J Med 2000;343:604-610.

17. Black DM, Cummings SR, Karpf DB, et al. Randomized trial of effect of alendronate on risk of fracture in women with existing vertebral fractures. Lancet 1996;348:1535-1541.

18. Harris ST, Watts NB, Genant HK, et al; Vertebral Efficacy with Risedronate Therapy (VERT) Study Group. Effects of risedronate treatment on vertebral and nonvertebral fractures in women with postmenopausal osteoporosis: a randomized, controlled trial. JAMA 1999;282:1344-1352.

19. Chesnut CH, Skag A, Christiansen C, et al. Effects of oral ibandronate administered daily or intermittently on fracture risk in postmenopausal osteoporosis. J Bone Miner Res 2004;19:1241-1249.

20. Chesnut CH, Silverman S, Andriano K, et al; PROOF Study Group. A randomized trial of nasal spray salmon calcitonin in postmenopausal women with established osteoporosis: the prevent recurrence of osteoporotic fractures study. Am J Med 2000;109:267-276.

21. Reeve J, Meunier PJ, Parsons JA, et al. Anabolic effect of human parathyroid hormone fragment on trabecular bone in involutional osteoporosis: a multicentre trial. Br Med J 1980;280:1340-1344.

22. Neer RM, Arnaud CD, Zanchetta JR, et al. Effect of parathyroid hormone$_{1-34}$ on fractures and bone mineral density in postmenopausal women with osteoporosis. N Engl J Med 2001;344:1434-1441.

23. Black DM, Delmas PD, Eastell R, et al. Once-yearly zoledronic acid for treatment of postmenopausal osteoporosis. N Engl J Med 2007;356:1809-1822.

24. Roux C, Reginster JY, Fechtenbaum J, et al. Vertebral fracture risk reduction with strontium ranelate in women with postmenopausal osteoporosis is independent of baseline risk factors. J Bone Miner Res 2006;21:536-542.

25. McClung MR, Lewiecki EM, Cohen SB, et al. Denosumab in postmenopausal women with low bone mineral density. N Engl J Med 2006;354:821-831.

Parkinson Disease 132

Nutan Sharma, MD, PhD

DEFINITION

Parkinson disease (PD) is a chronic, progressive neurodegenerative disease. On pathologic examination, it is characterized by preferential degeneration of dopaminergic neurons in the substantia nigra pars compacta and the presence of cytoplasmic inclusions known as Lewy bodies; clinically, it is characterized by a resting tremor, bradykinesia, and rigidity. It is important to distinguish PD from the disorders that are known collectively as the Parkinson-plus syndromes. These are relatively rare disorders that share some of the features of PD, such as rigidity and bradykinesia. However, the Parkinson-plus syndromes do not respond to medical treatment and have some unique clinical features as well.

The prevalence of PD, in industrialized countries, is estimated at 0.3% of the entire population and 1% of the population older than 60 years.[1] PD is clearly an age-related disease. Studies show that the prevalence of PD increases up to the ninth decade (ages 80 to 89 years) of life. Reliable information about the prevalence of PD beyond the ninth decade is not available. Some studies have reported a higher incidence of PD in men than in women, although other studies have refuted this finding.[2-4]

SYMPTOMS

The most common initial manifestations of PD are rest tremor and bradykinesia. Less common presenting complaints include hypophonia, gait difficulty, and fatigue.

It is not uncommon for one of these features to be present for months or even years before others develop.

Pain is also a part of PD. An aching pain in the initially affected limb may first be attributed to bursitis or arthritis. Additional symptoms, seen early in the course of PD, include a resting tremor and a sensation of stiffness. The resting tremor is suppressed by either purposeful movement or sleep and exacerbated by anxiety. The sensation of stiffness occurs in the affected arm or leg and may be accompanied by the perception that one is slow with movement.

As the disease progresses, there is marked difficulty in both initiating and terminating movement. There is difficulty in rising from a seated position, particularly when one is seated in a sofa or chair without armrests. Handwriting becomes smaller and more difficult to read. Friends and family members often complain that the patient's speech is more difficult to understand, particularly on the telephone. The symptom of a softer voice with a decline in enunciation is known as hypophonia.

PHYSICAL EXAMINATION

The most distinctive clinical feature is the rest tremor. It is typically present in a single upper extremity early in the course of the disease. As the disease progresses, the resting tremor may spread to both the ipsilateral lower limb and the contralateral limbs. Examination of motor tone reveals cogwheel rigidity in the affected limb. Motor strength, however, remains unaffected.

Additional features that must be evaluated in an examination include rapid, repetitive limb movements and gait. Examination of repetitive movements of the fingers or entire hand will reveal bradykinesia in the affected limb. Examination of gait will reveal decreased arm swing on the affected side, smaller steps, and an inability to pivot turn. Typically, patients make several steps to complete a turn because of some degree of postural instability. Deep tendon reflexes and sensation are not affected in PD.

In advanced PD, loss of postural reflexes becomes evident. Individuals are unable to maintain balance when turning. Other manifestations of advanced PD include freezing episodes and dysphagia.

In examination of someone who is taking medication for PD, it is important to record the time at which the last dose of medication was taken relative to the time at which the examination occurs. Medications for PD are particularly good at ameliorating the rest tremor and bradykinesia, particularly in the early stages of the disease. Typically, the rest tremor will subside for 1 to 3 hours after the last dose of medication. Other features, such as reduced arm swing, hypophonia, and loss of postural reflexes, do not respond to oral medication.

FUNCTIONAL LIMITATIONS

Functional limitations depend on which symptoms are most prominent in a particular patient. Early in the course of PD, the sole limitation may be in one's ability to write legibly. Affected individuals are still able to perform activities of daily living, although they may prefer to use the unaffected limb for tasks such as shaving and dressing. Although the rest tremor may result in a feeling of self-consciousness or embarrassment, it does not affect one's independence as it is suppressed with purposeful movement.

As the disease progresses, the ability to perform fine motor skills declines, and difficulty with standing and gait develops. An individual will have difficulty in buttoning a shirt or tying shoelaces. More time will be required to stand and initiate gait. Postural instability with a tendency to retropulse also develops. Thus, patients have difficulty in climbing stairs and walking safely and quickly. Slowed reaction times may also affect one's ability to drive safely. Decisions about whether someone should drive are often difficult and must be made on an individual basis. Marked hypophonia may make speaking on the telephone difficult as well. As the voice becomes more affected, dysphagia is likely to develop.

One aspect of PD that has historically gotten little attention from medical professionals is the effect it has on sexual activity. According to the National Parkinson Foundation, almost 81% of men and 43% of women with PD report experiencing diminished sexual activity. Men may experience erectile dysfunction. Women may experience a declining interest in sexual activity, abnormal sexual arousal, or reduced orgasm.

In end-stage PD, limitations include marked dysphagia and severe abnormalities of gait that require both devices and one or two persons for assistance. At this stage, help is necessary for all activities of daily living as well.

DIAGNOSTIC STUDIES

PD is a clinical diagnosis. Conventional laboratory investigations do not contribute to the diagnosis or management of PD. Computed tomography and magnetic resonance imaging scans of the brain do not reveal any consistent abnormalities. Positron emission tomography

with use of 6-[^{18}F]fluorolevodopa reveals reduced accumulation of radioisotope in the striata. There is greater loss contralateral to the side that is most affected clinically. These findings are consistent with the reduction of dopamine that occurs in PD. However, positron emission tomography remains an experimental rather than a diagnostic tool.

Differential Diagnosis

The differential diagnosis includes several diseases known collectively as the Parkinson-plus syndromes.

Multiple system atrophy: In addition to bradykinesia and rigidity, multiple system atrophy is characterized by ataxia and autonomic dysfunction that typically is manifested as episodes of flushing or palpitations.

Progressive supranuclear palsy: In addition to bradykinesia, rigidity, and rest tremor, progressive supranuclear palsy is characterized by the inability to voluntarily move the eyes upward and frequent falls that occur relatively early in the course of the disease.

Corticobasal degeneration: In addition to bradykinesia and rigidity, corticobasal degeneration is characterized by a loss of the ability to coordinate specific purposeful movements of the limbs (apraxia) and a sensation that one's limbs are not one's own (alien-limb syndrome).

Essential tremor: Essential tremor is an involuntary, rhythmic tremor of a body part. Essential tremor most commonly affects the arms and hands but can also involve the head, voice, tongue, trunk, or legs.

TREATMENT

Initial

The decision to initiate medical treatment is based on the degree of disability and discomfort that the patient is experiencing. Six classes of drugs are used to treat PD (summarized in Table 132-1). The selection of a particular drug depends on the patient's main complaint, which is usually either a rest tremor or bradykinesia. There is no evidence to suggest that expediting or delaying the onset of treatment for PD has any effect on the overall course of the disease. However, it is clear that those who do not receive treatment and are bradykinetic are at greater risk of falling and injuring themselves.

Anticholinergic agents are the oldest class of medications used in PD. They are most effective in reducing the rest tremor and rigidity associated with PD. However, the side effects associated with anticholinergic agents typically limit their usefulness. Amantadine is also used in the treatment of PD. Amantadine produces a limited improvement in akinesia, rigidity, and tremor.

Dopamine replacement remains the cornerstone of antiparkinson therapy. Levodopa is the natural precursor

TABLE 132-1 Classes of Antiparkinson Medications, Mechanisms of Action, Beneficial Effects, and Side Effects

Drug Class	Specific Agents	Mechanism of Action	Effective for	Side Effects
Anticholinergic	Benztropine	Muscarinic receptor blocker	Tremor, rigidity	Dry mouth, blurred vision, constipation, urinary retention, confusion, hallucinations, impaired concentration
Antiviral	Amantadine	Promotes synthesis and release of dopamine	Tremor, rigidity, akinesia	Leg edema, livedo reticularis, confusion, hallucinations
Dopamine replacement	Levodopa	Converted to dopamine	Tremor, rigidity, akinesia, freezing	Nausea, diarrhea, confusion, hallucinations
Dopamine agonists (D_1 and D_2)	Bromocriptine, pergolide	Dopamine analogues that bind to D_1 and D_2 receptors	Rigidity, akinesia	Leg edema, nausea, confusion, hallucinations
Dopamine agonists (D_2)	Ropinirole, pramipexole	Dopamine analogues that bind to D_2 receptors	Rigidity, akinesia	Leg edema, sleep attacks, nausea, confusion, hallucinations
Monoamine oxidase B inhibitors	Selegiline, rasagiline	Inhibit the metabolism of dopamine	Mild reduction in "wearing off" from levodopa	Nausea, hallucinations, confusion
Catechol O-methyltransferase inhibitor	Entacapone	Inhibits the metabolism of dopamine	Mild reduction in "wearing off" from levodopa	Dyskinesia, nausea, diarrhea

to dopamine and is converted to dopamine by the enzyme aromatic amino acid decarboxylase. To ensure that adequate levels of levodopa reach the central nervous system, levodopa is administered simultaneously with a peripheral decarboxylase inhibitor. In the United States, the most commonly used peripheral decarboxylase inhibitor is carbidopa. Levodopa is most effective in reducing tremor, rigidity, and akinesia. The most common side effects, seen with the onset of treatment, are nausea, abdominal cramping, and diarrhea. Long-term treatment with levodopa is associated with three types of complications: hourly fluctuations in motor state, dyskinesias, and a variety of psychiatric complaints including hallucinations and confusion. However, it is not clear whether the motor fluctuations are due to the levodopa treatment alone, the disease progression alone, or a complex interplay of imperfect dopamine replacement and the inexorable progression of disease. In summary, current evidence supports the use of dopamine replacement as soon as the symptoms of PD become troublesome to the individual patient. There is no evidence that supports withholding of treatment to minimize long-term motor complications.[5]

Dopamine agonists, which directly stimulate dopamine receptors, are also used in the treatment of PD. These agents can be used either as an adjunct to levodopa therapy or as monotherapy. The older dopamine agonists, which are relatively nonspecific and exert their effects at both D_1 and D_2 receptors, are bromocriptine and pergolide. In comparison to the side effects seen with levodopa, there is a lower frequency of dyskinesias and a higher frequency of confusion and hallucinations. The newer dopamine agonists pramipexole and ropinirole are more specific for D_2 receptors. These newer agents have been reported to cause excessive lethargy and sleep attacks.[6] All dopamine agonists can cause orthostatic hypotension, particularly when they are first introduced. It is best to start with a small dose of medication at bedtime and then slowly increase the total daily dose.

Inhibitors of dopamine metabolism are also used in the medical treatment of PD. Both selegiline and rasagiline inhibit monoamine oxidase B, which metabolizes dopamine in the central nervous system. Thus, inhibitors of monoamine oxidase B are thought to improve an individual's response to levodopa by alleviating the motor fluctuations that are seen with long-term levodopa treatment. Another agent that inhibits the metabolism of dopamine is entacapone. Entacapone inhibits catechol O-methyltransferase in the periphery. Entacapone is administered in conjunction with levodopa and, by inhibiting peripheral catechol O-methyltransferase activity, increases the amount of levodopa that reaches the central nervous system. The benefits of entacapone treatment include a reduction in total daily levodopa dose and an improvement in the length of time of maximum mobility.[7]

Constipation is a frequent complaint. Treatment includes increase in physical activity; discontinuation of anticholinergic drugs; and maintenance of a diet with intake of adequate fluids, fruit, vegetables, fiber, and lactulose (10 to 20 g daily).

Rehabilitation

The clinical pathologic process seen in PD reveals that patients tend to become more passive, less active, and less motivated as the disease progresses. The benefits to physical and occupational therapy are thus more far reaching than a simple improvement in motor function. The physical benefits include improvement in muscle strength and tone as well as maintenance of an adequate range of motion in the joints. The psychological benefits include enlistment of the patient as an active participant in treatment and provision of a sense of mastery over the effects of PD. Both physical therapy and occupational therapy focus on mobility, the use of adaptive equipment, and safety in both the home and community.

Because the symptoms of PD gradually worsen over time, individuals can benefit from periodic physical therapy training throughout the course of their illness. An emphasis on gait training is particularly helpful to prevent falls and injury. Gait training typically involves training an individual to be conscious of taking a longer stride and putting the foot down with each step. Another method is to use visual cues to maintain a regular size for each step. For example, one can put strips of masking tape on the floor, at a regular interval that is comfortable for one's height, weight, and gender. As PD progresses, episodes of frozen gait, in which the feet seem to be stuck to the floor, occur. Such freezing episodes can be broken by multiple techniques, such as visualizing that one is stepping over an imaginary line on the floor, counting in a rhythmic cadence, or marching in place.

Occupational therapy is particularly helpful in recommending adaptive devices or establishing new routines that allow people with PD to continue to live independently. For example, the use of a long-handled shoehorn reduces the need to bend over and thus eliminates the risk that a person with PD will fall while getting dressed. Other examples of adaptive equipment are a firmly secured grab bar in the bathtub and a relatively high toilet seat with armrests to minimize the risk of freezing while on the toilet.

Speech therapy plays a critical role for those PD patients who suffer from communication difficulties. Although dysarthria is difficult to treat, hypophonia can be overcome with training. Specifically, the Lee Silverman Voice Treatment program has been shown to be effective in improving both the volume and clarity of speech in those with PD.[8] Swallow evaluation and therapy are also helpful in the treatment of dysphagia, which occurs as PD progresses.

Procedures

Feeding tubes are sometimes used in individuals who have severe end-stage PD. Some patients elect hospice care, without artificial feeding at that point. Individuals who do get feeding tubes may need to have medication doses adjusted (e.g., carbidopa-levodopa will now bypass the esophagus and have a shortened time to onset of action).

Surgery

Although a large number of medications are available for the treatment of early and moderately advanced PD, they are of limited efficacy in those with advanced PD. Several surgical procedures are currently available for those with advanced PD. These procedures consist of either creation of a permanent lesion or insertion of an electrical stimulator in a specific nucleus of the brain.

Thalamotomy consists of introduction of a lesion in the ventral intermediate nucleus of the thalamus. Thalamotomy has been reported to produce a reduction in tremor of the contralateral limb in 80% of the patients who were treated.[9] There was no improvement in bradykinesia or in gait or speech abnormalities. Thalamotomy is recommended in PD patients with an asymmetric, severe, medically intractable tremor.

Unilateral pallidotomy consists of introduction of a lesion in the globus pallidus. The most striking benefits are a reduction in contralateral drug-induced dyskinesias, contralateral tremor, bradykinesia, and rigidity.[10,11] Unilateral pallidotomy is recommended in PD patients with bradykinesia, rigidity, and tremor who experience significant drug-induced dyskinesia despite optimal medical therapy. Few data are available about the cognitive effects of unilateral pallidotomy. Thus, neuropsychological evaluation is recommended in all patients both before and after surgery.

Deep brain stimulation (DBS) consists of high-frequency electrical stimulation in one of the following locations: the ventral intermediate nucleus of the thalamus, the globus pallidus, or the subthalamic nucleus. DBS requires surgery, in which the source of electrical stimulation is placed subcutaneously in the chest wall and the leads to which it is attached are placed in one of the locations listed. The advantage of DBS is that the degree of electrical stimulation can be easily adjusted, externally, once the DBS unit is in place. In contrast, both thalamotomy and pallidotomy result in permanent, fixed lesions in the brain. DBS of the ventral intermediate nucleus of the thalamus is effective in the treatment of a severe and disabling tremor that is unresponsive to medical therapy. DBS of the globus pallidus results in a marked reduction in dyskinesia. There are also improvements in bradykinesia, speech, gait, rigidity, and tremor. DBS of the subthalamic nucleus also results in marked improvement in tremor, akinesia, gait, and postural stability.[12]

For the symptoms of PD that no longer fully respond to medication, surgical treatment is an important therapeutic option. In carefully selected cases, thalamotomy and DBS of the thalamus can safely and effectively control contralateral tremor. Unilateral pallidotomy has been demonstrated to be an effective treatment of severe dyskinesias. Most commonly, DBS of the subthalamic nucleus improves motor function and reduces "off" time.[13] DBS of the ventral intermediate nucleus of the thalamus or the globus pallidus remains under investigation.

POTENTIAL DISEASE COMPLICATIONS

The true prevalence of depression in those with PD is unknown, but estimates vary from 7% to 75%.[14] It may be difficult to distinguish true depression from the apathy associated with PD. The crucial factor is to determine whether the patient has a true disturbance of mood, with loss of interest, sleep disturbance, and sometimes suicidal thoughts. The reasons for depression in PD are a subject of debate. There is a suspicion that the pathologic process of PD itself may predispose to depression. Regardless of the cause, recognition and treatment of depression may have a significant impact on the overall disability caused by the illness. Many PD patients have been treated safely and effectively with selective serotonin reuptake inhibitors, such as fluoxetine and paroxetine. Tricyclic antidepressants can be used, although their anticholinergic properties may limit their effectiveness.

Gastrointestinal complications also occur in PD. Dysphagia is typically due to poor control of the muscles of both mastication and the oropharynx. Soft food is easier to eat, and antiparkinson medication improves swallowing.

POTENTIAL TREATMENT COMPLICATIONS

The motor complications seen with pharmacologic treatment are divided into two categories: fluctuations (off state) and levodopa-induced dyskinesias. The off state consists of a return of the signs and symptoms of PD: bradykinesia, tremor, and rigidity. Patients may also experience anxiety, dysphoria, or panic during an off state.

The development of levodopa-induced dyskinesias appears to be related to the degree of dopamine receptor supersensitivity. As PD progresses, there is an increasing loss of dopamine receptors. This results in an increased sensitivity of the remaining dopamine receptors to dopamine itself. Thus, there is a greater chance for development of dyskinesias at a given dose of levodopa. Treatment options are to lower each dose of levodopa but with an increase in the frequency with which it is taken; to add or to increase the dose of a dopamine agonist while the dose of levodopa is decreased; and to add amantadine, which has been shown to be an antidyskinetic agent in some patients.[13,15] In addition, those patients who continue to experience an improvement in their mobility with levodopa but develop dyskinesias that become more pronounced as the day progresses are excellent candidates for DBS.

References

1. de Lau LML, Breteler MMB. Epidemiology of Parkinson's disease. Lancet Neurol 2006;5:525-535.
2. Benito-Leon J, Bermejo-Pareja F, Rodriguez J, et al; Neurological Disorders in Central Spain (NEDICES) Study Group. Prevalence of PD and other types of parkinsonism in three elderly populations of central Spain. Mov Disord 2003;18:267-274.
3. Mayeux R, Marder K, Cote LJ, et al. The frequency of idiopathic Parkinson's disease by age, ethnic group, and sex in northern Manhattan, 1988-1993. Am J Epidemiol 1995;142:820-827.
4. de Rijk MC, Tzourio C, Breteler MM, et al. Prevalence of parkinsonism and Parkinson's disease in Europe: the EUROPARKINSON Collaborative Study. European Community Concerted Action on the Epidemiology of Parkinson's disease. J Neurol Neurosurg Psychiatry 1997;62:10-15.
5. Goetz GC, Poewe W, Rascol O, Sampaio C. Evidence-based medical review update: pharmacological and surgical treatments of Parkinson's disease: 2001 to 2004. Mov Disord 2005;20:523-539.
6. Kaynak D, Kiziltan G, Kaynak H, et al. Sleep and sleepiness in patients with Parkinson's disease before and after dopaminergic treatment. Eur J Neurol. 2005;12:199-207.
7. Parkinson Study Group. Entacapone improves motor fluctuations in levodopa-treated Parkinson's disease patients. Ann Neurol 1997;42:747-755.
8. Ramig LO, Fox C, Sapir S. Parkinson's disease: speech and voice disorders and their treatment with the Lee Silverman Voice Treatment. Semin Speech Lang 2004;25:169-180.
9. Jankovic J, Cardoso F, Grossman RG, Hamilton WJ. Outcome after stereotactic thalamotomy for parkinsonian, essential, and other types of tremor. Neurosurgery 1995;37:680-687.
10. Fazzini E, Dogali M, Sterio D, et al. Stereotactic pallidotomy for Parkinson's disease: a long-term follow-up of unilateral pallidotomy. Neurology 1997;48:1273-1277.
11. Lang AE, Lozano AM, Montgomery E, et al. Posteroventral medial pallidotomy in advanced Parkinson's disease. N Engl J Med 1997;337:1036-1042.
12. Benabid AL, Chabardes S, Seigneuret E. Deep-brain stimulation in Parkinson's disease: long-term efficacy and safety—what happened this year? Curr Opin Neurol 2005;18:623-630.
13. Pahwa R, Factor SA, Lyons KE, et al. Practice Parameter: treatment of Parkinson disease with motor fluctuations and dyskinesia (an evidence-based review). Neurology 2006;66:983-995.
14. Veazey C, Aki SO, Cook KF, et al. Prevalence and treatment of depression in Parkinson's disease. J Neuropsychiatry Clin Neurosci 2005;17:310-323.
15. Metman LV, Del Dotto P, van den Munckhof P, et al. Amantadine as treatment for dyskinesias and motor fluctuations in Parkinson's disease. Neurology 1998;50:1323-1326.

Peripheral Neuropathies 133

Seward B. Rutkove, MD

Synonyms

Polyneuropathies
Neuropathies

ICD-9 Codes

356.2 Hereditary sensory neuropathy
356.4 Idiopathic progressive polyneuropathy
356.9 Idiopathic neuropathy, unspecified
357.1 Polyneuropathy in collagen vascular disease
357.2 Polyneuropathy in diabetes
357.3 Polyneuropathy in malignant disease
357.4 Polyneuropathy in other diseases classified elsewhere
357.5 Alcoholic polyneuropathy
357.6 Polyneuropathy due to drugs
357.7 Polyneuropathy due to other toxic agents
357.9 Inflammatory and toxic neuropathy, unspecified

DEFINITION

Peripheral neuropathies are a collection of disorders characterized by the generalized dysfunction of nerves. This group of diseases is heterogeneous, including those that predominantly affect the nerve axon, others that primarily affect the myelin sheath, and still others that involve both parts of the nerve simultaneously. In addition, some peripheral neuropathies affect only small, unmyelinated fibers, whereas others predominantly involve only large myelinated ones. Table 133-1 contains a list of the most frequently encountered forms of peripheral neuropathy.

Peripheral neuropathy is common; one Italian study suggested a prevalence of about 3.5% in the general population.[1] In diabetes, one study demonstrated clinical peripheral neuropathy affecting 8.3% of individuals compared with a control population, in whom 2.1% of individuals were affected.[2] After 10 years, 41.9% of the diabetic patients had developed peripheral neuropathy compared with 6% of the control subjects.

Defining peripheral neuropathy remains no simple task. Members of the American Academy of Neurology along with those from the American Association of Electrodiagnostic Medicine and the American Academy of Physi-cal Medicine and Rehabilitation have developed a formal case definition for distal symmetric polyneuropathy (the most common form).[3] The authors chose to use a combination of symptoms, signs, and electrodiagnostic testing results to formulate an ordinal ranking system to identify the likelihood of the disease in a given patient. Although it is a very useful tool for future research studies, the necessity of applying such a complex approach underscores the difficulty in attempting to define peripheral neuropathy in any simple fashion.

SYMPTOMS

Patients with peripheral neuropathy present with a number of specific sensory complaints, including decreased sensation often associated with pain, tingling (paresthesias), and burning. Some patients, usually with more advanced disease, will note thinning of the feet and some weakness, especially with the development of partial footdrop. Walking difficulties usually also develop once sensation is significantly impaired. Sensory symptoms in the hand (paresthesias and reduced tactile sensation) usually develop once an axonal peripheral neuropathy has progressed up to about the level of the knees. In patients with generalized demyelinating peripheral neuropathies, more generalized symptoms of weakness and sensory loss are often present, although distally predominant paresthesias often occur.

PHYSICAL EXAMINATION

The history includes a detailed past medical history, review of systems, and any prior exposure to toxins (Table 133-2).

The physical examination demonstrates distinct abnormalities that depend on the form of peripheral neuropathy present. Most commonly, patients present with a sensorimotor axonal peripheral neuropathy. In this condition, decreased sensation to pinprick, vibration, light touch, and temperature may be identified distally in the lower extremities with normal sensation more proximally. Some weakness of toe or foot extension and flexion may also be apparent. Deep tendon reflexes will

TABLE 133-1 Specific Disorders of Peripheral Nerves

Predominantly axonal disorders

Diabetic neuropathy

Alcoholic neuropathy

Medication-related neuropathy (e.g., metronidazole, colchicine, nitrofurantoin, isoniazid)

Systemic disease–related neuropathy (e.g., chronic renal failure, inflammatory bowel disease, connective tissue disease)

Thyroid neuropathy

Heavy metal toxic neuropathy (lead, arsenic, cadmium)

Porphyric neuropathy

Paraneoplastic neuropathy

Syphilitic, Lyme neuropathy

Sarcoid neuropathy

Human immunodeficiency virus–related neuropathy

Hereditary neuropathies (Charcot-Marie-Tooth, type 2; familial amyloid; mitochondrial)

Critical illness neuropathy

Predominantly demyelinating disorders

Idiopathic chronic inflammatory demyelinating polyradiculoneuropathy (CIDP)

CIDP associated with monoclonal proteins

Antimyelin-associated glycoprotein neuropathy (a form of CIDP)

Antisulfatide antibody–associated neuropathy (a form of CIDP)

Human immunodeficiency virus–associated CIDP

Guillain-Barré syndrome

Hereditary (Charcot-Marie-Tooth, types 1 and 3)

TABLE 133-2 Toxins Producing Peripheral Nerve Degeneration

Industrial chemicals

Affect peripheral nervous system preferentially

   Lead

   Acrylamide

   Organophosphates

   Thallium

Some effects on central nervous system

   Carbon disulfide

   Methylmercury

   Methyl bromide

Large amounts required

   Arsenic

   Trichloroethylene

   Tetrachloroethane

   2,4-dichlorophenoxyacetic acid (2,4-D)

   Pentachlorophenol

   DDT

Some effects on other than nervous tissue

   Carbon tetrachloride

   Carbon monoxide

Pharmaceutical substances

Arsenic

Arsenic-based chemicals

Clioquinol

Disulfiram

Gold

Hydralazine

Nitrofurantoin

Phenytoin

Sulfonamides

Thalidomide

Thallium

Vincristine

Modified from Gilliatt RW. Recent advances in the pathophysiology of nerve conduction. In Desmedt JE, ed. New Developments in Electromyography and Clinical Neurophysiology. Basel, Karger, 1973:2-18.

be hypoactive distally (e.g., ankle jerks decreased relative to knee jerks).

In patients with acquired demyelinating peripheral neuropathy, the examination may demonstrate marked generalized weakness with only mildly abnormal sensory findings, usually including decreased joint position sense. In this disorder, deep tendon reflexes may be reduced or diffusely absent. Patients with hereditary demyelinating polyneuropathies may demonstrate distal muscle atrophy in the feet and lower legs. Such patients may develop a pes cavus foot deformity, in which the foot is foreshortened and has a very high arch. A "champagne bottle" appearance to the legs (where muscular atrophy of the foreleg, especially the calf, is prominent) may also be present. As any peripheral neuropathy progresses, lower extremity sensory loss may lead to gait unsteadiness, and upper extremity sensory loss may produce decreased hand dexterity.

FUNCTIONAL LIMITATIONS

Patients with peripheral neuropathy face a number of potential functional limitations. In those individuals with a distal axonal peripheral neuropathy, limitations usually include problems with gait and unsteadiness, especially as the neuropathy progresses. If pain is a prominent symptom, the activities of daily living may be compromised to some extent. Pain may also be prominent at night, interfering with sleep. In those patients with very advanced axonal peripheral neuropathy or demyelinating forms, such as hereditary Charcot-Marie-Tooth disease, weakness can produce major functional limitations, restricting the patient's walking ability and in some cases leading to dyspnea and nocturnal hypoventilation. In patients with some chronic forms of demyelinating polyneuropathy, weakness of both proximal and distal muscles can become severe, limiting the performance of many activities of daily living. Sensory deficits can limit one's ability to button shirts, to zip pants, to turn a key in a lock, to tie shoelaces, or to type on a computer.

DIAGNOSTIC STUDIES

Electrodiagnostic studies (including electromyography and nerve conduction studies) remain the most important first tests in the evaluation of polyneuropathy.[4] Nerve conduction studies assist in determination of whether the peripheral neuropathy is mainly demyelinating, axonal, or mixed (Figs. 133-1 and 133-2) by evaluation of the amplitude and conduction velocities of the motor and sensory responses obtained.[5] Likewise, nerve conduction studies help determine the severity of the process as well. Although needle electromyography plays a more limited role in the diagnosis of peripheral neuropathy, a gradient of reinnervation, in which distal muscles are most abnormal and proximal muscles less affected, helps determine the degree of motor involvement. In addition, needle electromyography may assist in determining whether a superimposed problem, such as polyradiculopathy, is also contributing.

In general, a number of serologic tests are also performed to identify the cause of the peripheral neuropathy. These are outlined in Table 133-3.

Additional workup is occasionally necessary. For example, quantitative sensory testing can delineate the degree of sensory loss and the extent to which specific modalities are affected. In this technique, patients are asked to determine whether they can feel certain sensations generated by a probe touching the skin. By use of certain algorithms, the physician can obtain an accurate assessment of the severity of sensory deficit and the modalities affected. This form of testing can be especially help-

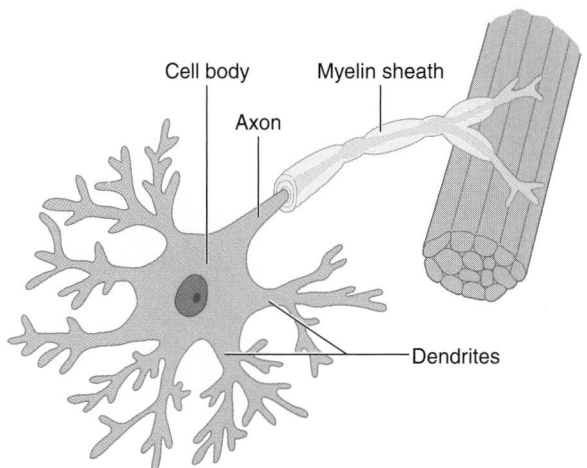

FIGURE 133-2. Schematic representation of a motor nerve extending from a cell body to the muscle it innervates.

ful in small-fiber peripheral neuropathies, as standard electrodiagnostic recording may be normal. Autonomic testing (such as tilt-table testing and heart rate variability to deep breathing) may also be helpful in delineating the involvement of the autonomic nervous system in the neuropathic process.

Sural nerve biopsy can be useful in determining the cause of the polyneuropathy for some conditions that are difficult to diagnose, such as amyloid neuropathy, as well as some other unusual forms of peripheral neuropathy. On occasion, muscle biopsy may also be helpful in this regard as well because vasculitic abnormalities or amyloid can also be identified. Lumbar puncture may aid in the determination of whether an acquired demyelinating peripheral neuropathy is present by the identification of a very elevated cerebrospinal fluid protein concentration and normal white blood cell count (so-called albuminocytologic dissociation). The analysis of cutaneous sensory fibers through the use of skin biopsy has also been introduced to identify small-fiber peripheral neuropathies.[6]

TREATMENT

Initial

If a cause of the axonal peripheral neuropathy is known or identified (which generally is achieved about 70% of the time), treatment geared toward the underlying disorder itself might help slow progression of the

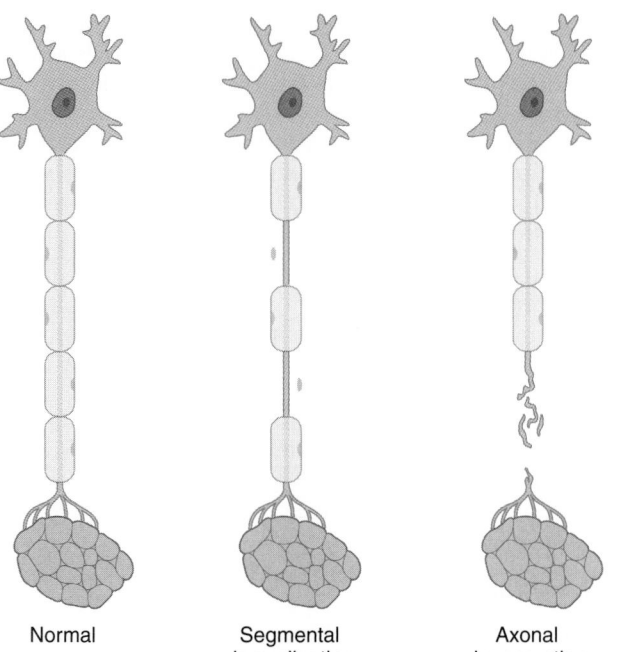

Normal   Segmental   Axonal
                demyelination   degeneration

FIGURE 133-1. Types of peripheral nerve damage.

Differential Diagnosis

Myelopathy (spinal cord compression)

Lumbosacral polyradiculopathy (lumbar stenosis)

Mononeuropathy multiplex

TABLE 133-3 Serologic Testing in Peripheral Neuropathy

Baseline testing

Vitamin B_{12}

Thyroid-stimulating hormone

Rapid plasma reagin (or VDRL test)

Serum glucose

Serum hemoglobin A_{1c}

Antinuclear antibody

Erythrocyte sedimentation rate

Serum protein electrophoresis

Urine protein electrophoresis

Some additional tests, depending on clinical suspicion

Serum protein immunophoresis

24-hour urine collection for heavy metals

24-hour urine collection for porphyrins

Glucose tolerance testing

Human immunodeficiency virus infection testing

Anti-Ro, anti-La antibodies (Sjögren syndrome)

Anti-Hu antibody (paraneoplastic neuropathy)

Additional antibody testing in certain demyelinating disorders

  Antimyelin-associated glycoprotein

  Antisulfatide antibody

Genetic testing (for disorders such as familial amyloidosis, Charcot-Marie-Tooth disease)

polyneuropathy. For example, improved glucose control can help improve neuronal function in diabetic neuropathy.[7] Likewise, in those people with a neuropathy secondary to toxin exposure, such as alcoholic neuropathy, decreased exposure to the toxin may, of course, be helpful.

In patients with axonal peripheral neuropathies, treatment is usually symptom based, with efforts toward reducing pain and dysesthesias. A number of drugs have proved useful in this regard.[8] The tricyclic antidepressants remain most effective (generally nortriptyline or amitriptyline, starting with 10 mg at bedtime and increasing as needed until improvement occurs). Gabapentin (starting at a dose of 100 to 300 mg three times daily) has also gained wide acceptance in the treatment of this disorder during the past several years.[9] Other medications, including carbamazepine, diphenylhydantoin, and more recently topiramate, have been used as well. Two new drugs have become available,[10,11] specifically approved for use in diabetic polyneuropathy: duloxetine (Cymbalta), at 30 mg or 60 mg daily; and pregabalin (Lyrica) at a dose of 50 mg three times daily, increasing to 100 mg if needed. However, it is not clear that either of these is more efficacious than previously available medications. Application of capsaicin ointment to the feet can also occasionally be helpful. In patients in whom these measures prove of limited value, the use of long-acting narcotic agents may be necessary.

In patients with certain forms of demyelinating peripheral neuropathy (such as chronic inflammatory demyelinating polyradiculoneuropathy), immunosuppressive or immunomodulating therapies can make a dramatic difference in the patient's symptoms and level of function. Drugs including corticosteroids, azathioprine, cyclosporine, and cyclophosphamide can be used.[12] Intravenous immune globulin and plasmapheresis are also widely used in this group of disorders.[13,14] Finally, in all patients with distal sensory loss due to peripheral neuropathy, regular podiatric care is extremely important in preventing the development of serious foot complications, such as ulcerations.

Rehabilitation

Physical therapy may be recommended to work on strength and balance and to improve mobility. In patients with moderate to severe peripheral neuropathy, gait training may consist of balance exercise and use of an assistive device, such as a cane or walker. Either a physical or occupational therapist can review falls precautions (e.g., avoiding throw rugs in the home, using a chair in the bath or shower). Some patients may benefit from an ankle-foot orthosis. However, in patients with compromised sensation, monitoring of the skin to prevent breakdown when a brace is used is critical. Patients can be taught to self-monitor their skin with use of a long-handled mirror to check the bottom of their feet. Custom shoes (e.g., extra depth and width) may be beneficial, as can custom shoe orthoses.

In patients with more advanced peripheral neuropathy, evaluation by an occupational therapist may help maximize the function of the hands and arms. The occupational therapist can provide the patient with information about adaptive equipment, such as elastic shoelaces, wide grip handles for cookware and utensils, and shoehorns. An occupational or physical therapist experienced in assistive technology can also be helpful in specialized equipment, such as voice-activated computer software, driving adaptations, and environmental control units.

If pain is an issue, both physical and occupational therapists can assist with modalities that may alleviate the pain. These may include instruction on use of transcutaneous electrical nerve stimulation, paraffin baths, and the like. It is important to caution the patient with impaired sensation not to use any heat or ice that may cause burns or frostbite. Individuals with impaired vascular status also should be advised not to use ice because of its vasoconstrictive properties.

Procedures

Patients with peripheral neuropathy are generally at increased risk for development of superimposed compressive neuropathies, such as carpal tunnel syndrome.

Treatment with local corticosteroid injections can be helpful for this problem (see Chapter 32).

Surgery

Surgery may be necessary for some associated conditions, including severe carpal tunnel syndrome, but it is usually more relevant to patients who develop infections of the distal lower extremities and require amputations. Other, less severe distal leg problems may also develop, requiring orthopedic or podiatric surgery. Although lower extremity nerve release surgeries are sometimes performed in the hope of treating neuropathic symptoms,[15] a review and position statement by the American Academy of Neurology reported that there is little evidence to support the use of these procedures to treat neuropathy.[16]

POTENTIAL DISEASE COMPLICATIONS

A number of potential foot complications can occur, including persistent, intractable pain, skin ulcerations, and foot trauma, possibly leading to amputations. Serious trauma secondary to increased gait unsteadiness is another potential problem. Finally, depression due to immobility and persistent pain also often plays a role in patients with more advanced peripheral neuropathy.

POTENTIAL TREATMENT COMPLICATIONS

The tricyclic antidepressants and other pain medications have the potential side effect of drowsiness. Dry mouth, constipation, and urinary retention also occur commonly with the tricyclic antidepressants. The seizure medications, but especially carbamazepine, have the potential of causing severe ataxia at higher doses and can make individuals feel groggy and inattentive. Rarely, a life-threatening idiosyncratic reaction to diphenylhydantoin characterized by skin defoliation and necrosis can occur (Stevens-Johnson syndrome). With narcotic use, addiction remains a concern. Side effects of duloxetine include dizziness, nausea, and constipation. Side effects of pregabalin include dizziness and somnolence.

Treatment of the autoimmune peripheral neuropathies poses significant risk, given the inherent toxicity of the medications employed. Patients using immunosuppressive medications are at increased risk for infection, malignant neoplasia, anemia, and multiple other side effects (e.g., liver toxicity with azathioprine, renal failure with intravenous immune globulin, hemorrhagic cystitis with cyclophosphamide).

Skin breakdown can occur with improper bracing.

References

1. Italian General Practitioner Study Group. Chronic symmetric symptomatic polyneuropathy in the elderly: a field screening investigation in two Italian regions. Neurology 1995;45:1832-1836.
2. Partanen J, Niskanen L, Lehtinen J, et al. Natural history of peripheral neuropathy in patients with non–insulin dependent diabetes mellitus. N Engl J Med 1995;333:89-94.
3. England JD, Gronseth GS, Franklin G, et al; American Academy of Neurology; American Association of Electrodiagnostic Medicine; American Academy of Physical Medicine and Rehabilitation. Distal symmetric polyneuropathy: a definition for clinical research: report of the American Academy of Neurology, the American Association of Electrodiagnostic Medicine, and the American Academy of Physical Medicine and Rehabilitation. Neurology 2005;64:199-207.
4. Dyck P, Dyck P, Grant I, Fealey R. Ten steps in characterizing and diagnosing patients with peripheral neuropathy. Neurology 1996;47:10-17.
5. Albers J. Clinical neurophysiology of generalized polyneuropathy. J Clin Neurophys 1993;10:149-166.
6. Hermann D, Griffin F, Hauer P, et al. Epidermal nerve fiber density and sural nerve morphometry in peripheral neuropathies. Neurology 1999;53:1634-1640.
7. Tron, W, Carta Q, Cantello R, et al. Peripheral nerve function and metabolic control in diabetes mellitus. Ann Neurol 1984;16:178-183.
8. Sindrup S, Jensen T. Pharmacologic treatment of pain in polyneuropathy. Neurology 2000;55:915-920.
9. Backonja M, Beydoun A, Edwards KR, et al. Gabapentin for the symptomatic treatment of painful neuropathy in patients with diabetes mellitus: a randomized controlled trial [see comments]. JAMA 1998;280:1831-1836.
10. Raskin J, Pritchett YL, Wang F, et al. A double-blind, randomized multicenter trial comparing duloxetine with placebo in the management of diabetic peripheral neuropathic pain. Pain Med 2005;6:346-356.
11. Shneker BF, McAuley JW. Pregabalin: a new neuromodulator with broad therapeutic indications. Ann Pharmacother 2005;39:2029-2037.
12. Barnett MH, Pollard JD, Davies L, McLeod JG. Cyclosporin A in resistant chronic inflammatory demyelinating polyradiculoneuropathy. Muscle Nerve 1998;21:454-460.
13. Hahn A, Bolton C, Zochodne D, Feasby T. Intravenous immunoglobulin treatment in chronic inflammatory demyelinating polyneuropathy. Brain 1996;119:1067-1077.
14. Hahn A, Bolton C, Pillay N, et al. Plasma-exchange therapy in chronic inflammatory demyelinating polyneuropathy. Brain 1996;119:1055-1066.
15. Aszmann OC, Kress KM, Dellon AL. Results of decompression of peripheral nerves in diabetics: a prospective, blinded study. Plast Reconstr Surg 2001;108:1452-1453.
16. Chaudhry V, Stevens JC, Kincaid J, So YT. Practice Advisory: utility of surgical decompression for treatment of diabetic neuropathy: report of the Therapeutics and Technology Assessment Subcommittee of the American Academy of Neurology. Neurology 2006;66:1805-1808.

Plexopathy—Brachial 134

Erik Ensrud, MD, and John C. King, MD

Synonyms

Brachial plexopathy
Neuralgic amyotrophy
Parsonage-Turner syndrome
Brachial amyotrophy
Idiopathic shoulder girdle neuropathy
Brachial plexitis
Erb palsy
Klumpke palsy

ICD-9 Codes

353.0   Brachial plexus lesions
353.5   Neuralgic amyotrophy
723.4   Brachial neuritis or radiculitis NOS
767.6   Birth trauma

DEFINITION

Brachial plexopathy is the pathologic dysfunction of the brachial plexus, a complex peripheral nerve structure in the proximal upper extremity. The brachial plexus starts just outside the spinal cord in the lower neck and extends to the axilla. The total average brachial plexus length is approximately 6 inches.[1] The plexus is divided into five sections: roots, trunks, divisions, cords, and branches or terminal nerves. The spinal nerves C5 through T1 classically supply anterior primary rami of the nerve roots, which then form the plexus. Variations in nerve root supply that involve other nerve roots are said to be expanded. When the C4 nerve root also supplies the brachial plexus and T1 contribution is minimal, the plexus is called prefixed. When the T2 nerve root supplies the brachial plexus and C5 contribution is minimal, the plexus is said to be postfixed.[2] The nerve roots combine to form the trunks behind the clavicle. There are three trunks, the upper, middle, and lower. The upper is formed from the C5 and C6 nerve roots, the middle is a continuation of C7, and the lower is formed from C8 and T1. The trunks then divide behind the clavicle into anterior and posterior divisions. Just inferior to the clavicle, the divisions coalesce into cords. The cords travel along the axillary artery, just inferior to the clavicle, and are named for their spatial relationship to the artery. The posterior cord is formed from the union of the three posterior divisions. The lateral cord is formed by the union of the anterior divisions of the upper and middle trunks. The medial cord is the continuation of the anterior division of the lower trunk. Nerve branches are the most distal elements of the brachial plexus and are the major nerves of the upper extremity. These branches begin in the distal axilla and other than the median nerve, which is formed by contributions from the medial and lateral cords, are continuations of the cords. There are also numerous peripheral nerves that arise directly from the roots, trunks, and cords (Fig. 134-1).

Brachial plexopathy can be due to wide-ranging causes, including idiopathic, autoimmune, traumatic, neoplastic, and hereditary. It can occur in any age group; but other than when it is secondary to obstetric trauma, it usually occurs from the ages of 30 to 70 years. Men are affected two to three times as often as women are, which is thought to be related to their more frequent participation in vigorous athletic activities that can lead to trauma. About half of the cases have no identified precipitating event; in others, brachial plexopathy follows an antecedent infection, trauma, surgery, or immunization.

SYMPTOMS

The brachial plexus is made up of motor and sensory peripheral nerve fibers that supply the entire upper extremity. Brachial plexopathy can result in symptoms of pain, weakness, and numbness, both at the level of the brachial plexus and distally in the supplied upper extremity. The area of pain and other symptoms correlates with the portion of the brachial plexus involved and the specific nerve elements from that area. Depending on the cause of the plexopathy, symptom onset can range from sudden to insidious. Because of the complex muscle suspension of the shoulder joint, chronic brachial plexopathy may result in glenohumeral subluxation and instability due to stretching of the shoulder capsule. Brachial plexopathy usually does not cause prominent neck pain. Some brachial plexopathies may occur bilaterally and therefore cause symptoms in both upper extremities.

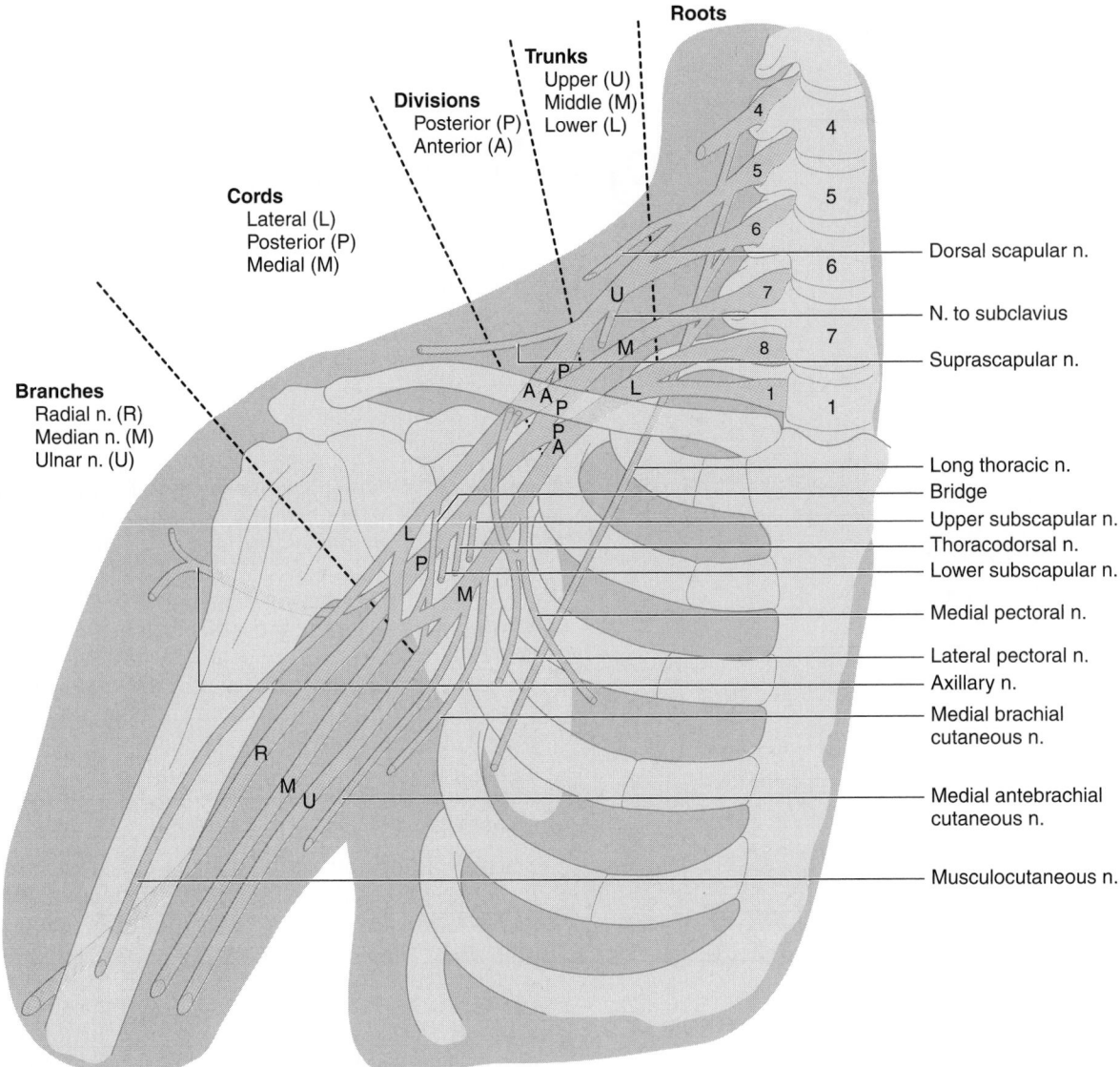

FIGURE 134-1. The brachial plexus. The clinician must be able to visualize this structure in performing electrodiagnostic examination so that an appropriate number of muscles and nerves are sampled to localize a lesion. (Reprinted with permission from Dumitru D, Amato A, Zwarts M. Electrodiagnostic Medicine, 2nd ed. Philadelphia, Hanley & Belfus, 2002.)

PHYSICAL EXAMINATION

The physical examination for brachial plexopathy must be thorough because of the complexity of its structure and function. The shoulder girdle and entire extremity need to be exposed during examination to allow close inspection of muscle bulk and fasciculations. Assessment of atrophy of muscles is often assisted by side-to-side comparisons. Muscle strength examination needs to be thorough and to include proximal muscles not commonly tested, such as infraspinatus, supraspinatus, rhomboids, and serratus anterior. Sensory testing also must be thorough, with both dermatomal and peripheral nerve sensory distributions examined. A musculoskeletal examination of the shoulder joint is helpful; joint disease can be both a possible primary cause of pain and a secondary effect of plexopathy. Shoulder range of motion and signs of tendinosis as well as reflexes and any muscle atrophy need to be

assessed. The lack of pain exacerbation with neck movement can help distinguish brachial plexopathy from cervical radiculopathy.[3] It is often not possible to determine the exact location of a brachial plexus lesion from physical examination, but the examination is usually helpful in focusing electrodiagnostic and radiologic testing.

FUNCTIONAL LIMITATIONS

Depending on whether the brachial plexopathy involves the upper plexus, lower plexus, or entire plexus, the proximal shoulder muscles, the distal muscles involved in fine finger movements, or the entire extremity can be weak or numb. Activities of daily living, such as dressing, feeding, and grooming, can be significantly affected. These impairments can result in disabilities in many activities, including computer use, writing, and driving. Brachial plexopathy secondary to birth trauma may subsequently cause difficulty for children and teens with sports and other recreational activity.

DIAGNOSTIC STUDIES

Electromyography (EMG) can be helpful in localizing the pathologic area in brachial plexopathy as well as in determining the severity of axonal injury and the potential for recovery. However, many brachial plexopathies cannot be definitely localized by EMG because of subtle findings encountered with incomplete nerve injury and the complexity of plexus-related innervation. The nerve conduction and needle EMG assessment is best directed by both symptoms and physical examination findings. Both nerve conduction studies and needle EMG are required for complete assessment. Sensory nerve conduction studies can help in localization by the pattern of abnormalities seen and in judging injury severity based on reductions of amplitudes or absence of potentials. The nerve conduction study may not detect abnormality if the lesion is mild in severity or too recent to allow axonal degeneration.

The following five basic sensory nerve conduction studies are suggested as a screen for brachial plexus evaluation: lateral antebrachial cutaneous, median recording from the thumb, median recording from the index finger, superficial radial, and ulnar recording from the little finger.[2] The presence of fibrillation potentials in EMG is particularly sensitive for motor axon loss and helps localize the site of lesions. The choice of muscles sampled on EMG is usually focused on the area of interest, but other areas are also included for the exclusion of wider disease. It is important to include paraspinal muscles of the relevant areas to investigate the possibility of radiculopathy (paraspinals are supplied by the posterior primary rami of the nerve roots, which do not supply the brachial plexus). EMG evaluation of the brachial plexus is complex and best performed by experienced electromyographers.

Radiologic studies of the plexus are helpful to evaluate the severity of trauma, the presence of mass lesions, and inflammation of the brachial plexus nerve elements.[4] Magnetic resonance imaging (MRI) has become the study of choice in evaluation of traumatic brachial plexus injuries.[5] More than 80% of traumatic nerve root avulsions will show pseudomeningoceles, which are tears in the meningeal sheath surrounding the nerve roots that allow extravasation of cerebrospinal fluid into nearby tissues. They appear bright on T2-weighted images.

MRI is also the most useful study for evaluation of other causes of brachial plexopathy. It is the most effective method of evaluating brachial plexus tumors, both secondary and primary.[6] An early MRI sign in Pancoast tumor is obliteration of the interscalene fat pad, which is best visualized on coronal T1-weighted MRI.[7] Inflammatory changes in the brachial plexus may be visualized with MRI, including brachial neuralgic amyotrophy.[8]

Chest radiographs are valuable for the evaluation of diaphragmatic paralysis in traumatic brachial plexopathy, which usually indicates an irreparable lesion of the brachial plexus.[9]

Differential Diagnosis

It is helpful to approach the differential diagnosis of brachial plexopathy by the common causes in the different anatomic regions where the brachial plexus is affected. The anatomic areas of interest are the supraclavicular, retroclavicular, and infraclavicular. There are also causes of brachial plexopathy that tend to produce more diffuse plexus injury.

Supraclavicular

Trauma usually involves the upper plexus and is especially seen with closed traction, as in "burner" sports injuries (sudden separation of the shoulder and head due to contact) and pressure from backpack straps. The roots can be stretched but remain continuous, tear, or avulse from the spinal cord.

Postoperative brachial plexopathy is secondary to arm positioning during surgery.[10]

Birth trauma is due to excessive lateral deviation of the head and neck to free the infant's shoulder, during both vaginal delivery and cesarean section. It is called Erb palsy when the C5-6 nerve roots are affected, resulting primarily in proximal arm weakness. When the C8-T1 roots are affected, the results are hand weakness, called Klumpke paralysis.

Neurogenic thoracic outlet syndrome is a rare condition in which a fibrous band extends from the lower cervical spine (cervical rib or transverse process) to the first rib. The T1 fibers are deflected and injured further by this fibrous band more than the C8 fibers.

Pancoast syndrome is direct extension of an apical lung tumor (usually small cell carcinoma) into the supraclavicular brachial plexus, often presenting with shoulder pain.[11]

Infraclavicular

Postirradiation injury follows radiation therapy directed at the axillary lymph nodes; it can occur months to years after radiation therapy. EMG studies may reveal evidence of conduction block and myokymia.

Secondary neoplastic injury is usually due to compression from enlargement of involved axillary lymph nodes.

In midclavicular fractures, brachial plexopathy can be secondary to the initial trauma and also result from the development of heterotopic ossification.[12]

Procedural—infraclavicular brachial plexus injury has been identified as a complication of axillary regional blocks.[13]

Retroclavicular

Retroclavicular brachial plexopathy is rare. It usually occurs in the context of widespread plexopathy.

Continued

Differential Diagnosis—cont'd

Diffuse localization

Neuralgic amyotrophy is a well-described syndrome of idiopathic monophasic brachial plexopathy that is also called Parsonage-Turner syndrome, brachial amyotrophy, idiopathic shoulder girdle neuropathy,[14] and brachial plexitis. Neuralgic amyotrophy was well characterized by a large case series.[15] The initial symptom of neuralgic amyotrophy is onset during a few hours of severe continuous proximal upper extremity pain, which occurred in 90% of patients in this case series. After onset of pain, weakness of the extremity usually develops within 2 weeks. Whereas sensory symptoms in the affected extremity are usually less pronounced than pain and weakness, they occur in 70% of patients. Pain decreases first, with an average pain duration of 28 days. Motor recovery begins within 6 months in most patients and with significant functional improvement; but in this case series, more than 70% of patients still had at least mild weakness detected on thorough strength examination at 3 years after weakness onset. Neuralgic amyotrophy can involve any part of the brachial plexus but tends to affect the upper plexus; 49% of patients have shoulder–proximal arm involvement. A similar condition with a genetic etiology is hereditary neuralgic amyotrophy, which is often autosomal dominant but is genetically heterogeneous.

Primary neoplastic peripheral nerve tumors can cause brachial plexopathies that occur anywhere in the brachial plexus but are rare and usually benign. Benign tumors are usually nerve sheath tumors, either schwannomas or neurofibromas (associated with neurofibromatosis type 1), and cause painless sensory loss and weakness.[2] In contrast, malignant peripheral nerve tumors in the brachial plexus are usually painful.[16,17]

TREATMENT

Initial

The treatment of brachial plexopathy needs to be customized to the individual patient and the cause of the brachial plexopathy. Pain can be the most disabling symptom but is usually effectively treated with neuropathic pain medications, such as gabapentin and tricyclic antidepressants, and analgesics, such as tramadol and opiates in cases of severe pain. Dosing is usually at the higher end of accepted ranges (such as gabapentin at 600 mg three times daily or more) secondary to the pain severity of acute plexopathy, although duration of therapy may be brief. Levetiracetam has been used successfully to reduce refractory brachial plexopathy pain and to decrease opioid need.[18]

Rehabilitation

When the muscles of the shoulder girdle are involved, therapy focused on positioning and shoulder range of motion can prevent secondary complications, such as adhesive capsulitis. Directed exercise can be beneficial, with the caveat that exercise of muscles with neurogenic weakness from brachial plexus lesions to full exhaustion may be counterproductive on the basis of findings in exercise in patients with peripheral neuropathy.[19] Occupational therapy is often indicated when weakness from brachial plexopathy results in loss of function. Adaptive aids can be very helpful when they are indicated, such as a shoulder sling to help reduce imbalance from proximal arm weakness from brachial plexopathy. Vocational rehabilitation may be indicated when the resultant disability from weakness affects the patient's ability to perform in the job setting.

Procedures

Brachial plexus blocks are rarely used but are possible for the treatment of severe pain from metastatic brachial plexopathy or severe acute brachial plexopathy.

Surgery

Surgery is an option in cases of traumatic plexopathy but has variable results. Surgical techniques such as nerve grafting, free muscle transfer, neurolysis, and neurotization are used. Surgeons who use these techniques frequently differ considerably in their approach to them, making conclusions about their efficacy difficult. Surgery is an option in brachial plexus birth injuries, usually when persistent severe motor deficits are present after 3 to 8 months of age. A case series found improvement in surgically treated patients on a shoulder motion scale.[20] The location of injury affects selection of patients for surgery and surgical outcome. For example, postganglionic nerve root avulsion injuries may do better with earlier surgery.[21] Preganglionic avulsions are difficult to repair, but direct implantation into the spinal cord may help some patients.[22]

POTENTIAL DISEASE COMPLICATIONS

Weakness from brachial plexopathy can result in joint instability or in joint and musculotendinous contractures of upper extremity joints. Complex regional pain syndrome may follow brachial plexopathy.[23] Secondary depression can be due to pain and loss of function. Insensate limbs are at risk for trauma neglect, infection, and amputation.

POTENTIAL TREATMENT COMPLICATIONS

Stretching and range of motion exercises for avoidance or treatment of contractures can acutely exacerbate neuropathic pain. Care to avoid shoulder impingement during range of motion exercises is important due to weak rotator cuff muscles. Insensate limbs become more susceptible to heat injuries, such as by hot packs or therapeutic ultrasound. Medicines used for brachial plexopathy pain can have side effects, which are specific to the particular medicine used. Surgery for brachial plexopathy may result in nerve or vascular injury.

References

1. Slinghuff CL Jr, Terzis CK, Edgerton MT. The quantitative microanatomy of the brachial plexus in man: reconstructive relevance. In Terzis JK, ed. Microreconstruction of Nerve Injuries. Philadelphia, WB Saunders, 1987:285-324.
2. Ferrante MA. Brachial plexopathies: classification, causes, and consequences. Muscle Nerve 2004;30:547-568.
3. Mamula CJ, Erhard RE, Piva SR. Cervical radiculopathy or Parsonage-Turner syndrome: differential diagnosis of a patient with neck and upper extremity symptoms. J Orthop Sports Phys Ther 2005;35:659-664.
4. Castillo M. Imaging the anatomy of the brachial plexus: review and self-assessment module. AJR Am J Roentgenol 2005;185:S196-S204.
5. Doi K, Otsuka K, Okamomo Y, et al. Cervical nerve root avulsion in brachial plexus injuries: magnetic resonance imaging classification and comparison with myelography and computerized tomography myelography. J Neurosurg Spine 2002;96:277-284.
6. Saifuddin A. Imaging tumors of the brachial plexus. Skeletal Radiol 2003;32:375-387.
7. Huang JH, Zagoul K, Zager EL. Surgical management of brachial plexus tumors. Surg Neurol 2004;61:372-378.
8. Sarikaya S, Sumer M, Ozdolap S, Erdem CZ. Magnetic resonance neurography diagnosed brachial plexitis: a case report. Arch Phys Med Rehabil 2006;86:1058-1059.
9. Belzberg AJ, Dorsi MJ, Strom PB, Moriarty JL. Surgical repair of brachial plexus injury: a multinational survey of experienced peripheral nerve surgeons. J Neurosurg 2004;101:365-376.
10. Wilbourn AJ. Iatrogenic nerve injuries. Neurol Clin 1998;16:55-82.
11. Huehnergarth KV, Lipsky BA. Superior pulmonary sulcus tumor with Pancoast syndrome. Mayo Clin Proc 2004;79:1268.
12. England JD, Tiel RL. AAEM case report 33: costoclavicular mass syndrome. American Association of Electrodiagnostic Medicine. Muscle Nerve 1999;22:412-418.
13. Tsao BE, Wilbourn AJ. Infraclavicular brachial plexus injury following axillary regional block. Muscle Nerve 2004;30:44-48.
14. Weaver K, Kraft GH. Idiopathic shoulder girdle neuropathy. Phys Med Rehabil Clin North Am 2001;12:353-364.
15. van Alfen N, van Engelen BG. The clinical spectrum of neuralgic amyotrophy in 246 cases. Brain 2006;129(pt 2):438-450.
16. Park JK. Peripheral nerve tumors. In Samuels MA, Feske SK, eds. Office Practice of Neurology, 2nd ed. Philadelphia, Churchill Livingstone, 2003:1118-1121.
17. Pacelli J, Whitaker C. Brachial plexopathy due to malignant peripheral nerve sheath tumor in neurofibromatosis type 1: case report and subject review. Muscle Nerve 2006;33:697-700.
18. Dunteman ED. Levetiracetam as an adjunctive analgesic in neoplastic plexopathies: case series and commentary. J Pain Palliat Care Pharmacother 2005;19:35-43.
19. Carter GT. Rehabilitation management of peripheral neuropathy. Semin Neurol 2005;25:229-237.
20. Grossman JA, DiTaranto P, Yaylali I, et al. Shoulder function following late neurolysis and bypass grafting for upper brachial plexus birth injuries. J Hand Surg Br 2004;29:356-358.
21. Waters PM. Update on management of pediatric brachial plexus palsy. J Pediatr Orthop B 2005;14:233-244.
22. Bertelli JA, Ghizoni MF. Brachial plexus avulsion injury repairs with nerve transfers and nerve grafts directly implanted into the spinal cord yield partial recovery of shoulder and elbow movements. Neurosurgery 2003;52:1385-1389.
23. de Carvalho M. Reflex sympathetic dystrophy precipitated by brachial plexitis. Electromyogr Clin Neurophysiol 1998;38:459-461.

Plexopathy—Lumbosacral 135

Hope S. Hacker, MD, and John C. King, MD

Synonyms

Lumbosacral plexitis
Neuralgic amyotrophy of the lumbosacral plexus
Lumbosacral plexus neuropathy
Lumbosacral radiculoplexus neuropathy
Diabetic amyotrophy

ICD-9 Codes

353.1 Lumbosacral plexus lesions
353.8 Other nerve root and plexus disorders
353.9 Unspecified nerve root and plexus disorder
907.3 Late effects of injury to nerve root, spinal plexus, and other nerve of trunk
953.5 Injury to lumbosacral plexus
953.8 Injury to multiple sites of nerve roots and spinal plexus
953.9 Injury to nerve root and spinal plexus, unspecified site

DEFINITION

Lumbosacral plexopathy is an injury to or involvement of one or more nerves that combine to form or branch from the lumbosacral plexus. This involvement is distal to the root level. The lumbar plexus originates from the first, second, third, and fourth lumbar nerves (Fig. 135-1). The fourth lumbar nerve makes a contribution to both the lumbar and the sacral plexus. There is typically a small communication from the twelfth thoracic nerve as well. As in the brachial plexus, these nerve roots divide into the dorsal rami and the ventral rami as they exit through the intervertebral foramina. The dorsal or posterior rami innervate the paraspinal muscles and supply nearby cutaneous sensation. The ventral or anterior rami for the lumbar plexus form the motor and sensory nerves to the anterior and medial sides of the thigh and the sensation on the medial aspect of the leg and foot. The undivided anterior primary rami of the lumbar and sacral nerves also carry postganglionic sympathetic fibers that are mainly responsible for vasoregulation of the lower extremities. The branches of the lumbar plexus include the iliohypogastric, ilioinguinal, genitofemoral, femoral, lateral femoral cutaneous, and obturator nerves.[1] The lumbar portion of the plexus lies just anterior to the psoas muscle.[2]

The sacral plexus innervates the muscles of the buttocks, posterior thigh, and leg below the knee and the skin of the posterior thigh and leg, lateral leg, foot, and perineum. It is formed from the lumbosacral trunk to include L5 and a portion of L4 as well as the S1 to S3 (or S4) nerve roots (Fig. 135-2). The anterior primary rami of S2 and S3 nerve roots carry parasympathetic fibers that mainly control the urinary bladder and anal sphincters. The triangular sacral plexus lies on the anterior surface of the sacrum, in the immediate vicinity of the sacroiliac joint and lateral to the cervix or prostate.[1] The branches of the sacral plexus include the superior and inferior gluteal nerves, the posterior cutaneous nerves of the thigh, the lumbosacral trunk that becomes the sciatic nerve with both tibial and peroneal divisions, and the pudendal nerve.

Etiology

Lumbosacral plexopathy has been recognized as a clinical entity or complication in a variety of surgical procedures, trauma, and obstetric surgery or delivery and as a clinical finding or sequela in treatment of pelvic tumors.

Pelvic fractures or pelvic ring fractures have a high incidence in traumatic injuries.[3] Sacral fractures have typically been considered of secondary importance in conjunction with pelvic trauma.[4] However, sacral fractures have become recognized as an essential consideration in pelvic trauma because of their high association with lumbosacral nerve deficits. This can have a profound influence on prognosis and level of functional recovery.[3,5] The more common sacral fractures are typically the compression or avulsion fractures of the sacral ala, which can occur in lateral compression and anterior-posterior compression pelvic fractures.[6] Fractures of the sacral neuroforamina or midline sacral fractures may also occur. Fractures of the sacrum can increase the incidence of neurologic injury in pelvic trauma to between 34% and 50% because of its proximity to the sacral nerve roots.[6] The highest incidence of neurologic injury has been reported in transverse fractures. Compression, avulsion, and traction injuries of the lumbosacral nerves or plexus may play some role in the pathophysiologic

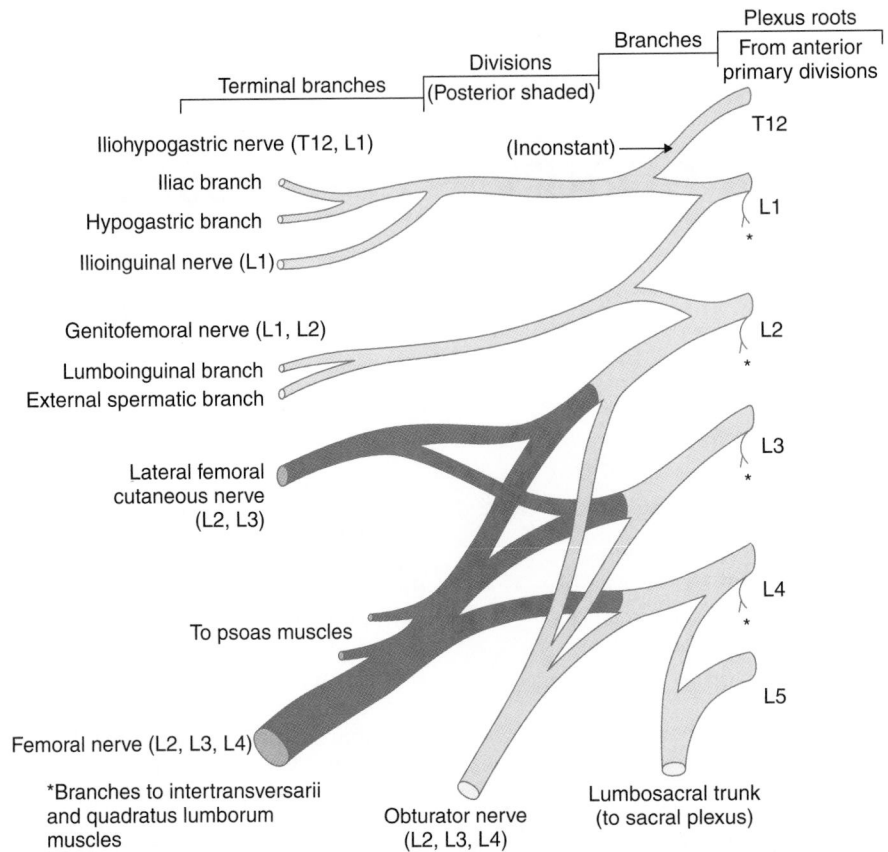

FIGURE 135-1. The lumbar plexus and its peripheral terminal branches. The shaded portions represent the posterior divisions of the ventral primary rami; those not shaded are either the ventral primary rami or their anterior branches. In this diagram, the nerve to the psoas major arises from the femoral nerve, as opposed to directly from the spinal nerve region. (Reprinted with permission from de Groot J, Chusid JG. Correlative Neuroanatomy, 21st ed. Norwalk, Conn, Appleton & Lange, 1991.)

process. It has been noted that midline sacral sagittal fractures have a significantly lower incidence of neurologic deficits, possibly because this type of fracture may protect the lumbosacral roots and plexuses from shear forces and compression.[6] Bowel and bladder injuries tend to occur in cases in which there is bilateral sacral root involvement. Sexual dysfunction has been documented in both bilateral and unilateral sacral injuries and pelvic trauma. Lumbosacral injuries are much more common in pelvic and sacral fractures but have been documented in acetabular fractures and midshaft femoral fractures as well.[3]

Gynecologic surgery is thought to be one of the most common causes of femoral nerve injury and lumbosacral plexus nerve injuries. Abdominal hysterectomy is the surgical procedure that has been most frequently implicated.[7,8] The second most common neuropathy documented after major gynecologic surgery is ilioinguinal or iliohypogastric nerve involvement. This has been noted especially with low transverse incisions.[9] The mechanisms of neurologic injury that have been established include improper placement or positioning of self-retaining or fixed retractors, incorrect positioning of the patient in lithotomy position preoperatively or prolonged lithotomy positioning without repositioning, and radical surgical dissection resulting in autonomic nerve disruption.[9] Lumbosacral injury has also been noted after appendectomy and inguinal herniorrhaphy. Patients who are thin, diabetic, or elderly are at increased risk for such an injury. Injury to the lumbosacral plexus with clinical findings occurs in up to 10% of hip replacement procedures, and injury that is subclinical but detected electromyographically occurred in up to 70% of patients.[10] Groin pain in the ilioinguinal region is frequent after herniorrhaphy. A review of 30 patients showed that subclinical motor involvement of the genitofemoral nerve is common after inguinal herniorrhaphy and can be documented by electrophysiologic testing.[11] Lateral femoral cutaneous nerve lesions have also been noted as a complication of pelvic surgery after an ilioinguinal approach.[12]

Trauma is a common cause of retroperitoneal hemorrhage, which can injure the lumbosacral plexus. In individuals receiving anticoagulant therapy or with acquired or congenital coagulopathies, hemorrhage may occur with no precipitating injury.[13,14] Retroperitoneal hematoma has also been documented as a rare but potentially serious complication after cardiac catheterization.[15,16] In a review of 9585 femoral artery catheterizations, a reported retroperitoneal hematoma rate of 0.5% occurred. In patients undergoing stent placement, there was evidence of lumbar plexopathy involving the femoral, obturator, and lateral femoral cutaneous nerves, and the condition was typically completely reversible.[17,18] A

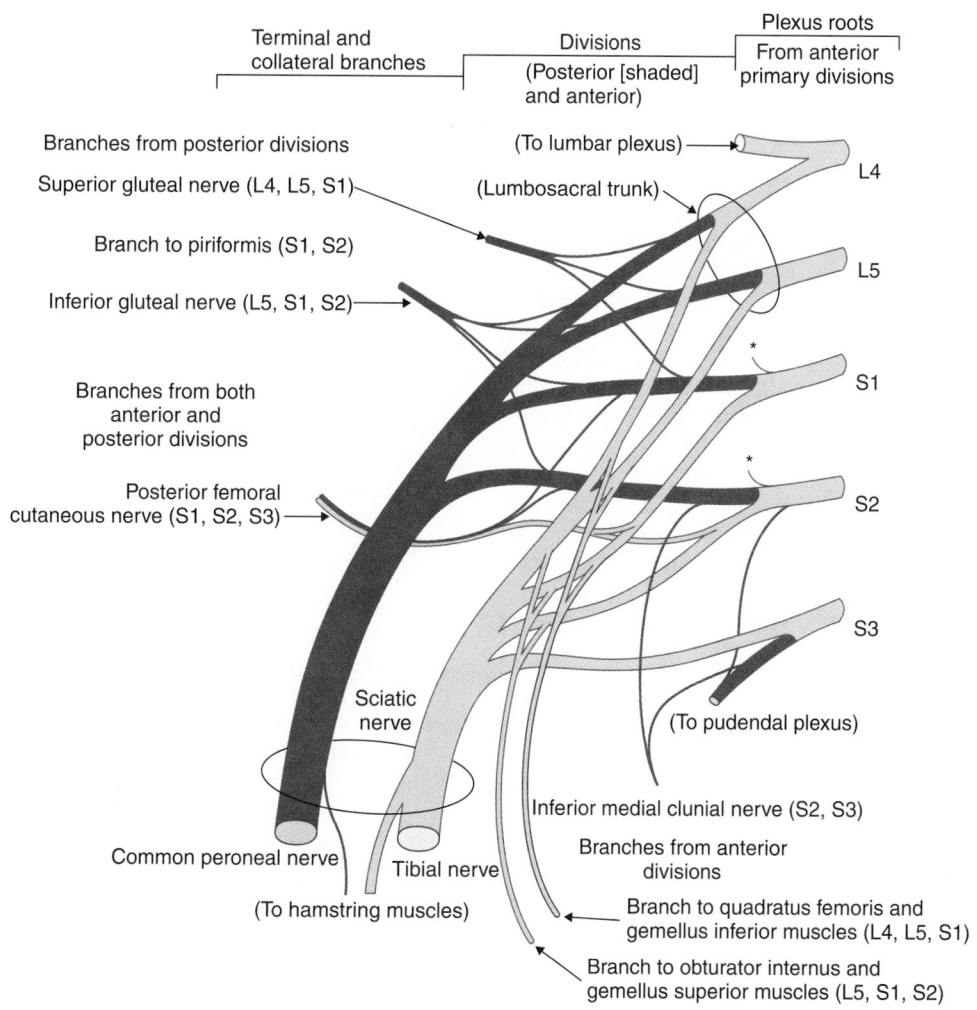

Terminal and collateral branches

Divisions (Posterior [shaded] and anterior)

Plexus roots From anterior primary divisions

Branches from posterior divisions

Superior gluteal nerve (L4, L5, S1)

Branch to piriformis (S1, S2)

Inferior gluteal nerve (L5, S1, S2)

Branches from both anterior and posterior divisions

Posterior femoral cutaneous nerve (S1, S2, S3)

(To lumbar plexus)

(Lumbosacral trunk)

L4

L5

S1

S2

S3

Sciatic nerve

(To pudendal plexus)

Common peroneal nerve

Tibial nerve

(To hamstring muscles)

Inferior medial clunial nerve (S2, S3)

Branches from anterior divisions

Branch to quadratus femoris and gemellus inferior muscles (L4, L5, S1)

Branch to obturator internus and gemellus superior muscles (L5, S1, S2)

FIGURE 135-2. Schematic representation of the sacral plexus. The shaded portions signify the posterior divisions of the ventral primary rami; the unshaded aspects are the anterior branches of the ventral primary rami. (Reprinted with permission from de Groot J, Chausid JG. Correlative Neuroanatomy, 21st ed. Norwalk, Conn, Appleton & Lange, 1991.)

delay in recognition of this complication may lead to delayed treatment and may have a significant effect on recovery. Femoral vein catheterization for dialysis has also been documented as a cause of hemorrhagic complications and retroperitoneal hemorrhage.[19]

The lumbosacral plexus may be compressed as a complication of labor and delivery. The incidence of neurologic injury that is reported in the literature for postpartum sensory and motor dysfunction is relatively low at 0.008% to 0.5%.[20,21] In 6000 women evaluated for prospective symptoms of neurologic injury in the lumbosacral spine or lower extremity the day after delivery, an incidence of 0.92% was reported. Factors associated with nerve injury were nulliparity and a prolonged second stage of labor; assisted vacuum or forceps vaginal delivery also had some positive association.[21] Women with nerve injury spent more time pushing in the semi-Fowler lithotomy position. Lateral femoral cutaneous neuropathies were the most common neurologic finding, followed by femoral neuropathy. Radiculopathies at L4, L5, or S1 were also noted.[22] During the second stage of labor, direct pressure of the fetal head may com-

press the lumbosacral plexus against the pelvic rim, which may result in nerve injury.[22,23] Footdrop during the third trimester of pregnancy or during labor has been documented in the literature as well.[24]

Both pelvic malignant neoplasms and treatment of pelvic tumors can damage the lumbosacral plexus. Lumbosacral radiculopathy is most common with gynecologic tumors, sarcomas, and lymphomas. Neoplastic plexopathy is characterized by severe and unrelenting pain, typically followed by weakness and sensory disturbances.[25] Pelvic radiation therapy may cause a delayed lumbosacral plexopathy that can occur 3 months to 22 years after completion of treatment; the median amount of time from the completion of treatment to onset of symptoms is about 5 years.[26-28] Chemotherapeutic agents can also cause symptoms of lumbosacral radiculopathy. Cisplatin, 5-fluorouracil, mitomycin C, and bleomycin have been implicated in the majority of these plexopathies.[2]

Metastatic or tumor extension into the lumbosacral plexus and malignant psoas syndrome have been described in the literature. Malignant psoas syndrome was first reported in 1990. It is characterized by proximal lumbosacral plexopathy, painful fixed flexion of the ipsilateral hip, and radiologic or pathologic evidence of ipsilateral psoas major muscle malignant involvement.[2]

Diabetic and nondiabetic lumbosacral radiculoplexus neuropathies have been documented in the literature. Diabetic lumbosacral radiculoplexus neuropathy is a subacute, painful asymmetric lower limb neuropathy that is associated with significant weight loss (at least 10 pounds), type 2 diabetes mellitus, and relatively recent diagnosis of diabetes with relatively good glucose control.[29] The underlying pathophysiologic mechanism is thought to be immune mediated with microvasculitis of the nerve rather than a metabolic issue caused by diabetes; nondiabetic lumbosacral radiculoplexus neuropathy has also been documented with similar clinical and pathophysiologic features.[29-33] The similar clinical symptoms, findings, and response to treatment suggest that the metabolic changes from diabetes may not be the cause of these symptoms, although impaired glucose tolerance has been noted in nondiabetic lumbosacral radiculoplexus neuropathy.[31]

The disease typically starts as an identifiable onset of asymmetric lower extremity symptoms that most typically involve the thigh and hip with pain that progresses to include weakness, which then becomes the main disabling symptom. In a few months, this usually evolves into bilateral symmetric weakness and pain with distal as well as proximal involvement. Whereas motor findings are prominent, sensory and autonomic nerves have also been shown to be involved.[29]

Gunshot wounds and motor vehicle accidents have long been recognized as a potential cause of lumbosacral plexus injuries. Electrodiagnostic studies have documented neurapraxia, axonotmesis, and neurotmesis as types of nerve injuries identified after gunshot wounds or motor vehicle accident.[34] In a retrospective comparison of patterns of lumbosacral plexus injury in motor vehicle crashes and gunshot wounds, individuals with gunshot wounds had a greater chance of involvement of the upper portion of the plexus in comparison to individuals who sustained a motor vehicle crash. Lower plexus injuries were more common in victims of motor vehicle accidents as opposed to gunshot wounds.[35]

Vascular causes of lumbosacral plexopathies may include diabetic amyotrophy and connective tissue diseases that may be associated with vasculitis, such as systemic lupus erythematosus, rheumatoid arthritis, and polyarteritis nodosa.[36] If a vascular cause is suspected, the aorta and iliac vessels must be evaluated for disease or occlusion.[37-39] The lumbosacral plexus receives its vascular supply from the aorta and the common iliac vessels, which then branch into the femoral artery.

SYMPTOMS

Plexopathies may vary considerably in their presentation, depending on the location and degree of involvement. A plexopathy involving the upper roots may primarily be manifested by femoral and obturator nerve symptoms. Femoral nerve injury typically is manifested with iliopsoas or quadriceps weakness, and there may be sensory deficits over the anterior and medial thigh as well as the anterior medial aspect of the leg.[7] Obturator injury has also been seen in upper plexus injuries with weakness of the hip adductors[21] and sensory changes in the upper medial thigh. Sensory changes are often seen in upper plexus injuries. Lateral femoral cutaneous neuropathy usually involves loss of sensation or dysesthesias to the anterolateral thigh. The genitofemoral nerve is a direct branch of the upper lumbar plexus (L1, L2) and may be involved with removal of large pelvic masses or lymph node biopsy[7]; sensory changes are relatively limited, with decreased sensation or paresthesias in the mons and labia majora. Abdominal wall surgical sites below the level of the anterior superior iliac spine may have the potential for ilioinguinal or iliohypogastric nerve involvement. Damage to these sensory nerves may have burning pain in the lower abdomen, upper medial thigh, or pelvic area and altered sensation in the inguinal area.[9] Clinical findings suggestive of this include hip flexion and forward flexion of the trunk and increased pain with coughing or sneezing. Local nerve block usually alleviates the pain. It is thought that the incidence of iliohypogastric and ilioinguinal injuries is underestimated in the literature because of the lack of recognition and reporting by physicians and patients.[9]

Lumbosacral plexopathy often begins with leg pain radiating to the low back and buttocks and progressing posterolaterally down the leg, soon followed by symptoms of numbness and weakness. Lumbosacral plexus injuries are often associated with a footdrop and sensory changes to the top of the foot. Symptoms of incontinence or sexual dysfunction are more likely to be seen with bilateral plexus involvement.[5,25]

PHYSICAL EXAMINATION

Clinical examination to evaluate for a lumbosacral plexopathy involves neurologic assessment to include motor strength testing, sensory testing, muscle stretch reflexes, tone, and bowel and bladder function. The pattern of sensory loss, asymmetric reflexes, or weakness is suggestive of multiple nerve or root level involvement. It is often important to differentiate this from single root level involvement, suggesting a radiculopathy or more generalized nerve changes consistent with peripheral neuropathy. Edema or swelling in one lower extremity may be suggestive of a pelvic mass or lumbosacral plexus involvement rather than a more global peripheral neuropathy[38] or possible retroperitoneal hematoma or pelvic malignant neoplasm.[2]

The lumbosacral plexus is more commonly evaluated in routine clinical practice, and it is important to look for a pattern of sensory loss or weakness involving more than one nerve root level. Footdrop or dorsiflexion weakness may be a sign of peroneal neuropathy, L5 radiculopathy, or lumbosacral plexus involvement.

Plantar flexion weakness is suggestive of tibial nerve or S1 level involvement. The Achilles tendon reflex may be diminished or absent. An upper lumbar plexopathy involving L3 or L4 is manifested by weakness of the hip flexors and knee extensors. Patellar tendon reflex may be diminished or absent.

FUNCTIONAL LIMITATIONS

Functional limitations depend on which portions of the lumbar or lumbosacral plexus have been injured and the severity of the injury. Patients frequently present with some type of difficulty with mobility and ambulation. Activities such as transferring from one surface to another, rising from a chair, ambulation, grooming, bathing, dressing, and cooking may potentially be affected. These functional limitations may have far-reaching consequences on one's ability to live independently and to continue in one's chosen vocation.

DIAGNOSTIC STUDIES

Electrodiagnostic Testing

The electrodiagnostic evaluation of lumbosacral plexopathy is one of the most effective tools available for differentiation of a specific pattern and severity of nerve involvement. Guided by a focused history and physical examination, the skilled electromyographer can use testing of both proximal and distal sensory and motor nerves as well as muscle needle examination to determine whether there is radicular involvement, lumbar or lumbosacral plexus involvement with multiple nerves involved but no paraspinal involvement, or a more generalized picture consistent with a peripheral neuropathy.

Testing for upper lumbar plexopathy may include lateral femoral cutaneous nerve, saphenous nerve, posterior femoral cutaneous sensory nerve, and femoral motor nerve studies. Side-to-side comparison is recommended to assess for asymmetry in these technically challenging studies. Sensory involvement without motor involvement suggests a lesion distal to the dorsal root ganglion. Studies to evaluate the lumbosacral plexus and lumbosacral roots include sural and superficial peroneal sensory studies, H reflex, and peroneal and tibial motor conduction studies. Depending on the timing of the injury, nerve conduction studies can demonstrate a decrease in amplitude for the sensory nerve action potentials starting at 5 to 6 days and for compound muscle action potentials starting at 2 to 4 days.[35]

The needle electromyographic examination is likely to be the most useful electrodiagnostic technique.[35] Careful examination of proximal and distal musculature demonstrates a pattern of muscle membrane instability in more than one peripheral nerve from different root levels without involvement of the paraspinal muscles. The pattern of muscle membrane instability indicates whether the injury appears to be a neurapraxia with conduction block, axonotmesis, or neurotmesis with

wallerian degeneration and poor prognosis for reinnervation. Increased insertional activity may be seen on rest activity in the involved musculature after 7 to 8 days, with positive waves and fibrillations starting at 10 to 30 days but being most prominent at 21 to 30 days after injury.[35] Decreased recruitment is noted immediately after injury, and this may be the only change on needle electromyographic examination in the first few days if the nerve is partially intact.

Imaging Studies

Computed tomography can be useful in determining the presence of a structural mass in the pelvic region. Computed tomographic scans, along with abdominal ultrasonography, may be used to diagnose a retroperitoneal hemorrhage. Both computed tomographic scanning and magnetic resonance imaging have been used to evaluate the lumbosacral plexus. Magnetic resonance imaging has been found to be more sensitive than computed tomography for diagnosis of cancer-related lumbosacral plexopathy.[40] High-resolution magnetic resonance neurography with T1-weighted fast spin echo and fat-saturated T2-weighted fast spin echo has been used to study the lumbosacral plexus and the sciatic nerve.[41] Plain radiographs are useful as a screening tool for suspected aneurysms or malignant disease.

Differential Diagnosis

Spinal cord injury

Cauda equina injury

Lumbosacral nerve root injury

Multiple peripheral nerve injuries

Anterior horn cell diseases

Myopathies

Occlusion of the aorta

TREATMENT

Initial

Initial treatment is based on both the presenting symptoms and the cause of the lumbosacral plexopathy. For example, many obstetric lumbosacral plexus symptoms are treated conservatively. Pelvic masses or a retroperitoneal hemorrhage may require surgical or medical intervention. Neoplastic or radiation-based plexopathy symptoms may need specific medical management, chemotherapy, or possibly surgery. If edema control is necessary, leg elevation and compressive stockings may be of some benefit. Medication for neuropathic pain might include gabapentin, duloxetine, or pregabalin. Tricyclic antidepressants may also be helpful. Opioids and nonsteroidal anti-inflammatory drugs may also provide pain relief. Use of nonsteroidal anti-inflammatory drugs is contraindicated, however, when hemorrhage is suspected. Controlled trials with immune modulation therapies are currently being evaluated for both diabetic and nondiabetic lumbosacral radiculoplexus neuropathies.[29,33] It is not clear at this time whether immunotherapy is of benefit in diabetic lumbosacral radiculoplexus neuropathy.

Rehabilitation

Rehabilitation aims to maximize mobility and functional independence. The goals of rehabilitation are preservation of joint range of motion and flexibility, joint protection, and pain management; these goals depend on a good physical examination to determine what neurologic and functional deficits are present.

One of the primary rehabilitation concerns in an individual with nerve involvement in the lumbar or lumbosacral plexus is safe mobility and ambulation. The patient should be evaluated for the need for an assistive device, such as a cane or a walker, with ambulation. Energy conservation techniques and care of insensate feet are key treatment tools. Symptoms of lumbosacral plexopathy may be subtle and may be difficult to appreciate in a clinical setting. Physicians need to address potentially sensitive issues such as work limitations, sexual functioning, and sensory changes in the pelvic and inguinal areas.

Procedures

Sympathetic nerve blocks and chemodenervation have both been used to ameliorate pain. This can be both diagnostic and treatment oriented in helping to confirm the suspected diagnosis. Sacral nerve stimulation has been evaluated for adjunctive treatment of lumbosacral plexopathy, but further research is required for its effectiveness to be determined.[13]

Surgery

Lumbosacral plexus injuries associated with pelvic or sacral fractures or with gynecologic surgery are often treated conservatively,[7] although it has been documented that long-term sequelae can occur. Nerve reconstruction including nerve grafting has been reported in an attempt to restore some lower extremity function.[42] Microsurgical treatment of lumbosacral plexopathies for neurolysis and nerve grafting has been used in the retroperitoneal space. In a series of 15 cases, the muscles that benefited the most from surgery were the gluteal and femoral innervated muscles. The more distal musculature did not seem to show much benefit.[43] Whereas motor improvement is an important consideration, pain is often extremely debilitating in patients with a lumbosacral plexopathy and may block or limit rehabilitation. Pain relief is one of the major goals for surgical intervention. Surgical resection of a tumor may also be indicated in certain cases with lumbosacral plexopathy.[25]

POTENTIAL DISEASE COMPLICATIONS

Potential complications of lumbosacral plexopathy include joint contractures, limited mobility, weakness, falls secondary to weakness or sensory loss, bowel or bladder incontinence, diminished or absent sensation, skin breakdown, sexual dysfunction, and significant decrease in functional independence from these complications.

POTENTIAL TREATMENT COMPLICATIONS

Treatment complications may include skin breakdown under orthoses and increased weakness if the rehabilitation program is too aggressive. Medication side effects are dizziness, somnolence, gastrointestinal irritation, and ataxia due to anticonvulsants; dry mouth, urinary retention, and atrioventricular conduction block due to tricyclic antidepressants; and dependence, dizziness, somnolence, and constipation due to opioid pain medications. Nonsteroidal anti-inflammatory drugs and analgesics can also have significant side effects that affect the gastrointestinal and renal systems as well as the liver.

References

1. Moore KL, Dalley AF, eds. Clinically Oriented Anatomy, 4th ed. Philadelphia, Lippincott Williams & Wilkins, 1999.
2. Agar M, Broadbent A, Chye R. The management of malignant psoas syndrome: case reports and literature review. J Pain Symptom Manage 2004;28:282-293.
3. Kutsy RL, Robinson LR, Routt ML. Lumbosacral plexopathy in pelvic trauma. Muscle Nerve 2000;23:1757-1760.
4. Medelman JP. Fractures of the sacrum: their incidence in fractures of the pelvis. Am J Roentgenol Radium Ther Nucl Med 1939;42:100-103.
5. Gibbons KJ, Soloniuk DS, Razack N. Neurological injury and patterns of sacral fractures. J Neurosurg 1990;72:889-893.
6. Bellabarba C, Stewart JD, Ricci WM, et al. Midline sagittal sacral fractures in anterior-posterior compression pelvic ring injuries. J Orthop Trauma 2003;17:32-37.
7. Irvin W, Andersen W, Taylor P, et al. Minimizing the risk of neurologic injury in gynecologic surgery. Obstet Gynecol 2004;103:374-382.
8. Fardin P, Benettello P, Negrin P. Iatrogenic femoral neuropathy. Considerations on its prognosis. Electromyogr Clin Neurophysiol 1980;20:153-155.
9. Whiteside JL, Barber MD, Walters MD, et al. Anatomy of ilioinguinal and iliohypogastric nerves in relation to trocar placement and low transverse incisions. Am J Obstet Gynecol 2003;189:1574-1578; discussion 1578.
10. Solheim LF, Hagen R. Femoral and sciatic neuropathies after total hip arthroplasty. Acta Orthop Scand 1980;51:531-534.
11. Bademkiran F, Tataroglu C, Ozdedeli K, et al. Electrophysiological evaluation of the genitofemoral nerve in patients with inguinal hernia. Muscle Nerve 2005;32:600-604.
12. de Ridder VA, de Lange S, Popta JV. Anatomical variations of the lateral femoral cutaneous nerve and the consequences for surgery. J Orthop Trauma 1999;13:207-211.
13. Chad DA, Bradley WG. Lumbosacral plexopathy. Semin Neurol 1987;7:97-107.
14. Rajashekhar RP, Herbison GJ. Lumbosacral plexopathy caused by retroperitoneal hemorrhage: report of two cases. Arch Phys Med Rehabil 1974;55:91-93.
15. Ozcakar L, Sivri A, Aydinli M, et al. Lumbosacral plexopathy as the harbinger of a silent retroperitoneal hematoma. South Med J 2003;96:109-110.

16. Kent KC, Moscucci M, Mansour KA, et al. Retroperitoneal hematoma after cardiac catheterization: prevalence, risk factors, and optimal management. J Vasc Surg 1994;20:905-910; discussion 910-913.
17. Lumsden AB, Miller JM, Kosinski AS, et al. A prospective evaluation of surgically treated groin complications following percutaneous cardiac procedures. Am Surg 1994;60:132-137.
18. Kent KC, Moscucci M, Gallagher SG, et al. Neuropathy after cardiac catheterization: incidence, clinical patterns, and long-term outcome. J Vasc Surg 1994;19:1008-1013; discussion 1013-1014.
19. Kaymak B, Ozcakar L, Cetin A, et al. Bilateral lumbosacral plexopathy after femoral vein dialysis: synopsis of a case. Joint Bone Spine 2004;71:347-348.
20. Holdcroft A, Gibberd FB, Hargrove RL, et al. Neurological complications associated with pregnancy. Br J Anaesth 1995;75:522-526.
21. Wong CA, Scavone BM, Dugan S, et al. Incidence of postpartum lumbosacral spine and lower extremity nerve injuries. Obstet Gynecol 2003;101:279-288.
22. Dawson DM, Krarup C. Perioperative nerve lesions. Arch Neurol 1989;46:1355-1360.
23. Feasby TE, Burton SR, Hahn AF. Obstetrical lumbosacral plexus injury. Muscle Nerve 1992;15:937-940.
24. Oei SG. Footdrop during pregnancy or labor due to obstetrical lumbosacral plexopathy [comment on Ned Tijdschr Geneeskd 2002;146:31-34]. Ned Tijdschr Geneeskd 2002;146:739-740; author reply 740.
25. Jaeckle KA. Neurological manifestations of neoplastic and radiation-induced plexopathies. Semin Neurol 2004;24:385-393.
26. Georgiou A, Grigsby PW, Perez CA. Radiation induced lumbosacral plexopathy in gynecologic tumors: clinical findings and dosimetric analysis. Int J Radiat Oncol Biol Phys 1993;26:479-482.
27. Taphoorn MJB, Bromberg JEC. Neurological effects of therapeutic irradiation. Continuum: Lifelong Learning in Neurology. Neuro-Oncology 2005;11:93-115.
28. Thomas JE, Cascino TL, Earle JD. Differential diagnosis between radiation and tumor plexopathy of the pelvis. Neurology 1985;35:1-7.
29. Fann A. Plexopathy—lumbosacral. In Frontera WR, Silver JK, eds. Essentials of Physical Medicine and Rehabilitation. Philadelphia, Hanley & Belfus, 2001:671.
30. Dyck PJB, Windebank AJ. Diabetic and nondiabetic lumbosacral radiculoplexus neuropathies: new insights into pathophysiology and treatment. Muscle Nerve 2002;25:477-491.
31. Dyck PJB, Norell JE, Dyck PJ. Non-diabetic lumbosacral radiculoplexus neuropathy: natural history, outcome and comparison with the diabetic variety. Brain 2001;124:1197-1207.
32. Kelkar P, Hammer-White S. Impaired glucose tolerance in non-diabetic lumbosacral radiculoplexus neuropathy [letter]. Muscle Nerve 2005;31:273-274.
33. Zochodne DW, Isaac D, Jones C. Failure of immunotherapy to prevent, arrest, or reverse diabetic lumbosacral plexopathy. Acta Neurol Scand 2003;107:299-301.
34. Musaev AV, Guseinova SG. Gunshot injuries of peripheral nervous system: the questions of classification and diagnostics [in Russian]. Zh Nevrol Psikhiatr Im S S Korsakova 2004;104:10-17.
35. Chiou-Tan FY, Kemp K, Elfenbaum M, et al. Lumbosacral plexopathy in gunshot wounds and motor vehicle accidents: comparison of electrophysiologic findings. Am J Phys Med Rehabil 2001;80:280-285.
36. Dumitru D, Zwarts MJ. Lumbosacral plexopathies and proximal mononeuropathies. In Dumitru D, Amato A, Zwarts M, eds. Electrodiagnostic Medicine, 2nd ed. Philadelphia, Hanley & Belfus, 2002:777-836.
37. van Alfen N, van Engelen BG. Lumbosacral plexus neuropathy: a case report and review of the literature. Clin Neurol Neurosurg 1997;99:138-141.
38. Frontera W, Silver JK, eds. Essentials of Physical Medicine and Rehabilitation. Philadelphia, Hanley & Belfus, 2001:671-677.
39. Larson WL, Wald JJ. Foot drop as a harbinger of aortic occlusion. Muscle Nerve 1995;18:899-903.
40. Taylor BV, Kimmel DW, Krecke KN, et al. Magnetic resonance imaging in cancer-related lumbosacral plexopathy. Mayo Clin Proc 1997;72:823-829.
41. Moore KR, Tsuruda JS, Dailey AT. The value of MR neurography for evaluating extraspinal neuropathic leg pain: a pictorial essay. Am J Neuroradiol 2001;22:786-794.
42. Tung TH, Martin DZ, Novak CB, et al. Nerve reconstruction in lumbosacral plexopathy. Case report and review of the literature. J Neurosurg 2005;102(Suppl):86-91.
43. Alexandre A, Coro L, Azuelos A. Microsurgical treatment of lumbosacral plexus injuries [abstract]. Acta Neurochir Suppl 2005;92:53-59.

Polytrauma Rehabilitation 136

Steven G. Scott, DO, Joel D. Scholten, MD, Gail A. Latlief, DO,
Faiza Humayun, MD, Heather G. Belanger, PhD,
and Rodney D. Vanderploeg, PhD

Synonyms

Blast injury
Multiple injuries
Multiple trauma

ICD-9 Codes

344.0	Quadriplegia and quadriparesis
344.1	Paraplegia
451.1	Phlebitis and thrombophlebitis of deep vessels of lower extremities
784.0	Headache
850	Concussion
854.0	Intracranial injury of other and unspecified nature without mention of open intracranial wound
854.1	Intracranial injury of other and unspecified nature with open intracranial wound
886	Traumatic amputation of other finger(s) (complete) (partial)
887	Traumatic amputation of arm and hand (complete) (partial)
895	Traumatic amputation of toe(s) (complete) (partial)
896	Traumatic amputation of foot (complete) (partial)
897	Traumatic amputation of leg(s) (complete) (partial)
905.0	Late effect of traumatic amputation
906.5	Late effect of burn of eye, face, head, and neck
906.6	Late effect of burn of wrist and hand
906.7	Late effect of burn of other extremities
906.8	Late effect of burn of unspecified site
907.0	Late effect of intracranial injury without mention of skull fracture
997.63	Infection (chronic)
V52	Fitting and adjustment of prosthetic device and implant

DEFINITION

Polytrauma literally means injury to multiple parts secondary to trauma. Because injury of multiple body parts or systems most typically includes traumatic brain injury, polytrauma can be defined in practice as injury to the brain in addition to other body parts or systems, resulting in physical, cognitive, psychological, or psychosocial impairments and functional disability. Injury to the brain is the impairment that typically guides the course of rehabilitation.[1,2] Other common disabling conditions include traumatic amputation, auditory and visual impairments, spinal cord injury, post-traumatic stress disorder, and other mental health disorders.

Because of recent military conflicts in the world (e.g., Iraq) as well as increasing terrorist and associated violence, the likelihood of polytraumatic injury is increasing for both military personnel and civilians. Polytrauma is frequently caused by exposure to high-energy blasts or explosions.[3] Currently, more than half of all combat injuries are the result of explosive munitions.[4] Blast-related injuries are divided into four categories: primary, secondary, tertiary, and quaternary or miscellaneous injuries. Individuals may sustain multiple injuries from one or more of these mechanisms. Primary blast injuries are caused by barotrauma—overpressurization from the "blast wave" followed by underpressurization; organ systems affected contain gas or have a gas-fluid interface (e.g., ears, lungs, bowel). Secondary blast injuries occur by fragments and other penetrating metal projectiles, which can cause soft tissue trauma and head injuries. Contamination from these fragments can also cause additional damage or infections. Tertiary blast injuries result from displacement of the whole body by combined pressure loads. Finally, there are miscellaneous blast-related injuries, such as burns and crush injuries from collapsed structures and displaced heavy objects.[5] Although explosions are a common military or terrorist cause of polytrauma, serious accidents like train derailments, severe motor vehicle accidents, and plane crashes can also result in polytrauma.

Polytrauma war-related injuries as well as civilian-based injuries occur more frequently in the younger population and predominantly in males. In noncombat conditions, active-duty men are 2.5 times more likely to have a traumatic brain injury. Statistics of the frequency of polytrauma injuries are not available at this time.[5,6]

SYMPTOMS

Most polytrauma patients present with obvious physical traumas or injuries from blasts with symptoms related to soft tissue or orthopedic injuries. Some symptoms related to traumatic brain injury, the signature wound of polytrauma, are immediately recognized; others are more subtle and may go unrecognized.[7] Symptoms related to damaged sensory organs, nervous system, and internal structures may be readily apparent or may be difficult to diagnose. Symptoms related to traumatic brain injury include cognitive, emotional, and physical symptoms (see Chapter 153).

Cognitive or mental symptoms may include difficulties with speech, thinking, memory, concentration, and judgment. Irritability, anxiety, depression, and emotional lability are common emotional sequelae. Physical symptoms include obvious issues, such as motor and sensory deficits, and more subtle symptoms, such as headache, dizziness, and fatigue. Balance and loss of equilibrium are common and may be overlooked.[8] There is frequently weakness and motor incoordination. Spasticity can also occur. Pain is common and arises from multiple causes, complicating pain management. Hearing loss with tinnitus is a hallmark symptom of blast-related polytrauma injuries. Vision is frequently impaired with visual field loss or unilateral blindness as a result of shrapnel or other penetrating injuries to the eye or brain. Almost half of polytrauma patients have communication problems, such as dysarthria and aphasia. Bladder and bowel dysfunction can affect a significant number of patients.

PHYSICAL EXAMINATION

A thorough physical examination is essential in the evaluation of a patient who has sustained polytrauma. A mechanism of injury–directed review of systems is suggested.[5] If the mechanism of injury is blast related, the examination emphasizes testing for typical sequelae. A thorough neurologic examination including assessment of cranial nerves, motor strength, sensation, and coordination and neuropsychological evaluation is mandatory.

Multiple specialty consultants are frequently needed to help in the assessment. Neuro-ophthalmologists, audiologists, and otolaryngologists are consulted to document functioning of specific senses. Wound specialists and plastic surgeons are also often needed to assist in evaluation of open wounds, burns, and skin grafts. In addition, special attention is paid to the assessment of skin and soft tissue for retained shrapnel.

FUNCTIONAL LIMITATIONS

Polytrauma patients have multiple functional limitations based on the severity and number of physical and cognitive impairments. Hearing and visual field deficits affect everyday life functions and can make educational and vocational goals difficult to achieve. Lower extremity muscle weakness often impairs ambulation and creates a safety risk from falls. Upper extremity weakness and spasticity impair the patient's ability to do everyday activities such as dressing, hygiene, and handwriting. Cognitive deficits affect the ability to work and to perform roles related to parenting and living independently.

Particularly in the early phase of recovery, some patients may require continuous surveillance to prevent wandering; chronologically later, driving can be achieved in some patients, but with modifications. Many will have social and relational problems. Traumatic brain injury, stress, and mental health–related issues predispose patients to depression, anger, and mood swings. Those with head injuries may experience significant personality changes, affecting their relationships.

DIAGNOSTIC STUDIES
Imaging Studies

Because of the complex nature of injuries, several different imaging modalities are used to assess the polytrauma patient. In general, central nervous system injury is assessed by a combination of computed tomography and magnetic resonance imaging. Because of retained ferrous shrapnel, magnetic resonance imaging may not be possible. Post-traumatic encephalomalacia, hydrocephalus, intracranial hemorrhage, diffuse axonal injury, cerebral contusions, mass effect, and degree of atrophy can be assessed by routine magnetic resonance or computed tomographic imaging of the brain. The same diagnostic studies can be applied to the spinal cord to determine an anatomic level of injury versus compression myelopathy.

Routine radiographs are often sufficient to assess for skeletal injuries and intra-thoracic and intra-abdominal disease. However, computed tomography can be used when more detailed examination is necessary. Bone scan is particularly useful for assessment of heterotopic ossification or recent injury or infection that is not readily apparent on radiographic examination.

Electrodiagnostics

Patients with multiple trauma often sustain damage to the peripheral nervous system. A review of 33 active-duty patients admitted to the Tampa Polytrauma Rehabilitation Center revealed multiple cases of plexopathies, single-nerve injuries, and multiple-nerve injuries related to blasts, penetrating wounds, crush injuries, and motor vehicle collisions.[9] Electromyography and nerve conduction studies should be used whenever a peripheral nerve injury is suspected.

In addition, electroencephalography is a useful tool in diagnosis of post-traumatic epilepsy or encephalopathy.

Vascular Studies

Thromboembolic disease is an unfortunate consequence of polytrauma and subsequent immobility after a blast injury. Venous Doppler ultrasonography is frequently employed to detect deep venous thrombosis in the extremities. More proximal testing can be done by computed tomographic angiography.

Arterial dissection has also been documented to occur secondary to blast. Traditional angiography and magnetic resonance angiography are both useful to explore the extent of dissection and superimposed thrombus after traumatic dissection.

Functional Testing

Quantitative gait analysis is useful in objective documentation of walking ability as well as in the identification of the underlying causes of walking abnormalities. It is helpful in determining the best course of treatment in patients with brain injury or neuromuscular injury.

Neuropsychological and Psychological Evaluations

A comprehensive battery of neuropsychological and psychological tests is necessary to determine the full spectrum of cognitive and psychological sequelae from polytrauma injuries. This is typically completed once the person is medically stable, in an acute rehabilitation program, and out of any postinjury confusional state such as post-traumatic amnesia. Evaluations may be repeated to address different clinical questions during the course of recovery. Initially, assessment helps identify cognitive and emotional impairments that should be a focus of treatment. Repeated evaluations may be useful in making decisions about additional treatment needs, residential placement independence capacity, and future vocational or educational endeavors.

TREATMENT

Initial

The initial treatment of soldiers wounded in war or of civilians injured in serious accidents is predominantly surgical. In the case of both civilian and war-related injuries, dramatic improvement in life expectancy has been attained by highly skilled emergency and surgical intervention; in the war-related injuries, this includes forward military surgical teams and then rapid evacuation to the continental United States. Massive quantities of blood products are often required during resuscitation of patients sustaining polytrauma in a combat situation. The concept of "hypotensive resuscitation" has now regained favor in the field. The combat wounded receive blood and blood products at a rate to keep a palpable distal radial pulse and systolic blood pressure at approximately 90 mm Hg.[10] This is thought to improve outcomes by preserving intravascular volume and diminishing risk of clot disruption, reducing dilutional coagulopathy, and minimizing hypothermia.[11] Serial abdominal closure is frequently used to treat patients with abdominal wounds in theater. Gore-Tex mesh is implanted and the abdomen is closed in several separate procedures, allowing the abdomen to remain decompressed and to protect the intra-abdominal components. This in turn allows earlier rehabilitation.[12]

Patients who may have sustained crush injuries in war and elsewhere may require fasciotomies because of

Differential Diagnosis

Conversion disorder

Somatoform disorder

Malingering

Some potential diagnoses are actually the traumas or injuries of polytrauma:

Dementia or cognitive disorder NOS

Normal pressure hydrocephalus

Toxic exposure

Fibromyalgia

Mycobacterial infection

Mycoplasmal infection

Infectious disease

Drug and alcohol abuse

Medication side effects

Others are potential differential diagnoses:

Progressive dementias

Sleep apnea

Multiple sclerosis

Neoplasms

Autoimmune disease (e.g., rheumatoid, lupus, vasculitis)

Other infectious diseases (Lyme disease, syphilis, poliomyelitis, human immunodeficiency virus infection, Epstein-Barr virus infection)

Differential diagnosis for patients sustaining polytrauma injuries is complex for seemingly simple problems. Even the cause of the injury is frequently debated. For example, brain injury can be caused by primary, secondary, and tertiary blast injuries or a combination of the three. A broad differential should be included when any problem with polytrauma patients is considered. The clinician must maintain a high index of suspicion for possible central nervous system infection when patients with a history of penetrating head injury present with such vague complaints as confusion, fatigue, and functional decline. Likewise, patients with a history of penetrating abdominal wounds may present with vague abdominal complaints, and an aggressive evaluation may be required for retained shrapnel and possible abscess. Musculoskeletal complaints may also be challenging, and evaluation for retained shrapnel causing impingement or nerve injury should be explored. Any complaint that does not respond to treatment as expected should be explored and the differential diagnosis widened in an effort to treat this challenging population of patients. In this regard, the potential for development of chronic pain or somatoform disorders, post-traumatic stress disorder, depression, or other psychological conditions should be considered.

impending compartment syndrome. Many patients who have sustained severe head trauma will require partial craniectomy both for removal of blood accumulation and for control of cerebral edema. The removed portion of the skull is frequently not able to be salvaged because of fragmentation injuries. If the skull plate is salvageable, it is either frozen or implanted into the abdominal wall for reimplantation at a later date.

Multiple surgeries are frequently required during the acute hospitalization phase. Multiple revisions of amputated limbs may be required as well as multiple interventions for burned patients, such as repeated skin grafting.

Infection control can also be a problem for returning wounded soldiers. Most casualties are initially placed in isolation status until surveillance cultures can be obtained, clearing them from isolation status.

Rehabilitation

The rehabilitation process begins in acute medical settings, such as military treatment facilities, with the initiation of individual physical, occupational, and speech therapy. Collaboration by video teleconferences has allowed earlier physiatric input into the care of these complex patients and helped coordinate a smooth transition from acute care facilities to rehabilitation units.

Successful rehabilitation of polytrauma patients requires both multidisciplinary medical care and interdisciplinary rehabilitation care. In addition to the physiatrist, the multidisciplinary team frequently includes specialists in medicine, surgery, infectious disease, neurology, psychiatry, burns, spinal cord injury, and others. The interdisciplinary rehabilitation team consisting of speech therapists, physical therapists, occupational therapists, nurses, blind rehabilitation specialists or certified low vision therapists, audiologists, recreational therapists, psychologists, social workers, rehabilitation counselors, and others work together to minimize disability, to maximize independence, and to support the family. There are also specialized rehabilitation teams to meet the needs of the ventilator-dependent, burn, and amputee polytrauma patients. The polytrauma patients, with their multiple impairments and disabilities, will need to be observed with a rehabilitation model of care consisting of transitional day programs and long-term rehabilitation care.

Procedures

During the rehabilitation process, various interventions may be used to augment the efforts of the multidisciplinary team. Botulinum toxin injection can help reduce spasticity and improve overall mobility, hygiene, pain, and function. Serial casting is often used to help slowly reduce contracture and to improve range of motion. Negative-pressure wound therapy with vacuum-assisted closure may be used for large or slowly healing traumatic or postsurgical wounds.

Surgery

Because of the complex nature of polytrauma patients, multiple surgical interventions may be required during the initial acute rehabilitation stay. Patients may also require frequent readmission to the hospital for more surgeries, and an additional stay in the rehabilitation unit may allow the attainment of further independence goals. Those patients with skull defects will eventually require cranioplasty for correction of the defect. Most surgeons recommend a wait of at least 3 to 6 months since the last major infection before cranioplasty is performed. Patients with hydrocephalus may require placement of a ventriculoperitoneal shunt. The patient's cognitive and functional status is carefully monitored; patients with penetrating head injuries with retained fragments appear to be at a higher risk for intracranial infections. Finally, reconstructive procedures for facial deformities, revision of skin grafts and scars, and resection of heterotopic ossification may be required in the late post–acute rehabilitation stage.

POTENTIAL DISEASE COMPLICATIONS

Explosions have the potential to inflict multiple and severe trauma that few U.S. health care providers outside the military and the Veterans Administration have experience treating. The acute complications vary according to the mechanism and pattern of trauma. Such complications can include air embolism, compartment syndrome, rhabdomyolysis, renal failure, seizures, hemorrhage, increased intracranial pressure, infections, meningitis, and encephalopathy. Early complications that follow major burns include bacterial infections, septicemia, deep venous thrombosis, pulmonary embolism, renal failure, hypovolemic shock, jaundice, glottic edema, and ileus.

From October 2001 through December 2005, 188 war-injured service members were treated at one of the four polytrauma rehabilitation centers.[13] Complications before admission to a polytrauma rehabilitation center and complications that occurred during the polytrauma rehabilitation program are listed in Table 136-1. During the acute rehabilitation stage of care, there is certainly overlap of potential complications; but some variable patterns emerge, depending on whether the major injury is traumatic brain injury, spinal cord injury, burn, or limb amputation. Complications in traumatic brain injury include seizures, meningitis, spasticity, contractures, heterotopic ossification, headache, and agitation. In the spinal cord–injured population, complications include urinary retention, decubitus ulcers, spasticity, heterotopic ossification, deep venous thrombosis, pulmonary embolism, osteopenia, fracture, and urinary tract infections. Complications in burns can include microstomia, contractures, heterotopic ossification, anemia, pain, and skin graft failure. Limb amputation complications include phantom pain, stump pain, contractures, sinus formation, heterotopic ossification, wound dehiscence, tissue necrosis, falls, fractures, wound infections, edema, and hematoma.

TABLE 136-1 Frequency and Percentage of Complications before and during PRC Treatment (N = 188)

Medical Condition	Pre-PRC	PRC
Anemia	22 (12%)	39 (21%)
Meningitis	19 (10%)	2 (1%)
Encephalitis	2 (1%)	1 (0.5%)
Decubitus ulcers	39 (21%)	34 (18%)
Deep venous thrombosis	30 (16%)	7 (4%)
Dermatologic problems	2 (1%)	25 (13%)
Encephalomalacia	8 (4%)	50 (26%)
Heterotopic ossification	4 (2%)	14 (7%)
Increased intracranial pressure	18 (10%)	0 (0%)
Methicillin-resistant *Staphylococcus aureus* infection	7 (4%)	16 (8%)
Nausea	8 (4%)	34 (18%)
Nutritional compromise	1 (0.5%)	129 (68%)
Pneumonia	37 (20%)	5 (3%)
Post-traumatic fatigue	1 (0.5%)	4 (2%)
Pulmonary embolism	16 (8%)	1 (0.5%)
Temporomandibular joint disorder	0 (0%)	8 (4%)
Thrush	6 (3%)	12 (6%)
Urinary tract infection	22 (12%)	26 (14%)
Acinetobacter infection	23 (12%)	7 (4%)
Other complications	83 (44%)	72 (38%)

PRC, polytrauma rehabilitation center.

Pain, ranging from traumatic, postsurgical, neuropathic, and burn-related headaches to chronic pain syndromes, is common in the polytrauma patient. Ninety-six percent of polytrauma rehabilitation center admissions experienced at least one pain problem.[14]

An often overlooked complication for almost all patients in rehabilitation is mental health status. Some of the more common challenges include depression, post-traumatic stress disorder and anxiety disorders, adjustment disorders, body image issues, and behavioral or emotional dysregulation. Any or all of these can have an impact on medication or treatment compliance and general recovery.

POTENTIAL TREATMENT COMPLICATIONS

The various pieces of exercise equipment, orthotics, prosthetics, ceiling lifts, and other medical or adaptive devices can sometimes result in complications, whether they are used correctly or incorrectly. For example, resting splints used in burn cases to prevent joint contractures can result in pressure ulcers. Compartment syndrome, nerve injury, and infections can develop under casts that are sometimes used to treat contractures in the

polytrauma population. An amputee may develop skin irritation, abrasions, ulcerations, or other skin changes from the prosthetic liner or socket. The polytrauma patient is at high risk for falls and injury during the rehabilitation treatment phase from multiple factors, including polypharmacy, deconditioning, altered cognition, impulsivity, agitation, limb loss, impaired balance, spasticity, bracing, weakness, and urinary incontinence.

With complex polytrauma often comes significant pain at one or more sites; 50% or more of these patients require opioids or nonsteroidal anti-inflammatories.[14] Complications of opioids have been well described and can include constipation, altered cognition, somnolence, nausea, vomiting, convulsions, hypothalamic effect, neuroendocrine effect, respiratory depression, tolerance, dependence, and addiction.[15] The principal side effects of nonsteroidal anti-inflammatory drugs are dyspepsia, peptic ulcer disease, renal dysfunction, altered liver function, gastrointestinal bleed, and impaired cartilage repair in osteoarthritis.

References

1. Brown A, Leibson C, Malec J, et al. Long-term survival after traumatic brain injury: a population-based analysis. Neurorehabilitation 2004;19:37-43.
2. Nolan S. Traumatic brain injury: a review. Crit Care Nurs Q 2005;28:188-194.
3. DePalma RG, Burris DG, Champion HR, Hodgson MJ. Blast injuries. N Engl J Med 2005;1335-1342.
4. Fox CJ, Gillespie DL, O'Donnell SD, et al. Contemporary management of wartime vascular trauma. J Vasc Surg 2005;41:638-644.
5. Belanger HG, Scott S, Scholten S, et al. Utility of mechanism-of-injury-based assessment and treatment: blast injury program case illustration. J Rehabil Res Dev 2005;42:403-412.
6. Scott SG, Vanderploeg RD, Belanger HG, Scholten J. Blast injuries: evaluating and treating the postacute sequelae. Fed Pract 2005;22:67-75.
7. Vanderploeg RD, ed. Traumatic Brain Injury. Birmingham, Alabama, Department of Veterans Affairs, Employee Education Resource Center, 2004.
8. Newton RA. Balance abilities in individuals with moderate and severe traumatic brain injury. Brain Injury 1995;9:445-451.
9. Merritt B, Humayun F, Tran H. Patterns of peripheral nerve injuries sustained by polytrauma active duty service members. Poster presented at the annual assembly of the American Academy of Physical Medicine and Rehabilitation, September 2007.
10. Holcomb JB, Jenkins D, Rhee P, et al. Damage control resuscitation: directly addressing the early coagulopathy of trauma. J Trauma 2007;62:307-310.
11. Covey DC. Combat orthopaedics: a view from the trenches. J Am Acad Orthop Surg 2006;14:S10-S17.
12. Vertrees A, Kellicut D, Ottman S, et al. Early definitive abdominal closure using serial closure technique on injured soldiers returning from Afghanistan and Iraq. J Am Coll Surg 2006;202:762-771.
13. Sayer N, Chiros C, Sigford B, et al. Characteristics and rehabilitation outcomes among patients with blast and other injuries sustained during the global war on terror. Arch Phys Med Rehabil 2008;89:163-170 .
14. Clark ME, Bair MJ, Buckenmaier CC III, et al. Pain and combat injuries in soldiers returning from Operations Enduring Freedom and Iraqi Freedom: implications for research and practice. J Rehabil Res Dev 2007;44:179-194.
15. Ballantyne JC, ed. The Massachusetts General Hospital Handbook of Pain Management, 3rd ed. Philadelphia, Lippincott Williams & Wilkins, 2005.

Post-Poliomyelitis Syndrome 137

Julie K. Silver, MD

Synonyms

Late effects of poliomyelitis
Post-poliomyelitis sequelae

ICD-9 Code

138   Late effects of acute poliomyelitis

DEFINITION

Poliomyelitis, a disease caused by an RNA virus, has been eradicated from the United States (with the exception of vaccine-related cases) since 1979. During the first half of the 20th century, however, there were major epidemics throughout the United States, and although accurate statistics are difficult to obtain, there may be as many as 1.5 million survivors of polio currently living in this country. There are many more millions of survivors worldwide, many of whom are children. In the United States, there are several historic reasons for the difficulty in tracking the number of survivors, including the fact that in the past, poliomyelitis was thought to be either "paralytic" or "nonparalytic." We are beginning to appreciate that people who might have had a very mild episode of poliomyelitis (perhaps clinically unappreciable and therefore not classified as paralytic poliomyelitis) may indeed have suffered some paralysis and may be at risk for post-poliomyelitis syndrome (PPS).[1]

PPS is a neurologic disorder defined by a collection of symptoms that occur in survivors of polio who experienced injury to the central nervous system (generally the anterior horn cells in the spinal cord) during their initial infection with the poliovirus. The symptoms of PPS typically occur many years after the initial episode, and the hallmark is new weakness. The new weakness may occur in muscles known to be previously affected or in muscles that were thought to be "normal." The majority of known survivors of paralytic poliomyelitis are reported to be affected (approximately 60%).[2] Although new weakness is the most defining symptom of PPS, other symptoms may include new muscle atrophy, pain, swallowing or breathing problems, cold intolerance, and fatigue.[3]

PPS is a diagnosis of exclusion and should fit specific criteria (Table 137-1).

The cause of PPS is uncertain. There is evidence to suggest that attrition of motor neurons is partially responsible.[4] An abnormality in acetylcholine transmission at the neuromuscular junction has also been suspected.[5] Metabolic factors may play a role.[6] Both the overuse of some muscles, leading to attrition of surviving neurons, and the disuse of other muscles are likely to contribute to new weakness.

Normal motor neurons (Fig. 137-1) are lost in acute poliomyelitis, and collateral sprouting of existing motor neurons occurs (Fig. 137-2A and B). Sprouts reinnervate denervated muscle fibers, resulting in larger than normal motor units (Fig. 137-2C). The burden on each of these remaining motor neurons is greater than under normal conditions because there are fewer motor units. As part of the aging process, there is gradual loss of some motor neurons.[7] Polio survivors may be more affected by this loss of motor neurons because they have fewer neurons.

SYMPTOMS

Weakness

The hallmark of PPS is new weakness; however, the progression of symptoms is usually slow and occurs during years rather than weeks to months.[8,9] Patients may report that they once were able to go up and down stairs using only one railing but now need two railings, or they may say that it has become more difficult or even impossible to lift a gallon of milk. They may give a history of falling as a result of knee buckling or tripping due to increased difficulty with clearing of the foot. Some patients may report that a limb or muscle looks smaller than it once did, which indicates new atrophy. It is important to glean from the history whether an individual has paresthesias, numbness, back or neck pain, or bowel and bladder symptoms that point to another cause (e.g., myelopathy or radiculopathy). Also, a history of progressive weakness during weeks to months may suggest an alternative diagnosis as well (e.g., thyroid myopathy, amyotrophic lateral sclerosis).

TABLE 137-1 Criteria for Post-Poliomyelitis Syndrome

History of old poliomyelitis, preferably with recent electrodiagnostic findings consistent with remote anterior horn cell disease[1]

A period of at least partial recovery from the initial illness and then a long stable period (more than 10 to 20 years)

New symptoms consistent with post-poliomyelitis syndrome that are not attributable to any other medical condition

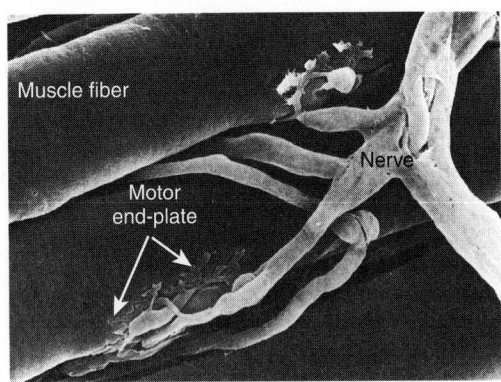

FIGURE 137-1. Normal neuromuscular junction. Note the nerve branching into several terminal axons, each innervating one muscle fiber. (Reprinted with permission from Fawcett DW. Bloom and Fawcett: A Textbook of Histology. Philadelphia, WB Saunders, 1986.)

Fatigue

Fatigue is the most common complaint, affecting 87% of polio survivors.[10] Typically, survivors of polio report that they feel refreshed in the morning but are exhausted later in the day. They may complain that they "hit a wall" or "a curtain comes down." In general, this fatigue improves with rest. Although patients may complain of problems with memory or word finding difficulty, true cognitive dysfunction is disputed.[11] For individuals who are tired first thing in the morning, an alternative diagnosis, such as depression, thyroid dysfunction, or sleep disorder, may be present.

Pain

Pain associated with PPS presents as aching, burning, or cramping in the muscles. Often, the pain is more prominent at the end of the day. Polio survivors are also susceptible to other types of pain resulting from muscle imbalance and stress. Pain may be due to a variety of factors, including osteoarthritis, which may occur earlier or more severely because of a lack of strong muscles to support the joints, and upper extremity neuropathies.

Respiratory Problems

New breathing problems are not uncommon in polio survivors, particularly those who had initial involvement of the respiratory muscles. The most common presentation is new weakness of the respiratory muscles, causing restrictive lung disease that is associated

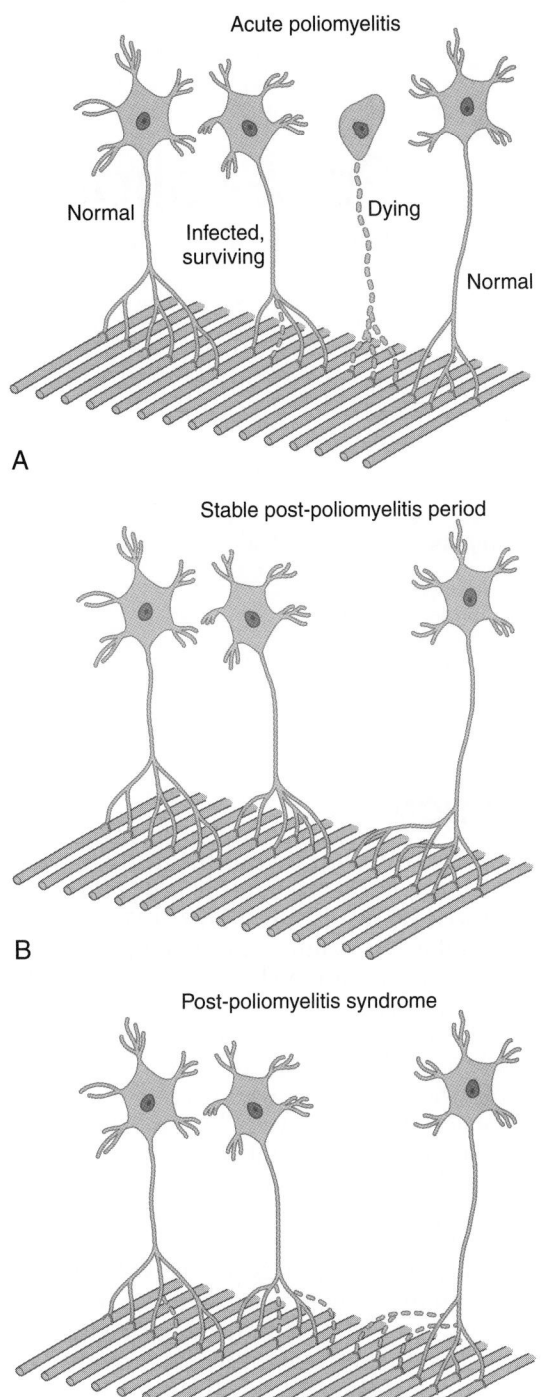

FIGURE 137-2. Poliomyelitis neuromuscular junction. **A,** In acute poliomyelitis, some neurons die, others are affected but survive, and still others are unaffected. **B,** In the stable post-poliomyelitis period, the surviving neurons cover more territory than they did before the poliomyelitis. **C,** In post-poliomyelitis syndrome, there is attrition of surviving axons and neurons.

with chronic alveolar hypoventilation. This restriction is worse in obese patients because of the excess weight over the thoracic cage and abdominal cavity. Patients may complain of shortness of breath, dyspnea on exertion, or chronic respiratory infections. Sleep-disordered breathing is also common in polio survivors, and patients may present with only a history of fatigue.[12,13]

Swallowing and Speaking Problems

New swallowing problems occur most commonly in patients who had "bulbar" poliomyelitis that affected the swallowing muscles during the initial infection. Patients may complain of choking, gagging, or coughing or just have vague complaints that they do not feel as comfortable eating as they once did. Some people will also complain of voice problems, especially dysphonia.[14]

Cold Intolerance

Cold intolerance often affects one or more limbs. Most often, limbs that were noticeably paralyzed are affected, but patients may complain of a general inability to thermoregulate. Cold intolerance may be exacerbated by other medical conditions, such as peripheral vascular disease.

PHYSICAL EXAMINATION

The musculoskeletal and neurologic examination findings should be consistent with a lower motor neuron disease process with absent or diminished reflexes, decreased muscle tone, and asymmetric atrophy and weakness or paralysis of the limbs or trunk. Sensation should be spared. Fasciculations are noted, and if they are pronounced and diffuse, an alternative diagnosis should be considered (e.g., amyotrophic lateral sclerosis). Because median and ulnar neuropathies are common in polio survivors, it is important to note sensory deficits and asymmetric muscle atrophy in the hands.[3,15,16] In some individuals, the findings on physical examination may be subtle.

Biomechanical abnormalities are also assessed. These can include lower extremity contractures due to muscle weakness (particularly at the hip and ankle), joint abnormalities (e.g., genu recurvatum at the knee due to weak quadriceps muscles), and loss of joint range of motion without apparent contributing weakness (common in the cervical spine and shoulders). Scoliosis and kyphosis may be due to muscle imbalance. It is important to identify leg length discrepancies as well.

When established testing protocols are followed, manual muscle testing is a useful measure of strength. Because this population of patients tends to use compensatory movements, proper stabilization and testing through the range are critical components of manual muscle testing. Proper positioning is also essential for assessment of grip and pinch strength with a dynamometer and a pinch gauge.

Specific areas that the patient reports as painful are evaluated (e.g., rotator cuff disease in someone who complains of shoulder pain).[17] Gait and seated posture are assessed because poor posture and biomechanical imbalances can contribute to painful sequelae.

With respect to fatigue, it is important to note the patient's mood and affect, assessing for depression. Blood pressure can be measured to determine whether orthostatic changes that may occur with anemia have taken place. Capillary refill with compression of the digits can be useful. Assessment of any underlying thyroid or respiratory conditions or chronic infections can help rule out alternative causes of fatigue.

Patients who complain of decreased endurance or shortness of breath are evaluated in the same manner as any patient with respiratory complaints; this includes vital signs and baseline pulse oximetry, if it is available. Pulmonary and cardiac auscultation is also important.

Swallowing problems are best assessed by a clinician who specializes in treatment of these disorders because they nearly always require technical examinations with specialized equipment to visualize the pharynx and larynx. Cold intolerance is assessed by noting the temperature and color of the extremities. Assessment of peripheral pulses and edema is also important.

FUNCTIONAL LIMITATIONS

Polio survivors lose strength at a rate greater than that associated with normal aging in both upper and lower extremity musculature.[18] New weakness can greatly affect mobility, including walking and transfers. Diminished strength can also affect the patient's ability to perform daily activities, such as gardening, grocery shopping, and even going to get the mail—which can significantly alter the level of independence. New leg weakness may also increase fall risk.[19]

Fatigue may be purely muscular or may affect cognition in terms of memory and concentration.[20] Post-poliomyelitis fatigue, which typically occurs most profoundly in the afternoon, may affect an individual's ability to work full-time. The need for a break or a nap may markedly limit what patients can accomplish during the day, and an early bedtime may limit social activities, resulting in social isolation. Poor sleep associated with anxiety or depression, sleep apnea, or periodic limb movement disorder may also contribute to fatigue and cognitive dysfunction.

Many polio survivors function well despite pain.[21] However, some people have such severe pain that they curtail their activities, particularly activities that exacerbate their symptoms, such as walking and lifting.

New breathing problems may limit the ability of patients to do their usual activities, particularly activities that require some physical endurance, such as walking. Reduction of activity can have the negative effect of contributing to muscle deconditioning, which can cause even greater breathing problems and decreased endurance. New swallowing problems, if severe, may cause social isolation; on the other hand, they may cause patients to feel as though they cannot be left alone when eating. Many people limit exposure to cold, such as avoiding going outside during cold weather. Some people may even choose to live in a warmer climate for comfort reasons. Others may turn up the furnace to accommodate their cold intolerance.

DIAGNOSTIC STUDIES

Weakness

Initial testing focuses on new weakness because it generally is the primary feature of PPS. Electrodiagnostic studies (electromyography and nerve conduction studies) are recommended to rule out other neuromuscular diseases and to help establish a previous history of poliomyelitis. Although a history of poliomyelitis cannot be proved by electrodiagnostic studies, some classic findings, such as very large motor unit action potentials, make the diagnosis much more likely if they are present and essentially rule out the diagnosis if they are absent.

If it is clinically appropriate to establish the correct diagnosis, imaging of the spine (e.g., magnetic resonance imaging or computed tomography with or without myelography) can help evaluate whether a myelopathy or radiculopathy is present. Useful laboratory studies may include thyroid function studies to rule out thyroid myopathy and muscle enzymes, which can be mildly elevated in PPS.

Paralysis in polio survivors, whether it is new or longstanding, contributes to decreased bone mineral density. That combined with a propensity to fall is a major source of increasing disability. Therefore, bone mineral density studies should be considered in all polio survivors; imaging focuses on the area of greatest paralysis.[22,23]

Fatigue

Patients presenting with fatigue should have a workup for anemia, thyroid dysfunction, depression, and sleep disorders. Sleep disorders are common in polio survivors and are often present as sleep apnea.[24] There should be a very low threshold for ordering a sleep study in a polio survivor complaining of fatigue.

Chronic conditions such as congestive heart failure, diabetes, and chronic infections can also contribute to fatigue and should lead to appropriate workup. Cancer and other serious alternative diagnoses should be ruled out. Respiratory etiology should also be considered (see the following discussion of respiratory problems).

Pain

Pain can be a result of many different causes and should be thoroughly investigated. Post-poliomyelitis pain is diagnosed by history and physical examination. However, diagnostic studies can be contemplated to rule out other conditions. Upper extremity neuropathies, such as carpal tunnel syndrome, should be considered and ruled out with electrodiagnostic studies. Plain radiographs can help in the diagnosis of osteoarthritis and spinal stenosis. Magnetic resonance imaging and computed tomography are performed to rule out alternative diagnoses.

Respiratory Problems

Respiratory problems are often manifested as chronic alveolar hypoventilation and can be initially evaluated with baseline pulmonary function tests. Chest radiography and laboratory studies (e.g., arterial blood gas analysis) may also be useful. Pulse oximetry (at rest, during exercise, and while sleeping) may provide additional information. Sleep studies are recommended for polio survivors with complaints of fatigue or difficulty with breathing.

Swallowing Problems

Swallowing disorders can be diagnosed by a variety of different imaging studies. The modified barium swallow study and the functional endoscopic evaluation of swallowing are most commonly performed.

Cold Intolerance

Cold intolerance is likely to be a result of a variety of factors, including alterations in the sympathetic nervous system and the paralysis of muscles in the extremities that are important in maintenance of dynamic blood flow. Diagnostic studies are generally not performed for this symptom except to rule out other conditions (e.g., peripheral vascular disease).

TREATMENT

Initial

Weakness

Intravenous immune globulin has been shown to increase strength in polio survivors.[25,26] In one double-blind study, the median increase was 8.3%.[26] This may translate into a more significant gain in functional status, although it is not clear at this time. Pyridostigmine, which is generally increased gradually to a dose of 60 mg three times daily, has been used with mixed results to improve strength.[27-29]

Fatigue

Fatigue is managed by treatment of any medical conditions that may be contributing to it. It is particularly important to address sleep disorders in polio survivors who have documented sleep apnea or periodic limb movement disorders.[30] Proper sleep hygiene is important (e.g., regular bedtimes, avoidance of caffeine late in the day). Underlying depression can be treated with medications or counseling or both. In addition, patients are encouraged to pace themselves, to take rest breaks during the day, and to avoid alcohol.

In patients with chronic debilitating fatigue, methylphenidate hydrochloride and bromocriptine have been tried with mixed results. More recently, modafinil has

Differential Diagnosis

Weakness

    Myopathy

    Amyotrophic lateral sclerosis

    Myelopathy (e.g., due to spinal stenosis, spinal tumors)

    Radiculopathy

    Peripheral neuropathy

    Deconditioning

    Multiple sclerosis

    Myasthenia gravis

    Parkinson disease

    Adult spinal muscular atrophy

Fatigue

    Sleep disorder

    Depression

    Thyroid dysfunction

    Anemia

    Deconditioning

    Cancer

    Chronic infections

    Respiratory dysfunction

    Cardiac dysfunction

    Chronic systemic disease (e.g., systemic lupus erythematosus, diabetes)

    Fibromyalgia

Pain

    Tendinitis

    Bursitis

    Osteoarthritis

    Radiculopathy

    Peripheral neuropathy

    Fibromyalgia

    Myofascial pain syndrome

Respiratory problems

    Cardiac disease

    Chronic obstructive pulmonary disease

    Asthma

    Anemia

    Deconditioning

Swallowing problems

    Gastroesophageal reflux disease

    Benign or malignant lesion

    Stricture

Cold intolerance

    Peripheral vascular disease

been used to treat fatigue pharmacologically, although the results have not been particularly encouraging.[31-33] The dose usually starts at 200 mg orally every morning and may be increased to 400 mg.

Pain

Pain is generally relieved when the underlying medical condition is addressed (e.g., carpal tunnel syndrome, arthritis). If medications are considered, nonsteroidal anti-inflammatory drugs and acetaminophen can be tried as analgesics. Tramadol as an oral analgesic and Lidoderm 5% patches placed regionally can be tried as well. Post-poliomyelitis myalgias can be treated and have been reported to respond to low-dose tricyclic antidepressants. However, keep in mind that these may exacerbate some sleep disorders.

Respiratory Problems

Respiratory problems, particularly sleep apnea, are often treated with significant improvement in symptoms by continuous positive airway pressure or bilevel positive airway pressure at night. Oxygen can exacerbate chronic alveolar hypoventilation and should be used with caution.

Swallowing Problems

Swallowing problems are generally amenable to conservative treatment with a speech and language pathologist. On occasion, surgical intervention is helpful. In rare instances, an alternative to oral feeding is required.

Cold Intolerance

Cold intolerance is treated symptomatically with layered clothing and thermal undergarments.

Rehabilitation

Rehabilitation focuses on education of the patient, therapeutic exercise, and adaptive equipment needs. Education of the patient includes knowledge of the diagnosis and appropriate precautions, pacing, falls precautions, postural education, ergonomics, pain management, home exercise program, and home safety. Home safety may include a home visit because recommendation of home modifications can markedly improve how safe people are in their homes.[34,35]

The exercise program should be individualized and address flexibility, strength, and conditioning.[36] A nonfatiguing protocol should be used for muscle groups affected by poliomyelitis. The conditioning program should be done gradually, with protocols similar to a walking program; it should work the individual's less involved muscle groups. Cross-training is a crucial exercise principle for this group because of muscle fatigability.

Equipment needs are addressed by the consideration of orthotic evaluation, walking aids, scooter or power wheelchair, chairlift, and driving adaptations. Orthotic evaluation should be comprehensive and may include both upper and lower extremity orthoses. For example, wrist splints may be prescribed for carpal tunnel syndrome and elbow pads for ulnar neuropathy. There are a variety of bracing options and materials; consider lightweight options, such as carbon fiber and Kevlar, for this population.[37]

A physical, occupational, or respiratory therapist skilled in treatment of respiratory disorders may be helpful in teaching the patient some breathing and postural techniques. In addition, knowledgeable therapists can help patients to conserve energy, which can decrease respiratory demands.

Speech and language pathologists can assist with swallowing difficulties by teaching the patient techniques to assist with swallowing and to prevent choking and aspiration. Also, the therapist can make recommendations about which foods or liquids to avoid. For safety, family members may be instructed in the Heimlich maneuver.

Procedures

On occasion, therapeutic procedures are recommended on the basis of specific symptoms. For instance, a wide variety of musculoskeletal conditions that are commonly found in polio survivors may be treated with injections (e.g., rotator cuff tendinitis, carpal tunnel syndrome, cervical myofascial pain syndrome).

Surgery

Surgery may be recommended for a variety of orthopedic conditions, such as joint replacements and carpal tunnel release. In some instances, individuals with severe swallowing problems are candidates for surgery or feeding tube placement.

POTENTIAL DISEASE COMPLICATIONS

PPS is characterized by slow progression of symptoms. One of the most significant complications of PPS is falling with subsequent injury. Of 233 polio survivors surveyed, 64% reported falling at least once within the last year.[38] This same study also correlated falls in polio survivors with a high incidence of fractures; 82 of 233 surveyed (35%) reported that they had a history of at least one fracture due to a fall. Because of osteopenia or osteoporosis in paralyzed limbs, polio survivors may be more susceptible to injuries.[39] Polio survivors will often report a decrease in functional ability after a serious fall.

Progressive respiratory compromise can also notably change functional status by decreasing endurance. Supplemental oxygen may even become necessary for an individual who has never needed it before.

Difficulty with swallowing can lead to aspiration pneumonia or malnutrition. These are serious and potentially life-threatening complications.

POTENTIAL TREATMENT COMPLICATIONS

There are three categories of treatment complications. Complications are related to medication side effects, falls, and inappropriate intervention.

Analgesics and nonsteroidal anti-inflammatory drugs have well-known side effects that most commonly affect the gastric, hepatic, and renal systems. The side effects of pyridostigmine are generally dose related and can be recalled by the acronym SLUD (increased salivation, lacrimation, urination, and defecation). Respiratory secretions may also be increased with this medication. Tricyclic antidepressants have cholinergic side effects, the most serious of which is the possibility of acute urinary retention in men (men with underlying prostate problems are generally at risk). The side effects of modafinil include headache, nausea, and nervousness. Modafinil may increase the circulating levels of diazepam, phenytoin, and propranolol.

In physical therapy, caution must be used in altering an individual's gait and movement patterns. During gait, a tight gastrocnemius can aid in creating a plantar flexion moment that will produce an extension moment at the knee, which will aid a weak quadriceps. If the gastrocnemius is stretched before bracing is addressed, the individual may be at increased risk for knee buckling. Heavy or inappropriate bracing or mobility devices may hinder mobility and can lead to falls.

Inappropriate interventions may adversely affect a survivor of polio. Overly aggressive exercise programs are thought to increase the risk for further weakness and may also result in disabling musculoskeletal injuries.

The bed rest associated with some surgeries seems to pose a significant recuperative problem for polio survivors. Postoperative rehabilitation is often necessary. Also, anecdotally, polio survivors have been reported to have difficulty with general anesthesia and may require larger than usual doses of postoperative pain medication. Careful consideration should be given to the risks and benefits of surgery for this population.

References
1. Halstead LS, Silver JK. Nonparalytic polio and postpolio syndrome. Am J Phys Med Rehabil 2000;79:13-18.
2. Gawne AC, Halstead LS. Post-polio syndrome: pathophysiology and clinical management. Crit Rev Phys Rehabil Med 1995;7:147-188.
3. Silver JK. Post-Polio. A Guide for Polio Survivors and Their Families. New Haven, Conn, Yale University Press, 2001.

4. Dalakas MC. Pathogenetic mechanisms of post-polio syndrome: morphological, electrophysiological, virological, and immunological correlations. Ann N Y Acad Sci 1995;753:167-185.

5. Maselli RA, Wollmann R, Roos R. Function and ultrastructure of the neuromuscular junction in post-polio syndrome. Ann N Y Acad Sci 1995;753:129-137.

6. Grimby G, Tollback A, Muller U, Larsson L. Fatigue of chronically overused motor units in prior polio patients. Muscle Nerve 1996;19:728-737.

7. Halstead LS. Managing Post-Polio: A Guide to Living Well with Post-Polio Syndrome. Washington, DC, NRH Press, 1998.

8. Nollet F, Beelen A, Twisk JW, et al. Perceived health and physical functioning in postpoliomyelitis syndrome: a 6-year prospective follow-up study. Arch Phys Med Rehabil 2003;4:1048-1056.

9. Stolwijk-Swuste JM, Beelen A, Lankhorst GJ, Nollet F. The course of functional status and muscle strength in patients with late-onset sequelae of poliomyelitis: a systematic review. Arch Phys Med Rehabil 2005;86:1693-1701.

10. Halstead LS, Rossi CD. New problems in old polio patients: result of survey of 539 polio survivors. Orthopedics 1985;8:845-850.

11. Ostlund G, Borg K, Wahlin A. Cognitive functioning in post-polio patients with and without general fatigue. J Rehabil Med 2005;37:147-151.

12. Chasens ER, Umlauf M, Valappil T, Singh KP. Nocturnal problems in postpolio syndrome: sleep apnea symptoms and nocturia. Rehabil Nurs 2001;26:66-71.

13. Schanke A-K, Stanghelle JK, Andersson S, et al. Mild versus severe fatigue in polio survivors: special characteristics. J Rehabil Med 2002;34:134-140.

14. Abaza MM, Sataloff RT, Hawkshaw MJ, Mandel S. Laryngeal manifestations of postpoliomyelitis syndrome. J Voice 2001;14:291-294.

15. Werner R, Waring W, Davidoff G. Risk factors for median mononeuropathy of the wrist in postpoliomyelitis patients. Arch Phys Med Rehabil 1989;70:464-467.

16. Veerendrakumar M, Taly AB, Nagaraja D. Ulnar nerve palsy due to axillary crutch. Neurol India 2001;49:67-70.

17. Klein MG, Whyte J, Keenan MA, et al. The relation between lower extremity strength and shoulder overuse symptoms: a model based on polio survivors. Arch Phys Med Rehabil 2000;81:789-795.

18. Klein MG, Whyte J, Keenan MA, et al. Changes in strength over time among polio survivors. Arch Phys Med Rehabil 2000;81:1059-1064.

19. Silver JK, Aiello DD. Polio survivors: falls and subsequent injuries. Am J Phys Med Rehabil 2002;81:567-570.

20. Bruno RL, Zimmerman JR. Word finding difficulty as a post-polio sequelae. Am J Phys Med Rehabil 2000;79:343-348.

21. Widar M, Ahlstrom G. Pain in persons with post-polio: the Swedish version of the Multidimensional Pain Inventory (MPI). Scand J Caring Sci 1999;13:33-40.

22. Silver JK, Aiello DD. Bone density and fracture risks in male polio survivors. Arch Phys Med Rehabil 2001;81:1329.

23. Silver JK, Aiello DD, MacNeil JR. Effect of fosamax on bone density in a male polio survivor: a case report. Arch Phys Med Rehabil 2001;81:1311.

24. Dean AC, Graham BA, Dalakas M, Sato S. Sleep apnea in patients with postpolio syndrome. Ann Neurol 1998;43:661-664.

25. Gonzalez H, Khademi M, Andersson M, et al. Prior poliomyelitis—IVIg treatment reduces proinflammatory cytokine production. J Neuroimmunol 2004;150:139-144.

26. Gonzalez H, Sunnerhagen KS, Sjorberg I, et al. Intravenous immunoglobulin for post-polio syndrome: a randomized controlled trial. Lancet Neurol 2006;5:493-500.

27. Seivert BP, Speier JL, Canine JK. Pyridostigmine effect on strength, endurance and fatigue in post-polio patients [abstract]. Arch Phys Med Rehabil 1994;75:1049.

28. Trojan DA, Collet JP, Shapiro S, et al. A multicenter, randomized, double-blind trial of pyridostigmine in post-polio syndrome. Neurology 1999;53:1225-1233.

29. Horesmans HLD, Nollet F, Beelen A, et al. Pyridostigmine in post-polio syndrome: no decline in fatigue and limited functional improvement. J Neurol Neurosurg Psychiatry 2003;74:1655-1661.

30. Hsu AA, Staata BA. "Post-polio" sequelae and sleep-related disordered breathing. Mayo Clin Proc 1998;73:216-224.

31. Kingshott RN, Vennelle M, Coleman EL, et al. Randomized, double-blind, placebo-controlled crossover trial of modafinil in the treatment of residual excessive daytime sleepiness in the sleep apnea/hypopnea syndrome. Am J Respir Crit Care Med 2001;163:918-923.

32. Mitler MM, Harsh J, Hiroshkowitz M, Guilleminault C. Long-term efficacy and safety of modafinil (Provigil) for the treatment of excessive daytime sleepiness associated with narcolepsy. Sleep Med 2000;1:231-243.

33. Chan KM, Strohschein FJ, Rydz D, et al. Randomized controlled trial of modafinil for the treatment of fatigue in postpolio patients. Muscle Nerve 2006;33:138-141.

34. Salkeld G, Cumming RG, O'Neill E, et al. The cost effectiveness of a home hazard reduction program to reduce falls among older persons. Aust N Z J Public Health 2000;24:265-271.

35. Cumming RG, Thomas M, Szonyi G, et al. Home visits by an occupational therapist for assessment and modification of environmental hazards: a randomized trial of falls prevention. J Am Geriatr Soc 1999;47:1397-1402.

36. Chan KM, Amirjani N, Sumrain M, et al. Randomized controlled trial of strength training in post-polio patients. Muscle Nerve 2003;27:332-338.

37. Silver JK, Aiello DD, Drillio RC. Lightweight carbon fiber and Kevlar floor reaction AFO in two polio survivors with new weakness [abstract]. Arch Phys Med Rehabil 1999;80:1180.

38. Silver JK, Aiello DD. Risk of falls in survivors of poliomyelitis [abstract]. Arch Phys Med Rehabil 2000;81:1272.

39. Silver JK. Aging, comorbidities, and secondary disabilities in polio survivors. In Halstead LS, ed. Managing Post-Polio: A Guide to Living Well with Post-Polio Syndrome. Washington, DC, NRH Press, 1998.

Post-Concussion Disorders 138

Mel B. Glenn, MD

DEFINITION

Post-concussion disorders are a set of symptoms commonly seen after concussion. The term *concussion* is generally used as a synonym for mild traumatic brain injury. One commonly used definition of mild traumatic brain injury is a traumatically induced physiologic disruption of brain function, manifested by at least one of the following:

- any period of loss of consciousness;
- any loss of memory for events immediately before or after the accident;
- any alteration in mental state at the time of the accident (e.g., feeling dazed, disoriented, or confused); and
- focal neurologic deficits that may or may not be transient;

but the severity of injury does not exceed the following:

- loss of consciousness of approximately 30 minutes or less;
- after 30 minutes, an initial Glasgow Coma Scale score of 13 to 15; and
- post-traumatic amnesia not longer than 24 hours.[1]

There are a number of classification schemes. Concussion can be graded according to the criteria established by the American Academy of Neurology, which are based on the occurrence and duration of loss of consciousness, confusion, and concussion symptoms. They were intended to guide the management of sports concussion[2] (Table 138-1). The approach developed by the 2nd International Symposium on Concussion in Sports,[3] including a more state-of-the-art set of guidelines for the treatment of sports concussion, is notable for its emphasis on outcome as well as the immediate sequelae of the injury. Simple concussion is defined as one that progressively resolves during a period of 7 to 10 days. A complex concussion involves persistent symptoms, specific sequelae (concussive seizure, loss of consciousness longer than 1 minute, prolonged cognitive impairment), or concussion previous to the one in question. (See also the section on treatment.)

SYMPTOMS

The most common post-concussive symptoms are headache, dizziness (vertigo), poor balance, forgetfulness, difficulty learning or remembering, difficulty concentrating, slowed thinking, hypersomnolence, fatigue, poor energy, insomnia, depression, anxiety, irritability, sensitivity to noise and light, and visual problems.[4-6]

Many of these symptoms may be related to events other than the cerebral insult. Symptoms may be present alone or in various constellations and as such do not constitute a true syndrome.[4] There may be a lag of days or weeks between the concussion and the patient's first complaints, and some related phenomena, such as depression and anxiety, may not become manifested until months after the initial injury. Although these symptoms can be seen with any severity of injury, they are often discussed in the context of mild traumatic brain injury. Over time, many people make a complete recovery.

Estimates of the numbers of people in the United States who have a mild traumatic brain injury each year range from 51 to 618 per 100,000 population.[7] Estimates and reports of the proportion of those who still have multiple symptoms 1 year after injury have ranged from less than 5%[8] to as high as 78%,[9] the latter number juxtaposed against a 47% incidence in a group of controls with orthopedic injuries. The difference in symptoms between the concussion group and the controls was largely due to complaints of dizziness, memory problems, and concentration problems. This study was done in Lithuania, where litigation is uncommon. One study found that up to 5 years after injury, the incidence of symptoms was higher among those with mild traumatic brain injury than among controls with other injuries.[10] The incidence of the symptoms

TABLE 138-1 American Academy of Neurology Concussion Classification

Grade of Concussion	Characteristics
Grade 1	Transient confusion
	All symptoms < 15 minutes
	Mental status changes < 15 minutes
Grade 2	Transient confusion
	Any symptoms > 15 minutes
	Mental status changes > 15 minutes
Grade 3a	Brief loss of consciousness (seconds)
Grade 3b	Prolonged loss of consciousness (minutes)

associated with post-concussion disorder is relatively high in healthy populations,[8] and there seems to be a tendency among people with mild traumatic brain injury to underestimate the extent of preinjury symptoms.[7,9] Most authors have not defined a particular time frame for the designation of "persistent" post-concussion disorder, although some have used 3 months as a cutoff.[11]

Most controlled studies indicate that cognitive deficits found on neuropsychological testing, largely in young adults, generally resolve within 3 months of mild traumatic brain injury.[7] Some studies have found subtle differences from controls.[12,13] Athletes who have had multiple concussions have been found to have a poorer performance on neuropsychological testing[14] and a greater prevalence of mild cognitive impairment in later life[15] than athletes who have not had a concussion. Although prospective studies are needed to clarify cause and effect, this suggests that a single concussion may result in some loss of brain function, possibly subclinical in most people.

The etiology of the various post-concussion symptoms is often multifactorial, and much of it is still not well understood. The usual inciting factors are mild traumatic brain injury with residual impairment of attention and memory, whiplash or other soft tissue injury to the head and neck, and at times disruption of the vestibular apparatus or central vestibular insult. Problems with attention, forgetfulness, and fatigue, coupled with the frequent development of headaches, insomnia, and vertigo, often lead to considerable anxiety and depression and a "shaken sense of self."[16] In those who develop persistent problems, a complex of symptoms often feed one on the other,[4] exacerbating the neuropsychological impairment, which may then take on a life of its own even as the underlying brain injury continues to recover.[16,17] A common scenario is one in which pain, anxiety (including, at times, post-traumatic stress disorder), and depression contribute to insomnia, which in turn exacerbates headaches, and all of these symptoms contribute to cognitive

impairment. Difficulty in concentrating can also result in headaches.

There is evidence to suggest that persistence of symptoms is associated with preexisting social, psychological, and vocational difficulties; age older than 40 years; being married; female gender; higher educational background; current student status; litigation; being out of work secondary to injury; motor vehicle crash as cause of injury; lack of fault for a collision; nausea; memory impairment; multiple painful areas after injury; preexisting physical impairment; and preexisting brain (including prior head injury) and other neurologic problems. However, studies vary with respect to some of these findings.[6-8,14,18,19]

Cognitive

The patient should be questioned about the inciting event with regard to whether there was a loss of consciousness, loss of anterograde or retrograde memory, other alteration in mental status, or focal neurologic findings. A patient's subjective feeling of being dazed or confused may or may not reflect actual brain injury. It is common for people to feel dazed because of the emotional shock experienced after an accident. There is often limited or no documentation of the patient's mental status immediately after the accident, and a clinician must do his or her best to reconstruct the situation largely on the basis of the history given by the patient. The observations of others may help clarify whether the patient was responding slowly or otherwise appeared confused. Emergency medical records should be obtained whenever possible but may or may not reflect the patient's mental status at the scene of the accident and may not pick up more subtle deficits if only orientation is evaluated.

Headaches

Tension, migraine, cervicogenic (musculoskeletal), and mixed headaches are the most frequent types seen after concussion. Pain from soft tissue injury at the site of impact, occipital neuralgic pain, and dysautonomic cephalgia can be seen as well. The patient should be questioned with respect to severity, quality, location and radiation, date at onset, duration, frequency, exacerbating or ameliorating factors, and frequency of medication use in addition to associated symptoms such as nausea, vomiting, visual phenomena, diaphoresis, rhinorrhea, and sensitivity to light and noise.[20-22]

Vestibular

Vertigo can be caused by cupulolithiasis or canalithiasis (benign paroxysmal positional vertigo), brainstem injury, perilymph fistula, endolymphatic hydrops, or labyrinthine concussion, or it may be cervicogenic. Perilymph fistula, endolymphatic hydrops, and labyrinthine concussion are usually associated with hearing loss and tinnitus as well. Nonvertiginous dizziness is not usually directly related to concussion; medication-induced dizziness (e.g., by nonsteroidal anti-inflammatory drugs and antidepressants) and other causes should be considered, including psychogenic dizziness.[23]

Other

The physician's history of the events surrounding the initial accident should also include exploration of other associated injuries, seizure, vomiting, and drug or alcohol intoxication. A preinjury medical, social, psychological, vocational, and educational history should be obtained, including any history of attention deficit disorder or learning disability.

PHYSICAL EXAMINATION

Cognitive

The examination of the individual with post-concussion disorder often elicits problems with attention, memory, and executive function on mental status evaluation. Memory problems are most often related to attention deficits or difficulty with retrieval.[24] The contribution of attention versus encoding versus retrieval problems to verbal memory can be evaluated with presentation of a word list followed by immediate recall, recall after 5 minutes, and then a multiple choice recognition task, which provides the structure needed to assist retrieval when information has been encoded. Mini-mental status test results may be normal; more extensive evaluation, and perhaps neuropsychological testing, including reaction time[13] and continuous performance tasks, may be necessary to reveal the deficits. Findings more severe than expected for a mild traumatic brain injury indicate that there are likely to be other contributing factors. Medications, anxiety, depression, insomnia, pain, and either conscious or unconscious symptom augmentation can exacerbate or cause problems with attention and memory.[6,16] A sleep history should be obtained.

Psychological

Assessment of mood and affect may reveal evidence of depression and anxiety. The Patient Health Questionnaire-9 is one approach to assessment of depression. It is a brief questionnaire that mirrors the diagnostic criteria of the *Diagnostic and Statistical Manual of Mental Disorders*, fourth edition, for major depression. It has been validated in people with traumatic brain injury.[25] Post-traumatic stress disorder should be suspected in individuals who have flashbacks, frequent nightmares, and anxiety for situations similar to those that caused the original injury (e.g., riding in a car).

Headaches

Examination of the head and neck often elicits restriction of motion, tender points, or trigger points radiating to the head. There may be tenderness at the site of the original head injury and occasionally pain elicited by compression of the occipital nerves.[21,22,26]

Vestibular

During acute vertigo, nystagmus will often be present, generally stronger with peripheral than with central vertigo. As adaptation begins to occur, nystagmus may be seen only with certain maneuvers (e.g., after 20 horizontal head shakes) or may not be seen at all. When benign paroxysmal positional vertigo is the cause, the Hallpike-Dix maneuver usually elicits vertigo and nystagmus. This maneuver is performed from the sitting position on a flat surface with the head rotated 45 degrees to either side. The patient is quickly lowered from the sitting to lying position, until the head, still rotated, is extended over the edge of the examining table. Vertigo is experienced and nystagmus is seen after a lag of up to 30 seconds.[23] Patients with vertigo may also have balance problems with difficulty with tandem walk, hopping, and other maneuvers involving movement of the head and eye-body coordination.

Visual

Some patients complain of a feeling of visual disorientation or intermittent blurred vision. The symptoms can be related to a need for changes in refraction, accommodative dysfunction,[27] or vascular, vestibular, attentional, or psychological problems. Frequently, nothing will be found on routine examination.

Olfactory

The sense of smell may be affected by damage to branches of the olfactory nerve as they pass through the cribriform plate or by focal cortical contusion.[26]

The examination findings of other cranial nerves, muscle strength, cerebellar test results, deep tendon reflexes, plantar stimulation, frontal signs, and sensation are usually normal.

FUNCTIONAL LIMITATIONS

The extent to which post-concussion disorders interfere with function varies with the extent of the associated pathologic process but depends also on the psychological reaction to the post-concussion impairments. The most common consequences of post-concussion disorder are limitations in home and community living skills and social, academic, or vocational disability. Patients may be forgetful and inattentive, have difficulty following conversations, and find crowded, noisy environments difficult to tolerate. Headaches are often exacerbated by attentional demands and other stresses. Vertigo causes difficulty in toleration of motion, including, for some, moving vehicles.

DIAGNOSTIC TESTING

If computed tomography was not performed acutely, a computed tomographic scan of the head should be obtained as soon as possible after injury to rule out intracranial hematoma in all patients with mild head injury who have had any question of loss of consciousness and who also have any of the following: focal neurologic findings, headache, vomiting, age older than 60 years, drug or alcohol intoxication, anterograde amnesia, physical evidence of trauma above the clavicles, or seizures.[28] Although definitive criteria have not been established for those who have had no loss of consciousness, it is probably wise to obtain a computed tomographic scan or magnetic resonance imaging study for anyone who continues to have significant problems (headaches, lethargy, confusion, or anterograde memory loss), has focal neurologic findings, and has not had any neuroimaging acutely. Functional neuroimaging has not yet been studied thoroughly enough to be used to answer clinical questions after mild traumatic brain injury.

Cervical spine radiography should be performed on patients with significant neck pain shortly after the accident to assess for fracture or subluxation.

Neuropsychological evaluation should be performed if forgetfulness and attention deficits persist, particularly when rehabilitation therapies are to be pursued. Testing can provide the patient and the treatment team with a more thorough understanding of the patient's neuropsychological strengths and weaknesses and in some instances can assist with understanding of the interplay between neurocognitive and other psychological contributions to cognitive disturbance. Tests for assessment of malingering and symptom magnification can be incorporated when necessary. It is useful for sports teams to have their players undergo at least brief baseline cognitive testing or, if the resources are available, formal neuropsychological testing so that any changes can be identified in cases of subtle symptoms after the concussion.[3]

A sleep study (polysomnography) is indicated to rule out sleep apnea and other disorders when excessive daytime sleepiness does not improve despite the absence of sedating medications. The threshold for obtaining polysomnography should be lower for obese patients and those who snore prominently.

When vestibular complaints are prominent or are not improving in the early months after the injury, a thorough vestibular evaluation, including electronystagmography, may be indicated. Audiologic evaluations should be done when hearing loss is suspected or when tinnitus persists.[23]

Ophthalmology or optometry evaluation by someone with particular expertise in visual problems related to brain injury should be considered when visual symptoms are present.

TREATMENT

Initial

Treatment depends on the specific constellation of symptoms and their severity. In general, if the patient is seen in the first few weeks after the injury, the major

Differential Diagnosis[6,18,26]

Depressive disorders

Anxiety disorders

Somatoform disorder

Whiplash injury with headache (myofascial pain syndrome)

Sleep apnea

Early progressive dementia

Malingering and symptom magnification

emphasis is placed on caring for acute problems with vertigo, headache, neck pain, and insomnia and on educating the patient and significant others. Explanations should integrate the physical, cognitive, and psychological dimensions of the symptoms in as clear and simple a manner as possible. This is no small task, given the diversity of symptoms and possible causes and our limited understanding of post-concussion disorders at this time. Some patients are very sensitive to discussions of psychological etiology and may not return if they think that this has been overemphasized. The patient's experience, including the psychological reactions, should be validated and normalized.[16] The patient should be told that improvement is to be expected; after milder concussions in young people with no history of previous concussion, attention deficit disorder, or learning disability, reasonable reassurance should be given that a good recovery is likely without dismissing what the patient is experiencing. Establishment of a reasonable expectation for recovery can be helpful in preventing persistent post-concussion disorder.[29] Anticipation of the psychological reactions to post-concussion symptoms that occur in some patients allows the patient to recognize these reactions if they begin and leaves the door open for the individual to seek psychological help. Follow-up should be planned and more extensive counseling provided at the first signs of significant distress and should be considered if substantial improvement is not seen within 3 months even without apparent psychological turmoil. Patients with significant symptoms should be instructed to take time off from work, school, or other taxing activities, as the attentional demands and accompanying psychological stresses of attempting to perform under these circumstances can exacerbate the symptoms.[18]

Athletes should not go back to competitive sports until they are free of symptoms and have gone through a program of graded exertion symptom free. Those with complex concussion should move through this program more slowly than those with simple concussion.[3] (See section on potential disease complications.)

Acute vertigo may require a few days of bed rest.[23] The management of acute neck pain is described in Chapter 5.

Rehabilitation

Cognitive

If symptoms persist, patients may benefit from speech or occupational therapy for cognitive restoration and/or to learn strategies for managing problems with arousal, attention, memory, and executive function. The timing of therapies depends on the severity of the disability and the pace of recovery, which can often be determined within the first 3 months after injury. There are no published data on the timing of these interventions, and no specific guidelines are available that address the use of restorative versus compensatory approaches. Therapies should address the specific functional tasks that the individual faces on a daily basis and may need to include community outings. Foam earplugs or sunglasses can be tried for those sensitive to noise and light, respectively.[26] Paper or electronic memory aids may be helpful. Psychostimulants (e.g., methylphenidate, 5 to 60 mg/day; amphetamines, 5 to 60 mg/day) and other drugs that treat attentional and arousal disorders (e.g., atomoxetine, 10 to 100 mg/day; donepezil, 5 to 10 mg daily; modafinil, 100 to 400 mg daily), including dopaminergic drugs and NMDA receptor blockers (e.g., amantadine, 100 to 400 mg/day; memantine, 5 to 20 mg/day) may be useful for reducing the extent of attention deficits and underarousal.[30] When sleep apnea is contributing to attentional or arousal problems, positive airway pressure therapy is indicated.

Psychological

If symptoms persist beyond a few months, psychological counseling is almost always indicated. Some individuals benefit from learning relaxation techniques and sleep hygiene. Education of the patient and significant others should continue to emphasize the interaction between the cognitive, psychological, and physical sequelae. It is important that the treatment team communicate on a regular basis for treatment planning and to ensure that all clinicians approach these issues from a common framework so that mixed messages are not delivered to the patient. Support groups are often useful as well and offer an opportunity for further education about the various contributing factors. Cognitive-behavioral therapy can be helpful in concert with other treatments[31] even when symptoms do not seem to be explained by the medical condition.[32] Family counseling should be offered when there is evidence of significant stress on family members or problematic family dynamics.

Depression and anxiety can also be addressed pharmacologically, usually simultaneously with counseling interventions. It is usually best to begin with nonsedating, non-anticholinergic agents, such as the selective serotonin reuptake inhibitors (e.g., citalopram, 20 to 60 mg/day) to avoid further exacerbation of neuropsychological problems.[30] Sedating agents such as trazodone (50 to 300 mg at bedtime), zolpidem (5 to 10 mg at bedtime), or eszopiclone (2 to 3 mg at bedtime) may be necessary for those with significant insomnia[20,30] if treatment of depression and anxiety and sleep hygiene approaches are not successful.

Headaches

Post-traumatic headaches can have a number of different causes and may be multifactorial.[17-23] They are therefore best addressed on multiple levels, with the emphasis depending on the headache type. Treatment of problems with attention, sleep disorders, and psychological stresses may reduce the tension component of headaches. Relaxation techniques, including electromyographic biofeedback, can be taught. When myofascial pain originating in the neck, upper back, or temporomandibular joints contributes, physical therapy including stretching and strengthening exercises, postural retraining, environmental modification, trigger point massage, modalities, electromyographic biofeedback, and massage should be tried (see Chapter 94). However, headaches often persist despite these interventions. Trigger point injections can be helpful, as can pharmacologic approaches. Patients with temporomandibular joint problems can be treated with myofascial techniques, mouth guards, and exercises (see Chapter 96). Those headaches with an apparent vascular component may respond to acetaminophen, nonsteroidal anti-inflammatory drugs, or vasoconstrictive agents commonly used to abort migraine headaches (e.g., sumatriptan). Overuse of these agents can cause rebound headaches. For prophylaxis, some β blockers (e.g., propranolol), calcium channel blockers (e.g., verapamil), antidepressants (e.g., amitriptyline, nortriptyline, venlafaxine), and anticonvulsants (particularly valproic acid) can be helpful. Tension headaches may respond to some of these agents as well, although not to calcium channel blockers. Injection of local anesthetics and corticosteroids can be considered for greater or lesser occipital neuralgia that does not respond to more conservative approaches. Injection should be done at the site along the nerve that replicates the headache when it is palpated.[20,21,33]

Vestibular

When vestibular symptoms persist beyond 3 months, vestibular rehabilitation may both encourage central nervous system accommodation under controlled circumstances and assist the patient in learning compensatory strategies.[34] Canolith repositioning maneuvers may bring relief from benign paroxysmal positional vertigo by displacing and dispersing calcium stones.[35] Suppressive medications (e.g., clonazepam, scopolamine, meclizine) should be used judiciously, if at all, when other approaches have failed.[23] The evidence for their efficacy is not strong, and they can cause worsening of problems with attention and memory. Cervicogenic dizziness can be treated by addressing the underlying cervical musculoskeletal problems (see Chapter 7).

Vocational

The extent to which an employer or academic institution is supportive after a mild traumatic brain injury can be crucial to successful return to work for those with persistent post-concussion disorder. Vocational counselors can facilitate communication between the patient and the workplace. Therapies should attempt to simulate workplace tasks. A gradual return to work can ease the transition.[16]

Procedures

Procedures are discussed in the previous sections.

Surgery

There is little that can be done surgically to manage post-concussion disorders. However, when a perilymph fistula is suspected as the cause of severe vertigo or disequilibrium, and it does not resolve with an extended period of activity restriction, surgical exploration and repair should be considered. The diagnosis is difficult to make and is largely dependent on history. Pressure-induced vertigo or disequilibrium should raise suspicion. Sensorineural hearing loss is often present as well. Surgery consists of a graft of fascia, perichondrium, or fat fixed to the opening in the round and/or oval window with a fibrin glue. Various materials and solutions are sometimes used to augment and buttress the graft. Limited activity and avoidance of lifting, bending, and straining are recommended for several weeks after the procedure. The literature on outcomes is limited to case series, with success rates ranging from 82% to 95% for vestibular symptoms and from 20% to 49% for hearing loss. Recurrence rates are reported at 8% to 27%, but others believe the recurrence rate is considerably higher, as much as 67%.[36-40]

POTENTIAL DISEASE COMPLICATIONS

Persistence of post-concussion disorders beyond a few months is a possible outcome. Such patients may present primarily as having a chronic pain problem or chronic depression.

Individuals who sustain a second concussion while still symptomatic from a recent concussion may be susceptible to cerebral edema and dangerous increases in intracranial pressure ("second impact syndrome"). Multiple concussions, even after apparent clinical recovery from earlier episodes, can result in cumulative brain injury. Thus, caution must be exercised by those responsible for returning athletes to play.[41]

POTENTIAL TREATMENT COMPLICATIONS

Those treating the patient with post-concussion disorders may contribute to the persistence of symptoms either by overemphasizing the role of brain injury in causing symptoms due to other etiologic factors or, conversely, by overemphasizing psychological factors when brain injury and other physiologic variables are prominent.[16,18] There is often a fine line to be walked, and each patient must be approached individually in this regard, although few data are available to guide the clinician.

Some of the complications related to medications can appear paradoxical. The frequent use of analgesics (nonsteroidal anti-inflammatory drugs, acetaminophen, and narcotics) can cause rebound headaches, as can the too frequent use of ergotamine and the "triptans." Although they are generally well tolerated, psychostimulants, dopaminergic agents, and antidepressants can lead to sedation, worsening attention, agitation, or psychosis. There are myriad other complications possible from the use of the medications mentioned.

References

1. Mild Traumatic Brain Injury Committee of the Head Injury Interdisciplinary Special Interest Group of the American Congress of Rehabilitation Medicine. Definition of mild traumatic brain injury. J Head Trauma Rehabil 1993;8:86-87.
2. Quality Standards Subcommittee of the American Academy of Neurology. Practice Parameter: the management of concussion in sports (summary statement). Neurology 1997;48:581-585.
3. McCrory P, Johnston K, Meeuwisse W, et al. Summary and agreement statement of the 2nd International Conference on Concussion in Sport, Prague 2004. Br J Sports Med 2005;39:196-204.
4. Cicerone KD, Kalmar K. Persistent postconcussion syndrome: the structure of subjective complaints after mild traumatic brain injury. J Head Trauma Rehabil 1995;10:1-17.
5. Alves W, Macciocchi SN, Barth JT. Postconcussive symptoms after uncomplicated mild head injury. J Head Trauma Rehabil 1993;8:48-59.
6. Mittenberg W, Strauman S. Diagnosis of mild head injury and the postconcussion syndrome. J Head Trauma Rehabil 2000;15:783-791.
7. Carroll LJ, Cassidy JD, Peloso PM, et al. Prognosis for mild traumatic brain injury: results of the WHO Collaborating Centre Task Force on Mild Traumatic Brain Injury. J Rehabil Med 2004;43 (Suppl):84-105.
8. Iverson GL. Outcome from mild traumatic brain injury. Curr Opin Psychiatry 2005;18:301-317.
9. Mickeviciene D, Schrader H, Obelieniene D, et al. A controlled prospective inception cohort study on the post-concussion syndrome outside the medicolegal context. Eur J Neurol 2004;11:411-419.
10. Masson F, Maurette P, Salmi LR, et al. Prevalence of impairments 5 years after a head injury, and their relationship with disabilities and outcome. Brain Inj 1996;10:487-497.
11. McHugh T, Laforce R Jr, Gallagher P, et al. Natural history of the long-term cognitive, affective, and physical sequelae of mild traumatic brain injury. Brain Cogn 2006;60:209-211.
12. Vanderploeg RD, Curtiss G, Belanger HG. Long-term neuropsychological outcomes following mild traumatic brain injury. J Int Neuropsychol Soc 2005;11:228-236.
13. Bleiberg J, Halpern EL, Reeves D, Daniel JC. Future directions for the neuropsychological assessment of sports concussion. J Head Trauma Rehabil 1998;13:36-44.
14. Collins MW, Grindel SH, Lovell MR, et al. Relationship between concussion and neuropsychological performance in college football players. JAMA 1999;282:964-970.
15. Guskiewicz KM, Marshall SW, Bailes J, et al. Association between recurrent concussion and late-life cognitive impairment in retired professional football players. Neurosurgery 2005;57:719-724.
16. Kay T. Neuropsychological treatment of mild traumatic brain injury. J Head Trauma Rehabil 1993;8:74-85.
17. Martelli MF, Grayson RL, Zasler ND. Post-traumatic headache: neuropsychological and psychological effects and treatment implications. J Head Trauma Rehabil 1999;14:49-69.
18. Alexander MP. Minor traumatic brain injury: a review of physiogenesis and psychogenesis. Semin Clin Neuropsychiatry 1997;2:177-187.

19. Fenton G, McClelland R, Montgomery A, et al. The postconcussional syndrome: social antecedents and psychological sequelae. Br J Psychiatry 1993;162:493-497.

20. Hines ME. Posttraumatic headaches. In Varney NR, Roberts RJ, eds. The Evaluation and Treatment of Mild Traumatic Brain Injury. Mahwah, NJ, Lawrence Erlbaum Associates, 1999:375-410.

21. Lew HL, Lin P-H, Fuh J-L, et al. Characteristics and treatment of headache after traumatic brain injury: a focused review. Am J Phys Med Rehabil 2006;85:619-627.

22. Zafonte RD, Horn LJ. Clinical assessment of post-traumatic headaches. J Head Trauma Rehabil 1999;14:22-33.

23. Tusa RJ, Brown SB. Neuro-otologic trauma and dizziness. In Rizzo M, Tranel D, eds. Head Injury and Postconcussive Syndrome. New York, Churchill Livingstone, 1996:177-200.

24. Nolin P. Executive memory dysfunctions following mild traumatic brain injury. J Head Trauma Rehabil 2006;21:68-75.

25. Fann JR, Dikmen S, Warms CA, Rau H. Validity of the Patient Health Questionnaire-9 in assessing depression following traumatic brain injury. J Head Trauma Rehabil. 2005;20:501-511.

26. Zasler ND. Neuromedical diagnosis and management of postconcussive disorders. Phys Med Rehabil State Art Rev 1992;6:33-67.

27. Leslie S. Accommodation in acquired brain injury. In Suchoff IB, Ciuffreda KJ, Kapoor N. Visual and Vestibular Consequences of Acquired Brain Injury. Santa Ana, Calif, Optometric Extension Program, 2001:56-76.

28. Haydel MJ, Preston CA, Mills TJ, et al. Indications for computed tomography in patients with minor head injury. N Engl J Med 2000;343:100-105.

29. Mittenberg W, Tremont G, Zielinski RE, et al. Cognitive-behavioral prevention of postconcussion syndrome. Arch Clin Neuropsychol 1996;11:139-145.

30. Glenn MB, Wroblewski B. Twenty years of pharmacology. J Head Trauma Rehabil 2005;20:51-61.

31. Andersson G, Asmundson GJ, Denev J, et al. A controlled trial of cognitive-behavior therapy combined with vestibular rehabilitation in the treatment of dizziness. Behav Res Ther 2006;44:1265-1273.

32. Smith RC, Lyles JS, Gardiner JC, et al. Primary care clinicians treat patients with medically unexplained symptoms: a randomized controlled trial. J Gen Intern Med 2006;21:671-677.

33. Bell KR, Kraus EE, Zasler ND. Medical management of posttraumatic headaches: pharmacological and physical treatment. J Head Trauma Rehabil 1999;14:34-48.

34. Wrisley DM, Pavou M. Physical therapy for balance disorders. Neurol Clin 2005;23:855-874.

35. White J, Savvides P, Cherian N, Oas J. Canalith repositioning for benign paroxysmal positional vertigo. Otol Neurotol 2005;26:704-710.

36. Hain TC. Perilymph fistula: dizziness-and-balance.com/disorders/unilat/fistula.html. Accessed December 30, 2007.

37. Goto F, Ogawa K, Kunihiro T, et al. Perilymph fistula: 45 case analyses. Auris Nasus Larynx 2001;28:29-33.

38. Gyo K, Kobayashi T, Yumoto E, Yanagihara N. Postoperative recurrence of perilymphatic fistulas. Acta Otolaryngol (Stockh) 1994; Suppl 514:59-62.

39. Black FO, Pesznecker S, Norton T, et al. Surgical management of perilymphatic fistulas: a Portland experience. Am J Otol 1992;13:254-262.

40. Seltzer S, McCabe BF. Perilymph fistula: the Iowa experience. Laryngoscope 1986;94:37-49

41. Kelly JP, Rosenberg J. Diagnosis and management of concussion in sports. Neurology 1997;48:575-580.

Psoriatic Arthritis 139

Mahboob U. Rahman, MD, PhD

Synonyms

Inflammatory arthritis associated with psoriasis
Spondyloarthropathy associated with psoriasis
Seronegative spondyloarthropathy

ICD-9 Code

696.0   Psoriatic arthropathy

DEFINITION

Psoriatic arthritis, a unique inflammatory arthritis associated with psoriasis, occurs in approximately 5% to 40% of patients with psoriasis and 0.3% to 1% of the general population.[1-3] Approximately 20% of patients with psoriatic arthritis develop a destructive and potentially disabling disease.[2] Several diagnostic criteria have been proposed for this disease; however, consensus is yet to be reached.[4] Patients generally present with an inflammatory arthritis, absence of rheumatoid factor, and psoriatic skin disease. Unlike with rheumatoid arthritis, there is an equal sex distribution. The onset of arthritis, however, can coincide with or precede the onset of skin disease.

Several patterns or subgroups of psoriatic arthritis are recognized: symmetric arthritis similar to rheumatoid arthritis; inflammatory arthritis confined to the distal interphalangeal joints of the hands and feet; arthritis mutilans; spondyloarthropathy (spondylitis and sacroiliitis); and oligoarticular arthritis.[5]

SYMPTOMS

Patients report a variety of constitutional, joint, eye, and skin symptoms.[5-9]

General

Morning stiffness is a prominent feature of psoriatic arthritis. Unlike the brief stiffness (5 to 10 minutes) that occurs in patients with osteoarthritis, the morning stiffness in psoriatic arthritis is longer than 30 to 60 minutes and often lasts for hours. Fatigue and generalized malaise are also common complaints.

Joint

Patients present with joint pain and swelling. Patients may also complain of loss of joint function, which may be due to joint inflammation or structural damage. Baker's cyst can develop and cause pain or swelling of the popliteal fossa. If the cyst ruptures, it causes pain, swelling, and erythema of the calf. Back pain and stiffness can be prominent features of the history. Enthesitis, inflammation at the site of tendon or ligamentous insertion onto bone, is common in psoriatic arthritis. Achilles enthesitis results in pain at the heel, and plantar fasciitis causes plantar foot pain that is typically most intense on rising in the morning.

Eye

Patients with conjunctivitis complain of red eyes. Iritis causes deep pain and tearing. As in rheumatoid arthritis, patients can have keratoconjunctivitis sicca (dry eyes) and relate a feeling of foreign body sensation, burning, or discharge.

Skin

Psoriasis is present in 90% of patients at the time of diagnosis of psoriatic arthritis. The arthritis, however, may precede the onset of skin disease. Patients who do not have psoriasis at the time of diagnosis may have had a history or a family history of psoriasis.[4]

PHYSICAL EXAMINATION

All joints are examined for swelling, warmth, effusion, range of motion, and deformity. Psoriatic arthritis can present in several different clinical patterns (Table 139-1).[5,6] Any joint can be involved. If patients do not relate a history of psoriasis, the examiner should perform a careful examination of the scalp, flexural regions, and nails (onycholysis, pitting, or hyperkeratosis).

In the hands, distal interphalangeal joint involvement is associated with psoriatic nail changes. Dactylitis is the result of digital joint and tendon sheath inflammation

TABLE 139-1 Joint Involvement

Pattern or Subgroup	Clinical Features
Symmetric polyarthritis (rheumatoid arthritis–like)	Small joints of hands and feet, wrists, ankles, elbows, or knees (may include distal interphalangeal joint, distinguishing it from rheumatoid arthritis)
	Seronegative
Distal interphalangeal joint involvement	Inflammatory changes in the distal interphalangeal joints
	High association with psoriatic nail changes (onycholysis and pitting)
Arthritis mutilans	Severe resorptive arthritis resulting in floppy or flail digits
	Shortening of the digits with skin folds that can be extended by the clinician (telescoping)
Spondyloarthropathy	Spondylitis
	Sacroiliitis
	Enthesitis
Oligoarthritis	Large joint (e.g., knee)
	One or two small joints of hands or feet
	Dactylitis (sausage digit)

and causes a diffusely swollen (sausage) digit. Inflammation of the Achilles tendon or its insertion site on the calcaneus can cause tenderness or thickening.

Patients with conjunctivitis will have red, injected sclera. Iritis causes pericorneal erythema (ciliary flush) and miosis.

FUNCTIONAL LIMITATIONS

Functional limitations depend on the location and severity of joint involvement. The criteria for the assessment of functional status that have been established for rheumatoid arthritis are also applied to patients with psoriatic arthritis (see Chapter 142). These criteria are based on activities of daily living, including self-care (dressing, feeding, bathing, grooming, and toileting) and vocational (work, school, and homemaking) and avocational (recreational and leisure) activities.[9]

DIAGNOSTIC STUDIES

Laboratory studies may reveal anemia of chronic disease and an elevated sedimentation rate. Joint fluid is inflammatory (more than 2000 white blood cells) with negative cultures and crystal examination. Rheumatoid factor is usually absent. In patients with rheumatoid factor, the coexistence of psoriasis and rheumatoid arthritis must be considered, especially if the pattern is a symmetric polyarthritis. Absence of anti–cyclic citrullinated peptide antibodies may also be helpful in increasing the diagnostic certainty in the appropriate patient.[3] In the spondylitic form, 25% of patients are HLA-B27 positive.[8]

Radiographs can assist in the evaluation of both axial and peripheral involvement.[6,10] Spine films may show syndesmophytes, although they often spare the thoracolumbar junction and are "chunky," helping to distinguish them from the changes of ankylosing spondylitis. Cervical spine views may show erosion of the odontoid and atlantoaxial subluxation. Radiologic evaluation of peripheral joints can help distinguish this form of arthritis from rheumatoid arthritis. Psoriatic changes include distal interphalangeal joint involvement, osteolysis (metacarpals and phalanges), joint ankylosis, periostitis, and pencil-in-cup deformity. Bone proliferation may be found in the pelvis and calcaneus, corresponding to enthesitis. Utility of magnetic resonance imaging in the management of psoriatic arthritis is being increasingly recognized.[11,12]

Differential Diagnosis

Other spondyloarthropathies

Enteropathic arthritis

Ankylosing spondylitis

Rheumatoid arthritis

Crystal-induced arthritis (especially with distal interphalangeal joint involvement)

  Gout

  Pseudogout

Asystemic lupus erythematosus

TREATMENT

Initial

The approach to treatment is generally the same as for other spondyloarthropathies.[13,14] Nonsteroidal anti-inflammatory drugs (NSAIDs) are effective in many patients. Cyclooxygenase 2 (COX-2)–specific anti-inflammatories may reduce the incidence of gastrointestinal symptoms in patients who have a history of bleeding or who are intolerant of traditional NSAIDs. For patients with inadequate response or progressive, erosive disease, disease-modifying antirheumatic drugs should be initiated. Antimalarials, intramuscular administration of gold, sulfasalazine, azathioprine, methotrexate, leflunomide, and cyclosporine have all been shown to be effective.[15-17] As with other inflammatory arthritides, combination therapy can be effective. Biologic agents such as anti–tumor necrosis factor antibodies (etanercept, infliximab, adalimumab) have been proven to be effective in the control of psoriatic skin lesions as well as signs and symptoms of arthritis and in the prevention of structural damage in involved joints.[15-18] Corticosteroids can be very useful and can be administered systemically as a bridge to therapy with disease-modifying antirheumatic drugs or intra-articularly for monarticular or oligoarticular involvement.

Photochemotherapy (PUVA) used by the dermatologist for skin disease can sometimes improve peripheral joint involvement but does not affect axial disease.[8]

Rehabilitation

Approaches to rehabilitation are identical to those in rheumatoid and other inflammatory arthritis. The role of occupational and physical therapy may be different in early or established disease and end-stage disease. In early disease, occupational therapy is directed toward education of the patient about how to minimize joint stress in performing activities of daily living. Splints may be employed to provide joint rest and to reduce inflammation. Splints may also allow functional use of joints that would otherwise be limited by pain. Paraffin baths can provide relief of pain and stiffness in the small joints of the hands. In end-stage disease, the occupational therapist plays an important role, providing aids and adaptive devices, such as raised toilet seats, special chairs and beds, and special grips, that can assist in self-care.

Physical therapy can be very helpful in reducing joint inflammation and pain. The therapist may employ a variety of techniques, including the application of heat or cold, transcutaneous nerve stimulation, and iontophoresis. Water exercise (hydrotherapy) is used to increase muscle strength without joint overuse. In patients with foot involvement, such as dactylitis, a high toe box or extra-depth shoe may decrease pain and provide a more normal gait. Shoe inserts are often used in Achilles tendinitis and plantar fasciitis. For patients with axial involvement, the goal of therapy is maintenance of a normal upright posture through stretching of paravertebral musculature and correction of the tendency toward kyphotic posture. In end-stage disease, the goals of therapy are to reduce joint inflammation, to loosen fixed position of joints, to improve the function of damaged joints, and to improve strength and general condition. Local immobilization may reduce inflammation and pain. Nonfixed contractures may be prevented or improved with periods of splinting combined with goal-oriented exercise. Muscle strength and overall conditioning may be improved by static, range of motion, and relaxation exercises. In recent years, aerobic and dynamic strengthening exercises have been used without detrimental effect to the joints. These dynamic exercises are more effective in increasing muscle strength, range of motion, and physical capacity.[19] The motivation and encouragement provided by the therapist should not be underestimated.

Procedures

For monarticular or oligoarticular involvement, local steroid injection may be used when NSAIDs fail to control joint inflammation.

Surgery

Orthopedic intervention, including joint replacement, tendon repair, and synovectomy, may be indicated. Patients with suspected or confirmed cervical spine involvement will need special consideration and handling during intubation for anesthesia.

POTENTIAL DISEASE COMPLICATIONS

Psoriatic arthritis can lead to progressive damage to joints, including ankylosis, resulting in lack of function. Ankylosis of the spine, together with osteoporosis, increases the susceptibility to fracture. Ruptured tendons result secondary to chronic enthesitis. Inflammatory eye disease sometimes results in visual loss.

POTENTIAL TREATMENT COMPLICATIONS

Medication side effects vary according to the drug used (Table 139-2).[20]

TABLE 139-2 Toxicities of Medications Used in Psoriatic Arthritis

Medication	Side Effects
NSAIDs	
Traditional	Dyspepsia, ulcer, or bleeding Renal insufficiency Hepatotoxicity Rash
COX-2 inhibitors	Same as traditional NSAIDs, but gastrointestinal side effects occur less often No platelet effect
Glucocorticoids	Increased appetite, weight gain Cushingoid habitus Acne Fluid retention Hypertension Diabetes Glaucoma, cataracts Atherosclerosis Avascular necrosis Osteoporosis Impaired wound healing Increased susceptibility to infection
Antimalarials	Dyspepsia Hemolysis (glucose-6-phosphate dehydrogenase–deficient patients) Macular damage Abnormal skin pigmentation Neuromyopathy Rash
Gold	Myelosuppression Proteinuria or hematuria Oral ulcers Rash Pruritus
Sulfasalazine	Myelosuppression Hemolysis (glucose-6-phosphate dehydrogenase–deficient patients) Hepatotoxicity Photosensitivity, rash Dyspepsia, diarrhea Headaches Oligospermia
Azathioprine	Myelosuppression Hepatotoxicity Pancreatitis (rarely) Lymphoproliferative disorders (long-term risk)
Methotrexate	Hepatic fibrosis, cirrhosis Pneumonitis Myelosuppression Mucositis Dyspepsia Alopecia
Cyclosporine	Renal insufficiency Hypertension Anemia
Biologic anti–tumor necrosis-α agents	Increased risk of infections, including tuberculosis

References

1. Espinoza LR, Cuellar MI, Silveira LH. Psoriatic arthritis. Curr Opin Rheumatol 1992;4:470-478.
2. Gladman DD, Antoni C, Mease P, et al. Psoriatic arthritis: epidemiology, clinical features, course, and outcome. Ann Rheum Dis 2005;64(Suppl 2):ii14.
3. Candia L, Marquez J, Gonzalez C, et al. Low frequency of anticyclic citrullinated peptide antibodies in psoriatic arthritis but not in cutaneous psoriasis. J Clin Rheumatol 2006;12:226-229.
4. Taylor W, Gladman D, Helliwell P, et al; CASPAR Study Group. Classification criteria for psoriatic arthritis: development of new criteria from a large international study. Arthritis Rheum 2006;54:2665-2673.
5. Pitzalis C, Pipitone N. Psoriatic arthritis. J R Soc Med 2000;93:412-415.
6. Helliwell PS, Wright V. Psoriatic arthritis: clinical features. In Klippel JH, Dieppe PA, eds. Rheumatology, 2nd ed. London, Mosby, 1998:21.1-21.8.
7. Moll JMH, Wright V. Psoriatic arthritis. Semin Arthritis Rheum 1973;3:55-78.
8. Boumpas DT, Tassiulas IO. Psoriatic arthritis. In Klippel JH, ed. Primer on the Rheumatic Diseases, 11th ed. Atlanta, Ga, Arthritis Foundation, 1997:175-179.
9. Hochberg MC, Chang RW, Dwosh I, et al. The American College of Rheumatology 1991 revised criteria for the classification of global functional status in rheumatoid arthritis. Arthritis Rheum 1992;35:493-502.
10. Resnick D, Niwayama G. Psoriatic arthritis. In Resnick D, Niwayama G, eds. Diagnosis of Bone and Joint Disorders, vol 2. Philadelphia, WB Saunders, 1981:1103-1129.
11. Marzo-Ortega H, McGonagle D, Rhodes LA, et al. Efficacy of infliximab on MRI determined bone oedema in psoriatic arthritis. Ann Rheum Dis 2007;66:778-781. Epub 2006 Dec 21.
12. Ghanem N, Uhl M, Pache G, et al. MRI in psoriatic arthritis with hand and foot involvement. Rheumatol Int 2007;27:387-393.
13. Gladman DD. Psoriatic arthritis: recent advances in pathogenesis and treatment. Rheum Dis Clin North Am 1992;18:247-256.
14. Haslock I. Ankylosing spondylitis: management. In Klippel JH, Dieppe PA, eds. Rheumatology, 2nd ed. London, Mosby, 1998:19.1-19.10.
15. Kavanaugh AF, Ritchlin CT; GRAPPA Treatment Guideline Committee. Systematic review of treatments for psoriatic arthritis: an evidence based approach and basis for treatment guidelines. J Rheumatol 2006;33:1417-1421.
16. Mease P. Psoriatic arthritis update. Bull NYU Hosp Jt Dis 2006;64:25-31.
17. Mease P. Management of psoriatic arthritis: the therapeutic interface between rheumatology and dermatology. Curr Rheumatol Rep 2006;8:348-354.
18. Mease PJ, Goffe BS, Metz J, et al. Etanercept in the treatment of psoriatic arthritis and psoriasis: a randomized trial. Lancet 2000;356:385-390.
19. van den Ende CH, Breedveld FC, le Cessie S, et al. Effect of invasive exercise on patients with active rheumatoid arthritis: a randomised clinical trial. Ann Rheum Dis 2000;59:615-621.
20. Cash JM, Klippel JH. Drug therapy: second-line drug therapy for rheumatoid arthritis. N Engl J Med 1994;330:1368-1375.

Pressure Ulcers 140

Chester H. Ho, MD, and Kath Bogie, DPhil

DEFINITION

The development of pressure ulcers due to tissue breakdown and cell necrosis is a significant secondary complication for many patients, including those with progressive neuromuscular disease, the elderly, and those with impaired mobility or paralysis. Tissue breakdown is referred to by many terms, including decubitus ulcers, pressure sores, ischemic sores, and bedsores. The term *pressure ulcer* is the most accurate nomenclature to describe both the cause and nature of chronic, nonhealing wounds due primarily to excessive applied pressure. This term is used throughout the chapter.

Staging of pressure ulcers describes the extent of tissue breakdown at initial examination. A widely accepted staging system based on the pathologic features of pressure ulcers was initially developed by Shea.[1] A modified version was recommended by the Agency for Health Care Policy and Research in the clinical practice guideline for treatment of pressure ulcers[2]:

Stage I nonblanchable erythema of intact skin, the heralding lesion of skin ulceration. In individuals with darker skin, discoloration of the skin, warmth, edema, induration, and hardness may also be indicators.

Stage II partial-thickness skin loss involving epidermis, dermis, or both. The ulcer is superficial and presents clinically as an abrasion, blister, or shallow crater.

Stage III full-thickness skin loss involving damage to or necrosis of subcutaneous tissue that may extend down to, but not through, underlying fascia. The ulcer presents clinically as a deep crater with or without undermining of adjacent tissue.

Stage IV full-thickness skin loss with extensive destruction; tissue necrosis; or damage to muscle, bone, or supporting structures (e.g., tendon, joint capsule). Undermining and sinus tracts also may be associated with stage IV pressure ulcers.

This staging system can be used *only* for initial description of the wound. It cannot be used for repeated assessments, primarily because it cannot characterize what is happening in a healing wound. Reepithelization will occur before lost muscle, subcutaneous fat, or dermis is replaced,[3] resulting in mistakes when healed wounds are staged again.

Care must also be taken in the evaluation of the skin of patients with darkly pigmented skin. Sprigle and colleagues[4] found that erythema in subjects with dark skin is more likely to be nonblanching and to have poor resilience. This indicates that clinicians should use persistence of erythema rather than blanching status to judge incipient pressure ulcers. The staging system defined here includes both visual and nonvisual indicators in the definition of a stage I ulcer, in part to address this issue.

The National Pressure Ulcer Advisory Panel has published recommendations that address limitations reported by clinicians with use of the Agency for Health Care Policy and Research staging system.[5,6] Differential description of pressure ulcers that develop subsequent to deep tissue damage under intact skin rather than by more superficial inflammatory responses should be included in the initial definition of the pressure ulcer and is relevant to both prognosis and clinical treatment.

The incidence of pressure ulcers among patients in acute care hospitals ranges from 1% to 33%, with prevalence rates of 3% to 69%.[7-13] Higher rates have been associated with increasing age and duration of hospital stay in the elderly.[14] In those with spinal cord injury, individuals with paraplegia are more likely to be rehospitalized because of pressure ulcers.[15] The prevalence of pressure ulcers on admission to skilled nursing facilities ranges between 15% and 25%.[16] A long-term study of pressure ulcer incidence in the State of Washington found that during the period 1987–2000, the incidence of pressure ulcers had more than doubled; however, the authors thought that this might be because pressure ulcers are now being reported in a more thorough manner.[17] In addition, Gunningberg and Ehrenberg[18] found that pressure ulcer prevalence determined by audit of clinical records is less than 50% of the rate found when the patient's skin is examined. This highlights the importance of accurate wound documentation. The use of electronic records may allow digital images of wounds to be incorporated into the patient's records routinely.

A consideration of the risk factors in pressure ulcer development is of vital importance because they contribute to the development of treatment and rehabilitation strategies. There are many factors that can lead to the development of pressure ulcers. These can be classified as extrinsic factors primarily related to the interface between the individual and the external environment and intrinsic factors related to the clinical and physiologic profile of the individual[1] (Table 140-1). Changes in clinical status over time can alter intrinsic factors and can increase the risk for pressure ulcer development. For example, urinary incontinence will alter the microenvironment of the skin surface and make it more susceptible to maceration and breakdown. Changes in environmental factors, such as the seating system used, will alter external factors that affect pressure ulcer risk status.

Intrinsic Risk Factors

Intrinsic risk factors in pressure ulcer development are a direct consequence of impairment. Reduced muscle activity and paralysis lead to loss of muscle bulk, thus reducing soft tissue coverage over the bone prominences of the pelvic region. As muscle bulk decreases, so regional vascularity diminishes and the proportion of avascular fatty tissue increases. Loss of normal muscle tone leads to abnormal responses to environmental stimuli, such as applied pressure, thus increasing the risk for blood flow to become compromised.

Motor paralysis will also directly affect a person's ability to respond unconsciously to potential noxious stimuli (e.g., fidgeting while sitting or turning while asleep). Reduced mobility also profoundly alters the individual's ability to consciously perform postural maneuvers necessary to relieve prolonged applied pressure, from weight shifting while sitting to walking. The loss or reduction of mobility may be further complicated by sensory impairment, leading to the absence or alteration of normal

perception of environmental stimuli, such as pain or temperature. Patients with impaired sensation or proprioception are at increased risk for pressure ulcer development because the individual cannot sense the warning signals that precede tissue damage.

The malnourished patient is at increased risk for pressure ulcer development and will also have an impaired response to healing. Normal tissue integrity depends on correct nitrogen balance and vitamin intake. Protein depletion will lead to decreased perfusion and impaired immune response. The presence of an exuding pressure ulcer will cause massive protein loss, and the patient will move into increasingly negative nitrogen balance. The severity of a pressure ulcer can be directly related to the degree of hypoalbuminemia.[19] Fluid balance must also be considered in conjunction with nutritional status because dehydration will decrease cellular nutrient delivery.

Extrinsic Risk Factors

The primary extrinsic risk factor in pressure ulcer development is external applied pressure. Body tissues can support high levels of hydrostatic pressure, such as in deep sea diving. When pressure is the same in all directions, there is no resulting tissue damage. However, nonuniform applied pressures cause tissue distortion, leading to localized tissue damage.[20] This will occur when a patient is in contact with an external load-supporting device, such as a bed or wheelchair. The pressure at the interface between the patient and the support surface must be maintained at a level such that the local blood supply and lymphatic circulation are not impaired. This threshold varies between individuals, and a specialized support system is often required in high-risk individuals, such as acute spinal cord–injured patients.

Any external load that can cause tissue distortion is also likely to cause shear stresses. When only shear forces are present, slipping occurs, and tissue damage will be minimized. However, shear and normal applied loads generally tend to occur together. The normal applied load required to occlude blood flow can be halved when shear forces are also present. Significant clinical problems can arise from propping patients up in bed at angles of less than 90 degrees. In contrast, in the side-lying position, it has been found that blood flow is severely impaired by fully lying on the trochanteric region; but at a partial 30-degree side-lying position, blood flow is maintained.[21]

SYMPTOMS

The primary symptom of a pressure ulcer is an area of persistent tissue breakdown involving the skin and underlying tissues. The severity of pressure ulcers has traditionally been characterized by the extent of breakdown, from grade I (least severe) to grade IV (most severe).[2]

All pressure ulcers are associated with some degree of bacterial colonization, which may or may not lead to local wound infection. The possible clinical signs and

TABLE 140-1 Risk Factors in Pressure Ulcer Development

Extrinsic Factors	Intrinsic Factors
Applied pressure	Reduced or absent sensation
Surface shear	Impaired mobility
Local microenvironment	Decreased blood flow
	Muscle atrophy
	Poor nutrition

symptoms of local infection include increasing pain in the wound; erythema, edema, and heat of the periwound area; foul odor; and purulent drainage.[22] Individuals with spinal cord injury may not have intact sensation; in such cases, infected wounds are painless but can cause systemic responses, such as autonomic dysreflexia.

Pressure ulcers also frequently exhibit wound drainage. However, this drainage is not necessarily due to wound infection, and unless it is clinically indicated, routine wound swab culture is not warranted[23] because this would give a false-positive result. On the other hand, in some cases, increased volumes of exudate may indicate wound infection.

Systemic infection may develop if the initial local wound infection is not adequately treated. In such cases, patients may exhibit fever, malaise, and chills. Cellulitis, osteomyelitis, and bacteremia may also develop.

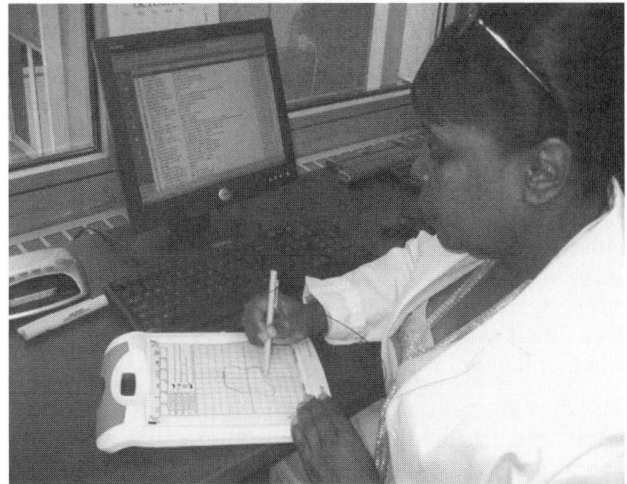

FIGURE 140-1. Visitrak wound measurement device. (Courtesy of Smith & Nephew, Largo, Fla.)

PHYSICAL EXAMINATION

Physical examination for a pressure ulcer starts with the overall assessment of the risk factors of the individual and his or her environment. On the general examination, evaluation of overall strength, muscle tone, spasticity, range of motion, and presence of contractures is important. Abnormalities in these areas can contribute to both the development and the persistence of pressure ulcers. In addition, it is important to note whether the individual is malnourished, anemic, incontinent of feces or urine, cognitively impaired, or immobile from medical conditions such as stroke or spinal cord injury as well as whether appropriate pressure-relieving surfaces for seating and sleeping have been used. The Braden Scale is a commonly used nursing risk assessment tool to determine whether an individual is at risk for pressure ulcer development.[24] An individual with a score of 18 or lower is found to be at risk.

A systematic approach to the examination of the pressure ulcer is necessary to provide accurate assessment and monitoring of the pressure ulcer. The following parameters are to be noted:

- Location of the ulcer
- Size of the pressure ulcer (length to be measured as the maximum measurement craniocaudally; width as the maximum measurement from side to side; depth to be measured at the deepest part of the wound perpendicular to the skin surface)
- Staging of the ulcer
- Presence of undermining or tunneling
- Ulcer bed appearance
- Presence of necrotic materials, slough, eschar, fibrous tissues
- Presence of rolled wound edges
- Presence and amount of drainage (exudate versus transudate)
- Presence of foul odor
- Tissue health of the periulcer tissues, including any surrounding erythema, maceration, edema, or associated fungal infection

Proper staging combined with the overall assessment forms the basis for institution of a treatment plan and monitoring of progress.[19]

Manual measurement of the wounds by length, width, and depth is the conventional method, but there is poor interrater reliability and the actual surface area of the wound is not known. Newer electronic technologies have allowed more accurate documentation and measurements of the surface areas. For instance, the Visitrak device allows easy measurement of wound surface area by a tracing method (Fig. 140-1); the VeV MD software provides digital imaging documentation of the wound as well as calculation of the surface area by planimetry (Fig. 140-2).

Once a pressure ulcer develops, it must be examined regularly for treatment progress to be monitored. At the minimum, weekly assessments should be performed to ensure that the treatment plan is having the desired effect.

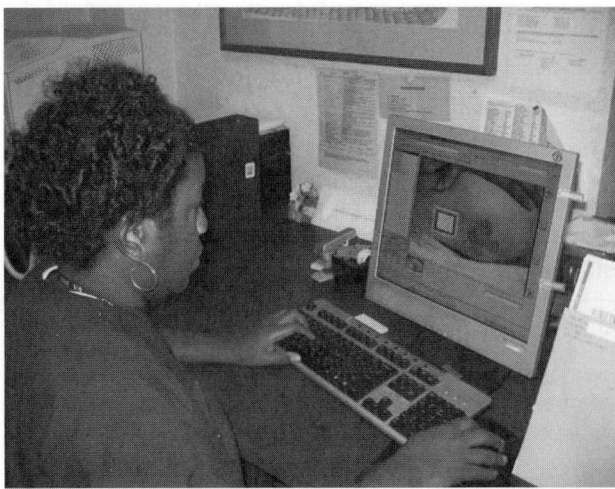

FIGURE 140-2. VeV MD wound measurement system. (Courtesy of Vista of Medical Ltd., Manitoba, Canada.)

FUNCTIONAL LIMITATIONS

If a pressure ulcer develops, functional limitations are generally exacerbated. For example, a wheelchair user who develops an ischial region pressure ulcer will lose mobility independence because treatment requires prolonged periods of total bed rest. Less obvious is a hemiplegic patient who always rolls and pivots to one side to get out of bed; if a greater trochanter pressure ulcer develops on the side that is aggravated by the pressure, shear, and friction of getting out of bed, either that individual will be limited in being able to get out of bed independently or a new technique must be explored.

The development and location of a pressure ulcer may sometimes give an indication of changes in the patient's mood and activity level. For example, an active wheelchair user may develop an ischial region pressure ulcer from sitting for long periods without adequate pressure relief. However, if that same individual presented with a trochanteric pressure ulcer, most likely due to lying in bed for long periods, the clinician would question whether the patient is depressed and not getting up and about. Changes in body mass should also be evaluated to determine whether the wheelchair and cushion are still appropriate; if a patient gains weight, the wheelchair and cushion can become too narrow, and increased pressures may develop at the greater trochanteric areas because of impingement.

The development of a pressure ulcer will affect many aspects of a patient's daily living activities. Patients in active rehabilitation programs may not be able to participate in therapy; independent mobility and transfers will be restricted, and it may not be possible for appropriate bracing or orthotics to be worn.

DIAGNOSTIC STUDIES

It is well accepted that malnutrition is linked to both the development of pressure ulcers and their ability to heal. A nutritional assessment that indicates malnutrition is a serum albumin level of less than 3.5 g/L, total protein level of less than 6.4 g/dL, or body weight decreased by more than 15% since the prior assessment. Prealbumin has a short half-life of only 2 or 3 days. Prealbumin concentration is an even more sensitive measure than serum albumin level and should be obtained in the determination of acute response to nutritional intervention. A nutritional assessment should be repeated every 12 weeks.[19] It has been proposed that the Mini Nutritional Assessment tool may be a reliable questionnaire-based approach to obtain repeated evaluations in the elderly.[25]

Anemia is another important factor that may affect pressure ulcer healing. Hemoglobin level below 12.0 g/dL has been associated with impaired wound healing because of reduced tissue oxygenation.[26]

Once a patient has a pressure ulcer, the determination of whether bacterial infection, underlying osteomyelitis, related abscess, or sinus tracts are hindering the healing process becomes important. There are many studies that can help us determine the diagnosis of osteomyelitis. High serum erythrocyte sedimentation rate and C-reactive protein level, although nonspecific, may be an indication of osteomyelitis. Plain radiography of the underlying bone, computed tomography, bone scan, and magnetic resonance imaging can all be used to better assess the underlying and surrounding tissue and bones for possible associated complications. The proper imaging for each patient depends on the history and desired focus of the study. The most definitive and yet most invasive diagnostic study is bone biopsy. This can be done either bedside with a needle or in the interventional radiology suite or the operating room. Culture of the bone biopsy specimen will give us the most accurate microbiologic diagnosis of the underlying osteomyelitis, allowing us to use the most specific antimicrobial agent for treatment. Routine swab culture of the wounds is not recommended because all wounds are colonized with bacteria; such cultures will only bring about false-positive results, leading to unnecessary and inappropriate antimicrobial treatments.

Differential Diagnosis

Ischemic ulcer

Diabetic ulcer

Venous stasis ulcer

Dermatologic neoplasms

Surgical wound dehiscence

Abscess

Abrasion

TREATMENT

Initial

Unfortunately, pressure ulcers remain one of the most common reasons for readmission to the hospital for many patients with impaired mobility. The patient with a major pressure ulcer will require an average of 180 days of nursing time.[27] Allman and colleagues[28] found that development of a nosocomial pressure ulcer was associated with significant and substantial increases in both hospital costs and length of stay in a group of patients admitted to the hospital with reduced mobility due to a primary diagnosis of hip fracture. Xakellis and Frantz[29] found that the cost of treating pressure ulcers was greatly increased when a patient required hospitalization. The cost to treat pressure ulcers was estimated to be in excess of $1.33 billion per annum in 1994.[30] With adjustment for inflation, this implies that current costs are around $1.89 billion per annum in the United States.

Both the European Pressure Ulcer Advisory Panel and the Consortium for Spinal Cord Medicine have issued clinical guidelines for the prevention and treatment of pressure ulcers.[31-33] When treating a pressure ulcer, the clinician should always keep in mind that the main precipitating factors are pressure, shearing forces, friction, and moisture and therefore focus treatment on minimizing these factors.[34] Figure 140-3 demonstrates the paradigm modified from Sibbald and coworkers[35]; it provides a helpful guideline for chronic wound preparation for treatment.

The comorbid conditions shown to delay ulcer healing are peripheral vascular disease, diabetes mellitus, immune deficiencies, collagen vascular diseases, malignant neoplasms, psychosis, smoking, and depression.[36] Identification and treatment of these conditions in patients with pressure ulcers are important.

If malnutrition is a factor, aggressive nutritional supplementation or support should be instituted to place the patient into a positive nitrogen balance. Nutritional support should occur only if it is consistent with the patient's wishes and is likely to change the patient's prognosis. Also, supplemental vitamins should be given if deficiencies are suspected by examination or confirmed by laboratory evaluation. Supplemental vitamin C and zinc have been used by many clinicians to enhance wound healing, even in the absence of clinical deficiency. Individual supplements up to 10 times the recommended dietary allowance for a particular water-soluble vitamin can be provided if it is found to be deficient.[2]

Pain should also be addressed and treated appropriately. Some pain may be eliminated or controlled by covering the wound and appropriate positioning. If the pain persists, analgesia is provided as needed during manipulations of the wound and for chronic wound pain.[37]

Once a pressure ulcer develops, therapy must focus on medical treatment of the ulcer while at the same time addressing the factors that led to ulcer formation. Apart from débridement, conservative treatment options, such as topical dressings, are employed whenever possible. Treatment is generally divided into four components: (1) débridement of necrotic tissue as needed (sharp, mechanical, enzymatic, or autolytic débridement); (2) cleaning of the wound initially and with each dressing change (normal saline is recommended; avoid antiseptic agents); (3) prevention of infection and diagnosis and treatment of an infection if one occurs; and (4) dressing of the ulcer to keep the ulcer bed moist and the surrounding tissue dry.[2] Many types of topical dressings and antibiotics can be employed to promote wound healing.[2] Promotion of a moist wound environment to facilitate wound healing is strongly indicated by evidence-based research.[38] Thus, the common goal is always to produce a moist wound environment that will promote cell proliferation.

Wound irrigation with normal saline must be done with adequate pressure to be effective for wound cleaning and mechanical débridement; the pressure of 4 to 15 psi has been found to be safe and nontraumatic to the wound bed. This can be achieved with an appropriate syringe or a pulsatile lavage device that produces irrigation pressure within this recommended range.

Positioning should be evaluated in both the lying and seated positions. Patients should be positioned to avoid direct pressure and shearing force on the ulcer area (see section on extrinsic factors). Immobile patients in bed should be turned on a scheduled basis, at least every 2 hours. If necessary, pillows or foam wedges can be used to help patients maintain a position that keeps the ulcer area pressure free. Multiple mattresses and overlays are available, depending on the patient, extent and location of the pressure ulcer, and goals of therapy. For the individuals who can tolerate lying prone, use of a prone cart allows the patient to be out of bed but avoids any pressure on the sacral area.

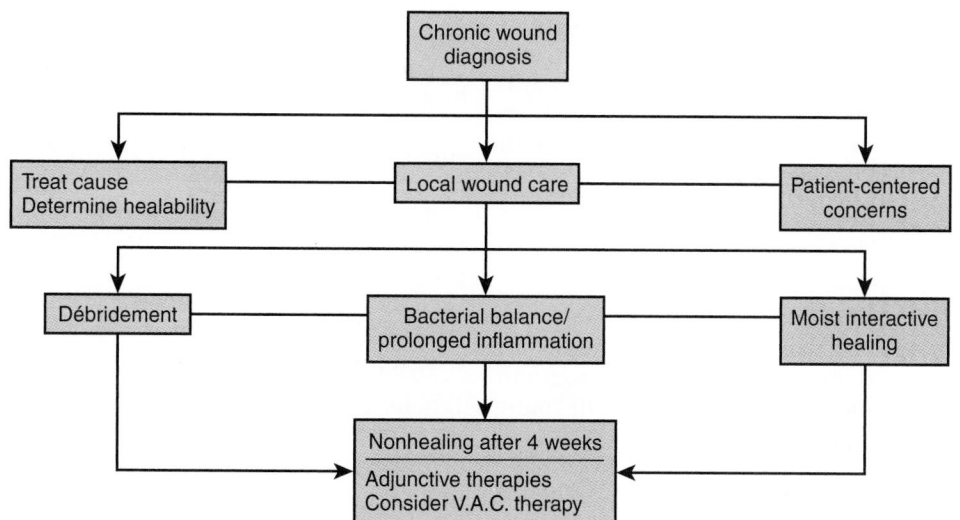

FIGURE 140-3. Standardized nonsurgical treatment paradigm for pressure ulcer therapy. V.A.C., vacuum-assisted closure.

Sitting should be avoided if pressure cannot be relieved from the ulcer area in the sitting position.

Within 1 to 2 weeks of the initiation of treatment, partial-thickness pressure ulcers should show signs of healing. Full-thickness ulcers should show reduction in size after 2 to 4 weeks of treatment.[37] This should be determined with some caution; pressure ulcers often appear to be initially larger after treatment because of the effect of débridement and cleaning, exposing the real extent of ulceration. There also appears to be a proportion of pressure ulcers that develop as the result of deep tissue damage, at the interface between the soft tissues and the bone rather than at the skin surface. These ulcers will often progress to full-thickness ulcers even when appropriate intervention is provided and should be treated more aggressively.

With this in mind, if the ulcer is truly not healing, the different aspects of the treatment plan previously outlined should be reviewed. In addition, adjuvant therapy (electrical stimulation, hyperbaric oxygenation, vacuum-assisted closure) and the possible need for surgical intervention for stage III and stage IV ulcers that are recalcitrant to standard therapy should be considered. Electrical stimulation has been shown in multiple studies to improve the rate and degree of healing when it is used in addition to standard interventions on recalcitrant ulcers.[33] Vacuum-assisted closure may also be very useful for the appropriate wounds. The guidelines for the use of vacuum-assisted closure are as follows[39]:

- There is no untreated, underlying osteomyelitis.
- The wound is free of fistulas to internal organs or body cavities.
- The wound has not decreased in size for 2 to 4 weeks, despite the use of best practices.
- The wound has been sufficiently débrided.
- The wound has not decreased in size by more than 30% 4 weeks after major débridement.

Many different therapeutic modalities for the treatment of pressure ulcers are being investigated, such as growth factors and tissue-engineered skin substitutes. Clinical research in the field of wound treatment is broadening the options for both the treatment and prevention of wounds through many different pathways. Some treatments and methodologies, such as platelet-derived growth factor (e.g., becaplermin, marketed as Regranex; collagen wound matrix dressings, such as Oasis), are closer to true widespread availability than others are.

Rehabilitation

Many of the major factors that increase susceptibility for ulcer development are interrelated intrinsic changes in body characteristics and functional abilities. In many conditions, these changes are irreversible. Nutritional status can be altered by adequate diet, but a complete spinal cord injury is permanent. Clinical approaches to pressure ulcer prevention generally focus on extrinsic factors that can be changed. These include educational methods, device-oriented methods, and comprehensive systems of preventive care. These approaches to pressure ulcer prevention are complementary and should be reviewed periodically.

It is critically important during initial rehabilitation that every patient and caregiver be thoroughly educated in the causes of pressure ulcers and what they should do to prevent them. Skills to be learned include the ability to carry out a pressure relief regimen, both through postural changes, when possible, and through the provision of appropriate equipment (e.g., cushions, wheelchairs, mattresses). The need for routine skin inspection and care must also be emphasized, with particular regard to pressure areas such as the ischii, sacrum, greater trochanters, heels, and occiput. Increased care contact time is associated with reduced pressure ulcer incidence,[40] although automated pressure relief systems can also provide an effective intervention during inpatient rehabilitation.[41] After initial rehabilitation, the at-risk patient must maintain a high level of skin care at all times to prevent the occurrence of pressure ulcers.

The provision of appropriate equipment for postural support and pressure relief, such as mattresses and wheelchair seating cushions, is an important component of rehabilitation. For a patient with impaired mobility who is being discharged to the community or to long-term care, this requires the selection of a wheelchair seating system, including both a wheelchair and a support cushion, to meet his or her individualized requirements. An inappropriate seating system can lead to poor posture, reduce functional abilities, and isolate the user from the environment. All these factors can in turn exacerbate the risk for pressure ulcer development in the rehabilitating patient.

Seating requirements of each patient must be thoroughly assessed during acute rehabilitation, and when he or she presents with a pressure ulcer, so that appropriate seating and other support surfaces can be recommended. Special seating and cushions are available to help distribute weight off of a pressure ulcer. Cushions can be divided into four categories: foam, viscoelastic foam, gel, and fluid flotation. Which cushion is best for a patient depends on pressure evaluation, lifestyle, postural stability, continence, and cost.[34] Pressure mapping can be very useful in the objective determination of the interface pressure between the seating surface and the skin, helping the clinician to choose the most appropriate seating surface with the best pressure-relieving properties. Pressure relief maneuvers should be done every 15 minutes while the patient is sitting to prevent the development of ischial region pressure ulcers.

Tertiary prevention of pressure ulcers seeks to decrease the number of patients who exhibit chronic recurrence of tissue breakdown. Device-oriented prevention techniques continue to be developed and refined. Active pressure relief mattresses often incorporate temperature sensors to control the microenvironment, and this type of technology is now starting to be applied in wheelchair cushions. Wheelchair cushions that can dynamically alter pressure distribution at the seating interface may provide a method for pressure ulcer prevention in individuals with compromised mobility. Advances in system components have increased the reliability and robustness of these cushions, although they remain relatively expensive. In addition, biofeedback systems have been developed that monitor the duration of applied pressure (i.e., static sitting time) and issue an alarm when the user should perform a pressure relief maneuver.[42]

Advanced technologies and new pharmacologic approaches are being explored that can affect the intrinsic clinical status of at-risk patients. The long-term application of implanted electrical stimulation devices offers a unique means to alter the intrinsic characteristics of paralyzed muscle, leading to sustained improvements in regional tissue health.[43] The use of anabolic steroids has also been investigated for both the treatment and prevention of pressure ulcers in the population with spinal cord injury.[44]

In addition to altering the intrinsic susceptibility of at-risk patients, the incidence of pressure ulcers may be decreased by ensuring effective delivery of care and education by a multidisciplinary clinical team, at all stages of rehabilitation. A survey of the prevalence of pressure ulcers in 5000 hospitalized patients throughout Europe, carried out by the European Pressure Ulcer Advisory Panel,[45] indicated that clinical expertise and standard treatment guidelines are not in themselves sufficient. They should be considered the starting point for effective prevention of pressure ulcers, rather than the endpoint. Personalized interactive programs have the potential to decrease readmission rates for high-risk individuals.[15,46] An increase in the involvement of the patient in his or her care whenever possible may also decrease susceptibility to pressure ulcer development.

Outpatients at risk for pressure ulcers, such as residents of long-term care facilities, often have restricted ease of community mobility that limits both their desire and ability to access clinical expertise. Telemedicine represents a relatively new model for health care delivery that can eliminate or greatly reduce the need for transportation of the patient and improve standard of care.

Procedures

Débridement of necrotic tissue from the wound is essential for healing to occur. Débridement can be accomplished by several different approaches. Sharp débridement is performed by a qualified clinician who uses a scalpel either at the bedside or in surgery. Mechanical débridement is commonly done with wet to dry dressings changed two or three times a day. Autolytic débridement permits the enzymes in the wound to dissolve the necrotic tissue by covering of the wound with a moisture-retentive dressing. Last, enzymatic débridement uses exogenous enzymes in commercial preparations, such as papain, to dissolve the necrotic tissue.[35] The determination of débridement method depends on the condition of the wound. Sharp débridement is often performed when there is a large amount of necrotic material; for instance, the presence of eschar tissue often leads to sharp débridement. This will allow efficient removal of necrotic materials from the wound. However, for chronic wounds that do not have easily removable necrotic tissues (e.g., adherent, yellow, necrotic tissues at the base of the wound), chemical débridement may be the method of choice, allowing nontraumatic débridement of the wound.

Surgery

A variety of surgical options are available to close stage III and stage IV pressure ulcers that do not heal by conservative means. Possible surgeries are as follows: direct closure, split- or full-thickness skin grafts, skin flaps, musculocutaneous flaps, and free flaps. The type of surgical repair depends on the location of the ulcer, the primary diagnosis of the patient, comorbid conditions, and the goals of treatment. The long-term outcomes of surgical intervention are variable.[47-49] Predictors of surgical success correlate with the compliance of the patient with postoperative bed rest as well as preoperative risk factors for wound healing.

POTENTIAL DISEASE COMPLICATIONS

The following complications are associated with pressure ulcers: bacteremia, osteomyelitis, cellulitis, amyloidosis, endocarditis, heterotopic bone formation, perineal-urethral fistula, pseudoaneurysm, septic arthritis, sinus tract or abscess, and squamous cell carcinoma in the ulcer.[2]

POTENTIAL TREATMENT COMPLICATIONS

Failure to heal and recurrence of pressure ulcers are potential treatment complications. The need to maintain pressure relief over the area of the ulcer may lead to the formation of another pressure ulcer in a different location.

Asymmetric sitting posture due to unilateral removal of necrotic bone may cause pressure ulcer development.

Prolonged bed rest and reduced activity levels will decondition the patient and may lead to or exacerbate other comorbidities.

Increased pain may occur with dressing changes and sharp or mechanical débridement.

Surgical complications of infection, bleeding, and wound dehiscence are possible. Medication side effects from nonsteroidal anti-inflammatory drugs, acetaminophen, and narcotics are well known and include gastric, renal, and liver toxicities. Drug dependency can also occur with long-term use of narcotics.

References

1. Shea JD. Pressure sores: classification and management. Clin Orthop Relat Res 1975;112:89-100.
2. Bergstrom N, Bennett MA, Carlson CE, et al. Treatment of Pressure Ulcers. Clinical Practice Guideline Number 15. Rockville, Md, U.S. Department of Health and Human Services, Public Health Service, Agency for Health Care Policy and Research, 1994. AHCPR publication 95-0652.
3. Xakellis GC Jr, Frantz RA. Pressure ulcer healing: what is it? What influences it? How is it measured? Adv Wound Care 1997;10:20-26.
4. Sprigle S, Linden M, Riordan B. Analysis of localized erythema using clinical indicators and spectroscopy. Ostomy Wound Manage 2003;49:42-52.
5. Ankrom MA, Bennett RG, Sprigle S, et al; National Pressure Ulcer Advisory Panel. Pressure-related deep tissue injury under intact skin and the current pressure ulcer staging systems. Adv Skin Wound Care 2005;18:35-42.
6. Doughty D, Ramundo J, Bonham P, et al. Issues and challenges in staging of pressure ulcers. J Wound Ostomy Continence Nurs 2006;33:125-130.
7. Bergstrom N, Braden B, Kemp M, et al. Multi-site study of incidence of pressure ulcers and the relationship between risk level, demographic characteristics, diagnoses, and prescription of preventive interventions. J Am Geriatr Soc 1996;44:22-30.
8. Brandeis GH, Morris JN, Nash DJ, Lipsitz LA. Incidence and healing rates of pressure ulcers in the nursing home. Decubitus 1989;2:60-62.
9. Gerson LW. The incidence of pressure sores in active treatment hospitals. Int J Nurs Stud 1975;12:201-204.
10. Staas WE Jr, LaMantia JG. Decubitus ulcers and rehabilitation medicine. Int J Dermatol 1982;21:437-444.
11. Tourtual DM, Riesenberg LA, Korutz CJ, et al. Predictors of hospital acquired heel pressure ulcers. Ostomy Wound Manage 1997;43:24-28, 30, 32-34.
12. Sternberg J, Spector WD, Kapp MC, Tucker RJ. Decubitus ulcers on admission to nursing homes: prevalence and residents' characteristics. Decubitus 1988;1:14-20.
13. Suriadi, Sanada H, Sugama J, et al. A new instrument for predicting pressure ulcer risk in an intensive care unit. J Tissue Viability 2006;16:21-26.
14. Chan EY, Tan SL, Lee CK, Lee JY. Prevalence, incidence and predictors of pressure ulcers in a tertiary hospital in Singapore. J Wound Care 2005;14:383-384, 386-388.
15. Cardenas DD, Hoffman JM, Kirshblum S, McKinley W. Etiology and incidence of rehospitalization after traumatic spinal cord injury: a multicenter analysis. Arch Phys Med Rehabil 2004;85:1757-1763.
16. The National Pressure Ulcer Advisory Panel. Pressure ulcers prevalence, cost and risk assessment: consensus development conference statement. Decubitus 1989;2:4-8.
17. Scott JR, Gibran NS, Engrav LH, et al. Incidence and characteristics of hospitalized patients with pressure ulcers: State of Washington, 1987 to 2000. Plast Reconstr Surg 2006;17:630-634.
18. Gunningberg L, Ehrenberg A. Accuracy and quality in the nursing documentation of pressure ulcers: a comparison of record content and patient examination. J Wound Ostomy Continence Nurs 2004;31:328-335.
19. Pinchcofsky-Devin GD, Kaminski MV Jr. Correlation of pressure sores and nutritional status. J Am Geriatr Soc 1986;34:435-440.
20. Scales JT. Pathogenesis of pressure sores. In Bader DL, ed. Pressure Sores—Clinical Practice and Scientific Approach. London, Macmillan, 1990:15-26.
21. Colin D, Abraham P, Preault L, et al. Comparison of 90 degrees and 30 degrees laterally inclined positions in the prevention of pressure ulcers using transcutaneous oxygen and carbon dioxide pressures. Adv Wound Care 1996;9:35-38.
22. National Pressure Ulcer Advisory Panel. Wound infection and infection control. Available at: http://www.npuap.org/woundinfection.html.
23. Folkedahl BA, Frantz R. Treatment of Pressure Ulcers. Iowa City, University of Iowa Gerontological Nursing Interventions Research Center, Research Dissemination Core, 2002.
24. Bergstrom N, Braden BJ, Laguzza A, Holman V. The Braden Scale for predicting pressure sore risk. Nurs Res 1987;36:205-210.
25. Langkamp-Henken B, Hudgens J, Stechmiller JK, Herrlinger-Garcia KA. Mini nutritional assessment and screening scores are associated with nutritional indicators in elderly people with pressure ulcers. J Am Diet Assoc 2005;105:1590-1596.
26. Salzberg CA, Byrne DW, Cayten CG, et al. A new pressure ulcer risk assessment scale for individuals with spinal cord injury. Am J Phys Med Rehabil 1996;75:96-104.
27. Hibbs P. King's Fund. Putting audit into practice. Nurs Stand 1990;5:55-56.
28. Allman RM, Goode PS, Burst N, et al. Pressure ulcers, hospital complications, and disease severity: impact on hospital costs and length of stay. Adv Wound Care 1999;12:22-30.
29. Xakellis GC, Frantz R. The cost of healing pressure ulcers across multiple health care settings. Adv Wound Care 1996;9:18-22.
30. Beckrich K, Aronovitch S. Hospital-acquired pressure ulcers: a comparison of costs in medical vs. surgical patients. Nurs Econ 1999;17:263-271.
31. European Pressure Ulcer Advisory Panel. Guidelines on prevention of pressure ulcers. Br J Nurs 1998;7:888-889.
32. European Pressure Ulcer Advisory Panel. Guidelines on treatment of pressure ulcers EPUAP Rev 1999;1:31-33.
33. Consortium for Spinal Cord Medicine. Pressure Ulcer Prevention and Treatment Following Spinal Cord Injury: A Clinical Practice Guideline for Health Care Professionals. Washington, DC, Paralyzed Veterans of America, 2000.
34. Kanj LF, Wilking SVB, Phillips TJ. Continuing medical education: pressure ulcers. J Am Acad Dermatol 1998;38:517-536.
35. Sibbald RG, Williamson D, Orsted HL, et al. Preparing the wound bed—débridement bacterial balance, and moisture balance. Ostomy Wound Manage 2000;46:14-35.
36. Lazarus GS, Cooper DM, Knighton DR, et al. Definitions and guidelines for assessment of wounds and evaluation of healing. Arch Dermatol 1994;130:489-493.
37. Van Rijswijk L, Braden BJ. Pressure ulcer patient and wound assessment: an AHCPR Clinical Practice Guideline Update. Ostomy Wound Manage 1999;45(Suppl 1A):56S-67S.
38. Helberg D, Mertens E, Halfens RJ, Dassen T. Treatment of pressure ulcers: results of a study comparing evidence and practice. Ostomy Wound Manage 2006;52:60-72.
39. Sibbald RG, Mahoney J; V.A.C. Therapy Canadian Consensus Group. A consensus report on the use of vacuum-assisted closure in chronic, difficult-to-heal wounds. Ostomy Wound Manage 2003;49:52-66.
40. Horn SD, Buerhaus P, Bergstrom N, Smout RJ. RN staffing time and outcomes of long-stay nursing home residents: pressure ulcers and other adverse outcomes are less likely as RNs spend more time on direct patient care [comments in Am J Nurs 2005;105:13, Am J Nurs 2006;106:15; author reply Am J Nurs 2006;106:15-16]. Am J Nurs 2005;105:58-70.
41. Catz A, Zifroni A, Philo O. Economic assessment of pressure sore prevention using a computerized mattress system in patients with spinal cord injury. Disabil Rehabil 2005;27:1315-1319.
42. Pressore Alert, Cleveland Medical Devices. Available at: http://www.clevemed.com/about_us/abtus_ulcermanagement_p_pressorealert.htm.
43. Bogie KM, Wang X, Triolo RJ. Long-term prevention of pressure ulcers in high-risk patients: a single case study of the use of gluteal neuromuscular electric stimulation. Arch Phys Med Rehabil 2006;87:585-591.
44. Spungen AM, Koehler KM, Modeste-Duncan R, et al. Nine clinical cases of nonhealing pressure ulcers in patients with spinal cord injury treated with an anabolic agent: a therapeutic trial. Adv Skin Wound Care 2001;14:139-144.
45. European Pressure Ulcer Advisory Panel. The prevalence of pressure ulcers in European hospitals. EPUAP Review 3, 2001. Available at: http://www.epuap.org/review3_3/index.html.
46. Maugham L, Cox R, Amsters D, Battistutta D. Reducing inpatient hospital usage for management of pressure sores after spinal cord lesions. Int J Rehabil Res 2004;27:311-315.

47. Gusenoff JA, Redett RJ, Nahabedian MY. Outcomes for surgical coverage of pressure sores in nonambulatory, nonparaplegic, elderly patients. Ann Plast Surg 2002;48:633-640.

48. Schryvers OI, Stranc MF, Nance PW. Surgical treatment of pressure ulcers: 20-year experience. Arch Phys Med Rehabil 2000;81:1556-1562.

49. Goodman CM, Cohen V, Armenta A, et al. Evaluation of results and treatment variables for pressure ulcers in 48 veteran spinal cord–injured patients. Ann Plast Surg 1999;42:665-672.

Pulmonary Rehabilitation **141**

John R. Bach, MD

Synonyms

None

ICD-9 Codes

E0450   Invasive mechanical ventilation
E0461   Noninvasive mechanical ventilation
E0482   Mechanical insufflation-exsufflation

DEFINITION

Pulmonary rehabilitation has been defined as "the art of medical practice wherein an individually tailored, multidisciplinary program is formulated through which accurate diagnosis, therapy, emotional support, and education stabilize or reverse both the physiopathology and psychopathology of pulmonary diseases in an attempt to return the patient to the highest possible functional capacity allowed by his or her pulmonary handicap and overall life situation."[1,2] Program goals are to reverse the cycle of dyspnea and deconditioning, to optimize airway secretion management and respiratory muscle function, to reduce frequency of hospitalizations and pulmonary complications, to address psychosocial factors to facilitate rehabilitation and community integration, and to improve daily function.[1-4] Candidates for outpatient pulmonary rehabilitation include pediatric and adult individuals who can benefit from these goals, who have respiratory muscle or pulmonary dysfunction that limits their activities or life expectancy, and whose conditions are sufficiently stable for outpatient management.

Overview of Contrasting Pathologic Processes and Approaches and Outcomes

In development of a prescription for an outpatient pulmonary rehabilitation program, it is essential to distinguish between pulmonary dysfunction due to lung or airways disease or oxygenation impairment and impairment of alveolar ventilation in the presence of essentially normal lung parenchyma. Patients with oxygenation impairment are often hypoxic with a normal carbon dioxide level. Patients with ventilatory impairment retain carbon dioxide from muscle dysfunction, activity overload, or central hypoventilation. With this classification scheme, a clinician can better generate a focused outpatient pulmonary rehabilitation prescription. Subsequently, this chapter outlines treatment based on this classification. Conditions associated with oxygenation impairment are listed in Table 141-1. Whereas either one or the other almost always predominates, when impairments overlap, the prescription must reflect approaches for both conditions.[5]

Potential outcomes of outpatient pulmonary rehabilitation include decreased hospitalization, decreased morbidity and mortality, decreased symptoms, improved quality of life, increased functional activity, improved neuropsychological condition, increased ability to work, and effective use of assistive respiratory technology. Each prescription is individual specific and is adjusted according to the patient's progress.

Incidence

The prevalence of chronic obstructive pulmonary disease (COPD) in the adult population is approximately 4% to 6% in men and 1% to 3% in women. In the 1996 National Health Interview Survey, approximately 14 million adults had chronic bronchitis. COPD is the fourth leading cause of death in the United States and the most common cause of oxygenation impairment.[6,7]

Respiratory failure associated with weakness of respiratory muscles (ventilatory impairment) has an incidence of 1 in 800, the approximate incidence of patients with neuromuscular diseases. However, both acute and chronic respiratory failure also results from respiratory muscle dysfunction associated with central nervous system diseases such as cerebrovascular disease and traumatic brain injury. Almost 50% of home mechanical ventilation users have primarily ventilatory impairment because their prognosis with ventilator use is much better than that of ventilator users with primarily oxygenation impairment. Attempts are being made to objectify the need for and prescription of ventilators for home use.[8]

TABLE 141-1 Conditions Associated with Oxygenation Impairment and Ventilatory Impairment

Conditions with predominant oxygenation impairment

Chronic obstructive pulmonary disease

Asthma

Emphysema and emphysema that follows lung volume reduction surgery

Cystic fibrosis

Bronchiectasis

Some restrictive diseases (e.g., pulmonary fibrosis, primary parenchymal disease)

Conditions with predominant ventilatory impairment

Myopathies

    Duchenne muscular dystrophy

    Becker muscular dystrophy

    Limb-girdle muscular dystrophy

    Emery-Dreifuss muscular dystrophy

    Facioscapulohumeral muscular dystrophy

    Congenital, autosomal recessive, myotonic muscular dystrophy

    Generalized nondystrophic myopathies

    Congenital, metabolic, inflammatory myopathies

    Myasthenia gravis

    Mixed connective tissue disease myopathies

Neurologic disorders

    Amyotrophic lateral sclerosis

    Spinal cord dysfunction

    Spinal muscular atrophies

    Motor neuron diseases

    Poliomyelitis

    Hereditary sensory motor neuropathies

    Phrenic nerve neuropathies, Guillain-Barré syndrome

    Multiple sclerosis

    Friedreich ataxia

    Myelopathies

    Botulism

Sleep-disordered breathing

    Central and congenital hypoventilation syndromes

    Hypoventilation associated with diabetic microangiopathy

    Down syndrome

    Familial dysautonomia

Musculoskeletal

    Thoracic wall deformities

    Kyphoscoliosis

    Ankylosing spondylitis

    Osteogenesis imperfecta

    Rigid spine syndrome

    Spondyloepiphyseal dysplasia congenita

Restrictive lung diseases

    Obesity hypoventilation

    Diseases of the pleura and chest wall

    Tuberculosis

    Milroy disease

SYMPTOMS

Symptoms of oxygenation impairment include dyspnea on exertion or during routine activities of daily living, anxiety, depression, headaches, and difficulty with concentration.[9] Patients may have chronic sputum production, coughing, wheezing, chest pains that vary with the respiratory cycle, weight loss, orthopnea, sleep disturbances, and low endurance. A constellation of allergy symptoms may also be seen. Associated symptoms may include fever and hemoptysis, as in patients with bronchiectasis.

Patients with predominant ventilatory impairment most commonly complain of fatigue. Other symptoms can include exertional dyspnea, weight loss, sleep disturbances, low endurance, morning headaches, and frequent arousals. For patients who use a wheelchair or scooter, minimal symptoms are common until anxiety or inability to fall asleep occurs during otherwise benign intercurrent respiratory tract infections—a harbinger of respiratory failure.[10] Episodes of acute respiratory failure are common for patients with neuromuscular weakness with an ineffective cough.

PHYSICAL EXAMINATION

Predominant Oxygenation Impairment

For patients with lung or airways disease, the physical examination depends on the underlying pathologic process (see Table 141-1). For patients with COPD, the examination may reveal plentiful sputum production, auxiliary respiratory muscle use, and "barrel" chest. Auscultation reveals wheezes, rales, or hyperresonant lung sounds. Evaluation with pulse oximetry during rest and exercise will often demonstrate worsening oxygenation impairment with activity.[6]

Predominant Ventilatory Impairment

All generalized neuromuscular diseases cause varying degrees of weakness of the inspiratory (breathing), expiratory (coughing), and bulbar-innervated (speech, swallowing, and air protection) muscles. Patients may have increased respiratory rate, shallow breathing, diaphragmatic or paradoxical breathing, accessory respiratory muscle use, nasal flaring, peribuccal or generalized cyanosis, flushing or pallor, drooling, difficulty in control of airway secretions, dysphagia, or nasality of speech.[5]

FUNCTIONAL LIMITATIONS

Baseline levels of function, including exercise tolerance and ability to perform activities of daily living, may be greatly diminished. There may be difficulty with control of airway secretions, difficulty with chewing and swallowing of food, and decreased social interaction. Many patients require ventilator use to rest inspiratory muscles to avoid or to diminish respiratory symptoms. Activities of daily life may be diminished by generalized muscle dysfunction or by specific impairment of respiratory muscles. For example, tachypnea does not allow patients sufficient time to chew and swallow. This results in malnutrition that further decreases respiratory function. Management with ventilatory assistance by a simple mouthpiece diminishes tachypnea and often results in better nutrition and improved strength (Fig. 141-1).

DIAGNOSTIC STUDIES

Diagnostic testing distinguishes between predominant ventilatory impairment and predominant oxygenation impairment. With predominant oxygenation impairment, patients have at least one of the following: respiratory limitation to exercise at 75% of predicted maximum oxygen consumption; irreversible airway obstruction with a forced expiratory volume in 1 second (FEV_1) of less than 2000 mL or an FEV_1 to forced vital capacity ratio (FEV_1/FVC ratio) of less than 60%; or pulmonary vascular disease with carbon monoxide diffusion capacity of less than 80% of predicted.

With predominant ventilatory impairment, patients have at least one of the following: hypercapnia; respiratory limitation to exercise at 75% of predicted maximum oxygen consumption; or diminished vital capacity with normal to high FEV_1/FVC ratio, diminished cough peak flows, decreased maximum inspiratory and expiratory pressures, and low lung volume measurements (i.e., total lung capacity, functional residual capacity, and residual volume). Many such patients have thoracic wall deformity. It is extremely important to measure unassisted as well as assisted cough flows for these patients because they most often develop respiratory failure as a result of ineffective coughing.[10] Assisted cough flows are created by air stacking consecutively delivered volumes of air provided through a manual resuscitator to the maximum volume that can be held with a closed glottis. At this point, an abdominal thrust is delivered in conjunction with glottic opening. The expelled air is measured as a cough flow into a peak flow meter.

Tests to Determine Candidates for Rehabilitation for Predominant Oxygenation Impairment

Active patients who are still able to walk several blocks but who have noted yearly decreases in exercise tolerance or who have recently begun to require ongoing medical attention for pulmonary symptoms or complications are ideal candidates for outpatient pulmonary rehabilitation.

Clinical exercise testing can best determine the extent of the patient's functional impairment due to pulmonary disease. It can diagnose and measure functional reserve and the capacity to perform exercise, the factors that limit exercise, and the reasons for exercise-related symptoms.[11-13] Clinical exercise testing permits the clinician to determine whether the primary disability is pulmonary, cardiac, or exercise-induced bronchospasm.[13] The last two diagnoses and even purely restrictive pulmonary syndromes are commonly mistaken for COPD. When it is performed both before and after the rehabilitation program, clinical exercise testing documents the patient's progress.

Vital signs, electrocardiography, oxygen consumption, carbon dioxide production, respiratory quotient, ventilatory equivalent, minute ventilation, and metabolic rate are monitored during clinical exercise testing, which is done with use of a treadmill, stationary bicycle, or upper extremity ergometry. All patients undergo a 3-, 6-, or 12-minute walk test. The patient is instructed to gradually increase speed and duration on subsequent walking exercise tests.[11-15] A clinical exercise test advances until oxygen consumption fails to increase; maximum allowable heart rate for age is reached; or electrocardiographic changes, chest pain, severe dyspnea, or fatigue occurs. Oximetry is performed to determine the need for supplemental oxygen therapy during reconditioning exercise (pulse oxyhemoglobin saturation [SpO_2] $SpO_2 < 90\%$ to 95%) or on a long-term basis ($PO_2 < 60$ mm Hg). When metabolic energy cost studies are not available, maximum exercise tolerance may be estimated from pulmonary function data.[11-13,16]

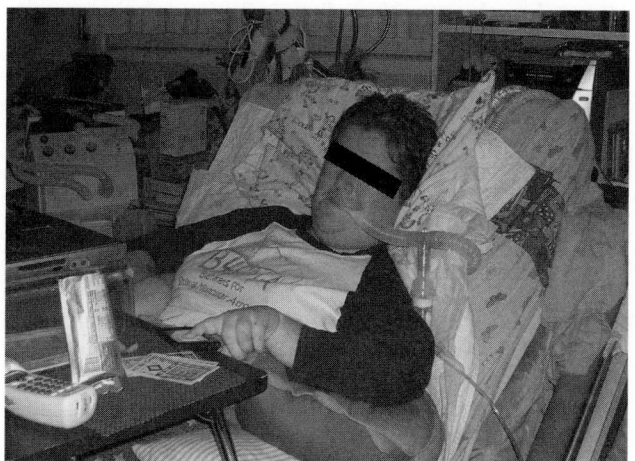

FIGURE 141-1. A 17-year-old girl with mild spinal muscular atrophy type 1 who is continuously ventilator dependent uses a mouthpiece during daytime hours and a nasal interface during sleep.

Predominant Ventilatory Impairment

Patients with primarily ventilatory impairment undergo spirometry to measure vital capacity in sitting and supine positions and maximum insufflation capacity, unassisted and assisted cough peak flows by peak flow meter, end-tidal carbon dioxide measurements, and pulse oximetry.[17] Sitting minus supine vital capacity greater than 20% provides a strong indication of diaphragm weakness out of proportion to accessory inspiratory muscle dysfunction. When the vital capacity is less than 80% of normal, the patient is trained to perform maximal insufflation techniques, such as air stacking as noted before. Air stacking along with manually and mechanically assisted coughing is aimed at maintaining adequate airway secretion clearance and preventing atelectasis and pneumonia. Cough peak flows of less than 270 L/min indicate initiation of the oximetry–respiratory aid protocol to be described later. Symptoms of nocturnal hypoventilation, end-tidal carbon dioxide above 45 mm Hg, or daytime or nocturnal oxygen desaturation below 95% warrant a nocturnal trial of noninvasive intermittent positive pressure ventilation.[17]

Differential Diagnosis

Deconditioning

Cardiac dysfunction

Pulmonary infection

Obesity

TREATMENT

Initial

Predominant Oxygenation Impairment

The main treatment for pulmonary rehabilitation is summarized in Table 141-2. The patient and caregivers are educated in preventive care measures. Smoking

---

TABLE 141-2   Pulmonary Rehabilitation

Basic outpatient pulmonary rehabilitation program

Initial assessment of

    Respiratory disease process

    Underlying medical disorder

    General medical condition

    Functional status

    Patient's goals

Select treatment goals

Interdisciplinary team management

Medication optimization

Adjustment of supplemental oxygen therapy

Airway secretion elimination techniques and devices

Smoking cessation program

Exercise program

    Ventilatory muscle training

    Endurance and strength training

Breathing retraining

Alternative breathing techniques

Energy conservation techniques

Therapeutic modalities

Adaptive devices and mobility equipment

Psychosocial counseling

Nutritional counseling

Patient and caregiver education

Maintenance program

---

cessation is emphasized to reduce chronic phlegm production and to decrease the rate of annual loss of FEV_1 to the level of nonsmokers.[18,19] Avoidance of atmospheric or vocational pollutants and of other aggravating factors, such as pollen, aerosols, excessive humidity, stress, large meals, and ill contacts with respiratory infections, is suggested. Adherence to medications as prescribed and reporting of any problems with medications to the clinician are encouraged. Recommended vaccinations include annual influenza vaccinations and the pneumococcal vaccinations, provided there are no contraindications.[19,20] Nutritional counseling reinforces good nutrition with adequate calorie intake, carbohydrate balance, and adequate hydration.[5,21,22]

Medical therapy involves optimal pharmacologic management of reversible bronchospasm when it is present, including the use of bronchodilators such as anticholinergics, methylxanthine derivatives, sympathomimetics, and combination medications (Table 141-3). An improvement in FEV_1 greater than 20% is significant with bronchodilator use. Inhaled adrenergics and anticholinergics appear to benefit many patients despite little objective evidence of improvement. Training for proper administration of nebulizers or inhalers is important to promote optimal medication deposition and to prevent inefficient use. Other medications, such as expectorants, mucolytics, corticosteroids, antibiotics, and disodium cromoglycate, are used along with humidification and bronchial toilet, as warranted, to prepare the patient for optimal participation in the therapeutic exercise program.

Respiratory secretion management is critical for treatment and preventive care. This involves training in the techniques of chest percussion, in postural drainage, and with huffing ventilatory and airway secretion clearance devices. In addition, autogenic drainage is a technique of breathing low tidal volumes between the functional residual capacity and residual volume, followed by taking increasingly larger tidal volumes and forced expirations to mobilize and to evacuate mucus. Positive end-expiratory pressure breathing techniques theoretically mobilize secretions by coughing or forced expirations with alveolar pressure and volume pushing behind mucous plugs. Flutter breathing with a flutter device applied to the mouth uses two mucus-evacuating techniques: positive end-expiratory pressure and oscillation. Devices that provide mechanical vibration or oscillation to the thorax include the Hayek Oscillator (Breasy Medical Equipment Inc., Stamford, Conn); ThAIRapy System (American Biosystems Inc., St. Paul, Minn); and intrapulmonary percussive ventilator, which provides aerosolized medications as high-flow percussive mini-bursts of air delivered to the airways (Percussionaire Corp. Sandpoint, Idaho).

Early medical attention for respiratory tract infections is very important. Broad-spectrum antibiotics and glucocorticoids should be considered. Home oxygen therapy is used for oxygenation-impaired patients with lung disease if the PO_2 is less than 60 mm Hg and when it remains so for more than 2 months after an acute exacerbation. This type of therapy decreases reactive pulmonary

TABLE 141-3 Commonly Prescribed Medications

Category	Representative Types	Main Respiratory Clinical Effects	Main Side Effects
Bronchodilator	Anticholinergics Sympathomimetics Methylxanthine derivatives Combinations	Relief of bronchospasm by relaxation of bronchial smooth muscle	See under specific medicines
Anticholinergics	Ipratropium	Relief of bronchospasm by relaxation of bronchial smooth muscle	Headache, dry mouth, dizziness, dyspnea, gastrointestinal disturbances
	Tiotropium	Relief of bronchospasm	Tachycardia, palpitations, gastrointestinal distress, nervousness, dry mouth, tremor

From Physicians' Desk Reference, 61st ed. Montvale, NJ, Medical Economics, 2007.

hypertension and polycythemia, improves cognition, prolongs survival, and may decrease hospitalizations. Transtracheal oxygen delivery avoids waste around the nose and mouth, avoids the "dead space" of the nasopharynx, and prevents discomfort and drying associated with nasal cannulas and facemasks. High-altitude travel may require 0.5 L/min of additional supplemental oxygen.

Patients with COPD have a high incidence of sleep-disordered breathing, that is, obstructive and central apneas, for which continuous positive airway pressure or bilevel positive airway pressure can be used. Bilevel positive airway pressure can also be useful to provide some ventilatory assistance, inspiratory muscle rest, and counter auto–positive end-expiratory pressure for hypercapnic COPD patients.

Predominant Ventilatory Impairment

Abdominal binders are useful for tetraplegic and thoracic-level paraplegic spinal cord patients to increase diaphragmatic excursion and vital capacity. However, whereas inspiratory muscle exercise has not been shown to increase respiratory muscle strength or vital capacity in patients with primarily ventilatory impairment, chest wall and lung mobilization has, and it is critical to maintain sufficient excursion to allow the increased lung volumes necessary for effective coughing.

Although bilevel positive airway pressure can be used by patients with primarily ventilatory impairment, it is appropriate only for those who do not have sufficient bulbar-innervated muscle function for air stacking. When bilevel positive airway pressure is used for these patients, polysomnographic titration is irrelevant. The bilevel positive airway pressure inspiratory-expiratory pressure span should be sufficient to rest inspiratory muscles, that is, be 18 to 20 cm H_2O. Any patients with bulbar-innervated musculature sufficient for air stacking should use volume-cycled ventilators rather than bilevel positive airway pressure machines. Modifications are made for mask discomfort and air leakage. Portable volume ventilators can provide greater inspiratory muscle assistance when it is needed, such as for patients with obesity hypoventilation.[5]

Psychosocial counseling addresses symptoms of depression, anxiety, and stress as well as social impediments to good progress. The goal is to break the influence of these psychosocial issues on the cycle of respiratory decline.[9]

Mechanical insufflation-exsufflation is used to assist expiratory muscles to increase cough flows to prevent pneumonia. It provides 10 L/sec of expiratory flow directly to the airways through the upper airway or through tracheostomy (CoughAssist, JH Emerson Co., Cambridge, Mass). Mechanically assisted coughing is used in conjunction with an exsufflation-timed abdominal thrust, combining the manual with the mechanical.[17]

Rehabilitation

An outpatient pulmonary rehabilitation program incorporates physical medicine interventions, evaluation for respiratory equipment, and rehabilitation by an interdisciplinary approach. The interdisciplinary team can include the patient, medical and nursing staff, respiratory therapists, physical therapists, occupational therapists, speech therapists, social workers, and a nutritionist. In addition, psychology or psychiatry services, recreational therapists, and vocational rehabilitation may be integrated as part of the team.

Exercise training for endurance, strength, and function-specific activities is prescribed (Table 141-4). The progress is monitored, and modifications to the prescription are made on the basis of the patient's increasing aerobic capacity with intensive exercise training. Scheduling for reevaluations of the prescription depends on each patient; the early stages of the program and any acute medical issues affect the need for possible prescription modifications. Frequency, duration, intensity, and specificity are general exercise components. Frequency of exercise is generally advised three to five times a week for a training effect to be seen.[13] Patients should also be taught about their respiratory equipment.

Predominant Oxygenation Impairment

Carefully prescribed exercise provides the greatest benefits for reducing dyspnea and respiratory rate and increasing exercise tolerance, maximum oxygen consumption, 6- and 12-minute walk distance, activities of daily living, work output, mechanical efficiency, and possibly gas exchange.[23-27] Anxiety and depression are

TABLE 141-4 Types of Exercise[1,2,8,12,13,24,25]

Type of Exercise	Example
Ventilatory muscle training	Inspiratory resistive exercise: maximum sustained ventilation, inspiratory resistive loading, inspiratory threshold loading, sustained hyperpnea
Strength training	Upper extremity exercise: pulleys, elastic bands, supervised circuit training, weightlifting with low resistance
	Lower extremity exercise: supervised circuit training, weightlifting with low resistance
Endurance training	Upper extremity exercise: unsupported upper extremity activities ranging from activities of daily living to athletic activities, supervised arm cycling, low-impact aerobics, pool therapy
	Lower extremity exercise: incremental treadmill program, supervised walking, cycling and stair climbing program, low-impact aerobics, pool therapy

also significantly decreased, and cognition and sense of well-being are improved.[9]

Low-intensity training can be prescribed on the basis of objective or subjective measures. Objective measures involve calculation of the maximal oxygen consumption or maximum heart rate. If open-circuit spirometry and metabolic cart are available, specific target intensity may be 50% of peak rate of oxygen uptake. Heart rate parameters may be most useful for patients with cardiac conditions. Several formulas are used. One is the desired exercise intensity multiplied by the maximum predicted heart rate. Hence, if the desired exercise intensity is defined as 60% of maximum predicted heart rate (HR), then

$$\text{Target HR} = 0.60 \times [\text{HR}_{max} = 220 - \text{age}]$$

Another is the Karvonen formula. For the target heart rate range for 50% to 85%:

$$\text{HR reserve} = [(\text{HR}_{max} - \text{HR}_{rest}) \times 0.50] + \text{HR}_{rest}$$
$$= [(\text{HR}_{max} - \text{HR}_{rest}) \times 0.85] + \text{HR}_{rest}$$

Initial targets can be 50% (range, 50% to 80%) of either objective measure or the level tolerated by the patient.[13]

When objective measures are not applicable, as in the case of patients taking negative chronotropic medications (e.g., β blockers or calcium channel blockers) and heart transplant recipients, subjective measures may be more predictive of exercise tolerance. In addition, because patients are often limited by exertional dyspnea, subjective measures may be more desirable.[13]

Subjective measures of exercise tolerance, such as the Borg rating of perceived exertion scale or dyspnea rating scales, allow patients to guide the program on the basis of their symptoms alone. The Borg rating of perceived exertion scale from 6 to 20 is linearly related to heart rate. This is illustrated by multiplying the chosen scale number by 10 to obtain the estimated predicted heart rate. For example, when the patient chooses the number 10 on the scale to describe exertion symptoms, heart rate is estimated by the following equation:

$$10 \times 10 = 100 \ (\pm 10)$$

The original Borg scale uses this method.[13,28]

Training specificity is determined by the patient's goal for daily activities and occupational pursuits. Daily activities in mobility and exercise programs are tailored accordingly. Depending on the patient's form of mobility and baseline level of function, specific mobility and endurance exercise programs can include walking, stair climbing, low-impact aerobics, stationary bicycling, and pool activities. For mobility, work, and recreational pursuits, assistive devices to improve daily activities may include wheelchair, walker, or cane. Strength training increases function in daily activities, mobility, and specific occupation-related tasks. Intermingled with endurance, strength, and task-specific training are energy conservation techniques that provide the patient with more energy efficient methods to perform daily activities. Increased endurance for exercise can occur independently of changes in ventilatory muscle endurance.

Review of the training program is made with the patient and caregiver. A plan is agreed on and is flexible to change, according to the patient's tolerance. The patient is made responsible for a progressive program to reinforce adherence and independence.

Breathing retraining exercises are used with the goals of modifying the breathing pattern to decrease the work of breathing and improving the cough mechanism. Pursed lip breathing and diaphragmatic breathing decrease the respiratory rate, coordinate the breathing pattern, and tend to prevent collapse of smaller bronchi. Air shifting is performed several times per hour. It involves a deep inspiration that is held with the glottis closed for 5 seconds. The air shifts to lesser ventilated areas of the lung and may help prevent microatelectasis. The subsequent expiration is through pursed lips. Pursed lip breathing aids in relaxation as well. Other relaxation exercises, such as Jacobson exercises and biofeedback, can be used to decrease tension and anxiety.[29,30]

For hypercapnic patients, interspersing periods of respiratory muscle rest with exercise of specific respiratory muscle groups is a principle of pulmonary rehabilitation. Rest can be achieved by overnight use of nasal bilevel positive airway pressure.[31,32] Improved daytime gas values, increased vital capacity, decreased fatigue, and increased well-being have been reported in such programs.

After the acute rehabilitation period, continued surveillance and attention to abstinence from smoking, bronchial hygiene (Table 141-5), breathing retraining, physical reconditioning, oxygen therapy, and airway secretion

TABLE 141-5 Pulmonary Hygiene Options[11,14,43]

Inhalers

Bronchodilators

Inhaled steroids

Leukotriene inhibitors

Mucolytics

Methods of airway secretion elimination

Oral, nasal, or transtracheal suctioning

Chest percussion and postural drainage

Positive expiratory pressure breathing

Flutter mucus clearance devices

Mechanical vibration devices to the chest wall

Intrapulmonary percussive ventilation with aerosolized medications

Mechanical insufflation-exsufflation applications

Autogenic drainage

Manual assisted cough

Abdominal binder

mobilization have been shown to reduce hospital admissions, length of hospital stays, and cost.[33,34] The benefits of pulmonary rehabilitation on exercise performance and quality of life are greatest during the first year and last up to 5 years.[26,27,35-37]

Predominant Ventilatory Impairment

The primary interventions for patients with generalized muscle weakness are the use of respiratory muscle aids and facilitation of "habilitation" to disability rather than "rehabilitation." Cough peak flows greater than 160 L/min are the minimum needed for airway secretion clearance and hence indicate safety for removal of a tracheostomy tube whether the patient is ventilator dependent or not. Ninety percent of episodes of acute respiratory failure are caused by ineffective coughing during otherwise benign upper respiratory tract infections; therefore, when assisted peak cough flows have decreased to less than 270 L/min, patients are prescribed oximeters and trained in air stacking of consecutively delivered volumes of air provided through mouth or nasal interfaces from a manual resuscitator (Ambu bag) to improve cough flows.[38] They are also taught manually assisted coughing (abdominal thrusts timed to glottic opening after maximal lung insufflation). They are introduced to mechanical insufflation-exsufflation (CoughAssist) provided at +35 to +50 to −35 to −50 cm H_2O pressure drops, with abdominal thrusts applied during exsufflations. Patients must have rapid (less than 2-hour) access to portable volume ventilators, CoughAssists, and various mouthpieces and nasal interfaces when they develop respiratory tract infections. In the respiratory muscle aid–oximetry protocol to prevent respiratory failure, patients and care providers are instructed to use continuous pulse oxyhemoglobin saturation (SpO_2) monitoring at the first sign of upper respiratory tract infection. Any decreases in SpO_2 of less than 95% indicate either hypoventilation or the presence of airway mucus accumulation that must be cleared to prevent atelectasis, pneumonia, and respiratory failure. Patients learn to use noninvasive ventilation or manually and mechanically assisted coughing to maintain sufficient alveolar ventilation and airway secretion clearance to keep SpO_2 at 95% or higher and thereby avoid respiratory failure. They are also told to use SpO_2 monitoring whenever fatigued, short of breath, or ill. They are instructed to use manually and mechanically assisted coughing, as needed, to maintain normal SpO_2 at all times.

When symptomatic, nocturnal SpO_2 decreases below 95% are common, and patients are encouraged to use nocturnal nasal intermittent positive-pressure ventilation for inspiratory muscle rest and symptom relief. Many patients use noninvasive intermittent positive-pressure ventilation for the first time to assist lung ventilation during chest infections and need it continuously during these episodes without requiring hospitalization.[17] Although muscle weakness may progress, patients may be maintained with noninvasive intermittent positive-pressure ventilation continuously without ever requiring hospitalization, in many cases despite having no measurable vital capacity for decades.[35,36]

Procedures

Training in the use of nebulizers, hand-held inhalers, chest percussion and postural drainage, and respiratory equipment is important during the outpatient pulmonary rehabilitation program. Self-directed patients should be independent in training their care providers in how to assist in airway secretion clearance and in how to change the settings of their ventilators and CoughAssist devices according to time of day and clinical situation.

Surgery

Lung volume reduction surgery is performed for patients with severe function-limiting emphysema with the goal of improving gas exchange, exercise capacity, lung function, and quality of life. Candidates for lung volume reduction surgery, patients who have had lung volume reduction surgery, and lung transplantation and post–lung transplantation patients may be prescribed an inpatient or outpatient pulmonary rehabilitation program, depending on the patient's goals and medical stability.[37,38]

Among patients with pulmonary dysfunction who have significant nutritional deficiencies by oral intake, alternative routes for nutrition, such as a percutaneous gastrostomy tube, are considered.

Patients with respiratory muscle impairment are taught the use of inspiratory and expiratory muscle aids (i.e., mouthpiece and nasal noninvasive mechanical ventilation and mechanically assisted coughing) before surgery so that they can be extubated to the use of these aids after surgery, even when they are not capable of independently ventilating their lungs.[39] Tracheostomy is needed only when bulbar-innervated muscle dysfunction is so severe that patients aspirate saliva to the extent that SpO_2 cannot be maintained at 95% or higher. In general, this occurs only for patients with advanced bulbar amyotrophic lateral sclerosis.[40]

POTENTIAL DISEASE COMPLICATIONS

Potential disease complications play a significant role in the outpatient pulmonary rehabilitation prescription. In generating a prescription, it is important to consider the patient's specific diagnosis and potential complications. Complications of chronic respiratory disease depend on the effects of progression of the primary pathologic process and natural aging on respiratory muscle function and lung tissues. Nutritional deficits, psychosocial issues, and comorbidities can also play an important role.

Predominant Oxygenation Impairment

Patients with primarily oxygenation impairment due to lung or airways disease often have intermittent exacerbations with episodes of acute respiratory failure. These often require acute hospitalization and invasive management. They are largely caused by inability to mobilize peripherally trapped airway secretions. There are many secretion mobilization systems to help mobilize airway secretions, but there is no clear evidence that one system works better than any other. The least expensive and simplest methods to supplement airway secretion mobilization efforts, such as use of a flutter valve, positive expiratory pressure mask, and chest vibrators, are probably as effective as expensive chest vibrating and oscillating devices.[41] Supplemental methods of respiratory therapeutic secretion mobilization that can be taught include chest percussion and postural drainage, huffing, and active cycle of breathing. The last is the most inexpensive technique of airway secretion mobilization because no assistive device is used. The patient simply breathes slowly and shallowly at lung volumes well below functional residual capacity; he or she gradually increases tidal volumes to approach functional residual capacity and, once reaching it, takes a deep breath and "huffs" out secretions. Other important strategies for these patients are to administer and to monitor compliance with antibiotics, bronchodilators, oxygen, mucolytics, and other medications.

Predominant Ventilatory Impairment

The evaluation for long-term "airway protection" with a tracheostomy is a common clinical scenario. However, because patients with no measurable vital capacity or any volitional skeletal muscle movement for more than 50 years do not require tracheostomy,[42,43] obviously one is not needed for inspiratory or expiratory muscle failure but rather for failure of bulbar-innervated muscula-

ture alone. Once aspiration of saliva causes the SpO_2 baseline value to decrease and to remain less than 95%, 90% of patients undergo tracheotomy or are deceased within 2 months.[40] This, however, occurs only for patients with advanced bulbar amyotrophic lateral sclerosis, for children with type 1 spinal muscular atrophy without sufficient home care,[44] for an occasional patient with facioscapulohumeral muscular dystrophy, and for very few others. Such patients almost invariably have maximum assisted peak cough flows of less than 160 L/min and are incapable of air stacking because of failure of glottic closure.[45]

POTENTIAL TREATMENT COMPLICATIONS

Potential treatment complications can result from oxygen toxicity, barotrauma from ventilator use, comorbidities such as concomitant cardiac or atherosclerotic peripheral vascular disease, and pharmacologic treatment. Routine evaluation of a patient's medication profile by the treating clinician is necessary. Immobility due to muscle weakness or acute illness can also exacerbate pulmonary secretion stasis and cause deep venous thromboses, cardiac deconditioning, skin ulceration, bone decalcification, and musculoskeletal contractures. Each individual's progress with mobilization, exercise, and daily activity facilitation programs is monitored, and prescriptions are modified accordingly.

References

1. Hodgkin J, Farrell M, Gibson S, et al. American Thoracic Society. Medical Section of the American Lung Association. Pulmonary rehabilitation. Am Rev Respir Dis 1981;124:663-666.
2. American Thoracic Society. Pulmonary rehabilitation—1999. Am J Respir Crit Care Med 1999;159:1666-1682.
3. American College of Chest Physicians and American Association of Cardiovascular and Pulmonary Rehabilitation. Pulmonary rehabilitation: joint ACCP/AACVPR evidence-based guidelines. ACCP/AACVPR Pulmonary Rehabilitation Guidelines Panel. Chest 1997;112:1363-1396.
4. Holden DA, Stelmach KD, Curtis PS, et al. The impact of a rehabilitation program on functional status of patients with chronic lung disease. Respir Care 1990;35:332-341.
5. Bach JR. Rehabilitation of the patient with respiratory dysfunction. In DeLisa JD, ed. Rehabilitation Medicine: Principles and Practice. Philadelphia, Lippincott-Raven, 2005:1843-1866.
6. Higgins MW, Thom T. Incidence, prevalence, and mortality: intra- and intercountry differences. In Hensley MJ, Saunders NA, eds. Clinical Epidemiology of Chronic Obstructive Pulmonary Disease. New York, Marcel Dekker, 1989:23-43.
7. Feinleib M, Rosenberg HM, Collins JG, et al. Trends in COPD morbidity and mortality in the United States. Am Rev Respir Dis 1989;140:S9-S18.
8. Koga T, Watanabe K, Sano M, et al. The breathing intolerance index for ventilator use. Am J Phys Med Rehabil 2006;85:24-30.
9. Smoller JW, Pollack MH, Otto MW, et al. Panic anxiety, dyspnea, and respiratory disease: theoretical and clinical considerations. Am J Respir Crit Care Med 1996;154:6-17.
10. Bach JR, Rajaraman R, Ballanger F, et al. Neuromuscular ventilatory insufficiency: the effect of home mechanical ventilator use vs. oxygen therapy on pneumonia and hospitalization rates. Am J Phys Med Rehabil 1998;77:8-19.
11. American College of Sports Medicine. Guidelines for Exercise Testing and Prescription, 5th ed. Philadelphia, Williams & Wilkins, 1995.

12. Jones NL. Current concepts: new tests to assess lung function. N Engl J Med 1975;293:541-544.

13. Jones NL, Campbell EJM. Clinical Exercise Testing, 2nd ed. Philadelphia, WB Saunders, 1982:158.

14. Guyatt GH, Thompson PJ, Berman LB, et al. How should we measure function in patients with chronic heart and lung disease? J Chronic Dis 1985;38:517-524.

15. American Association of Cardiovascular and Pulmonary Rehabilitation. Guidelines for Pulmonary Rehabilitation Programs, 2nd ed. Champaign, Ill, Human Kinetics, 1998.

16. Carlson DJ, Ries AL, Kaplan RM. Prediction of maximum exercise tolerance in patients with COPD. Chest 1991;100:307-311.

17. Gomez-Merino E, Bach JR. Duchenne muscular dystrophy: prolongation of life by noninvasive respiratory muscle aids. Am J Phys Med Rehabil 2002;81:411-415.

18. Camilli AE, Burrows B, Knudson RJ, et al. Longitudinal changes in forced expiratory volume in one second in adults. Effects of smoking and smoking cessation. Am Rev Respir Dis 1987;135:794-799.

19. Prevention of pneumococcal disease: recommendations of the Advisory Committee on Immunization Practices. MMWR Recomm Rep 1997;46(RR-8):1-24.

20. Bridges CB, Winquist AG, Fukuda K, et al. Prevention and control of influenza: recommendations of the Advisory Committee on Immunization Practices. MMWR Recomm Rep 2000;49(RR-3):1-38.

21. Wilson DO, Rogers RM, Wright EC, Anthonisen NR. Body weight in chronic obstructive pulmonary disease. Am Rev Respir Dis 1989;139:1435-1438.

22. Askanazi J, Weissman C, Rosenbaum SH, et al. Nutrition and the respiratory system. Crit Care Med 1982;10:163-172.

23. Gozal D. Nocturnal ventilatory supports in patients with cystic fibrosis: comparison with supplemental oxygen. Eur Respir J 1997;10:1999-2003.

24. Gimenez M, Servera E, Vergara P, et al. Endurance training in patients with chronic obstructive pulmonary disease: a comparison of high versus moderate intensity. Arch Phys Med Rehabil 2000;81:102-109.

25. Carter R, Nicotra B, Clark L, et al. Exercise conditioning in rehabilitation of patients with chronic obstructive pulmonary disease. Arch Phys Med Rehabil 1988;69:118-122.

26. Troosters T, Gosselink R, Decramer M. Short and long-term effects of outpatient rehabilitation in patients with chronic obstructive pulmonary disease: a randomized trial. Am J Med 2000;109:207-212.

27. Make B. Pulmonary rehabilitation and outcome measure. In Baum GL, Crapo JD, Celli BR, Karlinsky JB, eds. Textbook of Pulmonary Diseases, 6th ed. Philadelphia, Lippincott-Raven, 1998:987-1006.

28. Noble BJ, Borg GA, Jacobs I, et al. A category-ratio perceived exertion scale: relationship to blood and muscle lactates and heart rate. Med Sci Sports Exerc 1983;15:523-528.

29. Reina-Rosenbaum R, Bach JR, Penek J. The cost/benefits of outpatient based pulmonary rehabilitation. Arch Phys Med Rehabil 1997;78:240-244.

30. Khan AU. Effectiveness of biofeedback and counterconditioning in the treatment of bronchial asthma. J Psychosom Res 1977;21:97-104.

31. Elliot MW, Mulvey D, Moxham J, et al. Domiciliary nocturnal nasal intermittent positive pressure ventilation in COPD: mechanisms underlying changes in arterial blood gas tensions. Eur Respir J 1991;4:1044-1052.

32. Gay P, Hubmayr RD, Stroetz RW. Efficacy of nocturnal nasal positive pressure ventilation combined with oxygen therapy and oxygen monotherapy in patients with severe COPD. Am J Respir Crit Care Med 1996;154:353-358.

33. Hudson LD, Tyler ML, Petty T. Hospitalization needs during an outpatient rehabilitation program for chronic airway obstruction. Chest 1976;70:606-610.

34. Roselle S, D'Amico FJ. The effect of home respiratory therapy on hospital re-admission rates of patients with chronic obstructive pulmonary disease. Respir Care 1990;35:1208-1213.

35. Holle RH, Williams DV, Vandree JC, et al. Increased muscle efficiency and sustained benefits in an outpatient community hospital–based pulmonary rehabilitation program. Chest 1988;94:1161-1168.

36. Ilowite J, Niederman M, Fein A, et al. Can benefits seen in pulmonary rehabilitation be sustained long term? Chest 1991;100:182.

37. Mall RW, Medieros M. Objective evaluation of results of a pulmonary rehabilitation program in a community hospital. Chest 1988;94:1156-1160.

38. Bach JR, Gonzalves M, Paez S. Expiratory flow maneuvers of patients with neuromuscular diseases. Am J Phys Med Rehabil 2006;85:105-111.

39. Bach JR, Sabharwal S. High pulmonary risk scoliosis surgery: role of noninvasive ventilation and related techniques. J Spinal Disord Tech 2005;18:527-530.

40. Bach JR, Bianchi C, Aufiero E. Oximetry and prognosis in amyotrophic lateral sclerosis. Chest 2004;126:1502-1507.

41. Hardy KA. A review of airway clearance: new techniques, indications, and recommendations. Respir Care 1994;39:440-455.

42. Bach JR, Alba AS, Saporito LR. Intermittent positive pressure ventilation via the mouth as an alternative to tracheostomy for 257 ventilator users. Chest 1993;103:174-182.

43. Bach JR, ed. Noninvasive Mechanical Ventilation. Philadelphia, Hanley & Belfus, 2002.

44. Bach JR, Baird JS, Plosky D, et al. Spinal muscular atrophy type 1: management and outcomes. Pediatr Pulmonol 2002;34:16-22.

45. Kang SW, Bach JR. Maximum insufflation capacity. Chest 2000;118:61-65.

Rheumatoid Arthritis 142

Karen Atkinson, MD, MPH, and Jonas Sokolof, DO

DEFINITION

Rheumatoid arthritis is a chronic inflammatory disorder that primarily affects joints but may also have prominent extra-articular features. The arthritis is classically symmetric and affects the peripheral joints. The prevalence of rheumatoid arthritis is approximately 1% in white individuals, and it affects women about 2 to 2.5 times more often than men. Peak incidence of rheumatoid arthritis is in the third and fourth decades.[1-3] Classification criteria are available for rheumatoid arthritis and may be helpful in the evaluation of patients (Table 142-1). Many patients with early disease, however, will not fulfill these criteria.[4]

SYMPTOMS

Rheumatoid arthritis is a systemic disease, and symptoms vary according to the system involved.[5-7]

General

Morning stiffness is a prominent feature of rheumatoid arthritis. Unlike the brief stiffness (5 to 10 minutes) that occurs in patients with osteoarthritis, the morning stiffness in rheumatoid arthritis is longer than 30 to 60 minutes and often lasts for hours. Fatigue and generalized malaise are also common complaints.

Joint

Patients present with joint pain and swelling. Patients may also complain of loss of joint function, which may be due to joint inflammation or structural damage. Baker's cyst can develop and cause pain or swelling of the popliteal fossa. If the cyst ruptures, it causes pain, swelling, and erythema of the calf. If the cricoarytenoid joint is involved, patients may complain of laryngeal pain, hoarseness, or difficulty in swallowing.

Eye

Up to one third of patients will complain of dry eyes (keratoconjunctivitis sicca). These patients may also complain of foreign body sensation, burning, or discharge. Patients with episcleritis will complain of red, painful eyes.

Skin

Patients may note small, painless subcutaneous nodules, mainly over the extensor surfaces. Rheumatoid vasculitis will cause rash that may lead to ulceration. Patients with vasculitis may also complain of discoloration around the fingertips (digital infarcts).

Neurologic

Numbness and tingling are common symptoms of nerve involvement. Nerves can be affected in several ways. Nerve entrapment results from joint inflammation. The most common site is at the wrist, where median nerve involvement causes carpal tunnel symptoms. Mononeuritis mutiplex is the result of vasculitis and presents as weakness, numbness, or tingling in discrete nerve distributions (e.g., footdrop or wristdrop). Cervical spine instability may lead to myelopathy, causing sensory symptoms and weakness, most commonly in the upper extremities. This can occur in the absence of neck pain in patients with long-standing rheumatoid arthritis.

Cardiac

The incidence and prevalence of coronary artery disease are increased in any type of chronic inflammatory disorder, and this is especially evident in rheumatoid arthritis. Thus, patients may present with complaints of chest pain, shortness of breath, diaphoresis, and other symptoms consistent with cardiac ischemia. Because of the

TABLE 142-1 Classification Criteria for Rheumatoid Arthritis[*]

Criterion	Definition
Morning stiffness	Morning stiffness in or around the joints lasting at least 1 hour before maximal improvement
Arthritis of three or more joint areas	Soft tissue swelling or fluid in at least three joints observed by a clinician The 14 possible joints include right or left PIP, MCP, wrist, elbow, knee, ankle, and MTP joints.
Arthritis of the hand joints	At least one area swollen in a wrist, MCP, or PIP joint
Symmetric arthritis	Simultaneous involvement of the same joint areas on both sides of the body Involvement of the small joint groups (MCP joints, PIP joints, and metatarsophalangeal joints) is acceptable without absolute symmetry.
Rheumatoid nodules	Subcutaneous nodules occurring over bone prominences, extensor surfaces, or juxta-articular regions These must be observed by a clinician.
Serum rheumatoid factor	Abnormal amounts of serum rheumatoid factor by any method for which the result has been positive in < 5% of normal control subjects
Radiographic changes	Posteroanterior hand and wrist films that demonstrate erosion or unequivocal bone decalcification localized in or most marked adjacent to the involved joints

[*]A patient is said to have rheumatoid arthritis if he or she satisfies at least four of the seven criteria. Criteria one through four must have been present for at least 6 weeks.

overall lack of mobility in this population, it has been reported that prevalence of angina in patients with rheumatoid arthritis may actually be lower than observed. Other cardiac manifestations of rheumatoid arthritis include myocarditis, pericarditis, atrioventricular block, and cardiac rheumatoid nodules. Pericardial involvement is usually asymptomatic.

Pulmonary

Pleural inflammation or nodulosis may produce typical symptoms of pleurisy. Shortness of breath may occur secondary to pleural or interstitial disease.

PHYSICAL EXAMINATION

All joints are examined for swelling, warmth, effusion, range of motion, and deformity. Rheumatoid arthritis is a symmetric polyarthritis (involvement of more than four joints). Fingers, feet, wrists, and knees are most commonly involved. The distal interphalangeal (DIP) joints are usually spared. Any joint can be affected. In rare cases, patients will present with monarthritis (involvement of a single joint). Rheumatoid nodules are present in about 30% of patients and occur over bone prominences, over extensor surfaces, or in juxta-articular regions.[5]

In the hands, early rheumatoid arthritis causes fusiform swelling at the proximal interphalangeal (PIP) joint. Chronic inflammation may lead to subluxation of the metacarpophalangeal (MCP) joints with ulnar deviation of the fingers. Damage to collateral ligaments at the PIP joints results in the classic boutonnière (PIP joint flexion and DIP joint hyperextension) and swan-neck (PIP joint hyperextension and DIP joint flexion) deformities (Figs. 142-1 and 142-2).

Symmetric wrist swelling is usually present in rheumatoid arthritis. Subluxation results from synovitis and

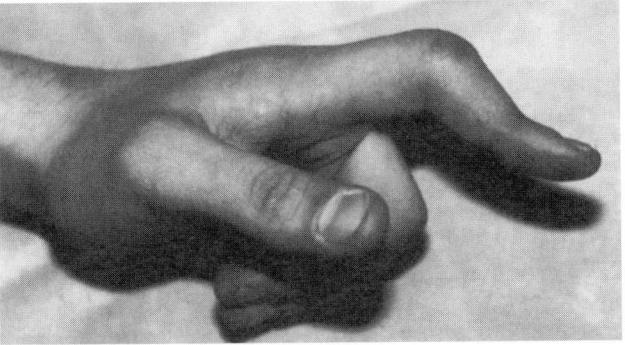

FIGURE 142-1. The boutonnière deformity, involving hyperextension of the DIP joint with flexion of the PIP joint, also is caused by a derangement of the extensor mechanism—typically a rupture of the central extensor tendon at its insertion in the middle phalanx. Early diagnosis and prolonged splinting of the PIP joint in extension are necessary for successful treatment of this difficult injury. (Reprinted with permission from Concannon MJ. Common Hand Problems in Primary Care. Philadelphia, Hanley & Belfus, 1999:151.)

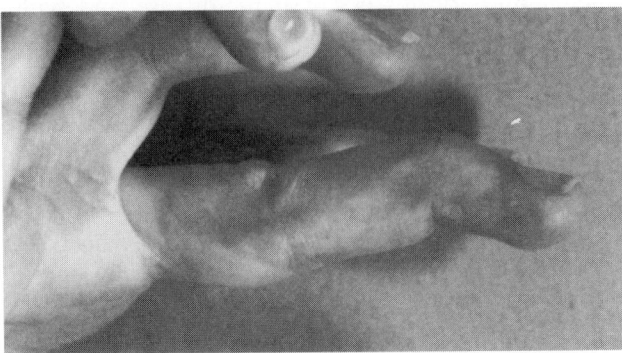

FIGURE 142-2. The swan-neck deformity (recurvatum) involves hyperextension of the PIP joint with flexion of the DIP joint. This is caused by a derangement in the extensor mechanism, with a dorsal migration of the lateral bands. (Reprinted with permission from Concannon MJ. Common Hand Problems in Primary Care. Philadelphia, Hanley & Belfus, 1999:151.)

weakening of the ligaments and causes prominence of the ulnar styloid.

Inflammation of the synovial tendon sheath is called tenosynovitis. This may occur in the flexor or extensor tendons of the fingers. Examination reveals that passive motion is greater than active motion. Crepitus is often felt when the hands are placed over the tendon sheaths and the fingers are flexed and extended. If the patient has a trigger finger, placement of one finger over the flexor tendon while the affected finger is flexed and extended will allow palpation of a nodule.

Elbow involvement is common. In early disease, inflammation and effusion cause decreased extension. Effusions can be palpated in the dimple (para–olecranon groove) found on either side of the olecranon process. With chronic inflammation and erosion of the cartilage between the radius and ulna, loss of extension and flexion occurs. Rheumatoid nodules are often found over the extensor aspect of the proximal ulna. The olecranon bursa may be enlarged and filled with fluid or nodules.

The shoulder may be involved in rheumatoid arthritis. Effusions are best seen on the anterior aspect of the shoulder below the acromion. Evaluation of rotator cuff strength is important because inflammation of the rotator cuff may result in destruction. A ruptured biceps tendon will cause a bulge in the biceps when it is flexed against resistance.

The cervical spine may have decreased range of motion or pain with range of motion. Physical examination is not adequate for assessment of stability. Patients with suspected cervical instability should have a thorough neurologic examination. Patients with cord involvement may demonstrate paresthesias, weakness, or pathologic reflexes. Tingling paresthesias that descend the thoracolumbar spine on flexion of the cervical spine are called Lhermitte sign (see Fig. 6-2).

The hip joint is deep, limiting evaluation for synovitis and effusion. An inflamed hip will cause groin pain on active and passive range of motion. Patients may walk with an antalgic gait, rapidly taking weight off the affected leg. Pain in the hip region may also result from trochanteric bursitis. Application of pressure over the lateral hip region reproduces the pain from the trochanteric bursa. Lateral hip pain and lack of groin pain distinguish trochanteric bursitis from joint inflammation. Iliopsoas bursitis may result in an inguinal mass.

The knee is commonly involved in rheumatoid arthritis. Small effusions can be detected by looking for a "bulge" sign. For the performance of this maneuver, the patient should be lying down. With one hand, the clinician makes an upward stroke to depress the medial synovial pouch. A downward stroke on the lateral aspect of the knee will result in a bulge of the medial pouch if a small effusion is present. A ballottable patella (patellar tap) indicates a larger effusion. Baker's cyst occurs as an extension of synovial fluid from the joint cavity (see Chapter 56). The cyst causes fullness in the popliteal fossa that can be seen when the patient is standing with his or her back facing the clinician. Erythema and

swelling of the calf may be seen if Baker's cyst has ruptured. Evaluation for hemorrhage below the malleoli of the ankle (the "crescent" sign) can distinguish this from thrombophlebitis.

The ankle may have synovitis, effusion, or decreased range of motion. Involvement of the hindfoot (subtalar and talonavicular joints) may result in valgus deformity and flatfoot. Metatarsophalangeal joint involvement is common. Synovitis causes pain and fullness with palpation. Hallux valgus deformity is also common. Progressive disease causes dorsal dislocation of the metatarsophalangeal joints and claw toes.

FUNCTIONAL LIMITATIONS

Functional limitations depend on the location and severity of joint and extra-articular involvement. Criteria for the assessment of functional status have been established (Table 142-2) and are based on activities of daily living, including self-care (e.g., dressing, feeding, bathing, grooming, and toileting) and vocational (e.g., work, school, and homemaking) and avocational (e.g., recreational and leisure) activities.[8]

Whereas radiologic changes have been shown to have only limited value in determining functional impairment and quality of life, disability from rheumatoid arthritis has been directly attributed to joint damage, disease activity, pain, and depressive symptoms.[9]

DIAGNOSTIC STUDIES

Laboratory histologic findings and radiographic findings may be suggestive of rheumatoid arthritis, but no test is diagnostic of the disease[5,10] (Figs. 142-3 and 142-4). Rheumatoid factor is present in the serum of 85% of patients.[7] However, because rheumatoid factor is often present in other inflammatory conditions, such as systemic lupus erythematosus, primary Sjögren syndrome, and chronic osteomyelitis, much debate exists about its utility in the diagnosis of rheumatoid arthritis as a result of low specificity.[11] Anti–cyclic citrullinated peptide antibodies have shown more promise as potential biologic markers because of sensitivities of 70% to 80% and specificities of 95% to 98% in patients with established rheumatoid arthritis.[12] Normochromic, normocytic anemia consistent with

TABLE 142-2	Criteria for Classification of Functional Status in Rheumatoid Arthritis
Class I	Able to perform all activities of daily living (self-care, vocational, and avocational)
Class II	Able to perform self-care and vocational activities, but limited in avocational activities
Class III	Able to perform usual self-care activities, but limited in vocational and avocational activities
Class IV	Limited in all activities of daily living (self-care, vocational, and avocational)

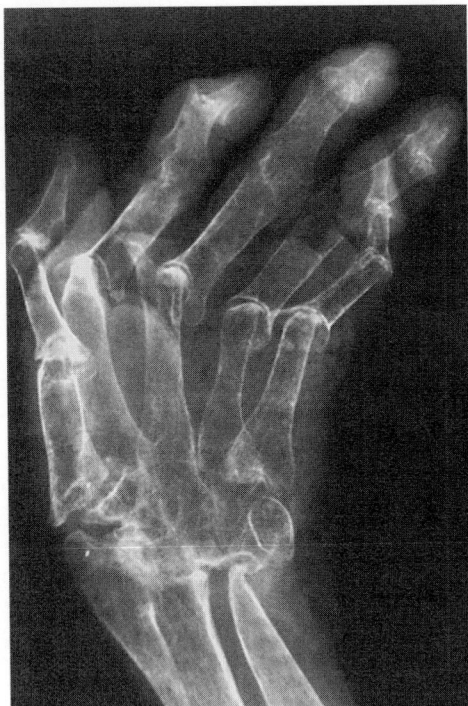

FIGURE 142-3. Advanced rheumatoid arthritis—hand and wrist. Bony ankylosis at the wrist, penciling of the distal ulna, and marked erosive changes at the MCP joints with ulnar deviation of the fingers are classic findings of rheumatoid arthritis. Also note the more severe involvement of the carpus and MCP joints; interphalangeal joints are typically less severely affected. (Reprinted with permission from Katz DS, Math KR, Groskin SA. Radiology Secrets. Philadelphia, Hanley & Belfus, 1998:273.)

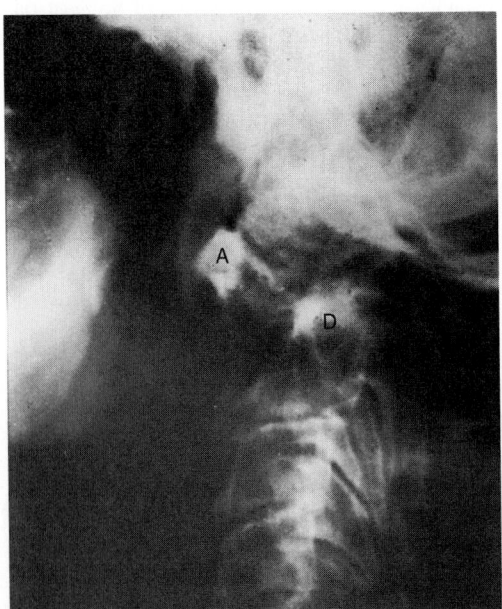

FIGURE 142-4. Atlantoaxial subluxation—rheumatoid arthritis. There is marked widening of the space between the anterior arch of the atlas (A) and the margin of the dens (D). (Reprinted with permission from Katz DS, Math KR, Groskin SA. Radiology Secrets. Philadelphia, Hanley & Belfus, 1998:273.)

chronic disease is often found, and the degree of anemia often correlates with disease activity. Acute-phase reactants, such as erythrocyte sedimentation rate, C-reactive protein concentration, and erythrocyte and platelet counts, are elevated. Eosinophilia may be found in patients with extra-articular manifestations. Patients with Felty syndrome (rheumatoid arthritis, splenomegaly, and leukopenia) exhibit low white blood cell counts and may have thrombocytopenia. A variant of Felty syndrome has been described in which patients have large granular lymphocytes in blood and bone marrow in addition to neutropenia. Liver enzymes including aspartate transaminase and alkaline phosphatase are often elevated in patients with active disease.

Evaluation of fluid taken from an affected joint will show an inflammatory cell count (more than 2000 white blood cells). Joint fluid should always be sent for culture to rule out infection and evaluated under a polarized microscope to exclude crystal disease. If pleurocentesis or pericardiocentesis is necessary, the fluid has a low complement concentration, a high protein concentration, and a predominance of lymphocytes. The glucose concentration is characteristically extremely low or may even be absent.

Characteristic changes on joint radiographs include periarticular osteopenia and marginal erosions. Early in the disease, however, joint films may be normal. Baseline hand and wrist films may aid in diagnosis and can be used to follow disease progression. Flexion and extension views of the cervical spine may demonstrate erosion of the odontoid and atlantoaxial subluxation. Pulmonary nodules or interstitial fibrosis can be seen on the chest radiograph. Echocardiography often reveals a small pericardial effusion, valvular thickening, or aortic root dilatation, but these are most often asymptomatic. Electrocardiography may reveal conduction abnormalities due to involvement of the cardiac conduction system by rheumatoid nodules.

Differential Diagnosis

Crystal-induced arthritis

Gout

Pseudogout

Spondyloarthropathies

Psoriatic arthritis

Ankylosing spondylitis

Enteropathic arthritis

TREATMENT

Initial

Nonsteroidal anti-inflammatory drugs (NSAIDs) are effective in some patients. Cyclooxygenase 2 (COX-2)–specific anti-inflammatories may reduce the incidence of gastrointestinal symptoms in patients who have a history of bleeding or who are intolerant of traditional NSAIDs.

For patients with inadequate response to NSAIDs or poor prognostic indicators, disease-modifying antirheumatic drugs (DMARDs) should be initiated. Poor prognostic factors include high-titer rheumatoid factor, early presence of bone erosion, many affected joints, extra-articular involvement, and considerable degree of physical disability at disease onset.[13]

DMARDs that are prescribed include antimalarials, intramuscular administration of gold, sulfasalazine, azathioprine, methotrexate, leflunomide, cyclosporine, and cyclophosphamide.[13,14] Anticytokine therapies include the anti–tumor necrosis factor-α agents etanercept, infliximab, and adalimumab and the interleukin-1 receptor antagonist anakinra. Other biologic agents currently available include abatacept (CTLA4-Ig) and rituximab, which is a B cell–depleting monoclonal antibody. Several studies support the use of combination DMARD therapy.[15] Anti–tumor necrosis factor-α agents used in combination with small-molecule DMARDs such as methotrexate will often halt disease activity and radiologic progression of joint destruction.[16] Corticosteroids can be very useful and can be administered systemically as a bridge to therapy with DMARDs or intra-articularly for monarticular or oligoarticular involvement.

Rehabilitation

The role of occupational and physical therapy may be different in early or established disease and end-stage disease.[17,18] In early disease, occupational therapy is directed toward education of the patient about how to minimize joint stress in performing activities of daily living. Splints may be used to provide joint rest and to reduce inflammation. Splints may also allow functional use of joints that would otherwise be limited by pain. Not all clinicians advocate this use. Paraffin baths can provide relief of pain and stiffness in the small joints of the hands. In end-stage disease, the occupational therapist plays an important role, providing aids and adaptive devices, such as raised toilet seats, special chairs and beds, and special grips, that can assist in self-care.

Physical therapy can be very helpful in reducing joint inflammation and pain. The therapist may employ a variety of techniques, including the application of heat or cold, transcutaneous nerve stimulation, and iontophoresis. Water exercise (hydrotherapy) is used to increase muscle strength without joint overuse. In patients with foot involvement, small alterations to footwear or inserts may decrease pain and provide a more normal gait. In end-stage disease, the goals of therapy are to reduce joint inflammation, to loosen fixed position of joints, to improve the function of damaged joints, and to improve strength and general condition. Local immobilization may be used to reduce inflammation and pain. Nonfixed contractures may be prevented or improved with periods of splinting combined with goal-oriented exercise. Muscle strength and overall conditioning may be improved by static, range of motion, and relaxation exercises. In recent years, aerobic and weight-bearing exercises have been used without detrimental effect to the joints. These dynamic exercises are more effective in increasing muscle strength, range of motion, and physical capacity.[19] However, high-intensity weight-bearing exercises have been shown to accelerate joint destruction in individuals with preexisting extensive large-joint damage from rheumatoid arthritis.[20] Thus, the exercise prescription must be appropriately tailored on the basis of the degree of disease present in each patient. The motivation and encouragement provided by the therapist should not be underestimated.

Procedures

For monarticular or oligoarticular involvement, local steroid injection may be used when oral medications fail to control joint inflammation.

Surgery

Orthopedic intervention including joint reconstruction or replacement (Fig. 142-5), tendon repair, and synovectomy may be indicated. Patients with suspected or confirmed cervical spine involvement will need special consideration and handling during intubation for anesthesia (Fig. 142-6). Cervical spine stabilization is usually not performed unless the patient has neurologic symptoms.

POTENTIAL DISEASE COMPLICATIONS

The most common complication is joint destruction with subsequent decreased functional use of affected joints. Neuropathy may be due to entrapment, pressure,

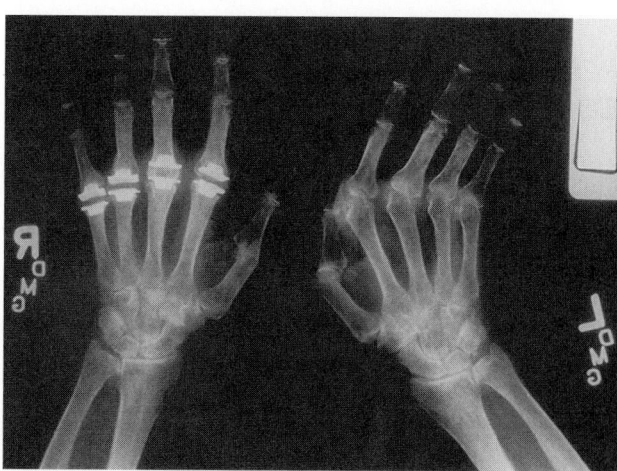

FIGURE 142-5. Hinged silicone prosthesis with grommets. Radiograph of implanted prostheses at the MCP joints of the index, middle, ring, and little fingers on the right hand. (Reprinted with permission from Weinzweig J. Plastic Surgery Secrets. Philadelphia, Hanley & Belfus, 1999:543.)

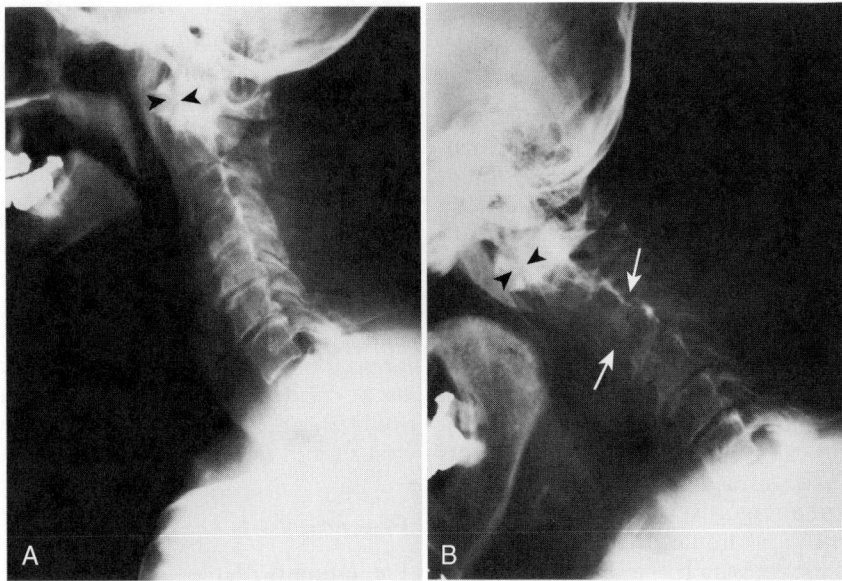

FIGURE 142-6. Subluxation of vertebrae in rheumatoid arthritis. The abnormal movement between vertebrae due to laxity of ligaments becomes more apparent in flexion of the cervical spine. Lateral flexion-extension views are requested if subluxation of cervical vertebrae is suspected. The radiograph in **A** is taken in the neutral position, and the one in **B** is taken in flexion. The arrowheads mark the distance between the anterior surface of the odontoid process and the posterior surface of the arch of the atlas. This space is increased in flexion because of subluxation of the arch of the atlas on the second vertebra. The arrows show anterior slippage of the third cervical vertebra on the fourth. In a normal cervical spine, the posterior surface of vertebral bodies forms a smooth curve that is convex anteriorly (lordosis). This curve is disturbed and a step-like deformity is seen *(arrows)* at the posteroinferior angle of the upper vertebra and the posterosuperior angle of the lower vertebra in subluxation. (Reprinted with permission from Mehta AJ. Common Musculoskeletal Problems. Philadelphia, Hanley & Belfus, 1997:149.)

or deposition of amyloid. Cervical instability can lead to myelopathy. Irregular bone edges may result in tendon rupture. Nodules may break down and ulcerate. Skin ulcerations may also occur in pressure points in the immobilized patient. The kidneys and gastrointestinal tract may be sites of deposition in patients who develop secondary amyloidosis. Scleritis may result in scleromalacia. As previously mentioned, cardiovascular disease is almost always present in aggressive or untreated cases.

POTENTIAL TREATMENT COMPLICATIONS

Medication side effects vary according to the drug (Table 142-3).[14]

Overly aggressive physical or occupational therapy can cause increased joint inflammation and pain.

TABLE 142-3 Side Effects of Medications Used to Treat Patients with Rheumatoid Arthritis

Medication	Side Effects
NSAIDs	
Traditional	Dyspepsia, ulcer, or bleeding
	Renal insufficiency
	Hepatotoxicity
	Rash
	Inhibit platelet function
COX-2 inhibitors	Same as traditional NSAIDs, but gastrointestinal side effects occur less often
	No platelet effect
Glucocorticoids	Increased appetite, weight gain
	Cushingoid habitus
	Acne
	Fluid retention
	Hypertension
	Diabetes
	Glaucoma, cataracts
	Atherosclerosis
	Avascular necrosis
	Osteoporosis
	Impaired wound healing
	Susceptibility to infection

Medication	Side Effects
Antimalarials	Dyspepsia
	Hemolysis (glucose-6-phosphate dehydrogenase–deficient patients)
	Macular damage
	Abnormal skin pigmentation
	Neuromyopathy
	Rash
Gold	Myelosuppression
	Proteinuria or hematuria
	Oral ulcers
	Rash
	Pruritus
Etanercept	Injection site reaction
	Exacerbation of infection
Cyclosporine	Renal insufficiency
	Hypertension
	Anemia
Sulfasalazine	Myelosuppression
	Hemolysis (glucose-6-phosphate dehydrogenase–deficient patients)
	Hepatotoxicity
	Photosensitivity, rash
	Dyspepsia, diarrhea
	Headaches
	Oligospermia
Azathioprine	Myelosuppression
	Hepatotoxicity
	Pancreatitis (rarely)
	Lymphoproliferative disorders (long-term risk)
Methotrexate	Hepatic fibrosis, cirrhosis
	Pneumonitis
	Myelosuppression
	Mucositis
	Dyspepsia
	Alopecia
	Increased rheumatoid nodules
Leflunomide	Hepatic fibrosis, cirrhosis
	Myelosuppression
	Dyspepsia
	Alopecia
Infliximab	Infusion reaction
	Exacerbation of infection
Cyclophosphamide	Dyspepsia, diarrhea
	Myelosuppression
	Alopecia
	Hemorrhagic cystitis
	Ovarian and testicular failure
	Teratogenicity
	Malignant neoplasia
	Opportunistic infection

References

1. MacGregor AJ, Silman AJ. Rheumatoid arthritis: classification and epidemiology. In Klippel JH, Dieppe PA, eds. Rheumatology, 2nd ed. London, Mosby, 1998:5.2.2-6.
2. Del Rincon I, Williams K, Stern MP, et al. High incidence of cardiovascular events in rheumatoid arthritis cohort not explained by traditional cardiac risk factors. Arthritis Rheum 2001;44: 2237-2245.
3. Maradit-Kremers H, Crowson CS, Nicola PJ, et al. Increased unrecognized coronary heart disease and sudden deaths in rheumatoid arthritis: a population-based cohort study. Arthritis Rheum 2005;52:402-411.
4. Arnet FC, Edworthy SM, Bloch DA, et al. The American Rheumatism Association 1987 revised criteria for the classification of rheumatoid arthritis. Arthritis Rheum 1988;31:315-324.
5. Fuchs HA, Sergent JS. Rheumatoid arthritis: the clinical picture. In Koopman WJ, ed. Arthritis and Allied Conditions: A Textbook of Rheumatology, 13th ed. Baltimore, Williams & Wilkins, 1997: 1041-1070.
6. Gordon AG, Hastings DE. Rheumatoid arthritis: clinical features of early, progressive and late disease. In Klippel JH, Dieppe PA, eds. Rheumatology, 2nd ed. London, Mosby, 1998:5.3.1-14.
7. Anderson RJ. Rheumatoid arthritis: clinical and laboratory features. In Klippel JH, ed. Primer on the Rheumatic Diseases, 11th ed. Atlanta, Arthritis Foundation, 1997:161-167.
8. Hochberg MC, Chang RW, Dwosh I, et al. The American College of Rheumatology 1991 revised criteria for the classification of global functional status in rheumatoid arthritis. Arthritis Rheum 1992;35:493-502.
9. Rupp I, Boshuizen HC, Dinant HJ, et al. Disability and health-related quality of life among patients with rheumatoid arthritis: association with radiographic joint damage, disease activity, pain, and depressive symptoms. Scand J Rheumatol 2006;35:175-181.
10. Matteson EL, Cohen MD, Doyt DL. Rheumatoid arthritis: clinical features and systemic involvement. In Klippel JH, Dieppe PA, eds. Rheumatology, 2nd ed. London, Mosby, 1998:5.4.1-7.
11. Symmons DP. Classification criteria for rheumatoid arthritis—time to abandon rheumatoid factor? Rheumatology (Oxford) 2007;46:725-726.
12. Avouc J, Gossec L, Dougados M. Diagnostic and predictive value of anti–cyclic citrullinated protein antibodies in rheumatoid arthritis: a systematic review. Ann Rheum Dis 2006;65: 845-851.
13. Paget SA. Rheumatoid arthritis: treatment. In Klippel JH, ed. Primer on the Rheumatic Diseases, 11th ed. Atlanta, Arthritis Foundation, 1997:168-173.
14. Cash JM, Klippel JH. Drug therapy: second-line drug therapy for rheumatoid arthritis. N Engl J Med 1994;330:1368-1375.
15. Perdriger A, Mariette X, Kuntz JL, et al. Safety of infliximab used in combination with leflunomide or azathioprine in daily clinical practice. J Rheumatol 2006;33:865-869.
16. Hyrich KL, Symmons DP, Watson KD, Silman AJ. Comparison of the response to infliximab or etanercept monotherapy with the response to cotherapy with methotrexate or another disease modifying antirheumatic drug in patients with rheumatoid arthritis: results from the British Society for Rheumatology Biologics Register. Arthritis Rheum 2006;54:1786-1794.
17. van Riel PL, Wijnands MJH, van de Putte LBA. Rheumatoid arthritis: evaluation and management of active inflammatory disease. In Klippel JH, Dieppe PA, eds. Rheumatology, 2nd ed. London, Mosby, 1998:5.14.1-12.
18. Hazes JMW, Cats A. Rheumatoid arthritis: management: end stage and complications. In Klippel JH, Dieppe PA, eds. Rheumatology, 2nd ed. London, Mosby, 1998:5.15.1-10.
19. van den Ende CH, Breedveld FC, le Cessie S, et al. Effect of intensive exercise on patients with active rheumatoid arthritis: a randomised clinical trial. Ann Rheum Dis 2000;59:615-621.
20. Munneke M, de Jong Z, Zwinderman AH, et al. Effect of a high-intensity weight-bearing exercise program on radiologic damage progression of the large joints in subgroups of patients with rheumatoid arthritis. Arthritis Rheum 2005;53:410-417.

Scoliosis and Kyphosis   143

Mark A. Thomas, MD, and Yumei Wang, MD

Synonyms

Scoliosis
Curvature of the spine
Curved spine
Crooked back
Kyphosis
Hunchback
Humpback
Roundback
Dorsum rotundum
Dowager's hump
Scheuermann disease
Postural roundback
Postural kyphosis
Gibbus deformity

ICD-9 Codes

732.0	Scheuermann disease
732.8	Other specified forms of osteochondropathy Adult osteochondrosis of spine
737.0	Adolescent postural kyphosis
737.10	Kyphosis (acquired) (postural)
737.11	Kyphosis due to radiation
737.12	Kyphosis, postlaminectomy
737.40	Curvature of spine, unspecified
737.41	Kyphosis
737.43	Scoliosis

DEFINITION

Scoliosis (Fig. 143-1) is a postural deformity of the spine resulting in a lateral (coronal) deviation or curve. Scoliosis is associated with rotation of the vertebral bodies located within the curve. It affects between 3% and 30% of the population; about 0.25% require treatment.[1] The incidence of scoliosis increases with age.[2] The scoliotic curve may be congenital, appearing during infancy (infantile scoliosis), or it may develop in childhood (juvenile scoliosis), adolescence (adolescent scoliosis), or adulthood (degenerative scoliosis). When the diagnosis of scoliosis is made in an adult patient, the curve should be defined as adult onset (usually degenerative) or adult presenting (most commonly an idio-

pathic adolescent curve that was not previously diagnosed). Scoliosis can result from congenital, degenerative, disease-related, iatrogenic, or, most commonly, idiopathic causes. There is increasing evidence that idiopathic curves relate to genetics; known candidates are chromosomes 6, 9, 16, and 17.[3] Less common causes include degenerative disc disease and spondylosis, congenital malformation of the vertebrae, tumor, neuromuscular disease, and connective tissue disease.

Kyphosis (Fig. 143-2) is a sagittal deviation in spinal alignment or backward curve exceeding normal values. Normal kyphosis in the thoracic spine varies between 20 and 40 degrees.[4-6] Pathologic kyphosis occurs in association with structural changes in the spine due to disease, such as osteoporotic compression fractures, tumor, and Scheuermann disease (juvenile kyphosis), and after radiation therapy.[7] It is caused by the resulting wedge deformity of the vertebral bodies.

SYMPTOMS

Scoliosis

The symptoms produced by scoliosis relate to the cause, location, and severity of the curve. The curve itself often does not produce symptoms or complaints, particularly a curve that does not exceed 20 degrees. When adult scoliosis is severe, pain and cosmetic deformities occur; pain is generally not recognized as a problem in children. Deformity, such as humping of the back, asymmetric shoulder or hip height, or asymmetry of breast size or waist contour, frequently produces psychosocial symptoms such as low self-esteem, anxiety, and depression, particularly among adolescents.[8] These may be the presenting complaints. Curves that exceed 60 to 80 degrees begin to affect other systems. They can produce shortness of breath due to restrictive lung disease and weakness, pain, paresthesia, or hypesthesia due to compression or impingement of thoracic or lumbar nerve roots, most commonly at the apex of the curve.[9] Activity tolerance can become limited by increased energy costs for maintaining trunk stability and ambulation (the determinants of gait are incompetent). Severe lumbar curves commonly produce low back pain,

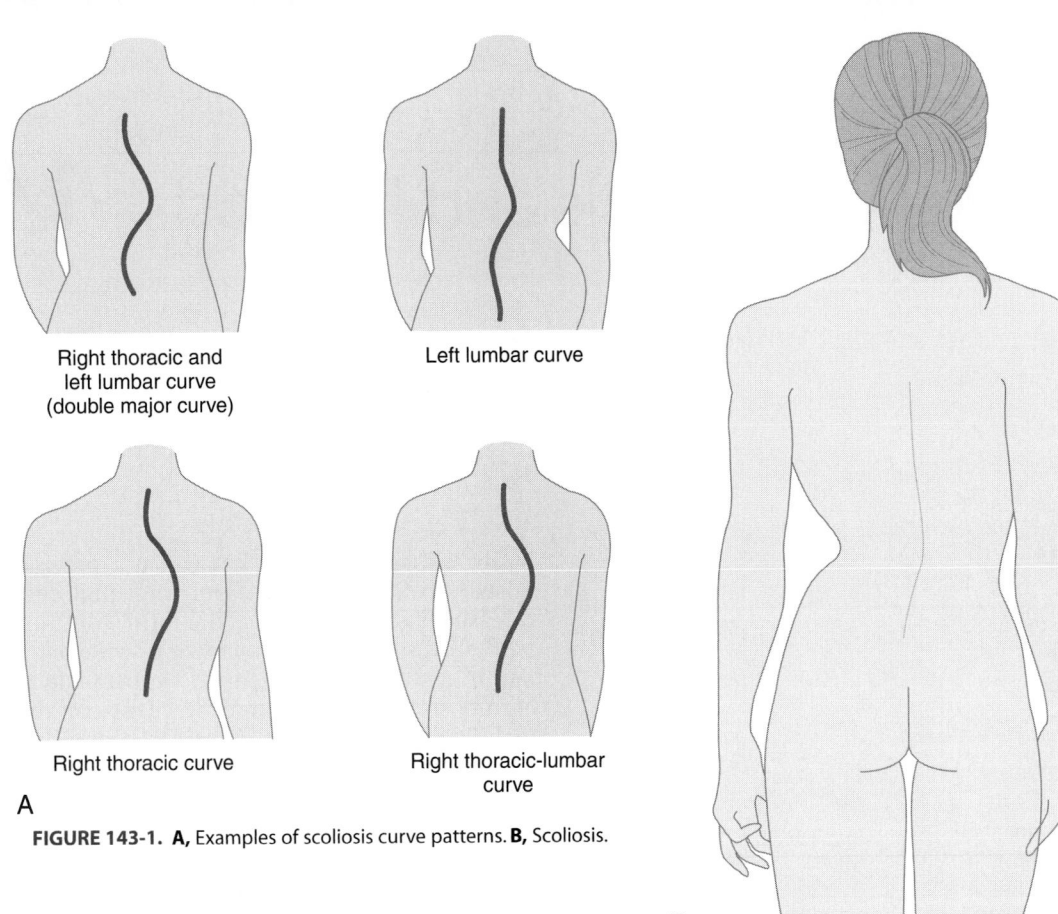

FIGURE 143-1. **A,** Examples of scoliosis curve patterns. **B,** Scoliosis.

Right thoracic and
left lumbar curve
(double major curve)

Left lumbar curve

Right thoracic curve

Right thoracic-lumbar
curve

A

B

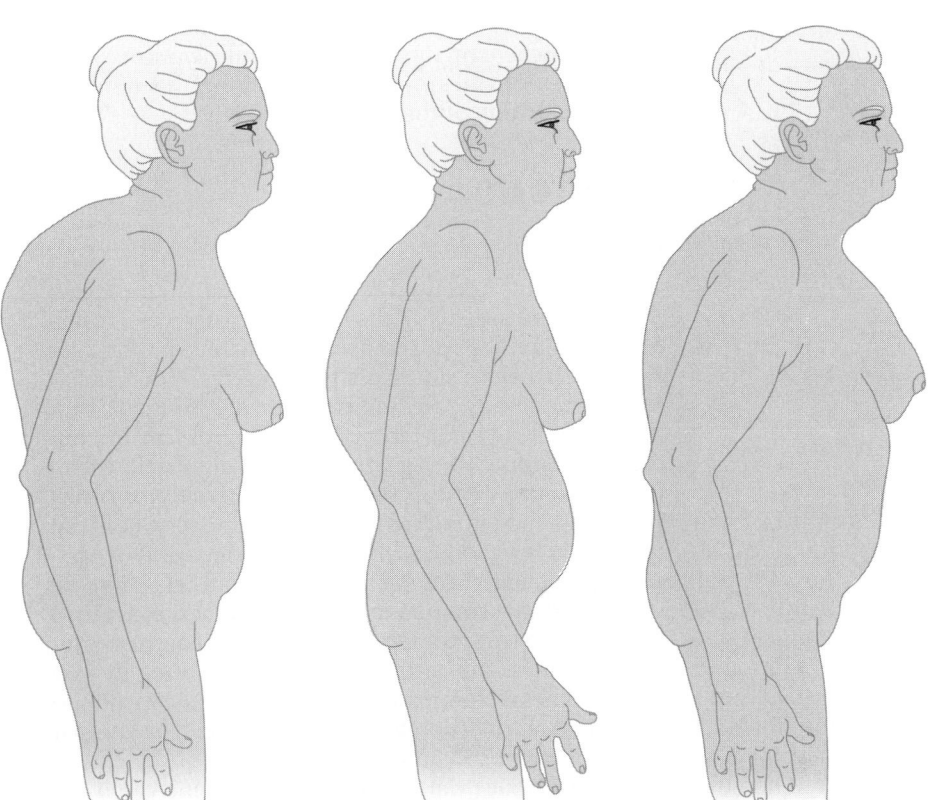

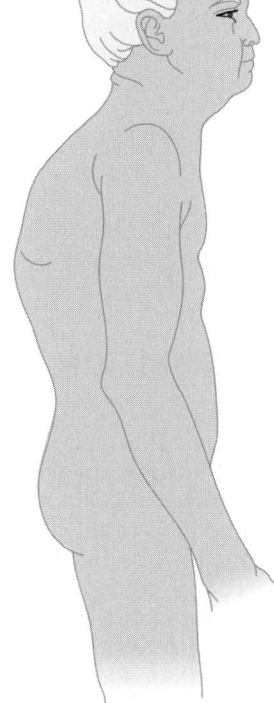

A

B

FIGURE 143-2. **A,** Kyphotic deformities. **B,** Kyphosis.

whereas severe thoracic curvature will most often result in psychosocial symptoms. Large curves, beyond 50 degrees, can affect childbearing.[1] If the onset of scoliosis is before 5 years of age, there is an association with plagiocephaly, congenital heart disease, inguinal hernia, and hip dysplasia. If such a curve exceeds 20 degrees, magnetic resonance imaging is warranted to rule out central nervous system lesions.[10]

Kyphosis

Complaints relate to the degree and location of the kyphos. Intermittent aching back pain and stiffness are the most usual presenting complaints and are most prominent at the apex of the curve. Pain and stiffness may be most severe when the patient is leaning forward. A compensatory increase in lumbar lordosis may be present and associated with low back pain.[4,11,12] Cardiopulmonary compromise, although unusual, can also develop in severe cases, causing shortness of breath, fatigue, and poor activity tolerance.

PHYSICAL EXAMINATION

Scoliosis

Minor curves are difficult to detect on inspection of the patient. An easy way to detect a subtle thoracic or lumbar curve is to drop a plumb line from the occiput, or C7 spinous process, and inspect the spine for lateral deviations from this line. For routine screening, have the patient bend forward. The rotation associated with scoliosis is most easily seen in this forward flexed position. Asymmetry of the back contour in this position is due to vertebral body or rib rotation and may be quantified. In idiopathic curves, a trunk rotation angle of 7 degrees roughly corresponds to a coronal curve of 20 degrees.

Subtle indicators that can be sought on physical examination are apparent (not actual) unequal breast size, asymmetry of the waist fold contour, and unequal iliac crest and shoulder height. Scoliosis should be suspected with café au lait spots (often associated with neurofibromatosis) or a leg length discrepancy exceeding 2.2 cm.[13,14] Thorough serial assessments are advisable every 6 to 12 months. These assessments usually include radiographs and focus on the degree of curvature, location and extent of the curve, degree of rotation, degree of skeletal maturity, correctability of the curve, height, vital capacity, and expiratory pulmonary function.

Patients with degenerative scoliosis should be examined for neurologic deficits. Lower extremity strength, sensation, and reflexes should be checked when the curvature exceeds 40 degrees or when the patient complains of weakness, paresthesias, or decreased sensation regardless of the cause of the scoliosis.

A full evaluation of a scoliotic curve necessitates identification of the cause of the curve for optimal treatment and prognostication. Curves may be idiopathic (juvenile, adolescent), functional (muscle spasm, posture), congenital (vertebral malformation), or degenerative or paralytic (motor unit disease). Scoliosis should be treated in the context of a patient's global status, and identification of the underlying or idiopathic causes of the curve allows care to be provided within the context of the patient's overall health.

Kyphosis

Increased thoracic kyphos results in a forward displacement of the head and neck and a compensatory increase in lumbar lordosis. These are apparent on inspection. The rounding of the back will not be fully corrected with trunk extension in a prone position, but the degree to which the curve reverses should be noted. Thoracolumbar and lumbar kyphoses are less readily appreciated on inspection. The clinician should note any prominence of the spinous processes, which indicates lower spine kyphosis.[15-18] Associated scoliosis should be sought and will be present in about one third of patients.[19-21] Restricted trunk extension results from either deformity or pain. Tenderness to palpation may be elicited over the spinous processes. Tightness of the hamstring and pectoralis muscles is common.

A neurologic examination should be performed when the patient complains of weakness, sensory changes, or gait abnormalities. Vital capacity, peak flow, and other expiratory respiratory parameters should be performed when the kyphosis exceeds 40 to 50 degrees.

FUNCTIONAL LIMITATIONS

The functional limitations related to scoliosis and kyphosis result from the loss of spinal motion.[15] A kyphosis-related restriction in upward gaze may affect driving and cause difficulty with lying prone or swimming in a prone position. Loss of shoulder range of motion, particularly forward flexion and abduction, may result from restricted scapular excursion over the thorax. This can interfere with overhead activities of daily living. Pain can result in limited sitting, standing, or walking tolerance.

The disruption of spinal balance that occurs will displace the center of gravity, particularly with severe kyphosis. This increases the energy costs for standing and ambulation. It can also impair balance. With severe deformity, cardiopulmonary compromise may decrease endurance. If the patient perceives cosmetic deformities as severe, social isolation can result.

DIAGNOSTIC STUDIES

Standing anteroposterior and lateral radiographs are useful in the evaluation of scoliosis and kyphosis. Bending or supine radiographs are not usually obtained but can help determine the flexibility or correctability of the curve. Radiographs can reveal congenital abnormalities of the vertebral body that cause spinal imbalance (block, bar, or butterfly vertebrae), evidence of Scheuermann disease (end-plate fluting), or lateral vertebral body wedging that is characteristic of idiopathic scoliosis.[22] Lordosis and pelvic obliquity correspond well to the pain experienced by the patient.[23]

Measurement of the scoliotic curve on plain films is done by either the Cobb or Risser method. The most common measurement, the Cobb angle, is determined by the intersection of two lines drawn perpendicular to the vertebral end plates that represent the maximal deviation of the spine (Fig. 143-3).

Plain films also allow assessment of vertebral body rotation and the growth centers in the ilium, vertebrae, and humerus. The degree of vertebral body rotation is gauged by the deviation from the midline of either the spinous process or pedicles. Rotation is graded 0 (no rotation) to 4 (rotation of 90 degrees or more). Epiphyseal closure can sometimes be assessed by plain films. Closure of the growth plates proceeds in a cephalad manner. Because vertebral growth plates are not consistently demonstrated on plain films, the iliac crest is a useful site for assessment of spine growth status. This is the Risser sign, which is graded 0 (no mineralization) to 5 (fusion of the growth plate).

Anterior-posterior films may demonstrate asymmetric disc degeneration; more than 20% of adult curves demonstrate unilateral disc disease. Scoliosis risk increases with asymmetric vertebral growth (e.g., after radiation therapy), vertebral height loss of more than 5 mm, or unilateral osteophyte formation.[24]

Magnetic resonance imaging is indicated for specific purposes, such as identification of a neurofibroma or diastematomyelia. If a neurologic deficit is present, magnetic resonance imaging should be performed.

Electrodiagnostic studies are a useful adjunct to these tests for grading the severity of a neurologic deficit. Somatosensory evoked potentials (tibial nerve) correlate with magnetic resonance imaging findings and offer another diagnostic option.[25] Curve severity parallels vertebral growth pattern and velocity of curve change. If growth velocity is high, there is increased electromyographic activity in the lower convex curve.[25] If surgery is being considered, preoperative magnetic resonance imaging or computed tomographic myelography is indicated.

Bone scans are helpful to exclude discitis or tumor as the cause of pain or spinal deformity. Bone densitometry demonstrates increased density on the convex side of the curve. This occurs even in osteoporotic patients.[26] Pulmonary function testing, particularly volume and expiratory studies, should be performed when curves exceed 60 degrees.

TREATMENT

Initial

In all patients, regardless of age, it is important to identify curves that are likely to progress. Curves that are large (degree of curvature), double (double major,

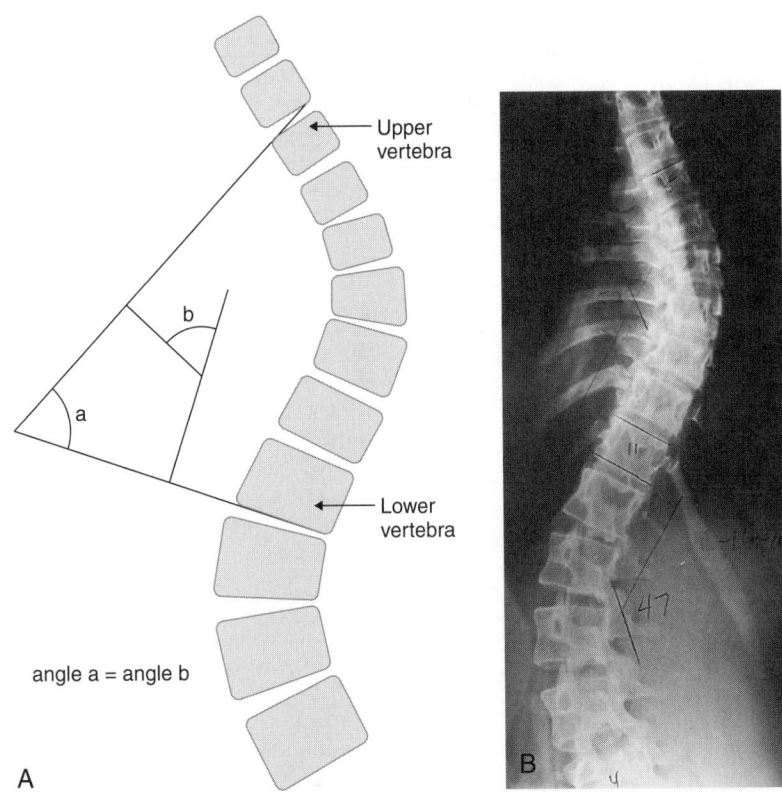

FIGURE 143-3. A, Measurement of idiopathic scoliosis by the Cobb angle. **B,** Idiopathic adolescent scoliosis. There is a primary thoracic dextroscoliosis (convexity to the right side) measuring 52 degrees and a compensatory lumbar levoscoliosis (convexity to the left side) measuring 47 degrees. (Reprinted with permission from Katz DS, Math KR, Groskin SA. Radiology Secrets. Philadelphia, Hanley & Belfus, 1998:321.)

Differential Diagnosis

Lateral listhesis

Spondylolisthesis

Morquio disease

Deformity resulting from other cause (fracture, tumor)

single major with a compensatory curve), closely packed (spanning a relatively small spinal segment), related to congenital vertebral body malformation, very rotated, or present in the immature spine are most likely to progress and require more frequent assessment and aggressive intervention.[24] In general, scoliotic curves of less than 20 degrees and kyphotic curves of less than 40 degrees are observed through serial assessments. Nonsteroidal anti-inflammatory drugs or analgesics may be used for pain management. Transcutaneous electrical nerve stimulation can be used for analgesia, but otherwise there is no clear role for electrical stimulation in the treatment of scoliosis.

If the scoliotic curve exceeds 20 degrees or the kyphosis exceeds 40 degrees, assess for bracing or surgery. The treatment goals for idiopathic curves are to limit progression of the scoliosis or kyphosis and to maintain full activity, independence, and comfort. This is best done with education of the patient, exercise, and bracing. Bracing for idiopathic adolescent curves provides the best correction effect, ranging between 42% and 92%. The best correction effect is seen with use of the nighttime wear orthoses, such as the Chênau, Charleston, and Providence braces.[27-29]

Rehabilitation

Exercise is beneficial for general well-being and flexibility and to improve posture. There is no clear evidence that exercise is a disease-modifying intervention for idiopathic scoliosis. Kyphosis may improve with cervicothoracic extension exercise, pelvic tilt to reduce lumbar lordosis, and stretching and strengthening exercise of the hamstring, hip flexor, and pectoralis muscles. Exercise, particularly spinal extension, abdominal strengthening, and hamstring stretch, is also helpful to reduce back pain.[15,19,30]

Bracing is an important part of the rehabilitation intervention. Without bracing, it is 20% to 40% more likely that the curve will progress than if a brace is used. There is no consensus regarding recommended brace wear time per day; recommendations range between 8 and 23 hours of daily wear. Some correction of the curvature may take place with conscientious use of the orthosis, although the goals of orthotic treatment are to reduce pain and to limit progression of the curve. The most common brace selection is a body jacket thoracolumbosacral orthosis, such as the Boston or Denver brace (Fig. 143-4). High thoracic and cervical curves

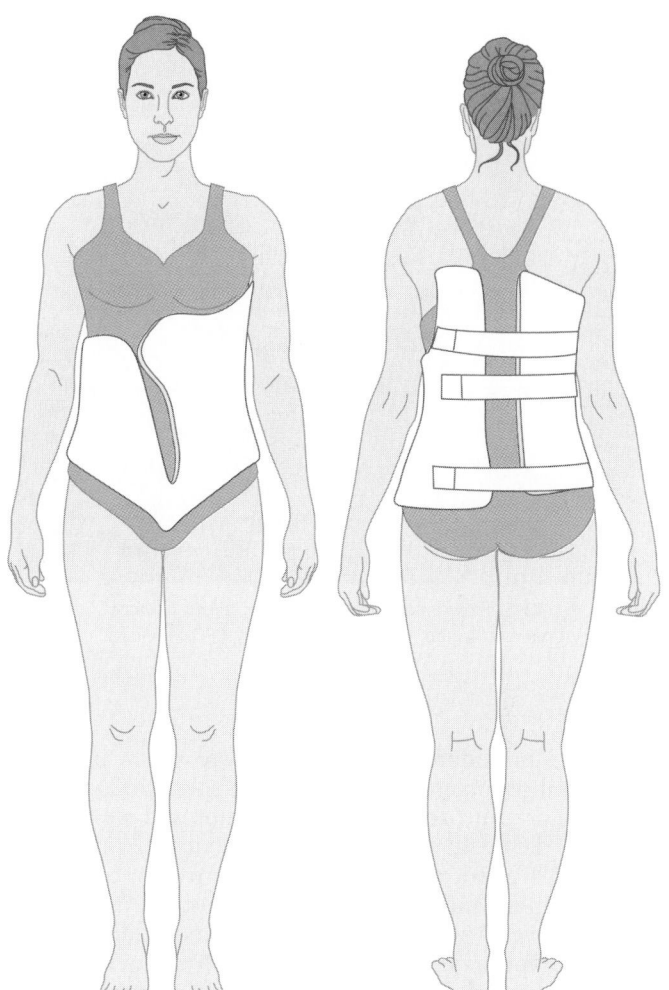

FIGURE 143-4. Body jacket thoracolumbosacral orthosis, posterior opening.

and kyphotic curves may require a Milwaukee cervicothoracolumbosacral orthosis. Bracing for idiopathic curves in a growing child or adolescent is maintained until spinal growth centers fuse. When a thoracolumbosacral body jacket or corset is used to decrease pain and to improve posture for patients with degenerative scoliosis, wear time depends on symptoms. Braces worn only at night (Providence and Charleston braces) offer an option that is effective and more attractive to the patient (Fig. 143-5).[27,28] Bracing is generally more effective for lower thoracic and lumbar curves.[25]

For scoliosis associated with neuromuscular diseases, bracing is often withheld if the patient is ambulatory. When a body jacket is provided, an abdominal window is needed to allow respiratory excursion. Contoured or custom-molded seating systems that align and support the trunk are useful. These allow the child, adolescent, or adult to maintain an upright posture while seated, improving head control and hand function.

Procedures

There are no invasive physiatric procedures indicated for the treatment of scoliosis or kyphosis.

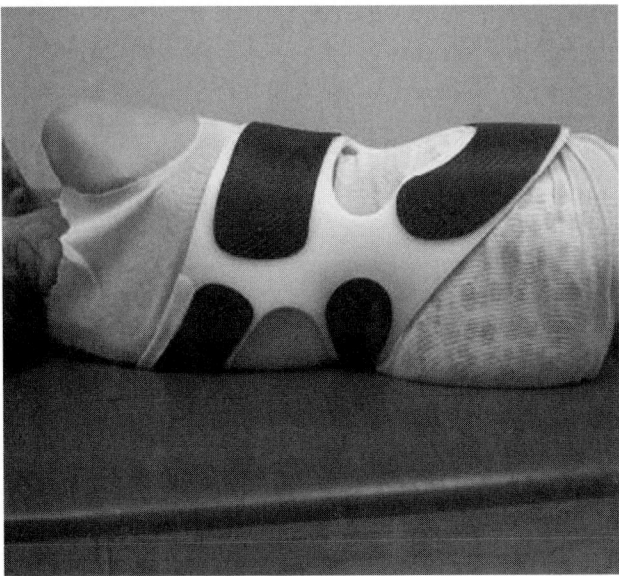

FIGURE 143-5. Providence nighttime brace. (From Scoliosis Research Society, Charles d'Amato, MD, and Barry McCoy, CPO, Providence, RI.)

Surgery

Surgical procedures attempt to restore spinal balance. The goal of surgery is to stabilize the spine through correction or control of the deformity. Improved cosmesis is a secondary goal. Restoration of lumbar lordosis is important.[31,32] Indications for surgical correction of scoliosis or kyphosis include progressive deformity, instability, progressive or new neurologic deficit, and cardiopulmonary compromise. Surgical stabilization of the spine for scoliosis associated with neuromuscular disease is performed earlier than for curves due to other causes. Pain, even when it is refractory to conservative management, is a controversial indication for surgery. Inability to use a brace and severe cosmetic deformity may be relative indications for surgery in specific instances.[6,15,33-36]

Scoliosis

Surgery addresses the coronal and rotational deformities by derotation and, less commonly, distraction. Any spinal instability is eliminated through compression or bone fusion.[36] Spine surgery may be complemented by rib resection in an attempt to improve appearance. The postoperative management of surgical patients varies according to the cause of the curve, age of the patient, and specifics of the surgery. Some patients may be placed in a cast or body jacket to immobilize the surgical segment until bone fusion occurs. Cotrel-Dubousset instrumentation and its various modifications that derotate the spine commonly do not require fusion, immobilization, or rib resection. Other surgical procedures, such as osteotomy and laminectomy, are done as appropriate.

Kyphosis

Various surgical approaches have been used, but anterior plus posterior instrumentation with fusion currently provides the highest success rate for lasting correction and pain relief.[6,37,38]

POTENTIAL DISEASE COMPLICATIONS

Complications of scoliosis or kyphosis result from the structural and degenerative changes that occur in the spine, along with secondary tightness or restriction due to soft tissue shortening. An increased incidence of spondylosis, facet arthropathy, spondylolisthesis, and spondylolysis is associated with large curves and correlates with the angle and rotation at the curve apex.[39-42] Such degenerative changes related to the curve are the most common causes of pain, but scoliosis can also produce discogenic pain.[43]

Foraminal, recess, or canal stenosis can occur with resulting neurologic compromise.[44,45] Root entrapment usually occurs on the concave side of the curve (rarely both convex and concave sides). Cauda equina compression has also been reported.[44] Lumbar spinal stenosis due to scoliosis can sometimes be differentiated from other types of stenosis because the disease and symptoms are more structural than positional. Patients often will not report relief of symptoms when sitting.[22]

Restrictive lung disease may occur as a complication of scoliotic curves exceeding 40 degrees or kyphosis in excess of 50 degrees, and cor pulmonale can complicate severe kyphosis or scoliotic curves in excess of 110 degrees.[39]

POTENTIAL TREATMENT COMPLICATIONS

Most treatment complications relate to surgery or bracing. Reported complications of bracing include skin breakdown, dermatitis due to an allergy to the orthotic material, hyperhidrosis, cutaneous infection, gastroesophageal reflux disease, esophagitis, and altered gastrointestinal motility. Psychosocial complications include low self-esteem, altered body image, and depression.[8]

Surgery may cause vascular or neurologic injury, pseudarthrosis, infection, graft donor site pain, progressive pelvic obliquity, painful degenerative changes in the segment adjacent to the level of fusion, instability, hardware prominence or failure, and thromboembolism.[31,37] Hardware complications include slippage of anchoring hooks, bending or fracture of a rod, wire pullout, and migration of the hardware. With instrumentation, there is a 10% to 29% incidence of reoperation.[46] Progression of the curve is possible despite surgical fixation. In the growing adolescent, the crankshaft phenomenon—progressive deformity resulting from continued growth of the anterior spine after posterior arthrodesis—may occur. This results in further loss of spinal balance but is usually not a problem. The patient with degenerative scoliosis who has undergone otherwise successful surgery may continue to experience pain or restricted mobility.

Exercise-related complications are less common but include overuse conditions of the soft tissues (tendinitis, bursitis, sprain, strain). Complications of nonsteroidal anti-inflammatory drug therapy are possible, particularly in the gastric, renal, and hepatic systems.

References

1. Asher MA, Burton DC. Adolescent idiopathic scoliosis: natural history and long term treatment effects. Scoliosis 2006;1:2.
2. Olgivie JW. Adult scoliosis: evaluation and nonsurgical treatment. Instr Course Lect 1992;41:251-255.
3. Miller NH, Justice CM, Marosy B, et al. Identification of candidate regions for familial idiopathic scoliosis. Spine 2005;30:1181-1187.
4. Lowe TG. Scheuermann's disease. J Bone Joint Surg Am 1990;72:940-945.
5. Tribus CB. Scheuermann's kyphosis in adolescents and adults: diagnosis and management. J Am Acad Orthop Surg 1998;6:36-43.
6. Esses SI. Textbook of Spinal Disorders. Philadelphia, JB Lippincott, 1995.
7. de Jonge T, Slullitel H, Dubousset J, et al. Late-onset spinal deformities in children treated by laminectomy and radiation therapy for malignant tumors. Eur Spine J 2005;14:765-771.
8. Sapountzi-Krepia D, Psychogiou M, Peterson D, et al. The experience of brace treatment in children/adolescents with scoliosis. Scoliosis 2006;1:8.
9. Kaplan PE, Segal V, Hughes R, et al. Neuropathy in thoracic scoliosis. Acta Orthop Scand 1980;52:263-266.
10. Gillingham BL, Fan RA, Akbarnia BA. Early onset idiopathic scoliosis. J Am Acad Orthop Surg 2006;14:102-112.
11. Sawark JF, Kramer A. Pediatric spinal deformity. Curr Opin Pediatr 1998;10:82-86.
12. Olgivie JW, Sherman J. Spondylolysis in Scheuermann's disease. Spine 1987;12:251-253.
13. Kann P, Schulz G, Schehler B, Beyer J. Backache and osteoporosis in perimenopausal women [in German]. Med Klin (Munich) 1993;88:9-15.
14. Papaiaonnou T, Stokes I, Kenwright J. Scoliosis associated with limb-length inequality. J Bone Joint Surg Am 1982;64:59-62.
15. Lonstein JE, Bradford DS, Winter RB, Olgivie JW. Moe's Textbook of Scoliosis and Other Spinal Deformities, 3rd ed. Philadelphia, WB Saunders, 1995.
16. Bradford DS. Kyphosis and postural roundback deformity in children and adolescents. Minn Med 1973;56:114-120.
17. Outland T. Juvenile dorsal kyphosis. Clin Orthop 1955;5:155.
18. Wassman K. Kyphosis juvenilis Scheuermann. Acta Orthop Scand 1951;21:65.
19. Ali RM, Green DW, Patel TC. Scheuermann's kyphosis. Curr Opin Pediatr 1999;11:70-75.
20. Sorenson KH. Scheuermann's Juvenile Kyphosis: Clinical Appearance, Radiography, Aetiology and Prognosis. Copenhagen, Munksgaard, 1964.
21. Bradford DS, Moe JH, Montalvo FJ. Scheuermann's kyphosis and roundback deformity. Results of Milwaukee brace treatment. J Bone Joint Surg Am 1974;56:740-758.
22. Grubb SA, Lipscomb HJ, Coonrad RW. Degenerative adult onset scoliosis. Spine 1988;13:241-245.
23. Schwab F, el-Fegoun AB, Gamez L, et al. A lumbar classification of scoliosis in the adult patient: preliminary approach. Spine 2005;30:1670-1673.
24. Kobayashi T, Atsuta Y, Takemitsu M, et al. A prospective study of de novo scoliosis in a community based cohort. Spine 2006;31:178-182.
25. Cheung J, Veldhuizen AG, Hallberts JP, et al. Geometric and electromyographic assessments in the evaluation of curve progression in idiopathic scoliosis. Spine 2006;31:322-329.
26. Routh RH, Rumancik S, Pathak RD, et al. The relationship between bone mineral density and biomechanics in patients with osteoporosis and scoliosis. Osteoporos Int 2005;16:1857-1863.
27. Weiss WR, Werkmann M, Stephan C. The ScoliOlogiC "Chênau light" brace—does the reduction of material affect the desired correction? Stud Health Technol Inform 2006;123:250-254.
28. Yrjonen T, Ylikoski M, Schlenzka D, Poussa M. Results of brace treatment of adolescent idiopathic scoliosis in boys compared to girls: a retrospective study of 102 patients treated with the Boston brace. Eur Spine J 2007;16:393-397. Epub 2006 Aug 15.
29. Yrjonen T, Ylikoski M, Schlenzka D, et al. Effectiveness of the Providence nighttime bracing in adolescent idiopathic scoliosis: a comparative study of 36 female patients. Eur Spine J 2006;15:1139-1143. Epub 2006 Jan 21.
30. Wenger DR, Frick SL. Scheuermann kyphosis. Spine 1999;24:2630-2638.
31. Manchesi DG, Aebi M. Pedicle fixation devices in the treatment of adult lumbar scoliosis. Spine 1992;17(Suppl):S304-S309.
32. Zurbriggen C, Markwalder TM, Wyss S. Long-term results in patients treated with posterior instrumentation and fusion for degenerative scoliosis of the lumbar spine. Acta Neurochir (Wien) 1999;141:21-26.
33. Lowe TG. Double L-rod instrumentation in the treatment of severe kyphosis secondary to Scheuermann's disease. Spine 1988;13:1099-1103.
34. Lowe TG. Scheuermann's disease. Orthop Clin North Am 1999;30:475-487.
35. Otsuka NY, Hall JE, Mah JU. Posterior fusion for Scheuermann kyphosis. Clin Orthop 1990;251:134-139.
36. Grubb SA, Lipscomb HJ, Suh PB. Results of surgical treatment of painful adult scoliosis. Spine 1994;19:1619-1627.
37. Bradford DS, Ahmed KB, Moe JH, et al. The surgical management of patients with Scheuermann's disease. J Bone Joint Surg Am 1980;62:705-712.
38. Herndon WA, Emans JB, Micheli LJ, Hall JE. Combined anterior and posterior fusion for Scheuermann's kyphosis. Spine 1981;6:125-130.
39. Kita N. Ultrastructural studies of articular cartilaginous degeneration in the facet joints of spinal scoliosis [in Japanese]. Nippon Seikeigeka Gakkai Zasshi 1994;68:184-195.
40. Richter DE, Nash CL Jr, Moskowitz RW, et al. Idiopathic adolescent scoliosis—a prototype of degenerative joint disease. The relation of biomechanic factors to osteophyte formation. Clin Orthop Relat Res 1985;193:221-229.
41. Hensiger RN, Green TL, Hunter L. Back pain and vertebral changes simulating Scheuermann's kyphosis. Spine 1982;5:341-342.
42. Tallroth K, Schlenzka D. Spinal stenosis subsequent to juvenile lumbar osteochondrosis. Skeletal Radiol 1990;19:203-205.
43. Grubb SA, Lipscomb HJ. Diagnostic findings in painful adult scoliosis. Spine 1992;17:518-527.
44. Benini A. Root compression in lumbar scoliosis—clinical picture and treatment based on 13 personal cases. Neurochirurgia (Stuttg) 1982;25:195-201.
45. Dick W. Surgical treatment of the degenerative lumbar spine in old age [in German]. Orthopade 1994;23:45-49.
46. Liljenqvist UR, Bullmann V, Schulte TL, et al. Anterior dual rod instrumentation in idiopathic thoracic scoliosis. Eur Spine J 2006;15:1118-1127. Epub 2006 Apr 12.

Spasticity **144**

Joel Stein, MD

DEFINITION

Spasticity is often defined as a velocity-dependent increase in muscle tone. This means that the faster the passive movement of the limb through its range, the greater the increase in muscle tone. The definition usually also includes clonus and flexor and extensor muscle spasms (involuntary sudden muscle contractions). Spasticity occurs in the context of an upper motor neuron lesion (brain or spinal cord disease) and in association with exaggerated deep tendon reflexes.

SYMPTOMS

The ability to move affected limbs actively or passively is reduced. Spasms may be a feature. Pain is present in some cases. Spasticity may be more evident during certain positions or activities (e.g., increased elbow flexor spasticity in a stroke survivor while walking; adductor spasticity in a paraplegic individual during urinary catheterization).

PHYSICAL EXAMINATION

Spasticity occurs in the presence of other signs and symptoms of upper motor neuron damage, including hyperreflexia, Babinski responses, reduced motor control, and other evidence of brain or spinal cord damage. Increased muscle tone in the absence of these findings should lead to consideration of alternative causes of increased muscle tone, such as dystonia, Parkinson disease, paratonia associated with Alzheimer disease, or pain-associated muscle spasm.

Contracture and spasticity frequently coexist, and it may be difficult in some cases to determine how much contracture is present in an individual with severe spasticity. The "clasp-knife" phenomenon, seen more commonly in spasticity of spinal origin, is characterized by a relaxation of the involved muscle after spasticity has been overcome. The presence and severity of ankle clonus, withdrawal reflexes, and extensor spasms should be noted. The skin should be inspected because abnormal positioning due to spasticity may directly cause skin injury (e.g., maceration of the palm due to a clenched fist) or contribute to decubitus ulcer formation.

FUNCTIONAL LIMITATIONS

Functional limitations include difficulty with ambulation or brace use, difficulty with positioning in a wheelchair, interrupted sleep, and difficulty with urinary catheterization or hygiene. Severe ankle inversion or ankle plantar flexor spasticity may interfere with the fit and function of a leg brace (e.g., ankle-foot orthosis). Spasms during transfers may affect functional independence for wheelchair users. Impaired sexual function may result from adductor muscle or other muscle spasms. In some cases, spasticity may interfere with volitional function; yet in others, it may serve as a partial substitute for voluntary muscle contraction. A common example of substitution for voluntary muscle function is the hip and knee extensor spasticity seen after stroke that may allow successful weight bearing through the weak leg and contribute to restoration of walking ability.

DIAGNOSTIC STUDIES

Spasticity is a clinical diagnosis, without any specific laboratory confirmation. Clinical measurement scales to quantify the severity of spasticity may be useful to monitor the efficacy of treatment. The most commonly used scales are the Ashworth scale (and a modified version of this scale),[1,2] which measures resistance of the muscle to passive stretch, and the Spasm Frequency scale, which characterizes the frequency of muscle spasms[3] (Tables 144-1 and 144-2).

849

TABLE 144-1 Modified Ashworth Scale[2]

0	No increase in muscle tone
1	Slight increase in muscle tone, manifested by a catch and release or by minimal resistance at the end range of motion when the part is moved in flexion or extension/abduction or adduction
1+	Slight increase in muscle tone, manifested by a catch, followed by minimal resistance throughout the remainder (less than half) of the range of motion
2	More marked increase in muscle tone through most of the range of motion, but the affected part is easily moved
3	Considerable increase in muscle tone, passive movement is difficult
4	Affected part is rigid in flexion or extension (abduction or adduction)

TABLE 144-2 Penn Spasm Frequency Scale[3]

How often are muscle spasms occurring?

0	No spasms
1	Spasms induced only by stimulation
2	Spasms occurring less than once per hour
3	Spasms occurring between 1 and 10 times per hour
4	Spasms occurring more than 10 times per hour

Differential Diagnosis

Dystonia

Rigidity (e.g., Parkinson disease)

Paratonia (as may be seen in Alzheimer disease)

Pain-associated muscle spasm

Contracture

TREATMENT

Initial

A change in previously well controlled spasticity should always lead to consideration of possible irritants or nociceptive stimuli that might be "triggering" the spasticity. Examples are urinary tract infections, skin breakdown, occult fractures, and an ingrown toenail in an insensate limb (e.g., in a paraplegic person).

Pharmacotherapy with oral medications (Table 144-3) is most effective in spasticity of spinal origin, as occurs in spinal cord injury or many cases of multiple sclerosis. Oral medications are often less effective in spasticity resulting from stroke or traumatic brain injury. Medications commonly used include baclofen, benzodiazepines,

tizanidine,[4,5] and dantrolene.[6] With the exception of dantrolene, these medications work centrally, at the GABA-A receptors (benzodiazepines), the GABA-B receptors (baclofen), or the α-adrenoreceptors (tizanidine). Dantrolene exerts its effects directly at the muscle, preventing calcium influx at the sarcoplasmic reticulum and thereby reducing muscle force.

Rehabilitation

Stretching and passive range of motion are key elements of spasticity management, regardless of cause. These activities serve to prevent contracture and temporarily to reduce increased muscle tone. Proper positioning can contribute to spasticity management and help prevent contracture. Ultrasound treatment has been used to facilitate stretching of contractures related to spasticity, although adequate clinical trials of efficacy have not been conducted. External cooling of a spastic limb may provide a temporary reduction in spasticity, but this modality is generally impractical as a long-term therapy.

Splinting is another critical aspect of a comprehensive rehabilitation program for spasticity and can include prefabricated splints, low-temperature thermoplastic custom splints, and plaster or fiberglass casts. Physical therapists can instruct the patient and caregivers in appropriate stretching techniques. Physical therapists with experience in casting can fabricate plaster or fiberglass casts or assist in selection of a prefabricated leg splint from a commercial vendor. If a sturdier device is needed (e.g., one that permits weight bearing through the device), an orthotist may be called on to fabricate a custom brace. Occupational therapists can similarly provide instruction in stretching and splinting of the upper extremity. Most occupational therapists are trained in fabrication of custom hand splints.

Procedures

Injections are an effective means of obtaining substantial reduction in spasticity in specific muscles with little risk of systemic side effects. Local anesthetic injections may be useful to assess the efficacy and benefits of more permanent injections. Intramuscular injection of botulinum toxin type A (Botox) provides local relief of spasticity for 3 to 4 months.[7,8] Therapeutic effects for spasticity may be seen in smaller muscles with doses of 10 to 25 units; larger muscles may require 200 units or more. For systemic toxicity to be avoided, total doses of botulinum toxin type A are generally limited to 6 units/kg; injection may be repeated every 3 months. Botulinum toxin type B (Myobloc) is probably effective as well, although it has not been studied as extensively.[9-11] The use of botulinum toxin type B for patients who have developed resistance to type A has yielded mixed results.[12] Perineural phenol injection may provide longer relief and may in some cases cause permanent reduction of spasticity.[13] Phenol doses are limited to 20 mL of a 5% aqueous solution during any single session; the rapid elimination of phenol from the body allows a subsequent injection within several days if it is needed.

TABLE 144-3 Commonly Used Oral Antispasticity Medications

Medication	Starting Dose	Maximum Dose	Common Side Effects	Relative Contraindications
Baclofen	5-10 mg tid	20 mg qid*	Sedation, rare hepatotoxicity	Cognitive impairment
Diazepam (other benzodiazepines have similar effects)	2 mg bid	10 mg qid	Sedation	History of benzodiazepine or other substance abuse
Tizanidine	2 mg tid	12 mg tid	Sedation, hypotension, hepatotoxicity	Cognitive impairment
Dantrolene	25 mg daily	100 mg qid	Weakness, hepatotoxicity, occasional sedation	Liver disease

*Approved by the U.S. Food and Drug Administration only up to 80 mg/day, but many clinicians exceed this in patients who tolerate this medication well but do not respond to smaller doses.

Surgery

Neurosurgical intervention involves the placement of an intrathecal baclofen pump, a highly effective treatment for individuals with intractable spasticity from spinal cord injury, multiple sclerosis, traumatic brain injury, or cerebral palsy.[14-16] Intrathecal baclofen therapy has also been shown to reduce spasticity and to increase gait velocity in hemiplegic stroke,[17,18] but its use remains less common for this condition.

Alternative neurosurgical procedures useful in carefully selected patients are rhizotomy and myelotomy. Orthopedic surgery including tendon lengthening, tenotomy, and joint fusion can be performed after failure of more conservative measures (e.g., stretching, casting, blocks) to provide adequate control of spasticity and contracture.

POTENTIAL DISEASE COMPLICATIONS

Permanent loss of range of motion can result from inadequately controlled spasticity or insufficient stretching and splinting. Contractures can hinder seating, contribute to skin breakdown, and interfere with hygiene, ambulation, and transfers. Spasticity can occasionally interfere with the expression of underlying motor control,[19] although the overall prevalence of this phenomenon remains unknown. The concern that spasticity might interfere with the restoration of motor control after stroke or other central nervous system injury remains unproven at this time.

POTENTIAL TREATMENT COMPLICATIONS

All of the centrally acting medications can cause significant sedation, which often determines the upper limit of the dose that can be tolerated. In individuals with preexisting cognitive impairments (e.g., stroke, traumatic brain injury), this maximally tolerated dose may be insufficient to control the symptoms of spasticity, and alternative therapies need to be considered.

In individuals with marginal motor function who may be relying in part on spasticity as a substitution for voluntary motor control, excessive reduction in spasticity may lead to reduced functional ability (e.g., loss of the ability to stand in a patient with paraparesis). Oral medication or intrathecal baclofen doses can generally be titrated to avoid this side effect; however, injected treatments (botulinum toxin, phenol) are more problematic if overtreatment occurs.

Abrupt discontinuation of oral antispasticity medications is inadvisable. Seizures have been described after abrupt discontinuation of baclofen, and rebound spasticity is a concern with all of these medications.

Phenol poses some risk of painful dysesthesia if peripheral nerves with cutaneous sensory representation are injected. Botulinum toxin is generally well tolerated in therapeutic doses, but transient (3 to 4 months) weakness of muscles adjacent to those targeted in treatment can be caused by diffusion of toxin. Dysphagia has been described after injection of the sternocleidomastoid and other cervical muscles. Injection of excessive doses of botulinum toxin could lead to symptoms of systemic botulism; this can be avoided by restricting injection to 6 units/kg of botulinum toxin type A or less within any 1-month period. Antibodies to botulinum toxin can develop after repeated injection, which can render treatment ineffective, although allergic or anaphylactic reactions have not been reported.

Intrathecal baclofen pump treatment can result in iatrogenic meningitis or infection of the external surface of the pump. Catheter failures can result in need for surgical intervention. Both overdosage due to programming errors and severe withdrawal symptoms due to pump failure have been described.[20]

References

1. Ashworth B. Preliminary trial of carisoprodol in multiple sclerosis. Practitioner 1964;192:540-542.
2. Bohannon RW, Smith MB. Interrater reliability of a modified Ashworth scale of muscle spasticity. Phys Ther 1986;67:206-207.
3. Penn RD, Savoy SM, Corcos D, et al. Intrathecal baclofen for severe spinal spasticity. N Engl J Med 1989;320:1517-1554.
4. Nance PW, Bugaresti J, Shellenberger K, et al. Efficacy and safety of tizanidine in the treatment of spasticity in patients with spinal cord injury. North American Tizanidine Study Group. Neurology 1994;44:S44-S45.

5. Smith C, Birnbaum G, Carter JL, et al. Tizanidine treatment of spasticity caused by multiple sclerosis: results of a double-blind, placebo-controlled trial. US Tizanidine Study Group. Neurology 1994;44:S34-S42.

6. Kita M, Goodkin DE. Drugs used to treat spasticity. Drugs 2000;59:487-495.

7. Simpson DM, Alexander DN, O'Brien CF, et al. Botulinum toxin type A in the treatment of upper extremity spasticity: a randomized, double-blind, placebo-controlled study. Neurology 1996;46:1306-1310.

8. Brashear A, Gordon MF, Elovic E, et al; Botox Post-Stroke Spasticity Study Group. Intramuscular injection of botulinum toxin for the treatment of wrist and finger spasticity after a stroke. N Engl J Med 2002;347:395-400.

9. Brashear A, McAfee AL, Kuhn ER, Ambrosius WT. Treatment with botulinum toxin type B for upper-limb spasticity. Arch Phys Med Rehabil 2003;84:103-107.

10. Brashear A, McAfee AL, Kuhn ER, Fyffe J. Botulinum toxin type B in upper-limb poststroke spasticity: a double-blind, placebo-controlled trial. Arch Phys Med Rehabil 2004;85:705-709.

11. Schwerin A, Berweck S, Fietzek UM, Heinen F. Botulinum toxin B treatment in children with spastic movement disorders: a pilot study. Pediatr Neurol 2004;31:109-113.

12. Barnes MP, Best D, Kidd L, et al. The use of botulinum toxin type-B in the treatment of patients who have become unresponsive to botulinum toxin type-A—initial experiences. Eur J Neurol 2005;12:947-955.

13. Glenn MB, Whyte J. The Practical Management of Spasticity in Children and Adults. Philadelphia, Lea & Febiger, 1990.

14. Van Schaeybroeck P, Nuttin B, Lagae L, et al. Intrathecal baclofen for intractable cerebral spasticity: a prospective placebo-controlled, double-blind study. Neurosurgery 2000;46:603-609.

15. Meythaler JM, Guin-Renfroe S, Grabb P, Hadley MN. Long-term continuously infused intrathecal baclofen for spastic-dystonic hypertonia in traumatic brain injury: 1-year experience. Arch Phys Med Rehabil 1999;80:13-19.

16. Francisco GE, Hu MM, Boake C, Ivanhoe CB. Efficacy of early use of intrathecal baclofen therapy for treating spastic hypertonia due to acquired brain injury. Brain Inj 2005;19:359-364.

17. Meythaler JM, Guin-Renfroe S, Brunner RC, Hadley MN. Intrathecal baclofen for spastic hypertonia from stroke. Stroke 2001;32:2099-2109.

18. Francisco GE, Boake C. Improvement in walking speed in post-stroke spastic hemiplegia after intrathecal baclofen therapy: a preliminary study. Arch Phys Med Rehabil 2003;84:1194-1199.

19. Cairns K, Stein J. Motor function improvement following intrathecal baclofen pump placement in a patient with locked-in syndrome. Am J Phys Med Rehabil 2002;81:307-309.

20. Reeves RK, Stolp-Smith KA, Christopherson MW. Hyperthermia, rhabdomyolysis, and disseminated intravascular coagulation associated with baclofen pump catheter failure. Arch Phys Med Rehabil 1998;79:353-356.

Speech and Language Disorders 145

Jason H. Kortte, MS, CCC-SLP, and Jeffrey B. Palmer, MD

Synonyms

Aphasia
Dysphasia
Dysarthria
Slurred speech
Dysphonia
Voice disturbance
Change in voice
Hoarseness
Hypernasality
Hyponasality

ICD-9 Codes

438.81   Apraxia
784.3   Aphasia
784.49   Dysphonia
784.5   Dysarthria

DEFINITIONS

Aphasia is a language processing disturbance that can involve the expression of language, the comprehension of language, or both. In acute stroke patients, aphasia is present in 21% to 38% of cases and is associated with high morbidity, mortality, and financial cost.[1] Aphasia is classified into specific syndromes according to the ability to produce, to understand, and to repeat language.[2] The ability to produce language is assessed in terms of fluency, which is defined as the rate of speech and the amount of effort in producing speech. Each syndrome of aphasia is associated with a particular set of language capabilities and disabilities. For example, an individual with Wernicke aphasia produces fluent language, has impaired auditory comprehension, and has poor repetition skills. In contrast, Broca aphasia is characterized by nonfluent language, relatively intact auditory comprehension, and poor repetition skills. Aphasia can be manifested in other modalities of language as well (e.g., reading, writing, and gestures). An overview of aphasia syndromes is presented in Table 145-1.

Apraxia of speech is a motor speech disorder that disrupts the motor programming of the volitional movements for speech.[3] Apraxia of speech is characterized by difficulties in orchestrating the movements of the lips, tongue, jaw, soft palate, vocal cords, and respiratory system for the production of speech. It can occur without muscle weakness or impairments in receptive and expressive language. Even though symptoms associated with apraxia of speech often occur with aphasia and dysarthria, apraxia of speech is a distinct motor speech disorder.[4]

Dysarthria is a group of motor speech disorders resulting from damage to the central or peripheral nervous system. Dysarthria is prevalent in 10% to 65% of cases of acquired brain injury, depending on type and extent of injury and time after onset.[5] Motor speech disorders may result from weakness, paralysis, or uncoordinated actions of the speech muscles and can impair articulation, respiration, resonance, and phonation (voice production). Dysarthria can be subdivided into different types according to the speech characteristics and underlying pathophysiologic process.[3] Dysarthria may be due to structural abnormalities, such as those found in cleft palate and after ablative surgery. The extreme form of dysarthria is anarthria, in which the individual is entirely incapable of producing articulated speech. Individuals with dysarthria often have dysphagia, or impaired swallowing, regardless of the primary cause and time elapsed since the onset.[6]

Dysphonia is a term used to describe faulty or abnormal phonation (voice production). Although prevalence rates are not well established, dysphonia is commonly associated with neurogenic motor disturbances (resulting in paresis, paralysis, or incoordination of the vocal cords) found in brainstem stroke, Parkinson disease, amyotrophic lateral sclerosis, Guillain-Barré syndrome, myasthenia gravis, and multiple sclerosis, among others.[3] A variety of secondary processes may alter the structure or function of the vocal cords, including vocal abusive behaviors (excessive talking, screaming, smoking), trauma (endotracheal or nasogastric intubation), surgery for laryngeal structures, and diseases (laryngeal cancer, reflux laryngitis).[7] Dysphonia is distinguished from dysarthria in that dysphonia involves only the sound of the voice,

TABLE 145-1 Aphasia Syndromes

Type of Aphasia	Speech	Comprehension	Repetition
Broca	Nonfluent	Intact	Poor
Wernicke	Fluent	Poor	Poor
Conduction	Fluent	Intact	Poor
Transcortical motor	Nonfluent	Intact	Intact
Transcortical sensory	Fluent	Poor	Intact
Anomic	Fluent	Intact	Intact

Modified from Damasio AR, Damasio H. Aphasia and the neuro basis of language. In Mesulam M, ed. Principles of Behavioral and Cognitive Neurology, 2nd ed. New York, Oxford University Press, 2000:294-315.

whereas dysarthria involves the overall sound of speech, including resonance and articulation.

Table 145-2 summarizes the speech and language disorders described in this chapter.

SYMPTOMS

Individuals with aphasia often complain of difficulty in speaking, reading, writing, or understanding speech. They often report difficulty in finding the word they wish to say and can become frustrated. Some aphasic individuals, however, are unaware of their deficits. People with motor speech disorders (e.g., dysarthria, dysphonia, and apraxia of speech) have no difficulty finding the words they wish to say but complain of difficulty in making their speech intelligible. These individuals report no

TABLE 145-2 Speech and Language Disorders

Disorder	Definition
Aphasia	Language processing disturbance that can involve the expression of language, the comprehension of language, or both Word finding errors and difficulty in understanding language are classic indicators of aphasia.
Dysarthria	Group of motor speech disorders associated with muscle paralysis, weakness, or incoordination Dysarthria often presents as slurred speech and does *not* involve language (receptive or expressive) processes.
Apraxia of speech	Motor speech disorder disrupting the motor programming of the volitional movements for speech Individuals struggle to find correct position of articulators (i.e., lips, tongue). It can occur without muscle weakness or impairments in receptive and expressive language.
Dysphonia	Faulty or abnormal phonation (voice production) Vocal quality may sound hoarse, harsh, strained, or breathy.

difficulties with reading, writing, or auditory comprehension. Patients with right hemispheric strokes may experience diverse right hemisphere syndromes, including abnormal visual-spatial perception, hemispatial neglect, memory loss, and disorders of prosody (the rhythm, rate, and inflection of speech).[8]

PHYSICAL EXAMINATION

During the initial interaction with the patient, it is important to attend to the patient's speech intelligibility, vocal quality, language fluency and content, and comprehension. Deficits in these areas may warrant a referral to a speech-language pathologist for comprehensive evaluation by standardized testing. In the rehabilitation setting, the Functional Independence Measure is a widely accepted scale used to measure functional abilities including communication.[9] Typical findings are described here for the four main categories of speech and language disorders.

Aphasia

Findings indicative of aphasia from the speech-language examination may vary greatly, depending on the location and size of the lesion in the brain (see Table 145-1). One classic sign of aphasia is difficulty in comprehending language (spoken, gestural, or written). Significant impairment can be characterized by difficulty in following simple commands, whereas milder impairments may be obvious only during lengthy or complicated messages. Individuals who are aphasic may also have deficits in verbal expression (producing meaningful speech), which may be manifested as a total loss of language, with the production of only jargon (multiple whole-word substitutions) or meaningless sounds. A person with less severe aphasia may be able to express basic wants and needs but have difficulty expressing complex ideas in conversation. The extent of impairment can vary for each modality of language and involve listening, reading, writing, recognition of numbers, and gesturing. Aphasia is *not* a result of decreased auditory or visual perceptual skills, disordered thought processes, impaired motor programming, or weakness or incoordination of speech musculature.[1]

Apraxia of Speech

The most common sign of apraxia of speech is a struggle to speak. This struggle is a direct result of the individual's having difficulty in finding the correct position of his or her articulators (i.e., lips, tongue). Speech is often halting and may contain sound substitutions, distortions, omissions, additions, and repetitions.[3] The individual is aware of his or her speech errors and will attempt to correct them with varying degrees of success. Severe forms of apraxia of speech may result in the inability to produce simple words. Interestingly, most people with apraxia of speech can produce common everyday phrases or sayings (e.g., *How are you? Have a nice day.* and *Thank you.*) without error. A symptom that commonly coincides with apraxia of speech is nonverbal oral apraxia, which is the inability to imitate or to follow commands to perform volitional movements with the mouth or tongue.[3] Apraxia of speech is not caused by muscle weakness, decreased tone, or incoordination, nor is it the result of linguistic disturbances as in aphasia. Sound level errors in apraxia of speech are thought to be a result of difficulty with motor execution and not with the selection of phonemes found in aphasia.[4] It differs from dysarthria in that apraxia of speech is not a result of paresis or paralysis or the uncoordinated movements of speech muscles. Rather, it is believed to reflect a disturbance in the programming of movements used for speech.[4] Errors heard in apraxia of speech are highly irregular; dysarthric errors are typically consistent and predictable.

Dysarthria

In dysarthria, speech is often characterized as being slurred; the predominant errors are distortions of speech sounds. Dysarthria may also be characterized by changes in a person's rate, volume, and rhythm of speech. Depending on the pathophysiologic process, the findings will vary greatly. Table 145-3 presents an overview of dysarthria classification.

Dysphonia

Dysphonia is characterized by a reduction or alteration in voice quality. Vocal quality may vary by degrees of loudness, breathiness, hoarseness, or harshness. A common example of dysphonia is the hoarse vocal quality of individuals with laryngitis. In the extreme form, aphonia, the individual is incapable of producing any voice but may be able to produce voiceless speech (e.g., whispering).

FUNCTIONAL LIMITATIONS

Functional limitations depend on the nature and severity of the communication impairment. Severe deficits may impair the person's ability to express daily wants and needs or to understand simple directions. He or she may not be able to effectively interact with family members or health care workers. Less severe deficits may allow the individual to express and to understand basic information but impair higher level activities. These may include the expression and understanding of complex and lengthy information to meet the person's vocational or social needs. Speech and language impairments may affect the individual's ability to read bills or newspapers and environmental signs, to use the telephone, to participate in conversations, to attend school, or to obtain employment. Speech and language impairments may result in frustration and can cause disruptions in personal relationships, community and religious participation, and vocational functioning.

DIAGNOSTIC STUDIES

A variety of standardized instruments can be administered by the speech-language pathologist or a neuropsychologist to diagnose aphasia. The aim of these instruments is to identify the pattern of symptoms to classify the aphasic syndrome, which is critical for the development of individualized interventions. Similarly, there are structured assessments for diagnosis of dysphonia, apraxia, and dysarthria. These in-depth assessments involve an oral-motor examination to identify the structure and function of oral musculature as well as the patient's speech characteristics (i.e., rate, volume, intelligibility). For determination of the etiology and pathophysiology of dysphonia, a referral to an otolaryngologist is warranted. Laryngoscopy may be necessary to evaluate both the structure and the function of the larynx. Biopsy is often indicated when mass lesions are seen. Stroboscopic examination of the larynx may reveal subtle abnormalities of the vocal fold motion. The voice spectrogram is sometimes useful for assessment of vocal features quantitatively.

TREATMENT

Initial

Treatment of speech and language disorders usually requires referral to a speech-language pathologist. Initial treatment depends on the nature and severity of the disorder. The treatment plans for aphasia, apraxia of speech, dysarthria, and dysphonia not only vary greatly for each disorder but also need to be individualized to meet the patient's communication needs. Initial intervention may include education of the patient and family about the communication impairment and effective compensatory strategies to facilitate communication.

TABLE 145-3 Classification of Dysarthria

Type	Localization	Motor Deficit
Flaccid	Lower motor neuron	Weakness, hypotonia
Spastic	Bilateral upper motor neuron	Spasticity
Ataxia	Cerebellum	Incoordination; inaccurate range, timing, direction; slow rate
Hypokinetic	Extrapyramidal system (basal ganglia circuit)	Variable speed of repetitive movements, rigidity
Hyperkinetic	Extrapyramidal system	Involuntary movements
Mixed	Multiple motor systems (amyotrophic lateral sclerosis, multiple sclerosis)	Weakness, reduced rate and range of motion

Modified from Duffy JR. Motor Speech Disorders: Substrates, Differential Diagnosis, and Management. St. Louis, Mosby, 1995.

Differential Diagnosis

Aphasia
Confusion, delirium

Schizophrenia

Apraxia of speech

Dysarthria

Neurogenic stuttering

Echolalia

Palilalia

Selective mutism

Depression

Apraxia of Speech
Dysarthria

Aphasia

Neurogenic stuttering

Dysarthria
Apraxia of speech

Aphasia

Depression

Abulia

Dysphonia
Acute and chronic laryngitis

Laryngeal hyperfunction (abuse and misuse)

Neurogenic disorders

Psychogenic disorders (i.e., conversion dysphonia)

Spasmodic dysphonia

Structural disorders of the larynx (congenital, traumatic, arthritic, neoplastic)

Rehabilitation

To maximize a patient's communication skills, a speech-language pathologist can offer specific strategies, exercises, and activities to regain functional communication abilities.

Aphasia

Intervention and activities involved in speech-language pathologist services in the stroke population have been well documented.[10] Intervention is largely based on the specific aphasia syndrome diagnosed. Common therapeutic activities may involve naming tasks that use hierarchical cueing techniques to improve language content and structure. Therapy may begin with having the client produce automatic speech, such as stating numbers or the days of the week. More difficult tasks may involve the individual's naming of objects and describing pictures. Written expression may be targeted through functional activities such as writing and copying biographical information. Common activities to improve auditory comprehension involve following simple or complex commands and answering spoken questions correctly. Therapy to improve reading comprehension may involve the client's matching objects to written words, following written directions, or reading functional information (bills, medication labels, environmental signs). Activities that involve problem solving and executive functioning skills were shown to have a positive effect on verbal expression and auditory comprehension.[11] Furthermore, collaboration between the speech-language pathologist and other skilled services, such as occupational therapy, can improve the patient's daily living skills.

The treatment plan for aphasia also includes education. It is important to teach the patient, family, and health care workers compensatory strategies to improve communication skills. Environmental modification and partner-facilitated approaches can dramatically improve communication success.[12-14] These can include turning off the television to reduce distractions, speaking slowly, using simple language, offering pen and paper, checking that you are understood, and paraphrasing. Volunteers can be trained in use of partner-facilitated techniques. Training of volunteers as conversation partners by the Supported Conversation for Adults with Aphasia intervention has been shown to be effective.[15]

Advances in computer technology have provided therapists with effective options in treating aphasia. Computer programs allow clinicians to easily design activities, to select stimulus items, to present cues, and to individualize reinforcements.[16] Software programs also can be used to turn a computer into a speech output communication device, allowing people with severe aphasia to produce phrases and sentences of varying degrees of complexity.[17]

Dysarthria

Rehabilitation for dysarthria also depends on the specific type diagnosed. Approaches to treatment include medical intervention, oral prosthetic devices, and behavioral management.[3] For example, dysarthric individuals with Parkinson disease may benefit from dopamine agonists. Palatal lifts and voice amplifiers are common prosthetics used to improve intelligibility. There has been reported success in improving speech intelligibility in a stroke patient with velopharyngeal incompetence by providing a palatal lift and augmentation prosthesis in conjunction with behavioral management by the speech-language pathologist.[18] Behavioral management of dysarthria involves muscle strengthening (e.g., lip closure, tongue protrusion, tongue elevation), improvement of breath support, and modification of posture. The individual is trained to use compensatory techniques to decrease rate of speech and to "overarticulate." As with aphasia, the family is educated in strategies to maximize communication. Treatment of severe expressive dysarthria or aphasia may include the development of an augmentative communication system in which the individual uses pictures, written words, or alphabet or pictograph boards to communicate wants and needs. Some individuals can be trained to use high-tech computerized systems that produce synthesized speech. These computer-based systems can offer the individual a wider variety of communication topics and can be personalized to the individual's needs.

Apraxia of Speech

Treatment of apraxia of speech involves techniques to elicit accurate voluntary speech production. The speech-language therapist incorporates multimodality cues, such as modeling mouth and lip movements, using verbal cues to describe accurate tongue and lip placement, and intoning words and sentences. Treatment approaches often incorporate the use of rate and rhythm control strategies.[4] For severe cases, alternative communication strategies, such as writing, drawing, and communication books, are used to augment or to replace speech.

Dysphonia

Management of dysphonia is based on the underlying disorder and the pathophysiologic process. Vocal hygiene education and proper voicing techniques can improve vocal quality for individuals with vocal nodules due to laryngeal hyperfunction (vocal abuse). Techniques to achieve firmer vocal fold approximation are useful in individuals with decreased vocal cord movement due to paresis. Laryngitis due to gastroesophageal reflux disease is treated with a vigorous antireflux regimen including proton pump inhibitors.

Procedures

Injection of a paralyzed vocal cord with Gelfoam or Teflon is sometimes performed to increase mass to bring the medial edge of the cord closer to the midline. This permits the mobile contralateral vocal cord to contact it, thereby improving phonation. This solution is usually only temporary, however. For cases of spasmodic dysphonia, an injection of botulinum toxin into the affected muscles can result in improved voice by correction of the motion impairment of the vocal folds.[19]

Surgery

Surgery is sometimes needed for treatment of voice disorders. Individuals with mass lesions of the larynx may need surgical excision. For individuals with unilateral vocal cord paralysis, there are several surgical procedures designed to bring the paralyzed cord closer to midline to achieve appropriate glottal closure. Implantation of a small device into the paralyzed hemilarynx, pushing the paralyzed cord toward the midline, can provide a lasting improvement in voice quality. Surgical treatment of other speech and language disorders depends entirely on the cause of the underlying disease process.

Structural lesions (e.g., cleft palate) or functional disorders (e.g., weakness of the palatal elevators) may cause inadequate seal of the velopharyngeal isthmus (the space between the soft palate and the pharyngeal walls). In either case, a surgical procedure can sometimes provide improved speech quality by narrowing or closing the defect.

POTENTIAL DISEASE COMPLICATIONS

Individuals with severe speech and language disorders may suffer extreme psychosocial consequences, including isolation, unemployment, depression,[20] alienation, ostracism, and inability to fulfill essential family roles. Aphasia has been shown to be a risk factor for disability after stroke and plays a significant role in quality of life issues.[21]

POTENTIAL TREATMENT COMPLICATIONS

Injection or surgical implant of the larynx may result in complications including infection, hemorrhage, and local tissue trauma. Injected material may gradually slip out of place and lose effectiveness, but this rarely leads to serious sequelae. Botulinum toxin injection rarely causes airway obstruction if the vocal folds become immobilized in the medial position. Leakage of the toxin into adjacent muscles may worsen the voice disorder or produce dysphagia.

References

1. Berthier ML. Poststroke aphasia: epidemiology, pathophysiology and treatment. Drugs Aging 2005;22:163-182.
2. Damasio AR, Damasio H. Aphasia and the neuro basis of language. In Mesulam M, ed. Principles of Behavioral and Cognitive Neurology, 2nd ed. New York, Oxford University Press, 2000:294-315.
3. Duffy JR. Motor Speech Disorders: Substrates, Differential Diagnosis, and Management. St. Louis, Mosby, 1995.
4. Ogar J, Slama H, Dronkers N, et al. Apraxia of speech: an overview. Neurocase 2005;11:427-432.
5. Wang YT, Kent RD, Duffy JR, Thomas JE. Dysarthria associated with traumatic brain injury: speaking rate and emphatic stress. J Commun Dis 2005;38:231-260.
6. Nishio M, Niimi S. Relationship between speech and swallowing disorders in patients with neuromuscular disease. Folia Phoniatr Logop 2004;56:291-304.
7. Prater RJ, Swift RW. Manual of Voice Therapy. Austin, Texas, Pro-Ed, 1984.
8. Jordan LC, Hillis AE. Aphasia and right hemisphere syndromes in stroke. Curr Neurol Neurosci Rep 2005;5:458-464.
9. Linacre JM, Heinemann AW, Wright BD, et al. The structure and stability of the Functional Independence Measure. Arch Phys Med Rehabil 1994;75:127-132.
10. Hillis AE. Cognitive neuropsychological approaches to rehabilitation of language disorders: introduction. In Chapey R, ed. Language Intervention Strategies in Aphasia and Related Neurogenic Communication Disorders, 4th ed. Baltimore, Lippincott Williams & Wilkins, 2001:513-523.
11. Hatfield B, Millet D, Coles J, et al. Characterizing speech and language pathology outcomes in stroke rehabilitation. Arch Phys Med Rehabil 2005;86:S61-S72.
12. Lubinski R. Environmental considerations for elderly patients. In Lubinski R, ed. Dementia and Communication. Philadelphia, BC Decker, 1991.

13. Lubinski R, Welland RJ. Normal aging and environmental effects on communication. Semin Speech Lang 1997;18:107-125.

14. Hengst JA, Frame SR, Neuman-Stritzel T, et al. Using others' words: conversational use of reported speech by individuals with aphasia and their communication partners. J Speech Lang Hear Res 2005;48:137-156.

15. Kagan A, Black SE, Duchan FJ, et al. Training volunteers as conversational partners using "Supported Conversation for Adults with Aphasia" (SCA): a controlled trial. J Speech Lang Hear Res 2001;44:624-638.

16. Katz RC, Hallowell B. Technological applications in the treatment of acquired neurogenic communication and swallowing disorders in adults. Semin Speech Lang 1999;20:251-268.

17. Koul R, Corwin M, Hayes S. Production of graphic symbol sentences by individuals with aphasia: efficacy of a computer-based augmentative and alternative communication intervention. Brain Lang 2005;92:58-77.

18. Ono T, Hamamura M, Honda K, Nokubi T. Collaboration of a dentist and speech-language pathologist in the rehabilitation of a stroke patient with dysarthria: a case study. Gerodontology 2005;22:116-119.

19. Blitzer A, Brin MF, Fahn S, et al. Localized injections of botulinum toxin for the treatment of focal laryngeal dystonia (spastic dysphonia). Laryngoscope 1988;98:193-197.

20. Kauhenen M, Korpelainen J, Hiltunen P, et al. Post stroke depression correlates with cognitive impairment and neurological deficits. Stroke 1999;30:1875-1880.

21. Flick CL. Stroke rehabilitation: stroke outcome and psychosocial consequences. Arch Phys Med Rehabil 1999;80:S21-S26.

Spinal Cord Injury (Cervical) 146

Sunil Sabharwal, MD

Synonyms

Tetraplegia
Quadriplegia

ICD-9 Codes

344.00 Quadriplegia, unspecified
344.01 C1-4, complete
344.02 C1-4, incomplete
344.03 C5-7, complete
344.04 C5-7, incomplete
344.09 Other

DEFINITION

Cervical spinal cord injury (SCI) results in tetraplegia. The term *tetraplegia* (preferred to quadriplegia) refers to an impairment or loss of motor or sensory function in the cervical segments of the spinal cord due to damage of neural elements within the spinal canal.[1] The result is impairment of function in the arms as well as in the trunk, legs, and pelvic organs. Impairment of sensorimotor involvement outside the spinal canal, such as brachial plexus lesions or injury to peripheral nerves, should not be referred to as tetraplegia.

In a complete SCI, sensory or motor function is absent in the lowest sacral segments S4-5 (i.e., no anal sensation or voluntary anal contraction is present). If sensory or motor function is partially preserved below the neurologic level and includes the lowest sacral segments, the injury is defined as incomplete.[1,2] The American Spinal Injury Association (ASIA) Impairment Scale is used in grading the degree of impairment (Table 146-1). Central cord syndrome is an incomplete SCI syndrome that applies almost exclusively to cervical SCI. It is characterized by greater weakness in the upper limbs than in the lower limbs and sacral sensory sparing.[1]

SCI primarily affects young men. However, the average age at injury has increased from 28.7 years in the 1970s to 38.0 years since 2000, and the prevalence of SCI in adults older than 60 years has increased from 4.7% to 11.5% in the same time period in the National Model Spinal Cord Injury Systems database.[3] Males account for about 80% of injuries. The most common cause is motor vehicle accidents, followed by falls, violence, and recreational sporting activities.[2,3] The proportion of injuries due to falls has increased over time. Cervical injuries occur more frequently than thoracic and lumbar injuries; cervical injuries accounted for 56.5% of the SCI database between 2000 and 2003. Since 2000, the most frequent neurologic category at discharge reported to the database is incomplete tetraplegia (34.1% of all SCI).

SYMPTOMS

Primary symptoms of cervical SCI are related to muscle paralysis, sensory impairment, and autonomic impairment (including bladder, bowel, and sexual dysfunction). The patient can present in the outpatient setting with a multitude of secondary conditions[4] and associated problems. Symptoms may be vague and nonspecific. For example, urinary tract infections may be manifested not with classic symptoms of urgency and dysuria but with increased spasticity, increased frequency of spontaneous voiding, and lethargy.[5] The patient with pneumonia may present with fever, shortness of breath, or increasing anxiety. Headache may be indicative of autonomic dysreflexia and may be the primary or only presentation of a variety of pathologic processes ranging from bladder distention, urinary infection, constipation, or ingrown toenail to myocardial infarction or acute abdominal emergencies.[6] Table 146-2 lists common presenting symptoms and underlying causes.

Because symptoms can reflect a variety of underlying conditions, these need to be evaluated carefully. For example, pain in cervical SCI may be multifactorial and needs to be further assessed by characteristics reported in the history, including quality, location, onset, timing, relieving and exacerbating factors, and associated symptoms. Various SCI pain classification systems have been described. In the Bryce-Ragnarsson classification (Table 146-3), the pain is first regionally localized relative to the level of SCI, that is, above level, at level, or

TABLE 146-1 American Spinal Injury Association (ASIA) Impairment Scale

Grade	Category	Description
A	Complete	No sensory or motor function is preserved in the sacral segments S4-5.
B	Sensory incomplete	Sensory but no motor function is preserved below the neurologic level including the sacral segments S4-5.
C	Motor incomplete*	Motor function is preserved below the neurologic level, and more than half of key muscles below the neurologic level have a muscle grade less than 3.
D	Motor incomplete*	Motor function is preserved below the neurologic level, and at least half of key muscles below the neurologic level have a muscle grade 3 or more.
E	Normal	Sensory function and motor function are normal; the patient may have abnormalities in reflex examination.

*There must be some sparing of sensory or motor function in S4-5 segments to be classified as motor incomplete.

below level. In the second tier of the classification, pain is identified as nociceptive or neuropathic, and then it is further stratified into subtypes of the regionally localized nociceptive or neuropathic pain types.[7]

PHYSICAL EXAMINATION

The neurologic examination is conducted by systematic examination of the dermatomes and myotomes (Tables 146-4 and 146-5) in accordance with *International Standards for Neurological and Functional Classification of Spinal Cord Injury* published by ASIA.[1]

Depending on the presentation, specific elements of the physical examination of various body systems that are relevant in evaluation of SCI-related conditions may include the following.

Neurologic

- Determine the level and completeness of the injury (Fig. 146-1). Conduct the examination in the supine position.
  - Sensory examination for pinprick and light touch sensation in key points bilaterally (see Table 146-4)
  - Motor examination for strength in key muscle groups bilaterally (see Table 146-5)
  - Neurologic rectal examination (voluntary anal contraction, deep anal sensation)
- Determine sensory, motor, and neurologic levels.
- Determine completeness of injury and ASIA Impairment Scale grade (see Table 146-1). If the ASIA Impairment Scale grade is A, determine the zone of partial preservation.
- Additional elements of neurologic examination:
  - Position and deep pressure sensation, testing of additional muscles
  - Muscle tone and spasticity
  - Muscle stretch reflexes, bulbocavernosus reflex, plantar reflex

Respiratory

- Assess respiratory effort, including effect of posture (e.g., sitting versus supine).
- Check for paradoxical respiration and chest expansion.

- Auscultate to assess for decreased breath sounds, rales, and wheeze.

Cardiac

- Low baseline blood pressure is often a "normal" finding in SCI.
- Look for orthostatic symptoms or excess fall in blood pressure with sitting.
- High blood pressure may indicate autonomic dysreflexia (Table 146-6).
- Examination of peripheral pulses may be especially important for identification of peripheral vascular disease in the absence of claudication and pain symptoms.

Abdomen

- Examine for abdominal distention; examine bowel sounds for evidence of ileus.
- Perform anorectal examination for hemorrhoids and fissures.

Spine

- Identify spinal deformity and tenderness.
- Observe spinal precautions if the examination is being conducted in the acute or postoperative state.

Extremities

- Examine for range of motion, contractures, and swelling.
- Identify nociceptive sources of pain; palpate for tenderness.
- Differentiate effects of SCI (pedal edema, cool extremities) from additional pathologic processes.

Skin

- Examine bone prominences for erythema or skin breakdown.
- Describe any pressure ulcers: location, appearance, size, stage, exudate, odor, necrosis, undermining, sinus tracts; evidence of healing in form of granulation and epithelialization; wound margins and surrounding tissues.[8]

TABLE 146-2 Etiology of Common Symptoms in Spinal Cord Injury

Symptom	Possible Cause
Fever	Infectious
	Urinary tract infection
	Pneumonia
	Infected pressure ulcer, cellulitis, osteomyelitis
	Intra-abdominal or pelvic infection
	Hot environment (due to poikilothermia)
	Deep venous thrombosis
	Heterotopic ossification
	Pathologic limb fracture
	Drug fever (e.g., from antibiotics or anticonvulsant pain medications)
Fatigue	Nonspecific, but could be the only symptom of serious illness
	Infection
	Respiratory or cardiac failure
	Side effect of medications
	Depression (inquire about associated dysphoric symptoms)
Daytime drowsiness	Side effect of medications (e.g., narcotics, antispasticity agents)
	Nocturnal sleep apnea
	Ventilatory failure with carbon dioxide retention
	Depression
Shortness of breath	Pneumonia
	Abdominal distention (e.g., postprandial, obstipation)
	Pulmonary embolus
	Ventilatory impairment (can be postural with sitting up if borderline)
	Cardiac causes
Diarrhea	Altered bowel management schedule
	Clostridium difficile infection
	Spurious diarrhea with bowel impaction
	Side effect of medications (antibiotic, excess laxative or stool softener)
Rectal bleeding	Hemorrhoids
	Trauma from bowel care
	Colorectal cancer
Hematuria	Urinary tract infection
	Urinary stones
	Traumatic bladder catheterization
	Bladder cancer
Headache	Autonomic dysreflexia; may be associated with any noxious stimulus below injury level
	Consider other causes in absence of increased blood pressure
Increased spasticity	Urine infection
	Pressure ulcer
	Bowel impaction
	Any noxious stimulus
	Syringomyelia
Pain	Multiple nociceptive and neuropathic causes (see Table 146-3)
Unilateral leg swelling	Osteoporotic fracture of the lower extremity
	Deep venous thrombosis
	Heterotopic ossification
	Cellulitis
	Hematoma
	Invasive pelvic cancer
New weakness or numbness	Syringomyelia
	Entrapment neuropathy (median at wrist, ulnar at elbow)

TABLE 146-3 Bryce-Ragnarsson Classification of Pain after Spinal Cord Injury

Location	Category	Type	Etiologic Subtype
Above level	Nociceptive	1	Mechanical, musculoskeletal
		2	Autonomic dysreflexia headache
		3	Other
	Neuropathic	4	Compressive neuropathy
		5	Other
At level	Nociceptive	6	Mechanical, musculoskeletal
		7	Visceral
	Neuropathic	8	Central
		9	Radicular
		10	Compressive neuropathy
		11	Complex regional pain syndrome
Below level	Nociceptive	12	Mechanical, musculoskeletal
		13	Visceral
	Neuropathic	14	General
		15	Other

TABLE 146-4 Key Sensory Points for Cervical Spinal Segments

Level	Key Sensory Point
C2	Occipital protuberance
C3	Supraclavicular fossa
C4	Top of the acromioclavicular joint
C5	Lateral side of the antecubital fossa
C6	Thumb, dorsal surface, proximal phalanx
C7	Middle finger, dorsal surface, proximal phalanx
C8	Little finger, dorsal surface, proximal phalanx
T1	Medial side of antecubital fossa

TABLE 146-5 Key Muscle Groups for Cervical Myotomes*

Level	Muscle Group
C5	Elbow flexors (biceps, brachialis)
C6	Wrist extensors (extensor carpi radialis longus and brevis)
C7	Elbow extensors (triceps)
C8	Finger flexors (flexor digitorum profundus) to the middle finger
T1	Small finger abductors (abductor digiti minimi)

*For those myotomes that are not clinically testable by manual muscle examination (e.g., C1 to C4), the motor level is presumed to be the same as the sensory level.

TABLE 146-6 Symptoms and Signs of Autonomic Dysreflexia

Sudden, significant increase in blood pressure

Pounding headache

Flushing of the skin above the level of the SCI, or possibly below

Blurred vision, appearance of spots in the patient's visual fields

Nasal congestion

Profuse sweating above the level of the SCI, or possibly below the level

Piloerection or goose bumps above the level of SCI, or possibly below

Bradycardia (may be a relative slowing only and still within normal range)

Cardiac arrhythmias

Feelings of apprehension or anxiety

Minimal or no symptoms, despite a significantly elevated blood pressure

FUNCTIONAL LIMITATIONS

Tetraplegia is associated with several functional limitations based on the level and completeness of injury.[9] Additional factors, such as age, comorbid conditions, pain, spasticity, body habitus, and psychosocial and environmental factors, can affect function after cervical SCI. A survey of individuals with tetraplegia conducted to rank seven functions in order of importance to their quality of life revealed that the greatest percentage ranked recovery of arm and hand function as their highest priority[10] (Table 146-7).

The Consortium for Spinal Cord Medicine has developed clinical practice guidelines on outcomes after SCI with expected functional outcomes for each level of injury in a number of domains.[9,11] Expected functional outcomes and equipment needs for each level of complete cervical SCI are summarized here.

Level C1-4

- Movement possible: neck flexion, extension, rotation (and preserved shoulder shrug with C4 level)
- Pattern of weakness: total paralysis of trunk, upper extremities, lower extremities
- Dependent on ventilator (most C4 and some C3 may be weaned off ventilator); unable to cough
- Expected functional outcomes:
- Independent in instructing others in care
  - Independent in power wheelchair with chin, head, or breath control
  - Independent in pressure relief in power chair with equipment
  - Total assist with bowel, bladder, bed mobility, transfers, eating, dressing, grooming, bathing, manual wheelchair propulsion, and transportation
- Equipment needed: ventilator and suction equipment; mouthstick; power or mechanical lift; power

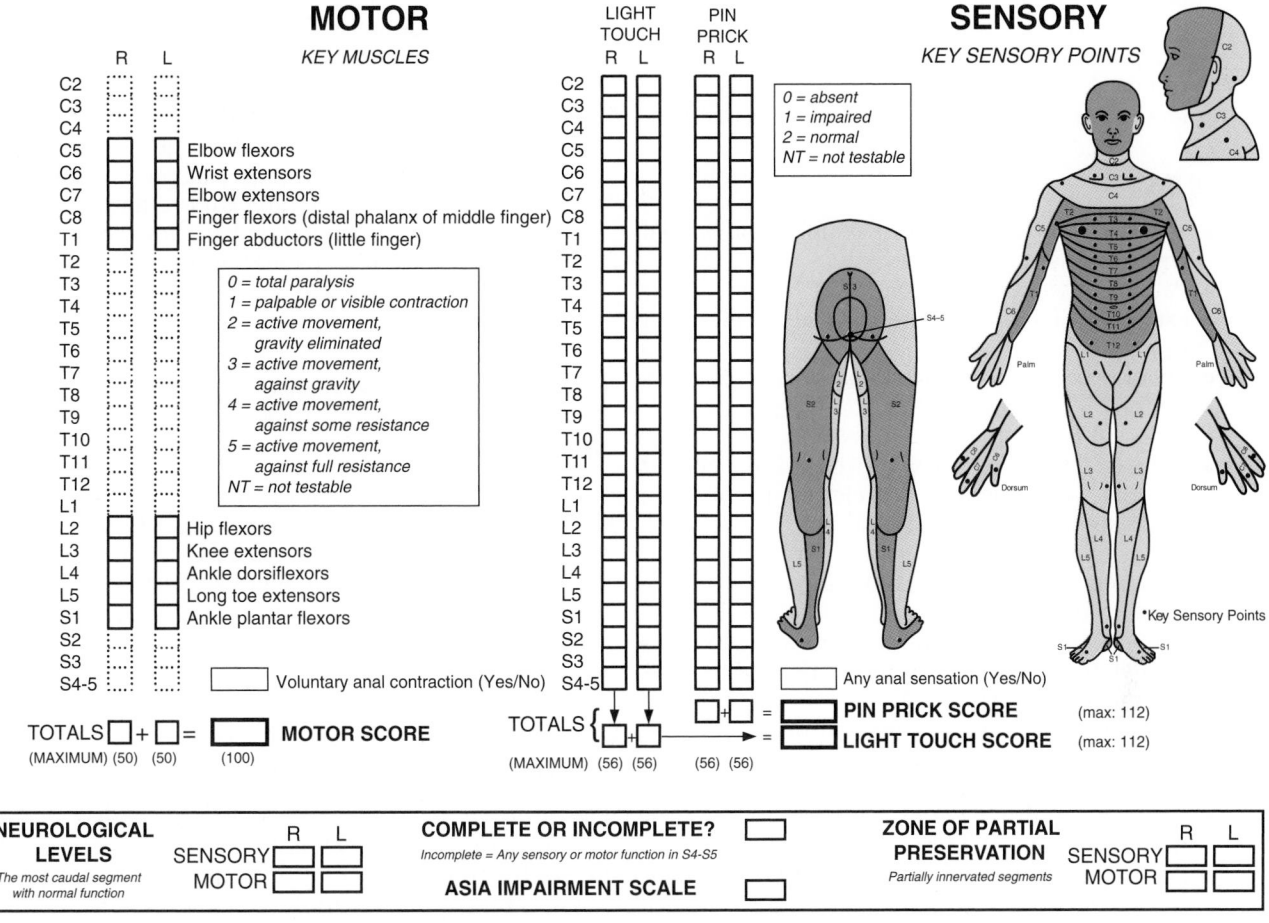

FIGURE 146-1. Standard neurologic classification of spinal cord injury. (Reprinted with permission from American Spinal Injury Association. International Standards for Neurologic Classification of Spinal Cord Injury. Chicago, American Spinal Injury Association, 1996.)

TABLE 146-7 Functional Recovery Priorities of Persons with Cervical Spinal Cord Injury

Area of Functional Recovery	Percentage Surveyed Ranking as the Most Important Item
Arm and hand function	48.7
Sexual function	13.0
Trunk stability	11.5
Bladder and bowel	8.9
Walking movement	7.8
Normal sensation	6.1
Chronic pain	4.0

From Anderson KD. Targeting recovery: priorities of the spinal cord–injured population. J Neurotrauma 2004;21:1371-1383.

wheelchair with tilt or recline (with postural support and head control devices as needed); pressure relief cushion; backup manual wheelchair; adapted feeding equipment; long-handled mirror; environmental control unit; reclining shower-commode chair; hospital bed; pressure relief mattress; attendant-operated van with tie-down

Level C5

- Movement possible: shoulder flexion, abduction, and extension; elbow flexion and supination
- Pattern of weakness: absent elbow extension, pronation, all wrist and hand movements; total paralysis of trunk and lower extremities
- Can get elbow flexion and forearm supination contractures due to unopposed biceps
- Low endurance and vital capacity; may require assistance to clear secretions
- Expected functional outcomes:
- Independent in power wheelchair mobility; independent to some assist with manual wheelchair indoors on non-carpet level surface; some to total assist outdoors
- Independent pressure relief and positioning with equipment
- Total assist in bowel, bladder, bathing, and lower extremity dressing
- Some assist with upper extremity dressing, bed mobility; independent eating with equipment after setup
- Can be independent in transportation in van with highly specialized equipment and lift
- Equipment: power wheelchair with tilt or recline; backup manual wheelchair; pressure relief cushion;

power or mechanical lift; long opponens splint (with pocket for inserting utensils); adapted feeding equipment; long-handled mirror; padded shower-commode chair or padded tub bench with commode cutout; hospital bed; pressure relief mattress

Level C6

- Movement possible: forearm supination, radial wrist extension
- Pattern of weakness: absent wrist flexion, elbow extension, hand movement; total paralysis of trunk and lower extremities
- Avoid overstretch of finger flexors to preserve tenodesis
- Expected functional outcomes:
- Independent in power wheelchair; independent indoors with manual wheelchair propulsion; needs some to total assist outdoors
- Independent pressure relief and positioning with equipment or adapted techniques
- Some to total assist for bladder and bowel
- Some assist for bed mobility; some assist to independent in level transfers, and some to total assist for uneven transfers
- Independent eating (except cutting); independent dressing and bathing upper body; assist for lower body
- Independent driving a modified van (with sensitized hand controls) from wheelchair
- Equipment: power wheelchair; lightweight manual wheelchair with modified rims; transfer board; mechanical lift; short opponens splint (with pocket for inserting utensils); adapted equipment for feeding, dressing, and grooming as needed; universal cuff; long-handled mirror; padded shower-commode chair or padded tub bench with commode cutout; hospital bed or full to king standard bed; pressure relief mattress

Level C7-8

- Movement possible: elbow extension, ulnar wrist extension, wrist flexion, finger flexion and extension; thumb flexion, extension, abduction
- Pattern of weakness: paralysis of trunk and lower extremities; limited grasp release and dexterity of hand due to intrinsic muscle weakness
- Expected functional outcomes:
- Independent in manual wheelchair propulsion; may need some assist with uneven terrain
- Independent in level transfer; may need some assist with uneven transfers
- Independent pressure relief and positioning
- Some to total assist for bowel, independent to some assist for bladder; males can perform intermittent catheterization
- Some assist for bed mobility; some assist to independent in level transfers, and some to total assist for uneven transfers
- Independent eating, grooming, dressing, and bathing upper body; may need assist for lower body

- Independent in light meal preparation and homemaking; assistance with heavy housekeeping
- Independent driving a modified van from captain's seat; independent car if independent with transfer and wheelchair loading
- Equipment: manual lightweight wheelchair; transfer board, if needed; adapted equipment for feeding, dressing, and grooming as needed; universal cuff; long-handled mirror; shower-commode chair or padded tub bench with commode cutout; hospital bed or full to king standard bed; pressure relief mattress

DIAGNOSTIC STUDIES

Spinal Imaging

Radiologic studies are performed to localize the site of the pathologic change. Magnetic resonance imaging is especially helpful because of its ability to visualize the soft tissues, including ligamentous structures, intravertebral discs, epidural or subdural hematomas, and hemorrhage or edema in the spinal cord. Magnetic resonance imaging with gadolinium is helpful in diagnosis of post-traumatic syringomyelia.

Electrodiagnostic Testing

Electromyography and nerve conduction studies may be helpful in distinguishing lesions of the peripheral nerves or brachial plexus from those of the spinal cord when patients present with neurologic worsening.[12]

Urologic Studies

Urodynamic studies assess neurogenic bladder and sphincter dysfunction. Tests to evaluate upper urinary tracts may be indicated on a periodic basis, but there currently is not a uniform consensus on the type or frequency of these tests.[4] Periodic cystoscopy may be indicated in those with chronic indwelling urinary catheters because of increased risk of bladder cancer.[13]

Pulmonary Function

Patients who are at high risk for pulmonary complications, such as those with high tetraplegia or with concomitant chronic obstructive airway disease, may require yearly measurements of forced vital capacity and repeated evaluations when new symptoms arise.[14] Chest radiographs will show evidence of pneumonia or atelectasis. Sputum culture and Gram stain will identify the involved pathogens and help guide antibiotic therapy.

Musculoskeletal Imaging

Radiographic evaluation may be needed in case of suspected fracture or to evaluate pain. Heterotopic ossification may be assessed with a bone scan in addition to plain radiographs.[11] If a pressure ulcer appears to involve the bone, magnetic resonance imaging or bone scan may be helpful to evaluate for osteomyelitis.[5]

TREATMENT

Initial

Initial management includes adequate immobilization and prevention of secondary injury. Physiatric consultation and intervention in an acute setting should address range of motion, positioning, bowel and bladder management programs, clearance of respiratory secretions, ventilatory management, consideration of venous thromboembolic prophylaxis, prevention of pressure ulcers, input about functional implications of options for surgery and spinal orthosis, and education of the patient and family.[15]

Rehabilitation

Information about potential for motor recovery can be used to set functional goals and to plan for equipment needs (as described for each level in the previous section on functional limitations), keeping in mind that individual factors and coexisting conditions may affect achievable goals.[9] Important elements of rehabilitation include an interdisciplinary approach, establishment of an individualized rehabilitation program with consideration of unique barriers and facilitators, and inclusion of the patient as an active participant in establishment of goals.[11]

In addition to the post-acute rehabilitation that follows the injury, lifelong rehabilitation interventions are often indicated to address changes in neurologic status, new goals, or functional decline associated with medical complications and comorbidities, changes in living situation, and aging.[16] Home modifications should be instituted to ensure accessability.[11]

Ongoing Management and Health Maintenance

There is general consensus that comprehensive preventive health evaluations for individuals with SCI are important,[4] although there is not uniform agreement about optimal frequency and specific elements. Because all body systems are potentially affected by cervical SCI, long-term management needs to be comprehensive as summarized here.

Respiratory Prompt identification and treatment of respiratory infections are important.[17] Measures such as smoking cessation and pneumonia and annual influenza vaccinations are vital in reducing respiratory problems.[4] Manually assisted cough methods can be taught to patients and caregivers. It is important to recognize and to address worsening ventilatory function if it occurs with aging or after other complications.

Cardiovascular Autonomic dysreflexia is a life-threatening emergency, and persons with tetraplegia can be at lifelong risk. Prompt identification and management are critical. The Consortium for Spinal Cord Medicine has published clinical practice guidelines for the acute management of autonomic dysreflexia.[6] If the patient has signs and symptoms of dysreflexia (see Table 146-6), the blood pressure is elevated, and the individual is supine, immediately sit the person up. Loosen any clothing or constrictive devices. Monitor the blood pressure and pulse frequently. Quickly survey for instigating causes, beginning with the urinary system. If an indwelling urinary catheter is not in place, catheterize the individual. Before the catheter is inserted, instill lidocaine jelly (if it is readily available) into the urethra. If the individual has an indwelling urinary catheter, check the system along its entire length for kinks, folds, constrictions, or obstructions and for correct placement of the indwelling catheter. If a problem is found, correct it immediately. Avoid manual compression of or tapping on the bladder. If the catheter is not draining and the blood pressure remains elevated, remove and replace the catheter. If the catheter cannot be replaced, consult a urologist. If acute symptoms of autonomic dysreflexia persist, including a sustained elevated blood pressure, suspect fecal impaction. If the elevated blood pressure is at or above 150 mm Hg systolic, consider pharmacologic management to reduce the systolic blood pressure without causing hypotension before checking for fecal impaction. Use an antihypertensive agent with rapid onset and short duration (e.g., nifedipine bite and swallow, 2% nitroglycerin ointment, or prazosin) while the causes of autonomic dysreflexia are being investigated, and monitor the individual for symptomatic hypotension. If fecal impaction is suspected, check the rectum for stool. If the precipitating cause of autonomic dysreflexia is not yet determined, check for other less frequent causes. Monitor the individual's symptoms and blood pressure for at least 2 hours after resolution of the autonomic dysreflexia episode to make sure that it does not recur. If there is poor response to the treatment specified or if the cause of the dysreflexia has not been identified, strongly consider admitting the individual to the hospital to be monitored, to maintain pharmacologic control of the blood pressure, and to investigate other causes of the dysreflexia. Document the episode in the individual's medical record. Once the individual with SCI has been stabilized, review the precipitating causes with the individual and caregivers and provide education as necessary.[6] Individuals with tetraplegia and their caregivers should be able to recognize and to treat autonomic dysreflexia and taught to seek emergency treatment if it is not promptly resolved.

Treatment of symptomatic orthostatic hypotension[11] addresses any exacerbating causes (e.g., medications, dehydration, or sepsis). Nonpharmacologic measures include postural challenges, abdominal binder, compression stockings, and increased salt intake. Pharmacologic treatment is administered if it is needed (e.g., with ephedrine, fludrocortisone, or midodrine).

Primary and secondary prevention of cardiovascular disease includes smoking cessation, diet and weight control, lipid management, screening for and treatment of hypertension and glucose intolerance or diabetes, and individualized exercise program.[18] For evaluation of coronary artery disease, a modified or pharmacologic stress test is often needed in these individuals, and if a cardiac rehabilitation program is required, it can be adapted for wheelchair users.

Genitourinary The goals of bladder management (Table 146-8) are to ensure low pressure and complete voiding, to minimize urinary tract complications, to preserve upper urinary tracts, and to be compatible with the individual's lifestyle.[13] Anticholinergics (e.g., oxybutynin, tolterodine) may be indicated for detrusor hyperreflexia and α-adrenergic blockers (prazosin, terazosin, tamsulosin) for detrusor-sphincter dyssynergia. Urinary infections should be identified and treated promptly, but antibiotics are generally not recommended for asymptomatic bacteriuria.[5] There is little role for prophylactic antibiotics, except before urologic procedures.

Counseling and education are key elements of managing sexual dysfunction. Phosphodiesterase type 5 inhibitors

(sildenafil, tadalafil, vardenafil) may be used to treat erectile impairment, although care needs to be taken to avoid simultaneous use of nitrate-based medications to treat autonomic dysreflexia, which could result in severe hypotension.[4] Other options include intracavernosal injections, devices, and implants. Advances in electroejaculation and fertility care have increased the fertility success rate for men with SCI. Female fertility is not affected once menses return, which typically occurs within 1 year of injury. Pregnancy and delivery in women with SCI carries risks, including autonomic dysreflexia, and close follow-up is recommended.[4]

Gastrointestinal The goals of bowel management are to facilitate predictable and effective elimination and to minimize bowel incontinence.[19] A scheduled individualized bowel program should be established, which typically includes reflex stimulation maneuvers, laxatives (stool softeners, stimulants), dietary interventions, and adequate fiber intake. Laxatives and enemas should be kept to a minimum. One should beware of fecal impaction presenting as spurious diarrhea and pay due attention to new bowel symptoms.

Skin Education of the patient, regular pressure relief practices, and prescription of pressure-reducing support surfaces are vital for prevention of pressure ulcers.[8] Daily comprehensive skin inspections should be carried out by the patient or caregiver, with particular attention to vulnerable insensate areas (e.g., sacrum-coccyx, ischii, trochanters, and heels). Adequate nutritional intake is important. Management of pressure ulcers is discussed further in Chapter 140.

Neurologic If spasticity is painful or continues to interfere with function after institution of a stretching and positioning program and treatment of any exacerbating factors, medications are often indicated.[20] Table 146-9 lists commonly used medications, although documented evidence of efficacy is insufficient for most.[21] Chapter 144

TABLE 146-8 Nonsurgical Options for Management of the Neurogenic Bladder in Spinal Cord Injury

Bladder Management	Indications
Intermittent catheterization	Often the first choice, if feasible Need sufficient hand skills or willing caregiver Must be willing and able to follow catheterization time schedule
Indwelling catheterization (urethral or suprapubic)	Consider for poor hand skills and lack of caregiver assistance Not able or willing to follow intermittent catheterization schedule High fluid intake Lack of success with less invasive measures Temporary management of vesicoureteral reflux Choose suprapubic with epididymo-orchitis, prostatitis
Credé and Valsalva	Generally avoided in cervical SCI (unless the patient had sphincterotomy)
Reflex voiding	Hand skills or willing caregiver to put on condom catheter, empty leg bag Confirmed small postvoid residual volumes, low voiding pressure Able to maintain condom catheter in place Need to also decrease detrusor-sphincter dyssynergia, if present (e.g., with α blocker, botulinum toxin injection, stent, sphincterotomy) Not an option for female patients

provides additional discussion about spasticity. Selective tightening (e.g., wrist extensors for tenodesis or back extensors for sitting balance) may be important for function in tetraplegia. Neurologic worsening (e.g., due to focal neuropathy, syringomyelia) should be investigated and addressed appropriately.[12]

Musculoskeletal Measures for upper extremity preservation after SCI should be instituted early and followed lifelong. These include optimization of equipment and wheelchair to minimize upper extremity stresses, activity modification to minimize repetitive or excessive upper extremity forces during daily activities and transfers, and individualized exercise program incorporating appropriate flexibility and strengthening components.[22]

It is important to recognize and to address contributing factors to pain, which is often multifactorial[7] (see Table 146-3). Pain medications (see Table 146-9) often do not provide complete or optimal relief.[20]

Heterotopic ossification is treated with etidronate sodium, nonsteroidals, and occasionally surgical resection, especially if it is interfering with function or comfort.[11] Pathologic fractures should be recognized and treated with padded splints or bivalved circular casts, monitoring of skin integrity, and often only a limited role for surgical treatment.[12] The role for pharmacologic treatment of osteoporosis in SCI is still evolving. Fall prevention (education, wheelchair lap belts) is important to prevent injuries.

Psychosocial It is important to address environmental barriers (physical and attitudinal), to promote self-efficacy, and to optimize participation and community integration in response to changes in the living situation and social support, functional decline, and aging. Depression should be identified and treated adequately, and substance abuse prevention and treatment programs should be offered.[23]

Procedures

Pressure Ulcers

Sharp débridement of pressure ulcers may be done at the bedside to remove necrotic tissue, although if it is extensive, débridement may need to be done in the operating room.

Spasticity

Motor point or nerve blocks with phenol or alcohol may be helpful in treating localized spasticity that interferes with positioning, mobility, or hygiene. Intramuscular injections of botulinum toxin are another option.

Pain

Shoulder pain due to subacromial bursitis may be temporarily responsive to local corticosteroid injections, as is the discomfort from carpal tunnel syndrome.[22]

TABLE 146-9 Medications Commonly Used for Spasticity and Pain in Spinal Cord Injury*

Problem	Drug Class	Medication
Spasticity	GABA related	Baclofen
		Gabapentin
	α₂ Agonist	Tizanidine
		Clonidine
	Benzodiazepine	Diazepam
		Clonazepam
	Calcium release inhibitor	Dantrolene
	Local injection	Botulinum toxin
		Phenol, alcohol
	Intrathecal agents	Baclofen
Pain	Nonopioid analgesic	Acetaminophen
		Tramadol
		Nonsteroidal anti-inflammatory drugs, salicylates
	Opioid	Morphine sulfate
		Oxycodone
		Hydrocodone
		Fentanyl (transdermal)
	Anticonvulsant	Gabapentin
		Carbamazepine
		Other (phenytoin, valproic acid, lamotrigine)
	Tricyclic antidepressant	Amitriptyline
		Nortriptyline
	Local anesthetic	Lidocaine patch
	Neuroblocking cream	Capsaicin
	Intrathecal agents	Morphine, clonidine

*The list is not meant to be exhaustive but includes examples of commonly used medications.

Surgery

Spine Surgery

When cervical spine injury is accompanied by mechanical instability, pain, deformity, or progressive neural impairment, surgical decompression and segmental instrumentation may be indicated for reconstruction of spinal alignment, stability, and early mobilization.[12,15]

Pressure Ulcers

Plastic surgery may be indicated for deep pressure ulcers. This includes excision of the ulcer and surrounding scar and muscle and musculocutaneous flap closure.[22]

Spasticity

If spasticity is not controlled with maximum dosages of oral medications, or if a patient is unable to tolerate the medications, the placement of an intrathecal baclofen pump may be considered.

Motor Function

Reconstructive surgery of the upper extremity with tendon transfers may improve motor function by one level, typically in those with a neurologic level at C5, C6, or C7. Depending on the level of injury, restoration of wrist extension, elbow extension, and key grip strength or improvement of active grasp and hand control may be an appropriate goal.[24]

Functional electrical stimulation has been used in SCI to improve motor function, including upper limb control, standing, and walking, as well as for electrophrenic respiration for ventilator-free breathing.[11]

Bladder Dysfunction

Surgical treatment of urolithiasis includes cystoscopic removal of bladder stones, lithotripsy, and percutaneous nephrolithotomy for larger renal stones. Endourethral stents or transurethral sphincterotomy may be considered in individuals with detrusor-sphincter dyssynergia.[13] Electrical stimulation and posterior sacral rhizotomy may be considered for individuals who have problems with catheterization, have good bladder contractions, have no extensive bladder fibrosis, and are willing to lose reflex erections.[13] Bladder augmentation may be indicated for intractable bladder contractions with incontinence and in those at high risk for upper tract deterioration. Urinary diversion may be an appropriate option for unsalvageable bladders secondary to urethral fistula and in individuals with bladder cancer requiring cystectomy.[13]

Bowel Dysfunction

Patients with neurogenic bowel who have significant difficulty or complications with typical bowel care may have improved quality of life after colostomy. Careful selection of patients and individualization are required in consideration of this surgery.[19]

Upper Extremity Pain

Surgery may occasionally be considered for chronic upper extremity overuse-related symptoms that are unresponsive to medical and rehabilitative treatment (e.g., for carpal tunnel syndrome or rotator cuff disease). Outcomes are often poor if upper extremity overuse continues.[22]

Post-traumatic Syringomyelia

Surgical placement of shunts may be indicated for post-traumatic syringomyelia associated with intractable pain or progressive neurologic decline.

POTENTIAL DISEASE COMPLICATIONS

Cervical SCI is associated with multiple complications that can involve every body system.

Respiratory

Respiratory problems include atelectasis, mucous plugs, and pneumonia secondary to impaired cough and retention of secretions; ventilatory failure with high tetraplegia; and sleep-disordered breathing.[17]

Cardiovascular

Patients with cervical SCI are prone to multiple cardiovascular complications throughout life.[18] Autonomic dysreflexia may occur in SCI above the T6 neurologic level and can be precipitated in response to any noxious stimulus below the level of injury. Symptomatic orthostatic hypotension often resolves after the first few months but may be persistent in some cases. Although venous thromboembolism risk is reduced after the initial months, it can increase even in chronic SCI in the setting of prolonged immobilization associated with medical illness or in the postsurgical state. Cardiovascular fitness is reduced and cardiovascular risk factors can be adversely affected (e.g., reduced high-density lipoprotein cholesterol, increased body fat and insulin resistance, decreased physical activity). Diagnosis of cardiovascular disease may be delayed because of confusing or absent symptoms and signs.[18]

Genitourinary

Neurogenic bladder is associated with loss of voluntary control, detrusor-sphincter dyssynergia, and incomplete bladder emptying. Complications include urinary tract infection, bladder and kidney stones, vesicoureteral reflux, and hydronephrosis with renal impairment. Bladder cancer risk is increased with chronic indwelling catheter, especially in smokers.[13] Erectile and ejaculatory dysfunction occurs, and sperm quality may be impaired.[4]

Gastrointestinal

There is loss of voluntary bowel control, anorectal dyssynergia, and reduced rectal expulsive force.[19] Fecal impaction may occur. Anorectal problems include hemorrhoids, fissures, proctitis, and prolapse. Gallstone risk is increased. Gastroesophageal reflux is common. False-positive results of examination for fecal occult blood may complicate colorectal cancer screening.

Skin

Pressure ulcers are common and may increase with duration of injury. Previous occurrence of a pressure ulcer is an important predictor of future pressure ulcers.[8]

Metabolic and Endocrine

Hyponatremia may be a persistent problem in some patients. Carbohydrate and lipid metabolism is affected, and there may be glucose intolerance associated with relative insulin resistance.[16] A reduction in bone mineral

TABLE 146-10 Pharmacokinetic Changes in Spinal Cord Injury

SCI-Related Change	Impact on Pharmacokinetics
Delayed gastric emptying	Rapid absorption of acidic drugs
	Delayed absorption of basic drugs
Reduced gastrointestinal motility	Increased absorption of drugs that undergo enterohepatic circulation
	Decreased bioavailability of drugs that are destroyed by gut bacteria
Reduced blood flow to skin and muscle	Less reliable transcutaneous, subcutaneous, and intramuscular drug absorption below injury level
Increased percentage of body fat	Effect on fat- and water-soluble drug distribution
Reduced plasma protein level	Increased free fraction of protein-bound drugs
Impaired kidney function	Reduced renal elimination of drugs

density with secondary osteoporosis is common in chronic SCI and affects both the upper and lower extremities in those with tetraplegia.

Neurologic

Neuropathic pain can be persistent and have a negative impact on quality of life. Entrapment neuropathies (median nerve at wrist, ulnar at elbow) and post-traumatic syringomyelia can result in neurologic deterioration.[12]

Musculoskeletal

Overuse syndromes include shoulder pain and rotator cuff problems.[12,22] Contractures may occur without due attention to range of motion and positioning. Heterotopic ossification, which is the development of ectopic bone within the soft tissues surrounding peripheral joints, occurs in SCI most commonly around the hip, followed by the knees, elbows, and shoulders.[11] It is further discussed in Chapter 123. Pathologic fractures may occur even with trivial injury because of severe osteoporosis.[12]

Psychosocial

SCI can increase the potential for stress, isolation, and depression.[23] Alcohol and substance abuse risk seems to be increased.

POTENTIAL TREATMENT COMPLICATIONS

Spinal pain at the surgical site may result from loosening, infection, or broken hardware. Instability or neurologic deterioration may be due to inadequate spinal immobilization. Surgical shunts can become blocked or infected, and intrathecal pumps or catheters may malfunction.

Complications of urethral catheterization include urethral trauma, erosions, strictures, urinary infections, and epididymitis.[13] Chronic indwelling catheters increase the risk of stones and squamous cell carcinoma of the bladder. Complications may occur with surgical procedures for SCI-related problems, such as neurogenic bladder. For example, transurethral sphincterectomy may be associated with significant intraoperative and perioperative bleeding and erectile and ejaculatory dysfunction. Posterior sacral rhizotomy done in conjunction with electrical stimulation of the bladder may result in loss of reflex erection and ejaculation and reduction of reflex defecation. Urinary diversion procedures may be followed by intestinal or urinary leak, infection, ureteroileal stricture, stomal stenosis, and intestinal obstruction due to adhesions.[13]

Because people with SCI are often prescribed multiple medications, drug-related side effects and complications are common. Cervical SCI can result in altered pharmacokinetics[25] in multiple ways (Table 146-10), which further increases unpredictability of side effects.

References

1. American Spinal Injury Association. International Standards for Neurological and Functional Classification of Spinal Cord Injury, revised 2002. Chicago, American Spinal Injury Association, 2002.
2. Ho CH, Wuermser LA, Priebe MM, et al. Spinal cord injury medicine. 1. Epidemiology and classification. Arch Phys Med Rehabil 2007;88(Suppl 1):S49-S54.
3. National Spinal Cord Injury Statistical Center. Spinal cord injury: facts and figures at a glance, June 2006. J Spinal Cord Med 2007;30:79.
4. Chiodo AE, Scelza WM, Kirshblum SC, et al. Spinal cord injury medicine. 5. Long-term medical issues and health maintenance. Arch Phys Med Rehabil 2007;88(Suppl 1):S76-S83.
5. Till M, Pertel P. Infections. In Green D, ed. Medical Management of Long-Term Disability. Boston, Butterworth-Heinemann 1996:233-262.
6. Consortium for Spinal Cord Medicine. Acute Management of Autonomic Dysreflexia: Individuals with Spinal Cord Injury Presenting to Health Care Facilities, 2nd ed. Washington, DC, Paralyzed Veterans of America, 2001. Available at: www.pva.org.
7. Bryce TN, Ragnarsson KT. Pain management in persons with spinal cord disorders. In Lin VW, ed. Spinal Cord Medicine: Principles and Practice. New York, Demos, 2003:441-460.
8. Consortium for Spinal Cord Medicine. Pressure Ulcer Prevention and Treatment Following Spinal Cord Injury. Clinical Practice Guidelines for Health Care Professionals. Washington, DC, Paralyzed Veterans of America, 2000. Available at: www.pva.org.
9. Consortium for Spinal Cord Medicine. Outcomes Following Traumatic Spinal Cord Injury. Clinical Practice Guidelines for Health Care Professionals. Washington, DC, Paralyzed Veterans of America, 1999. Available at: www.pva.org.

10. Anderson KD. Targeting recovery: priorities of the spinal cord–injured population. J Neurotrauma 2004;21:1371-1383.

11. Kirshblum SC, Priebe MM, Ho CH, et al. Spinal cord injury medicine. 3. Rehabilitation phase after acute spinal cord injury. Arch Phys Med Rehabil 2007;88(Suppl 1):S62-S69.

12. Little JW, Burns SP. Neuromusculoskeletal complications of spinal cord injury. In Kirshblum SC, Campagnolo D, DeLisa JE, eds. Spinal Cord Medicine. Philadelphia, Lippincott Williams & Wilkins, 2002:241-252.

13. Consortium for Spinal Cord Medicine. Bladder Management for Adults with Spinal Cord Injury. Clinical Practice Guidelines for Health Care Professionals. Washington, DC, Paralyzed Veterans of America, 2006. Available at: www.pva.org.

14. Consortium for Spinal Cord Medicine. Respiratory Management Following Spinal Cord Injury. Clinical Practice Guidelines for Health Care Professionals. Washington, DC, Paralyzed Veterans of America, 2005. Available at: www.pva.org.

15. Wuermser LA, Ho CH, Chiodo AE, et al. Spinal cord injury medicine. 2. Acute care management of traumatic and nontraumatic injury. Arch Phys Med Rehabil 2007;88(Suppl 1):S55-S59.

16. Bauman WA, Spungen AM, Adkins RH, Kemp BJ. Metabolic and endocrine changes in persons aging with spinal cord injury. Assist Technol 2001;11:88-96.

17. Lanig IS, Peterson WP. The respiratory system in spinal cord injury. Phys Med Rehabil Clin North Am 2000;11:29-43.

18. Sabharwal S. Cardiovascular dysfunction in spinal cord disorders. In Lin VW, ed. Spinal Cord Medicine: Principles and Practice. New York, Demos, 2003:179-192.

19. Consortium for Spinal Cord Medicine. Neurogenic Bowel Management in Adults with Spinal Cord Injury. Clinical Practice Guidelines for Health Care Professionals. Washington, DC, Paralyzed Veterans of America, 1998. Available at: www.pva.org.

20. Burchiel KJ, Hsu FP. Pain and spasticity after spinal cord injury: mechanism and treatment. Spine 2001;26(Suppl):S146-S160.

21. Taricco M, Pagliacci MC, Telaro E, Adone R. Pharmacological interventions for spasticity following spinal cord injury: results of a Cochrane Systematic Review. Eur Medicophys 2006;42:5-15.

22. Consortium for Spinal Cord Medicine. Preservation of Upper Limb Function Following Spinal Cord Injury. Clinical Practice Guidelines for Health Care Professionals. Washington, DC, Paralyzed Veterans of America, 2005. Available at: www.pva.org.

23. Consortium for Spinal Cord Medicine. Depression Following Spinal Cord Injury. Clinical Practice Guidelines for Health Care Professionals. Washington, DC, Paralyzed Veterans of America, 1998. Available at: www.pva.org.

24. Waters RL, Muccitelli LM. Tendon transfers to improve function of persons with tetraplegia. In Kirshblum SC, Campagnolo D, DeLisa JE, eds. Spinal Cord Medicine. Philadelphia, Lippincott Williams & Wilkins, 2002:424-437.

25. Richardson JS, Segal JL. Spinal cord injury: the role of pharmacokinetics in optimizing drug therapy. In Lin VW, ed. Spinal Cord Medicine: Principles and Practice. New York, Demos, 2003:247-256.

Spinal Cord Injury (Thoracic) 147

Jane Wierbicky, RN, BSN, and Shanker Nesathurai, MD

DEFINITION

Spinal cord injury (SCI) is a common cause of paralysis, particularly in young men (Table 147-1). Just more than one third of all injuries to the spinal cord occur at the thoracic level, most commonly at T12.[1] Compromise to the thoracic spinal cord typically results in paraplegia. Unlike paraplegia that results from compromise of the cauda equina associated with lumbar spine injuries, the clinical findings are consistent with upper motor neuron injury. However, lower limb paralysis is not the only impairment. The thoracic spinal cord also segmentally innervates the intercostal muscles as well as the upper and lower abdominal muscles. The intercostal muscles are innervated by the T1 to T12 spinal segments. The upper abdominal muscles are innervated by the T8 to T10 spinal segments; the T11 to T12 spinal segments innervate the lower abdominal muscles.[2]

A quantitative three-dimensional anatomy of the thoracic spine reveals three distinct zones: the cervical-thoracic transition zone, the middle region, and the thoracic-lumbar transition zone.[3,4] The T1-4 region is characterized by a narrowing of the vertebral end plate and spinal canal widths.[3] The middle thoracic region (T4-9) is notable for its relatively narrow end plate and small spinal canal. The rib articulations provide an increased degree of protection at this level. An enlargement of the spinal canal characterizes the lower thoracic region (T10-12).[3] There is also less rigidity of the spine at the T11 and T12 segments because of the lack of ventral attachment of the ribs.[3] Therefore, there is an increased vulnerability to SCI at the lower thoracic levels. Compared with the cervical and lumbar spinal levels, the blood supply is more tenuous in the thoracic spinal cord, and therefore

ischemia poses a greater threat to neurologic function in this area.[4]

Weakness, loss of sensation, and spasticity are the most common sequelae of a thoracic SCI. Issues commonly encountered in the outpatient clinic include pressure ulcer, urinary tract infection, dysreflexia, bowel irregularity, depression, sexual dysfunction, thrombosis, severe spasticity, heterotopic ossification, contractures, osteoporosis, and pain.

In an analysis of long-term medical complications among subjects enrolled in the National Spinal Cord Injury Statistical Center database, pressure ulcers were the most commonly reported postinjury complication. McKinley and colleagues[5] reported a 15.2% incidence of pressure ulcers in the first annual follow-up postinjury year. The rates increased steadily during all follow-up years in both complete and incomplete SCIs. Common sites for pressure ulcers are the sacrum, greater trochanter, and heels. The human and economic costs of pressure ulcers are enormous. Excessive pressure, shearing, friction, and maceration can increase the risk for pressure ulcers. Other risk factors include spasticity, impaired sensation, immobility, poor nutrition, weight gain, and incontinence.[6]

Neurogenic bowel and bladder are also complications of thoracic SCI. Most patients with thoracic-level SCI will have upper motor neuron bladder dysfunction. Low urinary volumes, high bladder pressures, bladder trabeculation, and diminished bladder compliance characterize upper motor neuron bladder dysfunction. Detrusor-sphincter dyssynergia (co-contraction of the bladder and sphincter) is common. Detrusor-sphincter dyssynergia can contribute to vesicoureteral reflux, which may result in hydronephrosis and subsequent chronic renal failure.

Sexual desire is not necessarily affected by SCI. However, associated depression, fears of inadequacy, and poor body image may consequently alter sexual desire. Sexual function (e.g., erection and ejaculation in men and lubrication in women) in patients with thoracic-level injuries may be altered. In general, patients with more complete lesions have more impairment. Men with thoracic-level lesions (with intact sacral reflexes)

TABLE 147-1 Demographic Comparison of Gunshot Spinal Cord Injury with Nonviolent Spinal Cord Trauma

	Gunshot SCI (%)	Nonviolent Traumatic SCI (%)
Gender		
Male	95.1	79.7
Female	4.9	20.3
Ethnicity		
White	9.8	51.5
Non-white	91.2	48.5
Marital status		
Never married	70.7	38.9
Married	19.5	44.3
Not married	9.8	16.8
Employment status		
Employed	41.5	75.4
Unemployed	58.5	24.5
Mean age	27.1	42.2

Modified from McKinley WO, Johns JS, Musgrove JJ. Clinical presentations, medical complications, and functional outcomes of individuals with gunshot wound–induced spinal cord injury. Am J Phys Med Rehabil 1999;78:102-107.

generally can achieve reflex erections with direct genital stimulation. However, many times, these reflex erections are of insufficient rigidity and duration for satisfactory vaginal penetration.[7]

SCI predisposes individuals to both deep venous thrombosis and pulmonary embolism. According to one study, the risk of death resulting from pulmonary embolism for patients with acute SCI is 210 times greater than for a similar healthy population.[8] The risk decreases to 19.1 times normal in postinjury years 2 to 5. The risk further decreases to 8.9 times normal for those who survive for more than 5 years.[8] Putative mechanisms include immobility as a result of paralysis and failure of the venous-muscle pump.

Osteoporosis among patients with SCI is common. Immobilization and the lack of weight-loading activities are among the chief causes of osteoporosis. Other factors may include alterations in blood circulation, lack of muscle traction on bone, and hormonal changes.[9] Osteoporosis in the lower extremities is the most common presentation in the individual with a thoracic-level lesion. The loss of bone density develops in the acute stage of injury, with demineralization occurring below the level of injury.[10] Patients with SCI are at significant risk for long bone fracture, and care must be taken to prevent fractures resulting from range of motion exercises and falls.

Heterotopic ossification, the development of bone in soft tissues (see Chapter 123), is most often seen in the first 6 months after injury in the spinal cord–injured population.[11] The incidence of heterotopic ossification among individuals with SCI ranges from 20% to 30%.

It is estimated that 18% to 37% of those developing heterotopic ossification will experience a significant loss of joint mobility.[12]

Psychosocial adaptation subsequent to SCI is a lifelong process. There is no single "classic" presentation of this phenomenon. Anger, hostility, anxiety, and depression often result from overwhelming losses confronting this population. Suicide is among the leading causes of death in these patients.

Individuals with SCI above the T6 level are also susceptible to autonomic dysreflexia as a result of the disruption of the autonomic nervous system pathways. Autonomic dysreflexia, which results in elevated blood pressure, is usually precipitated by noxious stimuli below the level of the lesion. The major splanchnic outflow exists at the T6 to L2 levels.[13] The afferent impulses generated by the noxious stimuli ascend in the cord, stimulating sympathetic neurons in the intermediolateral gray matter and initiating sympathetic vasoconstrictor reflexes.[13] This massive sympathetic outflow is unopposed by higher cortical modulating centers because of the lesion in the spinal cord. Baroreceptors in the aorta and carotid arteries detect the increased pressure and vagal stimulation occurs, resulting in bradycardia.[14] Autonomic dysreflexia is a medical emergency, and prompt medical intervention is required.[15] The Consortium for Spinal Cord Medicine has established clinical practice guidelines for the treatment of autonomic dysreflexia, published by the Paralyzed Veterans of America. If it is untreated, autonomic dysreflexia can lead to seizure, intracerebral hemorrhage, or even death.

SYMPTOMS

The presenting symptoms of thoracic SCI are consistent with the alteration to the motor, sensory, and autonomic pathways. The chief symptoms are weakness or paralysis of the abdominal and lower extremity musculature and loss of sensation in the lower limbs, thorax, and perineum. Altered bowel and bladder function and sexual dysfunction may also be expected. In the outpatient setting, the patient may complain of lower extremity spasticity, pain, and symptoms of autonomic dysreflexia (in patients with a thoracic cord lesion of T6 or higher). Patients with SCI are often insensate to the pain that accompanies deep venous thrombosis, and therefore both the clinician and the patient should be attentive to clinical signs such as edema, erythema, and increased tone. Heterotopic ossification may mimic deep venous thrombosis because the symptoms include swelling, decreased range of motion, erythema, increased spasticity, pain, and low-grade fever.

Pain originating from either musculoskeletal or neurologic sources is common. Neuropathic pain resulting from central or peripheral nervous disruption may be described as burning or shooting. An analysis of the National Model Spinal Cord Injury Systems database revealed an 80.5% overall prevalence of pain.[16] The prevalence of pain was greater in the respondents with paraplegia (64.5%) compared with people diagnosed with tetraplegia (58.7%).[16]

Autonomic dysreflexia is characterized by elevated systolic and diastolic blood pressure, pounding headaches, nasal congestion, anxiety, visual disturbances, pallor below the level of injury, and sweating and flushing above the level of injury. In patients with an old, stable injury who are experiencing new or progressive symptoms (e.g., increasing weakness, loss of sensation), the clinician should consider the possibility of a syrinx.

PHYSICAL EXAMINATION

The diagnosis of a thoracic-level SCI necessitates a thorough physical examination because of the multisystem complications that may ensue. The initial evaluation of the patient also includes the assessment of vital signs, respiratory function, skin integrity, and bowel and bladder function; an examination is performed for the presence of spasticity, pain, and contractures. In thoracic SCI, pressure ulcers are more common over bone prominences such as the sacrum, calcaneus, and greater trochanter.

New neurologic abnormalities on physical examination should alert the clinician to consider imaging studies to exclude a syrinx. Classic physical examination findings include change in sensory level, change in motor level, and reflex abnormality as well as increased muscle tone.

FUNCTIONAL LIMITATIONS

Persons who suffer from thoracic SCI can have significantly different levels of disability, depending on their degree of paralysis and associated potential complications (e.g., contractures, spasticity). A patient with high thoracic paraplegia (i.e., T2 level) typically has some component of truncal instability; as a result, the patient's wheelchair requires a high back. In contrast, a person with low thoracic paraplegia generally has preservation of most of the intercostal and abdominal muscles and could opt for a chair with a low back. Intercostal muscle impairment in patients with SCI in the upper thoracic region may cause an impaired cough and a decreased ability to mobilize secretions.

Functional goals for individuals with thoracic SCI include the ability to independently complete activities of daily living with or without the use of assistive equipment. Tasiemski and colleagues[17] have described a positive association of involvement in sports and recreational activities with increased life satisfaction in a community sample of people with SCIs. Numerous sports and recreational organizations offer adaptive sports programs for people with disabilities.

Bowel and bladder function may cause social embarrassment, leading to self-imposed social isolation. Sexual dysfunction may result in a loss of intimacy. The availability of partners is a concern for many patients because their disability and environmental and social barriers may preclude their involvement in some of the more typical dating activities.

Depression is common in patients with SCI; reported rates of depression in the newly injured range between 20% and 44%.[18] Depression has been associated with an increase in secondary complications and poor compliance with self-care activities.[18] Referral to mental health professionals is encouraged for patients at risk.

DIAGNOSTIC STUDIES

The diagnosis of thoracic SCI is often corroborated with magnetic resonance imaging. The stability of the injury is assessed by evaluation of the anterior, middle, and posterior columns of the spine. Magnetic resonance imaging is also the study of choice when a syrinx is suspected.

Urodynamic testing is commonly used to evaluate bladder function in the individual with SCI. Urodynamic studies involve filling of the bladder with fluid or gas and use of electromyographic and fluoroscopic techniques to evaluate voiding function. Annual evaluations often include an ultrasound examination to further assess the integrity of the renal system.

Patients with grade IV pressure ulcers may require a bone scan to detect osteomyelitis. The triple-phase bone scan is also used in the diagnosis of heterotopic ossification (see Chapter 123). Doppler surveillance studies are commonly performed to detect deep venous thrombosis in this highly susceptible population (see Chapter 118). Laboratory tests, such as elevated serum alkaline phosphatase level, are used to assess for heterotopic ossification. Routine colonoscopy and fecal occult blood testing may be appropriate for patients 50 years and older.[19] In patients susceptible to autonomic dysreflexia, appropriate precautions must be used during colonoscopy.

Differential Diagnosis

Amyotrophic lateral sclerosis

Post-traumatic syringomyelia

Guillain-Barré syndrome

Spinal cord infarction

Ischemic injury to spinal cord (i.e., secondary to abdominal and thoracic aneurysms)

Multiple sclerosis

Transverse myelitis

TREATMENT

Initial

Skin Management

The maintenance of skin integrity is an ever-present goal in patients with SCI. Pressure ulcer formation will lead to the development of scar tissue and an even greater likelihood of ulcer recurrence. Skin breakdown can be prevented by ensuring that seating and bedding surfaces are optimal. Seating surfaces should be reevaluated on a regular basis. A cushion that may have been satisfactory previously may currently be worn out. Patients with substantial weight changes should have their seating systems reevaluated.

Excessive pressure, shear forces, and moisture should be minimized. Patients are encouraged to perform daily skin examinations. Most paraplegic patients are able to independently perform pressure-relieving strategies, such as wheelchair pushups. These techniques should be performed every 15 minutes to minimize excessive pressure. Patients are encouraged to minimize pressure by turning frequently when in bed and using a pressure-relieving mattress.

Patients who develop a pressure ulcer must eliminate pressure to that area until the wound is healed. A variety of débridement methods are available for removal of necrotic debris from pressure ulcers. These methods include normal saline wet to dry gauze dressings, whirlpool therapy, irrigation, and chemical débridement agents (see Chapter 140).

Pain

In individuals who have pain, the specific condition should be addressed (e.g., rotator cuff tendinitis, lateral epicondylitis). The presentation of pain among the SCI population can be varied in nature; both neuropathic pain and pain resulting from abnormal mechanical stresses (e.g., tendinitis) are common. Non-narcotic analgesics and nonsteroidal anti-inflammatory drugs can be used to treat musculoskeletal causes of pain. Neuropathic pain generally is not responsive to these medications; however, tricyclic antidepressants and anti-seizure medications have been effective in its treatment but should be prescribed with caution.[20]

Bladder Management

Bladder management strategies should be individualized. In general, intermittent catheterization is the preferred treatment option. A typical intermittent catheterization program requires bladder emptying four to six times per day. Catheterization volumes should remain less than 500 mL. Most paraplegic patients have the manual dexterity to perform self-catheterization. However, some individuals, because of biologic or sociomedical factors, must use indwelling catheters (either suprapubic or urethral).

Indwelling catheters are associated with a higher incidence of bladder stones and bladder carcinoma.[21] In addition, in men, urethral catheters are associated with prostatitis, epididymitis, and urethral strictures.

The overriding goals of a bladder management program are to maintain socially acceptable continence and to minimize the long-term urologic sequelae of SCI. Detrusor-sphincter dyssynergia can be treated with medical interventions (see Chapter 129) that decrease bladder tone (e.g., oxybutynin) or decrease sphincter tone (e.g., terazosin).

Bowel Management

The patient with thoracic-level injuries will most likely suffer from constipation; therefore, a bowel program is necessary. A reasonable goal for a bowel regimen is to achieve socially acceptable fecal continence, with bowel evacuations at least three times per week. A bowel regimen may include medications (Table 147-2). In addition, bowel evacuation is scheduled after a meal to capitalize on the intrinsic increase in peristalsis after meals (i.e., the gastro-colic reflex). Bowel care programs done on a raised toilet seat use the benefits of gravity. Digital stimulation (gentle insertion of the finger) of the rectum or insertion of a suppository can activate the rectocolic reflex by stimulating peristalsis and promoting regular bowel movements. Glycerin and bisacodyl are colonic irritants that can be delivered by suppository, which can be a useful adjunctive agent in a bowel regimen. Enemas (Fleet, soapsuds) should not be part of a regular bowel program; however, these agents are useful in providing a clear gut before a bowel program is begun or for treating fecal obstipation.[19] The administration of an enema can precipitate autonomic dysreflexia in susceptible patients.

Mental Health

In individuals suffering from depression or other psychological sequelae, consultation with an appropriate mental health care professional is recommended. Continued follow-up is encouraged, when appropriate.

Sexual and Reproductive Function

Many patients with SCI have numerous questions and fears about sexuality and sexual function. Treatment should address concerns related to body image, dating,

TABLE 147-2 Oral Adjunctive Bowel Medications[19]

Medication	Brand	Mechanism of Action	Strength	Dose
Docusate sodium	Colace	Stool softener	100 mg (capsules)	1 tablet bid
Senna	Senokot	Colonic stimulant	8.6 mg (tablets)	1-2 tablets ghs
Bisacodyl	Dulcolax	Colonic irritant	5 mg (tablets)	2 tablets qd
Psyllium powder	Smooth Texture Sugar-Free Unflavored Metamucil	Bulk-forming agent	5.4 g per tsp	1 tsp qd-tid
Metoclopramide	Reglan	Prokinetic agent	10 mg (tablets)	1 tablet qid

Adapted from Bergman S. Bowel Management. In Nesathurai S, ed. The Rehabilitation of People with Spinal Cord Injury, 2nd ed. Malden, Mass, Blackwell Science, 2000:53-58.

and initiation and maintenance of intimate relationships. Peer counselors can share their experiences, and their advice can be beneficial. Peer counselors may be located through local independent living centers or through local chapters of the National Spinal Cord Injury Association. In addition, mental health professionals (e.g., psychologists, psychiatrists, social workers) can be a valuable resource to the patient and rehabilitation team.

Several options available to men with erectile dysfunction include oral medications (e.g., sildenafil), vacuum devices, penile injection programs (papaverine), and surgically implanted prostheses. Ejaculatory dysfunction is also common, including retrograde ejaculation into the bladder.[22] Chronic SCI is also associated with poor semen quality and decreased spermatogenesis.[23] Elevated scrotal temperatures (from chronic sitting) and frequent urinary tract infections may negatively affect semen quality. Although studies have indicated that less than 10% of men with SCI report ejaculation, fatherhood has become a possibility with use of semen retrieval methods such as penile vibrostimulation and electroejaculation along with improved assisted reproductive technology.[24] A chart review by Kafetsoulis and associates[25] revealed successful semen retrieval by electroejaculation or vibrostimulation in 95% of the SCI cases reviewed. The risk of autonomic dysreflexia exists among susceptible patients with an injury level of T6 and above; therefore, assisted semen retrieval should be initiated by medical teams well trained in semen retrieval methods and the treatment of autonomic dysreflexia.[26]

Women with thoracic-level lesions may note changes in vaginal lubrication. However, at this level, women may achieve reflex lubrication, much like men achieve reflex erection.[22] Direct stimulation of the genital region may result in sufficient lubrication. A water-soluble lubricant is recommended for patients with complaints of decreased vaginal lubrication.

Orgasm for both men and women after injury may be nonexistent, described as a primarily emotional event, or a pleasurable sensation in the pelvic region or sensory level with generalized muscle relaxation.[22]

Women with thoracic-level SCI remain fertile. Contraceptive options include barrier methods (condoms, diaphragm) and oral contraceptives. Intrauterine contraceptive devices are contraindicated because of the lack of sensation and the risk for development of pelvic inflammatory disease. Patients with SCI are at increased risk for the development of thromboembolism, and the administration of oral contraceptives further increases this risk.

The care of pregnant women with SCI has special challenges. Potential complications include premature labor, increased risk of urinary tract infection, increased spasticity, autonomic dysreflexia, and constipation. In pregnancy, autonomic dysreflexia presents most frequently during labor; therefore, hemodynamic monitoring is considered for all at-risk patients.[27]

Pregnant women with thoracic SCI levels above T10 may be unable to sense fetal movements and contractions. Therefore, uterine palpation, serial cervical examinations,

and fetal monitoring may be recommended. Regional anesthesia is preferred.[28]

Deep Venous Thrombosis

The patient with SCI is often administered fractionated or unfractionated heparin during the initial weeks after injury. Thigh-high compression stockings and pneumatic compression boots may also be used in the initial postinjury period. For more details on the prevention and treatment of deep venous thrombosis, see Chapter 118.

Spasticity Management

Spasticity should be treated when it results in significant pain, contributes to contractures, impairs hygiene, interferes with functional tasks, or obstructs nursing care. In the first instance, clinically significant spasticity should be treated by removal of noxious stimuli that may be contributing to the condition, such as urinary tract infection, ingrown toenails, and tight clothing. Second, physical interventions such as daily stretching of muscles with terminal sustained stretch can be considered. If these are unsuccessful, medications such as tizanidine and baclofen can be prescribed (see Chapter 144 for details).

Heterotopic Ossification

Treatment may include the administration of etidronate, which limits ossification, and physical therapy to maintain range of motion (see Chapter 123).

Osteoporosis

Supplementation with vitamin D is often recommended, although calcium supplementation remains controversial because of the associated risk of urinary calculi.[20] Others have investigated the use of alendronate and cyclical etidronate in the prevention of osteoporosis in this population[9] (see Chapter 131).

Autonomic Dysreflexia

To treat autonomic dysreflexia, it is necessary to remove the precipitating noxious stimulus. Patients should be placed in an upright position, if possible, to decrease blood pressure, and a search for a causative agent is initiated. The majority of cases of autonomic dysreflexia are related to bladder distention or bowel distention.[13] However, noxious stimuli such as ingrown toenails, pressure ulcer, and renal calculi are not uncommon. Vasodilating medications such as nitropaste may be required to decrease the blood pressure while the clinician seeks the causative factor.[29] Nitrates are contraindicated in individuals who have ingested sildenafil, as the nitrates can potentiate the hypotensive effects of sildenafil and cause severe hypotension.[26] For more details on the treatment of dysreflexia, see Chapter 129.

Rehabilitation

Rehabilitation focuses on helping the patient to function at optimal levels. Thus, supervised physical or occupational therapy should address improvement of strength in all active muscle groups and range of motion in all joints.

Mobility is a major issue that needs to be addressed both initially and then periodically as the patient's condition changes (e.g., women who become pregnant may require assistance with functional activities as the pregnancy progresses).

Adaptive equipment, such as long-handled shoehorns and reachers, can be recommended.

Passive interventions, such as therapeutic heat and cold as well as transcutaneous electrical nerve stimulation, may be beneficial in the management of pain. However, particular caution must be used with therapeutic heat or cold modalities over insensate areas.

Physical interventions, such as daily stretching of muscles with terminal sustained stretch, can be considered a first-line rehabilitative treatment for spasticity. Positioning as well as casting and splinting of the affected limbs can minimize spasticity.

Procedures

A number of procedures can be used to address issues such as spasticity and pain. Interventional approaches for the treatment of spasticity include botulinum toxin injection, motor branch blocks, and peripheral nerve blocks (see Chapter 144). To decrease sphincter tone in men, botulinum toxin can be injected into the sphincter. This treatment in women is associated with an unacceptably high incidence of urinary incontinence. A patient with dysreflexia caused by a bladder stone may require a urologic procedure for stone removal. For men with ejaculatory dysfunction, retrieval of sperm for insemination has been successfully accomplished by electroejaculation and vibrostimulation methods. These procedures may result in dysreflexia and are performed under medical supervision.

Surgery

Pressure ulcers that do not heal with conservative methods may require surgical closure. Direct closure, skin grafts, musculocutaneous flaps, and skin flaps are among the surgical treatments available for wound closure. Mobilization after surgical closure must be done under close supervision, with careful monitoring of the surgical wound.

A variety of surgical procedures are used in patients who cannot be satisfactorily maintained on an intermittent catheterization program. Sphincter tone can be reduced with a sphincterotomy for men. Men must wear external collection devices after this procedure because it results in continuous incontinence. Sphincterotomies may occasionally require revision because of the development of fibrosis that obstructs outflow. Sphincterotomies may result in erectile dysfunction in some men. In contemporary practice, sphincterotomies are performed less frequently.

Bladder augmentation is occasionally performed to increase bladder capacity. A piece of small bowel is interposed with the bladder tissue to increase vesical volume. Patients with chronic dysreflexia resulting from persistent bowel management difficulties, such as frequent impaction, may be candidates for ileostomy or colostomy procedures. Patients with hemorrhoids aggravated by digital stimulation occasionally require surgical consultation if the hemorrhoids are not relieved by more conservative methods (e.g., medicated suppositories or topical steroid creams).

On occasion, men with erectile dysfunction that is not amenable to lesser invasive therapies may opt for an implantable penile prosthesis. Again, with the introduction of medications to treat erectile dysfunction, these surgeries are less frequently performed. Surgical placement of an intrathecal morphine or baclofen pump may be beneficial for patients with severe pain or spasticity that is not responsive to noninvasive treatments. Surgical interventions are indicated in some cases of heterotopic ossification. Patients with functionally limited joint mobility or severe and chronic spasticity may benefit from surgical resection of the lesion.

POTENTIAL DISEASE COMPLICATIONS

The literature suggests that individuals with thoracic-level SCIs are more likely to suffer from serious associated injuries than are those with cervical or lumbosacral lesions. In one study, patients with thoracic cord injuries had a 46% occurrence of serious associated injuries, such as hemothorax, pneumothorax, and intra-abdominal injuries, compared with 12% of patients with cervical injuries and 22% of patients with lumbar or caudal injuries.[30]

Thoracic SCI may be associated with a lower life expectancy. The leading causes of death among people with SCI in the Collaborative SCI Survival Study database include respiratory, cardiovascular, and infectious diseases.[1] Complications arising from a thoracic-level injury result from immobility, changing sensory patterns, and alterations in autonomic nervous system function.

POTENTIAL TREATMENT COMPLICATIONS

The anticholinergic side effects of tricyclic antidepressants, including dry mouth, blurred vision, and urinary retention, can pose additional difficulties for the patient with SCI. Sphincterotomies, performed to alleviate detrusor-sphincter dyssynergia, may result in urinary incontinence and occasionally sexual dysfunction in men. Voiding by the Credé maneuver may lead to vesicoureteral reflux. The long-term use of indwelling catheters is associated with prostatitis, epididymitis, strictures, bladder stones, and bladder carcinoma.

Digital stimulation of the bowel can result in autonomic dysreflexia and hemorrhoids.

Medications used to treat autonomic dysreflexia can result in hypotension. The blood pressure must be closely monitored.

When the less invasive methods of treating spasticity are ineffective, botulinum toxin injections, motor branch blocks, or peripheral nerve blocks may be considered. Injections may result in bleeding or infection. Nerve blocks may result in dysesthesias and weakness. Patients with intrathecal baclofen pumps may experience drowsiness, weakness, catheter breakage, or infection.

References

1. 2005 Annual Report for the Model Spinal Cord Injury Care Systems. Birmingham, Alabama, National Spinal Cord Injury Statistical Center, 2005.
2. Nesathurai S. Functional outcomes by level of injury. In Nesathurai S, ed. The Rehabilitation of People with Spinal Cord Injury. Malden, Mass, Blackwell Science, 2000:37-38.
3. Panjabi M, Koichiro T, Goel V, et al. Thoracic human vertebrae: quantitative three-dimensional anatomy. Spine 1991;16:888-901.
4. Yashon D. Spinal Injury. New York, Appleton-Century-Crofts, 1978:96.
5. McKinley WO, Jackson AB, Cardenas DD, DeVivo MJ. Long-term medical complications after traumatic spinal cord injury: a regional model systems analysis. Arch Phys Med Rehabil 1999;80:1402-1410.
6. Glover M. Pressure ulcers. In Nesathurai S, ed. The Rehabilitation of People with Spinal Cord Injury, 2nd ed. Malden, Mass, Blackwell Science, 2000:59-65.
7. Ducharme S, Gill K. Sexuality After Spinal Cord Injury. Baltimore, Brookes, 1997.
8. Consortium for Spinal Cord Medicine. Prevention of Thromboembolism in Spinal Cord Injury, 2nd ed. Washington, DC, Paralyzed Veterans of America, 1999.
9. Pearson E, Nance P, Leslie W, et al. Cyclical etidronate: its effects on bone density in patients with acute spinal cord injury. Arch Phys Med Rehabil 1997;78:269-272.
10. Maimoun L, Fattal C, Micallef JP, et al. Bone loss in spinal cord–injured patients: from physiopathology to therapy. Spinal Cord 2006;44:203-210.
11. Garland D. Heterotopic ossification. In Nesathurai S, ed. The Rehabilitation of People with Spinal Cord Injury, 2nd ed. Malden, Mass, Blackwell Science, 2000:81-83.
12. Stover SL, Niemann KM, Tulloss JR. Experience with surgical resection of heterotopic bone in spinal cord injury patients. Clin Orthop 1991;263:71-77.
13. Consortium for Spinal Cord Medicine. Acute Management of Autonomic Dysreflexia: Individuals with Spinal Cord Injury Presenting to Health Care Facilities, 2nd ed. Washington, DC, Paralyzed Veterans of America, 2001.
14. Vapnek J. Autonomic dysreflexia. Top Spinal Cord Inj Rehabil 1997;2:54-69.
15. Consortium for Spinal Cord Medicine. Autonomic Dysreflexia: What You Should Know. Consumer Guideline. Washington, DC, Paralyzed Veterans of America, 1997.
16. Cardenas DD, Bryce TN, Shem K, et al. Gender and minority differences in the pain experiences of people with spinal cord injury. Arch Phys Med Rehabil 2004;84:1774-1781.
17. Tasiemski T, Kennedy P, Gardner BP, Taylor N. The association of sports and physical recreation with life satisfaction in a community sample of people with spinal cord injuries. NeuroRehabilitation 2005;20:253-265.
18. Dryden DM, Saunders LD, Rowe BH, et al. Depression following traumatic spinal cord injury. Neuroepidemiology 2005;25:55-61.
19. Bergman S. Bowel management. In Nesathurai S, ed. The Rehabilitation of People with Spinal Cord Injury, 2nd ed. Malden, Mass, Blackwell Science, 2000:53-58.
20. Roaf E. Aging and spinal cord injury. In Nesathurai S, ed. The Rehabilitation of People with Spinal Cord Injury, 2nd ed. Malden, Mass, Blackwell Science, 2000:95-101.
21. Hess MJ, Zhan EH, Foo DK, Yalla SV. Bladder cancer in patients with spinal cord injury. J Spinal Cord Med 2003;26:335-338.
22. Ducharme S. Sexuality and spinal cord injury. In Nesathurai S, ed. The Rehabilitation of People with Spinal Cord Injury, 2nd ed. Malden, Mass, Blackwell Science, 2000:89-94.
23. Monga M, Bernie J, Rajasekaran M. Male infertility and erectile dysfunction in spinal cord injury: a review. Arch Phys Med Rehabil 1999;80:1331-1337.
24. Elliott S. Sexual dysfunction and infertility in men with spinal cord disorders. In Lin V, ed. Spinal Cord Medicine: Principles and Practice. New York, Demos, 2003:349-365.
25. Kafetsoulis A, Brackett NL, Ibrahim E, et al. Current trends in the treatment of infertility in men with spinal cord injury. Fertil Steril 2006;86:781-789.
26. Elliott S. Sexual dysfunction and infertility in men with spinal cord disorders. In Lin V, ed. Spinal Cord Medicine: Principles and Practice. New York, Demos, 2003:349-365.
27. American College of Obstetricians and Gynecologists. ACOG Committee Opinion: Number 275, September 2002. Obstetric management of patients with spinal cord injuries. Obstet Gynecol 2002;100:625-627.
28. Kang AH. Traumatic spinal cord injury. Clin Obstet Gynecol 2005;48:67-72.
29. DeSantis N. Autonomic dysfunction. In Nesathurai S, ed. The Rehabilitation of People with Spinal Cord Injury, 2nd ed. Malden, Mass, Blackwell Science, 2000:71-74.
30. Ducker T, Saul T. The poly-trauma and spinal cord injury. In Tator C, ed. Early Management of Acute Spinal Cord Injury. New York, Raven Press, 1982:53-58.

Spinal Cord Injury (Lumbosacral) **148**

Sunil Sabharwal, MD

Synonyms

Paraplegia
Conus medullaris syndrome
Cauda equina syndrome

ICD-9 Codes

344.1   Paraplegia
344.6   Cauda equina syndrome
344.9   Paralysis, unspecified
806.4   Fracture of the vertebral column with spinal cord injury: lumbar
806.6   Fracture of the vertebral column with spinal cord injury: sacral

DEFINITION

Lumbosacral spinal cord injury (SCI) refers to impairment or loss of motor or sensory function in the lumbar or sacral segments of the spinal cord, secondary to damage of neural elements within the spinal canal.[1] With this level of injury, arm and trunk functions are spared, but the legs and pelvic organs are involved.

The terms *lumbosacral* SCI and *paraplegia* are also used in referring to cauda equina and conus medullaris injuries but not to impaired sensorimotor function due to neural involvement outside the spinal canal (as in lumbosacral plexus lesions or injury to peripheral nerves). Conus medullaris syndrome results from an injury to the sacral spinal cord (conus) and lumbar nerve roots within the spinal canal. Cauda equina syndrome refers to injury to the lumbosacral nerve roots within the neural canal.

Lumbosacral injuries account for about 11% of SCI cases in the National Model Spinal Cord Injury Systems database.[2] Overall, the most common cause is motor vehicle crashes, followed in order by falls, acts of violence, and recreational sporting activities.[3,4] There is an association between level of injury and cause of injury, and acts of violence are more often associated with paraplegia than with cervical injury and tetraplegia.[2]

Neurologic versus Skeletal Level of Injury

Lumbosacral SCI refers to the neurologic level of injury, which is different from the skeletal level of injury. Because of the discrepancy between the length of the spinal cord and the vertebral column, the L1-5 lumbar spinal cord segments are typically located at the T11-12 vertebral level, and the S1-5 sacral spinal cord segments are at the L1 vertebral level. The spinal cord ends between T12 and L2 (most often at L1 vertebra), and injury within the neural canal below that bony level involves the cauda equina. Lesions at the level of the lowermost thoracic and first lumbar vertebrae may result in mixed cauda equina and conus medullaris lesions.

SYMPTOMS

Lumbosacral SCI may present with weakness in the lower extremities, numbness and tingling, bladder and bowel disturbances (urinary retention, constipation, bladder or bowel incontinence), impotence, back pain, and burning perianal or lower extremity pain.

In the outpatient setting, patients may also present with secondary conditions and associated problems, such as urinary tract infections or pressure ulcers. Patients with SCI may have vague, atypical, or nonspecific symptoms. Classic symptoms of urinary tract infection, such as urinary frequency, urgency, and dysuria, may be absent, and patients may present instead with an increased frequency of spontaneous voiding or increased muscle spasms.[5] Fever and malaise may be indicative of a urinary tract infection but can also be due to other infections (such as osteomyelitis underlying a pressure ulcer) or noninfectious causes, such as osteoporotic long bone fracture, deep venous thrombosis, heterotopic ossification, or drug fever (e.g., due to antibiotics). Unilateral leg swelling may be the only presentation of osteoporotic lower limb fractures but could also be due to deep venous thrombosis, heterotopic ossification, hematoma, or cellulitis in the setting of SCI.[6]

Pain is a common symptom in people with SCI, and some studies suggest that pain prevalence may be even higher with paraplegia than with cervical injury and tetraplegia.[7,8] A comprehensive history of pain characteristics is needed to accurately determine the underlying cause, which may be mechanical, neuropathic, or a combination of both. New weakness or sensory deficits in the upper extremities may indicate post-traumatic syringomyelia extending into the cervical spinal cord or a peripheral nerve entrapment, such as the median nerve at the carpal tunnel or ulnar nerve at the elbow.[9] Patients with chronic SCI who present with extension or worsening of lower extremity weakness or numbness may have post-traumatic syringomyelia or spinal cord or nerve root compression due to progressive spinal deformity or instability.

Rectal bleeding is often caused by hemorrhoids but may be a manifestation of more sinister disease, such as colorectal cancer.[10] Similarly, hematuria may be due to urinary tract infection, stones, or catheter-induced trauma, but bladder cancer should be considered in the differential diagnosis, especially in smokers and those with chronic indwelling bladder catheters.[5]

Mood disturbances are common in SCI.[11] Depression may present with somatic symptoms such as appetite change and sleep disturbance, although symptoms like loss of energy may be difficult to interpret in the setting of SCI.[11,12] Because many medical diseases may produce similar somatic symptoms, it is helpful to inquire about specific symptoms typically associated with depression, such as suicidal thoughts, dysphoria, and feelings of hopelessness and worthlessness. Early morning awakening is suggestive of primary depression, and fatigue caused by depression is often worse in the morning.

PHYSICAL EXAMINATION

Spinal Inspection and Palpation

There may be reduced lumbar lordosis due to muscle spasm from pain. Spine fractures may result in deformity, and palpation may reveal areas of tenderness.

Evidence of Concurrent Injuries

Concurrent injuries, including head injury, extremity fractures, and abdominal visceral injury, may accompany lumbosacral SCI and should be considered during diagnostic examination.

Neurologic Examination

Neurologic examination is conducted in accordance with *International Standards for Neurological and Functional Classification of Spinal Cord Injury* published by the American Spinal Injury Association.[1] The neurologic findings may sometimes be subtle (e.g., limited to perineal anesthesia or urinary retention) and can be missed in the setting of acute trauma with routine placement of an indwelling catheter or drug-induced sedation, unless they are carefully considered.[13] The neurologic examination should be repeated at regular intervals to monitor for improvement or deterioration.[14]

Sensory Examination

The required portion of the sensory examination is completed through testing of key points in each dermatome on the right and left sides of the body (Table 148-1) for pinprick (tested with a disposable safety pin) and light touch sensation (tested with cotton). Pinprick and light touch sensation are separately scored at each key point on a 3-point scale: 0, absent; 1, impaired; and 2, normal. In testing for pinprick sensation, inability to distinguish dull from sharp sensation is graded 0.

Motor Examination

Muscle strength is graded on a 6-point scale of 0 to 5; 0 is no contraction and 5 is normal strength. For the lumbosacral myotomes, five key muscle groups are tested bilaterally (Table 148-2).

Neurologic Rectal Examination

Neurologic rectal examination includes determination of deep anal sensation and testing for voluntary contraction of the external anal sphincter around the examiner's finger (graded as present or absent). If there is

TABLE 148-1 Key Sensory Points for Lumbosacral Spinal Segments

Level	Key Sensory Point
T12	Inguinal ligament at midpoint
L1	Half the distance between T12 and L2
L2	Mid anterior thigh
L3	Medial femoral condyle
L4	Medial malleolus
L5	Dorsum of the foot at the third metatarsophalangeal joint
S1	Lateral heel
S2	Popliteal fossa in the midline
S3	Ischial tuberosity
S4-5	Perianal area (taken as one level)

TABLE 148-2 Key Muscle Groups for Lumbosacral Myotomes

Level	Muscle Group
L2	Hip flexors (iliopsoas)
L3	Knee extensors (quadriceps)
L4	Ankle dorsiflexors (tibialis anterior)
L5	Long toe extensors (extensor hallucis longus)
S1	Ankle plantar flexors (gastrocnemius, soleus)

voluntary contraction of the anal sphincter, the patient has a motor incomplete injury.

Additional Neurologic Examination

In addition to these required elements for neurologic classification of SCI, position and deep pressure sensation and muscle strength of additional lower extremity muscles, such as medial hamstrings and hip adductors, are also tested. Examination also includes assessment of muscle stretch reflexes, muscle tone, anal sphincter tone, bulbocavernosus reflex, and plantar reflexes.

Conus Medullaris and Cauda Equina Injuries

The examination will vary with the level of damage and the relative involvement of the conus and cauda equina and may include evidence of lower or upper motor neuron involvement. Patients with injury above the conus medullaris typically present with signs consistent with upper motor neuron or suprasacral SCI, whereas those with injury below this level present with a clinical picture consistent with lower motor neuron impairment. Lesions affecting the transition between the two regions (typically around L1 vertebral-level injury) can have a mixed picture. Conus medullaris lesions typically result in impaired sensation over the sacral dermatomes (saddle and perineal anesthesia), lax anal sphincter with loss of anal and bulbocavernosus reflexes, and sometimes weakness in the lower extremity muscles. Cauda equina involvement results in asymmetric atrophic, areflexic paralysis, radicular sensory loss, and sphincter impairment.[1,13]

Skin Examination

Skin examination is conducted with particular attention to the areas most vulnerable to pressure ulcer development. These include the sacrum-coccyx, heels, trochanters, and ischial tuberosities.[15]

FUNCTIONAL LIMITATIONS

Lumbosacral SCI can result in significant functional deficits. These include impaired mobility due to lower extremity paralysis and bladder, bowel, and sexual dysfunction due to autonomic dysregulation.

Expected Functional Outcomes

Predictions of function can be based on completeness and level of injury. The Consortium for Spinal Cord Medicine has developed clinical practice guidelines on outcomes after SCI with expected functional outcomes for each level of injury in a number of domains.[14] Expected outcomes for complete lumbosacral SCI are summarized in Table 148-3.

Ambulation

People with lumbosacral SCI should generally be independent at the wheelchair level and have the greatest potential for ambulation. If hip flexors and knee extensors demonstrate even minimal strength in the first few days after injury, functional recovery and community ambulation are likely. It has been reported that to ambulate independently after SCI,

TABLE 148-3 Expected Functional Outcomes for Motor Complete Lumbosacral Spinal Cord Injury

Domain	Expected Functional Outcome	Equipment
Bowel	Independent	Padded toilet seat
Bladder	Independent	
Bed mobility	Independent	Full to king size standard bed
Bed and wheelchair transfers	Independent	
Pressure relief	Independent	Wheelchair pressure relief cushion
Wheelchair propulsion	Independent indoor and outdoor	Manual lightweight wheelchair
Standing, ambulation	Standing: independent	Standing frame
	Ambulation: functional, some assist to independent	Knee-ankle-foot orthosis or ankle-foot orthosis
	L1-2: household ambulation	Forearm crutches or cane as indicated
	L3-S5: community ambulation	
Eating, grooming, dressing, bathing	Independent	Padded tub bench Hand-held shower
Communication	Independent	
Transportation	Independent in car, including loading and unloading wheelchair	Hand controls
Homemaking	Independent complex cooking and light housekeeping, some assist with heavy housekeeping	

Modified from Consortium for Spinal Cord Medicine. Outcomes Following Traumatic Spinal Cord Injury. Clinical Practice Guidelines for Health Care Professionals. Washington, DC, Paralyzed Veterans of America, 1999.

individuals need pelvic control, grade 3/5 (antigravity) hip extensor strength bilaterally to advance the lower extremities, and antigravity knee extensor strength on at least one side (so that no more than one knee-ankle-foot orthosis is needed).[16] There is individual variation and additional factors than have an impact on ambulation outcome, but patients with motor complete lumbosacral SCI at the L1-2 level can in general be expected to be household ambulators; community ambulation is an appropriate goal at L3-S5 levels.[16]

Bowel, Bladder, and Sexual Dysfunction

Bowel, bladder, and sexual dysfunction may be significantly disabling in these patients. SCI above the sacral segments is typically associated with an upper motor neuron or reflexic bowel; lesions involving the S2-4 anterior horn cells or cauda equina have areflexic or lower motor neuron bowel characterized by slow stool propulsion, dry and round stool referred to as scybalous, and risk of incontinence due to denervation of the external anal sphincter.[10,17] Depending on the location of injury and the extent of upper and lower motor neuron impairment, hyperreflexic, areflexic, or mixed type of neurogenic bladder may occur. Absent bulbocavernosus reflex and muscle stretch reflexes in the lower extremities suggest the likelihood of lower motor neuron impairment of the bladder and bowel. Sexual dysfunction is frequent.[18] Men with SCI at the sacral level often lose ability to have reflex erections, although psychogenic erections may be preserved in some. Ejaculation is often impaired, but it may be preserved in a higher proportion of those with incomplete lower motor neuron injuries.

Factors Affecting Functional Outcomes

Pain, whether nociceptive or neurogenic, may interfere with function.[7,19] Neuropathic pain is more common with cauda equina injuries than with injury limited to the conus medullaris. Age, concurrent injuries or comorbidities, body habitus, psychosocial and cultural factors, and personal goals and motivation can significantly affect functional outcomes.

DIAGNOSTIC STUDIES

Spinal Imaging

Radiologic and laboratory studies are used to localize the site of the pathologic change and the underlying cause.[13] Plain radiographs typically include anteroposterior, lateral, and oblique views. The entire spine should be visualized because multiple levels of injury are not unusual. Computed tomographic scanning allows optimal visualization of bone injury and canal occlusion due to bone fragments. Magnetic resonance imaging is especially helpful because of its ability to visualize the soft tissues, including ligamentous structures, intravertebral discs, epidural or subdural hematomas, and

hemorrhage or edema in the spinal cord. Magnetic resonance imaging with gadolinium is helpful in diagnosis of post-traumatic syringomyelia.

Electrodiagnostic Testing

Electromyography and nerve conduction studies may be helpful in distinguishing lesions of the spinal cord or cauda equina from those of the lumbar plexus or peripheral nerves.

Urologic Studies

Urodynamic studies are useful to assess the type and extent of neurogenic bladder and sphincter dysfunction. Periodic cystoscopy may be indicated in those with chronic indwelling urinary catheters because of increased risk of bladder cancer.[20] Studies to evaluate upper urinary tracts in patients with neurogenic bladder include renal ultrasonography, renal scan, abdominal radiography, intravenous pyelography, and abdominal computed tomography, but there currently is not a consensus on the type, indication, or frequency of these tests.

Differential Diagnosis

Lumbar spinal stenosis with spinal cord or cauda equina compression

Primary or metastatic spinal tumors

Spinal infections or abscess

Lesions of the lumbosacral plexus

Disorders involving multiple nerves (e.g., polyneuropathy, Guillain-Barré syndrome)

TREATMENT

Initial

Initial management[13] of anyone thought to have sustained spinal injury includes adequate immobilization, with placement on a board in the neutral supine position. Stabilization of the airway and hemodynamic status takes precedence in the setting of acute trauma. Methylprednisolone has been advocated in patients presenting within 8 hours of SCI, although effectiveness of this pharmacologic intervention is not uniformly accepted.

Rehabilitation

Information about potential for motor recovery can be used to set functional goals and to plan for equipment needs (see Table 148-3), keeping in mind that individual factors and coexisting conditions may affect achievable goals.[14] Important elements of rehabilitation include an interdisciplinary approach, establishment of an individualized rehabilitation program with consideration of unique barriers and facilitators, and inclusion of the patient as an active participant in establishment of goals.[16]

Bowel Management

An individualized bowel care program should be established.[10,17] For upper motor neuron (reflexic) bowel dysfunction, this includes digital rectal stimulation. For lower motor neuron (areflexic) bowel dysfunction, reflex stimulation will not be effective; digital manual evacuation by gloved lubricated fingers is needed, along with Valsalva maneuver or abdominal massage to increase pressure around the colon to push the stool out. Manual disimpaction is aided by use of bulking agents to keep stool consistency firm.

Bladder Management

Optimal bladder management minimizes urinary tract complications, preserves upper urinary tracts, and is compatible with the individual's lifestyle.[20] Because hand function is intact in individuals with lumbosacral injuries, they should be able to perform intermittent catheterization if it is needed for bladder management. If there is abnormal urethral anatomy, poor cognition or unwillingness to adhere to the catheterization schedule, or high fluid intake with consistently large bladder volumes, indwelling catheterization may be needed. Condom catheters can be an appropriate option for urinary drainage in men, provided low-pressure and complete voiding can be documented. For patients with lower motor neuron injuries with low outlet resistance, the use of Credé and Valsalva maneuvers may be considered.

In patients with suspected urinary tract infection, empirical antibiotic treatment may be started while waiting for urine culture results and modified as needed once results are available.[5] The presence of urinary tract obstruction, stones, reflux, abscess, or prostatitis should be considered if the patient fails to respond to antibiotic therapy or has a rapid recurrence with the same organism. Use of prophylactic antibiotics is usually not warranted but should be considered before urologic testing that involves instrumentation, especially in the presence of bacteriuria. Antibiotics to treat asymptomatic bacteriuria in patients with chronic indwelling bladder catheters are generally not indicated.

Pain and Spasticity

Nociceptive causes of pain should be identified and addressed.[19] Many medications, including anticonvulsants and tricyclic antidepressants, have been tried in management of neuropathic pain after SCI, but none has been shown to be consistently effective. Nonpharmacologic interventions and education of the patient are important and should not be ignored. Transcutaneous nerve stimulation may help pain originating at the level of injury. Opioid prescription may be needed for pain unresponsive to other measures. Minimization of extreme or potentially injurious positions at all joints, reduction in the frequency of repetitive upper extremity tasks, proper instruction in transfer techniques to minimize upper extremity injury, optimal

wheelchair selection and training, and incorporation of upper body flexibility and resistance exercises are important in preserving upper extremity function and reducing chronic pain due to upper extremity overuse.[21]

Spasticity is less of a problem in lumbosacral SCI than in cervical or high thoracic injuries. Management of spasticity[22] includes elimination of the underlying noxious stimulus, use of physical interventions, systemic medications, chemical denervation, intrathecal agents, and rarely orthopedic or neurosurgical procedures. Nonpharmacologic interventions include positioning and stretching (e.g., prone lying to stretch hip flexors and stretching of hamstrings and heel cords to prevent tightness and contractures). Several medications are used for treatment of SCI-related spasticity, including baclofen, tizanidine, gabapentin, and benzodiazepines, but a systematic review found insufficient evidence of effectiveness.[23]

Pressure Ulcer Prevention

Education of the patient is critical in this area. Avoidance of prolonged positional immobilization, institution of pressure relief, and prescription of pressure-reducing seating systems and support surfaces are important in prevention of pressure ulcers. Daily comprehensive skin inspections should be carried out with particular attention to vulnerable insensate areas (e.g., sacrum-coccyx, ischii, trochanters, heels). Adequate nutritional intake and smoking cessation should be stressed.[15]

Procedures

Spasticity

Motor point or nerve blocks with phenol or alcohol may be helpful in treatment of localized lower extremity spasticity (e.g., for hip adductors or ankle plantar flexors) that interferes with positioning, mobility, or hygiene. Intramuscular injections of botulinum toxin are another option.

Pain

Shoulder pain due to subacromial bursitis may be temporarily responsive to local corticosteroid injections, as is the discomfort from carpal tunnel syndrome.

Pressure Ulcers

Sharp débridement of pressure ulcers may be done at the bedside to remove necrotic tissue, although if it is extensive, débridement may need to be done in the operating room.

Surgery

Spine Surgery

When thoracolumbar fractures associated with lumbosacral SCI are accompanied by mechanical instability, pain, deformity, or progressive neural impairment, surgical decompression and segmental instrumentation may be indicated for reconstruction of spinal alignment, stability, and early mobilization.[13,24] The ideal timing of and indications for surgical intervention remain controversial.

Pressure Ulcers

Plastic surgery may be indicated for deep pressure ulcers. This includes excision of the ulcer and surrounding scar and muscle and musculocutaneous flap closure.[4]

Upper Extremity Pain

Surgery may sometimes be considered for chronic upper extremity overuse-related symptoms that are unresponsive to medical and rehabilitative treatment (e.g., for carpal tunnel syndrome or rotator cuff disease). Outcomes are often poor, especially if upper extremity overuse continues.[21]

Bladder and Bowel Dysfunction

Surgical treatment of urolithiasis includes cystoscopic removal of bladder stones, lithotripsy, and percutaneous nephrolithotomy for larger renal stones. Endourethral stents or transurethral sphincterotomy may be considered in individuals with detrusor-sphincter dyssynergia.[20] Patients with neurogenic bowel who have significant difficulty or complications with typical bowel care may be candidates for colostomy. This decision requires careful selection of the patient and individualization to make sure that it is appropriate.[17]

Post-traumatic Syringomyelia

Surgical placement of shunts may be indicated for post-traumatic syringomyelia associated with intractable pain or progressive neurologic decline.

POTENTIAL DISEASE COMPLICATIONS

Patients with lumbosacral SCI are prone to multiple complications. Urinary tract infections and pressure ulcers are two of the most common causes of hospitalization in individuals with paraplegia and can result in systemic sepsis.[25] Delayed neurologic deterioration may be due to spinal instability, progressive spinal deformity, or post-traumatic syringomyelia. Upper extremity overuse can result in shoulder pain due to rotator cuff injury or entrapment neuropathies, such as carpal tunnel syndrome.[21] Lower extremity joint contractures (e.g., of the heel cords) can interfere with mobility and with wheelchair positioning. Untreated high bladder pressure in patients with detrusor-sphincter dyssynergia or low bladder compliance may result in upper urinary tract damage. Potential complications of neurogenic bowel include anorectal problems (hemorrhoids, fissures), toxic megacolon, and colonic perforation.

POTENTIAL TREATMENT COMPLICATIONS

Neurologic deterioration may occur from inadequate spinal immobilization or as a complication of surgical instrumentation. Other surgical complications include

dural tears with cerebrospinal fluid leaks, infections at the surgical site, pseudarthrosis (which may cause progressive deformity), and chronic pain.

Because people with SCI are often prescribed multiple medications (e.g., to treat pain, spasticity, and bladder or bowel dysfunction), medication-related side effects and complications are common. Complications of urethral catheterization include urethral trauma, erosions, strictures, urinary infections, and epididymitis.[20] Chronic indwelling catheters increase the risk of stones and squamous cell carcinoma of the bladder.

References

1. American Spinal Injury Association. International Standards for Neurological and Functional Classification of Spinal Cord Injury, revised 2002. Chicago, American Spinal Injury Association, 2002.
2. DeVivo MJ. Epidemiology of traumatic spinal cord injury. In Kirshblum SC, Campagnolo D, DeLisa JE, eds. Spinal Cord Medicine. Philadelphia, Lippincott Williams & Wilkins, 2002:69-81.
3. National Spinal Cord Injury Statistical Center. Spinal cord injury: facts and figures at a glance. J Spinal Cord Med 2005;28:379-380.
4. Jackson AB, Dijkers M, DeVivo MJ, et al. Demographic profile of new spinal cord injury: changes and stability over 30 years. Arch Phys Med Rehabil 2004;85:1740-1748.
5. Till M, Pertel P. Infections. In Green D, ed. Medical Management of Long-Term Disability. Boston, Butterworth-Heinemann, 1996:233-262.
6. McKinley WO, Gittler MS, Kirshblum SC, et al. Spinal cord injury medicine. 2. Medical complications after spinal cord injury: identification and management. Arch Phys Med Rehabil 2002;83 (Suppl 1):S58-S64.
7. Cardenas DD, Bryce TN, Shem K, et al. Gender and minority differences in the pain experience of people with spinal cord injury. Arch Phys Med Rehabil 2004;85:1774-1781.
8. Rintala DH, Loubser PG, Castro J, et al. Chronic pain in a community-based sample of men with spinal cord injury: prevalence, severity, and relationship with impairment, disability, handicap, and subjective well-being. Arch Phys Med Rehabil 1998;79:604-614.
9. Little JW, Burns SP. Neuromusculoskeletal complications of spinal cord injury. In Kirshblum SC, Campagnolo D, DeLisa JE, eds. Spinal Cord Medicine. Philadelphia, Lippincott Williams & Wilkins, 2002:241-252.
10. Steins SA, Bergman SB, Goetz LL. Neurogenic bowel dysfunction after spinal cord injury: clinical evaluation and rehabilitative management. Arch Phys Med Rehabil 1997;78:S86-S100.
11. Consortium for Spinal Cord Medicine. Depression Following Spinal Cord Injury. Clinical Practice Guidelines for Health Care Professionals. Washington, DC, Paralyzed Veterans of America, 1998. Available at: www.pva.org.
12. Bombardier CH, Richards S, Krause JS, et al. Symptoms of major depression in people with spinal cord injury: implications for screening. Arch Phys Med Rehabil 2004;85:1749-1756.
13. Harrop JS, Hunt GE Jr, Vaccaro AR. Conus medullaris and cauda equina syndrome as a result of traumatic injuries: management principles. Neurosurg Focus 2004;16:19-23.
14. Consortium for Spinal Cord Medicine. Outcomes Following Traumatic Spinal Cord Injury. Clinical Practice Guidelines for Health Care Professionals. Washington, DC, Paralyzed Veterans of America, 1999. Available at: www.pva.org.
15. Consortium for Spinal Cord Medicine. Pressure Ulcer Prevention and Treatment Following Spinal Cord Injury. Clinical Practice Guidelines for Health Care Professionals. Washington, DC, Paralyzed Veterans of America, 2000. Available at: www.pva.org.
16. Kirshblum SC, Ho C, Druin E, at al. Rehabilitation after spinal cord injury. In Kirshblum SC, Campagnolo D, DeLisa JE, eds. Spinal Cord Medicine. Philadelphia, Lippincott Williams & Wilkins, 2002:275-298.

17. Consortium for Spinal Cord Medicine. Neurogenic Bowel Management in Adults with Spinal Cord Injury. Clinical Practice Guidelines for Health Care Professionals. Washington, DC, Paralyzed Veterans of America, 1998. Available at: www.pva.org.

18. Linsenmeyer TA. Sexual function and fertility following spinal cord injury. In Kirshblum SC, Campagnolo D, DeLisa JE, eds. Spinal Cord Medicine. Philadelphia, Lippincott Williams & Wilkins, 2002:322-330.

19. Bryce TN, Ragnarsson KT. Pain after spinal cord injury. Phys Med Rehabil Clin North Am 2000;11:157-168.

20. Consortium for Spinal Cord Medicine. Bladder Management for Adults with Spinal Cord Injury. Clinical Practice Guidelines for Health Care Professionals. Washington, DC, Paralyzed Veterans of America, 2006. Available at: www.pva.org.

21. Consortium for Spinal Cord Medicine. Preservation of Upper Limb Function Following Spinal Cord Injury. Clinical Practice Guidelines for Health Care Professionals. Washington, DC, Paralyzed Veterans of America, 2005. Available at: www.pva.org.

22. Kirshblum S. Treatment alternatives for spinal cord injury–related spasticity. J Spinal Cord Med 1999;22:199-217.

23. Taricco M, Pagliacci MC, Telaro E, Adone R. Pharmacological interventions for spasticity following spinal cord injury: results of a Cochrane Systematic Review. Eur Medicophys 2006;42:5-15.

24. McLain RF. Summary statement—thoracolumbar spine trauma. Spine 2006;31(Suppl):S103.

25. Cardenas DD, Hoffman JM, Kirshblum S, et al. Etiology and incidence of rehospitalization after traumatic spinal cord injury. Arch Phys Med Rehabil 2004;85:1757-1763.

Stroke 149

Joel Stein, MD

Synonyms

Cerebrovascular accident
Brain attack

ICD-9 Codes

430   Subarachnoid hemorrhage
431   Intracerebral hemorrhage
432   Other and unspecified intracranial hemorrhage
433   Occlusion and stenosis of precerebral arteries
434   Occlusion of cerebral arteries
435   Transient cerebral ischemia
436   Acute but ill-defined cerebrovascular disease
437   Other and ill-defined cerebrovascular disease
438   Late effects of cerebrovascular disease

DEFINITION

Stroke is an acquired injury of the brain caused by occlusion of a blood vessel or inadequate blood supply leading to infarction, or a hemorrhage within the parenchyma of the brain.

SYMPTOMS

Weakness, difficulty in speaking or swallowing, aphasia, cognitive disturbance, sensory loss, and visual disturbance are the most common presenting symptoms of stroke, and deficits in these areas often persist even after initial rehabilitation. Urinary urgency, increased muscle tone, fatigue, depression, and pain are symptoms that may be manifested after a stroke has already occurred. Reflex sympathetic dystrophy (also known as complex regional pain syndrome type I) may occur after stroke, although most post-stroke pain results from mechanical (e.g., joint subluxation) or central (e.g., thalamic pain syndromes) causes.

PHYSICAL EXAMINATION

A full neurologic examination is appropriate. This includes evaluation of mental status, cranial nerves, sensation, deep tendon reflexes, abnormal reflexes (e.g., Babinski), motor strength and coordination, muscle tone, and functional mobility (sitting, transfers, and ambulation). The protean manifestations of stroke can cause many different combinations of abnormalities in these aspects of the neurologic examination. An assessment of mood and affect is important, given the high prevalence of post-stroke depression. Range of motion in affected limbs should be measured; ankle plantar flexion contractures and upper limb contractures are common in hemiplegic stroke and interfere with rehabilitation efforts. Skin is examined for any areas of breakdown. Limb swelling is common and should be noted. The fit and function of leg braces, upper extremity splints, slings, wheelchairs, and ambulatory aids are assessed as part of the routine physical examination.

FUNCTIONAL LIMITATIONS

Difficulties in walking, performing activities of daily living, speaking, and swallowing are common manifestations of stroke. Cognitive impairments (memory, attention, visual-spatial perception) and impaired communication due to aphasia or dysarthria may be present. The impairments seen in stroke are based on the anatomy of the stroke; aphasia is generally a result of left hemisphere damage, and neglect and attentional deficits are more common with right hemisphere strokes. Impaired sexual function should be identified because patients may not volunteer functional impairments in this area unless the physician inquires.

As a result of these impairments, many individuals may be unable to drive or to use public transportation. Communication difficulties can lead to social isolation. Some individuals require ongoing supervision because of cognitive limitations. In severe cases, individuals with aphasia or cognitive impairments may not be able to live independently. Incontinence due to detrusor instability and urinary urgency can interfere with leaving the home and contribute to skin breakdown and social isolation.

Depression is common after stroke, affecting as many as 40% of stroke survivors. Depression should be identified as a treatable complication of stroke rather than accepted as a consequence of functional loss.

Among stroke survivors older than 65 years who were evaluated 6 months after a stroke, 30% were unable to walk without some assistance, 26% were dependent for activities of daily living, and 26% were institutionalized in a nursing home.[1]

DIAGNOSTIC STUDIES

In the acute setting, computed tomography is often the first diagnostic test performed because of the rapidity with which it can be obtained, its widespread availability, and its high sensitivity for cerebral hemorrhage. Magnetic resonance imaging provides greater anatomic resolution and avoids radiation exposure. With newer magnetic resonance imaging sequences, such as diffusion-weighted imaging, abnormalities can be demonstrated at an earlier stage than with computed tomography, providing important information for acute treatments such as thrombolysis.[2] Magnetic resonance angiography, computed tomographic angiography, noninvasive flow studies, Holter monitoring, and echocardiography are important studies to help determine the cause of a stroke and to determine the best treatment for prevention of recurrent stroke. In selected patients (particularly young individuals or those without typical risk factors), an evaluation for hypercoagulable states is indicated.

In patients with prior stroke, diagnostic studies are typically directed to complications of stroke, such as persistent dysphagia or urinary incontinence. Videofluoroscopic swallowing studies can be useful in swallowing disorders. Urodynamic studies may be useful in the assessment of urinary symptoms, particularly if initial treatment with anticholinergic medications is unsuccessful.

Differential Diagnosis

Hemiplegic migraine

Post-seizure (Todd) paralysis

Brain neoplasm

Multiple sclerosis

TREATMENT

Initial

When ischemic stroke is diagnosed within the first 3 hours, thrombolytic therapy has been shown to reduce disability.[3] In other cases, intravenous heparin is commonly administered when an embolic etiology is suspected. Aspirin (between 80 and 325 mg) has been found to be effective when it is used in the acute setting.

Secondary prevention depends on the cause of the stroke. Warfarin (Coumadin) is commonly used for the secondary prevention of embolic stroke, with the most extensive evidence for prevention of stroke in atrial fibrillation.[4] Antiplatelet agents, including aspirin, clopidogrel (Plavix), or a combination of aspirin and dipyridamole (Aggrenox), are used for prevention of most non-cardioembolic strokes or when anticoagulation is desirable but contraindicated because of comorbid conditions. Risk factor modification, including treatment of hypertension, diabetes, hyperlipidemia, and obesity as well as smoking cessation and exercise, should be addressed for all stroke survivors.[5]

Treatment of cerebral hemorrhage is based in part on the presumed cause. For hypertensive hemorrhages, control of blood pressure with antihypertensive medications is the mainstay of treatment. For all causes of cerebral hemorrhage, avoidance of anticoagulants, antiplatelet medications, and alcohol is important.[6]

Medications for the management of stroke and its complications on an outpatient basis are shown in Table 149-1. Anticholinergic medications are useful for bladder detrusor instability. Antispasticity medications are of limited efficacy in many cases (see Chapter 144). For sexual dysfunction in men, phosphodiesterase type 5 inhibitors may be effective. Treatment with selective serotonin reuptake inhibitors for post-stroke depression is widely employed, although a wide range of antidepressant medications can be effective. Psychostimulants may be useful for impaired attention. Anticonvulsants are used for central pain syndromes, but with variable benefit.

Rehabilitation

The rehabilitation program needs to be customized on the basis of the severity and nature of the impairments caused by the stroke. For individuals with moderate to severe stroke, a comprehensive multidisciplinary inpatient rehabilitation program in a rehabilitation hospital is often appropriate.[7] For these individuals, rehabilitation commonly continues through home care or outpatient services. Patients with more isolated and less severe deficits may be discharged directly from the acute care hospital to home and participate in an outpatient rehabilitation program.[8]

Exercise

Therapeutic exercise programs are usually functionally oriented, with an emphasis on restoration of functional mobility and ability to perform activities of daily living (Fig. 149-1). Instruction in compensatory techniques and family teaching are important in assisting individuals to return home. There is growing evidence of the impact of therapeutic exercise on cortical reorganization after stroke, with associated improvements in motor control and functional use.[9] Newer approaches being studied to enhance motor abilities include constraint-induced movement therapy, robot-assisted exercise training, virtual reality exercise training, and partial body weight–supported treadmill training.[10-15] These novel techniques appear to improve motor function, but the optimal exercise program to facilitate recovery remains to be defined.

TABLE 149-1 Medications Commonly Used for Treatment of Stroke and Its Complications

Class of Medication	Examples	Indication
Anticholinergics	Oxybutynin (Ditropan) Tolterodine (Detrol)	Bladder detrusor instability
Antispasticity	Baclofen (Lioresal) Tizanidine (Zanaflex) Diazepam (Valium) Dantrolene (Dantrium)	Muscle spasticity
Phosphodiesterase type 5 inhibitors	Sildenafil (Viagra) Vardenafil (Levitra)	Erectile dysfunction
Selective serotonin reuptake inhibitors	Fluoxetine (Prozac) Paroxetine (Paxil) Sertraline (Zoloft)	Post-stroke depression
Stimulants	Methylphenidate (Ritalin) Dextroamphetamine (Dexedrine)	Impaired attention, arousal
Anticonvulsants	Gabapentin (Neurontin) Carbamazepine (Tegretol)	Central pain syndromes, seizure disorders

Dysphagia

Management of dysphagia may include the use of nasogastric or gastrostomy tube feedings, modified diets (e.g., thickened liquids, pureed foods), and swallowing therapy (e.g., the use of compensatory strategies, such as "tucking" the chin during swallowing).

Communication

The rehabilitation of aphasia relies on extensive speech therapy as its mainstay; selected patients benefit from communication aids, such as a picture board. Speech therapy may provide significant benefit for dysarthria as well, with improved intelligibility resulting. Severely dysarthric or anarthric patients may benefit from the use of computer-based communication aids, including those with speech synthesis, as well as "low-tech" solutions such as spelling boards.

Cognition

Cognitive abilities are frequently affected by stroke; alterations in memory, attention, insight, and problem solving are common. Neuropsychological testing may be useful in defining the precise nature of these deficits and in helping to develop a remediation plan. Speech-language and occupational therapy approaches include both attempts at remediation and teaching of compensatory

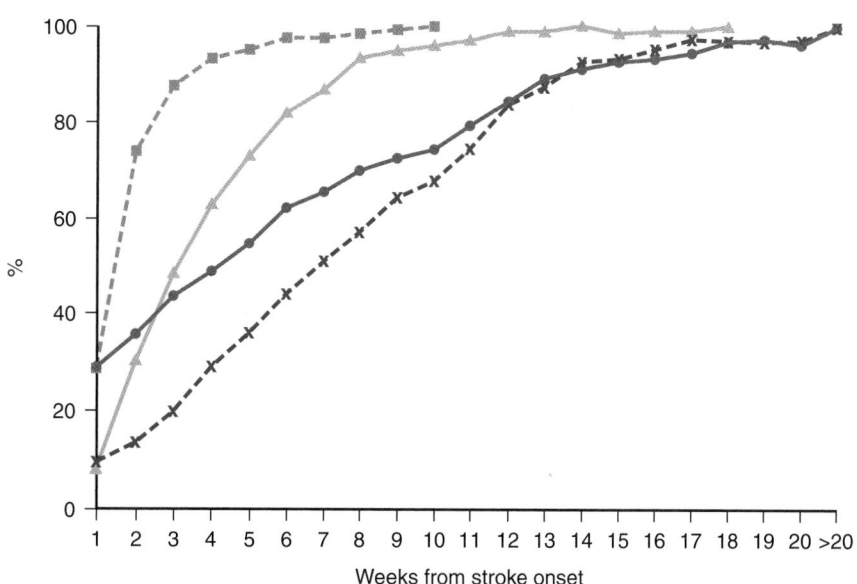

FIGURE 149-1. The time course of recovery after stroke is shown as the cumulative percentage of stroke survivors in each category who have reached their best function in activities of daily living relative to initial functional disability: ■, mild disability; ▲, moderate disability; ●, severe disability; and x, very severe disability. (Reprinted with permission from Jorgensen HS, Nakayama H, Raaschou HO, et al. Outcome and time course of recovery in stroke. Part II. Time course of recovery. The Copenhagen Stroke Study. Arch Phys Med Rehabil 1995;76:406-412.)

techniques. Family education and training are important components of cognitive rehabilitation. Recognition and treatment of post-stroke depression is very important because depression can contribute to reduced cognitive performance after stroke.[16]

Bracing

Lower extremity bracing is frequently helpful in restoration of mobility in hemiparetic stroke survivors. Most commonly, a plastic ankle-foot orthosis is used, although other braces are appropriate in selected circumstances. Bracing is helpful as a compensation for impaired ankle dorsiflexion, controlling ankle inversion and plantar flexor spasticity as well as providing some stabilization at the knee.

Ambulatory Aids and Wheelchairs

Because of hemiparesis, many stroke survivors require ambulatory aids, which may include a straight cane, a four-pronged ("quad") cane, a hemi-walker, or, in some cases, a conventional walker. Wheelchairs are often needed for more severely impaired stroke survivors or for moderately impaired stroke survivors for longer distance travel. A hemi-wheelchair is lower to the ground and allows use of the nonparetic leg to assist with propulsion. On occasion, a one-arm drive wheelchair is useful; it allows control of both wheelchair wheels from one side. Active, nonambulatory individuals may benefit from a power wheelchair.

Shoulder Subluxation

Shoulder subluxation commonly occurs in the setting of hemiplegia after stroke, although the presence of pain is highly variable. Arm boards and the selective use of slings help in reducing subluxation. Electrical stimulation may have a beneficial effect as well.[17]

Splints

Splints for proper positioning of the hemiplegic arm and ankle-foot are important to prevent contracture. These are particularly important when spasticity is present.

Vocational Rehabilitation

Although stroke is predominantly a disease of older individuals, a significant portion of stroke survivors are of working age. Once activities of daily living have been mastered, vocational counseling may assist individuals seeking to return to work. Coordination with the rehabilitation team is important because retraining for certain job tasks may involve a multidisciplinary effort. Accommodations in the workplace may be necessary, and the Americans with Disabilities Act may require the employer to provide reasonable accommodation for individuals with disabilities. See Chapter 150 for more details.

Procedures

Phenol or botulinum toxin injections may be useful in the management of spasticity after stroke. These injections are described in greater detail in Chapter 144.

Surgery

Selected patients require craniotomy in the acute phase for evacuation of a large intracerebral hematoma or for severe swelling with increased intracranial pressure. Carotid endarterectomy in appropriately selected patients has been shown to reduce the risk of recurrent stroke.[18] Carotid stenting is being studied as an alternative to endarterectomy for the treatment of carotid stenosis. Intrathecal baclofen has been found to be effective in treatment of post-stroke spasticity,[19,20] but it is infrequently used for hemiplegic stroke at this time. In patients with chronic impairments from stroke, tendon lengthening procedures are occasionally needed for contractures.

An experimental implantable cerebral cortical stimulator system has been found to facilitate motor recovery when it is used in conjunction with exercise therapy in pilot studies.[21] A multicenter study of this device is currently in progress.

POTENTIAL DISEASE COMPLICATIONS

Seizures can develop as an early or a late complication of stroke; strokes involving the cerebral cortex and hemorrhagic stroke carry greater risk. The risk of deep venous thrombosis is substantially elevated in hemiplegic stroke, and prophylactic treatment with subcutaneous heparin or low-molecular-weight heparin is advisable during the initial recovery phase.[22] The ideal duration of prophylaxis for deep venous thrombosis after stroke has not been established; in most cases, this is discontinued after a period of several weeks. Stroke recurrence is a feared complication of stroke, and individuals with a history of stroke remain at increased risk for recurrent stroke despite risk factor reduction. Aspiration pneumonia can occur as a complication of dysphagia, although this risk tends to abate over time except in the most severe cases.

POTENTIAL TREATMENT COMPLICATIONS

Both anticoagulants and antiplatelet medications can contribute to bleeding complications. Aspirin can cause gastritis. Clopidogrel has been associated with thrombotic thrombocytopenic purpura. The combined use of aspirin and clopidogrel appears to increase the risk of gastrointestinal hemorrhage without providing significant improvement in stroke prevention.[23]

Anticholinergic medications commonly cause dry mouth and may precipitate urinary retention. Antispasticity medications can cause sedation and may exacerbate cognitive impairments. Sildenafil is known to be hazardous when it is used concurrently with nitrates and should be avoided in patients receiving these medications. Selective serotonin reuptake inhibitors can cause gastrointestinal symptoms (especially nausea and anorexia) as well as interfere with libido and sexual function. Psychostimulants can cause anorexia, insomnia, anxiety, or agitation and should be slowly titrated upward. Gabapentin is usually well tolerated, although occasional sedation has been reported. Carbamazepine may cause leukopenia.

References

1. Kelley-Hayes M, Beiser A, Kase CS, et al. The influence of gender and age on disability following ischemic stroke: the Framingham study. J Stroke Cerebrovasc Dis 2003;12:119-126.
2. Lansberg MG, Albers GW, Beaulieu C, Marks MP. Comparison of diffusion-weighted MRI and CT in acute stroke. Neurology 2000;54:1557-1561.
3. Tissue plasminogen activator for acute ischemic stroke. The National Institute of Neurological Disorders and Stroke rt-PA Stroke Study Group. N Engl J Med 1995;333:1581-1587.
4. The Boston Area Anticoagulation Trial for Atrial Fibrillation Investigators. The effect of low-dose warfarin on the risk of stroke in patients with nonrheumatic atrial fibrillation. N Engl J Med 1990;323:1505-1511.
5. Stein J, Silver JK, Frates EP. Life After Stroke: The Guide to Recovering Your Health and Preventing Another Stroke. Baltimore, Johns Hopkins University Press, 2006.
6. Bronner LL, Kanter DS, Manson JE. Primary prevention of stroke. N Engl J Med 1995;333:1392-1400.
7. Kramer AM, Steiner JF, Schlenker RE, et al. Outcomes and costs after hip fracture and stroke: a comparison of rehabilitation settings. JAMA 1997;277:396-404.
8. Mayo NE, Wood-Dauphinee S, Cote R, et al. There's no place like home: an evaluation of early supported discharge for stroke. Stroke 2000;31:1016-1023.
9. Liepert J, Bauder H, Miltner WH, et al. Treatment-induced cortical reorganization after stroke in humans. Stroke 2000;31:1210-1216.
10. Dromerick AW, Edwards DF, Hahn M. Does the application of constraint induced movement therapy during acute rehabilitation reduce arm impairment after stroke? Stroke 2000;31:2984-2988.
11. Fasoli SE, Krebs HI, Stein J, et al. Effects of robotic therapy on motor impairment and recovery in chronic stroke. Arch Phys Med Rehabil 2003;84:477-482.
12. Stein J, Hughes R, Fasoli S, et al. Clinical applications of robots in rehabilitation. Crit Rev Phys Rehabil Med 2005;17:217-230.
13. Hesse S, Bertelt C, Jahnke MT, et al. Treadmill training with partial body weight support compared with physiotherapy in nonambulatory hemiparetic patients. Stroke 1995;26:976-981.
14. Hesse S, Bertelt C, Schaffrin A, et al. Restoration of gait in nonambulatory hemiparetic patients by treadmill training with partial bodyweight support. Arch Phys Med Rehabil 1994;75:1087-1093.
15. You SH, Jang SH, Kim YH, et al. Virtual reality–induced cortical reorganization and associated locomotor recovery in chronic stroke: an experimenter-blind randomized study. Stroke 2005;36:1166-1171.
16. Kimura M, Robinson RG, Kosier JT. Treatment of cognitive impairment after poststroke depression: a double-blind treatment trial. Stroke 2000;31:1482-1486.
17. Chantraine A, Baribeault A, Uebelhart D, Gremion G. Shoulder pain and dysfunction in hemiplegia: effects of functional electrical stimulation. Arch Phys Med Rehabil 1999;80:328-331.
18. Barnett HJ, Taylor DW, Eliasziw M, et al. Benefit of carotid endarterectomy in patients with symptomatic moderate or severe stenosis. North American Symptomatic Carotid Endarterectomy Trial Collaborators. N Engl J Med 1998;339:1415-1425.
19. Francisco GE, Boake C. Improvement in walking speed in poststroke spastic hemiplegia after intrathecal baclofen therapy: a preliminary study. Arch Phys Med Rehabil 2003;84:1194-1199.
20. Meythaler JM, Guin-Renfroe S, Brunner RC, Hadley MN. Intrathecal baclofen for spastic hypertonia from stroke. Stroke 2001;32:2099-2109.
21. Brown JA, Lutsep H, Cramer SC, Weinand M. Motor cortex stimulation for enhancement of recovery after stroke: case report. Neurol Res 2003;25:815-818.
22. Gresham G, Duncan PW, Stason WB; Post-Stroke Rehabilitation Guideline panel. Clinical Practice Guideline Number 16. Post-Stroke Rehabilitation. Rockville, Md, U.S. Department of Health and Human Services, Agency for Health Care Policy and Research, 1995.
23. Hankey GJ, Eikelboom JW. Adding aspirin to clopidogrel after TIA and ischemic stroke: benefits do not match risks. Neurology 2005;64:1117-1121.

Stroke in Young Adults 150

Randie M. Black-Schaffer, MD, MA

Synonyms

Cerebrovascular accident
Cerebral infarction
Intracerebral hemorrhage
Cerebral venous thrombosis
Subarachnoid hemorrhage

ICD-9 Codes

342.01 Flaccid hemiplegia, dominant side
342.02 Flaccid hemiplegia, non-dominant side
342.11 Spastic hemiplegia, dominant side
342.12 Spastic hemiplegia, non-dominant side
344.0   Quadriplegia, unspecified
438   Late effects of cerebrovascular disease
438.0   Cognitive deficits
438.10 Speech and language deficits, unspecified
438.11 Aphasia
438.12 Dysphasia
438.19 Other speech and language deficits
438.2   Hemiplegia/hemiparesis
438.20 Hemiplegia affecting unspecified side
438.21 Hemiplegia affecting dominant side
438.22 Hemiplegia affecting non-dominant side

DEFINITION

Four percent of strokes in the United States occur in adults younger than 45 years.[1] Although the 28,000 strokes in this age group are a small fraction of the 731,000 total events in the United States each year, stroke is an important cause of neurologic impairment in this group. Stroke occurs in those younger than 45 years more than twice as frequently as spinal cord injury (11,000 per year, all ages) or multiple sclerosis (11,000 per year, all ages), and yet there has been limited awareness in American society of stroke as a disease affecting younger adults. Before the age of 30 years, more women than men suffer strokes because of the risks of pregnancy, childbirth, and oral contraceptive use[2,3]; this trend reverses with advancing age. The incidence of stroke is two to five times higher in young ur-

ban blacks and twice as high in Hispanics than in whites in the United States.[4] Strokes in young adults are particularly devastating events because they often occur in otherwise healthy-seeming individuals who are in the prime of life and fully involved with family, community, and workplace responsibilities. Young adults also have high expectations of recovery and consequent difficulty in adjusting to residual disability.

Although more than 60 different disorders causing stroke in young adults have been identified, they can be grouped into several broad categories. Atherosclerotic disease accounts for approximately 20%; cardiac emboli, 20%; arteriopathies (particularly large-vessel dissection), 10%; coagulopathy, 10%; and peripartum cerebrovascular accidents, 5%. Another 20% may be related to mitral valve prolapse, migraine, and oral contraceptive use, and 15% remain unexplained after full evaluation.[5] In American studies, illicit drug use has been associated with stroke in 4% to 12% of cases.[4,6] Approximately 75% of patients younger than 65 years will survive 5 years or more after their stroke.[1] Individual survival, of course, depends on the specific cause of the stroke and its treatment. Two thirds of young survivors achieve good functional recovery, although a history of diabetes mellitus, severe deficit at presentation, or stroke involving the total anterior circulation may reduce that likelihood. Overall, the risk for recurrence in those who have suffered a first stroke averages 5% per year and varies with the survivor's burden of risk factors.[7-9]

SYMPTOMS

The presenting neurologic symptoms of stroke are the same in young as in elderly patients and are reviewed in Chapter 149. The clinician caring for young adult stroke survivors in the post-acute phase is likely to encounter, in addition to neurologic residua of the stroke, a number of secondary symptoms that will require ongoing management. The most common of these are emotional effects, pain, muscle stiffness due to spasticity, bladder dysfunction, sexual dysfunction, and fatigue. These symptoms may also occur in older stroke patients; however, this chapter focuses on the impact they have on the young stroke survivor.

Emotional Effects

The common emotional consequences of stroke are depression, emotional lability, and anxiety. Clinical depression occurs in approximately 40% of patients after stroke; its incidence peaks 6 months to 2 years after the ictus. It is more likely in those with a prior history of alcoholism or depression and in patients who have suffered a severe stroke.[10,11]

Depression can be difficult to identify in aphasic patients who cannot respond reliably to questions about mood and in patients with motor aprosodia (loss of emotional tone in facial expression and voice) due to right hemispheric stroke. Patients tend to become more socially isolated after stroke because of language, cognitive, and physical deficits. Loss of social interaction and support increases the likelihood of depression. Stress related to marital role reversal after a stroke in one member of a couple is common, as is depression in caregivers.[11]

Neurologically mediated emotional lability, also known as pseudobulbar affect or emotional incontinence, in which the patient has abrupt episodes of crying or laughing in response to mention of an affectively charged topic, may be a source of distress to the patient and family. It may also complicate evaluation of the patient's true emotional state.

Patients may experience heightened anxiety chronically after stroke. In some cases, specific triggers of the anxiety, such as fear of falling while walking with a cane or fear of being left alone, can be identified in the history.

Pain

Pain is a common problem after stroke in young patients. It usually affects the hemiparetic extremities and may be centrally or peripherally mediated. Shoulder pain occurs in up to 85% of stroke patients, usually during the first 6 to 12 months after stroke.[12] The history should address its many potential causes[13] (Table 150-1). In addition, younger individuals with partially recovered motor function may develop secondary sprains, tendinitis, skin breakdown, and nerve palsies in the paretic extremities as these are pushed beyond their physiologic limits in the effort to resume normal activities. The normal arm and leg may suffer similar overuse injuries in the course of compensating for the weak side. Heavy use of assistive devices, including canes, walkers, braces, and splints, may contribute to these injuries and consequent pain.

TABLE 150-1 Post-Stroke Shoulder Pain[7]

Disorder	Inferior Subluxation	Rotator Cuff Tear	CRPS I (Shoulder-Hand)	Frozen Shoulder	Impingement Syndrome	Biceps Tendinitis
Examination	Acromiohumeral separation Flaccid	Positive abduction test result Positive drop arm test result Flaccid or spastic	Metacarpophalangeal joint compression test Skin color changes Flaccid or spastic	External rotation <15 degrees Early scapular motion Spastic	Pain with abduction of 70-90 degrees End range pain with forward flexion Spastic	Positive Yergason test result Flaccid or spastic
Diagnostic Test	Standing scapular plane x-ray	Arthrography Subacromial injection of lidocaine Magnetic resonance imaging	Triple-phase bone scan Stellate ganglion block	Arthrography	Subacromial injection of lidocaine	Tendon sheath injection of lidocaine
Treatment						
Initial	Analgesics, nonsteroidals	Nonsteroidals, analgesics	Oral corticosteroids	Analgesics	Nonsteroidals, analgesics	Nonsteroidals, analgesics
Rehabilitation	Harris sling or wheelchair arm board	AAROM Electrical stimulation to supraspinatus	AAROM Heat modalities	PROM Manipulation	AAROM Scapular mobilization	AAROM
Procedures		Steroid injection Surgical repair	Stellate ganglion block	Subacromial, intra-articular steroids Débridement Reduction of internal rotator tone	Subacromial steroids Reduction of internal rotator tone	Tendon sheath injection of steroids

AAROM, active-assisted range of motion; CRPS I, chronic regional pain syndrome type I; PROM, passive range of motion.

Muscle Stiffness due to Spasticity

Stiffness and heaviness of muscles and joints are common complaints of young stroke patients in the post-acute setting. These symptoms are often due to the evolution of muscle tone from the flaccid to the spastic state that occurs during the first several months that follow a stroke. Although it is occasionally helpful in allowing weight bearing on a leg with little voluntary motor return, spasticity more often complicates the patient's efforts to resume normal motor function. In middle cerebral territory strokes, hypertonicity in the upper extremity typically occurs in a pattern of flexion, adduction, internal rotation, and pronation, involving variable combinations of the muscles subserving these movements. In the lower extremity, the usual pattern is extensor with reduced knee flexion, heightened thigh adduction, increased plantar flexion and inversion of the ankle, and toe curling. This extensor pattern becomes apparent during gait and contributes to the slow speed and increased energy cost of hemiplegic gait. The reader is referred to Chapter 144 for further discussion of spasticity symptoms.

Joint stiffness may also be due to contracture, which is shortening of the muscles, ligaments, or tendons around a joint due to rheologic changes in the tissues. This is common in the finger joints of the affected hand. Frozen shoulder, with contracture of the glenohumeral joint capsule, also occurs.

Bladder Dysfunction

Chronically diminished bladder control with urge incontinence occurs commonly in younger stroke patients. The history should ascertain chronicity and frequency of the problem, diurnal pattern, and presence or absence of the sensation of needing to void; a relationship to coughing, laughing, or straining is noted. The patient is queried about abdominal pain and pain on urination.

Sexual Dysfunction

Whether the physiologic process of sexual function changes as a result of stroke, and if so, how it changes, has not been scientifically established. Nonetheless, a majority of patients report diminished sexual function after stroke. This may involve diminished libido or decreased erectile or ejaculatory function. Decreased libido may correlate with the presence of depression and reduced physiologic sexual function with medical comorbidity. Neither clearly relates to size or location of stroke. There is evidence that patients' partners play a significant role in the decline of sexual activity, through fear of relapse, anguish, and lack of excitation. A small number of patients report increased libido after stroke, and rarely, troublesome hypersexuality appears.[14,15] The history should note change in interest and frequency of sexual activity, alteration in ability to achieve erection or ejaculation in men and lubrication or orgasm in women, and presence of depression or active

medical comorbidities that may influence sexual activity level. Medications are reviewed for antihypertensives, antidepressants, and others that may hinder sexual function and possibly fertility, although there is little research on this topic.

Fatigue

Increased fatigue after stroke has been reported in 39% to 68% of patients in published series. It is frequently influenced by coexisting depression. Young adults who never before needed naps now do. Patients become fatigued, physically and mentally, with less effort than before the stroke. Return to active work and family life may be limited by fatigue.[16,17] The history should document a change in fatigue level after the stroke and probe the daily pattern of fatigue and sleep for symptoms of insomnia, sleep apnea, and the many medical conditions that produce fatigue. Medications are reviewed to identify sedative agents. Depression and loss of physical conditioning may affect energy levels, as may the increased energy cost of hemiplegic gait.[18]

PHYSICAL EXAMINATION

In the post-acute setting, the examination of the younger patient after a stroke includes neurologic and functional status for evidence of improvement or deterioration.

Improved motor control in the affected leg may allow trimming back of a brace and progression in gait training to a less supportive assistive device. Worsening motor or sensory function, on the other hand, may signal not only further cerebral events but also intercurrent systemic illness, medication intolerance, new peripheral nerve injuries related to positioning or assistive devices, or worsening neuropathy.

Confrontation testing for visual fields and double sensory stimulation tests for visual and tactile neglect provide important information to the patient and physician about suitability for community mobility, particularly driving. Clock drawing, target cancellation, line bisection, and reading from a magazine can be quickly performed in the office and provide additional information about neglect and attention. The Mini Mental State Examination is a rapid and helpful cognitive screen.[19,20] The affected arm and leg should be inspected for skin breakdown. Maceration of the palm in a tightly flexed hand and friction marks on the dorsum of the foot and calf of patients using ankle-foot orthoses are common. Ulnar palsy and olecranon bursitis related to a constantly flexed spastic elbow can occur. It is particularly important to identify and to treat these problems early in patients with diminished sensation.

Signs of unusual causative entities should be sought if the etiology of the stroke is unclear. These may include the skin laxity and hypermobility of Ehlers-Danlos syndrome, the ipsilateral ptosis and miosis (partial Horner syndrome) associated with carotid dissection, the multiple venipuncture marks of intravenous drug abuse, the livedo reticularis of Sneddon syndrome, the vasculitic rash of connective tissue diseases, and the arachnodactyly and tall habitus of Marfan syndrome.

Emotional Effects

Mood should be evaluated for signs of depression, lability, and anxiety. For patients with intact verbal function, the two questions *During the past 2 weeks, have you felt down, depressed, or hopeless?* and *During the past 2 weeks, have you felt little interest or pleasure in doing things?* may be as helpful as more extensive screening tools, such as the depression screening criteria of the *Diagnostic and Statistical Manual of Mental Disorders.*[21,22] In severely aphasic patients, the screen must, of necessity, consider facial expression, gestures, and posture and the reports of caretakers regarding appetite, sleep, and mood. If the caretaker shows signs of depression, it may be helpful to offer him or her referral for further evaluation. Lability can often be elicited by discussing affectively relevant topics, such as children or spouse. Physical examination signs of chronic anxiety may include hunched posture, fleeting eye contact, cold or moist hands, mild tachycardia, rapid and hypophonic speech, and ready startle reaction.

Pain

The examination addresses appearance, tenderness, pain pattern, and range of motion of the painful regions, looking for signs of specific medical and musculoskeletal disorders. See Table 150-1 for helpful physical examination signs in the diagnosis of post-stroke shoulder pain.

Muscle Stiffness due to Spasticity

Muscle tone at the shoulder adductors, elbow flexors and extensors, wrist and finger flexors, knee extensors, and ankle plantar flexors should be assessed and recorded at each visit with use of the Ashworth scale (Table 150-2). Pain encountered on range of motion is recorded. Reflexes are evaluated, assessing for sustained

clonus, which at the ankle and knee can compromise gait and at the wrist and fingers may be mistaken for seizure activity.

Bladder Dysfunction

Palpatory examination of the abdomen may reveal suprapubic tenderness due to cystitis or an enlarged bladder indicative of retention with overflow incontinence.

Sexual Dysfunction

Full gynecologic and urologic examinations will screen for infectious, traumatic, neoplastic, and hormonal causes of sexual dysfunction in young stroke survivors. The neurologic examination may reveal a neuropathy (manifested by decreased sensation in the feet or hands, decreased ankle and knee reflexes, and occasionally distal weakness) that may be affecting sexual function.

Fatigue

Idiopathic post-stroke fatigue is a diagnosis of exclusion. The examination must screen the patient for the many illnesses that cause fatigue. Among the more prominent of these in this population are Epstein-Barr viral disease, sleep apnea, allergic rhinitis, anemia, dehydration, cerebral hypoperfusion, hypothyroidism, depression, malignant neoplasia, and medications.

FUNCTIONAL LIMITATIONS

Driving

In most communities in the United States, return to driving is a necessary step for return to a normal lifestyle and avoidance of social isolation. Once they have been discharged home, young adult stroke patients are generally eager to resume driving. Many rehabilitation clinics offer written tests of driving ability. Although these have not been shown to be adequate predictors of on-the-road performance, they serve a useful screening purpose. Recent work with a computerized driving simulator suggests that these may be helpful and safe tools for retraining of driving skills.[23] A number of factors have been shown to predict driving performance after stroke; right hemisphere location of stroke, visual-perceptual deficits, reduced sustained and selective attention, impulsivity, poor judgment, and lack of organizational skills all correlate with poor performance behind the wheel. Aphasia, although it may have a negative impact on performance on written and road tests because of compromised processing of verbal instructions, does not always interfere with self-directed driving.

Physicians are often consulted about a patient's readiness to resume driving; visual acuity and fields can be readily screened in an office setting, but evaluation for impulsivity, judgment, and selective and divided attention is more difficult. An on-the-road test performed either by a driving instructor or by the state licensing agency remains the "gold standard" for assessment of driving ability.

TABLE 150-2	Modified Ashworth Scale for Measurement of Spasticity
0	No increase in muscle tone
1	Slight increase in muscle tone, manifested by a catch and release or by minimal resistance at the end range of motion
1+	Slight increase in muscle tone, manifested by a catch, followed by minimal resistance throughout the remainder (less than half) of the range of motion
2	More marked increase in muscle tone through most of the range of motion, but the affected part is easily moved
3	Considerable increase in muscle tone, passive movement difficult
4	Affected part is rigid in flexion or extension

Return to Work

The ability to perform valued work is central to self-esteem and an important goal for most young stroke patients. Between 11% and 81% of patients achieve this goal; the wide range reported in this literature is due to differing age ranges, definitions of work, and disability compensation systems. Of those who return to work after stroke, 70% do so at a reduced level. Factors predictive of success in return to work include pure motor or no hemiparesis, good self-care and mobility function at completion of rehabilitation, no aphasia or apraxia, advanced education, and a white collar job. Barriers to successful vocational rehabilitation include, in addition to the reverse of these factors, cognitive impairment, visual-perceptual impairment, age older than 55 years, and economic disincentives related to disability and retirement benefits.

In the outpatient setting, the rehabilitation physician is often asked to certify that the young stroke patient is "medically cleared" to return to work. This may simply mean indicating that the patient has sufficient cardiovascular capacity to perform the job; but more often, a detailed evaluation of the patient's cognitive and physical capacities as they relate to specific job tasks is desired. This assessment is complex and is ideally accomplished with the assistance of a coordinated multidisciplinary team including physical therapist, occupational therapist, speech therapist, neuropsychologist, and vocational rehabilitation counselor.

Patients who are able to resume work after a stroke on average do so within the first 6 months. The 1990 Americans with Disabilities Act has had a positive impact on employers' responsiveness to the requests of stroke survivors for job accommodations, not only regarding physical access and equipment but also for personal assistance, schedule flexibility, and task modification.[24-26] The majority of patients return to their previous employer, although young stroke survivors with minimal cognitive impairment may be able to take on new jobs.

Parenting

The young adult stroke survivor who needs to return to parenting faces particular challenges in the performance of child bathing, dressing, feeding, and transporting tasks. Problem solving of these tasks can be done with the assistance of other adult family members, home care occupational therapists, or hired child-care assistants. Many helpful items of equipment are readily available (paper disposable diapers with easy to close tabs, microwaves for heating bottles, baby tub inserts). Even when frequent assistance is needed, the patient should be encouraged to assume the supervisory role in child-care.

DIAGNOSTIC STUDIES

Because the use of illicit drugs has been linked to strokes in younger individuals, ongoing drug screening in the post-acute setting may occasionally be indicated. For other diagnostic testing, see Chapter 149.

Differential Diagnosis

Brain infection (abscess, encephalitis)

Brain neoplasm

Cranial nerve palsy

Peripheral nerve palsy

Hemiplegic migraine

Multiple sclerosis

Progressive multifocal leukoencephalopathy

Positional vertigo

Post-seizure (Todd) paralysis

Toxic metabolic encephalopathy

Conversion disorder

TREATMENT

The post-acute setting affords an excellent opportunity for the young stroke survivor and his or her physician to review the cause of the patient's stroke, to identify modifiable risk factors for recurrence, and to jointly develop a plan to minimize these. The patient's motivation to comply with treatment for hypertension and diabetes, to develop a habit of compliance with newly prescribed anticoagulation therapy, to quit smoking, to avoid excessive alcohol intake, and to turn away from the use of street drugs will be maximal in the months that follow the stroke.

The remainder of this section discusses specific treatment of the secondary symptoms previously detailed.

Emotional Effects

Initial

Post-stroke depression responds to antidepressant medications of several classes. The lower cardiac risk profile of selective serotonin reuptake inhibitors makes them an attractive option for patients with arrhythmia. They should be used with caution in patients with sexual dysfunction. The sedative and urinary retentive properties of tricyclic antidepressants may be helpful for patients with concomitant neuropathic pain, excessive salivation, and sleep disturbance or urge incontinence. All of the major classes of antidepressants have the potential to lower seizure threshold.

The family and community, including local and national stroke support and education groups, are important resources for the young patient who is struggling with emotional adjustment to residual disability and altered lifestyle. Referral to a psychiatrist, psychologist, home care social worker, or psychiatric nurse is often helpful. Emotional lability often responds to selective serotonin reuptake inhibitors and usually diminishes over time.[27,28] Management of anxiety in cognitively impaired young stroke patients should emphasize the less sedating anxiolytics, counseling, and environmental manipulation to reduce known triggers.

Rehabilitation

Neurologic and functional improvement is perhaps the best antidote to post-stroke depression. A multidisciplinary stroke rehabilitation program, by providing graded and progressive activities in many areas, gives the patient the opportunity to make and to appreciate numerous improvements in parameters of mobility, self-care, language, and cognition. Therapists are skilled at providing encouragement and positive reinforcement for successes, large and small, in the targeted activities. The rehabilitation therapy environment provides substantial psychological support to the patient, and it is common for depression first to become evident, or to worsen, at the time outpatient therapy finishes and this support system is withdrawn.

Procedures

Electroconvulsive therapy may be indicated for refractory depression.

Pain

Initial

Measures for soft tissue–based pain include non-narcotic analgesics and nonsteroidal anti-inflammatory drugs, with care taken to consider the cardiac, renal, hepatic, and gastrointestinal risks. When narcotic medication for pain relief is required, the fentanyl transdermal patch is a useful option. Neuropathic and central pain syndromes often respond to gabapentin. See Table 150-1 for treatment options for the several varieties of post-stroke shoulder pain.

Rehabilitation

Rehabilitation treatment of pain syndromes is useful both in itself and because it allows close monitoring by a qualified therapist of the patient's symptoms and response to treatments. Soft tissue injuries often respond to stretching and strengthening, positioning, electrical stimulation of the affected muscles, and heat modalities including hot packs and ultrasound when sensation is adequate to allow their use. Transcutaneous electrical nerve stimulation and functional electrical stimulation to the supraspinatus and upper trapezius are often helpful in poorly defined shoulder pain, as are arm slings, such as the Harris hemi-sling, that promote optimal glenohumeral alignment.

Procedures

Acupuncture can be beneficial for central pain syndromes, and subacromial bursa steroid injection will help approximately half of patients with post-stroke shoulder pain. Botulinum toxin and phenol injections provide relief when pain is due to spasticity in specific muscles.

Surgery

In post-stroke shoulder pain, surgical repair may be considered when rotator cuff tear can be established as the cause. Surgical débridement may be required for severe, unremitting frozen shoulder.

Muscle Stiffness due to Spasticity

Initial

The management of muscle stiffness due to spasticity is discussed in detail in Chapter 144. Intercurrent infections, localized sores, stress, and anxiety can worsen spasticity and should be treated before other interventions are added. Sedation in this cognitively fragile population is to be avoided and limits dosage titration of all the available antispasticity agents. Tizanidine and gabapentin, because of their analgesic as well as muscle relaxant actions, are logical choices for painful spasticity. Selective serotonin reuptake inhibitors occasionally exacerbate spasticity.

Rehabilitation

Mild post-stroke spasticity in the heel cord and finger and wrist flexors can often be adequately controlled with a stretching program performed two or three times per day by the patient. Range of motion in a spastic ankle or hand can be preserved with nighttime use of custom fabricated resting splints.

Procedures

Injection of spastic muscles with botulinum toxin and of peripheral motor nerves with phenol can enhance gait pattern and hand function and reduce pain in young stroke survivors. Once a pattern of useful response to injection to specific muscles and nerves has been established, consideration should be given to surgical referral for more permanent intervention.

Surgery

Tendon lengthening, sectioning, and transfers infrequently performed in elderly stroke patients because of limited life expectancy and medical risks should be considered in younger patients when the pattern of hypertonicity has stabilized. Achilles tendon lengthening may allow improved heel strike in patients with chronic equinovarus posturing due to spastic triceps surae. Sectioning of short toe flexors can reduce painful toe clawing, and splitting and lateral reattachment of a portion of the anterior tibial tendon (SPLATT procedure) can rebalance a varus foot. Electrophysiologic evaluation of the extremity in a gait laboratory can provide useful information to supplement the physical examination and help ensure that the optimal muscles are targeted for surgical intervention.

Bladder Dysfunction

Initial

For the stroke survivor with urge incontinence due to spastic neurogenic bladder, helpful medications are available. The anticholinergics oxybutynin and tolterodine are first-line agents for management of detrusor instability. In addition, tricyclic antidepressants provide mild anticholinergic stimulation and can be used to increase bladder capacity.

Rehabilitation

Urinary incontinence can be successfully managed in the inpatient rehabilitation setting or at home with timed voiding (every 2 hours while awake), timed fluid intake (none after supper), use of padded clothing or condom catheter, and a commode or urinal by the bedside.

Pelvic floor strengthening exercises are helpful for stress incontinence. There are no specific rehabilitation treatments for detrusor instability, although the patient's therapists are often in a position to observe and to document the extent of the problem.

Surgery

Bladder suspension surgery may be indicated for stress incontinence.

Sexual Dysfunction

Initial

Treatment of depression with medications such as bupropion, mirtazapine, and nefazodone, which do not hinder sexual function,[29] and of active concurrent medical illnesses can promote improved sexual function. Elimination of other medications that compromise ejaculatory or orgasmic function will obviously help as well. Treatment with testosterone to enhance libido and with sildenafil to improve erection or estrogen to improve lubrication may be considered.

Fatigue

Initial

Efforts to ensure a normal sleep-wake cycle should be made. These include maintenance of a consistent and appropriate bedtime, avoidance of stimulant beverages late in the day, and use of hypnotic agents at bedtime, if needed. For the patient who sleeps well at night but remains easily fatigued during the day, a trial of methylphenidate on arising and at noon may be considered. Loss of initiation due to frontal lobe disease may be perceived as fatigue and occasionally responds to amantadine. For the depressed patient with fatigue, a nonsedating antidepressant should be chosen. Short daytime naps in patients with normal nighttime sleep pattern should not be discouraged.

Rehabilitation

A tailored cardiovascular conditioning program is helpful to maximize the patient's aerobic capacity and physical stamina. Patients with significant physical impairment will benefit from a physical therapist's assistance in designing an adapted conditioning program, which may emphasize use of a stationary bicycle, arm ergometer, and therapeutic pool. Patients with limiting cardiovascular

comorbidities will require the physician's input for heart rate and blood pressure guidelines. Appropriate bracing and use of assistive devices and gait training by an experienced physical therapist can help reduce the energy cost of hemiplegic gait. For some patients, wheelchair propulsion is less fatiguing than walking.

POTENTIAL DISEASE COMPLICATIONS

The spectrum of neurologic and medical complications of stroke in young adults is similar to that in older stroke patients. See Chapter 149.

POTENTIAL TREATMENT COMPLICATIONS

Complications of stroke treatment are similar in young and older adults. They are discussed in Chapter 149.

References

1. Weinfeld FD. National survey of stroke. Stroke 1981;12(pt 2, Suppl 1):I1-I90.
2. Lidegaard O, Soe M, Andersen MV. Cerebral thromboembolism among young women and men in Denmark 1977-1982. Stroke 1986;17:670-675.
3. Naess H, Nyland HI, Thomassen L, et al. Incidence and short-term outcome of cerebral infarction in young adults in western Norway. Stroke 2002;33:2105-2108.
4. Chong JY, Sacco RL. Epidemiology of stroke in young adults: race/ethnic differences. J Thromb Thrombolysis 2005;20:77-83.
5. Hart RG, Miller VT. Cerebral infarction in young adults: a practical approach. Stroke 1983;14:110-114.
6. Adams HP, Kappelle LJ, Biller J, et al. Ischemic stroke in young adults. Arch Neurol 1995;52:491-495.
7. Naess H, Nyland HI, Thomassen L, et al. Long-term outcome of cerebral infarction in young adults. Acta Neurol Scand 2004;110:107-112.
8. Nedeltchev K, der Maur TA, Georgiadis D, et al. Ischaemic stroke in young adults: predictors of outcome and recurrence. J Neurol Neurosurg Psychiatry 2005;76:191-195.
9. Sacco RL. Risk factors and outcomes for ischemic stroke. Neurology 1995;45(Suppl 1):S10-S14.
10. Sobel RM, Lotkowski S, Mandel S. Update on depression in neurologic illness: stroke, epilepsy, and multiple sclerosis. Curr Psychiatry Rep 2005;7:396-403.
11. Dennis M, O'Rourke S, Lewis S, et al. Emotional outcomes after stroke: factors associated with poor outcome. J Neurol Neurosurg Psychiatry 2000;68:47-52.
12. Gresham G, Duncan PW, Stason WB; Post-Stroke Rehabilitation Guideline panel. Clinical Practice Guideline Number 16. Post-Stroke Rehabilitation. Rockville, Md, U.S. Department of Health and Human Services, Agency for Health Care Policy and Research, 1995:125.
13. Black-Schaffer RM, Kirsteins AE, Harvey RL. Stroke rehabilitation. 2. Co-morbidities and complications. Arch Phys Med Rehabil 1999;80:S8-S16.
14. Korpaelainen JT, Nieminen P, Myllyla VV. Sexual functioning among stroke patients and their spouses. Stroke 1999;30:715-719.
15. Carod J, Egido J, Gonzalez JL, et al. Poststroke sexual dysfunction and quality of life. Stroke 1999;30:2238-2239.
16. Schepers VA, Visser-Meily AM, Ketelaar M, Lindeman E. Poststroke fatigue: course and its relation to personal and stroke-related factors. Arch Phys Med Rehabil 2006;87:184-188.
17. Naess H, Nyland HL, Thomassen L, et al. Fatigue at long-term follow-up in young adults with cerebral infarction. Cerebrovasc Dis 2005;20:245-250.

18. Waters RL, Mulroy S. The energy expenditure of normal and pathologic gait. Gait Posture 1999;9:207-223.

19. Folstein MF, Folstein SE, McHugh PR. "Mini-mental state," a practical method for grading the cognitive state of patients for the clinician. J Psychiatr Res 1975;12:189-198.

20. Azouvi P, Samuel C, Louis-Dreyfus A, et al. Sensitivity of clinical and behavioural tests of spatial neglect after right hemisphere stroke. J Neurol Neurosurg Psychiatry 2002;73:160-166.

21. Whooley MA, Avins AL, Miranda J, Browner WS. Case-finding instruments for depression: two questions are as good as many. J Gen Intern Med 1997;12:439-445.

22. American Psychiatric Association. Diagnostic and Statistical Manual of Mental Disorders, 4th ed. Washington, DC, American Psychiatric Association, 1994.

23. Akinwuntan AE, DeWeerdt W, Feys H, et al. Effect of simulator training on driving after stroke: a randomized controlled trial. Neurology 2005;65:843-850.

24. Gresham GE, Fitzpatrick TE, Wolf PA, et al. Residual disability in survivors of stroke. The Framingham study. N Engl J Med 1975;293:954-956.

25. Black-Schaffer RM, Lemieux L. Vocational outcome after stroke. Top Stroke Rehabil 1994;1:74-86.

26. Wozniak MA, Kittner SJ. Return to work after ischemic stroke: a methodological review. Neuroepidemiology 2002;21:159-166.

27. Robinson RG, Schultz SK, Castillo C, et al. Nortriptyline versus fluoxetine in the treatment of depression and in short-term recovery after stroke: a placebo-controlled, double-blind study. Am J Psychiatry 2000;157:351-359.

28. Choi-Kwon S, Han SW, Kwon SU, et al. Fluoxetine treatment in poststroke depression, emotional incontinence, and anger proneness: a double-blind, placebo-controlled study. Stroke 2006;37:156-161.

29. Hirschfield RM. Care of the sexually active depressed patient. J Clin Psychiatry 1999;60(Suppl 17):32-35; discussion 46-48.

Systemic Lupus Erythematosus 151

Mahboob U. Rahman, MD, PhD

DEFINITION

Systemic lupus erythematosus (SLE) is an autoimmune multisystem disorder of unknown etiology with variable clinical and laboratory manifestations, course, and prognosis. The manifestations of SLE can vary from mild rashes and musculoskeletal symptoms to potentially life-threatening involvement of major organ systems, including the kidneys, lungs, and heart and the hematopoietic, gastrointestinal, and central nervous systems. Many other organs and systems can be involved alone or in combination. The characteristic laboratory manifestation is the presence of autoantibodies directed against the various components of the nucleus of a cell and thus termed antinuclear antibodies.

Although SLE is primarily a disease of young women of reproductive age, pediatric and geriatric cases are also encountered. The female-to-male ratio in the peak incidence age group (15 to 40 years) is approximately 5:1. The prevalence among the general population is approximately 1 in every 2000 persons, but it varies according to race, ethnicity, and socioeconomic background.

Classification criteria, which are essential for clinical trials and may provide a useful reference for clinical practice, have been proposed (Table 151-1). Both the sensitivity and specificity of these criteria for the diagnosis of SLE are 95% (i.e., 5% of patients who have SLE will not meet these criteria, and 5% of patients who do not have SLE may meet these criteria).

The severity of the disease is also extremely variable, and a waxing and waning clinical course is common. The disease can be mild enough or can be controlled in most cases to allow an essentially normal life with jobs and children. Pregnancy, however, can be complicated and requires close monitoring by a high-risk obstetrician. Patients with SLE are at a much higher risk for development of atherosclerotic disease than is the general population.

SYMPTOMS

The presentation varies widely according to the organ systems involved.[1,2] Most patients present with musculoskeletal and mucocutaneous symptoms, Raynaud phenomenon, and chronic fatigue. The first noticeable symptom may be the classic "butterfly rash" across the nose. It is not uncommon to have a life-threatening illness and severe disability due to involvement of major organ systems early in the course of the disease.

Pain, weakness, and generalized fatigue are common symptoms of SLE (Table 151-2).

PHYSICAL EXAMINATION

Because so many organ systems may be involved, it is important to conduct a thorough physical examination (see Table 151-2).

Constitutional signs may include fever, tachycardia, bradycardia, tachypnea, and conjunctival pallor. Rashes include the typical maculopapular erythematous malar or butterfly rash and discoid and other rashes, including purpura. Oral and nasal ulcerations, lymphadenopathy, heart murmur, pleural or pericardial rub and other signs of heart failure and pleural effusion, diffuse abdominal tenderness, hepatosplenomegaly, stigmata of deep venous thrombosis or arterial thrombosis including pulmonary embolism, and peripheral edema can be detected during physical examination.

The musculoskeletal system is commonly involved and may cause stiffness, swelling, pain in joints and periarticular structures, and weakness of muscles from acute and chronic inflammation. Examination may reveal symmetric swelling, tenderness, warmth, erythema, and decreased range of motion of joints.

Although the arthritis in SLE is usually nonerosive, damage of periarticular structures can lead to tendon rupture and reducible joint deformities or subluxation (Jaccoud arthropathy) and may compromise hand function. The joints usually lack the exuberant synovitis seen in rheumatoid arthritis, and joint tenderness is often out of proportion to physical and radiologic findings. Muscle tenderness and weakness and fibromyalgia tender points can also be seen.

Focal neurologic signs and change in mental status may indicate central nervous system involvement by SLE.

FUNCTIONAL LIMITATIONS

Functional limitations vary widely, depending on the severity of the disease and which organ systems are involved. Some patients may have no limitations. If musculoskeletal or joint involvement is present, pain, weakness, and loss of range of motion can limit hand, arm, and leg function. Typically, patients have difficulty in dressing, bathing, doing household chores, working, and participating in recreational activities. Mobility, including walking and running, may also be affected. Cardiac or pulmonary involvement may affect endurance. Central nervous system sequelae can be particularly devastating, and limitations depend on the part of the brain affected.

DIAGNOSTIC STUDIES

The wide variation in the manifestation of SLE often makes both the diagnosis and management of the condition a challenge. Diagnosis of SLE requires a careful and elaborate history, a meticulous physical examination, and diagnostic studies that depend on disease manifestations. The classification criteria (see Table 151-1) can also be a useful guide in making the diagnosis.

Some of the common but nonspecific laboratory findings include anemia; positive Coombs test result; elevated erythrocyte sedimentation rate and C-reactive protein concentration; increased transaminase, creatine kinase, aldolase, amylase, and lipase activities; and elevated blood urea nitrogen and creatinine levels. Proteinuria, dysmorphic red blood cells, and red and white blood cell casts on urinalysis indicate kidney involvement. When suspicion for SLE is high on clinical grounds, some of the following more specific tests are usually ordered to establish the diagnosis of SLE[3,4]:

- Antinuclear antibodies and antibodies to extractable nuclear antigens, which include Ro, La, Sm, and U1RNP (Table 151-3).
- Anticardiolipin antibodies, lupus anticoagulant, and false-positive results of nonspecific tests for syphilis (e.g., VDRL test) may confirm the presence of SLE-associated antiphospholipid antibody syndrome.
- Elevated serum concentrations of immune complexes and evidence of complement consumption (e.g., decreased serum concentrations of complement split products, such as C4b, C5a, and SC5b-9) can be a good indicator of SLE disease activity.

Radiographs of involved joints may reveal periarticular osteopenia without bone erosion and may also show signs of advanced osteonecrosis. Radiographs of the chest can show pleural effusion, increased interstitial markings, prominent pulmonary vessels, consolidations, and cardiomegaly. High-resolution computed tomography of the chest may be needed when pulmonary hemorrhage or active interstitial lung disease is suspected. Computed tomography and ultrasonography may help diagnose lupoid hepatitis and pancreatitis. Magnetic resonance imaging can detect early osteonecrosis.

Biopsy of involved tissues (commonly the skin and kidneys), lumbar puncture, and cultures are often needed to rule out other possible diagnoses.

Differential Diagnosis

Other autoimmune disorders and overlap syndrome (e.g., mixed connective tissue disease, polymyositis or dermatomyositis, scleroderma, Raynaud disease, spondyloarthropathies, rheumatoid arthritis)

Dermatitis

Hematologic disorders (e.g., idiopathic thrombocytopenic purpura)

Neurologic disorders (e.g., epilepsy, multiple sclerosis)

Psychiatric disorders

TABLE 151-2 Signs and Symptoms of Systemic Lupus Erythematosus

Organ System	Signs and Symptoms
Constitutional	Fatigue, malaise, fever, anorexia
Skin and mucous membrane	Rashes (including the typical malar or butterfly rash, discoid and other rashes)
	Photosensitivity (develop rash and constitutional symptoms)
	Oral and nasal ulcerations (typically painless at the onset)
Musculoskeletal system	Joint pain
	Polyarthralgia (symmetric joint pain)
	Polyarthritis (symmetric joint pain with swelling, warmth, erythema, and morning stiffness)
	Osteonecrosis (usually the ends of the long bones, and thus joint pain)
	Muscles
	Myalgia (muscle aches or pain)
	Myositis (muscle aches or pain and weakness)
Serosal	Pleuritis (pleuritic chest pain, shortness of breath)
	Pericarditis (chest pain, rarely associated with hemodynamic compromise)
	Peritoneal inflammation (often presents with diffuse abdominal pain)
Cardiovascular	Raynaud phenomenon
	Myocarditis, endocarditis (chest pain, shortness of breath, peripheral edema)
	Vasculitis—small vessel (variable presentation, depending on organs involved)
Pulmonary	Interstitial disease, "shrinking lung syndrome" (cough, shortness of breath)
	Pneumonitis, pulmonary hemorrhage (shortness of breath, cough, hemoptysis)
	Pulmonary hypertension (shortness of breath, syncope)
Hematologic	Lymphadenopathy (swollen glands)
	Thrombocytopenia (easily bruised, purpuric rash)
	Hemolytic anemia (fatigue, weakness, pallor)
Renal and urologic	Lupus nephritis (peripheral edema, dark urine)
	Lupoid cystitis (urgency, frequency, and dysuria with sterile urine)
Neuropsychiatric	Neurologic
	Headache (particularly refractory migraine-like headaches)
	Seizures
	Cerebral vascular accidents
	Peripheral neuropathy
	Cranial neuropathy
	Transverse myelitis
	Psychiatric
	Cognitive dysfunction
	Depression
	Psychosis

TREATMENT

Initial

Determination of disease activity and severity is required to develop an effective therapeutic regimen.[5] Disease activity indicates the degree of inflammation; severity indicates the degree of organ damage and dysfunction. It is important to determine both, as disease activity warrants immunosuppressive therapy, whereas organ damage without evidence of active inflammation may not require immunosuppressive therapy. Disease activity can be evaluated by a combination of a careful history, physical examination, and clinically indicated organ-specific labora-tory investigation and other tests (e.g., high-resolution computed tomography to evaluate pulmonary involvement; renal biopsy, anti-double-stranded DNA antibody, complement levels, and urinalysis to monitor renal involvement; and erythrocyte sedimentation rate, radiography, and magnetic resonance imaging to evaluate arthritis).[6-9] Several new laboratory measures of disease activity have been reported and are being adopted in clinical practice, such as antibodies to nucleosomes, complement activation products, soluble T-cell activation markers, cytokine levels, antigenic factors, adhesion molecules, gene expression profiling, and proteomic approaches.[10,11] A number of research instruments have been developed:

TABLE 151-3 Serologic Tests Commonly Used for Systemic Lupus Erythematosus

Antibody	Sensitivity for SLE*	Specificity for SLE†	Clinical Correlation
Antinuclear	95	+	Screening test; specificity, 60%
			Also present in other autoimmune, rheumatic, and inflammatory disorders; in infections; and in approximately 8% of the normal population
			Patterns of antinuclear antibodies are usually nonspecific except for certain antibodies:
			Peripheral nuclear pattern (anti–double-stranded DNA), seen in SLE
			Centromere pattern (anticentromere), seen in 75% of patients with CREST
			(calcinosis, *R*aynaud phenomenon, *e*sophageal dysmotility, *s*clerodactyly, and *t*elangiectasia) syndrome
			Nucleolar pattern (antinucleolar), usually seen in scleroderma
Anti–double-stranded DNA	60-90	++	Glomerulonephritis; titers may correlate with disease activity
Antihistone	50-70	+	Drug-induced lupus
Anti-Ro (SS-A)	20-60	+	Subacute cutaneous lupus; neonatal SLE and congenital heart block; anti-Ro in 60% and anti-La in 50% of patients with Sjögren disease; "antinuclear antibody–negative SLE"
Anti-La (SS-B)	15-40	+	
Anti-Sm	10-30	++	Nephritis, central nervous system involvement; titers may correlate with disease activity‡
Anti-RNP	10-30	+	Mixed connective tissue disease‡
Anti-U1RNP	10	+	Mixed connective tissue disease‡
Anti-P	10-15	++	Central nervous system lupus, lupus psychosis
Anti-cardiolipin	10-30	−	Thrombosis, fetal loss, thrombocytopenia

*The sensitivity of the test depends on the frequency at which the antibodies are detected in patients with SLE.
†++, highly specific; +, antibody present in other autoimmune disorders; −, antibody present in other inflammatory diseases.
‡An overlap syndrome of SLE, polymyositis, and scleroderma occurs at higher frequency in patients with anti-RNP and anti-Sm antibodies. The presence of anti-U1RNP antibodies is a requirement for the diagnosis of mixed connective tissue disease.

the University of Toronto SLE Disease Activity Index (SLE-DAI), the Systemic Lupus Activity Measure (SLAM), the British Isles Lupus Assessment Group (BILAG) scale, and a European Consensus Lupus Activity Measurement (ECLAM); these may eventually be useful for clinical practice also.[12-15]

Treatment depends on the particular manifestations for a given patient (see Table 151-2). Some general principles of management include education of the patient and psychosocial interventions, avoidance of sun exposure (which is well known to cause exacerbation of SLE), assiduous treatment of hypertension, treatment of clotting diatheses, prompt evaluation of unexplained fever (because these patients are immunocompromised as a result of either disease activity or the medication used to treat SLE), immunizations with influenza and pneumococcal vaccines, and antibiotic prophylaxis for any invasive procedures such as dental work (if the patient is taking immunosuppressive medications). Finally, a reliable means of family planning is needed because pregnancy can cause flare-up of disease. These patients need close monitoring by a high-risk obstetrician, especially because they are often taking medications for which safety in pregnancy has not been established. Patients with musculoskeletal symptoms or serositis frequently respond to nonsteroidal anti-inflammatory drugs. Analgesics may also be used for pain control.

Antimalarials, especially hydroxychloroquine, are the most commonly used second-line agent for such symptoms and are also used for SLE skin lesions. Ideally, corticosteroids should be reserved for major organ system involvement and life-threatening situations; they are, however, widely used for many manifestations of SLE. For skin disease, topical steroid preparations may suffice. For patients who require high doses of steroids for long periods, immunosuppressive drugs such as cyclophosphamide, azathioprine, methotrexate, cyclosporine, and mycophenolate mofetil may be used as steroid-sparing agents. Depending on disease manifestations, hormonal therapies (danazol, prolactin secretion inhibition by bromocriptine, dehydroepiandrosterone), plasma exchange, intravenous immune globulin (for thrombocytopenia and pulmonary hemorrhage), and dapsone (cutaneous disease) may also be useful. A number of other therapies for organ-specific manifestations are being studied, including but not limited to autologous stem cell transplantation,[16] anti-B cell antibodies (e.g., rituximab, epratuzumab),[17,18] and recombinant human interleukin-1 receptor antagonist (anakinra).[19]

Rehabilitation

Depending on the manifestations of the disease, patients may benefit from skilled physical and occupational therapy.

Although the arthropathy of SLE is usually mild and non-aggressive and can be adequately controlled by general medical treatment, therapists can assist with the fabrication of splints and the performance of gentle range of motion and strengthening exercises. In an acutely inflamed joint, aggressive movement is avoided and strengthening is typically done statically. Modalities such as paraffin baths can also help decrease pain and improve range of motion. Even with treatment, nonerosive SLE arthropathy can still lead to reducible subluxation or deformities with ulnar deviation and swan-neck deformities of the hands (Jaccoud arthropathy) that resembles rheumatoid arthritis.

Patients with severe involvement of the hands may benefit from adaptive equipment, such as elastic (no tie) shoelaces, reachers, and wide-handled tools (e.g., scissors, knives). For individuals who use the computer, voice-activated software or a foot computer mouse may be beneficial.

Patients with severe pulmonary and cardiac manifestations and extreme fatigue may also benefit from physical or occupational therapy to learn pacing strategies, breathing exercises, and relaxation techniques. Gentle conditioning exercises may be appropriate in some individuals to improve cardiovascular endurance.[20-26] Inactivity due to various manifestations of SLE can lead to rapid loss of muscle mass and stamina and thus worsening of the fatigue. In such patients, a regimen of graded exercise may be beneficial.[27] If mobility is affected, physical therapy can be ordered to specifically address walking and transfers. Appropriate assistive devices, such as canes and walkers, can be provided by the physical therapist, who will also instruct the patient in how to use the device. Patients who have significant lower extremity weakness may benefit from bracing. In some cases, wheelchairs or scooters may be necessary.

Procedures

Depending on disease manifestations, patients may benefit from corticosteroid injections of joints, bursae, tendon sheaths, and tender points. Patients may also require thoracentesis, pericardiocentesis, pleurodesis and pleural stripping, pericardial window, bronchoscopy, lumbar puncture, and biopsy of involved tissue for both diagnostic and therapeutic purposes. Patients with end-stage lupus nephropathy are managed with dialysis or kidney transplantation.[20,28-34]

Surgery

SLE is a multisystem organ disease and surgery may rarely be required for management of the disease manifestations or complications (e.g., osteonecrosis, ischemic bowel).

POTENTIAL DISEASE COMPLICATIONS

Depending on disease manifestations, complications may range from reducible joint deformities or subluxations (Jaccoud arthropathy) to life-threatening renal, pulmonary, cardiac, vasculitic, thrombotic, gastrointestinal, and central nervous system complications—some of which could be irreversible.

POTENTIAL TREATMENT COMPLICATIONS

Side effects of medications commonly used in SLE are listed in Table 151-4.[20,28-34]

TABLE 151-4 Side Effects of Medications Commonly Used in Systemic Lupus Erythematosus

Medication	Side Effects
Nonsteroidal anti-inflammatory drugs	
Traditional	Dyspepsia
	Peptic ulcer
	Gastrointestinal bleeding
	Platelet dysfunction
	Renal insufficiency
	Hepatotoxicity
	Rash
	Aseptic meningitis
Cyclooxygenase 2 selective	Dyspepsia
	Renal insufficiency
	Hepatotoxicity
	Rash
Gluocorticoids	Increased appetite, weight gain
	Cushingoid habitus
	Acne
	Fluid retention
	Hypertension
	Diabetes
	Glaucoma, cataracts
	Atherosclerosis
	Avascular necrosis
	Osteoporosis
	Impaired wound healing
	Increased susceptibility to infection
Antimalarials	Dyspepsia
	Macular damage
	Abnormal skin pigmentation
	Neuromyopathy
	Rash
Cyclophosphamide	Dyspepsia, diarrhea
	Myelosuppression
	Myeloproliferative disorders, other malignant neoplasms
	Hemorrhagic cystitis
	Infertility
	Alopecia

Continued

TABLE 151-4 Side Effects of Medications Commonly Used in Systemic Lupus Erythematosus —cont'd

Medication	Side Effects
Azathioprine	Myelosuppression
	Hepatotoxicity
	Pancreatitis
	Lymphoproliferative disorders (long-term risk)
Methotrexate	Hepatic fibrosis, cirrhosis
	Pneumonitis
	Myelosuppression
	Mucositis
	Dyspepsia
	Alopecia
Mycophenolate mofetil	Dyspepsia
	Diarrhea, vomiting
	Myelosuppression
	Leukopenia
	Infection, sepsis
	Hypertension
	Tremor
Cyclosporine	Renal insufficiency
	Hypertension
	Anemia
	Hirsutism
	Tremor
	Gum hyperplasia

References

1. Tan EM, Cohen AS, Fries JF, et al. The 1982 revised criteria for the classification of systemic lupus erythematosus. Arthritis Rheum 1982;25:1271-1277.
2. Boumpas DT, Austin HA, Fessler BJ, et al. Systemic lupus erythematosus: renal, neuropsychiatric, cardiovascular, pulmonary, and hematologic disease. Ann Intern Med 1995;122:940-950.
3. Maddison PJ. Autoantibody profile. In Maddison PJ, Isenberg DJ, Woo P, Glass DN, eds. Oxford Textbook of Rheumatology, 2nd ed. New York, Oxford University Press, 1998:665-676.
4. Elkon KB. Autoantibodies in SLE. In Klippel JH, Dieppe PA, eds. Rheumatology, 2nd ed. Philadelphia, Mosby, 1998:7.5.1.
5. Gladman DD, Ibanez D, Urowitz MB. Systemic lupus erythematosus disease activity index 2000. J Rheumatol 2002;29:288-291.
6. Illei GG, Tackey E, Lapteva L, Lipsky PE. Biomarkers in systemic lupus erythematosus. I. General overview of biomarkers and their applicability. Arthritis Rheum 2004;50:1709-1720.
7. Liu CC, Manzi S, Ahearn JM. Biomarkers for systemic lupus erythematosus: a review and perspective. Curr Opin Rheumatol 2005;17:543-549.
8. Linnik MD, Hu JZ, Heilbrunn KR, et al. Relationship between anti–double-stranded DNA antibodies and exacerbation of renal disease in patients with systemic lupus erythematosus. Arthritis Rheum 2005;52:1129-1137.
9. Liu CC, Manzi S, Danchenko N, Ahearn JM. New measurement of complement activation: lessons of systemic lupus erythematosus. Curr Rheumatol Rep 2004;6:375-381.
10. Li QZ, Xie C, Wu T, et al. Identification of autoantibody clusters that best predict lupus disease activity using glomerular proteomic arrays. J Clin Invest 2005;115:3428-3439.
11. Ronnblom L, Eloranta ML, Alm GV. The type I interferon system in systemic lupus erythematosus. Arthritis Rheum 2006;54:408-420.
12. Haq I, Isenberg DA. How does one assess and monitor patients with systemic lupus erythematosus in daily practice? Best Pract Res Clin Rheumatol 2002;16:181-194.
13. Merrill JT. Measuring disease activity in systemic lupus erythematosus: progress and problems. J Rheumatol 2002;29:2256-2257.
14. Rahman A, Hiepe F. Anti-DNA antibodies—overview of assays and clinical correlations. Lupus 2002;11:770-773.
15. Illei GG, Tackey E, Lapteva L, Lipsky PE. Biomarkers in systemic lupus erythematosus. II. Markers of disease activity. Arthritis Rheum 2004;50:2048-2065.
16. Burt RK, Traynor A, Statkute L, et al. Nonmyeloablative hematopoietic stem cell transplantation for systemic lupus erythematosus. JAMA 2006;295:527-535.
17. Ng KP, Leandro MJ, Edwards JC, et al. Repeated B cell depletion in treatment of refractory systemic lupus erythematosus. Ann Rheum Dis 2006;65:942-945.
18. Dörner T, Kaufmann J, Wegener WA, et al. Initial clinical trial of epratuzumab (humanized anti-CD22 antibody) for immunotherapy of systemic lupus erythematosus. Arthritis Res Ther 2006;8:R74.
19. Ostendorf B, Iking-Konert C, Kurz K, et al. Preliminary results of safety and efficacy of the interleukin 1 receptor antagonist anakinra in patients with severe lupus arthritis. Ann Rheum Dis 2005;64:630-633.
20. Di Cesare PE, Zuckerman JD. Articular manifestations of systemic lupus erythematosus. In Lahita RG, ed. Systemic Lupus Erythematosus, 3rd ed. New York, Academic Press, 1999:793.
21. Forte S, Carlone S, Vaccaro F, et al. Pulmonary gas exchange and exercise capacity in patients with systemic lupus erythematosus. J Rheumatol 1999;26:2591-2594.
22. Kipen Y, Briganti EM, Strauss BJ, et al. Three year follow-up of body composition changes in pre-menopausal women with systemic lupus erythematosus. Rheumatology (Oxford) 1999;38:59-65.
23. Daltroy LH, Robb-Nicholson C, Iversen MD, et al. Effectiveness of minimally supervised home aerobic training in patients with systemic rheumatic disease. Br J Rheumatol 1995;34:1064-1069.
24. Robb-Nicholson LC, Daltroy L, Eaton H, et al. Effects of aerobic conditioning in lupus fatigue: a pilot study. Br J Rheumatol 1989;28:500-505.
25. Jonsson H, Nived O, Sturfelt G, et al. Lung function in patients with systemic lupus erythematosus and persistent chest symptoms. Br J Rheumatol 1989;28:492-499.
26. Labowitz RJ, Challman J, Palmeri S. Aerobic exercise in the management of rheumatic diseases. Del Med J 1988;60:659-662.
27. Tench CM, McCarthy J, McCurdie I, et al. Fatigue in systemic lupus erythematosus: a randomized controlled trial of exercise. Rheumatology (Oxford) 2003;42:1050-1054.
28. Spalton DJ, Verdon Roe GM, Hughes GR. Hydroxychloroquine, dosage parameters and retinopathy. Lupus 1993;2:355-358.
29. Wilson K, Abeles M. A 2 year open-ended trial of methotrexate in systemic lupus erythematosus. J Rheumatol 1994;21:1674-1677.
30. Waltz-LeBlanc BA, Dagenais P, Urowitz MB, Gladman DD. Methotrexate in systemic lupus erythematosus. J Rheumatol 1994;21:836-838.
31. Klippel JH. Is aggressive therapy effective for lupus? Rheum Dis Clin North Am 1993;19:249-261.
32. Wang CL, Wang F, Bosco JJ. Ovarian failure in oral cyclophosphamide treatment for systemic lupus erythematosus. Lupus 1995;4:11-14.
33. Khamashta MA, Ruiz-Irastorza G, Hughes GR. Therapy of systemic lupus erythematosus: new agents and new evidence. Expert Opin Investig Drugs 2000;9:1581-1593.
34. Chan TM, Li FK, Tang CS, et al. Efficacy of mycophenolate mofetil in patients with diffuse proliferative lupus nephritis. Hong Kong–Guangzhou Nephrology Study Group. N Engl J Med 2000;343:1156-1162.

Transverse Myelitis **152**

Peter A. C. Lim, MD

Synonyms

Transverse myelitis
Acute transverse myelitis
Idiopathic transverse myelitis
Myelitis

ICD-9 Codes

323.9   Unspecified cause of encephalitis
344.11   Chronic paraplegia
         (Paraplegia NOS)
344.12   Acute paraplegia

DEFINITION

Transverse myelitis is an inflammation across the width of the spinal cord along one or more levels. The inflammation can damage nerve cell fiber myelin, resulting in disruption of nervous system conduction.[1] Associated words include *acute,* indicating brief and severe, and *idiopathic,* implying that no specific viral or bacterial agent or any known inflammatory cause can be found.[2] There are few population-based studies of transverse myelitis available. In the United States, the incidence has been reported to be 4.6 cases per million per year in Albuquerque, New Mexico; 45% of the cases were parainfectious, 21% were connected with multiple sclerosis, 12% were connected with spinal cord ischemia, and 21% were idiopathic.[3] A study of acute transverse myelitis in Israel showed an average yearly incidence of 1.34 per million population during a 20-year period.[4]

The onset of transverse myelitis is variable, and up to 45% of cases worsen maximally within the first 24 hours; others do so during a few weeks.[1,5,6] The presentation may be subacute (progressing during days to weeks, ascending, and associated with a good to fair prognosis) or acute and catastrophic (associated with back pain and a poorer outcome).[7] Parainfectious transverse myelitis tends to be manifested with greater weakness and is more likely to have spinal shock than is transverse myelitis associated with multiple sclerosis or spinal ischemia. Parainfectious transverse myelitis also has a greater tendency for back and interscapular pain, ascending spinal cord dysfunction over more segments, and cord swelling on magnetic resonance imaging; 73% of this group had a preceding upper respiratory tract illness, 13% gastroenteritis, and 13% generalized influenza-like syndrome.[3]

Recovery is often related to clinical presentation and may or may not be complete. More than one third of patients with acute transverse myelitis make good recovery, another third have fair recovery, and the rest either fail to improve or die.[4] If no recovery has occurred by 1 to 3 months, complete recovery is less likely.[3,4,7]

SYMPTOMS

Patients with transverse myelitis may present with back or neck pain, girdle sensations around the trunk, other sensory abnormalities (temperature, pain, light touch, position, vibration), weakness in the arms or legs, fever, and influenza-like symptoms. Many report sensations of tight bands and dysesthesias around the trunk at the levels of the lesion.[6] Difficulty with bowel or bladder function is common. Inflammation of the cord may cause partial or complete paralysis, with a posterior column syndrome, anterior spinothalamic tract syndrome, hemicord syndrome, nonspecific pattern, or complete spinal cord injury.[5] In one study, transverse myelitis most commonly affected the cervical region, followed by the upper thoracic region.[8] However, others report that the sensory level or demyelination usually occurs at the thoracic level.[1,3]

Careful questioning may reveal symptoms consistent with infection, immunocompromise, autoimmune disease, space-occupying lesion, multiple sclerosis, or vitamin deficiencies. These conditions have particular characteristics, and details should be thoroughly explored. The season may determine which virus is more likely (e.g., tick-borne infections are more common in spring and early summer).[2] History of exposure to certain environments or pets and the travel, past medical, and family history can provide clues. A careful social history may reveal sexual exposure or exercise routines traumatic to the spine or nerves.

A full review of organ systems will include questions about upper respiratory tract illnesses, cough, chest pain, and difficulty breathing. Inquiries should be made about recent vaccinations, animal bites, tick bites, rashes, joint aches and muscle pain, vision changes, nausea, diarrhea, constipation, and difficulty with voiding. Particular attention should be paid to details pointing to potentially ameliorable or reversible conditions (e.g., those responsive to antimicrobials or surgical decompression).

With increasing numbers of physiatrists performing invasive blocks for pain management, there should be an awareness of injury to the spinal cord as a possible complication. Cases of acute paraplegia with sensory, bowel, and bladder dysfunction have been reported after epidural steroid injections and lumbosacral nerve root blocks. Inadvertent direct cord injury may occur, or vascular injury resulting in cord infarction may be the cause.[9-11] One postulate was damage to an abnormally low artery of Adamkiewicz as it travels with the nerve root through the neural foramen. This dominant radiculomedullary artery arises between T9 and L2 levels in 85% of people, but it may come from the lower lumbar region to as low as S1.[11] There has also been a report of transverse myelitis resulting from the infected catheter tip of an intrathecal morphine pump placed for chronic pain.[12]

PHYSICAL EXAMINATION

Most infections or autoimmune illnesses affecting the spinal cord also affect other systems. Vital sign abnormalities like temperature elevations may point to an infectious etiology, and tachypnea can suggest a problem with oxygenation or blood flow. The physical examination should be systematic, with an evaluation of the skin and joints and the cardiovascular, respiratory, gastrointestinal, and genitourinary systems. An in-depth neurologic examination is essential. Involvement of cognitive function or cranial nerves is generally not seen with idiopathic transverse myelitis and suggests another diagnosis. A full evaluation of the motor strength, tone, coordination, muscle stretch reflexes, and sensory perception (for pinprick, light touch, vibration, position sense, or temperature) will help determine the level of involvement and focus for diagnostic testing.[6]

FUNCTIONAL LIMITATIONS

As with any spinal cord injury, functional limitations in transverse myelitis depend on the level of injury and muscles that continue to be innervated. Debilitation and deconditioning from associated illnesses and prolonged recumbence will also affect function.

Individuals with only C4 innervation will be dependent for most self-care activities, although environmental control can be achieved by sip-and-puff, head, cheek, or tongue switches or by infrared or voice-activated devices. A C5 level allows self-feeding and grooming with equipment, independent use of a power wheelchair, and possibly driving of a specially adapted van. C6 innervation allows independence with upper extremity dressing, bathing with equipment, use of a manual wheelchair indoors, perhaps transfers with a sliding board, and self-catheterization with appropriate aids. A C7 level potentially allows independence in all self-care activities with equipment, and the patient may be able to live alone. T1 innervation allows independent use of a manual wheelchair and self-catheterization in most cases.

Further upper thoracic innervation allows easier use of manual wheelchairs and independence in bladder and bowel self-care. Some ambulation with knee-ankle-foot orthoses may be attempted for exercise, but independent bipedal ambulation is not realistic unless the patient has some upper lumbar innervation.[13] Each additional lumbar and sacral innervation increases the ease of ambulation. Incomplete spinal injuries will present with different combinations of functional abilities.

DIAGNOSTIC STUDIES

When transverse myelitis is suspected, magnetic resonance imaging is generally performed to rule out potentially treatable causes, such as tumor, abscess, or other lesions causing compressive myelopathy.[6] Contrast material can be given to better highlight lesions,[14] and myelography may be done if magnetic resonance imaging is not available.[6] Although they are not definitive, there are magnetic resonance imaging features that help differentiate transverse myelitis from other disorders, such as multiple sclerosis. Transverse myelitis is more likely to have high signal intensity on T2-weighted images extending longitudinally over more segments.[8,14] The number of segments involved may be one or two to as many as 11 and may even affect the entire cord or sometimes only the medulla.[8,14-16] In transverse myelitis, the lesion appears more likely to affect the central region of the cord and involve more than two thirds of the cord diameter. In multiple sclerosis, the lesion appears more peripheral and generally involves less than half of the diameter of the cord.[14] The lesion in transverse myelitis is more likely to resemble a spinal cord tumor, and biopsy may even be mistakenly performed.[8,14]

Magnetic resonance imaging of the brain with contrast enhancement is often performed to help determine whether the patient's condition is a prelude to multiple sclerosis rather than "idiopathic" transverse myelitis. A study that does not show brain lesions translates to the likelihood of evolving multiple sclerosis at 5% to less than 20%. When brain abnormalities are seen, however, the chance for development of multiple sclerosis increases to 50% to 90%.[5,6] Asymmetric motor or sensory symptoms and absence of peripheral nervous system involvement at presentation suggest acute myelopathic multiple sclerosis, whereas symmetric symptoms and neurophysiologic evidence of peripheral nervous system involvement suggest acute transverse myelitis.[17,18]

Other tests include blood counts and chemistry; tests for autoimmune conditions, such as antinuclear antibodies, anti–double-stranded DNA antibodies, anti-Sm antibodies, and erythrocyte sedimentation rate; SS-A antibody for Sjögren disease; immunoglobulin levels; and VDRL test. Vitamin B_{12} levels may be tested, and *Mycoplasma pneumoniae* or *Mycobacterium* cultures may be performed. Lyme titers and titers for various viruses including human immunodeficiency virus, West Nile virus, poliovirus, hepatitis virus, Epstein-Barr virus, cytomegalovirus, and enteric cytopathic human orphan virus may be elevated.

A lumbar puncture allows the assessment of central nervous system pressure as well as obtains cerebrospinal fluid for cell count, determination of protein and glucose concentrations, measurement of immunoglobulins, and protein electrophoresis. In one study, cerebrospinal fluid oligoclonal bands were present in three of five patients with multiple sclerosis–associated transverse myelitis but in none of four patients with parainfectious transverse myelitis.[3] Vascular flow studies or clotting parameters may be needed if spinal hematoma, thrombosis, or vasculitis is suspected.

Electrodiagnostic studies, including somatosensory and motor evoked potentials, may be useful for both diagnostic purposes and monitoring of treatment progress.[19] Cardiac stress testing may be appropriate for certain patients because of enormous stresses placed on the heart when mobility is impaired. A urinary evaluation may include cystography, voiding cystourethrography, and cystoscopy. A baseline renal ultrasound and urodynamic evaluation has been recommended because of the very high rates of persistent long-term bladder dysfunction.[20,21] Bowel evaluation may require radiography, computed tomography, magnetic resonance imaging, or colonoscopy to rule out obstruction.

TREATMENT

Initial

Hospitalization may be necessary to monitor vital signs, to manage respiratory status and bowel or bladder complications, and to carry out investigations.[6,13,20,32] Various medications have been tried for idiopathic transverse myelitis without clear success in changing the course. Intravenous methylprednisolone has been advocated to prevent further damage to the spinal cord as a result of swelling.[5,15,16,22] Cyclophosphamide in combination with methylprednisolone has some success on lupus-related lesions.[16,23] Immunosuppressive agents, antiviral agents, antibacterial agents, and surgical decompression may also be useful, depending on whether a specific cause has been identified.[22] Timely management of compressive lesions may reverse neurologic injury to the cord.[6]

Rehabilitation

Rehabilitation is a crucial component of the treatment for any spinal cord injury,[33] and more severe cases of transverse myelitis will usually require a comprehensive multidisciplinary rehabilitation program led by a

Differential Diagnosis[1-6,9-12,14-16,22-31]

Postinfectious

Viral: Epstein-Barr virus, herpes simplex, varicella-zoster, cytomegalovirus, human immunodeficiency virus, enteroviruses (poliovirus, coxsackievirus, enteric cytopathic human orphan virus, echovirus), mumps, adenovirus, rubella, measles, angiotropic large-cell lymphoma, leukemia virus, influenza, rabies, West Nile virus

Bacteria: Lyme borreliosis, syphilis, tuberculosis, pneumonia (*Mycoplasma pneumoniae*), cat-scratch disease (*Bartonella henselae*), histoplasmosis

Multiple Sclerosis Associated

Multiple sclerosis
Neuromyelitis optica (Devic disease)

Autoimmune

Systemic lupus erythematosus
Sjögren syndrome
Sarcoidosis
Behçet disease
Mixed connective tissue disease

Spinal Cord Ischemia or Injury

Space-occupying lesions: tumors, herniated nucleus pulposus, spinal abscess, hematoma, spinal stenosis

Vascular: atherosclerosis, thrombosis of spinal arteries, arteriovenous malformations, vasculitis in heroin abuse, iatrogenic

Others

Idiopathic
Post-vaccination (measles, mumps, chickenpox, rabies)
Paraneoplastic syndrome

physiatrist. Physical and occupational therapists on the team can work with patients on strengthening, endurance, balance, coordination, joint range of motion, reconditioning, mobility, and independence with activities of daily living. If pain is present, appropriate medications or heat, cold, and electrical modalities may be helpful. An orthotist can improve mobility with bracing devices, such as an ankle-foot orthosis or knee-ankle-foot orthosis. An assessment for appropriate equipment (e.g., wheelchair and other assistive devices) is needed. Education of the patient and family about the disease, resultant impairments, potential complications, and plans for rehabilitation is important. The psychological state of the patient should not be neglected, and there should be monitoring for depression. Discharge planning and community reintegration need to be assessed.

Transverse myelitis may or may not be a transient condition. Recovery may occur, and it is important to minimize the effects of even temporary denervation. All muscles and joints should be kept as active as possible, and putting joints through a full range of motion daily will help prevent contractures. Passive and active exercises and, at times, electrical stimulation are methods to keep muscle as flexible and strong as possible. If respiration is compromised, exercises for muscles of inspiration may be started, glossopharyngeal breathing is taught, and electrical stimulation of the diaphragm may need to be considered.[32]

Spasticity may be a complication, as with other upper motor neuron lesions. Regular stretching and antispasticity medications, such as baclofen, diazepam, and tizanidine, can minimize and decrease joint contractures. Checking the skin thoroughly on a daily basis can potentially avoid skin breakdown and associated infections. Insensate areas of high pressure should be relieved with special cushions and mattresses (e.g., egg crate foam, alternating pressure overlays), and pressure-relieving ankle-foot orthoses may be helpful.

Bladder and bowel programs should be started immediately because a neglected neurogenic bowel or bladder may lead to stool obstruction or kidney damage. An indwelling catheter can initially be used for bladder drainage, but intermittent catheterization is commonly instituted whenever possible. Long-term follow-up of 2 to 10 years in pediatric patients with transverse myelitis showed that residual bladder dysfunction is common, even with improvement of paraparesis and lack of urologic symptoms. In a study, 86% had persistent bladder dysfunction and 77% had persistent bowel dysfunction.[21]

A bowel program includes adequate fluids, proper diet, activity, and scheduled bowel movements. Upper motor neuron bowels may need a stool softener (e.g., docusate), osmotic laxative (lactulose), or stimulant laxative (senna or bisacodyl) for evacuation. Digital stimulation of the rectum is often effective and needs to be taught. With areflexic lower motor neuron bowels, use of bulk laxatives like psyllium or methylcellulose to obtain formed stools may help in digital manual evacuation. Bowel training is often started daily in the hospital, but it can be extended to every 2 or 3 days once an individual returns home.

Individuals who require assistive devices for mobility must be trained in use of a wheelchair, walker, crutches, or cane, including maneuvering over steps and curbs. If transfers and ambulation require assistance, training of family members or assistants becomes crucial. For patients with transverse myelitis at the cervical level, various types of equipment and temporary or permanent orthoses can be provided to help with self-care activities. Proper bathroom equipment and modifications, such as a tub bench, commode, hand-held shower, raised toilet seat, and grab bars, may make the difference between dependence and independence.

Selection of appropriate aids is essential to maximize function, and many are expensive. Timing of these purchases may need to be carefully considered in this possibly transient condition. Despite a reasonable prognosis for eventual recovery, it is important to keep an individual as functionally independent as possible throughout the entire recovery period.

Procedures

Procedures in transverse myelitis are determined by systems affected by the spinal cord injury. Renal ultrasound and urodynamic evaluations are almost routine procedures for these patients to monitor bladder dysfunction. Intramuscular botulinum toxin injections or alcohol and phenol nerve or motor point blocks may be needed for spastic limbs. An intrathecal baclofen pump may be effective in intractable cases. Other procedures include implantation of diaphragmatic electrodes (phrenic nerve stimulation) when respiratory muscles have been affected. Some patients receive functional electrical stimulation systems to help maintain fitness or to increase hand and ambulatory function. Anterior sacral root stimulators may be effective for bladder management.

Surgery

There is no specific surgical procedure for idiopathic transverse myelitis. However, compressive abnormalities, such as abscess, herniated nucleus pulposus, spinal stenosis, and tumor, may need surgery as soon as possible to relieve pressure from the spinal cord. Complications stemming from spinal cord dysfunction that may require surgical intervention include skin breakdown, accidental injury including fractures from lack of sensation in muscles and joints, development of kidney stones, and infections. Tendon transfers may be considered at a later stage to increase an individual's functioning.

POTENTIAL DISEASE COMPLICATIONS

Potential disease complications resulting from spinal cord injury are generally similar irrespective of the cause. Common complications are deep venous thrombosis, pulmonary embolism, and pressure ulceration of skin if pressure relief is not done regularly. There may be varying degrees of respiratory muscle weakness; when it is severe, mechanical ventilatory assistance may be required. Patients are at increased risk for pneumonia or sleep apnea from the illness, compounded by any sedating medications or respiration-depressing narcotics given. Spasticity and joint contractures may result over time. Heterotopic ossification may surround a joint, further promoting contracture. Gastrointestinal complications may begin with an acute ileus and follow with chronic constipation.

Urinary tract infections are common because retained urine and instrumentation both increase the likelihood of infection. Autonomic dysreflexia may occur, especially for lesions above T6. Pain is a frequent complaint after spinal cord injury and in some studies affects more than 90% of individuals. This is often attributed to "central" or neurogenic pain, although some are believed to have a psychogenic component. Treatment initiated for this pain includes tricyclic antidepressants, anticonvulsants, analgesics, and nonsteroidal anti-inflammatory drugs.

Overuse syndromes can result because muscles and joints are commonly stressed in trying to maintain or to learn new functions. Shoulder pain is a prominent issue, and the problem—tendinitis, arthritis, rotator cuff tear, impingement, or contracture—must be properly identified and rehabilitated. Often, use of proper transfer techniques or specific adaptive equipment is helpful. Pressure from resting too long on superficial nerves can also cause pain or weakness. There may be difficulty with reproduction and fertility issues as well; techniques for sexual fulfillment need to be addressed.

POTENTIAL TREATMENT COMPLICATIONS

Treatment complications may result from side effects of medications and equipment required to treat the disease. Skin complications may result from ill-fitting devices or poorly applied dressings. Strictures or tracheal inflammation can result from tracheostomy tubes, and if mechanical ventilation is required, failure of equipment can result in hypoxia. Respiratory infections occur frequently with prolonged mechanical ventilation in high tetraplegia. High-dose steroids used to treat initial inflammation may cause gastritis, ulceration, or hemorrhage in the gastrointestinal tract. Deep venous thrombosis prophylaxis and anticoagulant treatment may exacerbate bleeding complications. Catheterization may cause urinary tract infections or false passages in the urethra, making further catheterization difficult, with possible development of strictures. If bowel programs are not well managed, anal irritation may go on to skin maceration and breakdown around the sacral region.

ACKNOWLEDGMENT

This is an update of the chapter on transverse myelitis by Deborah Reiss Schneider, M.D., from the first edition of this book.

References

1. National Institute of Neurological Disorders and Stroke. Transverse Myelitis Fact Sheet. Available at: http://www.ninds.nih.gov/disorders/transversemyelitis/detail_transversemyelitis.htm. Accessed Jan 8, 2007.
2. Griffin DE. Approach to the patient with infection of the central nervous system. In Gorbach SL, Bartlett JG, Blacklow NR. eds. Infectious Diseases, 2nd ed. Philadelphia, WB Saunders, 1998:1378-1379.
3. Jeffery DR, Mandler RN, Davis LE. Transverse myelitis: retrospective analysis of 33 cases, with differentiation of cases associated with multiple sclerosis and parainfectious events. Arch Neurol 1993;50:532-535.
4. Berman M, Feldman S, Alter M, et al. Acute transverse myelitis: incidence and etiological considerations. Neurology 1981;31:966-971.
5. Hauser SL. Diseases of the spinal cord. In Braunwald E, Fauci AS, Kasper DL, et al, eds. Harrison's Principles of Internal Medicine, 15th ed. New York, McGraw-Hill, 2001:2425-2434.
6. Transverse Myelitis: Symptoms, Causes and Diagnosis. Available at: http://www.myelitis.org/tm.htm. Accessed Jan 8, 2007.
7. Ropper AH, Poskanzer DC. The prognosis of acute and subacute transverse myelopathy based on early signs and symptoms. Ann Neurol 1978;4:451-459.
8. Bakshi R, Kinkel PR, Mechtler LL, et al. Magnetic resonance imaging findings in 22 cases of myelitis: comparison between patients with and without multiple sclerosis. Eur J Neurol 1998;5:35-48.
9. Glaser SE, Falco F. Paraplegia following a thoracolumbar transforaminal epidural steroid injection. Pain Physician 2005;8:309-314.
10. Tripathi M, Nath SS, Gupta RK. Paraplegia after intracord injection during attempted epidural steroid injection in an awake patient. Anesth Analg 2005;101:1209-1211.
11. Houten JK, Errico TJ. Paraplegia after lumbosacral nerve root block: report of three cases. Spine J 2002;2:70-75.
12. Ubogu EE, Lindenberg JR, Werz MA. Transverse myelitis associated with *Acinetobacter baumanii* intrathecal pump catheter-related infection. Reg Anesth Pain Med 2003;28:470-474.
13. Cardenas DD, Burns SP, Chan L. Rehabilitation of spinal cord injury. In Grabois M, Garrison SJ, Hart KA, Lehmkuhl LD, eds. Physical Medicine and Rehabilitation: The Complete Approach. Malden, Mass, Blackwell Science, 2000:1305-1324.
14. Murthy JM, Reddy JJ, Meena AK, Kaul S. Acute transverse myelitis: MR characteristics. Neurol India 1999;47:290-293.
15. Manabe Y, Sasaki C, Warita H, et al. Sjögren's syndrome with acute transverse myelopathy as the initial manifestation. J Neurol Sci 2000;176:158-161.
16. Kovacs B, Lafferty TL, Brent LH, et al. Transverse myelopathy in systemic lupus erythematosus: an analysis of 14 cases and review of the literature. Ann Rheum Dis 2000;59:120-124.
17. Scott TF, Bhagavatula K, Snyder PJ, Chieffe C. Transverse myelitis. Comparison of spinal cord presentations of multiple sclerosis. Neurology 1998;50:429-433.
18. Harzheim M, Schlegel U, Urbach H, et al. Discriminatory features of acute transverse myelitis: a retrospective analysis of 45 patients. J Neurol Sci 2004;217:217-223.
19. Kalita J, Guptar PM, Misra UK. Clinical and evoked potential changes in acute transverse myelitis following methyl prednisolone. Spinal Cord 1999;37:658-662.
20. Cheng W, Chiu R, Tam P. Residual bladder dysfunction 2 to 10 years after acute transverse myelitis. Paediatr Child Health 1999;35:476-478.
21. Tanaka ST, Stone AR, Kurzrock EA. Transverse myelitis in children: long-term urological outcomes. J Urol 2006;175:1865-1868.
22. Andersen O. Myelitis. Curr Opin Neurol 2000;13:311-316.
23. Neumann-Andersen G, Lindgren S. Involvement of the entire spinal cord and medulla oblongata in acute catastrophic-onset transverse myelitis in SLE. Clin Rheumatol 2000;19:156-160.
24. Wakatsuki T, Miyata M, Shishido S, et al: Sjögren's syndrome with primary biliary cirrhosis, complicated by transverse myelitis and malignant lymphoma. Intern Med 2000;39:260-265.
25. Weatherby SJ, Davies MB, Hawkins CP, Dawes P. Transverse myelopathy, a rare complication of mixed connective tissue disease: comparison with SLE related transverse myelopathy [letter]. J Neurol Neurosurg Psychiatry 2000;68:532-533.
26. Muranjan MN, Deshmukh CT. Acute transverse myelitis due to spinal epidural hematoma—first manifestation of severe hemophilia. Indian Pediatr 1999;36:1151-1153.
27. Renard JL, Guillamo JS, Ramirez JM, et al. Acute transverse cervical myelitis following hepatitis B vaccination. Evolution of anti-HBs antibodies. Presse Med 1999;28:1290-1292.
28. Bohr L, Paerregaard A, Valerius NH. Acute transverse myelitis caused by enterovirus. Ugeskr Laeger 1999;161:2817-2818.
29. Giobbia M, Carniato A, Scotton PG, et al. Cytomegalovirus-associated transverse myelitis in a non-immunocompromised patient. Infection 1999;27:228-230.
30. Caldas C, Bernicker E, Nogare AD, Luby JP. Case report: transverse myelitis associated with Epstein-Barr virus infection. Am J Med Sci 1994;307:45-48.
31. Smith R, Eviatar L. Neurologic manifestations of *Mycoplasma pneumoniae* infections: diverse spectrum of diseases. A report of six cases and review of the literature. Clin Pediatr 2000;39:195-201.
32. Alba AS. Concepts in pulmonary rehabilitation. In Braddom RL, ed. Physical Medicine and Rehabilitation, 2nd ed. Philadelphia, WB Saunders, 2000:687-701.
33. Frost FS. Spinal cord injury medicine. In Braddom RL, ed. Physical Medicine and Rehabilitation, 2nd ed. Philadelphia, WB Saunders, 2000:1230-1282.

Traumatic Brain Injury 153

David Burke, MD, MA

Synonyms

Head injury
Acquired brain injury
Concussion

ICD-9 Codes

854.0   Intracranial injury of other and unspecified nature
without mention of open intracranial wound
854.1   Intracranial injury of other and unspecified nature with
open intracranial wound
907.0   Late effect of intracranial injury without mention of
skull fracture

DEFINITION

Traumatic brain injury is an insult to the brain stemming from an external physical force and resulting in either temporary or permanent impairment, functional disability, or psychosocial maladjustment. Brain injuries occur twice as frequently in males as in females. There is a peak incidence among those 15 to 24 years old and again among those 75 years and older.[1] Brain injuries usually occur as a consequence of motor vehicle accidents, falls, violence, and sports. In the United States, an average of 1.4 million traumatic brain injuries occur each year, including 1.1 million emergency department visits, 235,000 hospitalizations, and 50,000 deaths.[2-4] However, routinely reported U.S. national data underestimate the true burden of traumatic brain injury for several reasons. First, they do not include persons treated for traumatic brain injury in other settings, including outpatient settings and physicians' offices. Second, patients seen in military facilities both in the United States and abroad are not recorded. Finally, the number of those who receive medical care but for whom the traumatic brain injury is not diagnosed or who sustain a traumatic brain injury but do not seek care is not known.[2]

The pathophysiologic process of brain injury is usually divided into primary injury, which is the injury to the brain that results at the time of the insult, and secondary injury, which can be thought of as the biochemical or physiologic damage that develops during a period of hours, days, weeks, and perhaps months after the primary injury. Secondary insults include intracranial hemorrhage, swelling, hypoxia, brain shift, herniation, and numerous neurochemical and cellular events.[5] Some of these have yet to be well described or their significance well elucidated.

SYMPTOMS

Symptoms may vary according to the severity of the injury and the stage of recovery. The history should include a detailed summary of the injury, comorbid conditions, initial Glasgow Coma Scale score (Table 153-1), length of the coma (if any), and length of post-traumatic amnesia. A review of important relationships both in the home and in the community is helpful in determining the prognosis for the patient's recovery. If regression in function has occurred since the injury, the clinician should review for potential metabolic insults, such as infection, side effects of medications, or lack of nutrients including hydration and oxygen.

Patients with severe injury and extremely altered levels of arousal often have no subjective symptoms. After the acute phase of recovery, the clinician can expect symptoms to include seizures, contractures, spasticity, altered vision, vertigo or dizziness, and altered sense of smell. These may be the result of cranial nerve injuries or of central processing dysfunction. Symptoms of dysautonomia may still be seen at outpatient follow-up and may be characterized by increased body temperatures, tachycardia, tachypnea, increased posturing or tone, and profuse sweating.[6]

Common late symptoms may include memory deficits (especially those of short-term memory to long-term memory transfer), higher level executive dysfunction, headaches, difficulty with sleep-wake cycles, labile mood, depression, apathy, difficulty with attention, social disinhibition, sexual dysfunction, anxiety, impulsivity, fatigue, and difficulties with fine and gross motor control.[1,7]

PHYSICAL EXAMINATION

A thorough neurologic examination, including a neuropsychological evaluation, is important to assess the consequences of a brain injury. The neurologic

913

TABLE 153-1 Glasgow Coma Scale	
Patient Response	**Score**
Eye opening	
Eyes open spontaneously	4
Eyes open when spoken to	3
Eyes open to painful stimuli	2
Eyes do not open	1
Motor	
Follows commands	6
Makes localized movements to painful stimuli	5
Makes withdrawal movements to painful stimuli	4
Demonstrates flexor posturing to painful stimuli	3
Demonstrates extensor posturing to painful stimuli	2
No motor response to pain	1
Verbal	
Oriented to place and date	5
Converses but is disoriented	4
Utters inappropriate words, though not conversing	3
Makes incomprehensible nonverbal sounds	2
Not vocalizing	1

examination evaluates mental status, cranial nerve function, vision, hearing, deep tendon reflexes, and abnormal reflexes. The examination should also evaluate muscle strength, tone, and coordination and assess gait or mobility in a wheelchair. It is important to make a thorough neuropsychological profile with the assistance of a neuropsychologist. This should be done to determine both physical abilities and the cognitive and emotional issues that will affect the patient's function.

FUNCTIONAL LIMITATIONS

Motor

Patients may have difficulty with mobility and self-care as a result of isolated motor weakness or coordination of either the upper or the lower extremities. Safe mobility may also be impeded by poor cognition, including deficits with planning and poor impulse control.

Behavior

Individuals often experience subtle or dramatic personality changes that alter relationships with others. These may include problems in the initiation of responses, verbal or physical aggression, altered emotional control, social disinhibition, depression, apathy, decreased sense of self-worth, and altered sexual function.

Social

Patients often are unable to return to work at the previous level of function. As a consequence, they may suffer significant economic strain and may have difficulty with their relationships, including their marriage. Family members may be helpful in pointing out issues of social isolation, depression, and anger.

DIAGNOSTIC STUDIES

Imaging Studies

As a rule, computed tomography or magnetic resonance imaging is helpful for the initial assessment of intracranial bleeding as well as the shifting of fluids and tissues, but these studies are poor in their ability to estimate the actual volume and location of injured tissue.[8] More sophisticated testing has been introduced, including single-photon emission computed tomography, functional magnetic resonance imaging, and positron emission tomography, but for the most part, these are of little use in assessing the functional limitations caused by the injury. At the time of outpatient follow-up, it may be necessary to remind the patient and his or her caregivers of the extreme limitations of these studies and to focus on that patient's functional abilities as the more important measure of the extent of the injury. In general, follow-up radiologic examinations are useful tools if the patient has excessively slow progress or has demonstrated a decline in function. These may be helpful in determining new or expanding lesions. Otherwise, these are generally of limited utility.

Functional Assessment Tools

One of the best diagnostic tools is the Glasgow Coma Scale, which is used for the initial evaluation of the severity of the patient's injury (see Table 153-1). A review of this initial score will help in the determination of the extent of the injury and thus with prognostication. Later, as a review of function in the outpatient setting, progress can be measured by the Glasgow Outcome Scale or the Disability Rating Scale. Post-traumatic amnesia is important for prognostication as well and can be assessed by the Galveston Orientation Assessment Test. To characterize the current level of functional recovery, the Rancho Los Amigos Scale is helpful in assessing the patient's awareness and interaction with the environment.

Neuropsychological Testing

This battery of tests, performed by a neuropsychologist, is the best means of determining the full spectrum of cognitive, affective, and emotional function of the individual. This may be done early in the course of recovery but should be repeated when a change in function needs to be documented. This testing may provide the clinician with critical information needed to understand the ability of the patient to progress toward more independence or responsibility at home or at work. This also may be a critical assessment tool for the documentation of the injury for insurance purposes.

Differential Diagnosis

Anoxic brain injury

Metabolic encephalopathy

Affective disorder

Depression

Whiplash-associated disorder

TREATMENT

Initial

The initial focus of treating a patient with a brain injury is to reduce the magnitude of the secondary head injury. If the initial injury is of sufficient severity, computed tomography or magnetic resonance imaging is needed to determine the need for surgical intervention. The scans are reviewed for signs of excessive bleeding, edema, and shifting of the brain. If these signs are absent, medical intervention addresses the possible secondary injury that may result. Although it is still unclear as to how long a window of opportunity exists to affect the extent of secondary injury, it is generally accepted that this opportunity is likely to exist within the time of the initial acute hospitalization.[2] For this reason, there is little opportunity to affect this process in the outpatient setting.

Initially, metabolic issues such as blood pressure, electrolytes, hydration and nutrition, infectious processes, sleep apnea, and medications need to be addressed. Any imbalance in these may inhibit the function of the surviving brain tissue. Hydration and nutrition should be well maintained. An individual with a brain injury may be unable or unwilling to take nutrients by mouth, and this may necessitate either intravenous or direct gastrointestinal feedings. This may be a significant issue well into the post-acute phase of recovery.

A survey for possible infectious processes includes, at a minimum, the pulmonary and genitourinary systems. Even infections that a clinician may otherwise label subclinical can disrupt the function of a damaged brain. For this reason, such infections should be treated as potentially symptomatic.

Medications can have exaggerated effects among those with a brain injury and thus need to be reviewed carefully to eliminate any that may interfere with cognitive function. The list is long, but the most common offenders include antiseizure medications, antihypertensive medications, antispasticity medications, neuroleptics, sedatives, hypnotics, and gastrointestinal medications. Some of these may be unnecessary, whereas others may have less disruptive alternatives.[9-11]

In addition to neuropsychological testing of the cognitive performance of the patient, psychological services are important in the assessment and treatment of affective disorders, which may include depression, apathy, and post-traumatic stress disorder. It is important to consider psychology services as being useful for the family and support system because the stress on these individuals may be tremendous. Psychologists and behavior specialists may be helpful for the intervention into behavior issues.

After the metabolic status has been optimized, the clinician should focus on the remaining physical and cognitive deficits to determine whether medications will be useful to enhance the function of the individual.

Arousal

Arousal will fluctuate throughout the day for a person with brain injury. Fatigue and endurance will be long-standing issues. Frequent rests and naps may be needed, even at more than 1 year after injury. Medical intervention may be initiated for hypoarousal and excessive fatigue. This includes amantadine, bromocriptine, carbidopa-levodopa, methylphenidate, modafinil, atomoxetine, amphetamine, nortriptyline, and protriptyline.[12]

Attention

Neuropharmacologic agents for attention are similar to those used for arousal. These include neurostimulants, such as methylphenidate, pemoline, modafinil, and atomoxetine, and dopaminergic agents, including amantadine, bromocriptine, and carbidopa-levodopa. Antidepressants include a long list of mixed as well as selective serotonin reuptake inhibitors; these will be especially useful if there is an element of depression interfering with cognition.

Agitation

Because agitation is a common and often troubling issue among those recovering from a brain injury, a careful selection of agents is important to prevent injury, to allow focus on rehabilitation, and to reduce the stress on caregivers. In general, the agents that are preferred help control behavior while producing the least reduction in cognition. Because benzodiazepines are thought to have the potential of interfering with the recovery of the injured brain, these are often not recommended in the early stages of recovery. Other medications are therefore used as first-line agents. As an anxiolytic, buspirone seems preferable. A clinician may use antiseizure medications as a mood stabilizer (e.g., divalproex sodium, carbamazepine), newer antipsychotic medications (e.g., risperidone, quetiapine), β blockers (e.g., propranolol), and antidepressants for anxious or agitated patients. Because poor attention to the environment may result in behavioral agitation, stimulants such as amantadine and methylphenidate should also be considered useful agents.

Memory

Because memory requires both arousal and attention, the medications previously discussed may produce improvements in the ability to learn. In addition, there have been limited reports of positive results through the use of donepezil, memantine, and other similar medications. Memory can be more certainly enhanced, however, through the use of compensatory strategies and services. Speech pathologists can be useful for the introduction of and training in some of these strategies. There are portable computers that can be preprogrammed with important information, and these memory aids can be frequently updated for individuals whose brain injury precludes the programming of the electronic memory aids.

Seizures

There is a reasonable body of literature to suggest that the use of antiseizure medications is not warranted if no seizure occurs within the first week after the brain injury. If the patient experiences a seizure after 1 week, the use of anticonvulsant agents is probably warranted for an extended period. Recommended agents depend on seizure type and usually include carbamazepine, valproic acid, and gabapentin.[10]

Spasticity

Spasticity is a common problem among patients with brain injury. Patients may also have hyperactive muscle stretch reflexes and clonus. If these problems are not addressed, early contracture of joints may result. The modified Ashworth scale (see Table 144-1) can be used to measure the degree of spasticity. As a first step of intervention, the clinician should look for noxious stimuli, including anything that may produce pain. Infectious issues, positioning, and seating should be addressed as potential offenders. Stretching should be initiated and may necessitate serial casting and splinting. If medications are needed, these may include tizanidine, clonidine, dantrolene, diazepam, and baclofen. All of these agents have potential side effects and should be used judiciously. Dantrolene is unique in its lack of central effect but often results in acute liver dysfunction.

Rehabilitation

The rehabilitation of patients with brain injury begins during the acute stage of treatment when the issues of secondary brain injury are the greatest. After the acute phase, it is important that the clinician review the potential pharmacologic management and combine this with an interdisciplinary group of therapies, depending on the specific deficits of the patient.

Physical Therapy

Physical therapy is important for the restoration of range of motion of the lower extremities and, if needed, through the use of serial casting. This may be aided by neurolysis or blocks at the neuromuscular junction. Later, issues of wheelchair preparation and propulsion may be important for those with sufficient impairment of mobility. Ambulation training with the appropriate assistive device should be frequently reviewed as the patient progresses with ambulation. Safety must always be considered because the patient with brain injury may be endangered by impulsivity or poor planning and judgment.

Occupational Therapy

Occupational therapy addresses the preservation of joints when a lack of strength or an excess in tone or spasticity threatens a joint. As strength and ataxia are often issues in the first year, these should be addressed individually. The issues of self-care, including daily activities such as dressing, bathing, and grooming, must be addressed and emphasize the need for a planning strategy for the patient. Cooking and driving evaluations may be needed to advise the patient before his or her return to the home.

Speech Pathology

Early in the care of the patient, the ability to swallow safely may need to be addressed. In addition, the speech pathologist, ideally working with the neuropsychologist, identifies focal cognitive needs of the patient and addresses these over a length of time.[13] These often involve memory strategies and pragmatics for return to independence in the home.

Vocational Rehabilitation

Many patients will have difficulty in returning to their previous level of employment. Vocational rehabilitation counselors can evaluate a patient's skills and determine the need for training.

Procedures

For spasticity, local injections may be preferable to oral medications. These may include nerve root blocks, nerve blocks, motor unit blocks (all with phenol), and neuromuscular junction blocks (with botulinum toxin). When spasticity is severe and not responsive to these interventions, an intrathecal pump may be considered for continuous infusion of baclofen into the cerebrospinal fluid (refer to Chapter 144).

Surgery

Patients with new-onset hydrocephalus may need a shunt placed to reduce the pressure load at the brain. If medications and other measures fail to control spasticity and contractures result, surgery may be an option. If joint contractures occur, a surgical release by an orthopedic surgeon may be indicated.

POTENTIAL DISEASE COMPLICATIONS

Seizures can result from a brain injury. The risk is highest early after the injury but persists for years. Soon after the injury, patients are at risk for aspiration pneumonia and, if their swallowing is impaired, for malnutrition and dehydration. Sleep apnea is a frequent early issue; it may, if not treated, exacerbate the symptoms of the brain injury. Continuous positive airway pressure may be an effective treatment. As with all trauma patients, there is a risk for deep venous thrombosis. This must be treated with prophylactic heparin or, if hemorrhage is a risk, with pneumatic compression devices or an inferior vena cava filter.

POTENTIAL TREATMENT COMPLICATIONS

Medications that are used to treat attention and arousal may lead to excess arousal and agitation. This may also present as somatic complaints or delirium. Medications for agitation and seizures may slow the patient's recovery over time and may reduce the patient's function while the medications are taken. Refer to Table 153-2.

References

1. Rutland-Brown W, Langlois JA, Thomas KE, Xi YL. Incidence of traumatic brain injury in the United States, 2003. J Head Trauma Rehabil 2006;21:544-548.
2. Langlois JA, Rutland-Brown W, Wald MM. The epidemiology and impact of traumatic brain injury: a brief overview. J Head Trauma Rehabil 2006;21:375-380.
3. Finkelstein E, Corso P, Miller T. The Incidence and Economic Burden of Injuries in the United States. New York, Oxford University Press, 2006.
4. Langlois JA, Rutland-Brown W, Thomas KE. Traumatic Brain Injury in the United States: Emergency Department Visits, Hospitalizations, and Deaths. Atlanta, Centers for Disease Control and Prevention, National Center for Injury Prevention and Control, 2004.
5. Burke DT, Kamath A. Management of post-traumatic seizure disorders. In Woo BH, Nesathurai S, eds. The Rehabilitation of People with Traumatic Brain Injury. Malden, Mass, Blackwell Science, 2000.
6. Baguley IJ, Nicholls JL, Felmingham KL, et al. Dysautonomia after traumatic brain injury: a forgotten syndrome? J Neurol Neurosurg Psychiatry 1999;67:39-43.
7. Burke D, et al. Sleep-wake patterns in an acute inpatient rehabilitation hospital setting. J Appl Res 2004;4:240-244.

TABLE 153-2 Medications Used to Treat Patients with Traumatic Brain Injury

Symptoms	Medication	Initial Dose	End Dose
Arousal	Amantadine	50 mg 8 AM and 2 PM	100 mg 8 AM and 2 PM
	Bromocriptine*	1.25 mg 8 AM and 2 PM	50 mg 8 AM and 2 PM
	Carbidopa-levodopa*	10 mg/100 mg tid	25 mg/100 mg tid
	Methylphenidate	2.5 mg AM and 2 PM	20 mg AM and 2 PM
	Modafinil	100 mg qd	100 mg 8 AM and 2 PM
	Dextroamphetamine (Dexedrine)	5 mg qd	30 mg AM and 2 PM
	Nortriptyline	10 mg tid	25 mg tid
	Protriptyline	5 mg tid	20 mg tid
Attention	Methylphenidate	2.5 mg AM and 2 PM	20 mg AM and 2 PM
	Adderall	5 mg bid	20 mg bid
	Pemoline	37.5 mg AM	50 mg bid
	Modafinil	100 mg AM	100 mg AM and PM
	Amantadine	100 mg AM	150 mg AM and 2 PM
	Bromocriptine*	1.25 mg AM	50 mg 8 AM and 2 PM
	Carbidopa-levodopa*	10 mg/100 mg tid	25 mg/100 mg tid
	Sertraline (Zoloft)	50 mg qd	200 mg qd
	Citalopram (Celexa)	20 mg qd	60 mg qd
	Donepezil (Aricept)	2.5 mg qd	5 mg bid
	Memantine (Namenda)	5 mg qd	10 mg qd
	Atomoxetine (Strattera)	20 mg qd	60 mg qd
Agitation	Buspirone	7.5 mg bid	30 mg bid
	Carbamazepine	200 mg bid	600 mg bid
	Risperidone	1 mg bid	16 mg/day
	Morphine	10 mg q4h	10 mg q4h
	Propranolol	10 mg qd	Limited by heart rate and blood pressure
	Quetiapine (Seroquel)	25 mg qd	800 mg qd

*Limited by hypotension.

8. Chesnut RM, Carney N, Maynard H, et al. Rehabilitation for Traumatic Brain Injury. Evidence Report Number 2. Rockville, Md, Agency for Health Care Policy and Research, 1999.

9. Kaplan M. Neuropharmacology after traumatic brain injury. In Woo BH, Nesathurai S, eds. The Rehabilitation of People with Traumatic Brain Injury. Malden, Mass, Blackwell Science, 2000.

10. Massagli TL. Neurobehavioral effects of phenytoin, carbamazepine, and valproic acid: implications for use in traumatic brain injury [see comments]. Arch Phys Med Rehabil 1991;72:219-226.

11. Perna R. Brain injury: benzodiazepines, antipsychotics and functional recovery. J Head Trauma Rehabil 2006;21:82-84.

12. Gordon WA, Zafonte R, Cicerone K, et al. Traumatic brain injury rehabilitation: state of the science. Am J Phys Med Rehabil 2006;85:343-382.

13. Stringer, A. Ecologically Oriented Neurorehabilitation of Memory. Los Angeles, Western Psychological Services, 2007.

Index

Note: Page numbers followed by f refer to figures; page numbers followed by t refer to tables.

A

Abatacept, in rheumatoid arthritis, 162
Abduction stress test, in medial collateral ligament sprain, 320, 320f
Abduction–external rotation test, in thoracic outlet syndrome, 499
Abductor pollicis brevis, strength testing of, 205–206
Acetaminophen. See also Nonsteroidal anti-inflammatory drugs (NSAIDs)
  in hip arthritis, 273
  in knee arthritis, 347, 348t
  in lumbar spinal stenosis, 261
  in stress fracture, 395
  in thoracic compression fracture, 214
Achilles tendinitis, 407–409, 408f
Achillodynia, 415–420, 416t, 417t, 418t, 419t
Acromioclavicular joint injury, 41–46, 42f, 42t, 43f, 44f, 45f, 46f
Acromioclavicular resisted extension test, 42, 43f
Active compression test, 42, 43f
Activity relearning, in rotator cuff tendinitis, 75
Acupuncture
  in chronic fatigue syndrome, 640
  in epicondylitis, 107
  in fibromyalgia, 526
  in knee arthritis, 350
  in osteoarthritis, 749
  in thoracic sprain/strain, 227
Acute coronary syndrome, vs. costosternal syndrome, 546
Acute-phase reactants, in rheumatoid arthritis, 162
Acyclovir, in postherpetic neuralgia, 562
Adalimumab, in rheumatoid arthritis, 162
Adduction stress test, in lateral collateral ligament sprain, 320, 320f
Adhesive capsulitis, 49–54, 50f, 50t, 51f
Adson test, 499
Adult spinal muscular atrophy, 705–711, 706f, 707t, 708t
Agitation, in traumatic brain injury, 915
Alar scapula, 83–88, 84t, 86f, 87t
Albert disease, 415–420, 416t, 417t, 418t, 419t
Albuminocytologic dissociation, 769
Alendronate, in osteoporosis, 755t, 756–757
Alkaline phosphatase, in heterotopic ossification, 693
Allen test, 150–151, 151f
Alzheimer dementia. See Dementia
Alzheimer disease, 665–671, 666t
Amantadine, in Parkinson disease, 715, 763t
Ambulation
  after hip replacement, 299
  in ankle sprain, 424
  in lower limb amputation, 600–601, 602t, 603
  in lumbosacral spinal cord injury, 881–882, 881t
  in metatarsalgia, 462
  in Parkinson disease, 762
  in stress fracture, 395, 396
  in stroke, 890

Amenorrhea, exercise-induced, 393, 395
Amitriptyline
  in cervical sprain/strain, 25
  in complex regional pain syndrome, 514t, 515
  in intercostal neuralgia, 552
  in occipital neuralgia, 488, 489t
Amputation
  in burns, 612
  lower limb, 599–603, 602t, 603f, 673
  upper limb, 595–598
β-Amyloid plaque, 666
Amyotrophic lateral sclerosis, 705–711, 706f, 707f, 708t
Amyotrophy
  brachial, 773–777, 774f
  lumbosacral, 779–784, 780f, 781f
Anabolic steroids, in burns, 611
Anal manometry, in coccydynia, 573
Anemia
  chronic kidney disease and, 648
  hip replacement and, 297–298
  knee replacement and, 401
  pressure ulcer and, 816
Anesthetic injection
  in acromioclavicular joint injury, 45, 46f
  in carpal tunnel syndrome, 175
  in cervical facet arthropathy, 7, 8, 8f, 9
  in cervicogenic vertigo, 34, 34f
  in coccydynia, 573–574
  in costosternal syndrome, 547–548, 547f
  in glenohumeral instability, 67, 68f
  in lateral femoral cutaneous neuropathy, 285, 285f, 286
  in lumbar facet joint disease, 239
  in Morton neuroma, 467, 467f
  in rotator cuff tendinitis, 72–73, 75
  in sacroiliac joint dysfunction, 269
  in shoulder arthritis, 93–94, 93f, 94f
  in spasticity, 850
  in spondylolysis, 257
  in Tietze syndrome, 559
  in trapezius strain, 39, 39f
  in trochanteric bursitis, 305
Angina, vs. costosternal syndrome, 546
Angiography
  in heterotopic ossification, 693
  in polytrauma, 788–789
  in stroke, 888
Angioplasty, in diabetes mellitus, 675–676
Angiotensin-converting enzyme inhibitors, in chronic kidney disease, 646, 648–649
Angiotensin receptor blocker, in chronic kidney disease, 646
Ankle. See also Foot (feet)
  adhesive bursitis of, 420
  anatomy of, 416f, 422f
  bursitis of, 415–420, 416t, 417t, 418t, 419t
  chronic instability of, 433–436, 434f
  examination of, 422, 423f
  ganglion cyst of, 445–447, 446f
  osteoarthritis of, 411–413, 412f

Ankle (Continued)
  rheumatoid arthritis of, 835
  sprain of, 421–425, 422f, 423f
Ankle-brachial index, 674
Ankle-foot orthosis, 412
Ankylosing spondylitis, 605–607, 606f
Ankylosis. See Contracture
Anserine bursitis, 355
Anterior chest wall syndrome, 545–548, 546f, 547f
Anterior cruciate ligament, 381, 382f
  tear of, 307–312, 308f, 309f, 310t, 311t
Anterior drawer test
  in ankle sprain, 422
  in anterior cruciate ligament tear, 308, 309f
  in medial collateral ligament sprain, 320
Anterior interosseous syndrome, 109–113, 110f, 111f, 112f, 113f
Antibiotics
  in extensor tendon injury, 140
  in hand osteoarthritis, 158
  in olecranon bursitis, 117
Antibodies
  in systemic lupus erythematosus, 902, 904t
  in transverse myelitis, 908–909
Anticholinergics
  in bladder dysfunction, 723, 737t, 740, 740t
  in Parkinson disease, 715, 762, 763t
  in pulmonary rehabilitation, 826, 827t
Anticoagulants
  prophylactic, 297, 660–661, 661t, 662
  in stroke, 888, 890
Anticonvulsants
  in arachnoiditis, 567, 567t, 568
  in complex regional pain syndrome, 514t, 515
  in femoral neuropathy, 279
  in fibromyalgia, 526
  in intercostal neuralgia, 552–553
  in lumbar radiculopathy, 244
  in multiple sclerosis, 723
  in occipital neuralgia, 487, 488, 489t
  in peroneal neuropathy, 378
  in phantom limb pain, 576t, 577
  in traumatic brain injury, 915
  in trigeminal neuralgia, 494, 495t
  in ulnar neuropathy, 190
Antidepressants
  in arachnoiditis, 567, 567t, 568
  in chronic fatigue syndrome, 639
  in complex regional pain syndrome, 514t, 515
  in dementia, 670
  in fibromyalgia, 526
  in hyperreflexic bladder, 737t
  in intercostal neuralgia, 552
  in lumbar stenosis, 261
  in motor neuron disease, 709
  in myofascial pain syndrome, 533
  in occipital neuralgia, 487, 488, 489t
  in peripheral neuropathy, 770, 771
  in peroneal neuropathy, 378
  in phantom limb pain, 576t, 577

Antidepressants (Continued)
   in repetitive strain injury, 542
   in trapezius strain, 38, 39–40
Antimalarials
   in psoriatic arthritis, 811
   in rheumatoid arthritis, 837
   side effects of, 689t
   in systemic lupus erythematosus, 904
Antinuclear antibodies, in systemic lupus
      erythematosus, 902, 904t
Antioxidants, in amyotrophic lateral sclerosis, 707
Antiplatelet agents, in stroke, 888
Antivirals, in postherpetic neuralgia, 562
Anxiety
   motor neuron disease and, 709
   stroke and, 894, 896
Aortic aneurysm, 232t
Aphasia, 854t, 855, 856, 857, 859, 889
Apicitis, patellar, 367–369, 369f
Apley grind test, 361, 362f
Apophyseal joint pain, 7–9, 8f
Apprehension relocation test, in glenohumeral
      instability, 64, 66f
Apprehension test, 64, 65f, 72
Apraxia, speech, 853, 854–855, 854t, 857
Arachnoiditis, 565–569, 566f, 566t, 567t
Arcade of Struthers, ulnar nerve entrapment at,
      125
Arnold neuralgia, 485–489, 486f, 488f, 489t
Arterial insufficiency, lower extremity, 673–676
Arteriovenous fistula, 647, 649
Arteriovenous graft, 647, 649
Arthritis. See also Osteoarthritis and at specific joints
   bowel-associated, 685–689, 686f, 687f, 689t
   inflammatory. See Rheumatoid arthritis
   psoriatic, 809–812, 810f
   reactive, 685–689, 686f, 687f, 689t
   rheumatoid. See Rheumatoid arthritis
   seronegative, 605–607, 606f
   spinal. See Cervical spine, degenerative disease
      of; Cervical spine, facet arthropathy of;
      Lumbar spine, degenerative disease of
Arthrocentesis
   after knee replacement, 403
   in cruciate ligament injury, 309, 384
Arthrodesis
   in costosternal syndrome, 548
   in elbow arthritis, 101–102
   in hammer toe, 455
   in hand osteoarthritis, 158
   in hand rheumatoid arthritis, 163
   in Kienböck disease, 169
   in lumbar degenerative disease, 234
   in lumbar spinal stenosis, 263
   in mallet toe, 459
   in mucous cyst, 158
   in shoulder arthritis, 94–95
   of wrist, 200, 200f, 208, 209f, 210f
Arthrofibrosis. See Contracture
Arthrography
   in adhesive capsulitis, 51, 51f
   in Baker's cyst, 316
   in biceps tendinitis, 57
   in chronic ankle instability, 434, 434f
   in epicondylitis, 106
   in lumbar facet arthropathy, 238, 238f
   in rotator cuff tear, 79
Arthroplasty
   in ankylosing spondylitis, 607
   in cerebral palsy, 633
   disc, 234
   in elbow arthritis, 100–102
   in hammer toe, 455
   in hand osteoarthritis, 158–159
   in hand rheumatoid arthritis, 164
   of hip, 274–275, 295–301

Arthroplasty (Continued)
   of knee, 351–352, 399–405, 402t, 404t
   in lumbar degenerative disease, 234
   in mallet toe, 459
   in osteoarthritis, 94, 100–102, 158–159,
      749–750
   in shoulder arthritis, 94
   in wrist arthritis, 199–200
Arthroscopy
   diagnostic
      in biceps tendinitis, 57
      in wrist osteoarthritis, 206
   therapeutic
      in anterior cruciate ligament tear, 312
      in elbow arthritis, 100
      in ganglion cyst, 152
      in knee arthritis, 351, 351t
      in osteoarthritis, 749
      in shoulder arthritis, 94
Aspiration
   in anterior cruciate ligament tear, 311
   in Baker's cyst, 316, 317
   in ganglion cyst, 151, 152, 158
   in meniscal tear, 362, 363–364
   in olecranon bursitis, 116–118, 118f
Aspirin, in stroke, 888
Assistive devices
   in cancer-related fatigue, 624
   in cerebral palsy, 632
   in cervicogenic vertigo, 34
   in knee arthritis, 349
   in motor neuron disease, 710
   in multiple sclerosis, 724
   in myopathy, 732
   in osteoarthritis, 157, 157t, 749
   in peripheral neuropathy, 770
   in post-poliomyelitis syndrome, 798
   in stroke, 890
   in transverse myelitis, 910
   in trapezius strain, 38
Ataxia, in multiple sclerosis, 724
Atherosclerosis
   coronary, 833–834
   peripheral, 673–676
Athetosis, 714
Austin Moore endoprosthesis. See Hip,
      replacement of
Autonomic dysreflexia, 860, 862t, 872, 873
   treatment of, 740, 865–866, 875
Autonomic testing, in peripheral neuropathy,
      769
Avascular necrosis, lunate, 167–170, 168f, 168t,
      169f, 170f
Avoidance behavior, in chronic fatigue syndrome,
      636–637
Azathioprine
   in peripheral neuropathy, 770
   side effects of, 689t

B

Babinski sign, 4
Back pain. See also Low back strain/sprain;
      Lumbar spine, stenosis of
   axial, 247–248
   differential diagnosis of, 232t–233t
   in lumbar degenerative disease, 229–230,
      247
   in lumbar facet arthropathy, 237,
      247–248
   myofascial, 248
   radicular, 248
   referred, 248
   in scapular winging, 85–86
   in spondylolysis, 254
   thoracic, 223–227

Baclofen
   in lumbar degenerative disease, 233t
   in multiple sclerosis, 723, 725
   in neurogenic bladder, 737t
   in spasticity, 851, 851t
   in trigeminal neuralgia, 494, 495t
Baker's cyst, 315–317, 316f, 833
Balanitis, circinate, 686
Bath Ankylosing Spondylitis Functional Index, 606
Beatty maneuver, 531
Bed rest
   joint contracture and, 651, 652f
   in lumbar radiculopathy, 243
   in post-poliomyelitis syndrome, 798
   in thoracic sprain/strain, 226
Bedsores. See Pressure ulcers (sores)
Benzodiazepines
   in amyotrophic lateral sclerosis, 709
   in movement disorders, 716
   in multiple sclerosis, 723
   in neurogenic bladder, 737t
   in spasticity, 850, 851t
Benzopyrones, in lymphedema, 700
Benztropine, in Parkinson disease, 762, 763t
Bernhardt-Roth syndrome, 283–286, 284t
Bethanechol, in areflexic bladder, 737t
Biceps brachii
   corticosteroid injection of, 57, 58f
   rupture of, 59–61, 60f
Biceps tendon
   rupture of, 59–61, 60f
   tendinitis of, 55–58, 56f, 58f
Biceps tenodesis, in biceps tendinitis, 57–58
Bicipital groove, palpation of, 55, 56f
Bicipital strain, 59–61, 60f
Bilevel positive airway pressure, 827
   in amyotrophic lateral sclerosis, 711
Biofeedback therapy
   in dysphagia, 681–682
   in phantom limb pain, 577
Biologic therapy
   in psoriatic arthritis, 811
   in rheumatoid arthritis, 162, 837
Biopsy
   in myopathy, 731
   in peripheral neuropathy, 769
   in pressure ulcers, 816
   in systemic lupus erythematosus, 902
Birmingham hip resurfacing. See Hip,
      replacement of
Bisphosphonates
   in heterotopic ossification, 693–694
   in osteoporosis, 755t, 756–757
Bladder
   areflexic, 734, 735t, 738f, 739
   control of, 733–734
   drug effects on, 734, 737t
   dysfunction of
      after stroke, 895, 896, 898–899
      in cervical spinal cord injury, 868
      in lumbosacral spinal cord injury, 882,
         883, 884
      in multiple sclerosis, 723
      in Parkinson disease, 734
      in thoracic spinal cord injury, 877
      in transverse myelitis, 910
   neurogenic, 733–742
      examination of, 735–736, 738f, 739f
      symptoms of, 733–735, 735t, 736f
      treatment of, 737–742, 737t, 740t, 741f,
         866, 866t, 868
Blast injury, 787–791, 791t
Blood clot. See Deep venous thrombosis
Blood flow
   pressure ulcer formation and, 814
   in repetitive strain injury, 539–540

Blood pressure, ankle/foot, 674
Bone
    brittle (thin). *See* Osteoporosis
    injury to. *See* Fracture
Bone mineral density, 754–755, 755t
    in post-poliomyelitis syndrome, 796
Bone scan
    in cancer, 622–623
    in hip disease, 297
    in quadriceps contusion, 292
    in scoliosis, 844
    in spondylolysis, 255–256, 256f
    in thoracic spinal cord injury, 872
    in Tietze syndrome, 558
    in trochanteric bursitis, 304
Borg exertion scale, 618, 619f, 828
Botulinum toxin injection
    in cerebral palsy, 633
    in cervical dystonia, 581–582
    in cervicogenic vertigo, 34
    in coccydynia, 574
    in epicondylitis, 107
    in headache, 522
    in movement disorders, 716
    in multiple sclerosis, 724–725
    in myofascial pain syndrome, 529, 530
    in neurogenic bladder, 737t
    in piriformis syndrome, 288, 530
    in postherpetic neuralgia, 563
    in spasmodic dysphonia, 857
    in spasticity, 850, 851
    in thoracic spinal cord injury, 876
    in thoracic sprain/strain, 227
    in trapezius strain, 39, 40
Boutonnière deformity, 141, 142t, 161, 162f,
    164, 834, 834f
Bowel-associated arthritis, 685–689, 686f, 687f,
    689t
Bowel dysfunction
    in cervical spinal cord injury, 865–866, 868
    in lumbosacral spinal cord injury, 882, 883,
        884
    in multiple sclerosis, 720, 722, 723–724
    neurogenic bladder and, 738–739
    in Parkinson disease, 763
    in thoracic spinal cord injury, 874, 874t,
        877
    in transverse myelitis, 910
Brace
    after knee replacement, 404
    in ankle sprain, 424
    in cerebral palsy, 632
    in chronic ankle instability, 434
    in epicondylitis, 106
    in joint contracture, 653
    in knee arthritis, 349
    in patellofemoral syndrome, 372
    in scapular winging, 87–88
    in spinal deformity, 845, 846, 846f
    in stroke, 890
    in thoracic compression fracture, 214, 215f
    in thoracic radiculopathy, 221
Brachial plexopathy, 773–777, 774f
Brachial plexus, 497, 498f, 773, 774f
Brachialgia, 17–21, 18f, 18t, 19f
Bragard sign, 249t
Brain attack. *See* Stroke
Brain injury. *See* Post-concussion disorders;
    Traumatic brain injury
Break-dancer's thumb, 183–185
Breast cancer
    exercise in, 623–624
    lymphedema in, 697, 699f
    mastectomy-related pain in, 589–590
Breathing retraining exercises, 828
Brittle bones. *See* Osteoporosis

Bromocriptine, in Parkinson disease, 715, 763,
    763t
Bronchodilators, 826, 827t
Brunelli test, 129
Bucket-handle injury, 360, 361, 361f
Bunion, 427–429, 428f, 429f
Bunionette, 429–430
Bupropion
    in cardiac rehabilitation, 617
    in complex regional pain syndrome, 514t
Burn contracture. *See* Burns
Burns, 609–613, 610t, 611f
Bursectomy, in olecranon bursitis, 118
Bursitis
    foot and ankle, 415–420, 416f, 416t, 417t,
        418t, 419f
    knee, 355–358, 356f, 357f
    olecranon, 115–118, 116f, 118f
    septic, 115–117, 116f, 118, 118f, 420
    trochanteric, 232t–233t, 303–305, 304f

C

C-reactive protein, in heterotopic ossification, 693
Calcaneus altus. *See* Foot (feet), bursitis of
Calcifications, in trochanteric bursitis, 304
Calcitonin
    in osteoporosis, 755t, 757
    in thoracic compression fracture, 214
    in Tietze syndrome, 559
Calcium, in osteoporosis, 755–756
Calculi, renal, 736
Calf, edema of, 657
Calf hypertension. *See* Compartment syndrome
Callosity, of toe, 441–443, 442f, 443f
Cancer
    breast, 589–590, 623–624, 697, 699f
    fatigue with, 621–625
    lumbosacral plexopathy with, 781–782
    lymphedema with, 697, 699f
Cane, in arthritis, 274, 349
Capsaicin
    in complex regional pain syndrome, 514t
    in intercostal neuralgia, 552
    in knee arthritis, 347, 348t
Capsulitis. *See also* Contracture
    adhesive, 49–54, 50f, 50t, 51f
Carbamazepine
    in brain injury, 915
    in complex regional pain syndrome, 514t, 515
    in occipital neuralgia, 488, 489t
    in peripheral neuropathy, 770
    in phantom pain, 577
    in spinal cord injury, 867, 867t
    in trigeminal neuralgia, 494, 495t
Cardiac rehabilitation, 615–620, 617t, 618t, 619t
Cardiovascular disease
    chronic kidney disease and, 648
    rehabilitation in, 615–620, 617t, 618t, 619t
    rheumatoid arthritis and, 833–834
Caregiver support, in dementia, 669t, 670
Carisoprodol, in lumbar degenerative disease,
    233t
Carotid endarterectomy, 890
Carpal cyst. *See* Ganglion cyst
Carpal tunnel
    corticosteroid injection of, 199
    release of, 176
Carpal tunnel syndrome, 173–177, 174f, 175f,
    176f
    in rheumatoid arthritis, 195, 198
Carpectomy
    in Kienböck disease, 169
    in osteoarthritis, 207–208, 208f, 209f, 210
Carpometacarpal joint, corticosteroid injection
    of, 157, 158f

Cast
    in joint contracture, 653, 654f, 655
    in lower limb amputation, 601, 602t
    in posterior tibial dysfunction, 477
    in spasticity, 850
    in ulnar collateral ligament sprain, 184
Catechol *O*-methyltransferase inhibitor, in
    Parkinson disease, 763, 763t
Catheterization
    femoral artery, 780–781
    urinary
        intermittent, 734, 739, 874
        suprapubic, 741, 741f
Cauda equina syndrome. *See* Spinal cord injury,
    lumbosacral
Causalgia, 511–516, 513t, 514t
Celiac disease, 686, 687, 688
Cellulitis, lymphedema and, 701, 702f
Cerebral infarction. *See* Stroke, young adult
Cerebral palsy, 627–633, 630f
    mortality from, 627–628
    types of, 627
Cerebral venous thrombosis. *See* Stroke, young
    adult
Cerebrospinal fluid analysis
    in peripheral neuropathy, 769
    in transverse myelitis, 909
Cerebrovascular accident, 887–891, 889t,
    893–899, 894t, 896t. *See also* Stroke,
    young adult
Cervical collar
    in radiculopathy, 20, 21
    in spondylotic myelopathy, 5
Cervical dystonia, 579–582, 582t
Cervical migraine, 485–489, 486f, 488f, 489t
Cervical rib syndrome. *See* Thoracic outlet
    syndrome
Cervical rotation–lateral flexion test, 499–500,
    500f
Cervical spine. *See also* Spinal cord injury, cervical
    aging-related changes in, 3, 11
    canal diameter in, 3, 4, 5f
    decompression and fusion of, 14
    degenerative disease of, 11–15, 12t, 13f
    examination of, in rotator cuff tear, 77
    facet arthropathy of, 7–9, 8f
    facet joint of, 7
    neurocentral joints of, 11, 12f
    palpation of, in facet arthropathy, 7
    radiculopathy of, 17–21, 18f, 18t, 19f
    rheumatoid arthritis of, 835, 836f, 837, 837f
    spondylotic myelopathy of, 3–6, 5f
    sprain/strain of, 23–25, 24f
    stenosis of, 27–31, 28f, 29f
    traction on
        in cervical stenosis, 30, 31
        in degenerative disease, 14
Cervicogenic vertigo, 33–35, 34f
Chamay procedure, 200
Cheiralgia paresthetica, 121–124, 122f, 123f
Chest pain
    atypical, 545–548, 546f, 547f
    in cardiac rehabilitation, 615
    differential diagnosis of, 551t, 558t
    in Tietze syndrome, 555
Chlorzoxazone, in lumbar degenerative disease,
    233t
Choking, 679
Cholinesterase inhibitors, in dementia, 669, 671
Chondritis, costal, 555–560, 556f, 557f, 558f
Chondrodynia
    costosternal, 545–548, 546f, 547f
    parasternal, 555–560, 556f, 557f, 558f
Chondroitin sulfate, 347, 348t, 748
Chondromalacia, patellar, 371–374, 372f, 373f,
    374f

Chondropathia tuberosa, 555–560, 556f, 557f, 558f
Chorea, 714
Chronic fatigue syndrome, 635–640, 637t, 638t
Chronic obstructive pulmonary disease, 823. *See also* Pulmonary rehabilitation
Chronic pain syndrome, 505–509, 506t, 507t, 508t, 522. *See also* Pain
Chronic paroxysmal hemicrania, 494t
Chronic venous insufficiency, fasciotomy and, 329
Cigarette smoking
    cessation of
        in cardiac rehabilitation, 617
        in osteoporosis, 756
    diabetes and, 675
Cilostazol, in diabetes mellitus, 675
Citalopram, in complex regional pain syndrome, 514t
Clasp-knife phenomenon, 849
Claudication
    neurogenic, 260. *See also* Lumbar spine, stenosis of
    vascular, 673–676
Clavicle, distal, atraumatic osteolysis of, 41–46, 42f, 42t, 43f, 44f, 45f, 46f
Clavus, 441–443, 442f, 443f
Claw toe, 437–440, 438f, 439f
Clonazepam
    in complex regional pain syndrome, 514t
    in trigeminal neuralgia, 494, 495t
Clonidine, in complex regional pain syndrome, 514t
Cluster headache, 519, 522
Cobb angle, 844, 844f
Coccydynia, 571–574, 572f, 573f
Coccygectomy, 574
Coenzyme Q10, in amyotrophic lateral sclerosis, 707
Cognitive-behavioral therapy
    in chronic fatigue syndrome, 639
    in myofascial pain syndrome, 532–533
Cognitive impairment/deficit, 667, 667t, 668, 669f. *See also* Dementia
    in cancer, 623
    in cerebral palsy, 630
    in multiple sclerosis, 721, 724
    in post-concussion disorders, 802, 803, 805
    in stroke, 889
Cognitive testing, in dementia, 667–668
Cognitive training, in dementia, 670–671
Cold intolerance, in post-poliomyelitis syndrome, 795, 796, 797
Cold therapy
    in Achilles tendinitis, 408
    in acromioclavicular joint injury, 44
    in ankle sprain, 424
    in biceps tendinitis, 57
    in cervical stenosis, 30
    in costosternal syndrome, 547
    in foot and ankle bursitis, 419
    in hammer toe, 454
    in hamstring strain, 333
    in intercostal neuralgia, 553
    in mallet toe, 458
    in plantar fasciitis, 471
    in quadriceps contusion, 292
    in repetitive strain injury, 542
    in rotator cuff tear, 79
    in trapezius strain, 38
    in trochanteric bursitis, 305
    in wrist osteoarthritis, 207
Collateral ligament sprain, 319–322, 320f, 321f
Communication disorders, 853–857, 854t

Compartment syndrome
    in biceps tendon rupture, 61
    lower extremity, 325–329
        acute, 325–329, 325f, 326f
        chronic, 325–329, 327f
        pressure measurements in, 327–328, 327f
Complex regional pain syndrome, 511–516, 513t, 514t
    stages of, 511–512
    treatment of, 513–516, 513t, 514t
Compression devices/garments
    in burn-related scarring, 611
    in deep venous thrombosis prophylaxis, 660
    in lymphedema, 700–701
Compression test, in sacroiliac joint dysfunction, 268
Computed tomographic myelography
    in cervical degenerative disease, 13
    in cervical spondylotic myelopathy, 4
Computed tomography (CT)
    in cerebral palsy, 631
    in cervical radiculopathy, 20
    in chronic ankle instability, 434
    in dementia, 668
    in glenohumeral arthritis, 92
    in heterotopic ossification, 693
    in lumbar degenerative disease, 231
    in lumbar radiculopathy, 243, 244f
    in lumbar spinal stenosis, 262t
    in lumbosacral plexopathy, 783
    in lumbosacral spinal cord injury, 882
    in occipital neuralgia, 486
    in polytrauma, 788
    in post-concussion disorders, 803–804
    in scapular winging, 87
    in spondylolysis, 255, 255f, 256f
    in stroke, 888
    in thoracic sprain/strain, 225
    in Tietze syndrome, 558
    in traumatic brain injury, 914
    in wrist osteoarthritis, 206
Concussion, 801, 802t. *See also* Post-concussion disorders; Traumatic brain injury
Conjunctivitis, in psoriatic arthritis, 809
Constipation
    in cerebral palsy, 629
    in multiple sclerosis, 720, 723–724
    in Parkinson disease, 763
    in spinal cord injury, 874, 882, 883
Continent diversion, in neurogenic bladder, 742
Continuous passive motion, after total knee replacement, 401, 402t, 403
Continuous positive airway pressure, 827
Contracture, 651–655, 652t, 654f
    bed rest and, 651, 652f
    in burns, 611, 611f, 612
    in cerebral palsy, 633
    in compartment syndrome, 326, 328
    Dupuytren, 133–136, 134f
    lower extremity, 652–653, 654f
    in lower limb amputation, 600
    physical examination in, 652, 653f
    spasticity and, 849
    spinal cord injury and, 651
    stroke and, 869, 895
    upper extremity, 652
Contusion
    hamstring, 331–335, 332f, 333f, 334f
    quadriceps, 291–293
Conus medullaris syndrome, 780t, 781t, 879–884
Corns, 441–443, 442f, 443f
Coronary heart disease
    rehabilitation in, 615–620, 617t, 618t, 619t
    in rheumatoid arthritis, 833–834
Corticobasal degeneration, 762

Corticosteroids
    injection of
        in acromioclavicular joint injury, 45, 46f
        in adhesive capsulitis, 51
        in ankylosing spondylitis, 607
        in biceps tendinitis, 57, 58, 58f
        in carpal tunnel syndrome, 175, 176, 176f
        in cervical radiculopathy, 20–21
        in cervical stenosis, 30, 31
        in chronic ankle instability, 435
        in coccydynia, 573–574
        in costosternal syndrome, 547–548, 547f
        in de Quervain tenosynovitis, 131
        in degenerative disease, 14
        in Dupuytren contracture, 135
        in elbow arthritis, 100, 101f
        in epicondylitis, 106–107, 107f
        in foot and ankle bursitis, 419, 420
        in foot and ankle ganglia, 446
        in glenohumeral instability, 67, 68f
        in hammer toe, 455
        in hand osteoarthritis, 157, 158f
        in hip arthritis, 274, 274f
        in iliotibial band syndrome, 341–342, 342f
        in intercostal neuralgia, 553
        in jumper's knee, 369
        in knee arthritis, 350, 350f, 350t
        in knee bursitis, 357, 357f
        in lateral femoral cutaneous neuropathy, 285, 285f, 286
        in lumbar degenerative disease, 234
        in lumbar disc disease, 250
        in lumbar facet joint disease, 239
        in lumbar radiculopathy, 245
        in lumbar spinal stenosis, 263
        in mallet toe, 458
        in Morton neuroma, 467, 467f, 468
        in myofascial pain syndrome, 533–534
        in olecranon bursitis, 118
        in osteoarthritis, 749
        in piriformis syndrome, 288, 534
        in plantar fasciitis, 472, 472f, 473
        in postherpetic neuralgia, 563
        in quadriceps tendinitis, 388
        in rotator cuff tendinitis, 75
        in sacroiliac joint dysfunction, 269
        in shoulder arthritis, 93–94, 93f, 94f
        in Tietze syndrome, 559
        in trigger finger, 181, 181f
        in trochanteric bursitis, 305
        in ulnar neuropathy, 191, 191f
        in wrist osteoarthritis, 207
        in wrist rheumatoid arthritis, 198–199
    intravenous, in cervical sprain/strain, 25
    oral
        in carpal tunnel syndrome, 175
        in cervical degenerative disease, 14
        in cervical stenosis, 30
        in complex regional pain syndrome, 515
        in median neuropathy, 175
        in multiple sclerosis, 722–723
        in rheumatoid arthritis, 162, 837, 838t
        side effects of, 689t, 838t
        in thoracic radiculopathy, 221
Corticotropin-releasing hormone, in fibromyalgia, 530
Costal chondritis, 555–560, 556f, 557f, 558f
Costochondral junction syndrome, 555–560, 556f, 557f, 558f
Costochondritis, 545–548, 546f, 547f
Costoclavicular syndrome. *See* Thoracic outlet syndrome
Costosternal chondrodynia, 545–548, 546f, 547f
Costosternal joints, in thoracic sprain/strain, 224–225
Costosternal syndrome, 545–548, 546f, 547f

Costotransverse joints, in thoracic sprain/strain, 224–225
Costovertebral joints, in thoracic sprain/strain, 224–225
Cough therapy
　in cervical spinal cord injury, 865
　in ventilatory impairment, 829
Coughing, in dysphagia, 679, 680t
Coumadin. See Warfarin
Creatine kinase
　in heterotopic ossification, 693
　in myopathy, 731
Creatinine, serum, in chronic kidney disease, 645
Creatinine clearance, in chronic kidney disease, 645
Credé maneuver, 739
Crest pad
　in corns, 442, 442f
　in mallet toe, 458
Crohn disease, 685, 686, 686f, 688–689
Cross-body adduction test, 42, 42f
Cruciate ligament
　anterior, 381, 382f
　　tear of, 307–312, 308f, 309f, 310t, 311t
　posterior, 381, 382f
　　sprain of, 381–385, 382f, 382t, 383f, 384f
Crutches, in ankle sprain, 424
Cryotherapy. See Cold therapy
Cubital tunnel syndrome, 98, 99, 125–127, 126f
Cucumber heel. See Foot (feet), bursitis of
Cumulative trauma disorder, 539–543
Cyclobenzaprine
　in lumbar degenerative disease, 233t
　in myofascial pain syndrome, 533
Cyclooxygenase 2 inhibitors. See Nonsteroidal anti-inflammatory drugs (NSAIDs)
Cyclosporine, 689t
Cyst(s)
　Baker's, 315–317, 316f, 809, 833
　ganglion
　　foot and ankle, 445–447, 446f
　　hand and wrist, 149–153, 150f, 151f
　　paralabral, 92
　　popliteal, 315–317, 316f
　　synovial, 149
Cystoscopy
　in cervical spinal cord injury, 864
　in lumbosacral spinal cord injury, 882
　in neurogenic bladder, 736

D

D-dimer assay, in deep venous thrombosis, 658–659
Dantrolene
　in multiple sclerosis, 723
　in neurogenic bladder, 737t
　in spasticity, 851t
Darifenacin, 740, 740t
Darrach procedure, 199, 200f
De Quervain tenosynovitis, 129–131, 130f
Débridement
　in ankle arthritis, 412
　in elbow arthritis, 100, 102
　in knee arthritis, 351, 351t
　in pressure ulcers, 819
　in shoulder arthritis, 94
Debulking surgery, in lymphedema, 701, 701f
Decubitus ulcers, 813–819, 814t, 815f, 817f
　in cerebral palsy, 630
　in cervical spinal cord injury, 866, 867
　in lumbosacral spinal cord injury, 883, 884
　in thoracic spinal cord injury, 872–873, 876
Deep brain stimulation
　in cervical dystonia, 582
　in Parkinson disease, 764

Deep venous thrombosis, 657–662, 658t, 659f, 659t, 661t, 662f
　hip replacement and, 297
　knee replacement and, 401, 404
　spinal cord injury and, 872, 875
　stroke and, 890
Degenerative joint disease. See Osteoarthritis
Deglutition disorder. See Dysphagia
Delirium, 668t
Dementia, 665–671, 666t, 669f, 669t
Denosumab, in osteoporosis, 757
Denture pain, 493t
Deprenyl, in Parkinson disease, 715
Depression
　after stroke, 887, 894, 896, 897–898
　in cardiac rehabilitation, 616
　vs. dementia, 668t
　dementia and, 670, 671
　in motor neuron disease, 709
　in Parkinson disease, 764–765
　in post-concussion disorders, 803, 805
　in thoracic spinal cord injury, 872
　in traumatic brain injury, 915
　in upper limb amputation, 598
Desensitization therapy
　in complex regional pain syndrome, 515
　in postherpetic neuralgia, 562
Desipramine, in complex regional pain syndrome, 514t
Detrol, 740, 740t
Detrusor hyperactivity, 723, 735t
Detrusor-sphincter dyssynergia, 723, 734, 735t, 737t, 739f
Dextromethorphan, in phantom limb pain, 577
Diabetes mellitus
　lumbosacral plexopathy in, 779–784, 780f, 781f
　peripheral arterial disease in, 673–676
　polyneuropathy in, 770
　polyradiculopathy, 233t
　thoracic radiculopathy in, 219
Dialysis, 647
Dialysis elbow, 115–118, 116f, 118f
Diarrhea, in multiple sclerosis, 724
Diazepam. See Benzodiazepines
Diet
　in cardiac rehabilitation, 617, 617t
　in chronic kidney disease, 649
　in dysphagia, 680, 681
　in multiple sclerosis, 723–724
Diffuse idiopathic skeletal hyperostosis, 229, 232t
Digital flexor tenosynovitis, 179–182, 180f, 181f
Disc. See Intervertebral disc
Discography, in lumbar degenerative disease, 231
Disease-modifying drugs, in rheumatoid arthritis, 837
Disseminated sclerosis. See Multiple sclerosis
Distraction test, in sacroiliac joint dysfunction, 268
Ditropan, 740, 740t
Diuretics, in lymphedema, 700
Dizziness
　cervicogenic, 33–35, 34f
　post-concussion, 802–803, 805, 806
Donepezil, in dementia, 669
Dopamine agonists, in Parkinson disease, 763, 763t
Dorsal rhizotomy
　in cerebral palsy, 633
　in occipital neuralgia, 487
Dorsal scapular nerve palsy, 84
Dossifying fibromyopathy/fibromyositis. See Heterotopic ossification
Double-crush syndrome, 12, 500
Dowager's hump. See Kyphosis

Doxepin, in complex regional pain syndrome, 514t
Draftsman's elbow, 115–118, 116f, 118f
Drawer test
　anterior
　　in ankle sprain, 422
　　in anterior cruciate ligament tear, 308, 309f
　　in medial collateral ligament sprain, 320
　posterior
　　in posterior cruciate ligament sprain, 381, 383f
Dressing
　in hip replacement, 297
　in lower limb amputation, 601–602, 602t, 603f
Driving
　dementia and, 671
　lower limb amputation and, 601–602
　stroke and, 896
Drop arm test, 72
Drugs. See also specific drugs and classes of drugs
　myopathy with, 729, 730t
　peripheral neuropathy with, 768t
Dual-energy x-ray absorptiometry, 754–755, 755t
Duloxetine
　in arachnoiditis, 567, 567t
　in complex regional pain syndrome, 514t
Duodenal ulcer, 232t
Dupuytren contracture (disease), 133–136, 134f
Durkan test, 195
Dysarthria, 853, 854t, 855, 855t, 856–857
　in dysphagia, 679
　in motor neuron disease, 710
　in multiple sclerosis, 721, 724
　in Parkinson disease, 715, 761
　in stroke, 889
Dyskinesia, 713–717
Dysphagia, 679–683, 680t, 681t, 682t
　in motor neuron disease, 710
　in multiple sclerosis, 721, 724
　in post-poliomyelitis syndrome, 795, 796, 797
　in stroke, 889
Dysphonia, 679, 853–854, 854t, 855, 857
　in post-poliomyelitis syndrome, 795
Dyspnea
　in cancer, 621, 622
　in cardiac rehabilitation, 616
　in post-poliomyelitis syndrome, 794–795
　in pulmonary disease, 823, 824
　in spinal cord injury, 860, 861t
Dysreflexia, autonomic, 740
Dystonia, 714, 715, 716
　spastic. See Spasticity

E

Echocardiography, in rheumatoid arthritis, 836
Edema. See also Lymphedema
　calf, 657
　hip replacement and, 297
　lower limb amputation and, 601, 602t
　pulmonary, 644
Effusion, in rheumatoid arthritis, 98, 835
Eichoff test, 129
El Escorial criteria, 706–707, 706f
Elastic bandage, in lower limb amputation, 601, 602t
Elbow
　amputation below/above, 595–598
　bursitis of, 115–118, 116f, 118f
　immobilization of, in biceps tendon rupture, 61
　injection of, 100, 101f
　osteoarthritis of, 97–102, 98t, 99f, 100f, 101f
　rheumatoid arthritis of, 835
　tennis/pitcher's/golfer's, 105–107, 107f
　ulnar neuropathy at, 125–127, 126f

Electrical stimulation
   in cervical sprain/strain, 25
   in knee arthritis, 349
   in lateral femoral cutaneous neuropathy, 285
   in lumbosacral plexopathy, 784
   in myofascial pain syndrome, 532
   in neurogenic bladder, 741
   in occipital neuralgia, 487–488, 488f
   in osteoarthritis, 749
   in Parkinson disease, 764
   in phantom limb pain, 577
   in postherpetic neuralgia, 562
   in shoulder arthritis, 93
Electroacupuncture, in Tietze syndrome, 559
Electrocardiography
   in cardiac rehabilitation, 616
   in rheumatoid arthritis, 836
Electrodiagnostic testing
   in biceps tendinitis, 57
   in brachial plexopathy, 775
   in carpal tunnel syndrome, 175
   in cerebral palsy, 631
   in cervical radiculopathy, 20
   in cervical spinal cord injury, 864
   in cervical spondylotic myelopathy, 4
   in femoral neuropathy, 278
   in lumbar degenerative disease, 231
   in lumbar radiculopathy, 243
   in lumbar spinal stenosis, 262t
   in lumbosacral plexopathy, 783
   in lumbosacral spinal cord injury, 882
   in median neuropathy, 111
   in myopathy, 731
   in peripheral neuropathy, 769
   in peroneal neuropathy, 377
   in piriformis syndrome, 288
   in polytrauma, 788
   in post-poliomyelitis syndrome, 796
   in radial neuropathy, 122
   in repetitive strain injury, 541
   in rotator cuff tendinitis, 72
   in scapular winging, 87
   in scoliosis, 844
   in thoracic radiculopathy, 220
   in transverse myelitis, 909
   in ulnar neuropathy, 126, 189
Electromyography
   in brachial plexopathy, 775
   in carpal tunnel syndrome, 175
   in cerebral palsy, 631
   in cervical radiculopathy, 20
   in cervical spinal cord injury, 864
   in femoral neuropathy, 278
   in lateral femoral cutaneous neuropathy, 284
   in lumbar radiculopathy, 243
   in lumbar spinal stenosis, 262t
   in lumbosacral plexopathy, 783
   in lumbosacral spinal cord injury, 882
   in median neuropathy, 111
   in myopathy, 731
   in peripheral neuropathy, 769
   in peroneal neuropathy, 377
   in radial neuropathy, 122
   in scapular winging, 87
   in thoracic radiculopathy, 220
   in ulnar neuropathy, 126, 189–190
Electrotheraphy, in myofascial pain syndrome, 532
Electrothermal therapy, in lumbar degenerative disease, 234
Elephantiasis, 699–700, 701, 701f
Elevated arm stress test, 499
Embolectomy, 661

Embolism, pulmonary. See also Deep venous thrombosis
   knee replacement and, 404
   spinal cord injury and, 872
Emotional lability/incontinence
   after stroke, 894
   in motor neuron disease, 709
Encephalomyelitis, myalgic. See Chronic fatigue syndrome
Endometriosis, 232t
Endoscopy, in dysphagia, 681–682
Enoxaparin, prophylactic, for hip replacement, 297
Entacapone, in Parkinson disease, 763, 763t
Enteropathic arthritis, 685–689, 686f, 687f, 689t
Epicondylitis, 105–107, 107f
   vs. radial neuropathy, 123
Epoetin, in chronic kidney disease, 648
Erb palsy, 773–777, 774f
Erectile dysfunction, in thoracic spinal cord injury, 875, 876
Ergonomics, in repetitive strain injury, 542–543
Erysipelas, lymphedema and, 701, 702f
Erythropoietin, in chronic kidney disease, 648
Esophagectomy, 682
Esophagoscopy, in dysphagia, 680
Esophagus, dilatation of, 681
Etanercept, in rheumatoid arthritis, 162
Etidronate disodium, in heterotopic ossification, 693–694
Exercise(s)
   in Achilles tendinitis, 409
   in acromioclavicular joint injury, 45
   in adhesive capsulitis, 51–52, 53f
   after hip replacement, 275, 299
   in ankle sprain, 424
   in ankylosing spondylitis, 607
   in anterior cruciate ligament injury, 310, 310t, 311, 311t
   in arachnoiditis, 567–568
   in biceps tendinitis, 57
   in biceps tendon rupture, 61
   in brachial plexopathy, 776
   in burns, 611
   in cancer-related fatigue, 623–624
   in cardiac rehabilitation, 618–619, 618t, 619f, 619t
   in cerebral palsy, 632
   in cervical degenerative disease, 14
   in cervical facet arthropathy, 8
   in cervical sprain/strain, 25
   in chronic ankle instability, 435
   in chronic fatigue syndrome, 639
   in collateral ligament sprain, 322
   in diabetes mellitus, 675
   in dysphagia, 681, 682f
   in epicondylitis, 106
   in flexor tendon injury, 147–148, 147t
   in foot and ankle bursitis, 418–419, 419t
   in glenohumeral instability, 66–67, 67t
   in hammer toe, 454
   in hamstring strain, 334, 335f
   in hand osteoarthritis, 157
   in heterotopic ossification, 694
   in hip arthritis, 273
   in iliotibial band syndrome, 340–341, 341f
   in jumper's knee, 368–369, 369f
   in knee arthritis, 347, 349
   in knee bursitis, 357
   in kyphosis, 845
   in low back pain, 250
   in lumbar radiculopathy, 244
   in lumbar spondylolysis and spondylolisthesis, 257
   in lumbar stenosis, 262

Exercise(s) (Continued)
   in lymphedema, 701
   in mallet toe, 458
   in meniscal injury, 363
   in metatarsalgia, 463
   in motor neuron disease, 709–710
   in movement disorders, 716
   in myofascial pain syndrome, 532
   in myopathy, 732
   in occipital neuralgia, 487
   in osteoarthritis, 748–749
   in osteoporosis, 756
   in Parkinson disease, 716
   in patellofemoral syndrome, 373, 373f, 374f
   in peroneal neuropathy, 378
   in piriformis syndrome, 288
   in plantar fasciitis, 471
   in post-poliomyelitis syndrome, 797–798
   in post-thoracotomy pain, 587
   in posterior cruciate ligament sprain, 384
   in posterior tibial dysfunction, 477
   in psoriatic arthritis, 811
   in pulmonary rehabilitation, 827, 828t
   in quadriceps contusion, 292–293
   in quadriceps tendinitis, 388
   in rheumatoid arthritis, 837
   in rotator cuff tear, 79–80, 80
   in rotator cuff tendinitis, 74
   in scapular winging, 88
   in shin splints, 391
   in shoulder arthritis, 93
   in spondylolysis, 257
   in stroke, 888, 889f
   in thoracic outlet syndrome, 501–502, 501f
   in thoracic sprain/strain, 226
   in tibial neuropathy, 481
   in Tietze syndrome, 559
   in trapezius strain, 38, 39
   in trochanteric bursitis, 305
   in ulnar collateral ligament sprain, 185
   in ulnar neuropathy, 190
Exercise testing
   in cardiac rehabilitation, 616, 617–618, 620
   in pulmonary rehabilitation, 825
Extensor brevis tendon lengthening, 455
Extensor digitorum longus lengthening, 455
Extensor tendon injury, 139–143, 140f, 141t, 142t, 143t
Extensor tendon reconstruction, in rheumatoid arthritis, 163
External rotation recurvatum test, 320, 321f
Extracorporeal shock wave therapy, in plantar fasciitis, 472
Extrapyramidal disease. See Movement disorders

F
Facet joints
   cervical, disease of, 7–9, 8f
   lumbar
      disease of, 237–239, 238f
      injection of, 234, 235, 239
Facial pain, 491–496, 493t–494t, 495f, 495t
FAIR test, in piriformis syndrome, 288
Falls
   in post-poliomyelitis syndrome, 798
   prevention of, 756
   in tarsal tunnel syndrome, 480
Famciclovir, in postherpetic neuralgia, 562
Familial lymphedema. See Lymphedema
Far-out syndrome, 259–260
Fasciectomy, in Dupuytren contracture, 136
Fasciitis
   gluteal, 232t–233t
   plantar, 469–473, 470f, 472f

Fasciotomy
in Dupuytren contracture, 135, 136
in lower extremity compartment syndrome, 328–329
Fatigue
after stroke, 895, 896, 899
in brain injury, 913, 915
in cancer, 621–625
chronic, 635–640, 637t, 638t
in multiple sclerosis, 721, 724, 724t
in post-poliomyelitis syndrome, 794, 795, 796
in systemic lupus erythematosus, 901
in traumatic brain injury, 915
Fatigue fracture, 393–396, 394f, 395f
Feeding
in cerebral palsy, 629
in dysphagia, 681
in motor neuron disease, 711
in Parkinson disease, 764
Felty syndrome, 836
Femoral artery catheterization, 780–781
Femoral nerve, 277, 278f, 279f
injury to, 780, 782
traction testing on, 280f
Femoral neuropathy, 277–280, 278t, 280f
Femur, stress fracture of, 393–397, 394f, 395f
Fertility, thoracic spinal cord injury and, 875, 876
Fibroblast, in Dupuytren disease, 133
Fibroma, perineural, 461–462, 465–468, 466f, 467f
Fibromatosis, plantar, 469–473, 470f, 472f
Fibromyalgia, 232t, 525–527, 526f, 530. See also Myofascial pain syndrome
definition of, 37, 525
trapezius, 37–40, 39f
Fibrositis, 525–527, 526f. See also Myofascial pain syndrome
humeroscapular, 49–54, 50f, 50t, 51f
trapezius, 37–40, 39f
Filariasis, 697
Finger. See also Hand; Thumb
amputation of, 595–598
extensor injury of, 139–143, 140f, 141t, 142t, 143t
flexor injury of, 145–148, 146f, 147f, 147t
trigger (locked), 179–182, 180f, 181f
Finkelstein test, 129, 130f
First dorsal interosseus, strength testing of, 206
Fistula, arteriovenous, in chronic kidney disease, 647, 649
Flatfoot deformity, 475–477, 476f
Flexor digitorum longus lengthening, in claw toe, 439
Flexor digitorum longus tendon transfer, in hammer toe, 455
Flexor digitorum longus transfer, in posterior tibial dysfunction, 477
Flexor hallucis longus lengthening, in claw toe, 439
Flexor hallucis longus tendon transfer, in claw toe, 439
Flexor tendon injury, 145–148, 146f, 147f, 147t
Flexor tendon reconstruction, in rheumatoid arthritis, 163
Flexor tenosynovitis, in rheumatoid arthritis, 163
Flutter breathing, 826
Focal sclerosis. See Multiple sclerosis
Foot (feet). See also Ankle
adhesive bursitis of, 420
bursae of, 415, 416f
bursitis of, 415–420, 416t, 417t, 418t, 419t
care of, in diabetes mellitus, 675
corns of, 441–443, 442f, 443f
diabetic, 673–676
examination of, in cerebral palsy, 630

Foot (feet) (Continued)
flat-, 475–477, 476f
ganglion cyst of, 445–447, 446f
hallux valgus of, 427–429, 428f, 429f
innervation of, 481f
Morton neuroma of, 461–462, 465–468, 466f, 467f
ulcer of
in claw toe, 439
in corns, 441
in diabetes, 673–676
in hammer toe, 453
in mallet toe, 457
in tibial neuropathy, 482
Footdrop
in compartment syndrome, 326
in peroneal neuropathy, 375, 376–377, 378
Footwear. See Shoe(s)
Forced vital capacity, in cervical spinal cord injury, 864–865
Forearm band, in epicondylitis, 106
Fracture
hip, 754
humeral, 46
osteoporotic, 758
sacral, 779–780
stress (insufficiency, fatigue, march), 393–396, 394f, 395f
thoracic, 213–217, 214f, 215f, 216f
wrist, 203, 204f, 754
Freiberg sign, 287, 531
Froment sign, 125–126, 126f
Frozen shoulder, arthritic, 91–95, 92f, 93f, 94f

G
Gabapentin
in arachnoiditis, 567, 567t
in complex regional pain syndrome, 514t, 515
in intercostal neuralgia, 552–553
in multiple sclerosis, 723
in occipital neuralgia, 487, 489t
in peripheral neuropathy, 770
in phantom pain, 576t, 577
in post-thoracotomy pain, 586
in repetitive strain injury, 542
in spinal cord injury, 867, 867t
in trigeminal neuralgia, 494, 495t
Gaenslen test, 249t, 268, 605, 606f
Gait
in cerebral palsy, 630, 631
in cervical spondylotic myelopathy, 3, 4
in femoral neuropathy, 279
in hamstring strain, 332
in hip disease, 272, 295
in lower limb amputation, 603
in osteoarthritis, 746
in Parkinson disease, 761, 764
in polytrauma, 789
Galantamine, in dementia, 669
Galeazzi sign, 629–631, 630f
Gamekeeper's thumb, 183–185
Ganglion cyst
foot and ankle, 445–447, 446f
hand and wrist, 149–153, 151f, 155, 158
paralabral, 92
Gapping test, in sacroiliac joint dysfunction, 268
Garrod nodes, 133
Gastrostomy tube
in cerebral palsy, 629
in motor neuron disease, 711
Genetic testing, in myopathy, 731
Genitofemoral nerve, injury to, 780, 782
Geste antagoniste, 580, 581

Giant cell arteritis, 494t
Gibbus deformity, 232t, 841–846, 842f
Girdlestone flexor tendon transfer
in claw toe, 439
in hammer toe, 455
Glasgow Coma Scale, 914, 914t
Glenohumeral joint
injection of, 67, 68f, 93–94, 93f, 94f
instability of, 63–68, 64f, 65f, 66f, 67t, 68f
osteoarthritis of, 91–95, 92f, 93f, 94f
Glomerular filtration rate, in chronic kidney disease, 643, 644, 644t
Glossopharyngeal neuralgia, 493t
Glucosamine
in knee arthritis, 347, 348t
in osteoarthritis, 748
Gold therapy
in psoriatic arthritis, 811
in rheumatoid arthritis, 837
side effects of, 689t
Golfer's elbow, 105–107, 107f
Goniometry, 652, 653f
Graft
in anterior cruciate ligament tear, 312
arteriovenous, in chronic kidney disease, 647, 649
in post-concussion disorders, 806
Great toe
bunion of, 427–429, 428f, 429f
clawed, 437–440, 438f, 439f
osteoarthritis of, 449–451, 450f, 451f
Greater trochanteric pain syndrome, 303–305, 304f
Gross Motor Function Classification System (GMFCS), 630
Gunshot wound, lumbosacral plexopathy with, 782
Guyon canal
corticosteroid injection into, 191, 191f
ulnar nerve entrapment in, 187–192, 188f, 188t, 189f, 190f

H
H reflex, 288
Haglund deformity, 415, 418. See also Foot (feet), bursitis of
Hallpike-Dix maneuver, 803
Hallux rigidus, 449–451, 450f, 451f
Hallux valgus, 427–429, 428f, 429f
Hammer toe, 453–455, 454f
Hamstrings, 331, 332f
strain of, 331–335, 332f, 333f, 334f
stretch of, 334, 335f
Hand. See also Finger; Thumb; Wrist
amputation of, 595–598
deformity of, in rheumatoid arthritis, 161, 162f, 164, 194
extensor tendon injury of, 139–143, 140f, 141t, 142t, 143t
flexor tendon injury of, 145–148, 146f, 147f, 147t
ganglia of, 149–153, 150f, 151f
osteoarthritis of, 155–159, 156f, 157f, 158f
rheumatoid arthritis of, 161–164, 162f, 194, 834–835, 836f, 837, 837f
in thoracic outlet syndrome, 498, 498f
Hatchet-shaped heel. See Foot (feet), bursitis of
Hauser neuroma, 465
Head injury. See Post-concussion disorders; Traumatic brain injury
Headache, 494t, 519–523, 520t
cervicogenic, 485–489, 486f, 488f, 489t
cluster, 519, 522
migraine, 519, 520t, 521–522

Headache, 494t, 519–523, 520t (Continued)
  occipital, 485–489, 486f, 488f, 489t
  post-concussion, 802, 803, 805
  tension-type, 520, 522
Heart disease
  rehabilitation in, 615–620, 617t, 618t, 619t
  in rheumatoid arthritis, 833–834
Heart rate, 828
Heat therapy
  in cervical stenosis, 30
  in costosternal syndrome, 547
  in degenerative disease, 14
  in osteoarthritis, 748
  in piriformis syndrome, 288
  in thoracic sprain/strain, 225–226
  in trapezius strain, 38
  in trochanteric bursitis, 305
Heberden nodes, 155, 156f, 272
Heel cord tendinitis, 407–409, 408f
Heel lift
  in bursitis, 418
  in knee arthritis, 349
Heel wedge, in chronic ankle instability, 435
Heloma, 441–443, 442f, 443f
Hematoma, quadriceps, 291–293
Hemodialysis, 647
Hemorrhage
  cerebral. See Stroke
  retroperitoneal, 780–781
Heparin
  prophylactic, 660–661, 661t, 662
  in stroke, 888
Herpes zoster, 561–563
Herpes zoster ophthalmicus, 561
Heterotopic ossification, 610, 612, 691–695, 692f, 872, 875
Heuter neuroma, 465
High-prow heel. See Foot (feet), bursitis of
Hip
  bursitis of, 303–305, 304f
  in cerebral palsy, 629–631, 630f
  flexion contracture of, 296, 296f
  flexion maneuver for, in low back strain/ sprain, 249t
  fracture of, 754
  osteoarthritis of, 271–275, 272f, 274f
  replacement of, 295–301, 296f, 297f, 299t, 300f, 301f
  rheumatoid arthritis of, 835
  snapping, 338
Hip pocket neuropathy, 287–289, 288f
Hippotherapy, in cerebral palsy, 632
HLA-B27, 607
Hoffmann response, in cervical spondylotic myelopathy, 4
Homocysteine, in atherosclerosis, 675
Horizonal flexion test, 546, 546f
Hormone replacement therapy
  dementia and, 670
  in osteoporosis, 756
Horner syndrome, 895
Housemaid's knee, 355
Humeroscapular fibrositis, 49–54, 50f, 50t, 51f
Humerus, fracture of, 46
Huntington chorea, 715
Hutchinson sign, 562
Hyaluronan, in osteoarthritis, 207, 350, 749
Hydrocephalus, 671
Hydrotherapy
  in enteropathic arthritis, 688
  in joint contracture, 653
  in psoriatic arthritis, 811
  in rheumatoid arthritis, 837
Hyperabduction test, in thoracic outlet syndrome, 499
Hyperkeratosis, of toe, 441–443, 442f, 443f

Hyperkinesia, 713–717
Hypertrophic scarring from burns. See Burns
Hypnosis, in myofascial pain syndrome, 533
Hypoalbuminemia, in chronic kidney disease, 646
Hypokinesia, 713–717

I
Ibandronate, in osteoporosis, 755t, 757
Iceland disease, 635–640, 637t, 638t
Idiopathic torsion dystonia, 579–582, 582t
Ileovesical conduit, in neurogenic bladder, 742
Iliac gapping test, in low back strain/sprain, 249t
Iliohypogastric nerve, injury to, 780
Ilioinguinal nerve, injury to, 780
Iliotibial band, 337, 338f
  stretch of, 341, 341f
Iliotibial band syndrome, 337–342, 339f, 340f, 341f, 342f
Imaging. See Computed tomography (CT); Magnetic resonance imaging (MRI); Radiography; Ultrasonography
Imipramine, in occipital neuralgia, 488, 489t
Immobility, pressure ulcer and, 814
Immune globulin, intravenous, in post- poliomyelitis syndrome, 796
Impingement sign, 64, 64f, 72
Impingement syndrome, 71–75, 72f, 73f, 74t
Infection
  arthroplasty and, 102, 275, 352
  lymphedema and, 701, 702f
  in neurogenic bladder, 740–741, 742
  varicella-zoster virus, 561–563
Inflammatory bowel disease, 685, 686, 686f, 688–689
Inflammatory myopathy, 729, 730t
Infliximab, in rheumatoid arthritis, 162
Inhalers, in pulmonary rehabilitation, 829
Injection. See Anesthetic injection
Insomnia. See Sleep disturbance
Insufficiency fracture, 393–396, 394f, 395f
Insular sclerosis. See Multiple sclerosis
Intercostal nerve, 549, 550f
  blockade of, 547, 553, 553f
Intercostal neuralgia, 549–554, 550f, 551t, 552t
Interferon, in multiple sclerosis, 723, 725
Intermetatarsal nerve entrapment, 461–462, 465–468, 466f, 467f
Intermittent positive-pressure ventilation, 829
International Classification of Functioning, Disability, and Health, 637–638
Interphalangeal joint
  arthrodesis of, 163
  corticosteroid injection of, 157, 158f
  osteoarthritis of, 155, 156f, 158
  rheumatoid arthritis of, 161–164, 162f
Intervertebral disc
  aging-related changes in, 3, 229
  cervical
    aging-related changes in, 3
    degeneration of, 3–6, 5f, 11–15
    herniation of, 17–21, 18f, 18t, 19f
    replacement of, 14
  lumbar
    degeneration of, 247–250, 248t, 249t
    herniation of, 241–245, 242f, 242t, 244f
    thoracic, herniation of, 219–221, 220f
Intestinal bypass, 686, 687, 688
Intracerebral hemorrhage. See Stroke, young adult
Intraosseous cyst. See Ganglion cyst
Intravenous immune globulin, in post- poliomyelitis syndrome, 796
Inulin clearance, in chronic kidney disease, 645
Inversion stress test, in ankle sprain, 422, 423f
Iritis, in psoriatic arthritis, 809

Ischemia, cardiac, in cerebral palsy, 629
Iselin neuroma, 465

J
Jersey finger, 145–148, 146f, 147f, 147t
Joint disease. See Arthritis; Contracture; Osteoarthritis and specific joints
Joints of Luschka, 11, 12f
Jones procedure, 439
Jumper's knee, 367–369, 369f

K
Karvonen formula, 828
Kennedy disease, 705–711, 706f, 707t, 708t
Keratoconjunctivitis sicca, 833
Keratoderma blennorrhagicum, 686
Kidney disease, chronic, 643–649, 644t, 646t
Kidney stones, 736
Kidney transplantation, 647–648, 649
Kienböck disease, 167–170, 168f, 168t, 169f, 170f, 205, 206
Klumpke palsy, 773–777, 774f
Knee
  amputation below/above, 599–603, 602t, 603f
  arthroscopic débridement of, 351, 351t
  aspiration of
    in anterior cruciate ligament tear, 311
    in meniscal tears, 362, 363–364
  Baker's cyst of, 315–317, 316f, 833
  bursitis of, 355–358, 356f, 357f
  cartilage tears of, 359–364, 360f, 361f, 362f, 363f
  collateral ligament sprain of, 319–322, 320f, 321f
  housemaid's, 355
  jumper's, 367–369, 369f
  meniscal injury of, 359–364, 360f, 361f, 362f, 363f
  osteoarthritis of, 345–352, 346t, 347f, 348t, 350f, 350t, 351t
    collateral ligament sprain and, 322
  osteophytes of, 347, 347f
  osteotomy of, 351, 351t
  posterior cruciate ligament sprain of, 381–385, 382f, 382t, 383f, 384f
  replacement of, 351–352
  rheumatoid arthritis of, 835
  total replacement of, 399–405, 402t, 404t
  vicar's, 355
Knee bend exercise, 373, 373f
Knobby heel. See Foot (feet), bursitis of
Kyphoplasty, in thoracic compression fracture, 216
Kyphosis, 232t, 841–846, 842f

L
Labor, lumbosacral plexus injury with, 781
Lachman test
  in anterior cruciate ligament tear, 308
  in posterior cruciate ligament sprain, 381, 383f
Laminectomy
  in cervical spondylotic myelopathy, 6
  in lumbar spinal stenosis, 263
  in thoracic radiculopathy, 221
Laminoplasty, in cervical spondylotic myelopathy, 6
Lamotrigine
  in complex regional pain syndrome, 514t, 515
  in trigeminal neuralgia, 494, 495t
Lasègue sign, 249t
Late effects of burn injury. See Burns
Lateral collateral ligament, 319, 320f
  sprain of, 319–322, 320f, 321f

Lateral femoral cutaneous nerve, 283, 284f
Lateral femoral cutaneous neuropathy, 283–286, 284t
Laterolisthesis, 253
Latissimus dorsi, in post-thoracotomy pain, 587
Ledderhose disease, 133
Leflunomide, in rheumatoid arthritis, 162
Leptomeningitis, chronic, 565–569, 566f, 566t, 567t
Levator ani syndrome, 272f, 273f, 571–574
Levator scapulae muscles, 84, 85f
Levetiracetam
    in complex regional pain syndrome, 514t
    in multiple sclerosis, 723
Levodopa, in Parkinson disease, 715, 762–763, 763t, 765
Lewy bodies, dementia with, 665–671, 666t
Lhermitte sign
    in cervical spondylotic myelopathy, 4
    in cervical stenosis, 27, 28f
    in multiple sclerosis, 719, 724
Lidocaine
    in adhesive capsulitis, 52
    in coccydynia, 573–574
    in complex regional pain syndrome, 514t, 515
    in trigeminal neuralgia, 494–495, 495t
Lift-off test, 64, 64f, 72
Lipid-lowering therapy, 675
Liposuction, in lymphedema, 701
Little's disease. See Cerebral palsy
Load and shift maneuver, 64
Local anesthetic injection. See Anesthetic injection
Long thoracic nerve, 83, 85f
Long thoracic nerve palsy, 83–88, 84t, 86f, 87t
Loose bodies
    in ankle arthritis, 411
    in knee arthritis, 347
Lou Gehrig's disease, 705–711, 706f, 707f, 708t
Low back strain/sprain, 247–250, 248t, 249t. See also Back pain
Low-molecular-weight heparin, 660–661, 661t, 662
Ludington test, 59, 60f
Lumbar plexus, 780f
Lumbar spine, 260f. See also Spinal cord injury, lumbosacral
    degenerative disease of, 229–235, 230t, 231f, 232t–233t, 233t
    facet disease of, 237–239, 238f, 247–248
    muscle stabilization program for, 234, 250
    radiculopathy of, 241–245, 242f, 242t, 244f
    spondylolisthesis of, 253–257, 254f
    spondylolysis of, 253–257, 254f, 255f, 256f
    stenosis of, 259–264, 260t, 262t
    strain/sprain of, 247–250, 248t, 249t
Lumbosacral plexopathy, 779–784, 780f, 781f
Lumbosacral spinal fibrosis, 565–569, 566f, 566t, 567t
Lunate
    Kienböck disease of, 167–170, 168f, 168t, 169f, 170f, 205, 206
    revascularization of, 169
Lung disease, rehabilitation for, 826t, 827t, 829t, 832–830
Lung volume reduction surgery, 829
Lupus, 901–906, 902t, 903t, 905t–906t
Luschka, joints of, 11, 12f
Lymph node dissection, lymphedema and, 701
Lymphangioscintigraphy, 700
Lymphatic system, 697, 698f
    manual drainage of, 700

Lymphedema, 697–702, 698f, 699f, 699t, 701f, 702f
    malignant, 701, 702
    prevention of, 700
Lymphoscintigraphy, 700

M

Magnetic resonance imaging (MRI)
    in Achilles tendinitis, 408
    in acromioclavicular joint injury, 44
    in adhesive capsulitis, 51, 52f
    in ankle arthritis, 411
    in ankle sprain, 423
    in anterior cruciate ligament tear, 309
    in arachnoiditis, 566, 566f
    in Baker's cyst, 316
    in biceps tendon rupture, 60
    in brachial plexopathy, 775
    in cerebral palsy, 631
    in cervical degenerative disease, 13, 14f
    in cervical radiculopathy, 19
    in cervical spondylotic myelopathy, 4, 5f
    in cervical stenosis, 29, 29f
    in chronic ankle instability, 434
    in claw toe, 438
    in complex regional pain syndrome, 513
    in dementia, 668
    in elbow arthritis, 98
    in epicondylitis, 106
    in foot and ankle ganglia, 445, 446f
    in glenohumeral instability, 65
    in hamstring strain, 333, 334f
    in hip arthritis, 273
    in hip disease, 297
    in iliotibial band syndrome, 339
    in intercostal neuralgia, 551–552
    in jumper's knee, 368
    in Kienböck disease, 167–168, 168f, 170f
    in knee arthritis, 347
    in low back strain/sprain, 250
    in lumbar degenerative disease, 231
    in lumbar radiculopathy, 243
    in lumbar spinal stenosis, 262t
    in lumbosacral plexopathy, 783
    in lumbosacral spinal cord injury, 882
    in meniscal injury, 362, 363f
    in Morton neuroma, 466
    in multiple sclerosis, 722
    in myopathy, 731
    in occipital neuralgia, 486
    in olecranon bursitis, 117
    in peroneal neuropathy, 377
    in plantar fasciitis, 470
    in polytrauma, 788
    in posterior tibial dysfunction, 476
    in quadriceps contusion, 292
    in repetitive strain injury, 541
    in rheumatoid arthritis, 162
    in rotator cuff tear, 78–79, 78f
    in rotator cuff tendinitis, 72
    in scapular winging, 87
    in scoliosis, 844
    in shin splints, 390
    of shoulder, 78–79, 78f
    in shoulder arthritis, 92
    in spondylolysis, 255
    in stress fracture, 394–395, 395f
    in stroke, 888
    in thoracic outlet syndrome, 500
    in thoracic spinal cord injury, 872
    in thoracic sprain/strain, 225
    in transverse myelitis, 908
    in traumatic brain injury, 914
    in trigeminal neuralgia, 492

Magnetic resonance imaging (MRI) (Continued)
    in trigger finger, 179
    in trochanteric bursitis, 304
Mallet finger, 140–141, 141t
Mallet toe, 457–459, 458f
Malnutrition
    cerebral palsy and, 629
    pressure ulcer and, 814, 816, 817
    renal failure and, 644, 646
Mandible, osteomyelitis of, 493t
Manipulation, after knee replacement, 403
Mannerfelt syndrome, 161, 195
Manual Ability Classification System, in cerebral palsy, 630–631
Manual therapy
    in cervical facet arthropathy, 8
    in cervical sprain/strain, 25
    in degenerative disease, 14
    in lumbar spinal stenosis, 262–263
    in occipital neuralgia, 487
    in sacroiliac joint dysfunction, 269
    in thoracic sprain/strain, 226–227
March fracture, 393–396, 394f, 395f
Mastectomy
    lymphedema after, 697, 699f
    pain after, 589–590
McConnell taping, in patellofemoral syndrome, 372
McMurray test, 361, 361f
MDRD (Modification of Diet in Renal Disease) equation, 645–646, 646t
Medial collateral ligament, 319, 320f
    bursitis of, 355
    sprain of, 319–322, 320f, 321f
Medial tibial stress syndrome, 389–392, 390f
Median nerve
    blockade of, 112, 113f
    compression of
        in biceps tendon rupture, 61
        in rheumatoid arthritis, 194
Median neuropathy
    elbow, 109–113, 110f, 111f, 112f, 113f
    wrist, 173–177, 174f, 175f, 176f
Memantine
    in dementia, 669
    in phantom limb pain, 577
Memory
    after traumatic brain injury, 916
    impairment of, 667, 667t. See also Cognitive impairment/deficit; Dementia
    types of, 667
Meniscus (menisci)
    anatomy of, 359, 360f
    excision of, 364
    injury to, 359–364, 360f, 361f, 362f, 363f
Mental status examination, in chronic fatigue syndrome, 636
Meralgia paresthetica, 283–286, 284t
Metabolic myopathy, 729, 730t
Metacarpophalangeal joint
    osteoarthritis of, 155
    rheumatoid arthritis of, 163
    splinting of, 180
    stenosing tenosynovitis at, 179–182, 180f, 181f
Metatarsal neuralgia, 461–462, 465–468, 466f, 467f
Metatarsalgia, 461–463, 462f
    bunion and, 427
    claw tow and, 438
    hammer toe and, 453
Methocarbamol, in lumbar degenerative disease, 233t

Methotrexate
    in rheumatoid arthritis, 162
    side effects of, 689t
Methylprednisolone
    in cervical degenerative disease, 14
    in cervical sprain/strain, 25
    in thoracic radiculopathy, 221
Mexiletine
    in complex regional pain syndrome, 514t
    in occipital neuralgia, 488, 489t
    in trigeminal neuralgia, 494, 495t
Microsurgery, in lymphedema, 701
Micturition reflex, 733–734
Middle finger test, in epicondylitis, 105
Migraine, 519, 520t, 521–522
    cervical, 485–489, 486f, 488f, 489t
Miner's elbow, 115–118, 116f, 118f
Mitochondrial myopathy, 729
Mitrofanoff procedure, 742
Mixed dementia, 665–671, 666t
Moberg procedure, 450
Modified Ashworth Scale, 849, 850t
Mononeuritis multiplex, 833
Morton neuroma, 461–462, 465–468, 466f, 467f
Motor function
    in cervical radiculopathy, 18–19, 18t
    in cervical spinal cord injury, 860, 862t
    in cervical spondylotic myelopathy, 3–4
    in complex regional pain syndrome, 512
    in lumbosacral spinal cord injury, 880, 880t
Motor neuron, 793, 794f
Motor neuron disease, 705–711, 706f, 707t, 708t
Movement disorders, 713–717
Mucous cyst, hand-wrist, 149–153, 150f, 155, 158
Mulder test, 465–466, 466f
Multi-infarct dementia. See Dementia
Multiple sclerosis, 491, 719–725, 720t, 721t, 724t
Multiple system atrophy, 762
Muscle relaxants
    in cervicogenic vertigo, 34
    in lumbar degenerative disease, 233, 233t
    in lumbar stenosis, 261
    in movement disorders, 715
    in multiple sclerosis, 723
    in myofascial pain syndrome, 533
    in spasticity, 850, 851t
    in trapezius strain, 38, 39
Muscle transfer, in scapular winging, 88
Muscular dystrophy, 729, 730–731, 730t, 732
Myalgic encephalomyelitis. See Chronic fatigue syndrome
Myelitis, transverse, 907–911
Myelopathy, cervical, 27–31, 28f, 29f
    spondylotic, 3–6, 5f
Myocardial infarction
    vs. costosternal syndrome, 546
    rehabilitation after, 615–620, 617t, 618t, 619t
Myoclonus, 714
Myofascial pain syndrome, 529–535. See also Chronic pain syndrome
Myofasciitis, trapezius, 37–40, 39f
Myogelosis. See Myofascial pain syndrome
Myopathy, 729–732, 730t
Myositis, trapezius, 37–40, 39f
Myositis ossificans, 610, 691–695, 692f, 872, 875
Myotonia, 729–730, 730t

N

Nebulizers, in pulmonary rehabilitation, 829
Neck. See also Cervical spine
    bending maneuver for, in low back strain/sprain, 249t
    range of motion of, in cervical spondylotic myelopathy, 4

Necrosis, avascular, of lunate, 167–170, 168f, 168t, 169f, 170f
Nephrolithiasis, 232t
Nerve block
    in adhesive capsulitis, 52
    in complex regional pain syndrome, 515–516
    in headache, 522–523
    in intercostal neuralgia, 553, 553f
    in lower limb amputation, 601
    in lumbosacral plexopathy, 784
    in median neuropathy, 112, 113f
    in multiple sclerosis, 724
    in myofascial pain syndrome, 533
    in occipital neuralgia, 486, 487, 488f
    in phantom limb pain, 576
    in post-mastectomy pain, 590
    in post-thoracotomy pain, 587
    in thoracic radiculopathy, 221
    in trigeminal neuralgia, 495, 495f
Nerve conduction study
    in brachial plexopathy, 775
    in carpal tunnel syndrome, 175
    in cerebral palsy, 631
    in cervical spinal cord injury, 864
    in femoral neuropathy, 278
    in lumbosacral plexopathy, 783
    in lumbosacral spinal cord injury, 882
    in median neuropathy, 111
    in myopathy, 731
    in peripheral neuropathy, 769
    in peroneal neuropathy, 377
    in radial neuropathy, 122
    in scapular winging, 87
    in ulnar neuropathy, 126, 189–190
Nerve graft, in lumbosacral plexopathy, 784
Nerve roots
    cervical, 17. See also Cervical spine, radiculopathy of
    lumbar, 241, 242f. See also Lumbar spine, radiculopathy of
Neuralgia. See also Pain
    intercostal, 549–554, 550f, 551t, 552t
    Morton (metatarsal, plantar), 461–462, 465–468, 467f
    occipital, 485–489, 486f, 488f, 489f
    postherpetic, 561–563
    trigeminal, 491–496, 493t–494t, 495f, 495t
Neurasthenia. See Chronic fatigue syndrome
Neuritis
    occipital, 485–489, 486f, 488f, 489t
    ulnar, 125–127, 126f
    wallet, 287–289, 288f
Neuroalgodystrophy. See Complex regional pain syndrome
Neurocentral joints (joints of Luschka), 11, 12f
Neurocompression test, in cervical sprain/strain, 24
Neurofibrillary tangles, 666
Neurogenic bladder, 733–742, 735t, 736f, 740t, 741f, 866, 866t, 868
Neuroleptics, in movement disorders, 715
Neuroma
    intercostal, 549–554, 550f, 551t, 552t
    Morton (interdigital, intermetatarsal, metatarsal), 461–462, 465–468, 466f, 467f
    postamputation, 602
Neuromodulatory therapy, in sacroiliac joint dysfunction, 269
Neuromuscular junction, 794f
Neuropathy, peripheral. See Peripheral neuropathy
Neuropsychological testing, in traumatic brain injury, 914–915, 914t
Noble compression test, 338, 341f

Nodules
    flexor tendon, 179, 180f
    in rheumatoid arthritis, 833, 834t, 835, 836, 838
Noninvasive positive-pressure ventilation, in motor neuron disease, 711
Nonsteroidal anti-inflammatory drugs (NSAIDs)
    in acromioclavicular injury, 44, 46
    in adhesive capsulitis, 51, 54
    in ankle arthritis, 412
    in ankylosing spondylitis, 607
    in arachnoiditis, 567
    in biceps tendinitis, 57, 58
    in carpal tunnel syndrome, 175
    in cervical degenerative disease, 13–14
    in cervical facet arthropathy, 8
    in cervical radiculopathy, 20, 21
    in cervical sprain/strain, 25
    in cervical stenosis, 30, 31
    in cervicogenic vertigo, 35
    in De Quervain tenosynovitis, 131
    in femoral neuropathy, 279
    in glenohumeral instability, 66, 67t
    in hamstring strain, 333
    in headache, 522
    in heterotopic ossification, 693, 694
    in Kienböck disease, 169
    in knee arthritis, 347, 348t
    in lateral femoral cutaneous neuropathy, 285
    in low back strain/sprain, 250
    in lumbar radiculopathy, 243
    in lumbar stenosis, 261, 263
    in median neuropathy, 112, 113, 175
    in myofascial pain syndrome, 533
    in occipital neuralgia, 487, 488, 489t
    in olecranon bursitis, 117, 118
    in osteoarthritis, 748, 750
    in plantar fasciitis, 471, 473
    in post-thoracotomy pain, 586
    in psoriatic arthritis, 810–811
    in quadriceps contusion, 292
    in repetitive strain injury, 542
    in rheumatoid arthritis, 162, 836–837, 838t
    in rotator cuff tendinitis, 73, 74t
    in sacroiliac joint dysfunction, 269
    side effects of, 689t
    in stress fracture, 395, 396
    in thoracic compression fracture, 214
    in thoracic radiculopathy, 220–221
    in Tietze syndrome, 559
    in trapezius strain, 38, 39
    in wrist osteoarthritis, 207
Noone-Milroy-Meige syndrome. See Lymphedema
Normal pressure hydrocephalus, 671
Nortriptyline. See Tricyclic antidepressants
Numbness, in carpal tunnel syndrome, 173, 174f
Nutrition
    in cerebral palsy, 629
    in motor neuron disease, 710, 711
    in renal failure, 644, 646

O

Ober test, 338, 340f
O'Brien test, 56, 64
Obturator nerve injury, 782
Occipital nerve, 485, 486f
    blockade of, 487, 488f, 522–523
    electrical stimulation of, 487–488, 488f
Occipital neuralgia, 485–489, 486f, 488f, 489t
Occupational overuse syndrome, 37, 539–543
Occupational therapy
    after amputation, 601–602
    after stroke, 896–897

Occupational therapy (Continued)
  after traumatic brain injury, 916
  in cerebral palsy, 632
  in cervical stenosis, 30
  in dementia, 670
  in lower limb amputation, 601–602
  in osteoarthritis, 748
  in Parkinson disease, 764
  in peripheral neuropathy, 770
Odontalgia, atypical, 494t
OK sign, 110–111, 111f
Olecranon bursitis, 115–118, 116f,
    118f
  septic, 115–117, 116f, 118, 118f
Olfaction, post-concussion, 803
Ondansetron, in cervicogenic vertigo, 34
Oophorectomy, in migraine headache,
    523
Opioids
  after knee replacement, 401
  in arachnoiditis, 567
  in cancer-related pain, 623
  in complex regional pain syndrome, 515
  in intercostal neuralgia, 553
  in low back strain/sprain, 250
  in lumbar radiculopathy, 243–244
  in lumbar stenosis, 261
  in phantom limb pain, 597
  in post-thoracotomy pain, 586
  in sacroiliac joint dysfunction, 269
Optic neuritis, 563
Orbital apex syndrome, 563
Orphenadrine, in lumbar degenerative disease,
    233t
Orthosis
  in ankle arthritis, 412
  in ankle sprain, 424
  in ankylosing spondylitis, 607
  in bunion, 428
  in claw toe, 438
  in hammer toe, 454
  in knee bursitis, 357
  in lumbar degenerative disease, 233
  in mallet toe, 458
  in peroneal neuropathy, 378
  in posterior tibial dysfunction, 477
  in shin splints, 391
  in spondylolysis, 256
  in tarsal tunnel syndrome, 481
  in thoracic compression fracture, 214, 215f,
    217
  in transverse myelitis, 909
Osgood-Schlatter disease, 367
Ossifying fibromyopathy/fibromyositis, 610,
    612, 691–695, 692f, 872, 875
Osteoarthritis, 745–750, 747f. See also at specific
    joints
  complications of, 750
  diagnosis of, 746–747, 747t
  functional limitations in, 746
  pathogenesis of, 745, 747f
  physical examination in, 746
  primary, 745
  risk factors for, 745, 746t
  secondary, 745, 746t
  symptoms of, 745–746
  treatment of, 748–750
Osteodystrophy. See also Complex regional pain
    syndrome
  in chronic kidney disease, 648
Osteoma, neurogenic. See Heterotopic
    ossification
Osteomalacia, 233t, 753
Osteonecrosis, lunate, 167–170, 168f, 168t,
    169f, 170f, 205, 206

Osteophytes
  of cervical spine, 17
  of great toe, 449
  of knee, 347, 347f
Osteoporosis, 233t, 753–758, 754t, 755t
  post-traumatic. See Complex regional pain
    syndrome
  spinal cord injury and, 872, 875
Osteotomy
  in ankylosing spondylitis, 607
  in knee arthritis, 351, 351t
  in osteoarthritis, 749
Overuse syndromes, 37, 539–543
Oxcarbazepine
  in complex regional pain syndrome, 514t
  in trigeminal neuralgia, 494, 495t
Oximetry, transcutaneous, 674
Oxybutynin, 740, 740t
Oxycodone, in osteoarthritis, 347, 348t, 748
Oxygen therapy, 826–827
  in cluster headache, 522
  in motor neuron disease, 710–711
Oxygenation impairment, 823–826, 824t. See
    also Pulmonary rehabilitation
  in amyotrophic lateral sclerosis, 710–711
  rehabilitation in, 827–829, 827t
  treatment of, 826–827
Oxytrol, 740, 740t

P
Pace sign, 287, 531
Paget disease, 233t
Pain. See also Neuralgia
  Achilles tendon, 407
  after knee replacement, 401
  after stroke, 894, 894t
  ankle
    in arthritis, 411
    in sprain, 421
  antecubital fossa, in biceps tendon
    rupture, 59
  in arachnoiditis, 565
  back. See Back pain
  in brachial plexopathy, 773
  burn-related, 611–612
  buttock, 531
  in cerebral palsy, 628
  cervical. See Cervical spine, degenerative
    disease of; Cervical spine, facet
    arthropathy of; Cervical spine,
    spondylotic myelopathy of
  in cervical dystonia, 580
  in cervical spinal cord injury, 859–860, 861t,
    867, 867t, 868, 869
  chest. See Chest pain
  chest wall, 545, 549
  chronic. See Chronic pain syndrome
  in chronic fatigue syndrome, 636
  coccygeal, 273f, 571–574, 572f
  complex regional, 511–516, 513t, 514t
  dental, 493t
  elbow
    in arthritis, 97
    in epicondylitis, 105
  in femoral neuropathy, 277
  in fibromyalgia, 525
  foot
    in bursitis, 416, 418
    in plantar fasciitis, 469
    in posterior tibial dysfunction, 475
  forefoot, 461–463, 462f
    bunion and, 427
    claw toe and, 438
    hammer toe and, 453

Pain (Continued)
  groin, in hip arthritis, 271
  hand
    in carpal tunnel syndrome, 173
    in rheumatoid arthritis, 161
  head. See Headache
  hip, in arthritis, 271–272
  intractable. See Chronic pain syndrome
  knee
    anterior. See Patellofemoral syndrome
    in anterior cruciate ligament tear, 307
    in arthritis, 345–346
    in collateral ligament sprain, 319
    differential diagnosis of, 348
    in iliotibial band syndrome, 338
    in jumper's knee, 367
    in peroneal neuropathy, 375–376
  in lateral femoral cutaneous neuropathy, 283
  leg
    in compartment syndrome, 325–326
    in diabetes mellitus, 673–674
    in hip disease, 295
    in lumbosacral plexopathy, 782
    in lumbar radiculopathy, 241, 242t
    in lumbosacral spinal cord injury, 879–880,
      883, 884
    in motor neuron disease, 710
    in multiple sclerosis, 719, 721t, 724
  myofascial, 529–535
  myopathic, 730
  neck
    in cervical sprain/strain, 23–25, 24f
    in degenerative disease, 11–12
    in facet arthropathy, 7
    prevalence of, 11
    in radiculopathy, 17
  in Parkinson disease, 761
  patellar, 371–374, 372f, 373f, 374f
  in peripheral neuropathy, 770
  phantom limb, 575–577, 576t, 597, 599–600
  in piriformis syndrome, 287
  post-mastectomy, 589–590
  in post-poliomyelitis syndrome, 794, 796,
    797
  post-stroke, 894, 894t, 896, 898
  post-thoracotomy, 585–587, 586t
  pupal, 493t
  in repetitive strain injury, 540
  sacroiliac joint, 267–268
  shoulder
    in acromioclavicular joint injury, 41
    in adhesive capsulitis, 49–50, 51t
    in arthritis, 91
    in biceps tendinitis, 55
    in glenohumeral instability, 63
    post-stroke, 894, 894t, 896
    in rotator cuff tear, 77, 79
    in rotator cuff tendinitis, 71
    in scapular winging, 85–86
  stump, 600
  thigh, in hamstring strain, 332
  thoracic, benign, 223–227
  in thoracic compression fracture, 214
  in thoracic outlet syndrome, 498, 499
  in thoracic radiculopathy, 219, 220, 220f
  in thoracic spinal cord injury, 872, 874
  tibial, 389, 390f
  toe, 437–438, 453, 465
  in transverse myelitis, 910, 911
  trapezius, 37–38
  trochanteric, 303
  in ulnar collateral ligament sprain, 184
  wrist, in osteoarthritis, 203
Painful phantom sensation, 575–577, 576t
Pallidotomy, in Parkinson disease, 764

Palmar oblique ligament, in trapeziometacarpal joint arthritis, 158
Palmaris brevis sign, 190
Pancoast syndrome, 775
Pancreatitis, 232t
Paraffin bath
    in joint contracture, 653
    in wrist rheumatoid arthritis, 198
Paralysis agitans. See Parkinson disease
Paraosteoarthropathy, 610, 612, 691–695, 692f, 872, 875
Paraplegia. See Spinal cord injury, lumbosacral; Spinal cord injury, thoracic
    heterotopic ossification in. See Heterotopic ossification
Paraplegic disc, 245
Parasternal chondrodynia, 555–560, 556f, 557f, 558f
Parathyroid hormone, in osteoporosis, 757
Parenting, after stroke, 897
Paresthesias
    in carpal tunnel syndrome, 173, 174f
    in cervical radiculopathy, 17
    in multiple sclerosis, 719
Parkinson disease, 713–717, 761–765
    treatment of, 715–717, 762–764, 763t
    urinary dysfunction in, 734
Paroxetine, in complex regional pain syndrome, 514t
Pars interarticularis, stress fracture in, 253. See also Lumbar spine, spondylolysis of
Parsonage-Turner syndrome, 773–777, 774f
Patella
    arthroplasty-related disorders of, 404
    malalignment of, 349
    Q angle of, 371, 372f
    tracking of, 371, 372f
Patellar ligament, partial rupture of, 367–369, 369f
Patellar tendinitis, 367–369, 369f
Patellectomy, 352
Patellofemoral syndrome, 371–374, 372f, 373f, 374f
Patrick test (FABER test)
    in hip arthritis, 272, 272f
    in low back strain/sprain, 249t
    in sacroiliac joint dysfunction, 268
Paxinosis sign, 42, 43f
Pellegrini-Stieda disease, 322
Pelvic examination, in neurogenic bladder, 735
Pelvic inflammatory disease, 232t
Pelvic rock maneuver, 249t
Pelvic tension myalgia, 272f, 273f, 571–574
Pelvic tumor, 781
Pendulum exercise, in adhesive capsulitis, 53f
Penn Spasm Frequency Scale, 849, 850t
Perceived exertion, 618, 619f
Percutaneous endoscopic gastrostomy, in motor neuron disease, 711
Percutaneous transluminal angioplasty, in diabetes mellitus, 675–676
Pergolide, in Parkinson disease, 715, 763, 763t
Periarticular ossification, 610, 612, 691–695, 692f, 872, 875
Pericardiocentesis, in cancer, 624
Perineural fibroma, 461–462, 465–468, 466f, 467f
Periodontitis, 493t
Periostitis, tibial, 389–392, 390f
Peripheral neuropathy, 767–771
    axonal, 767–768, 768t, 770
    in burns, 612
    complications of, 771
    definition of, 767
    demyelinating, 768, 768t, 770

Peripheral neuropathy, 767–771 (Continued)
    diagnosis of, 769, 769f, 770t
    femoral, 277–280, 278t, 280f
    functional limitations in, 768–769
    lateral femoral cutaneous, 283–286, 283f, 284f, 285f
    median, 109–113, 122f, 123f, 173–177, 174f, 175f, 176f
    peroneal, 375–379, 376f, 377f
    physical examination in, 767–768, 768t
    radial, 121–124, 122f, 123t
    in rheumatoid arthritis, 833, 837–838, 837f
    symptoms of, 767
    tibial, 479–482, 480f, 481f
    treatment of, 769–771
    ulnar, 125–127, 126f, 187–192, 188f, 189f, 190f, 191f
Peritendinitis, de Quervain, 129–131, 130f
Peritendinosis, Achilles, 407–409, 408f
Peroneal neuropathy, 375–379, 376f, 377f
    knee replacement and, 404
Pes planus, 475–477, 476f
Peyronie disease, 133
Phalen test, 174, 175f, 195
Phantom limb pain, 575–577, 576t, 597, 599–600, 602–603
Phantom limb sensation, 599, 601
Phenol injection
    in cerebral palsy, 633
    in spasticity, 850, 851
Phenoxybenzamine, in complex regional pain syndrome, 515
Phentolamine, in complex regional pain syndrome, 515
Phenytoin
    in complex regional pain syndrome, 514t, 515
    in trigeminal neuralgia, 494, 495t
Phlebothrombosis. See Deep venous thrombosis
Photochemotherapy, in psoriatic arthritis, 811
Piriformis muscle, 287, 288f
Piriformis syndrome, 232t, 287–289, 288f, 530, 531, 534
Pitcher's elbow, 105–107, 107f
Pivot shift test, 308, 308f
Plantar fasciitis, 469–473, 470f, 472f
Pleurisy, 834
Pleurocentesis, in cancer, 624
Plexopathy
    brachial, 773–777, 774f
    lumbosacral, 779–784, 780f, 781f
    neoplastic, 781–782
Pneumatic compression
    in deep venous thrombosis prophylaxis, 660
    in lymphedema, 700–701
Poliomyelitis, 793–798, 794f, 794t
Polymyalgia rheumatica, 232t
Polysomnography, in post-concussion disorders, 804
Polytrauma, 787–791, 791t
Popliteal cyst, 315–317, 316f
Post-concussion disorders, 801–806, 802t
Post-mastectomy pain syndrome, 589–590
Post-poliomyelitis syndrome, 793–798, 794f, 794t
Post-thoracotomy pain syndrome, 585–587, 586t
Post-thrombotic syndrome, 662, 662f
Post-traumatic dystrophy, 511–516, 513t, 514t
Post-traumatic stress disorder, 803
Post-viral fatigue syndrome, 635–640, 637t, 638t
Posterior cruciate ligament, 381, 382f
    sprain of, 381–385, 382f, 382t, 383f, 384f
Posterior drawer test, 381, 383f
Posterior element disorder, 7–9, 8f
Posterior interosseous nerve dysfunction, in wrist rheumatoid arthritis, 195

Posterior sag test, 381–382, 384f
Posterior tibial dysfunction, 475–477, 476f
Postherpetic neuralgia, 493t, 561–563
    vs. intercostal neuralgia, 551
Postmastectomy lymphedema. See Lymphedema
Postural roundback (kyphosis), 232t, 841–846, 842f
Posture
    examination of, 224
    poor, 223–224
    in thoracic sprain/strain, 226
Pramipexole, in Parkinson disease, 763, 763t
Prednisone. See Corticosteroids
Pregabalin
    in arachnoiditis, 567, 567t
    in complex regional pain syndrome, 514t
    in fibromyalgia, 526
Pregnancy
    deep venous thrombosis during, 661
    ectopic, 232t
    thoracic spinal cord injury and, 875
Pressure, compartment, 327–328, 327f
Pressure ulcers (sores), 813–819, 814t, 815f, 817f
    in cerebral palsy, 630
    in cervical spinal cord injury, 866, 867
    in lumbosacral spinal cord injury, 883, 884
    in thoracic spinal cord injury, 872–873, 876
PRICE (protect, reset, ice, compression, elevation)
    in ankle sprain, 424
    in collateral ligament sprain, 321
    in hamstring strain, 333
    in knee arthritis, 347
    in plantar fasciitis, 471
    in posterior cruciate ligament sprain, 382
    in stress fracture, 395
Primary lateral sclerosis, 705–711, 706f, 707t, 708t
Primary lymphedema. See Lymphedema
Proctalgia fugax, 272f, 273f, 571–574
Progressive bulbar palsy, 705–711, 706f, 707t, 708t
Progressive muscular atrophy, 705–711, 706f, 707t, 708t
Progressive supranuclear palsy, 762
Prolotherapy
    in coccydynia, 574
    in sacroiliac joint dysfunction, 269
Pronator teres syndrome, 109–113, 110f, 112f, 113f
Propoxyphene, in thoracic compression fracture, 214
Proprioceptive neuromuscular facilitation, in quadriceps contusion, 293
Proprioceptive training
    in ankle sprain, 424
    in rotator cuff tear, 80
    in rotator cuff tendinitis, 74
Prostatitis, 232t
Prosthesis
    in lower limb amputation, 601-602, 602t, 603
    in upper limb amputation, 597
Proteinuria, in chronic kidney disease, 646
Prow beak deformity. See Foot (feet), bursitis of
Proximal row carpectomy, 207–208, 208f, 209f, 210
Pruritus, burn-related, 612
Pseudobulbar affect
    after stroke, 894
    in motor neuron disease, 709
Pseudoclaudication, 260. See also Lumbar spine, stenosis of
Pseudoneuroma (Morton neuroma), 461–462, 465–468, 466f, 467f
Psoas syndrome, 782
Psoriatic arthritis, 809–812, 810t, 812t

Psychological counseling, in post-concussion disorders, 805
Psychological disorders
    in cerebral palsy, 629, 630
    in chronic fatigue syndrome, 636
Psychological testing
    in polytrauma, 789
    in post-concussion disorders, 804
Psychological therapy
    in burns, 612, 613
    in chronic pain syndrome, 507
    in myofascial pain syndrome, 532–533
    in post-concussion disorders, 805
    in Tietze syndrome, 559
Psychosocial problems, spinal cord injury and, 869, 872
Psychostimulants, in post-concussion disorders, 805
Puborectalis syndrome, 272f, 273f, 571–574
Pudendal nerve, 733
Pulled upper back, 223–227
Pulmonary embolism. See also Deep venous thrombosis
    knee replacement and, 404
    spinal cord injury and, 872
Pulmonary hygiene, 826, 828–829, 829t, 830
Pulmonary rehabilitation, 823–830, 826t, 827t, 829t
    diagnostic studies for, 825–826
    disease complications in, 830
    for oxygenation impairment, 826–827, 827t
    for ventilatory impairment, 827
Pulpitis, 493t
Pump bump, 415–420, 416t, 417t, 418t, 419t

Q
Q angle, 371, 372f
Quadriceps contusion, 291–293
Quadriceps tendinitis, 367–369, 369f, 387–388
Quadriceps testing, 277
Quadriplegia. See Spinal cord injury, cervical

R
Radial deviation, in rheumatoid arthritis, 194
Radial nerve, 121, 122f
    decompression of, 124
    lesions of, 105, 121–124, 122f, 123t
Radial pulse, in thoracic outlet syndrome, 499
Radial shortening, in Kienböck disease, 169
Radial tunnel syndrome, 121–124, 122f, 123t
Radiation therapy, in heterotopic ossification, 694
Radiculopathy
    cervical, 17–21, 18f, 18t, 19f
    lumbar, 241–245, 242f, 242t, 244f
    thoracic, 219–221, 220f
Radiculoplexus neuropathy, lumbosacral, 779–784, 780f, 781f
Radiography. See also Computed tomography (CT); Magnetic resonance imaging (MRI); Ultrasonography
    in acromioclavicular joint injury, 44, 44f
    in adhesive capsulitis, 51, 51f
    in ankle arthritis, 411–412, 412f
    in ankle sprain, 423
    in anterior cruciate ligament tear, 309
    in Baker's cyst, 315, 316
    in biceps tendinitis, 56–57
    in biceps tendon rupture, 60
    in brachial plexopathy, 775
    in bunion, 428, 429f
    in carpal tunnel syndrome, 173, 174f
    in cerebral palsy, 631

Radiography (Continued)
    in cervical degenerative disease, 13
    in cervical facet arthropathy, 7–8, 8f
    in cervical radiculopathy, 19–20
    in cervical spinal cord injury, 864–865
    in cervical spondylotic myelopathy, 4
    in cervical sprain/strain, 24, 24f
    in cervical stenosis, 28–29, 29f
    in chronic ankle instability, 434, 434f
    in coccydynia, 572f, 573
    in collateral ligament sprain, 321
    in complex regional pain syndrome, 513
    in costosternal syndrome, 546
    in diffuse idiopathic skeletal hyperostosis, 229
    in elbow arthritis, 98, 98t, 99f, 100f
    in enteropathic arthritis, 687, 687f
    in extensor tendon injury, 139
    in foot and ankle bursitis, 417–418, 418t
    in foot and ankle ganglia, 445
    in ganglion cyst, 151
    in glenohumeral instability, 65
    in hallux rigidus, 449–450, 450f, 451f
    in hamstring strain, 333
    in hand osteoarthritis, 156
    in heterotopic ossification, 692–693, 692f
    in hip arthritis, 272–273, 273f
    in hip disease, 296–297, 297f
    in iliotibial band syndrome, 339
    in jumper's knee, 368
    in Kienböck disease, 167, 168f, 169f
    in knee arthritis, 346–347
    in knee bursitis, 356
    in kyphosis, 843–844
    in low back strain/sprain, 248, 250
    in lumbar degenerative disease, 231, 231f
    in lumbar facet arthropathy, 238, 238f
    in lumbar radiculopathy, 243, 244f
    in lumbar spinal stenosis, 262t
    in lumbosacral spinal cord injury, 882
    in meniscal injury, 362
    in Morton neuroma, 467
    in occipital neuralgia, 486
    in olecranon bursitis, 116, 116f
    in osteoarthritis, 746–747
    in patellofemoral syndrome, 372
    in post-concussion disorders, 804
    in post-poliomyelitis syndrome, 796
    in posterior tibial dysfunction, 476, 476f
    in psoriatic arthritis, 810
    in quadriceps contusion, 292
    in repetitive strain injury, 541
    in rheumatoid arthritis, 162, 834t, 836, 836f
    in rotator cuff tear, 78, 78f
    in rotator cuff tendinitis, 72
    in sacroiliac joint dysfunction, 269
    in scapular winging, 87
    in scoliosis, 843–844, 844f
    in shin splints, 390
    in shoulder arthritis, 92, 92f
    in spondylolysis, 255, 255f
    in systemic lupus erythematosus, 902
    in thoracic compression fracture, 213, 214f
    in thoracic outlet syndrome, 500
    in thoracic sprain/strain, 225
    in Tietze syndrome, 556
    in trochanteric bursitis, 304
    in ulnar collateral ligament sprain, 184
    in ulnar neuropathy, 126, 188
    in wrist osteoarthritis, 204f, 205f, 206
    in wrist rheumatoid arthritis, 196–198, 196f, 196t, 197f
Raloxifene, in osteoporosis, 755t, 756
Ramisectomy, in cervical dystonia, 582

Ramsay Hunt syndrome, 561
Range of motion
    ankle
        in arthritis, 411
        in sprain, 422
    cervical spine, 224
        in radiculopathy, 18
        in spondylotic myelopathy, 4
        in sprain/strain, 23
        in trapezius strain, 38
    elbow, 98
    hamstring, 333, 333f
    hip, 296
        in arthritis, 272
        in lower limb amputation, 600
    knee
        after replacement surgery, 404–405, 404t
        in cerebral palsy, 630
        in lower limb amputation, 600
        in meniscal injury, 363
        in quadriceps contusion, 291, 293
    shoulder
        in acromioclavicular injury, 41–42
        in adhesive capsulitis, 49, 52
        in arthritis, 91
        in biceps tendinitis, 55–56
        in glenohumeral instability, 64
        restoration of, 74
        in rotator cuff tear, 79–80
        in rotator cuff tendinitis, 71–72, 74
    thoracic spine, 219, 224
Rasagiline, in Parkinson disease, 763, 763t
Rash
    in rheumatoid arthritis, 833
    in systemic lupus erythematosus, 901, 902t, 903t
Reactive arthritis, 685–689, 686f, 687f, 689t
Rectum
    bleeding from, 880
    examination of, 735, 880–881
Reflex(es)
    in cerebral palsy, 630
    in cervical degenerative disease, 12, 12t
    in cervical radiculopathy, 18t, 19
    micturition, 733–734
    in multiple sclerosis, 721
    in neurogenic bladder, 735–736
    in thoracic sprain/strain, 224
Reflex myoclonus, 714
Reflex sympathetic dystrophy, 511–516, 513t, 514t
Reiter syndrome, 685–689, 686f, 687f, 689t
Relaxation therapy, in cardiac rehabilitation, 617
Relocation test, 64
    in rotator cuff tendinitis, 72, 73f
Renal calculi, 736
Renal failure, chronic, 643–649, 644t, 646t
Renal transplantation, 647–648, 649
Repetitive strain injury, 37, 539–543
    trapezius, 37–40, 39f
Residual limb stump, 599–603, 602t, 603f
Respiration. See also Pulmonary rehabilitation
    in post-poliomyelitis syndrome, 794–795, 796, 797
Respiratory failure
    in motor neuron disease, 710–711
    in multiple sclerosis, 725
Retinacular cyst, 149–153, 150f
Retrocalcaneal bursitis, 415–420, 416t, 417t, 418t, 419t
Retrolisthesis, 253
Revascularization procedure, in Kienböck disease, 169
Reverse pivot shift test, 382, 384f

Reverse straight-leg raising, 249t
Rheumatism, nonarticular. See Trapezius
    muscle, strain of
Rheumatoid arthritis, 833–839, 834t, 835t,
    836f, 838t
    definition of, 161, 833, 834t
    of hand, 161–164, 162f, 194, 834–835,
        836f, 837, 837f
    nodules in, 833, 834t, 835, 836, 838
    pathophysiology of, 193–194
    treatment of, 836–837
    of wrist, 203–211, 204f, 205f, 206f, 207f,
        210f, 834–835, 836f
Rheumatoid factor, 834t
Rhizotomy
    in cerebral palsy, 633
    in occipital neuralgia, 487
Rib(s)
    cervical, 497
    first, 497–498, 501, 501f
    in thoracic sprain/strain, 225
Rigid dressing, in lower limb amputation, 601,
    602t, 603f
Riluzole, in amyotrophic lateral sclerosis, 707
Risedronate, in osteoporosis, 755t, 757
Rituximab, in rheumatoid arthritis, 162
Rivastigmine, in dementia, 669
Romberg test, in cervical spondylotic
    myelopathy, 4
Roos test, in thoracic outlet syndrome, 499
Ropinirole, in Parkinson disease, 763, 763t
Rotator cuff
    functions of, 77
    impingement test of, 64, 64f
    muscles of, 78f
    tear of, 77–81, 78f
    tendinitis of, 71–75, 72f, 73f, 74t
Roundback, 232t, 841–846, 842f
Royal Free disease, 635–640, 637t, 638t
Rucksack palsy, 83–88, 84t, 86f, 87t
Running program, in plantar fasciitis, 471–472

S

Sacral plexus, 781f
Sacral sulcus pressure test, 268
Sacroiliac joint, 267
    compression maneuver for, in low back
        strain/sprain, 249t
    dysfunction of, 267–270
Sacrum
    fracture of, 779–780
    pressure ulcers of, 883, 884
Saline injection, in adhesive capsulitis, 52
Saphenous nerve, 277, 279f
Saturday night palsy, 121–124, 122f, 123t
Sauvé-Kapandji procedure, 200
Scalene muscles, activation of, 501, 501f
Scalenotomy, in thoracic outlet syndrome, 502
Scalenus anticus syndrome. See Thoracic outlet
    syndrome
Scaphoid shift test, 205
Scapula, 83
    stabilization of, in rotator cuff tear, 80
    winging of, 83–88, 84t, 86f, 87t
Scapular winging, 83–88, 84t, 86f, 87t
Scapulothoracic fusion, 88
Scar
    in burns, 611, 612
    in post-thoracotomy pain, 587
Scarf test, 56
Schober maneuver, 686, 686f
Schober test, 605
Sciatic nerve, 287, 288f
Sciatica, 241–245, 242f, 242t, 244f

Sclerosis, disseminated. See Multiple sclerosis
Scoliosis, 232t–233t, 841–846, 842f, 845f, 846f
Secondary lymphedema. See Lymphedema
Second impact syndrome, 806
Seizures
    after stroke, 890
        after traumatic brain injury, 916
Selective estrogen receptor modulators, in
    osteoporosis, 755t, 756
Selective serotonin-norepinephrine reuptake
    inhibitors, in complex regional pain
    syndrome, 514t
Selective serotonin reuptake inhibitors, in
    complex regional pain syndrome, 514t
Selegiline, in Parkinson disease, 715, 763, 763t
Semimembranosus bursitis, 355
Senile dementia. See Dementia
Sensorineural hearing loss, 806
Sensory discrimination training, in phantom
    limb pain, 577
Sensory function
    in arthritic wrist, 206
    in cervical degenerative disease, 12, 12t
    in cervical radiculopathy, 18–19, 18t
    in cervical spinal cord injury, 860, 862t
    in cervical spondylotic myelopathy, 3–4
    in complex regional pain syndrome, 512
    in diabetic foot, 674
    in lateral femoral cutaneous neuropathy, 283
    in lumbar radiculopathy, 242, 242t
    in lumbosacral spinal cord injury, 880,
        880t
    in multiple sclerosis, 721
    in peroneal neuropathy, 376, 376f, 377f
    in thoracic sprain/strain, 224
    in ulnar neuropathy, 188
Sentinel node biopsy, 701
Sepsis, in olecranon bursitis, 115–117, 116f,
    118, 118f
Seronegative spondyloarthropathy, 605–607,
    606f. See also Enteropathic arthritis
Serratus anterior, 83
    in post-thoracotomy pain, 587
Sexual activity, in cardiac rehabilitation, 617
Sexual dysfunction
    after stroke, 895, 896, 899
    in multiple sclerosis, 721, 723
    in Parkinson disease, 762
Shaker exercise, in dysphagia, 681, 682f
Shaking palsy. See Parkinson disease
Shin splints, 389–392, 390f
Shingles, 561–563
Shoe(s)
    in ankle sprain, 424
    in bunion, 428
    in bunionette, 430
    in claw toe, 438
    in enteropathic arthritis, 688
    in foot and ankle bursitis, 418
    in foot and ankle ganglia, 446
    in hallux rigidus, 450
    in hammer toe, 454, 455
    in knee arthritis, 349–350
    in knee bursitis, 357
    in mallet toe, 457–458
    in plantar fasciitis, 472
    in psoriatic arthritis, 811
    in shin splint, 391
    in stress fracture, 396
Shoe wedge, in knee arthritis, 349
Shoulder
    adhesive capsulitis of, 49–54, 50f, 50t, 51f, 710
    anatomy of, 50f
    dislocation/instability of, 63–68, 64f, 65f,
        66f, 67t, 68f

Shoulder (Continued)
    injection of, in arthritis, 93–94, 93f, 94f
    magnetic resonance imaging of, 78–79, 78f
    movement of, 55
    osteoarthritis of, 91–95, 92f, 93f, 94f
    pain in
        in arthritis, 91
        in biceps tendinitis, 55
        in glenohumeral instability, 63
        myofascial, 37–40, 39f
        in rotator cuff tear, 77, 79
        in scapular winging, 85–86
    post-mastectomy dysfunction of, 590
    post-thoracotomy dysfunction of, 587
    range of motion of
        in arthritis, 91
        in biceps tendinitis, 55–56
        in glenohumeral instability, 64
        in rotator cuff tear, 79–80
    rheumatoid arthritis of, 835
    separated, 41–46, 42f, 42t, 43f, 44f, 45f, 46f
    stretching of, in biceps tendinitis, 57
    subluxation of, 63–68, 64f, 65f, 66f, 67t, 68f
        after stroke, 890
    tear of, 77–81, 78f
Shoulder abduction release, in cervical degener-
    ative disease, 12, 14
Shoulder-hand syndrome. See Complex re-
    gional pain syndrome
Shunt, in normal pressure hydrocephalus, 671
Sialorrhea, in motor neuron disease, 709, 711
SIGECAPS screen, in cerebral palsy, 630
Silicone sleeve, in corns, 442, 442f
Single photon emission computed tomography
    in cervical facet arthropathy, 8
    in complex regional pain syndrome, 513
    in spondylolysis, 256
Sitting root test, in low back strain/sprain, 249t
Skier's thumb, 183–185, 184f
Skin
    anatomy of, 609, 610f
    in lower limb amputation, 600, 603
    pressure ulcers (sores) of, 813–819, 814t,
        815f, 817f
        in cerebral palsy, 630
        in cervical spinal cord injury, 866
        in lumbosacral spinal cord injury, 883, 884
        in thoracic spinal cord injury, 872–873, 876
Skin graft
    in burns, 612
    in Dupuytren contracture, 136
    in pressure ulcers, 819
SLAC (scapholunate advanced collapse) wrist,
    203, 204f, 205f, 206
SLE. See Systemic lupus erythematosus
Sleep disturbance
    in brain injury, 917
    in cerebral palsy, 629
    in chronic fatigue syndrome, 637
    in chronic pain syndrome, 506
    in repetitive strain injury, 540
Sling
    in acromioclavicular joint injury, 44
    in elbow arthritis, 99
    in glenohumeral instability, 66
    in scapular winging, 87
Slipped vertebra. See Lumbar spine, spondyloly-
    sis; Lumbar spine, spondylolisthesis
Smoking
    cessation of
        in cardiac rehabilitation, 617
        in osteoporosis, 756
    diabetes and, 675
SNAC (scaphoid nonunion advanced collapse)
    wrist, 203, 204f, 206

Snapping hip, 338. *See also* Iliotibial band syndrome
Solifenacin, 740, 740t
Somatosensory evoked potentials
  in lateral femoral cutaneous neuropathy, 284
  in thoracic outlet syndrome, 500
Spasmodic torticollis, 579–582, 582t
Spasticity, 849–851, 850t, 851t
  after stroke, 894–895, 896, 896t, 898
  after traumatic brain injury, 916
  in cervical spinal cord injury, 866, 867–868, 867t
  in lumbosacral spinal cord injury, 883
  in motor neuron disease, 709
  in multiple sclerosis, 719, 721, 722, 723, 725
  in myofascial pain syndrome, 530
  in thoracic spinal cord injury, 875, 877
  in transverse myelitis, 910
Speech/language disorders, 853–857, 854t
  after traumatic brain injury, 916
  in amyotrophic lateral sclerosis, 706
  in Parkinson disease, 764
  in stroke, 889
Speed test, 56, 56f, 59
Sphincterotomy, transurethral, 741–742
Spinal accessory nerve, 83, 85f
Spinal accessory nerve palsy, 83–88, 84t, 86f, 87t
Spinal adhesive arachnoiditis, 565–569, 566f, 566t, 567t
Spinal canal, diameter of, 259–260
Spinal cord injury
  cervical, 859–869
    abdominal examination in, 860
    autonomic dysreflexia in, 860, 862t, 865–866, 868
    bladder management in, 865–866, 866t, 868
    bowel management in, 866–867, 868
    C5, 863–864, 863f
    C6, 863f, 864
    C1-4, 862–863, 863f
    C7-8, 863f, 864
    cardiac examination in, 860, 862t, 866
    complications of, 868–869, 869t
    compressive, 3, 11, 13, 13f, 27
    extremity examination in, 860
    fracture in, 860
    functional limitations in, 862–864, 863t
    heterotopic ossification in, 867
    motor function in, 868
    neurologic examination in, 860, 862f, 862t
    pain in, 859–860, 861t, 867, 867t, 868
    pharmacokinetics in, 869, 869t
    physical examination in, 860, 862, 862t, 863f
    pressure ulcers in, 867
    psychosocial factors in, 867
    respiratory examination in, 860
    skin examination in, 862, 866
    spasticity in, 866, 867, 867t
    symptoms of, 859–860, 860t, 861t
    treatment of, 865–868, 866t, 867t
  lumbosacral, 879–884
    bladder dysfunction in, 882, 883, 884
    bowel dysfunction in, 882, 883, 884
    complications of, 884
    functional limitations in, 881–882, 881t
    neurologic examination in, 880–881, 880t
    pain in, 883, 884
    physical examination in, 880–881, 880t
    pressure ulcers in, 883, 884
    rectal examination in, 880–881
    sexual dysfunction in, 882
    skeletal level of, 879
    skin examination in, 881

Spinal cord injury *(Continued)*
    spasticity in, 883
    symptoms of, 879–880
    treatment of, 882–884
  thoracic, 871–877
    autonomic dysreflexia in, 872, 873, 875
    bladder management in, 874, 876
    bowel management in, 874, 874t, 876
    complications of, 871–872, 876–877
    death from, 876
    deep venous thrombosis in, 875
    definition of, 871–872, 872t
    depression in, 872, 874
    drug effects in, 876
    erectile dysfunction in, 876
    functional limitations in, 873
    heterotopic ossification in, 875
    osteoporosis in, 875
    pain in, 872, 874
    physical examination in, 873
    pressure ulcers in, 872–873, 876
    sexual function in, 874–875, 876
    spasticity in, 875, 877
    symptoms of, 872–873
    treatment of, 873–876, 874t
Spinal cord stimulation
  in arachnoiditis, 568, 568f, 569
  in intercostal neuralgia, 553
Spinal manipulation, in occipital neuralgia, 487
Spinal muscular atrophy, 705–711, 706f, 707t, 708t
Spine. *See also* Cervical spine; Lumbar spine; Thoracic spine
  cord injury to. *See* Spinal cord injury
  deformity of. *See* Kyphosis; Scoliosis
  neoplasia of, 233t, 248
Spinobulbar muscular atrophy, 705–711, 706f, 707t, 708t
Spirometry, for pulmonary rehabilitation, 825–826
SPLATT procedure, 898
Splint
  in Achilles tendinitis, 409
  after stroke, 890
  in anterior interosseous syndrome, 112, 112f
  in biceps tendon rupture, 61
  in carpal tunnel syndrome, 175
  in de Quervain tenosynovitis, 131
  in Dupuytren contracture, 135
  in elbow arthritis, 99
  in enteropathic arthritis, 688
  in epicondylitis, 106
  in extensor tendon injury, 140–141, 141t, 142–143, 142f, 142t, 143t
  in flexor tendon injury, 147, 147f, 147t
  in ganglion cyst, 152
  in hand osteoarthritis, 157
  in joint contracture, 653, 655
  in Kienböck disease, 169
  in median neuropathy, 175
  in peroneal neuropathy, 378
  in plantar fasciitis, 472
  in pronator teres syndrome, 112, 112f
  in psoriatic arthritis, 811
  in radial neuropathy, 123
  in rheumatoid arthritis, 837
  in spasticity, 850
  in trigger finger, 180
  in ulnar neuropathy, 190
  in wrist osteoarthritis, 207
  in wrist rheumatoid arthritis, 198
Spondyloarthropathy, seronegative, 232t, 605–607, 606f
Spondylolisthesis, lumbar, 253–257, 254f

Spondylolysis, lumbar, 253–257, 254f, 255f, 256f
Spondylosis, cervical, 3–6, 5f
Spondylosis deformans, 229
Sprain
  ankle, 421–425, 422f, 423f
  cervical, 23–25, 24f
  lateral collateral ligament, 319–322, 320f, 321f
  low back, 247–250, 248t, 249t
  medial collateral ligament, 319–322, 320f, 321f
  posterior cruciate ligament, 381–385, 382f, 382t, 383f, 384f
  thoracic, 223–227
  ulnar collateral ligament, 183–185, 184f, 185f
  washerwoman's, 129–131, 130f
Spurling maneuver, 249t, 486
Spurling test
  in cervical degenerative disease, 12
  in cervical radiculopathy, 19, 19f
  in cervical stenosis, 27
Squeeze test, in ankle sprain, 422, 423f
Standing cable column exercise, 373, 374f
Stenosing tenosynovitis
  of finger, 179–182, 180f, 181f
  of wrist, 129–131, 130f
Stenosis
  cervical, 27–31, 28f, 29f
  lumbar, 259–264, 260t, 262t
Stenting, carotid, 890
Sternocleidomastoid muscle injection, 34, 34f
Stevens-Johnson syndrome, 771
Stewart-Treves syndrome, 699
Straight-leg raising, 242, 249t
  in chronic pain syndrome, 506
Strain
  bicipital, 59–61, 60f
  cervical, 23–25, 24f
  hamstring, 331–334, 332f, 333f, 334f
  low back, 247–250, 248t, 249t
  quadriceps, 291–293
  repetitive, 539–543
  thoracic, 223–227
  trapezius, 37–40, 39f
Strength testing
  in cerebral palsy, 630
  in glenohumeral instability, 64, 64f
Strengthening exercise. *See* Exercise(s)
Stress fracture, 393–396, 394f, 395f
Stress response, in myofascial pain syndrome, 533
Stretching exercise. *See* Exercise(s)
Stroke, 887–891, 889t
  young adult, 893–899, 894t, 896t
Strontium ranelate, in osteoporosis, 757
Student's elbow, 115–118, 116f, 118f
Stump neuroma, 600
Stump shrinker, 601, 602t
Subarachnoid hemorrhage. *See* Stroke, young adult
Subscapularis, lift-off test of, 64, 64f, 72
Substance P, in fibromyalgia, 530
Sudeck atrophy (Sudeck syndrome), 511–516, 513t, 514t
Sulcus sign, in glenohumeral instability, 64
Sulfasalazine, 689t
SUNCT, 494t
Supinator syndrome, 121–124, 122f, 123t. *See* Radial nerve, lesions of
Supraspinatus muscle tests, 72
Sural nerve biopsy, 769

Swallowing
    disorders of, 679–683, 680t, 681t, 682t
        in cerebral palsy, 629
        in motor neuron disease, 710
        in multiple sclerosis, 721, 724
        in post-poliomyelitis syndrome, 795, 796,
            797
        in stroke, 889
    videofluorographic study of, 680, 681f
Swan-neck deformity, 161, 162f, 164, 834, 834f
Sweet criteria, 491
Swimming, in thoracic sprain/strain, 226
Syme's amputation, 599–603, 602t
Sympathetic nerve block
    in complex regional pain syndrome, 515–516
    in lumbosacral plexopathy, 784
    in post-amputation phantom pain, 602
Sympathetically maintained pain. See Complex
    regional pain syndrome
Synovectomy
    in elbow arthritis, 102
    metacarpophalangeal, 163
    in wrist arthritis, 199
Synovial fluid analysis
    in osteoarthritis, 747
    in rheumatoid arthritis, 836
Synovium, rheumatoid hypertrophy of. See
    Wrist, rheumatoid arthritis of
Syringomyelia, post-traumatic, 868, 884
Systemic lupus erythematosus, 901–906, 902t,
    903t, 905t–906t

T

Tactile stimulation, in phantom limb pain, 577
Tailor's bunion, 429–430
Talar tilt test, 422, 423f
Taping
    in claw toe, 438–439, 439f
    in patellofemoral syndrome, 372
    in ulnar collateral ligament sprain, 184, 185,
        185f
Tardive dyskinesia, 714, 715–716
Tarsal tunnel syndrome, 479–482, 480f, 481f
Temperature, skin, in complex regional pain
    syndrome, 512
Tender points, in fibromyalgia, 37, 525, 526f
Tender spots, in cervical degenerative disease, 12
Tendinitis/tendinosis
    Achilles, 407–409, 408f
    biceps, 55–58, 56f, 58f
    de Quervain, 129–131, 130f
    patellar, 367–369, 369f
    plantar, 469–473, 470f, 472f
    quadriceps, 367–369, 369f, 387–388
    rotator cuff, 71–75, 72f, 73f, 74t
Tendon transfer, in wrist rheumatoid arthritis,
    199
Tennis elbow, 105–107, 107f
Tenosynovectomy
    in posterior tibial dysfunction, 477
    in rheumatoid arthritis, 163
Tenosynovitis
    de Quervain, 129–131, 130f
    extensor, 163
    flexor, 163
    posterior tibial, 475–477, 476f
    in rheumatoid arthritis, 163, 835
Tension neckache, 37–40, 39f
Tension-type headache, 520, 522
Teriparatide, in osteoporosis, 755t, 757
Tetraplegia. See Spinal cord injury, cervical
Thalamotomy, in Parkinson disease, 764
Thermal capsulorrhaphy, in shoulder arthritis,
    94–95

Thermal injury. See Burns
Thermoregulation, in burns, 613
Thin bones. See Osteoporosis
Thomas test, 296, 296f, 338, 339f
Thompson test, 408, 408f
Thoracentesis, in cardiac rehabilitation, 619
Thoracic outlet syndrome, 497–502, 498f, 500f,
    501f, 775
Thoracic outlet syndrome index, 499
Thoracic spine
    compression fracture of, 213–217, 214f, 215f,
        216f
        vs. thoracic radiculopathy, 219
    radiculopathy of, 219–221, 220f
        vs. intercostal neuralgia, 550–551
    range of motion of, 219
    sprain/strain of, 223–227
Thoracic wedge, in thoracic sprain/strain, 226
Thoracochondralgia, 555–560, 556f, 557f, 558f
Thoracolumbosacral orthosis, 845, 845f
Thoracotomy, pain after, 550, 585–587, 586t
Thrombectomy, 661
Thromboembolism, venous. See Deep venous
    thrombosis
Thrombolytic therapy
    in deep venous thrombosis, 661
    in stroke, 888
Thrombophlebitis. See Deep venous thrombosis
Thromboprophylaxis, after hip arthroplasty,
    275
Thrombosis, venous. See Deep venous
    thrombosis
Thumb. See also Finger; Hand
    gamekeeper's, 183–185
    rheumatoid arthritis of, 164
    skier's, 183–185, 184f
Thumb spica splint, in de Quervain
    tenosynovitis, 131
Tiagabine, in complex regional pain syndrome,
    514t
Tibial nerve transplantation, in peroneal neu-
    ropathy, 378
Tibial neuropathy, 479–482, 480f, 481f
Tibial pain syndrome. See Compartment
    syndrome
Tibialis posterior tendon insufficiency, 475–477,
    476f
Tic douloureux, 491–496, 492f, 493t–494t,
    495f
Tics, 714, 715
Tietze syndrome, 545, 555–560, 556f, 557f,
    558f
Tinel sign, 480, 481f
    in carpal tunnel syndrome, 174
    in elbow arthritis, 98
    in radial neuropathy, 121
    in ulnar neuropathy, 125
    in wrist rheumatoid arthritis, 195
Tizanidine
    in complex regional pain syndrome, 514t
    in multiple sclerosis, 723
    in spasticity, 851t
Toes
    bunion of, 427–429, 428f, 429f
    claw, 437–440, 438f, 439f
    corns of, 441–443, 442f, 443f
    hammer, 453–455, 454f
    mallet, 457–459, 458f
    osteoarthritis of, 449–451, 450f, 451f
Tolterodine, 740, 740t
Tooth
    crack/fracture of, 493t
    phantom, 494t
Topiramate, in complex regional pain syn-
    drome, 514t

Torg-Pavlov ratio
    in cervical spondylotic myelopathy, 4
    in cervical stenosis, 29
Torsion dystonia, idiopathic, 579–582, 582t
Torticollis, spasmodic, 579–582, 582t
Tourette syndrome, 714
Toxins, peripheral neuropathy with, 768t
Tracheostomy, in motor neuron disease, 711
Traction
    cervical, in degenerative disease, 14
    on femoral nerve, 280f
Tram-tracking, in deep venous thrombosis,
    659f
Tramadol
    in complex regional pain syndrome, 514t
    in knee arthritis, 347, 348t
    in low back strain/sprain, 250
    in thoracic compression fracture, 214
Transcutaneous electrical nerve stimulation. See
    Electrical stimulation
Transverse myelitis, 907–911
Trapeziometacarpal joint, osteoarthritis of, 156,
    158–159
Trapezius muscle, 83–84, 85f
    strain of, 37–40, 39f
Trauma, multiple, 787–791, 791t
Traumatic brain injury, 913–917, 914t, 917t
Treadmill testing, in cardiac rehabilitation,
    616
Tremor, 713–714, 715, 716
    essential, 714, 762
    intention, 714
    in multiple sclerosis, 720, 724
    in Parkinson disease, 761, 762
Trendelenburg sign, 296, 296f, 303, 304f
Tricyclic antidepressants
    in arachnoiditis, 567, 567t, 568
    in cervical sprain/strain, 25
    in chronic fatigue syndrome, 639
    in complex regional pain syndrome, 514t,
        515
    in fibromyalgia, 526
    in intercostal neuralgia, 552
    in motor neuron disease, 709
    in occipital neuralgia, 487, 488, 489t
    in peripheral neuropathy, 770
    in peroneal neuropathy, 378
    in phantom limb pain, 576t, 577
    in repetitive strain injury, 542
    in trapezius strain, 38, 39–40
Trigeminal nerve, 491
    blockade of, 495, 495f
Trigeminal neuralgia, 491–496, 493t–494t,
    495f, 495t
Trigger finger, 179–182, 180f, 181f
Trigger point(s)
    in chronic fatigue syndrome, 640
    in myofascial pain syndrome, 529, 531
Trigger point injection
    in cervical sprain/strain, 25
    in cervicogenic vertigo, 34, 34f
    in fibromyalgia, 526
    in headache, 522
    in myofascial pain syndrome, 534, 535
    in thoracic sprain/strain, 227
    in trapezius strain, 39, 39f, 40
Trihexyphenidyl, in Parkinson disease, 715
Trochanteric bursitis, 303–305, 304f
Trospium, 740, 740t
Tumor necrosis factor antagonists, in rheuma-
    toid arthritis, 162
Two-flight stair test, in cardiac rehabilitation,
    617
Two-point sensory discrimination test, in carpal
    tunnel syndrome, 173–174

U

Ulcer(s)
  duodenal, 232t
  foot
    in claw toe, 439
    in corns, 441
    in diabetes, 673–676
    in hammer toe, 453
    in mallet toe, 457
    in tibial neuropathy, 482
  pressure (decubitus), 813–819, 814t, 815f, 817f
    in cerebral palsy, 630
    in cervical spinal cord injury, 866
    in lumbosacral spinal cord injury, 883, 884
    in thoracic spinal cord injury, 872–873, 876
  skin, in diabetes mellitus, 673–676
Ulcerative colitis, 685, 686, 686f, 688–689
Ulna bursa, injection of, in carpal tunnel syndrome, 176, 176f
Ulnar claw, 188
Ulnar collateral ligament complex, 183
Ulnar collateral ligament sprain, 183–185, 184f, 185f
Ulnar neuropathy
  elbow, 107, 125–127, 126f
  wrist, 187–192, 188f, 188t, 189f, 190f
Ultrasonography. See also Ultrasound therapy
  in acromioclavicular joint injury, 44
  in Baker's cyst, 315, 316
  in biceps tendinitis, 57
  in cerebral palsy, 631
  in deep venous thrombosis, 658
  in glenohumeral arthritis, 92
  in heterotopic ossification, 693
  in iliotibial band syndrome, 339
  in jumper's knee, 368
  in knee arthritis, 347
  in Morton neuroma, 466, 466f
  in neurogenic bladder, 736
  in osteoporosis, 755
  in plantar fasciitis, 470
  in polytrauma, 788
  in posterior tibial dysfunction, 476
  in quadriceps contusion, 292
  in rheumatoid arthritis, 162
  in rotator cuff tear, 79
  in Tietze syndrome, 556–557, 557f, 558f
  in trochanteric bursitis, 304
Ultrasound therapy
  in biceps tendinitis, 57
  in cervical sprain/strain, 25
  in joint contracture, 653
  in knee bursitis, 357
  in piriformis syndrome, 288
  in plantar fasciitis, 471
  in postherpetic neuralgia, 562
  in rotator cuff tear, 80
  in spasticity, 850
Urea, blood, in chronic kidney disease, 645
Uremia, 644–645

Urethral sphincter, 733
Urinary catheterization, 734, 739
  intermittent, 874
  suprapubic, 741, 741f
Urinary incontinence
  in cerebral palsy, 629
  in cervical spondylotic myelopathy, 4
  in multiple sclerosis, 721, 722
Urinary tract infection, in neurogenic bladder, 740–741, 742
Urodynamic testing
  in cervical spinal cord injury, 864
  in lumbosacral spinal cord injury, 882
  in neurogenic bladder, 736–737, 738f, 739f
  in thoracic spinal cord injury, 872

V

Vacuum-assisted closure, in pressure ulcers, 818
Valacyclovir, in postherpetic neuralgia, 562
Valproate, in trigeminal neuralgia, 494, 495t
Valproic acid, in complex regional pain syndrome, 514t
Varicella-zoster virus infection, 561–563
Vascular access, in chronic kidney disease, 647
Vascular dementia, 665–671, 666t
Vasculitis, in rheumatoid arthritis, 833
Vastus medialis obliquus strengthening, in patellofemoral syndrome, 373
Vaughan-Jackson syndrome, 161, 195
Vena cava filter, 661
Venlafaxine, in complex regional pain syndrome, 514t
Venography, in deep venous thrombosis, 658, 659f
Ventilation, in myopathy, 732
Ventilatory impairment, 823–826, 824t
  complications of, 830
  rehabilitation for, 827
Vertebral crush fracture, 213–217, 214f, 215f, 216f
  vs. radiculopathy, 219
Vertebroplasty, in thoracic compression fracture, 216, 216f
Vertigo
  cervicogenic, 33–35, 34f
  post-concussion, 802–803, 805, 806
Vicar's knee, 355
Videofluorography, of swallowing, 680, 681f
Viking disease, 133–136, 134f
Virchow's triad, 657
Viscosupplementation injection, in arthritis, 274, 350
Vision disorders
  in cerebral palsy, 628
  in multiple sclerosis, 719–720, 721, 724
  post-concussion, 803
  in psoriatic arthritis, 809
  in stroke, 895
Vitamin C
  in amyotrophic lateral sclerosis, 707
  in knee arthritis, 347, 348t
Vitamin D, in osteoporosis, 756

Vitamin E, 670
  in amyotrophic lateral sclerosis, 707
Vocal cord injection, 857
Vocational therapy. See also Occupational therapy
  after stroke, 890
  in post-concussion disorders, 805–806
Volar carpal ligament, 173, 174f
Volkmann ischemia. See Compartment syndrome

W

Waddell signs
  in lumbar degenerative disease, 230, 230t
  in lumbar radiculopathy, 242
Walk test, for pulmonary rehabilitation, 825
Walker, in knee arthritis, 349
Walking program, in plantar fasciitis, 471–472
Wallet neuritis, 287–289, 288f
War-related injury. See Polytrauma
Warfarin
  in hip replacement, 297
  in knee replacement, 401
  in stroke, 888
Wartenberg sign, 125
Washerwoman's sprain, 129–131, 130f
Well-leg compartment syndrome, 325
Wells prediction rules, in deep venous thrombosis, 658, 659t
Whiplash injury, 23–25, 24f
Whipple disease, 685, 686, 687, 688
Winter heel. See Foot (feet), bursitis of
Work-related upper limb disorder. See Repetitive strain injury
Wrist. See also Finger; Hand
  de Quervain tenosynovitis of, 129–131, 130f
  fracture of, 754
  fusion of, 200, 200f, 208, 209f, 210f
  ganglia of, 149–153, 150f, 151f
  malunited fracture of, 203, 204f
  osteoarthritis of, 193–201, 194f, 195f, 198f, 199f, 200f
  palpation of, 205
  rheumatoid arthritis of, 203–211, 204f, 205f, 206f, 207f, 210f, 834–835, 836f
  treatment of, 198–200, 200f
  swelling of, 204–205, 205f
Wristdrop neuropathy, 121–124, 122f, 123t

Y

Yeoman test, in low back strain/sprain, 249t
Yergason test, 56, 56f, 59
Yuppi flu, 635–640, 637t, 638t

Z

Z-joint pain, 7–9, 8f
Zoledronic acid, in osteoporosis, 757
Zygapophyseal joint pain, 7–9, 8f